AACN Essentials of Critical Care Nursing
Fifth Edition

Sarah A. Delgado, MSN, RN, ACNP
Clinical Practice Specialist
American Association of Critical-Care Nurses
Aliso Viejo, California

New York   Chicago   San Francisco   Athens   London   Madrid   Mexico City
Milan   New Delhi   Singapore   Sydney   Toronto

ISBN 978-1-264-26988-4
MHID 1-264-26988-9

NOTICE

Medicine is an ever-changing science. As new research and clinical experience broaden our knowledge, changes in treatment and drug therapy are required. The authors and the publisher of this work have checked with sources believed to be reliable in their efforts to provide information that is complete and generally in accord with the standards accepted at the time of publication. However, in view of the possibility of human error or changes in medical sciences, neither the authors nor the publisher nor any other party who has been involved in the preparation or publication of this work warrants that the information contained herein is in every respect accurate or complete, and they disclaim all responsibility for any errors or omissions or for the results obtained from use of the information contained in this work. Readers are encouraged to confirm the information contained herein with other sources. For example and in particular, readers are advised to check the product information sheet included in the package of each drug they plan to administer to be certain that the information contained in this work is accurate and that changes have not been made in the recommended dose or in the contraindications for administration. This recommendation is of particular importance in connection with new or infrequently used drugs.

This book was set in Minion Pro by KnowledgeWorks Global Ltd.
The editors were Sydney Keen Vitale and Christina M. Thomas.
The production supervisor was Richard Ruzycka.
Project management was provided by Nitesh Sharma, KnowledgeWorks Global Ltd.
The cover designer was W2 Design.

This book is printed on acid-free paper.

Library of Congress Control Number: 2023936554

Contents

Contents in Detail

Contributors

Anna M. Alder, MS, RN, PCCN, CCRN, NPD-BC
Clinical Instructor
University of Utah College of Nursing
Salt Lake City, Utah
Chapter 14: Gastrointestinal System

Earnest Alexander, PharmD, BCCCP, FCCM
Assistant Director, Clinical Pharmacy Services
Tampa General Hospital
Tampa, Florida
Chapter 7: Pharmacology

John C. Bazil, RN, BSN, BSEE
Registered Nurse
UT Southwestern Medical Center
Dallas, Texas
Chapter 12: Neurologic System
Chapter 21: Advanced Neurologic Concepts

Elizabeth J. Bridges, PhD, RN, CCNS, FCCM, FAAN
Professor
University of Washington School of Nursing
Clinical Nurse Researcher
University of Washington Medical Center
Seattle, Washington
Chapter 4: Hemodynamic Monitoring
Chapter 24: Hemodynamic Monitoring Troubleshooting
  Guide

Jie Chen, RN, CMSN, ACNP-BC
Harrisburg, Pennsylvania
Chapter 15: Renal System

Yvonne D'Arcy, MS, APRN, CNS, FAANP
Pain Management and Palliative Care Nurse Practitioner
Retired Suburban Hospital Johns Hopkins Medicine
Ponte Vedra Beach, Florida
Chapter 6: Pain, Sedation, and Neuromuscular Blockade
  Management

John J. Gallagher, DNP, RN, CCNS, CCRN, TCRN, CHSE, RRT, FCCM
Professor/Clinical Nurse Specialist
University of Pittsburgh School of Nursing
Pittsburgh, Pennsylvania
Chapter 20: Advanced Respiratory Concepts:
  Modes of Ventilation

Danya Garner, PhD, RN, OCN, CCRN-K, NPD-BC
Associate Director, Continuing Professional Education
The University of Texas MD Anderson Cancer Center
Houston, Texas
Chapter 13: Hematologic and Immune Systems

Sonya M. Grigsby, DNP, APRN, AGACNP-BC, FNP-BC, EMBA-HCM, CCRN
Nurse Practitioner
Christus Mother Frances Hospital
Tyler, Texas
Chapter 11: Multisystem Problems

Kiersten Henry, DNP, ACNP-BC, CCNS, CCRN-CMC
Chief Advanced Practice Provider
MedStar Montgomery Medical Center
Olney, Maryland
Chapter 10: Respiratory System

Carol Jacobson, MN
Partner, Cardiovascular Nursing Education Associates
Cardiovascular Nursing Education Associates
Seattle, Washington
Chapter 3: Interpretation and Management of Basic Cardiac
  Rhythms
Chapter 18: Advanced ECG Concepts
Chapter 25: Cardiac Rhythms, ECG Characteristics, and
  Treatment Guide

Robert E. St. John, MSN, RN, RRT
Senior Clinical Director – Patient Monitoring
Medtronic
St. Louis, Missouri
Chapter 5: Airway and Ventilatory Management

Mary Jo Kelly, DNP, RN, ARNP, CCNS, ACNS-BC, CCRN
Clinical Nurse Specialist
Providence Swedish Health Care System
Seattle, Washington
Chapter 4: Hemodynamic Monitoring
*Chapter 24: Hemodynamic Monitoring Troubleshooting
    Guide*

Sara Knippa, MS, RN, ACCNS-AG, CCRN, PCCN
Critical Care Clinical Nurse Specialist
UCHealth
Aurora, Colorado
*Chapter 6: Pain, Sedation, and Neuromuscular Blockade
    Management*

Christopher Kolokythas, MS, AGACNP-BC, ACCNS-AG
Senior Nurse Practitioner
R Adams Cowley Shock Trauma Center
Baltimore, Maryland
Chapter 17: Trauma

Janet Lee, RN, DNP, AGACNP-BC, ACCNS-AG, CRNP
R Adams Cowley Shock Trauma Center at University of
    Maryland Medical Center
Baltimore, Maryland
Chapter 17: Trauma

**Barbara Leeper, MN, APRN CNS-MS, CCRN-K,
    CV-BC, FAHA**
Clinical Nurse Specialist, Cardiovascular and Critical Care
Dallas, Texas
Chapter 9: Cardiovascular System
Chapter 19: Advanced Cardiovascular Concepts

DaiWai M. Olson, RN, PhD, FNCS
Professor
University of Texas Southwestern
Dallas, Texas
Chapter 12: Neurologic System
Chapter 21: Advanced Neurologic Concepts

Heather Roff, MS, AGACNP-BC, ACCNS-AG, CCRN
Critical Care Nurse Practitioner
University of California San Francisco
San Francisco, California
Chapter 16: Endocrine System

**Maureen A. Seckel, MSN, APRN, ACNS-BC, CCRN,
    CCRN-K, FCCM, FCNS, FAAN**
Critical Care Clinical Nurse Specialist and Sepsis
    Coordinator
ChristianaCare
Newark, Delaware
Chapter 5: Airway and Ventilatory Management
Chapter 10: Respiratory System

Maxine Wanzer, MSN, AGACNP
Critical Care APP & Fellowship Advisor
OhioHealth
Columbus, Ohio
*Chapter 1: Assessment of Critically Ill Patients and
    Their Families*
*Chapter 2: Planning Care for Critically Ill Patients and
    Their Families*

Laura Webster, D.Be, RN, HEC-C, CEN
Pacific NW Division VP of Ethics – CommonSpirit Health
Affiliate Faculty – University of Washington School
    of Medicine Department of Bioethics and Humanities
Seattle, Washington
Chapter 8: Ethical and Legal Considerations
Chapter 23: Implementing Crisis Standards of Care

Peer Reviewers

Janet Ahlstrom, MSN, APRN, ACNS-BC, NEA-BC
Clinical Nurse Specialist
University of Kansas Health System
Kansas City, Kansas

Markie Baxter, BSN, RN
Nurse Professional Development Specialist
Virginia Mason Medical Center
Seattle, Washington

Linda Bell, MSN, RN
Clinical Practice Specialist
American Association of Critical-Care Nurses (AACN)
Tryon, North Carolina

Naomi Colón, MSN, RN, CCRN, PCCN, TNS
Clinical Nurse Educator
Bethesda Butler Trihealth Hospital
Hamilton, Ohio

Stephanie Gregory, FNP-C, BMTCN
Lead Nurse Practitioner
Northside Hospital BMT unit
Atlanta, Georgia

Lindsey A. Hart, DNP, AGPCNP-BC
Nurse Practitioner Coordinator, Structural Heart Program
Maimonides Medical Center
Brooklyn, New York

Carrie Judd, MSN, APRN, FNP-C
Clinical Instructor
The University of Texas at Tyler
Longview, Texas

Mary Beth Flynn Makic, PhD, RN, CCNS, CCRN-K, FAAN, FNAP, FCNS
Professor
Adult-Gerontology Clinical Nurse Specialist
  Program Director
University of Colorado
College of Nursing
Aurora, Colorado

Gail Markowski, DNP, ANP-C, ACNP-C, CCRN
Clinical Assistant Professor
State University of New York at Buffalo
Buffalo, New York

Karen Marzlin, DNP, CCNS, ACNPC-AG, CCRN-CMC, CHFN
Acute Care Nurse Practitioner, Clinical Nurse Specialist, Educator, Consultant
Kidney and HTN Consultants, Cardiovascular Nursing
  Education Associates, Key Choice
Canton, Ohio

Georgina Morley, PhD, MSc, RN, HEC-C
Nurse Ethicist
Cleveland Clinic
Cleveland, Ohio

Nancy Munro, RN, MN, CCRN, ACNP-BC, FAANP
Nurse Practitioner
Pulmonary Hypertension Service, NIH
Bethesda, Maryland

Heather Przybyl, DNP, RN, CCRN
RN Certified Specialist
Banner University Medical Center Phoenix
Phoenix, Arizona

Brenda Pun, DNP, RN, FCCM
Director of Data Quality
Vanderbilt University Medical Center
Nashville, Tennessee

Gina Riggi, PharmD, BCCCP, BCPS
Clinical Coordinator, Trauma ICU Clinical Specialist
Jackson Memorial Hospital
Miami, Florida

Magally Rolen, MSN, RN, PCCN
Intensive Care Unit – Registered Nurse
Texas Health Resources
Fort Worth, Texas

Kristin E. Sandau, PhD, RN, FAHA, FAAN
Professor of Nursing
Bethel University
St. Paul, Minnesota

Mary A. Stahl, MSN, RN, CCNS, CCRN-K
Clinical Practice Specialist
American Association of Critical-Care Nurses
Parkville, Missouri

Daniel N. Storzer, DNP, ACNP, CCRN, EMT-P, FCCP, FCCM
Intensivist
ThedaCare
Neenah, Wisconsin

Scott Carter Thigpen, DNP, RN, MSN, CCRN-K
Professor of Nursing
South Georgia State College, School of Nursing
Douglas, Georgia

Terri Townsend, MA, RN, CCRN-CMC
Clinical Educator, Ret.
Community Hospital Anderson, Ret.
Anderson, Indiana

Maxine Wanzer, MSN, AGACNP
Critical Care APP & Fellowship Advisor
OhioHealth
Columbus, Ohio

Catherine A. Wolkow, PhD, BSN, RN, CCRN
Critical Care Nurse
UWMC-Northwest (University of Washington Medical Center – Northwest)
Seattle, Washington

Susan Yeager, DNP, RN, CCRN, ACNP-BC, FNCS
Advanced Practice Provider Neurocritical Care Educator
The Ohio State University Wexner Medical Center
Columbus, Ohio

Preface

This text provides the reader with evidence-informed content about the care of critically ill patients and their families. Written by nursing experts, this book sets a standard for critical care nursing education, supports preparation for national certifications, and can be a resource to address uncertainty in patient care delivery. The organization of the text recognizes the learner's need to assimilate foundational knowledge before attempting to master more complex critical care nursing concepts. In addition, the American Association of Critical-Care Nurses affirms this book's value to the AACN community and especially to clinicians at the point of care. As the editor, I am grateful for the time and effort that AACN's team put forth in providing this validation. The title continues to carry AACN's name, as it has since the first edition.

AACN Essentials of Critical Care Nursing is divided into four parts:

- Part I: The Essentials presents core information that clinicians must understand to provide safe, competent nursing care to all critically ill patients, regardless of the setting or diagnoses. This part includes content on assessment, diagnosis, planning, and interventions common to critically ill patients and their families; interpretation and management of cardiac rhythms; hemodynamic monitoring; airway and ventilatory management; pain, sedation, and neuromuscular blockade management; pharmacology; and ethical and legal considerations. Chapters in Part I provide the critical care clinician with information to develop foundational competence.
- Part II: Pathologic Conditions covers pathologic conditions and management strategies commonly encountered in critical care units, closely paralleling the blueprint for the CCRN certification examination. Chapters in this part are organized by body systems and selected critical care conditions, such as cardiovascular, respiratory, multisystem, neurologic, hematologic and immune, gastrointestinal, renal, endocrine, and trauma.

- Part III: Advanced Concepts in Caring for the Critically Ill Patient presents advanced critical care concepts or pathologic conditions that are more complex and represent expert level information. Specific advanced chapter content includes ECG concepts, cardiovascular concepts, modes of ventilation, and neurologic concepts.
- Part IV: Key Reference Information contains selected reference information including laboratory and diagnostic values that apply to the content cases in the text; cardiac rhythms, ECG characteristics and treatment guide and hemodynamic troubleshooting. New in this edition is a table that demonstrates how conventional, contingency, and crisis standards of care are implemented. Content in part IV is presented primarily in table format for quick reference.

Each chapter in Parts I, II, and III, begins with "Knowledge Competencies" that can be used to guide informal or formal teaching and to gauge the learner's progress. In addition, each of the chapters provide "Essential Content cases" that focus on key information presented in the chapters in order to assist clinicians in understanding the chapter content and how to best assess and manage conditions and problems encountered in critical care. The case studies are also designed to enhance the learners understanding of the magnitude of the pathologic problems/conditions and their impact on patients and families. Questions and answers are provided for each case so that learners may test their knowledge of the essential content.

The design of this text demonstrates the expertise of the first edition editors, Marianne Chuley and Suzanne M. Burns. Both are outstanding leaders with boundless nursing expertise, and I am honored and humbled to contribute to their tradition. The world of critical care nursing has shifted dramatically since they published the first edition. The prevalence of e-learning programs, including AACN's Essentials of Critical Care Orientation, as well as webinars, podcasts, and other platforms offers nurses many ways to advance or confirm the knowledge that informs patient care.

Technology has also changed our interventions and the way we document them. New evidence has altered old practices and changed our interpretation of clinical data. The COVID-19 pandemic has profoundly altered the delivery of critical care, and the lives of those who provide it. While the complexity of critical care requires collaboration among team members who each bring unique expertise, it is nurses who provide a continual and compassionate presence for patients.

As critical care continues to evolve, the skills and knowledge that nurses leverage will also change. The constant element will be nurses' profound commitment to learning and translating that learning to optimal patient outcomes. This 5th edition, like its predecessors, meets nurses in their journey to learn, supports their pursuit of validation through certification, and offers a resource for direct patient care. As the book's editor, I hope it also serves to honor the profound contributions that nurses make every moment of every day and every night in the lives of patients, families, and their communities.

In gratitude for the profession of nursing,

Sarah A. Delgado, MSN, RN, ACNP

The Essentials

I

ASSESSMENT OF CRITICALLY ILL PATIENTS AND THEIR FAMILIES

1

Maxine Wanzer

KNOWLEDGE COMPETENCIES

1. Discuss the importance of a consistent and systematic approach to the assessment of critically ill patients and their families.
2. Identify the assessment priorities for different stages of a critical illness:
   • Prearrival assessment
   • Admission quick check

• Comprehensive admission assessment
• Ongoing assessment(s)
3. Describe how the assessment is altered based on the patient's clinical status.

The assessment of critically ill patients and their families is an essential competency for critical care nurses. Information obtained from an assessment identifies the immediate and future needs of the patient and their family so a plan of care can be initiated and revised to address or resolve these needs. In this text, the term family refers to a person or persons with whom the patient shares a valued relationship.

Traditional approaches to patient assessment include a complete evaluation of the patient's history, review of systems, and a comprehensive physical examination of all body systems. This approach, although ideal, rarely is possible in critical care due to life-threatening situations during admission, and nurses must balance the need to gather data while simultaneously prioritizing and providing care. Traditional approaches and techniques for assessment are modified to balance the need for information, while considering the critical nature of the patient and family's situation.

This chapter outlines an assessment approach that recognizes the emergent and dynamic nature of a critical illness. This approach emphasizes the collection of assessment data in phases consistent with patient care priorities, and can be used as a generic template for assessing most critically ill patients and their families. The assessment can then be individualized to address specific aspects of the patient diagnosis.

The components of the assessment appropriate to particular disease states are identified in subsequent chapters.

Crucial to developing competence in assessing critically ill patients and their families is a consistent and systematic approach. Without this approach, it would be easy to miss subtle signs or details that may identify an actual or potential problem and also indicate a patient's changing status. Assessments focus first on the patient, then on the technology. The patient is the focal point of the critical care practitioner's attention, with technology augmenting the information obtained from the direct assessment.

There are two standard approaches to assessing patients: the head-to-toe approach and the body systems approach. Most critical care nurses use a combination, a systems approach applied in a "top-to-bottom" manner. The admission and ongoing assessment sections of this chapter are presented with this combined approach in mind.

ASSESSMENT FRAMEWORK

Assessing the critically ill patient and family begins from the moment the nurse is made aware of the pending admission of the patient and continues until transitioning to the next phase of care. The assessment process can be viewed as four distinct stages: (1) prearrival, (2) admission quick check ("just the basics"), (3) comprehensive initial, and (4) ongoing assessment(s).

Prearrival Assessment

A prearrival assessment begins the moment the information is received about the upcoming admission of the patient. This notification comes from the initial healthcare team contact. The contact may be paramedics in the field reporting to the emergency department (ED), a transfer from another facility, or a transfer from other areas within the hospital such as the ED, operating room (OR), progressive care unit, or medical/surgical nursing unit. The prearrival assessment paints the initial picture of the patient and allows the critical care nurse to begin anticipating the patient's physiologic and psychological needs. This prearrival assessment also allows the critical care nurse to determine the appropriate resources that are needed to care for the patient. Technology may be used to augment the prearrival assessment as well. Using the electronic health records (EHRs), basic information may be gathered quickly; such as chief complaint, past medical history, allergies, etc. Based on the information received in the prearrival phase, the critical care nurse prepares the environment to meet the individual needs of the patient and family.

Admission Quick Check

An admission quick check assessment is obtained immediately upon arrival and is based on assessing the parameters represented by the ABCDE acronym (Table 1-1). The admission quick check assessment is a quick overview of the adequacy of ventilation and perfusion to ensure early intervention for any life-threatening situations. Energy is also focused on exploring the chief complaint and obtaining essential diagnostic tests to supplement physical assessment findings. The admission quick check is a high-level view of the patient, which validates that basic neurologic, cardiac, and respiratory function are sufficient.

Comprehensive Initial Assessment

A comprehensive initial assessment is performed as soon as possible, with the timing dictated by the degree of physiologic stability and emergent treatment needs of the patient. If the patient is being admitted directly to the intensive care unit (ICU) from outside the hospital, the comprehensive assessment is an in-depth assessment of the past medical, surgical, and social history and a complete physical examination of

TABLE 1-1. ABCDE ACRONYM

Airway
Breathing
Circulation, Cerebral perfusion, and Chief complaint
Drugs and Diagnostic tests
Equipment

each body system. If the patient is being transferred to the ICU from another area in the hospital, the comprehensive assessment includes a review of the admission assessment data and comparison to the current state of the patient. The comprehensive assessment is vital to successful outcomes because it provides valuable insight into proactive interventions that may be needed.

Ongoing Assessment(s)

After the baseline comprehensive initial assessment is completed, ongoing assessments and an abbreviated version of the comprehensive initial assessment are performed at varying intervals according to unit protocol and the individual needs of the patient. The assessment parameters outlined in this section are usually completed for all patients, in addition to other ongoing assessment requirements related to the patient's specific condition, treatments, and response to therapy.

Patient Safety Considerations in Admission Assessments

Admission of an acutely ill patient can be a chaotic and fast-paced event with multiple disciplines involved in many activities. It is at this time, however, that healthcare providers must be particularly cognizant of accurate assessments and data gathering to ensure the patient is cared for safely with appropriate interventions. Obtaining inaccurate information on admission can lead to ongoing errors that may not be easily rectified or discovered and lead to poor patient outcomes.

Obtaining information from a critically ill patient may be difficult, if possible at all. If the patient is unable to supply information, other sources must be utilized such as family members or friends, EHRs, past medical records, transport records, the transport team, or information from the patient's belongings. Of particular importance at admission is obtaining accurate patient identification, as well as past medical history including any known allergies. Obtaining current medication regimens as soon as possible is essential as they can provide clues to the patient's medical condition and any potential contributing factors to the current condition and ensures medication reconciliation to continue appropriate medications and avoid medication interactions.

EHRs can facilitate timely access to patient's past and current health information. Critical care providers may have access to both inpatient and outpatient records within the same healthcare system, assisting them in quickly identifying the patient's most recent medication regimen and laboratory and diagnostic results. In addition, many healthcare systems within the same geographic locations are working together to make access available to intersystem medical records of patients being treated at multiple healthcare institutions. This is particularly beneficial in the critical care setting where patients may be unable to articulate imperative medical information, including advance directives, allergies, next of kin, or their current plan of care with outpatient providers. By filling these gaps, the EHR can improve continuity of care.

Careful physical assessment on admission to the critical care unit is pivotal in the prevention and/or early treatment for complications associated with critical illness. Of particular importance is the assessment of risk for pressure injury, infection, falls and/or delirium. Patients who develop delirium during their ICU stay have a high risk of developing post–intensive care syndrome (PICS). This syndrome is defined as cognitive, psychological, and physical signs and symptoms that may persist for months or years after discharge from the ICU. Patients who develop PICS have a decreased quality of life and may not be able to return to employment or their previous level of activity and cognitive acuity. Family members are also at risk for a similar syndrome. There are interventions that have been shown to prevent delirium and PICS. The ABCDEF bundle, the framework from the Society of Critical Care Medicine's ICU Liberation initiative, consists of preventative measures and standards of care for ICU patients at risk for developing delirium and PICS.

Risks associated with accurate patient identification never lessen, particularly as these relate to interventions such as performing invasive procedures, medication administration, blood administration, advance directives, and collection of laboratory tests. Nurses need to be cognizant of safety issues as treatments begin. For example, accurate programming of pumps infusing high-risk medications is essential. It is imperative that nurses use all safety equipment available to them such as preprogrammed drug libraries in infusion pumps and bar-coding technology. Healthcare providers must also ensure the safety of invasive procedures that need to be performed emergently.

PREARRIVAL ASSESSMENT: BEFORE THE ACTION BEGINS

A prearrival assessment begins when information is received about the pending arrival of the patient. The prearrival report, although abbreviated, provides key information about the chief complaint, diagnosis, or reason for admission, pertinent history details, and physiologic stability of the patient (Table 1-2). The gender and age of the patient, information on the presence of invasive tubes and lines, medications being administered, other ongoing treatments, and pending or completed laboratory or diagnostic tests are also included. This information assists the clinician in anticipating the patient's physiologic and emotional needs prior to admission and in ensuring that the bedside environment is set up to provide all monitoring, supply, and equipment needs prior to the patient's arrival.

It is also important to consider the need for isolation precautions, neutropenic precautions, or special respiratory isolation. For example, depending on local transmission rates, testing for SARS-CoV-2 (the virus that causes COVID-19) may be required on admission to the ICU. If COVID-19 testing is in process, the patient should be placed in the appropriate isolation while waiting to confirm results. A negative air flow room may be required by your institution.

TABLE 1-2. SUMMARY OF PREARRIVAL AND ADMISSION QUICK CHECK ASSESSMENTS

Prearrival Assessment
- Abbreviated report on patient (age, gender, chief complaint, diagnosis, pertinent history, physiologic status, invasive devices, equipment, and status of laboratory/diagnostic tests)
- Allergies
- Complete room setup, including verification of proper equipment functioning
  - Do Not Resuscitate (DNR) Status
  - Isolation Status

Admission Quick Check Assessment
- General appearance (patient's size and level of consciousness)
- *Airway:*
Patency
Position of artificial airway (if present)
- *Breathing:*
Quantity and quality of respirations (rate, depth, pattern, symmetry, effort, use of accessory muscles)
Breath sounds
Presence of spontaneous breathing
- *Circulation and Cerebral Perfusion:*
Electrocardiogram (ECG) (rate, rhythm, and presence of ectopy)
Blood pressure
Peripheral pulses and capillary refill
Skin, color, temperature, moisture
Presence of bleeding
Level of consciousness, responsiveness
- *Chief Complaint:*
Primary body system
Associated symptoms
- *Drugs and Diagnostic Tests:*
Drugs prior to admission (prescribed, over-the-counter, illicit)
Current medications
Review diagnostic test results
- *Equipment:*
Patency of vascular and drainage systems
Appropriate functioning and labeling of all equipment connected to patient

Being prepared for isolation needs prevents potentially serious exposures to the patient or the healthcare providers. If the patient requires isolation, special consideration needs to be made regarding limiting the number of staff and the number of times in and out of the patient's room. This helps to preserve personal protective equipment (PPE) and to limit staff exposure to infectious pathogens. Gather all required equipment and supplies and appoint a staff member to be a runner for additional supplies you may need. Consider ways to communicate without leaving isolation, such as writing messages on a whiteboard.

Many critical care units have a standard room setup, guided by the major diagnosis-related groups of patients each unit receives. The standard monitoring and equipment list for each unit varies; however, there are certain common requirements (Table 1-3). The standard room setup is modified for each admission to accommodate patient-specific needs (eg, additional equipment, intravenous [IV] fluids, medications). Proper functioning of all bedside equipment is verified prior to the patient's arrival and demographic information is entered into the bedside monitor.

TABLE 1-3. EQUIPMENT FOR STANDARD ROOM SETUP

- Bedside ECG and invasive pressure monitor with appropriate cables
- ECG electrodes
- Blood pressure cuff
- Pulse oximeter
- End-tidal CO_2
- Thermometer
- Suction gauges and canister setup
- Suction catheters
- Bag-valve-mask device
- Oxygen flowmeter, appropriate tubing, and appropriate oxygen delivery device
- IV poles and infusion pumps
- Bedside supplies to include alcohol swabs, nonsterile gloves, syringes, bedpads, and dressing supplies
- Admission kit that usually contains bath basin and general hygiene supplies
- Bedside computer and/or paper admission documentation forms

Prearrival setup also includes preparing the medical record or bedside computer to enter data including vital signs, intake and output, medication administration, patient care activities, and patient assessment. The prearrival report may suggest pending procedures, necessitating the organization of appropriate supplies at the bedside. Having the room prepared and all equipment available facilitates a rapid, smooth, and safe admission of the patient. If the ICU is partnering in a tele-ICU (e-ICU) model, inform the e-ICU hub of the pending admission so they can also prepare to begin surveillance of the critically ill patient upon arrival.

Prior to arrival, the critical care nurse also plans for the patient's family, who often arrive with the patient or even prior to the patient's arrival in the ICU. If visitation limitations are in place, prepare to call them as soon as possible after the patient arrives at the ICU. A healthcare worker can be designated to connect with family members by phone or on their arrival, answering questions, giving them a brief orientation or verbal overview to the unit, showing them to a place where they can comfortably wait if applicable, providing them specific information as to when they will be able to see their loved one, reviewing the visitation policy, and offering support.

ADMISSION QUICK CHECK ASSESSMENT: THE FIRST FEW MINUTES

From the moment the patient arrives in the ICU setting, their general appearance is immediately observed and assessment of ABCDEs is quickly performed (see Table 1-1). On arrival, the nurse verifies any urgent changes in patient condition or equipment in use since the prearrival report. The presenting problems are prioritized so that life-threatening emergent needs can be addressed first. The patient is connected to monitoring and support equipment, critical medications are administered, and essential laboratory and diagnostic tests are ordered. Simultaneous with the ABCDE assessment, the nurse must validate that the patient is appropriately identified through self-identification, a hospital wristband, personal identification documents, and/or family identification. In addition, the patient's allergy status is determined, including the type and severity of reaction that occurs as well as what, if any, treatment has been used to alleviate the allergic response in the past.

There may be other healthcare professionals present to receive the patient and assist with admission tasks. The critical care nurse, however, is the leader of the receiving team. The patient's nurse directs the team in completing delegated tasks, such as changing over to the ICU equipment or attaching monitoring cables. The leadership of the critical care nurse is vital to a smooth admission, preventing fragmented care and ensuring that vital assessment clues are not overlooked.

The critical care nurse rapidly assesses the ABCDEs in the sequence outlined in this section. If any aspect of this preliminary assessment deviates from normal, interventions are immediately initiated to address the problem before continuing with the admission quick check assessment. Additionally, regardless of the patient's level of consciousness (LOC), talking to them through the admission process, is an essential element of care.

ESSENTIAL CONTENT CASE

Prearrival Assessment

The charge nurse notifies Terry that they will be receiving a 26-year-old man from the ED who was involved in a motor vehicle crash. The ED nurse caring for the patient has called to give Terry a report following the hospital's standardized report format.

The patient was an unrestrained driver in a low-speed head-on collision and has sustained a closed-head injury and thoracic trauma with collapsed left lung. The patient was intubated and placed on a mechanical ventilator. IV access was obtained, and a left chest tube was inserted. The ED nurse provides the latest trend of the patient's vital signs

and neurologic assessments and how he has responded to the administered pain medication. After a computed tomographic (CT) scan of the head, chest, and abdomen is obtained, the patient will be transferred to the ICU. Terry questions the ED nurse regarding whether the patient has been agitated, had a Foley catheter and nasogastric (NG) tube placed, and whether family had been notified of the accident.

Terry goes to check the patient's room prior to admission and begins to do a mental check of what will be needed. "The patient is intubated so I'll connect the bag valve to the oxygen source, check for suction catheters, and make sure the suction systems are working. I'll notify respiratory therapy to update them on the admission and coordinate to ensure that the pulse oximetry, end-tidal CO_2, and the ventilator are ready to go. I have an extra suction gauge to connect to the chest tube system. I'll also turn on the ECG monitor and have the ECG electrodes ready to apply. An arterial line kit is at the bedside, and the flush system and transducer are also ready to be connected. The IV infusion devices are set up. This patient has an altered LOC, which means frequent neuro checks and potential insertion of an ICP catheter for monitoring. I will prepare to perform a neuro exam during handoff with the ED RN. I have my pen light handy, but I better check to see if we have all the equipment to insert the ICP catheter in case the physician wants to perform the procedure here after the CT scan. The computer in the room is on and ready for me to begin documentation. I think I'm ready."

Case Question 1: What basic information will Terry want to know from the prearrival communication with the ED nurse?

Case Question 2: What patient issues are likely to need immediate assessment and/or intervention on arrival to the ICU to ensure the appropriate equipment is set up in the room?

Case Question 3: What information is included in the more formal handoff between the ED nurse and Terry after the patient is admitted to the ICU?

Answers

1. Patient name/age; type and timing of accident; extent of accident injuries; pertinent medical history, allergies, vital signs, and significant assessment information; placement of tubes and lines; medications being administered; significant laboratory results; anticipated plan on admission; presence of family; and any other special instructions.

2. Vital signs, neurologic status, and information such as whether the ventilator is adequately addressing the patient's ventilation needs, medications are appropriately infusing, and whether the patient is agitated or experiencing extensive pain.

3. Using an SBAR (situation-background-assessment-recommendation) format, the ED nurse can give more detailed information about the injuries from the car accident, the patient's complete medical history as known, reiteration of known allergies, a system by system assessment review; diagnostic test results, confirmation of all invasive lines and equipment settings, the anticipated plan for ongoing assessments and interventions, and any pertinent family information. Terry can also clarify any remaining questions she might have.

Airway and Breathing

Patency of the patient's airway is verified by having the patient speak, if their voice is normal and clear, then the airway is patent. If the airway is compromised, reposition the head using the head tilt-chin lift or jaw thrust maneuver to prevent the tongue from occluding the airway and inspect the upper airway for the presence of blood, vomitus, and foreign objects. Insert an oral or nasal airway, if indicated (see Chapter 5, Airway and Ventilatory Management). If the patient already has an artificial airway, such as an endotracheal (ET) tube or tracheostomy, assess that it is secured properly and note the position and size of the airway. For ET tubes, note the marking closest to the teeth, lips, or nares to assist with future comparisons for proper placement. Suction the upper airway, either through the oral cavity or artificial airway to ensure that the airway is free from secretions. Observe and document the amount, color, and consistency of any secretions that are removed.

Assessment of the patient's breathing also includes observation of the rate, depth, pattern, and symmetry of breathing; the effort of breathing; use of accessory muscles; and, if mechanically ventilated, synchrony with the ventilator. Do not overlook nonverbal signs of respiratory distress including restlessness, anxiety, or change in mental status. Auscultate the chest for presence of bilateral breath sounds, quality of breath sounds, and bilateral chest expansion. Optimally, both anterior and posterior breath sounds are auscultated; if patient condition or time limitations exist, the anterior chest only is assessed. Check the noninvasive oxygen saturation and quickly analyze the result. If the patient is receiving assistive breaths from a bag valve mask or mechanical ventilator, evaluate the presence of spontaneous breaths and the amount of pressure required for inspiration.

If present, pleural and mediastinal chest tubes are also assessed in the initial quick check. Ensure that they are connected to suction, if appropriate, and are not clamped or kinked. In addition, assess whether the chest tubes are functioning properly (eg, air leak, fluid fluctuation in the water seal chamber with respiration) and review the amount and character of the drainage. Stop assessment here if intervention is warranted to maintain or establish a patent airway.

Circulation and Cerebral Perfusion

The initial assessment of circulation includes quickly palpating a pulse and viewing the electrocardiogram (ECG) monitor for the heart rate, rhythm, and presence of ectopy. Assess the patient's blood pressure and temperature and assess peripheral perfusion by evaluating the color, temperature, and moisture of the skin along with capillary refill. Based on the prearrival report and reason for admission, there may also be a need to inspect the body for any signs of blood loss and determine if active bleeding is occurring.

Evaluating cerebral perfusion in the admission quick check assessment is focused on determining the functional integrity of the brain as a whole, which is done by rapidly evaluating the gross LOC. Assess whether the patient is alert and oriented, and what level of stimulus, verbal or painful, elicits a response or whether the patient is unresponsive. Observing the response of the patient during movement from the stretcher to the ICU bed can supply additional information about the LOC. For example, does the patient follow simple commands such as "Place your hands on your chest" or "Slide your hips over?" If the patient is unable to talk because of trauma or the presence of an artificial airway, note whether their head nods appropriately to questions or their eyes follow events in the room. Note that a depressed LOC may indicate that rapid intervention is warranted.

Chief Complaint

Optimally, the description of the chief complaint is obtained from the patient, but this may not be realistic. Data may need to be gathered from family, friends, bystanders, and/or prehospital personnel. For patients with whom you face a language barrier, an approved hospital translator can assist with the interview and subsequent evaluations and communication. Steer clear of using family or friends as translators in order to protect the patient's privacy, avoid the likelihood that family will not understand appropriate medical terminology for translation, and to eliminate well-intentioned but potential bias in translating for the patient. In the absence of a history source, practitioners must depend on physical findings (eg, presence of medication patches, permanent pacemaker, or old surgery scars), knowledge of pathophysiology, access to prior electronic medical records (EMRs), and transport records to identify the chief complaint.

Assessment of the chief complaint focuses on determining the body systems involved and the extent of associated symptoms. Additional questions explore the time of onset, precipitating factors, and severity. Although the admission quick check phase is focused on obtaining a quick overview of the key life-sustaining systems, a more in-depth assessment of a particular system may need to be done at this time. For example, in the prearrival case study scenario presented, completion of the ABCDEs is followed quickly by more extensive assessment of both the neurologic and respiratory systems.

Drugs and Diagnostic Tests

Information about medications and diagnostic tests is integrated into the admission quick check. If IV access is not already present, it is immediately obtained and input and output records are started. If IV medications are infusing, check the medication to verify the name and concentration, and check the pump to verify that this information was correctly selected and that the medication is infusing at the desired dosage and rate. Obtain ordered critical diagnostic tests and augment basic screening tests (Table 1-4) by additional tests appropriate to the underlying diagnosis and chief complaint. Review available laboratory diagnostic data for abnormalities or indications of potential problems requiring immediate intervention. The abnormal laboratory and diagnostic data for specific pathologic conditions will be covered in subsequent chapters.

Equipment

The last phase of the admission quick check is an assessment of the equipment in use. Quickly evaluate all vascular

TABLE 1-4. COMMON DIAGNOSTIC TESTS OBTAINED DURING ADMISSION QUICK CHECK ASSESSMENT

Serum electrolytes
Glucose
Complete blood count with platelets
Coagulation studies
Blood type, screen, and crossmatch
Arterial blood gases
Drug screen and toxicology
Chest x-ray
ECG
Serum troponins

and drainage tubes for location and patency and connect to appropriate monitoring or suction devices. Note the amount, color, consistency, and odor of drainage secretions. Verify the appropriate functioning of all equipment attached to the patient and label as required. While connecting the monitoring and care equipment, it is imperative that the nurse continue to assess the patient's respiratory and cardiovascular status until it is clear that all equipment is functioning appropriately and can be relied on to transmit accurate patient data.

The admission quick check assessment is accomplished in a matter of a few minutes. After completion of the ABCDE assessment, the comprehensive initial assessment begins. Any instability identified during the admission quick check is addressed before proceeding to the comprehensive admission assessment.

After the admission quick check assessment is completed, and if the patient requires no urgent intervention, there may now be time for a more thorough report from the healthcare team transferring the patient to the ICU. It is important to note that handoffs with transitions of care are intervals when safety gaps may occur. Omission of pertinent information or miscommunication at this critical juncture can result in patient care errors. Use of a standardized handoff format—such as the SBAR format, which includes communication of the **S**ituation, **B**ackground, **A**ssessment, and **R**ecommendations—can minimize the potential for miscommunication. Use the handoff as an opportunity to confirm observations such as dosage of infusing medications, abnormalities found on the quick check assessment, the patient's neurologic examination, confirmation of equipment settings, and any potential inconsistencies between the quick arrival assessment and the prearrival report. It is easier to clarify questions while the transporters are still present if possible.

This may also be an opportunity for the first interactions with the patient's family. The relationship between the family and the healthcare team begins with a professional introduction, reassurance, and confirmation of the intent to give the patient the best care possible (Table 1-5). If feasible, allow the family to briefly see the patient. If this is not feasible, give them an approximate time frame when they can expect to receive an update on the patient's condition. Enlisting the assistance of other health team members

TABLE 1-5. EVIDENCE-BASED PRACTICE: FAMILY NEEDS ASSESSMENT

Quick Assessment
- Offer realistic hope
- Give honest answers and information
- Give reassurance

Comprehensive Assessment
- Use open-ended communication and assess their communication style
- Assess family members' level of anxiety
- Assess perceptions of the situation (knowledge, comprehension, expectations of staff, expected outcome)
- Assess family roles and dynamics (cultural and religious practices, values, spokesperson)
- Assess coping mechanisms and resources (what do they use, social network and support)

TABLE 1-6. SUMMARY OF COMPREHENSIVE ADMISSION ASSESSMENT REQUIREMENTS

Past Medical History
- Medical conditions, surgical procedures
- Psychiatric/emotional problems
- Hospitalizations
- Medications (prescription, over-the-counter, herbal or alternative supplements, illicit drugs) and time of last medication dose
- Allergies
- Review of history by body system (see Table 1-7)

Social History
- Age, gender, and self-identified gender
- Ethnic origin
- Height, weight
- Highest educational level completed
- Preferred language
- Occupation
- Marital status
- Primary family members/significant others/decision makers
- Religious affiliation
- Advance Directive, Durable Power of Attorney for Health Care, Medical Orders for Life-Sustaining Treatment (MOLST)
- Substance use/abuse (alcohol, illicit or prescription drugs, caffeine, tobacco)
- Domestic abuse or vulnerable adult screen

Psychosocial Assessment
- General communication
- Coping styles
- Anxiety and stress
- Expectations of critical care unit
- Current stresses
- Family needs

Spirituality
- Faith/spiritual preference
- Healing practices

Physical Assessment[a]
- Nervous system
- Cardiovascular system
- Respiratory system
- Renal system
- Gastrointestinal system
- Endocrine, hematologic, and immune systems
- Integumentary system

[a]Pain may need to be assessed in each body system rather than as a stand-alone assessment—see Table 1-9.

such as social workers and chaplains as family support during the stressful admission period can be invaluable and can set the stage for assessment of the ongoing support family members may need. Identify the primary point of contact, obtain their contact information, and explain visitation policies. Ensure the contact person is updated as soon as possible and involved in daily or shift updates or as your institution has specified. See Chapter 2 for further discussion of family visitation.

COMPREHENSIVE INITIAL ASSESSMENT

Comprehensive initial assessments determine the physiologic and psychosocial baseline to which future changes can be compared to determine whether the status is improving or deteriorating. The comprehensive initial assessment also defines the patient's pre-event health status, determining problems or limitations that may impact patient status during this admission as well as potential issues for future transitions of care. The content presented in this section is a template to screen for abnormalities or determine the extent of injury to the patient. Any abnormal findings or changes from baseline warrant a more in-depth evaluation of the pertinent system.

The comprehensive initial assessment includes review of the patient's medical and brief social history, and physical examination of each body system. The comprehensive admission assessment of the critically ill patient is similar to admission assessments for non-critically ill patients with a few exceptions. This section describes only those aspects of the assessment that are unique to critically ill patients or require more extensive information than is obtained from a non-critical care patient assessment. The entire assessment process is summarized in Tables 1-6 and 1-7.

An increasing proportion of patients in critical care units are older adults, requiring assessments that incorporate the effects of aging. Although assessment of older adults does not differ significantly from that of younger adults, understanding how aging alters the physiologic and psychological status of the patient is important. Key physiologic changes pertinent to the critically ill older adult are summarized in Table 1-8.

Additional emphasis must also be placed on the past medical history as older adults may have coexisting chronic conditions and may be taking multiple prescription and over-the-counter medications. Social history includes addressing issues related to home environment, support systems, and self-care abilities. The interpretation of clinical findings in the older adult must also take into consideration their diminished reserves and the greater risk for rapid physiologic deterioration than in younger adults.

Past Medical History

Besides the primary event that led to the hospital admission, it is important to determine prior medical and surgical conditions, hospitalization, medications, and symptoms (see Table 1-7). In reviewing medication use, ensure assessment

TABLE 1-7. SUGGESTED QUESTIONS FOR REVIEW OF PAST HISTORY CATEGORIZED BY BODY SYSTEM

Body System	History Questions
Neurological	• Have you ever had a seizure? • Have you ever had a stroke? • Have you ever fainted, blacked out, or experienced alcohol withdrawal symptoms? • Do you ever have numbness, tingling, or weakness in any part of your body? • Do you have any difficulty with your hearing, vision, or speech? • Has your daily activity level changed due to your present condition? • Do you require any assistive devices such as canes? • Have you fallen in the past 6 months?
Cardiovascular	• Have you experienced any heart problems or disease such as heart attacks or heart failure? • Do you have any problems with extreme fatigue? • Do you have an irregular heart rhythm? • Do you have high blood pressure? • Do you have a pacemaker or an implanted defibrillator?
Respiratory	• Do you ever experience shortness of breath? • Do you have any pain associated with breathing? • Do you have a persistent cough? Is it productive? • Have you had any exposure to environmental agents that might affect the lungs? • Do you have sleep apnea?
Renal	• Have you had any change in frequency of urination? • Do you have any burning, pain, discharge, or difficulty when you urinate? • Have you had blood in your urine?
Gastrointestinal	• Has there been any recent weight loss or gain? • Have you had any change in appetite? • Do you have any problems with nausea or vomiting? • Do you have any difficulty swallowing? • How often do you have a bowel movement and has there been a change in the normal pattern? Do you have blood in your stools? • Do you have dentures? • Do you have any food allergies?
Integumentary	• Do you have any problems with your skin?
Endocrine	• Have you had a change in your energy level? • Do you have a history of diabetes? Thyroid disease?
Hematologic	• Do you have any problems with bleeding?
Immunologic	• Do you have problems with chronic infections? • Have you recently been exposed to a contagious illness? • Have you recently traveled outside the country?
Psychosocial	• Do you have any physical conditions which make communication difficult (hearing loss, visual disturbances, etc)? • How do you best learn? Do you need information repeated several times and/or require information in advance of teaching sessions? • What are the ways you cope with stress, crises, or pain? • Who are the important people in your "family" or network? Who do you want to make decisions with you, or for you? • Have you had any previous experiences with critical illness? • Have you ever been hurt, or threatened verbally, with physical harm? • Do you feel safe in your home? • Have you ever experienced trouble with anxiety, irritability, being confused, mood swings, or suicidal thoughts or attempts? • What are the cultural practices, religious influences, and values that are important to you or your family? • What are family perceptions and expectations of the critical care staff and the setting?
Spiritual	• What is your faith or spiritual preference? • What practices help you heal or deal with stress? • Would you like to see a chaplain, priest, or other spiritual guide?

of over-the-counter medication use as well as any herbal or alternative supplements. For every positive symptom response, additional questions are asked to explore the characteristics of that symptom (Table 1-9).

Social History

The social history includes asking about caffeine, alcohol, tobacco, illicit drugs, or prescription medications such as opioids. Because the use of these agents may impact

treatment during critical illness, the history also includes the frequency, amount, and duration of any substance use. Keep in mind the information provided regarding alcohol and substance use may not always be honest. Alcohol use is common in all age groups, and acknowledging this fact may be helpful in obtaining an accurate answer (eg, "How much alcohol do you drink?" vs "Do you drink alcohol and how much?"). Family may be helpful in providing additional information about substance use. The information revealed

TABLE 1-8. PHYSIOLOGIC EFFECTS OF AGING

Body System	Effects
Neurological	Diminished hearing and vision, short-term memory loss, altered motor coordination, decreased muscle tone and strength, slower response to verbal and motor stimuli, decreased ability to synthesize new information, increased sensitivity to altered temperature states, increased sensitivity to sedation (confusion or agitation), decreased alertness levels
Cardiovascular	Increased effects of atherosclerosis of vessels and heart valves, decreased stroke volume with resulting decreased cardiac output, decreased myocardial compliance, increased workload of heart, diminished peripheral pulses
Respiratory	Decreased compliance and elasticity, decreased vital capacity, increased residual volume, less effective cough, decreased response to hypercapnia
Renal	Decreased glomerular filtration rate, increased risk of fluid and electrolyte imbalances
Gastrointestinal	Increased presence of dentition problems, decreased intestinal mobility, decreased hepatic metabolism, increased risk of altered nutritional states
Endocrine, hematologic, and immunologic	Increased incidence of diabetes, thyroid disorders, and anemia; decreased antibody response and cellular immunity
Integumentary	Decreased skin turgor, increased capillary fragility and bruising, decreased elasticity
Miscellaneous	Altered pharmacokinetics and pharmacodynamics, decreased range of motion of joints and extremities
Psychosocial	Difficulty falling asleep and fragmented sleep patterns, increased incidence of depression and anxiety, cognitive impairment disorders, difficulty with change

during the social history can often be verified during the physical assessment through the presence of signs such as skin lesions concerning for injection sites, discoloration on teeth and fingers concerning for nicotine use, or the smell of alcohol on the breath.

Patients are also asked about physical and emotional safety in their home environment in order to uncover potential abuse. It is best if patients can be assessed for vulnerability when they are alone., Ask questions such as "Is anyone hurting you?" or "Do you feel safe at home?" in a non-threatening manner. Suspicion of abuse or vulnerability is reason for a consultation with a social worker and possible reporting to protective services.

Physical Assessment by Body System

In this section, the physical assessment sequence is the combination of the system-based and head-to-toe approach. Although content is presented as separate components,

TABLE 1-9. IDENTIFICATION OF SYMPTOM CHARACTERISTICS

Characteristic	Sample Questions
Onset	How and under what circumstances did it begin? Was the onset sudden or gradual? Did it progress?
Location	Where is it? Does it stay in the same place or does it radiate or move around?
Frequency	How often does it occur?
Quality	Is it dull, sharp, burning, throbbing, etc?
Intensity	Rate intensity on a scale (numeric, word description, FACES)
Quantity	How long does it last?
Setting	What are you doing when it happens?
Associated findings	Are there other signs and symptoms that occur when this happens?
Aggravating and alleviating factors	What things make it worse? What things make it better?

generally the history questions are integrated into the physical assessment. The physical assessment section uses the techniques of inspection, auscultation, percussion, and palpation.

Pain assessment is generally linked to each body system rather than considered as a separate system category. For example, if the patient has chest pain, assessment and documentation of that pain is incorporated into the cardiovascular assessment. Rather than have general pain assessment questions repeated under each system assessment, they are presented here.

Pain and discomfort are clues that alert both the patient and the critical care nurse that something is wrong and needs prompt attention. Pain assessment includes differentiating acute from chronic pain, determining related physiologic symptoms, and investigating the patient's perceptions and emotional reactions to the pain. Explore the qualities and characteristics of pain by using the questions listed in Table 1-9. Pain is a subjective assessment and critical care practitioners sometimes struggle with applying their own values when attempting to evaluate the patient's pain. To resolve this dilemma, use the patient's own words and descriptions of the pain whenever possible and use a patient-preferred pain scale (see Chapter 6, Pain, Sedation, and Neuromuscular Blockade Management) to objectively and consistently evaluate pain levels. If the patient is nonverbal, there are several validated tools that can be used to assess pain beyond physiologic signs such as the critical care pain observation tool (CPOT) or the behavioral pain scale (BPS).

Neurological System

The neurological system is the "master computer" of all the systems and is divided into the central and peripheral nervous systems. With the exception of the peripheral nervous system's cranial nerves, almost all attention in the critically ill patient is focused on evaluating the central nervous system (CNS). The physiologic and psychological impact of critical illness, in addition to pharmacologic interventions, frequently alters CNS functioning. The single most important indicator of cerebral functioning is the LOC. The LOC is assessed in the critically ill patient using a standardized scale (see Chapter 12, Neurologic System).

Additional neurological assessment includes evaluating the patient's pupils for size, shape, symmetry, and reactivity to direct light. Certain medications such as atropine, morphine, or illicit drugs may affect pupil size. A baseline pupil and neurologic assessment is important even in patients without a neurologic diagnosis because some individuals have unequal or unreactive pupils normally. If pupils are not checked as a baseline, a later check of pupils during an acute event could inappropriately attribute pupil abnormalities to a pathophysiologic event.

LOC and pupil assessments are followed by motor function assessment of the upper and lower extremities for symmetry and quality of strength. Traditional motor strength exercises include having the patient raise two fingers or show a thumbs up, and plantar flexing and dorsiflexing of the patient's feet. If the patient cannot follow commands, an estimate of strength and quality of movements can be inferred by observing activities such as pulling against restraints or thrashing around. If the patient has no voluntary movement or is unresponsive, check reflexes including but not limited to the gag, cough, and corneal reflexes. If head trauma is involved or suspected, check for evidence of fluid leakage around the nose or ears, differentiating between cerebral spinal fluid and blood (see Chapter 12, Neurologic System).

Now is a good time to assess mental status if the patient is responsive. Assess orientation to person, place, and time. Ask the patient to state their understanding of what is happening. As they answer questions, observe for eye contact, pressured or muted speech, and rate of speech. Rate of speech is usually consistent with the patient's psychomotor status. Underlying cognitive impairments such as dementia and developmental delays are typically exacerbated during critical illness due to physiologic changes, medications, and environmental changes. The patient should be screened for delirium regularly, at least once a shift, ideally using a standardized tool such as the Confusion Assessment Method for the ICU (CAM-ICU). The family may be able to provide information about the patient's baseline level of functioning.

Laboratory data pertinent to the nervous system include serum glucose, ammonia, thyroid function, electrolytes, urine osmolarity, and specific gravity. Drug toxicology and alcohol levels may be evaluated to rule out potential sources of altered LOC. If the patient has an intracranial pressure (ICP) monitoring device in place, note the type of device (eg, ventriculostomy, epidural, subdural) and analyze the baseline pressure and waveform. Check all diagnostic values and monitoring system data to determine whether immediate intervention is warranted.

Cardiovascular System

The cardiovascular system assessment is directed at evaluating central and peripheral perfusion. Revalidate your admission quick check assessment of the blood pressure, heart rate, and rhythm. Assess the ECG for T-wave abnormalities and ST-segment changes, and determine the PR, QRS, QT intervals, and the QTc measurements (see Chapter 3, Interpretation and Management of Basic Cardiac Rhythms). Note any abnormalities or indications of myocardial damage, electrical conduction problems, and electrolyte imbalances. Note the pulse pressure. If treatment decisions will be based on the cuff pressure, blood pressure is taken in both arms to determine if there is a difference. If different, a decision about which to use is made to ensure consistency. Consider obtaining a manual pressure to confirm an abnormal pressure. If an arterial pressure line is in place, use a fast flush test to assess the dynamic response and accuracy. Determine which pressure will be used for ongoing monitoring. Switching between cuff and arterial line methods may lead critical care teams to inappropriately attribute fluctuations in blood pressure to physiologic changes rather than anatomic differences.

Note the color and temperature of the skin, with particular emphasis on lips, mucous membranes, and distal extremities. Visualize the chest wall for surgical scaring, presence of pacing wires, and invasive tubes. Also evaluate nail color and capillary refill. Inspect for the presence of edema, particularly in the dependent parts of the body such as feet, ankles, and sacrum. Measurement scales to quantify the severity of peripheral edema vary between sources and institutions. Nurses are encouraged to follow institutional policy, as appropriate, to ensure consistency.

Auscultation of heart sounds includes assessment of S_1 and S_2 quality, intensity, and pitch and the presence of extra heart sounds, murmurs, clicks, or rubs. Listen to one sound at a time, consistently progressing through the key anatomic landmarks of the heart each time. Note whether there are any changes with respiration or patient position.

Palpate the peripheral pulses for amplitude and quality, and rate using the 0 to +4 scale (Table 1-10). Check bilateral pulses simultaneously, except the carotid, comparing each pulse to its partner. If the pulse is difficult to palpate, an ultrasound (Doppler) device is used. To facilitate finding a weak pulse for subsequent assessments, mark the location of the pulse with a permanent marker. It is also helpful to compare quality of the pulses to the ECG to evaluate the perfusion of heart beats.

Electrolyte levels, complete blood counts (CBCs), coagulation studies, and lipid profiles are common laboratory

TABLE 1-10. PERIPHERAL PULSE RATING SCALE

- 0 Absent pulse
- +1 Palpable but thready; easily obliterated with light pressure
- +2 Normal; cannot obliterate with light pressure
- +3 Full
- +4 Full and bounding

tests evaluated for abnormalities of the cardiovascular system. Cardiac biomarkers (troponin, creatine kinase-MB, B-natriuretic peptide) are obtained for any complaint of chest pain, suspected chest trauma, or a concern for heart failure. Drug levels of commonly used cardiovascular medications, such as digoxin, may be warranted for certain types of arrhythmias. A 12-lead ECG is typically evaluated on all adult patients with cardiovascular symptoms or risk factors (eg, with complaints of chest pain, irregular rhythms, syncope, dizziness or suspected myocardial contusion from trauma).

Note the type, size, and location of IV catheters, and verify their patency. If continuous infusions of medications such as vasopressors or antiarrhythmics are being administered, ensure the dose matches current orders. Also check to see that they are being infused into an appropriately sized vessel in accordance with hospital policies. If two medications or solutions are infusing through the same line, check to ensure they are compatible.

Verify that all monitoring system alarm parameters are active with appropriate limits set. Note the size and location of invasive monitoring lines such as arterial, central venous, and pulmonary artery (PA) catheters. Confirm that the appropriate flush solution is hanging and that the correct amount of pressure is applied. Level the invasive line to the appropriate anatomic landmark and zero the monitor as needed. For PA catheters, note the size of the introducer and the length (in centimeters), marking where the catheter exits the introducer. Interpret hemodynamic pressure readings in relation to normal value ranges and the patient's underlying pathophysiology. Assess waveforms to determine the quality of the waveform and whether the waveform appropriately matches the expected characteristics for the anatomic placement of the invasive catheter (see Chapter 4, Hemodynamic Monitoring). For example, a right ventricular waveform for a central venous pressure line indicates a problem with the position of the central venous line that needs to be corrected. If the PA catheter has continuous mixed venous saturation (SvO_2) capabilities or continuous cardiac output data, these numbers are also evaluated in conjunction with vital sign data and any concurrent pharmacologic and/or volume infusions.

Evaluate any cardiovascular devices as feasible, such as a pacemaker (internal or external), an implantable cardioverter defibrillator (ICD), automated external defibrillator (AED), or any ventricular assist device. Verify and document equipment settings, appropriate function of the device, and the patient's response to the device's function.

Respiratory System

Oxygenation and ventilation are the focus of respiratory assessment parameters. Reassess the rate and rhythm of respirations and the symmetry of chest wall movement. If the patient has a productive cough or secretions are suctioned from an artificial airway, note the color, consistency, and amount of secretions. Evaluate whether the trachea is midline or shifted. Inspect the thoracic cavity for shape,

anterior-posterior diameter, structural deformities (eg, kyphosis or scoliosis), and presence of scars. Palpate for equal chest excursion, presence of crepitus, and any areas of tenderness or fractures. If the patient is receiving supplemental oxygen, verify the mode of delivery and percentage of oxygen and compare to provider orders.

Auscultate upper and lower lobes anteriorly and posteriorly for bilateral breath sounds to determine the presence of air movement and adventitious sounds such as crackles or wheezes. Note the quality and depth of respirations, and the length and pitch of the inspiratory and expiratory phases.

Arterial blood gases (ABGs) are frequently used to assess oxygenation, ventilatory status, and acid-base balance. Hemoglobin and hematocrit values are interpreted for their impact on oxygenation and fluid balance. If the patient's condition warrants, the oxygen saturation values may be continuously monitored via connection to a noninvasive oxygen saturation monitor or via SvO_2 through a PA catheter device. Continuous end-tidal CO_2 is often integrated into the respiratory assessment, particularly during cardiac arrest, intubation, in postoperative patients, or after moderate sedation.

If the patient is intubated, note the size of the ET tube and record the centimeter marking at the teeth or nares to assist future comparisons for proper placement. Note mechanical ventilator settings including the ventilatory mode, tidal volume, respiratory rate, positive end-expiratory pressure (PEEP), pressure support, and percentage of oxygen and compare to prescribed settings. Observe whether the patient has spontaneous breaths, noting both the rate and the average tidal volume of each breath and whether those breaths are in synchrony. Note the amount of pressure required to ventilate the patient for later comparisons to determine changes in pulmonary compliance. For patients placed on noninvasive positive pressure breathing devices (eg, continuous positive airway pressure [CPAP] or bilevel positive airway pressure [BiPAP]), assess breathing patterns, including the rate and depth of respirations as well as tolerance to the ventilator support mechanism.

If chest tubes are present, palpate the area around the insertion site for crepitus. Ensure all connections are secured and intact, note the amount and color of drainage, and whether fluctuations occur with respiration and if an air leak is present. Verify whether the chest tube drainage system is under water seal or connected to suction.

Renal System

Urine characteristics, amount of urine output, both serum and urine electrolyte status as well as blood urea nitrogen (BUN) and creatinine are important parameters used to evaluate kidney function. In conjunction with the cardiovascular system, the renal system's impact on fluid volume status is also assessed.

For patients with indwelling urinary catheters in place, note the amount, clarity, and color of the urine and, if warranted, obtain a sample for urinalysis to assess for the abnormal presence of glucose, protein, and blood. Inspect the external genitalia and urethral meatus for signs or trauma or infection, that is, bleeding, inflammation, swelling, ulcers, and abnormal drainage. Determine if the patient meets criteria for an indwelling catheter or if a noninvasive urinary collection device can be used instead, to reduce the risk of catheter-associated infection and still monitor urinary output. If suprapubic tubes or a ureterostomy are present, note the position as well as the amount and characteristics of the drainage. Observe whether any drainage is leaking around the drainage tube and assess the tube site for signs of complication.

Gastrointestinal System

Key factors when reviewing the gastrointestinal system are assessment of the abdomen, nutritional status, and fluid balance. Inspect the abdomen for overall symmetry, noting whether the contour is flat, round, protuberant, or distended. Note the presence of trauma, wounds, scars, ecchymosis, visibly dilated abdominal veins, discoloration, or striae. Nutritional status is evaluated by looking at the patient's weight and muscle tone, the condition of the oral mucosa, and laboratory values such as serum albumin, prealbumin, and transferrin.

Auscultation of bowel sounds is performed in all four quadrants in a clockwise order, noting the frequency and presence or absence of sounds. Bowel sounds are usually rated as absent, hypoactive, normal, or hyperactive. Before noting absent bowel sounds, listen for at least 60 to 90 seconds. Characteristics and frequency of the sounds are noted. After listening for the presence of normal sounds, determine if any adventitious bowel sounds such as friction rubs, bruits, or hums are present.

Light palpation of the abdomen identifies masses, areas of fluid or ascites, rigidity, tenderness, pain, and guarding or rebound tenderness. Remember to auscultate before palpating because palpation may change the frequency and character of the patient's peristaltic sounds. The abdomen is percussed, checking for tympanic or dull sounds over hollow and solid organs.

Assess the location and function of any drainage tubes, and note the characteristics of their drainage. Make sure to validate the proper placement and patency of the NG tube. Check emesis and stool for occult blood as appropriate and if ordered. Evaluate ostomies for location, color of the stoma, and color and consistency of their output. If indicated, evaluate for abdominal compartment syndrome by measuring intraabdominal pressure via the urinary catheter.

Endocrine, Hematologic, and Immune Systems

The endocrine, hematologic, and immune systems often are overlooked when assessing critically ill patients. The assessment parameters used to evaluate these systems are included under other system assessments, but consciously considering these systems when reviewing these parameters is essential. Assessing the endocrine, hematologic, and immune systems is based on a thorough understanding of the primary function of each of the hormones, blood cells, or immune components of each of the respective systems.

Assessment of the endocrine system is challenging because symptoms of changes in hormone secretion are similar to symptoms that occur due to disorders in the other systems. The patient's history may help differentiate the source, but any abnormal assessment findings detected regarding fluid balance, metabolic rate, altered LOC, color and temperature of the skin, electrolytes, glucose, and acid-base balance require the critical care nurse to consider the potential involvement of the endocrine system. For example, are the signs and symptoms of hypervolemia related to acute kidney injury or excessive amounts of antidiuretic hormone? Is hypotension due to cardiac dysfunction or due to adrenal insufficiency? Serum blood tests for specific hormone levels may be required to rule out or confirm the involvement of the endocrine system.

Assessment parameters specific to the hematologic system include laboratory evaluation of the red blood cells (RBCs) and coagulation studies. Diminished RBCs may affect the oxygen-carrying capacity of the blood, which is evidenced by pallor, cyanosis, light-headedness, tachypnea, and tachycardia. Check the patient for bruising, oozing of blood from puncture sites or mucous membranes, or overt bleeding, which may indicate low platelet count or a deficiency in clotting factors. See Chapter 13 (Hematologic and Immune Systems) for additional discussion of the hematologic and immunologic assessment.

The immune system's primary function of fighting infection is assessed by evaluating the white cell and differential counts from the CBC, and assessing puncture sites and mucous membranes for drainage, inflammation, and redness. Spiking or persistent low-grade temperatures often are indicative of underlying infections. The absence of these symptoms, however, may not indicate the absence of infection. Many critically ill patients have impaired immune systems and the normal response to infection, such as purulent drainage around an insertion site or elevated temperature and white blood cell count (WBC), may not be evident. If infection is suspected, consider the potential sources that can be readily addressed, such as the length of time an invasive line or urinary catheter has been in place.

Integumentary System

The skin is the first line of defense against infection so assessment parameters are focused on evaluating the intactness of the skin. Assessing the skin can be undertaken while performing other system assessments. For example, while listening to breath sounds or bowel sounds, the condition of the thoracic cavity or abdominal skin can be observed, respectively. It is important that a thorough head-to-toe, anterior, posterior, and between skin folds assessment is performed and documented on admission to identify any preexisting skin integrity concerns that need to be immediately addressed, and to establish a baseline for comparison with future assessments.

Inspect the skin for overall integrity, color, temperature, and turgor. Note the presence of rashes, striae, discoloration, scars, or lesions. For any abrasions, lesions, pressure injury, or wounds, note the size, depth, and presence or absence of drainage. Consider use of a skin integrity risk assessment tool to determine immediate interventions that are needed to prevent development of further loss of skin integrity and/or pressure injury.

Psychosocial Assessment

The rapid physiologic and psychological changes associated with critical illnesses, coupled with pharmacologic and biological treatments, can profoundly affect behavior. Patients may suffer from illnesses that lead to predictable psychological responses, and, if untreated, may threaten recovery or life. To avoid making assumptions about how a patient or family feels, ask them directly. Educate families about the psychological symptoms that critically ill patients may experience and encourage their emotional support of the patient. As dictated by institution policy, assess the risk for self-harm and suicide and implement precautions accordingly.

General Communication

Factors that affect communication include culture, developmental stage, physical condition, stress, perception, neurocognitive deficits, emotional state, and language skills. The nature of a critical illness, coupled with pharmacologic and airway technologies, interferes with the patients' usual methods of communication. It is essential to determine pre-illness communication abilities and identify methods and styles to ensure optimal communication with the critically ill patient and family. The inability of many critically ill patients to communicate verbally necessitates that critical care practitioners become expert at assessing nonverbal clues. Important assessment data include body gestures, facial expressions, eye movements, involuntary movements, and changes in physiologic parameters, particularly heart rate, blood pressure, and respiratory rate.

Anxiety and Stress

Anxiety is both psychologically and physiologically exhausting. Being in a prolonged state of arousal is hard work and uses adaptive reserves needed for recovery. The critical care environment is very stressful, full of constant auditory, visual, and tactile stimuli, and may contribute to a patient's anxiety level. The critical care setting may force isolation from social supports, dependency, loss of control, trust in unknown care providers, helplessness, and an inability to solve or attend to a problem. Restlessness, distractibility, hyperventilation, and unrealistic demands for attention are warning signs of escalating anxiety.

Medications such as interferons, corticosteroids, angiotensin-converting enzyme inhibitors, and vasopressors can induce anxiety. Abrupt withdrawal from benzodiazepines, caffeine, nicotine, and narcotics, as well as akathisia from phenothiazines, may mimic anxiety. Additional etiologic variables associated with anxiety include pain, sleep loss, delirium, hypoxia, ventilator synchronization or weaning, fear of death, loss of control, high-technology equipment, and a dehumanizing setting. Admission to or repeated transfers to the critical care unit may also induce anxiety.

Coping Styles

Individuals cope with a critical illness in different ways and understanding their pre-illness coping style, personality traits, or temperament allows the nurse to anticipate coping styles in the critical care setting. Include the patient's family when assessing previous resources, coping skills, or defense mechanisms. For instance, some patients want to be informed of everything that is happening with them in the ICU. Providing information reduces their anxiety and gives them a sense of control. Other patients prefer to have others receive information and make decisions for them. Giving them detailed information only exacerbates their level of anxiety and diminishes their ability to cope. Understanding the meaning that the patient and family assign to this illness event is also crucial in evaluating their ability to cope. Does the coping resource fit with the event and meet the patient's and family's need?

Assessment of spiritual beliefs may reveal an additional tool to support coping. Minimally, patients are asked whether they have a faith or spiritual preference and offered the support of a chaplain, or other spiritual guide. In addition, patients are asked about spiritual and cultural healing practices that are important to them to determine whether those can be continued during their ICU stay.

Patients and families use different modes of interacting and coping to feel safe. Some may remain stoic and avoid interacting while others may seek attention from the healthcare team. Efforts to cope may present as impulsive behaviors, a low tolerance for frustration, or a general avoidance of rules or limits. Others may cope by withdrawing and actually requesting use of sedatives and sleeping medications to blunt the stimuli and stress of the environment.

Fear has an identifiable source and plays an important role in the ability of the patient to cope. Treatments, procedures, pain, and separation are common objects of fear. The dying process elicits specific fears, such as fear of the unknown, loneliness, loss of body, loss of self-control, suffering, pain, loss of identity, and loss of everyone loved by the patient. The family, as well as the patient, experiences the grieving process, which may include the phases of denial, shock, anger, bargaining, depression, and acceptance.

Family Needs

Family is not defined by social or legal boundaries but rather by the nature of the patients' relationship with others. Ideally the patient is asked to identify those they view as their family, and to select who receives information and makes decisions if they become unable to make decisions on their own. Advanced directive, Medical/Physician Orders for Life-sustaining Treatment (MOLST or POLST) forms provide insight as to the patient's wishes about their care and may also provide guidance as to who the patient defines as their family. Critical care teams need to take into account traditional legal requirements of "next of kin" as well as the patient's wishes surrounding "next of kin" so that communication is extended to, and sought from, surrogate decision makers and patient designates.

Families can have a positive impact on patients' abilities to cope with and recover from a critical illness. Open visitation practices with policies and protections in place to address violence and incivility are encouraged. Each family system is unique and varies by culture, values, religion, previous experience with crisis, socioeconomic status, psychological integrity, role expectations, communication patterns, health beliefs, and ages. It is important to assess the family's needs and resources to develop interventions that will optimize the impact of the family on the patient and support the family's collaboration with the healthcare team. Areas for family needs assessments are outlined in Table 1-5.

Family Visitation

Limitations on family visitation may be imposed due to exceptional circumstances such as those created by the COVID-19 pandemic. Visitation policies must balance the risks to the community of spreading a communicable disease with the benefits that family presence offers. Ideally, visitation policies promote patient access to visitors whom they have identified as a source of support. Visitation restrictions may be appropriate in some circumstances and should be imposed on a case-by-case basis or only applied to nonessential visitors during periods of high community transmission. Strategies for connecting families with patients if their access is limited include:

- Designating a family member as the contact person.
- Establishing a time every day and a method for communication for regularly connecting with the family.
- Identifying language barriers or translation needs.
- Leveraging, the healthcare team, eg, social workers, chaplains, and other team members, to also provide communication and support to the patient's family.
- Exploring the use of cellphones and tablets for video calls. If you are using visual communication, explain what they will see in the patient's room
- Video or audio recordings of family members' voices may also provide a sense of their presence.

Unit Orientation

It is important that the critical care nurse takes time to educate the patient (if alert) and family about the ICU environment. Explain the equipment being used in the care of the patient, visitation policies, the routines of the unit, and how the patient and family can communicate their needs to the unit staff. Provide the unit telephone number and the names of the key individuals including nurse leaders, the charge nurse, and the team members caring for the patient. Explain to the patient and family how they will be involved in the patient's care and describe opportunities to ask any questions.

TABLE 1-11. EXAMPLES OF POTENTIAL REFERRALS NEEDED FOR CRITICALLY ILL PATIENTS

Referral	Resources Needed
Social work	• Financial needs/resources for patient and/or family • Coping resources for patient and/or family
Nutrition	• Nutritional status at risk and in need of in-depth nutritional assessment • Altered nutritional status on admission
Therapies	• Physical therapy for maintaining or improving physical flexibility and strength • Occupational therapy for assistive devices • Speech therapy for assessment of ability to swallow or communication needs
Pastoral care	• Spiritual guidance for patient and/or family • Coping resources for patient and/or family
Wound ostomy continence (WOC) nursing	• Stoma assessment and needs • Wound vacuum management • In-depth skin integrity needs
Ethics committee	• Decisions involving significant ethical complexity • Decisions involving disagreements over care between care providers or between care providers and patient/family • Decisions involving withholding or withdrawing life-sustaining treatment not adequately addressed in policy
Care coordinator	• Anticipated transition needs throughout and post-hospitalization

Referrals

After completing the comprehensive initial assessment, the critical care nurse analyzes the information gathered and determines the need to make referrals to other healthcare providers and resources (Table 1-11). To ensure appropriate and timely discharge, maintain continuity of care and promote appropriate resource management, referrals are initiated as soon as possible.

ONGOING ASSESSMENT

After the admission quick check and the comprehensive admission assessments, all subsequent assessments are used to determine trends, evaluate response to therapy, and identify new potential problems or changes from the comprehensive baseline assessment. Ongoing assessments become more focused and the frequency is driven by the stability of the patient; however, routine periodic assessments are the norm. For example, ongoing assessments may occur every few minutes for extremely unstable patients, though unit protocols may require an assessment every 2 to 4 hours. Additional assessments are made when any of the following situations occur:

- Caregivers change
- Before and after a procedural intervention, such as intubation or chest tube insertion
- Before and after transport out of the critical care unit for diagnostic procedures or other events
- Deterioration in physiologic or mental status
- Initiation of any new therapy

As with the admission quick check, the ongoing assessment section is offered as a generic template that can be used as a basis for all patients (Table 1-12). More in-depth and system-specific assessment parameters are added based on the patient's diagnosis and pathophysiologic problems.

TABLE 1-12. ONGOING ASSESSMENT TEMPLATE

Body System	Assessment Parameters
Neurological	• LOC • Pupils • Motor strength of extremities
Cardiovascular	• Blood pressure • Heart rate and rhythm • Heart sounds • Capillary refill • Peripheral pulses • Patency of IVs • Verification of IV solutions and medications • Hemodynamic pressures and waveforms • Cardiac output data • Pacemaker or implanted defibrillator function
Respiratory	• Respiratory rate and rhythm • Breath sounds • Color and amount of secretions • Noninvasive technology information (eg, pulse oximetry, end-tidal CO_2) • Mechanical ventilatory parameters • Type, patency, and function of chest tubes • Arterial and venous blood gases
Renal	• Intake and output • Color and clarity of urinary output • Blood urea nitrogen (BUN)/creatinine values
Gastrointestinal	• Bowel sounds • Contour of abdomen • Position and patency of drainage tubes • Position of feeding tube • Color and amount of secretions • Bilirubin and albumin values
Endocrine, hematologic, and immunologic	• Fluid balance • Electrolyte and glucose values • CBC and coagulation values • Temperature • WBC with differential count
Integumentary	• Color and temperature of skin • Risk for pressure injury • Skin integrity • Areas of redness
Pain/discomfort	• Assessed in each system • Response to interventions
Psychosocial	• Mental status and behavioral responses • Reaction to critical illness experience (eg, stress, anxiety, coping, mood) • Presence of cognitive impairments (dementia, delirium), depression, or demoralization • Family functioning and needs • Ability to communicate needs and participate in care • Sleep patterns

PRINCIPLES OF MANAGEMENT

- There are four distinct components in the assessment of a critically ill patient: (1) the prearrival assessment, (2) the admission quick check, (3) the comprehensive initial assessment, and (4) ongoing assessments.
- The admission quick check is systematic so as not to miss subtle signs or cues. It is also used to ensure that patients' urgent needs are met. For instance, the patient's mental status can be observed during transfer from stretcher to hospital bed and addressed quickly.
- A common standard assessment approach is a combination of a body systems and a head-to-toe approach. A consistent process is applied to ensure complete information is gathered, while additional attention is given to certain systems according to the patient's presenting pathology.
- Assessment focuses first on the patient, and then on technology.

SELECTED BIBLIOGRAPHY

Critical Care Assessment

American Association of Critical-Care Nurses. *Practice Alert: Assessment and Management of Delirium Across the Lifespan.* Aliso Viejo, CA: AACN; 2016. https://www.aacn.org/clinical-resources/practice-alerts/assessment-and-management-of-delirium-across-the-life-span

American Association of Critical-Care Nurses. *Practice Alert: Ensuring Accurate ST Monitoring.* Aliso Viejo, CA: AACN; 2016. https://www.aacn.org/clinical-resources/practice-alerts/st-segment-monitoring

American Association of Critical-Care Nurses. *Practice Alert: Obtaining Accurate Non-Invasive Blood Pressure Measurements in Adults.* Aliso Viejo, CA: AACN; 2016. https://www.aacn.org/clinical-resources/practice-alerts/obtaining-accurate-noninvasive-blood-pressure-measurements-in-adults

Bickley LS. *Bates' Guide to Physical Examination and History Taking.* 13th ed. Philadelphia, PA: Lippincott Williams & Wilkins; 2020.

Diepenbrock N. *Quick Reference to Critical Care.* 5th ed. Philadelphia, PA: Lippincott, Williams, & Wilkins; 2016.

Good VS, Kirkwood PL. *Advanced Critical Care Nursing.* 2nd ed. St. Louis, MO: Elsevier; 2018.

Hartjes TM. *AACN Core Curriculum for High Acuity, Progressive, and Critical Care.* St. Louis, MO: Elsevier; 2018.

Wiegand DLM. *AACN Procedure Manual for High Acuity, Progressive, and Critical Care.* 7th ed. Philadelphia, PA: Elsevier; 2017.

Evidence-Based Practice

Ahn J, Jang H, Son Y. Critical care nurses' communication challenges during handovers: a systematic review and qualitative meta-synthesis. *J Nurs Manag.* 2021;May 29(4):623-634.

American Heart Association. 2020 American Heart Association guidelines for cardiopulmonary resuscitation and emergency cardiovascular care. *Circulation.* 2020;142(16):S337-S357.

Balas MC, Weinhouse GL, Denehy L, et al. Interpreting and implementing the 2018 pain, agitation/sedation, delirium, immobility, and sleep disruption clinical practice guideline. *Crit Care Med.* 2018;46(9):1464-1470.

Bialek K, Sadowski M. Stress, anxiety, depression and basic hope in family members of patients hospitalised in intensive care units—preliminary report. *Anaesthesiol Intensive Ther.* 2021;53:2.

Buckley P, Andrews T. Intensive care nurses' knowledge of critical care family needs. *Intensive Crit Care Nurs.* 2011;27(5):263-272.

Davidson JE, Harvey MA. Patient and family post-intensive care syndrome. *AACN Adv Crit Care.* 2016;27(2):184-186.

Devlin JW, Skrobik Y, Gélinas C, et al. Clinical practice guidelines for the prevention and management of pain, agitation/sedation, delirium, immobility, and sleep disruption in adult patients in the ICU. *Crit Care Med.* 2018;46(9):e825-e873.

Hansen L, Rosenkranz SJ, Mularski RA, Leo MC. Family perspectives on overall care in the intensive care unit. *Nurs Res.* 2016;65(6):446-454.

Hilligoss B, Cohen MD. The unappreciated challenges of between-unit handoffs: negotiating and coordinating across boundaries. *Ann Emerg Med.* 2013;61(1):15-160.

Inoue S, Hatakeyama J, Kondo Y, et al. Post-intensive care syndrome: its pathophysiology, prevention, and future directions. *Acute Med Surg.* 2019;Jul 6(3):233-246.

Kotfis K, Roberson SW, Wilson JE, Dabrowski W, Pun BT, Ely EW. COVID-19: ICU delirium management during SARS-CoV-2 pandemic. *Crit Care.* 2020;24:176.

Kowitlawakul Y, Leong, BSH, Lua A, et al. Observation of handover process in an intensive care unit (ICU): barriers and quality improvement strategy. *Int J Qual Health Care.* 2015;27(2):99-104.

Marmo S, Milner KA. From open to closed: COVID-19 restrictions on previously unrestricted visitation policies in adult intensive care units. *Am J Crit Care.* 2022;Sep 30:e1-e11. doi:10.4037/ajcc2023365

Sandau KE, Funk M, Auerbach A, et al. Update to practice standards for electrocardiographic monitoring in hospital settings: a scientific statement from the American Heart Association. *Circulation.* 2017;136(19):e273-e344.

Society of Critical Care Medicine. ICU Liberation Bundle. https://www.sccm.org/Clinical-Resources/ICULiberation-Home/ABCDEF-Bundles

Spooner AJ, Corley A, Chaboyer W, Hammond NE, Fraser JF. Measurement of the frequency and source of interruptions occurring during bedside nursing handover in the intensive care unit: an observation study. *Aust Crit Care.* 2015;28(1):19-23.

Turner-Cobb JM, Smith PC, Ramchandani P, Begen FM, Padkin A. The acute psychobiological impact of the intensive care experience on relatives. *Psychol Health Med.* 2016;21(1):20-26.

US Preventative Services Task Force. Cardiovascular Disease Risk: Screening with Electrocardiography. June 12, 2018. https://www.uspreventiveservicestaskforce.org/uspstf/recommendation/cardiovascular-disease-risk-screening-with-electrocardiography

PLANNING CARE FOR CRITICALLY ILL PATIENTS AND THEIR FAMILIES

2

Maxine Wanzer

KNOWLEDGE COMPETENCIES

1. Discuss the importance of an interprofessional plan of care for optimizing clinical outcomes.

2. Describe interventions for prevention of common complications in critically ill patients:
   - Venous thromboembolism
   - Infection
   - Sleep pattern disturbances
   - Pressure injury
   - Delirium

3. Discuss interventions to maintain psychosocial integrity and minimize anxiety for the critically ill patient and family members.

4. Describe interventions to promote family-centered care and patient and family education.

5. Identify necessary equipment and personnel required to safely transport the critically ill patient within the hospital.

6. Describe transfer-related complications and preventive measures to be taken before and during patient transport.

The achievement of optimal clinical outcomes in the critically ill patient requires a coordinated approach to care delivery by interprofessional team members. Experts in nutrition, respiratory therapy, physical therapy, social work, pharmacy, palliative medicine, critical care nursing and medicine, as well as other disciplines, work collaboratively to effectively and efficiently provide optimal care.

The following section provides an overview of interprofessional plans of care. In addition, this chapter discusses approaches to patient needs that are not diagnosis specific, but common to a majority of critically ill patients, such as sleep deprivation, pressure injury, and patient and family education. Additional discussion of these needs or problems is also presented in other chapters if related to specific disease management.

INTERPROFESSIONAL PLAN OF CARE

An *interprofessional plan of care* is a set of expectations for the major components of care a patient receives during hospitalization to manage a specific medical or surgical problem. Other types of plans include *clinical pathways*, *protocols*, and *care maps*. The interprofessional plan of care expands on the concept of a medical or nursing care plan and provides a comprehensive blueprint for patient care that includes the roles of multiple team members. The result is a diagnosis-specific plan of care that focuses the entire care team on expected patient outcomes.

The interprofessional plan of care outlines the tests, medications, care, and treatments needed to transition the patient to the next stage of care in a timely manner with all patient needs met. These plans have a variety of benefits to both patients and the hospital system:

- Improved patient outcomes (eg, morbidity and mortality)
- Increased quality of care
- Continuity of care
- Improved communication and collaboration between team members
- Identification of hospital system problems
- Coordination of necessary services
- Prioritization of interventions

Teams of individuals who closely interact with a specific patient population develop interprofessional plans of care. The process of multiple disciplines communicating and collaborating around the needs of the patient benefits patients. Representatives of disciplines commonly involved in developing plans of care include providers, nurses, pharmacists, respiratory therapists, physical, occupational and speech therapists, social workers, and dietitians. The format for the interprofessional plans of care typically includes the following categories:

- Patient goals (eg, pain control, activity level, absence of complications)
- Assessment and evaluation
- Consultations
- Diagnostic studies
- Medications
- Nutrition
- Activity
- Education
- Discharge planning and expected outcomes

The suggested activities within each of these categories may be divided into daily activities or grouped into phases of the hospitalization (eg, pre-, intra-, and postoperative phases). This team approach in development and utilization optimizes communication, collaboration, coordination, and commitment in using the plan of care to achieve patient outcomes.

With the use of electronic health records, interprofessional plans of care are evolving into many different forms. Some electronic formats mimic the paper version. Other institutions may incorporate pieces of the plan of care into varied electronic flow sheets (eg, orders, assessments, interventions, education, outcomes, specific plans of care). Each individual who assesses progress toward patient goals and implements various aspects of the plan of care is accountable for documenting on the care plan in the approved format. Specific patient goals on the plan of care can then be evaluated and tracked to determine whether they are met, not met, or not applicable.

Goals on the plan of care that are not completed typically are termed *variances*, which are deviations from the expected activities or goals outlined. Goal outcomes outlined on the plans of care that occur early are termed *positive variances*.

Negative variances are planned outcomes that are not accomplished on time. Negative variances typically include outcomes not completed or achieved due to the patient's condition, hospital system challenges (such as diagnostic studies or therapeutic interventions not completed within the optimal time frame), or lack of orders. Assessing patient progression on the plan of care helps caregivers to have an overall picture of patient recovery as compared to the goals and can be helpful in early recognition and resolution of problems. It is important to remember that individual discipline documentation on the plan of care does not preclude the need for ongoing direct communication and collaboration between disciplines to facilitate optimal patient care and achievement of goals.

PLANNING CARE THROUGH STAFFING CONSIDERATIONS

Planning care for critically ill patients begins with ensuring each nurse caring for a patient has the corresponding competencies and skills to meet the patient's needs. The American Association of Critical-Care Nurses (AACN) has developed the AACN Synergy Model for Patient Care to delineate core patient characteristics and needs that drive the core competencies of nurses required to care for patients and families (Table 2-1).

All eight competencies identified in the AACN Synergy Model are essential for the critical care nurse's practice, though the extent to which any particular competency is needed on a daily basis depends on the patient's needs at that point in time. One strategy for optimizing staffing assignments is to assess the priority needs of the patient and assign a nurse who has the proficiencies to meet those patient needs. By matching the competencies of the nurse with the needs of the patient, synergy occurs resulting in optimal patient outcomes.

PATIENT SAFETY CONSIDERATIONS IN PLANNING CARE

Intensive care units (ICUs) are high-technology, high-intervention environments with multiple disciplines caring for the patient. The critical care nurse is thoughtful of minimizing the safety risks inherent in such an environment. ICUs are constantly working to optimize care and minimize risks to patients.

Acutely ill patient conditions can change quickly so ongoing awareness and vigilance is required even when the patient appears to be stable or improving. The ICU environment itself may present various safety issues. Consider that inappropriate use of medical gas equipment, improperly grounded electrical devices, certain types of restraints, bedside rails, cords, and tubing lying on the floor may all be hazardous to the patient. In addition, with so many healthcare disciplines involved in the care of each patient, it is imperative that communication remain accurate and timely. Use of a standardized handoff communication tool (ie, SBAR; see Chapter 1) is a fundamental step in preventing errors related to poor communication among healthcare providers.

TABLE 2-1. CORE PATIENT CHARACTERISTICS AND NURSE COMPETENCIES AS DEFINED IN THE SYNERGY MODEL

Patient Characteristics	Description
Resiliency	The capacity to return to a restorative level of functioning using compensatory/coping mechanisms
Vulnerability	Susceptibility to actual or potential stressors that may adversely affect patient outcomes
Stability	The ability to maintain a steady-state equilibrium
Complexity	The intricate entanglement of two or more systems
Resource availability	Extent of resources (technical, fiscal, personal, psychological, and social) the patient/family bring to the situation
Participation in care	Extent to which patient/family engages in aspects of care
Participation in decision making	Extent to which patient/family engages in decision making
Predictability	Characteristic that allows one to expect a certain course of events or course of illness

Nurse Competencies	Description
Clinical judgment	Clinical reasoning (clinical decision making, critical thinking, and global understanding of situation) coupled with nursing skills (formal and informal experiential knowledge and evidence-based practice)
Advocacy and moral agency	Working on another's behalf and representing concerns of patients/families and nursing staff
Caring practices	Activities that create a compassionate, supportive, and therapeutic environment
Collaboration	Working with others in a way that promotes each person's contributions toward achieving optimal patient/family goals
Systems thinking	Body of knowledge that allows the nurse to manage environment and system resources for patients, families, and staff
Response to diversity	The sensitivity to recognize, appreciate and incorporate differences into the provision of care. Differences may include, but are not limited to, cultural differences, spiritual beliefs, gender, race, ethnicity, lifestyle, socioeconomic status, age, and values
Facilitation of learning	Ability to facilitate learning for patients, families, and staff
Clinical inquiry	Ongoing process of questioning and evaluating practice and providing informed practice

Data from American Association of Critical-Care Nurses. The AACN Synergy Model for Patient Care. Aliso Viejo, CA: AACN.

ESSENTIAL CONTENT CASE

Synergy Between Patient Characteristics and Nurse Competencies

MG is an 83-year-old woman with a history of coronary heart disease and metastatic breast cancer who is admitted to the hospital with worsening shortness of breath. She requires intubation and sedation and is on a vasopressor for periods of hemodynamic instability. It has been determined the shortness of breath and respiratory failure are due to a large pleural effusion. MG is widowed with three children who are very supportive but all live at least 5 hours away and are unsure about their mother's wishes regarding medical treatment or her goals of care.

Case Question 1: Based on the AACN Synergy Model (see Table 2-1), what four priority patient characteristics would the charge nurse consider in making a nurse assignment for MG?

Case Question 2: The charge nurse assigns Rebecca to care for MG. What particular skills will Rebecca use in caring for MG during the upcoming shift?

Answers
1. MG's priority characteristics include instability, minimally resilient, vulnerable, and currently unable to fully participate in decision making.
2. Clinical judgment, advocacy and moral agency, and caring practices.

Finally, planning the care of critically ill patients includes measures to prevent hospital-acquired conditions such as ventilator-associated events, central line-associated bloodstream infections, catheter-associated urinary tract infections (CAUTIs), *Clostridium difficile* infections, and multidrug-resistant organisms (MDROs). In addition to meticulous infection prevention techniques, nurses participate in and may lead daily discussions with the healthcare team about the use of invasive lines and catheters. Removing all lines, tubes, and drains as soon as clinically appropriate is the first step in preventing related complications.

PREVENTION OF COMMON COMPLICATIONS

The development of a critical illness, regardless of its cause, predisposes the patient to a number of physiologic and psychological complications. A major focus when providing care to critically ill patients is the prevention of complications associated with critical illness. The following content describes some of the most common complications.

Physiologic Instability

Ongoing assessments and monitoring of critically ill patients (see Table 1-12) are key to early identification of physiologic changes and to ensuring that the patient is progressing to the identified transition goals. After each assessment, the data obtained is reviewed in totality as they relate to the status of the patient. When an assessment changes in one body system, rarely does it remain an isolated issue, but rather it frequently impacts, or is a result of, changes in other systems.

By considering all the findings together, the nurse can monitor trends and anticipate appropriate interventions.

When assuming care of the patient, the nurse identifies specific achievable goals related to physiologic status that can be attained by the end of the shift. This strategy prevents a narrow focus on individual tasks and interventions and encourages a broader consideration of the patient's overall progress. In addition, this broader view allows the nurse to anticipate the potential patient responses to interventions. For instance, the nurse may set a goal related to blood glucose management and then notice that the patient requires an increase in the insulin infusion every morning at the same time. When looking at the whole picture, the nurse realizes that the patient is receiving several medications in the early morning that are mixed in a dextrose diluent. Recognition of this pattern helps the nurse intervene appropriately to stabilize fluctuations in blood glucose.

Venous Thromboembolism

Critically ill patients are at increased risk of venous thromboembolism (VTE) due to their underlying condition and immobility. Routine interventions can prevent this potentially devastating complication from occurring. Increased mobility is a key step. Early and progressive mobility of patients in the critical care unit to decreases the risk of VTEs, improves respiratory function, increases muscle strength, reduces pressure injury risk, and prevents delirium. It takes a team effort to fully implement early mobility protocols, including nurses, physical therapists, respiratory therapists, and providers. An example of progressive mobility involves beginning with having the patient sit on the side of the bed for a specific interval, then assisting them in transferring to a chair, and later ambulating in the hall.

Other strategies to reduce VTE risk include the use of sequential compression devices (described in Chapter 10), ensuring adequate hydration, avoiding groin or lower extremity vascular access lines, and chemical prophylaxis, such as low-dose unfractionated heparin or enoxaparin low-molecular-weight heparin (LMWH). There is evidence showing a significantly lower risk of death in patients who receive VTE prophylaxis during critical illness. While mobility does not eliminate the need for chemical prophylaxis, patients on full anticoagulation for concurrent diseases may not need additional treatment for VTE prophylaxis. Some conditions such as obesity may be indications for a higher than standard dose for VTE prophylaxis. Active bleeding or thrombocytopenia are often contraindications in the use of chemical prophylaxis for VTE.

Hospital-Acquired Infections

Critically ill patients are especially vulnerable to infection due to the use of multiple invasive devices and the frequent presence of debilitating underlying diseases. Hospital-acquired infections (HAI) increase the patient's length of stay (LOS) and hospitalization costs, and can markedly increase mortality rates depending on the type and severity of the infection and the underlying disease. CAUTIs are the second most commonly observed HAI according to recent data from the CDC, accounting for 15% of reported HAIs. These rates have dropped in recent years due to prevention campaigns, including nurse-led interventions, put into action across the country.

Hospital-acquired pneumonia (HAP) is another common HAI. HAP carries a significant mortality, with documented rates as high as 70%. Details of specific risk factors and control measures for the prevention of HAP are presented in Chapter 10 (Respiratory System). Other frequent infections include bloodstream and surgical site infections. In addition, *C. difficile* and MDRO infections have become a large burden to the healthcare system. This is particularly concerning as there are very limited options for treating MDROs. It is imperative for critical care practitioners to understand the processes that contribute to these potentially lethal infections and their role in preventing these untoward events.

Infection Prevention and Control

Standard precautions, sometimes referred to as "universal precautions" or "body substance isolation," signify the basic precautions that are to be used on all patients, regardless of their diagnosis. The general premise of standard precautions is that all body fluids have the potential to transmit any number of infectious diseases, both bacterial and viral. Certain basic principles are followed to prevent direct and indirect transmission of these organisms. Nonsterile examination gloves are worn when performing venipuncture, touching nonintact skin or mucous membranes, or contact with body fluid including urine, stool, saliva, emesis, sputum, and blood. Other personal protective equipment (PPE), such as face shields and protective gowns, are worn whenever there is a risk of splashing blood or body fluids into the face or onto clothing. This not only protects the healthcare worker (HCW) but also prevents contamination between patients via healthcare personnel.

Other infection prevention and control measures are transmission-based, meaning that strategies are designed around current understanding of how the disease spreads. Table 2-2 provides examples of isolation precaution categories and the types of infections for which they are instituted. For transmission-based precautions that include the use of PPE, placing PPE before entering the patient's room is imperative. The COVID-19 pandemic demonstrated the importance of appropriate infection prevention and control measures as everyone caring for patients with this disease faced the risk of contracting it. In addition to PPE, administrative controls such as grouping patients with the same infection in the same unit, and engineering controls such as negative pressure rooms are essential in keeping HCWs and patients safe. To align with Occupational and Safety Health Administration (OSHA) standards, all HCWs should have access to appropriate protective equipment when caring for patients. The manner in which PPE is used should not be adjusted to conserve supplies unless an actual shortage of supplies exists.

TABLE 2-2. ISOLATION CATEGORIES AND RELATED INFECTION EXAMPLES

Isolation Categories	Infection Examples When Used
Standard precautions	Apply to the care of all patients and includes hand hygiene, and gloves for contact with blood and body fluids
Airborne precautions	Tuberculosis, measles (rubeola), varicella (includes use of an N95 or equivalent respiratory protection)
Droplet precautions	*Neisseria meningitidis, Haemophilus influenzae,* pertussis, mumps, whooping cough (includes use of a medical-surgical face mask)
Contact precautions	Vancomycin-resistant enterococcus (VRE), methicillin-resistant *Staphylococcus aureus* (MRSA), *Clostridium difficile,* scabies, impetigo, varicella, respiratory syncytial virus (includes use of a gown and gloves for all interactions; for patients with *C. difficile* soap and water are required for hand hygiene)
Transmission-based precautions for known or suspected COVID-19	A NIOSH-approved N95 or equivalent or higher-level respirator, gown, gloves, eye protection. CDC guidance includes strategies used when supplies are short. Resource-limited settings may use a medical-surgical facemask. N95 or equivalent protection must be worn for aerosol-generating procedures

Data from Transmission-Based Precautions. Centers for Disease Control and Prevention and Infection Control Guidance for Healthcare Professionals about Coronavirus (COVID-19). Centers for Disease Control and Prevention.

Some interventions to prevent HAI are similar regardless of the site or source of infection. These strategies include:

- Maintaining glycemic control in both diabetic and nondiabetic patients.
- Removing invasive lines or tubes as soon as possible. Such lines are never kept in place for staff convenience or patient preference.
- Using closed drainage systems whenever possible and avoiding breaks in systems such as urinary drainage systems, IV lines, and ventilator tubing.
- Applying aseptic technique when breaks in these systems are necessary.
- Performing hand hygiene before and after patient care activities.

Interventions to reduce the occurrence of CAUTIs include the following:

- Impregnation of antimicrobial agents in catheters
- Use of daily checklists, algorithms, and nurse-driven protocols for catheter removal
- Staff education and implementation of consistent perineal care practices
- Adherence to aseptic technique for insertion and manipulation of catheters
- Bundled intervention approaches including utilization of electronic health record tools
- Avoiding placement of catheters when alternatives are available

Strategies to prevent HAP in critically ill patients, particularly in patients at risk for aspiration which is a risk factor for HAP, include the following:

- Maintaining the head of the bed at greater than or equal to 30°
- Use of a specialized endotracheal tube (ETT), which removes subglottic secretions above the ETT cuff
- Standardized, consistent oral care
- In patients on enteral feeding, assess tolerance and intervene to promote stomach emptying, such as increasing gut motility, or adjusting feeding rates as appropriate
- Hand hygiene before and after contact with patient secretions or respiratory equipment (refer to Chapters 5 and 14 for specific content related to those recommendations, and to the Clinical Practice Guidelines by the Infectious Diseases Society of America)

Interventions to prevent infection associated with vascular access devices include:

- Removing or replacing peripheral lines in accordance with hospital policy
- Monitoring patients with central venous catheters (CVC) for signs and symptoms of infection and removing or replacing lines when infection from the line is suspected
- Replace CVC as soon as possible when aseptic technique during insertion is uncertain (such as in an emergency situation)
- Keep dressings over CVC insertion sites dry and intact and change at the first signs of being damp, soiled, or loosened. Impregnated dressings should be applied in accordance with institutional policy
- Change IV tubing in accordance with unit policy and with specific consideration when administering blood products or lipid-based solutions

Hand hygiene is one of the most important defenses to prevent infection. Hand hygiene is defined by the CDC as using hand washing (soap and water), antiseptic hand wash, antiseptic hand rub (alcohol-based hand sanitizer including foam or gel), or surgical hand antisepsis. *Hand washing technique* is described by the CDC as vigorous rubbing together of lathered hands with soap and water for 15 seconds followed by a thorough rinsing under a stream of running water. Particular attention is paid around rings and under fingernails. It is best to keep natural fingernails well-trimmed and unpolished. Hand washing with soap and water is performed when hands are visibly soiled, after exposure to a patient with known or suspected *C. difficile* or norovirus, before eating, and after using the restroom. Use of alcohol-based waterless cleansers is convenient and effective when no visible soiling or contamination has occurred and after all other activities. Hand hygiene is performed prior to donning examination gloves to carry out patient care activities and after removing examination gloves.

Frequent hand washing, especially with antimicrobial soap, can lead to extremely dry skin. The use of latex examination gloves has been associated with increased sensitivities and allergies, causing an additional risk to skin integrity. This may put the healthcare provider at risk for blood-borne pathogen transmission, as well as for colonization or infection with bacteria. Hospital-approved lotions and emollients are used to promote skin integrity.

It has been estimated that HCWs cleanse their hands as much as 50% fewer times than necessary. It is important to involve all disciplines in encouraging and reminding each other to perform hand hygiene when it is overlooked. Some institutions also encourage patients and families to be partners in hand hygiene efforts by asking care providers if they have cleansed their hands prior to patient contact.

Pressure Injury

Pressure and shear injury is a major risk in critically ill patients due to immobility, poor nutrition, invasive lines, surgical sites, poor circulation, edema, and incontinence issues. Skin can become very fragile and can easily tear. Pressure injuries may begin to occur in as little as 2 hours. Healthy people constantly reposition themselves, even in their sleep, to relieve areas of pressure. Critically ill patients cannot reposition themselves and rely on caregivers to assist them. Pay particular attention to pressure points that are most prone to pressure injury, namely, heels, elbows, coccyx, and occiput. When receiving critically ill patients following prolonged surgical procedures, ask the perioperative providers about the patient's positioning during the procedure. This will help determine the need for close monitoring of the related pressure points for early indication of deep tissue injury. Also be cognizant of equipment that may contribute to pressure injury such as tube stabilizers and even bed rails if patients are positioned in constant contact with them. As the patient's condition changes, so does the risk of developing a pressure injury. Routine use of a risk assessment tool alerts the caregiver to increasing or decreasing risk of pressure injury and the need for changes in interventions. Chapter 11 provides a full discussion of assessment of pressure injuries.

Interventions to promote skin integrity include:

- Repositioning the patient minimally every 2 hours, particularly if they are not spontaneously moving
- Using pressure-reduction mattresses for all critically ill patients
- Elevating heels off the bed using pillows placed under the calves or using heel protectors and/or elbow pads
- Avoiding long periods of sitting in a chair without repositioning
- Using a skin care protocol with ointment barriers for patients experiencing incontinence to prevent skin irritation
- Avoiding use of inflatable cushions (donuts) that increase pressure on surrounding skin surfaces
- Using polyurethane foam dressings prophylactically over bony prominences that may be exposed to shear and friction

TABLE 2-3. FACTORS CONTRIBUTING TO SLEEP DISTURBANCES IN CRITICAL CARE

Illness
- Metabolic changes
- Underlying diseases (eg, cardiovascular disease, chronic obstructive pulmonary disease [COPD], dementia)
- Pain
- Anxiety, fear
- Delirium

Medications
- Analgesics
- Antidepressants
- Beta-blockers
- Bronchodilators
- Benzodiazepines
- Corticosteroids

Environment
- Noise, such as from medical equipment
- Staff conversations
- Television/radio
- Equipment alarms
- Frequent care interruptions
- Lighting, too dark during the day or too bright at night
- Lack of usual bedtime routine
- Room temperature
- Uncomfortable sleep surface
- Visitors
- Bad odors

Sleep Pattern Disturbance

All critically ill patients experience altered sleep patterns and this affects healing and exacerbates the risk for delirium. Table 2-3 identifies the many reasons patients may experience sleep deprivation. The priority of sleep in the hierarchy of patient needs is often misperceived though survivors of critical care often note that lack of sleep is a major stressor along with the discomfort of unrelieved pain. The vicious cycle of undertreated pain, anxiety, and sleeplessness continues unless clinicians intervene to break the cycle with simple, but essential, individualized patient interventions. Psychological changes in sleep deprivation include confusion, irritability, and agitation. Physiologic changes include depressed immune and respiratory systems and a decreased pain threshold.

Enhancing patients' sleep potential in the critical care setting involves knowledge of how the environment, including noise, lights, and frequent monitoring affects the patient. A nighttime sleep protocol where patients are closely monitored but untouched from 1 to 5 AM is an excellent example of eliminating hourly disturbances to the critically ill. Encouraging blocks of time for sleep and careful assessment of the quantity and quality of sleep are important to patient well-being. Table 2-4 details basic recommendations for sleep assessment, and modifying the internal and external environments to promote sleep. When these activities are incorporated into standard practice routines, critically ill patients receive optimal opportunity to achieve sleep.

TABLE 2-4. EVIDENCE-BASED PRACTICE: SLEEP PROMOTION IN CRITICAL CARE

- Assess patient's usual sleep patterns
- Minimize effects of underlying disease process as much as possible (eg, reduce fever, eliminate pain, and minimize metabolic disturbances)
- Avoid medications that disturb sleep patterns
- Consult with providers to continue behavioral medications as appropriate
- Mimic patients' usual bedtime routine as much as possible
- Minimize environmental impact on sleep as much as possible
- Utilize complementary therapies to promote sleep as appropriate
- Implement nighttime quiet hours
- Provide earplugs and sleep masks
- Encourage lights on during the day and lights off at night, open window blinds during the day for natural light exposure
- Minimize nocturnal sleep interruptions; cluster nighttime care activities
- Maximize daytime nursing care goals to increase daytime activity
- Employ interventions for cognitive stimulation; place clocks in room, update wall calendar
- Reduce sedation in daytime hours where clinically appropriate
- Address pain, anxiety, and fear
- Avoid caffeine intake in afternoon hours and at night
- Provide early progressive mobility
- Notify medical provider for signs/symptoms of sleep disturbance (ie, cognitive problems, delirium, emotional distress, or anxiety related to sleep).

Psychosocial Impact

Basic Tenets

The time spent in the ICU can have long-term physical, mental, and cognitive changes, impacting patients and families for years following the illness. These long-term effects are often referred to as postintensive care syndrome (PICS) and include impaired functional status, cognitive impairment, and clinically significant psychiatric morbidity, including posttraumatic stress disorder (PTSD), depression, and/or anxiety symptoms. About 25% of critical illness survivors experience PTSD, 34% experience depression, and 40% develop anxiety within the first 6 months after ICU discharge. While evidence is still emerging on interventions to prevent and treat PICS, there are basic interventions that can be done. These include:

- encouraging family participation in care;
- promoting a proper sleep-wake cycle;
- encouraging communication, and empowering the patient to participate in decisions as appropriate;
- providing patient and family education about unit expectations and rules, procedures, medications, and the patient's physical condition;
- ensuring pain relief and comfort;
- providing continuity of care providers.
- keeping sensory and physical aids available including glasses and hearing aids;
- encouraging family to bring in familiar items or photographs.

In addition, ICU diaries, written by staff members and families, support patients' understanding of what occurred and may alleviate their psychological suffering. The use of diaries in the ICU can be helpful after discharge in providing context for patients about their experiences when their memories may be minimal or confusing.

Critical illness can also have long-term effects on family members, this is called post ICU syndrome-family (PICS-F). Family members can experience both psychiatric sequelae such as anxiety, depression, PTSD, and complicated grief and physical symptoms such as sleep disturbance, fatigue, and exacerbation of preexisting physical problems. If family members develop any of these symptoms, they can negatively impact their quality of life.

To reduce these risks, rehabilitation bundles should incorporate

- family-centered care
- promotion of sleep hygiene
- open visitation policies (when possible)
- family involvement in rounds
- informational brochures
- ICU diaries

The use of ICU diaries by families can provide an emotional outlet for family members when they make entries or when they reflect back and review the diary.

Delirium

Delirium is evidenced by disorientation, confusion, perceptual disturbances, restlessness, distractibility, and sleep-wake cycle disturbances. Assessment of delirium should be routine in the critical care unit, and there are several valid and reliable tools that can be used to identify delirium, including the Brief Confusion Assessment Method (bCAM) and Confusion Assessment Method for Intensive Care Units (CAM-ICU). Due to the nature of most critical care units, it is the rare patient that is not at risk for development of confusion and subsequently delirium. Treatment of delirium is a challenge and therefore prevention is ideal. Delirium is most common in postsurgical and elderly patients and is the most common cause of disruptive behavior in the critically ill. It is common for providers to suspect delirium in critically ill, confused, and restless patients. However, in reality, there are different subtypes of delirium: hyperactive (restlessness, agitation, irritability, aggression); hypoactive (slow response to verbal stimuli, psychomotor slowing); and mixed delirium (both hyperactive and hypoactive behaviors).

Sensory overload is a common risk factor that contributes to delirium in the critically ill. Medications that may also play a role in the development of delirium include prochlorperazine, diphenhydramine, famotidine, benzodiazepines, opioids, corticosteroids, and antiarrhythmic medications. Other factors that contribute to delirium include metabolic disturbances, polypharmacy, immobility, infections (particularly urinary tract and respiratory infections), dehydration, electrolyte imbalances, and sensory impairment.

The best approaches to preventing delirium are multimodal, employing a variety of interventions simultaneously, often referred to as a "bundle" of care. A typical

TABLE 2-5.   THE ABCDEF OR "A2F" BUNDLE FOR DELIRIUM PREVENTION

A. Assess and Manage Pain, using validated tools
B. Both Spontaneous Awakening Trials & Spontaneous Breathing Trials
C. Choice of analgesia and sedation
D. Delirium: assess, prevent and manage—using validated tools
E. Early mobility and exercise
F. Family engagement and empowerment

Data from Vanderbilt University Medical Center https://www.icudelirium.org/medical-professionals/overview.

bundle to prevent delirium might include frequent reorientation, addressing pain, breathing trails to facilitate removal of mechanical ventilation, implementing early mobility, ensuring adequate sleep with sleep hygiene, providing assistive devices such as glasses and hearing aids to address sensory deficits and minimizing the use of medications that contribute to delirium. Family involvement in reorienting the patient and providing familiar faces and voices is also helpful in preventing delirium. The ICU Delirium website offers a bundled approach called A2F or ABCDEF bundle. See Table 2-5 for the components of the bundle. Additional discussion of delirium prevention can be found in Chapters 5 and 6.

Once delirium develops, the first priority is to identify the cause. Is there a physiologic change such as an electrolyte abnormality, hypoxemia, or an adverse reaction to a medication? Are the patient's underlying health problems, such as heart failure, poorly controlled? Could the patient have a new infection? Is the patient in pain? The THINK pneumonic, in Table 2-6, is one strategy for considering different causes of delirium. Once a cause is identified, collaborate with providers in the selection of an appropriate treatment plan. Medication for managing delirium is best reserved for those cases in which behavioral interventions have failed. Restraints are discouraged and tend to increase agitation.

If the patient demonstrates a paranoid element in their delirium, avoid confrontation and remain at a safe distance. Accept bizarre statements calmly, without agreement. Explain to the family that the behaviors are symptoms that will most likely resolve with time, resumption of normal sleep patterns, and addressing the underlying cause. Delirious patients usually remember the events, thoughts, conversations, and provider responses that occur during delirium. The recovered patients may feel embarrassment and guilt if they were combative during their illness.

TABLE 2-6.   THE THINK PNEUMONIC FOR CONSIDERING CAUSES OF DELIRIUM

T: Toxic situations—CHF, shock, dehydration, delirogenic medications (tight titration), new organ failure (kidney/liver)
H: Hypoxemia
 I: Infection/sepsis (hospital acquired), immobilization
N: Nonpharmacologic interventions—hearing aids, glasses reorient, sleep protocols, music noise control, ambulation
K: K+ or electrolyte problems

Adapted with permission from Marta Render, MD – Deparmtent of Veteran Affairs Inpatient Evaluation Center (IPEC).

Depression

Depression occurring with a medical illness affects long-term recovery by lengthening the course of the illness and increasing morbidity and mortality. Risk factors that predispose for depression with medical disorders include social isolation, recent loss, pessimism, financial pressures, history of mood disorder, alcohol or substance use/withdrawal, previous suicide attempts, and pain. Many patients arrive in the ICU with a history of depression that can be exacerbated by the critical illness crisis. It is important that healthcare providers maintain the patient's psychiatric medication regimen if at all possible in order to avoid worsening of the patient's psychological status.

The best way to assess for depression is to ask directly. Allow the patient to direct the conversation. If negative distortions about illness and treatment are communicated, it is appropriate to correct, clarify, and reassure with realistic information to promote a more hopeful outcome. Consistency in care providers promotes trust in an ongoing relationship and enhances recovery. Educating the patient and family that depression is not an unusual phenomenon during critical illness and providing reassurance that it is usually temporary are also important steps. If depressive symptoms require new pharmacologic intervention, a psychiatric consult may be warranted. Keep in mind that it may take several weeks for antidepressants to reach their full effectiveness.

A patient who has attempted suicide or is suicidal can be frightening to hospital staff. Assessing for suicidal ideation (the thought of self-harm) and suicidal intent (a plan for self-harm) are appropriate nursing interventions. Do not avoid asking such questions as they do not promote suicidal thoughts. The communication of feeling suicidal may indicate a desire to discuss fear, pain, or loneliness. A psychiatric referral is recommended in these situations for further evaluation and intervention. Suicide precautions such as increased monitoring, removing objects that can be used for self-harm, and frequent patient observations may also be instituted, in accordance with hospital and unit policy.

Anxiety

Medical disorders can cause anxiety and panic-like symptoms, which are distressing to the patient and family and may exacerbate the medical condition. Treatment of the underlying medical condition may decrease the concomitant anxiety. Both pharmacologic and nonpharmacologic interventions can be helpful in managing anxiety during critical illness. Pharmacologic agents for anxiety are discussed in Chapters 6 (Pain, Sedation, and Neuromuscular Blockage Management) and 7 (Pharmacology). Goals of pharmacologic therapy are to titrate the drug dose to maintain patient's cognition and ability to interact with staff, family, and environment; complement pain control; and assist in promoting sleep. The lowest effective dose is the ideal regimen. There are also a variety of nonpharmacologic interventions to decrease or control anxiety:

- *Breathing techniques*: These techniques target somatic symptoms and include deep and slow abdominal breathing patterns. It is important to demonstrate and do the breathing with patients, as their heightened anxiety decreases their attention span. Practicing this technique may decrease anxiety and promote synchrony for patients whom you anticipate may need ventilator support.

- *Muscle relaxation*: Reduce psychomotor tension with muscle relaxation. Again, the patient will most likely need cues for this and it may be an excellent opportunity for the family to participate in care. Cuing might be, "The mattress under your head, elbow, heel, and back feels heavy against your body, press harder, and then try to drift away from the mattress as you relax." Mobile applications and websites with commercial relaxation techniques are available but are not as useful as the cuing by a familiar voice.

- *Imagery*: Interventions targeting cognition, such as imagery techniques, depend on the patient's capacity for attention, memory, and processing. Visualization imagery involves recalling a pleasurable, relaxing situation, for example, a hot bath, lying on a warm beach, listening to waves, or hearing birds sing. Guided imagery and hypnosis are additional therapies but require some competency to be effective; thus, a referral is suggested. Patients who practice meditation as an alternative for stress control are encouraged to continue but the environment may need modification to optimize the effects.

- *Preparatory information*: Providing the patient and family with preparatory information is extremely helpful in controlling anxiety. Allowing the patient and family to control some aspects of the patient's care can be comforting to families.

- *Distraction techniques*: These techniques may also interrupt the anxiety cycle. Methods for distraction include listening to familiar music, watching videos, or counting backward from 200 by 2 rapidly.

- *Use of previous coping methods*: Identify how the patient and family have dealt with stress and anxiety in the past and suggest they use the approach if feasible. Supporting previous coping techniques may well be adaptive.

PATIENT AND FAMILY EDUCATION

Patient and family education in the critical care environment is essential and includes providing information regarding diagnosis, prognosis, treatments, and procedures. In addition, appropriate education puts fears and concerns in perspective so that patients and family members can become active members in the decisions made about their care.

Providing patient and family education in critical care is challenging; multiple barriers (eg, environmental factors,

TABLE 2-7. ASSESSMENT OF LEARNING READINESS

General Principles
• Do the patient and the family have questions about the diagnosis, prognosis, treatments, or procedures?
• What do the patient and the family desire to learn about?
• What is the knowledge level of the individuals being taught? What do they already know about the issues that will be taught?
• What is their current situation (condition and environment) and have they had any prior experience in a similar situation?
• Do the patient or the family have any communication barriers (eg, language, illiteracy, culture, listening/comprehension deficits)?
• What is patient's or family members' preferred method of learning?

Special Considerations in Critical Care
• Does the patient's condition allow you to assess this information from them (eg, physiologic/psychological stability)?
• Is the patient's support system/family/significant other available or ready to receive this information?
• What environmental factors (including time) present as barriers in the critical care unit?
• Are there other members of the healthcare team who may possess vital assessment information?

patient stability, patient and family anxiety) are overcome, or adapted, to provide this essential intervention. The importance of education, coupled with the barriers common in critical care, necessitates that education be a continuous ongoing process engaged in by all members of the team. Some education of the patient and family is subtle, occurring with each interaction between the patient, family, and members of the healthcare team.

Assessment of Learning Readiness

Assessment of the patient's and family's learning needs focuses primarily on learning readiness. *Learning readiness* refers to that moment in time when the learner is able to comprehend and synthesize the shared information. Without learning readiness, teaching may not be useful. Questions to assess learning readiness are listed in Table 2-7.

Strategies to Address Patient and Family Education

Prior to teaching, the information gathered in the assessment is prioritized and organized into a format that is meaningful to the learner (Table 2-8). Next, the outcome of the teaching is established along with appropriate content, and then a decision is made about how to share the information. The next step is to teach the patient, family, and significant others (Table 2-9). Although this phase often appears to be the easiest, it is actually the most difficult. It is crucial during the communication of the content, regardless of the type of communication vehicle used (video, pamphlet, discussion) to listen carefully to the needs expressed by the learner and to provide clear and precise responses to those needs. Use of teach-back is a simple method to ensure the patient and family members comprehend the information provided. Teach-back involves asking the patient or family member to

TABLE 2-8. PRINCIPLES FOR TEACHING PLANS

General Principles
• Establish the outcome of the teaching.
• Determine what content needs to be taught, given the assessment.
• Identify what support systems are in place to support your educational efforts (eg, unit leadership, education department, standardized teaching plans, teaching materials such as pamphlets, computer applications, brochures, videos).
• Familiarize yourself with the content and teaching materials.
• Contact resources to clarify and provide consistency in information and additional educational support and follow-up.
• Determine the most appropriate teaching strategy (video, written materials, computer applications, discussion) and to whom (patient or family) it should be directed.

Special Considerations in Critical Care
• Plan the teaching strategy carefully. Patients and families in the critical care environment are stressed and an overload of information adds to their stress. When planning education, consider content and amount based on the assessment of the patient, nature, and severity of the patient's illness, availability of significant others, and existing environmental barriers.

relay back, in their own words, what they need to do or know. This allows the healthcare provider to clarify or re-explain the content if learners have misunderstood or not comprehended the information relayed.

Principles for Educational Outcome Monitoring

Following educational interventions, it is essential to determine if the educational outcomes have been achieved

TABLE 2-9. PRINCIPLES FOR EDUCATIONAL SESSIONS

General Principles
• Consider the time needed to convey the information and the support systems available.
• Consider the situation the patient is currently experiencing. Postponement may need to be considered.
• Be aware of the amount of content and the patient's and the family's ability to process the information.
• Be sensitive in the delivery of the information. Make sure it is conveyed at a level that the patient and the family can understand.
• Refer to and involve resources as appropriate.
• Convey accurate and precise information. Make sure this information is consistent with previous information given to the patient.
• Listen carefully and solicit feedback during the session to guide the discussion.
• Use teach-back to ensure the patient and family understood and comprehend the information provided. Re-explain and clarify any potential misinterpretations.

Special Considerations in Critical Care
• Keep the time frame of educational sessions short to optimize learning. Education must be episodic due to the nature of the patient's condition and the environment.
• Provide repetition of the information. Stress and the critical care environment can alter comprehension: for this reason, repetition is necessary.
• Avoid details unless the patient or family specifically requests them. Often, details can cloud the information given. Details can come later in the hospitalization, if necessary.

TABLE 2-10. PRINCIPLES FOR EDUCATIONAL OUTCOMES MONITORING

General Principles
• Measure the outcome. Was the outcome met? Was the outcome unmet?
• Communicate the outcome verbally and in the healthcare record to other members of the healthcare team.
• Provide necessary follow-up and reinforcement of the teaching.
• Make referrals that may have been identified in or as a result of patient and family education.
• Evaluate the teaching process for barriers or problems, and then address those areas and be aware of these for future interactions.

Special Considerations in Critical Care
• Recognize that repetition of information is the rule, not the exception. Be prepared to repeat information previously given, many times if necessary.

(Table 2-10). Even if the outcome appears to have been achieved, it is common for the learners to not retain all the information. Patients and families experience a great deal of stress while in the critical care environment; reinforcement is often necessary and is important to anticipate.

FAMILY-CENTERED CARE

There is a strong evidence that family presence and involvement in the ICU aids in the recovery of critically ill patients. Family members can help patients cope, reduce anxiety, and provide a resource for the patient. Families also need support and encouragement to meet their own needs to be a positive influence for the patient. Developing a partnership and a trusting relationship with the family is in everyone's best interest. Research shows that there can frequently be disagreement between the nurse and family about the type or priorities of family needs. Therefore, it is important to discuss family needs and perceptions directly with each family and tailor interventions based on those needs (Table 2-11).

TABLE 2-11. EVIDENCE-BASED PRACTICE: FAMILY INTERVENTIONS

Planning
• Determine what the family sees as priority needs.
Interventions
• Determine spokesperson and contact person.
• Establish optimum methods to contact and communicate with family, and make communication routine.
• Make referrals for support services as appropriate (eg, palliative care, social work, spiritual support).
• Provide information according to family needs.
• Include family in direct care and decision making as appropriate.
• Provide a comfortable environment.
• Consider development of a program for families to keep an "ICU diary" of events and emotions.
• Encourage family presence and active participation during team rounds.
Evaluation
• Evaluate achievement of meeting family needs through multiple methods (eg, feedback, satisfaction surveys, care conferences, follow-up after discharge).

Data from Leske JS. Interventions to decrease family anxiety. Crit Care Nurse. 2002;22(6):61-55 and Coombs M, Puntillo KA, Franck LS, et al: Implementing the SCCM Family-Centered Care Guidelines in Critical Care Nursing Practice. AACN Adv Crit Care. 2017;28(2):138-147.

TABLE 2-12. EVIDENCE-BASED PRACTICE: FAMILY VISITATION IN CRITICAL CARE

- Establish ways for families to have access to the patient (eg, open visitation, contract visitation, unit phone numbers).
- Ask patients their preferences related to visiting.
- Promote access to patients with consistent unit policies and procedures with options for individualization.
- Prepare families for visit.
- Model interaction with patient.
- Give information about the patient's condition, equipment, and technology being used.
- Monitor the response of the patient and family to visitation.

Research has consistently identified the following major areas of family needs.

Receiving Assurance

Family members need reassurance that the best possible care is being given to the patient. This instills confidence and a sense of security. It can also assist in either maintaining hope or can be helpful in redefining hope to a more realistic goal when appropriate.

Remaining Near the Patient

Family members need to have consistent access to their loved ones. Of primary importance to the family is the unit visiting policy. Specifics to be discussed include the number of visitors allowed at one time, and any recommendations related to the age of visitors (Table 2-12). Restrictions on visitation during a crisis should be evaluated frequently for the benefit and risk they confer. There is evidence to support the presence of a family member with the patient during invasive procedures, as well as during cardiopulmonary resuscitation (CPR). Written policies developed through an interprofessional approach promote implementing family presence at CPR or procedures.

Receiving Information

It is important that communication with the patient and family is open and honest. Keep promises (be thoughtful before making promises), describe expectations, acknowledge inconveniences and mistakes, and maintain confidentiality. Avoid contracting for secrets or eliciting care provider preferences. Use concise, simplistic explanations without medical jargon (eg, "road trip" transporting the patient to a diagnostic site or procedure area) or alphabet shorthand (eg, positive end-expiratory pressure [PEEP], intra-aortic balloon pump [IABP] to facilitate understanding). Contact interpreters, as appropriate, when language barriers exist.

Evaluate the effectiveness of communication by asking the patient and family for their understanding of the message, its content and intent. When conflict occurs, find a private place for discussion. Avoid taking the confrontation personally. Consider what the issue is and what needs to occur to reach resolution. If too much emotion is present, agree to address the issue at a later time, if possible.

It is helpful to establish a communication tree by designating one family member to be called if there are changes in the patient's condition and consider establishing a time for that person to call the unit for updates. Unit expectations and rules can be conveyed in a pamphlet for the family to refer to over time. Content that is helpful includes orientation about the philosophy of care; routines such as shift changes and provider rounds; the varied roles of personnel who work with patients; and information to address the family's needs such as food services, bathrooms, waiting areas, chapel services, transportation, and lodging. Some critical care units invite family members to medical rounds for the discussion of their loved one's care. Adequate communication can decrease anxiety, increase a sense of control, and assist in decision-making by families.

Being Comfortable

Available space, in or near the ICU, is necessary to meet comfort needs of the family. This space may include comfortable furniture, access to phones and restrooms, and assistance with finding overnight accommodations. Encourage the family to admit when they are overwhelmed, take breaks, go to meals, rest, sleep, and connect with other family and friends. Helping the family with basic comfort needs helps to decrease their distress and maintain their reserves and coping mechanisms. This improves their ability to be a valuable resource for the patient.

Having Support Available

Utilize all potential resources in meeting family needs. Relying on nurses to fulfill all family needs while they are trying to care for a critically ill patient can create tension and frustration. Assess the family for their own resources that can be maximized. Use hospital referrals that can assist in family support such as chaplains, social workers, palliative care, and child-family life departments as available.

Family Visitation

There is an abundance of evidence demonstrating that unrestricted access of the patient's support network (family, significant others, trusted friends) benefits the patient by providing emotional and social support; improving the healthcare team's understanding of the patient's goals of care; increasing communication; and increasing patient and family satisfaction. There may be circumstances where open visitation is not appropriate due to medical, therapeutic, or safety considerations (eg, disruptive behavior, infectious disease concerns, patient privacy, or per patient request). Limitations on visitation imposed for these reasons should offer the minimal necessary restrictions to maintain safety and be lifted when feasible. Decisions about visitation restrictions due to concerns about COVID-19 transmission require careful weighing of risks and benefits and must include consideration of community levels of transmission and the individual patient circumstances.

For the family, the critical care setting symbolizes a variety of hopes, fears, and beliefs that range from hope of a cure to end-of-life care. A family-centered approach can promote coping and cohesion among family members and minimize the isolation and anxiety for patients. Anticipating family needs, focusing on the present, fostering open communication, and providing information are vital to promoting psychological integrity for families.

TRANSPORTING THE CRITICALLY ILL PATIENT

Preventing common complications and maintaining physiologic and psychosocial stability is a challenge even when in the controlled environment of the critical care unit. It is even more challenging when transporting the critically ill patient to other areas of the hospital for diagnostic and therapeutic purposes. The decision to transport the critically ill patient out of the well-controlled environment of the critical care unit elicits a variety of responses from clinicians. It is not uncommon to hear phrases like these: "She's too sick to leave the unit!" "What if something happens en route?" "Who will take care of my other patients while I'm gone?" Responses like these underscore the clinicians' understanding of the risks involved in transporting critically ill patients.

Safe patient transport requires thoughtful planning, organization, and interprofessional communication and cooperation. The goal during transport is to maintain the same level of care, regardless of the location in the hospital. The transfer of critically ill patients always involves some degree of risk to the patient. The decision to transfer, therefore, is based on an assessment of the potential benefits of transfer weighed against the potential risks.

The reason for moving a critically ill patient is typically the need for care, technology, or specialists not available in the critical care unit. Whenever feasible, diagnostic testing or simple procedures are performed at the patient's bedside within the critical care unit. If the diagnostic test or procedural intervention under consideration is unlikely to alter management or outcome of the patient, then the risk of transfer may outweigh the benefit. It is imperative that every member of the healthcare team assist in clarifying what, if any, benefit may be derived from transport.

Assessment of Risk for Complications

Prior to initiating transport, a patient's risk for development of complications during transport are systematically assessed. The switching of life support technologies in the critical care unit to portable devices may lead to undesired physiologic changes. In addition, complications may arise from environmental conditions outside the critical care unit that are difficult to control, such as body temperature fluctuations or inadvertent movement of invasive devices (eg, ET,

TABLE 2-13. POTENTIAL COMPLICATIONS DURING TRANSPORT

Pulmonary
- Changes in oxygenation
- Hyperventilation
- Hypoventilation
- Airway obstruction
- Aspiration
- Recurrent pneumothorax
- Arterial blood gas changes
- Inadequate ventilation, particularly if portable ventilator does not provide the same support

Cardiovascular
- Hypotension
- Hypertension
- Arrhythmias
- Decreased tissue perfusion
- Cardiac ischemia
- Pulmonary edema
- Peripheral ischemia
- Interruption of vasoactive medications

Neurologic
- Increased intracranial pressure
- Cerebral hypoxia
- Cerebral hypercarbia
- Inadequate immobilization for patients with cranial or vertebral fracture

Gastrointestinal
- Nausea
- Vomiting

Pain
- Anxiety

chest tubes, IV devices). Common complications associated with transportation are summarized in Table 2-13.

Level of Care Required During Transport

During transport, there should be no interruption in the monitoring or maintenance of the patient's vital functions. It is necessary to ensure that the equipment used during transport, as well as the skill level of accompanying personnel, are equivalent with the interventions required or anticipated in the critical care unit (Table 2-14). Intermittent and continuous monitoring of physiologic status (eg, cardiac output and rhythm, blood pressure, oxygenation, ventilation) continues during transport and while the patient is away from the critical care unit (Table 2-15).

Questions that need to be answered to prepare for transfer include the following:

- What is the current level of care (equipment, personnel)?
- What will be needed during the transfer or at the destination to maintain that level of care?
- What additional therapeutic interventions may be required before or during transport (eg, analgesic and sedative agents or titration of vasoactive or inotropic agents)?

Preparation

Before transfer, the plan of care for the patient during and after transfer is coordinated to ensure continuity of care and

TABLE 2-14. TRANSPORT PERSONNEL AND EQUIPMENT REQUIREMENTS

Personnel
- A minimum of two people should accompany the patient.
- One of the accompanying personnel should be a critical care nurse with Advanced Cardiac Life Support certification.
- Additional personnel may include a respiratory therapist, registered nurse, or provider. A respiratory therapist should accompany all patients requiring mechanical ventilation.

Equipment
The following minimal equipment should be available:
- Cardiac monitor/defibrillator.
- Airway management equipment and resuscitation bag of proper size and fit for the patient.
- Oxygen source of ample volume to support the patient's needs for the projected time out of the ICU, with an additional 30-minute reserve.
- Standard resuscitation drugs: epinephrine, atropine, amiodarone.
- Blood pressure cuff (sphygmomanometer) and stethoscope.
- Ample supply of the IV fluids and continuous infusion medications (regulated by battery-operated infusion pumps) being administered to the patient.
- Additional medications to provide the patient's scheduled intermittent medication doses and to meet anticipated needs (eg, sedation) with appropriate orders to allow their administration if a provider is not present.
- For patients receiving mechanical support of ventilation, a device capable of delivering the same volume, pressure, PEEP, and a Fio_2 equal to or greater than what the patient is receiving in the ICU. For practical reasons, in adults a Fio_2 of 1.0 is most feasible during transfer because this eliminates the need for an air tank and air-oxygen blender. During neonatal transfer, Fio_2 should be precisely controlled.
- Resuscitation cart and suction equipment need not accompany each patient being transferred but such equipment should be stationed in areas used by critically ill patients and be readily available by a predetermined mechanism for emergencies that may occur en route.

Data from Day D. Keeping patients safe during intrahospital transport. Crit Care Nurse. 2010;30(4):18-32.

TABLE 2-15. MONITORING DURING TRANSFER

- If technologically possible, patients being transferred should receive the same physiologic monitoring during transfer that they were receiving in the ICU.
- Minimally, all critically ill patients being transferred must have continuous monitoring of ECG and pulse oximetry and intermittent measurement and documentation of blood pressure, respiratory rate, and pulse rate.
- In addition, selected patients, based on clinical status, may benefit from monitoring by capnography; continuous measurement of blood pressure, PAP, and ICP; and intermittent measurement of CVP, Pao_2, and CO.
- Intubated patients receiving mechanical support of ventilation should have end-tidal carbon dioxide and airway pressure monitored. If a transfer ventilator is used, it should have alarms to indicate disconnects or excessively high airway pressures.

Data from Day D. Keeping patients safe during intrahospital transport. Crit Care Nurse. 2010;30(4):18-32.

TABLE 2-16. PRETRANSFER COORDINATION AND COMMUNICATION

- Provider-to-provider and/or nurse-to-nurse communication regarding the patient's condition and treatment preceding and following the transfer should be documented in the medical record when the management of the patient will be assumed by a different team while the patient is away from the ICU.
- The area to which the patient is being transferred (x-ray, operating room, nuclear medicine, etc) must confirm that it is ready to receive the patient and immediately begin the procedure or test for which the patient is being transferred.
- Ancillary services (eg, security, respiratory therapy, escort) must be notified as to the timing of the transfer and the equipment and support needed.
- The responsible provider must be notified either to accompany the patient or to be aware that the patient is out of the ICU at this time and may have an acute event requiring the provider's response to provide emergency care in another area of the hospital.
- Documentation in the medical record must include the indication for transfer, the patient's status during transfer, and whether the patient is expected to return to the ICU.

Data from Day D. Keeping patients safe during intrahospital transport. Crit Care Nurse. 2010;30(4):18-32.

availability of appropriate resources (Table 2-16). The receiving units are contacted to confirm whether there is access to necessary resources, for instance, plugs for equipment with limited battery power and wall suction if required. Communication between team members delineates the current status of the patient, management priorities, and the process to follow in the event of untoward events (eg, unexpected hemodynamic instability or airway problems).

After assessing the patient's risk for transport complications, prepare the patient for transfer, both physically and mentally. Explain the transfer process to the patient and family. The explanation includes a description of the sensations the patient may expect, an estimate of the procedure's length, and the role of individual members of the transport team. It is important to allay any patient or family anxiety by identifying current caregivers who will accompany the patient during transport. The availability of emergency equipment and medications and how communication is handled during transportation also may be information that will reassure the patient and family.

Transport

Once preparations are complete, the actual transfer can begin. Ensure that the portable equipment has adequate battery life to last well beyond the anticipated transfer time in case of unanticipated delays. Connect each of the portable monitoring devices prior to disconnection from the bedside equipment, if possible. This enables a comparison of hemodynamic values with the portable equipment.

Once hemodynamic pressure and noninvasive oxygenation monitors are in place and values verified, disconnect the patient from the mechanical ventilator or bedside oxygen source, and begin portable ventilation and oxygenation. Assess for clinical signs and symptoms of respiratory distress and changes in ventilation and oxygenation. It may be easier to transfer the patient on the bed if it fits in elevators and spaces in the receiving area. Check IV lines, pressure lines, monitor cables, NG tubes, chest tubes, urinary catheters, or drains of any sort to ensure proper placement during transport and to guard against accidental removal during transport.

During transport, the critical care nurse is responsible for continuous assessment of cardiopulmonary status (electrocardiograph, blood pressure, respirations, oxygenation, end-tidal CO_2, etc) and interventions as required to ensure stability. Throughout the time away from the critical care environment, vigilant monitoring to evaluate the patient's response to the transport and to the procedure or therapeutic intervention is imperative. Alterations in drug administration, particularly analgesics, sedatives, and vasoactive drugs, are frequently needed during the time away from the critical care unit to maintain physiologic stability. Documentation of assessment findings, interventions, and the patient's responses continues throughout the transport process.

Following return to the critical care unit, monitoring systems and interventions are reestablished and the patient is reassessed. Often, some adjustment in pharmacologic therapy or ventilator support is required following transport.

Allowing for some uninterrupted time for the family to be at the patient's bedside and for the patient to rest is another important priority following return to the unit.

TRANSITIONING TO THE NEXT STAGE OF CARE

Planning for the transition of the patient to the next stage of care begins soon after the patient is admitted to the ICU. It involves assessing minimally where and with whom the patient lives, what external resources were being used prior to admission, and what resources are anticipated to be required on transfer out of the critical care unit. Complex patients require extensive preplanning in achieving a successful transition. As the patient stabilizes and improves, the thought of leaving the ICU may be frightening as it is perceived as moving to a level of care where there are fewer staff to monitor the patient. Reinforce the positive aspect of

TABLE 2-17. RECOMMENDATIONS FOR END-OF-LIFE CARE

Domain	Main recommendations
EOL decision-making	If possible, decisions to withhold or withdraw life-sustaining treatment should be made together with the patient, and the patient's wishes and values should be included.
	Families should be continuously involved in assessment of the patient's situation. Family involvement in decision-making depends on legal practice in each country.
	EOL decisions should include all members of the interprofessional team.
	EOL decisions should be documented.
	A do-not-resuscitate order does not automatically mean that other therapies should be withheld.
Place to die	If in any way possible, the patient should be allowed to die in the ICU.
	Single rooms are preferred.
	If discharging the patient from the ICU is necessary, information and reasons should be given as early as possible.
	It may be possible to let patients go home to die.
Patient comfort	When life-sustaining treatments are withdrawn, palliative care becomes the main goal.
	Patient comfort entails frequent assessment of needs and individually tailored use of medical and nonmedical methods.
	Comforting patients at the EOL is about being aware of and sensitive to factors at play in each different situation.
	Great effort should be made to identify and honor the patient's wishes regarding visits, catering, spiritual support, etc.
	For the patient without family, the nurse is an important substitute for relatives.
Family presence in the ICU	Free access throughout the day and night for close family and friends (if the patient wants it) is the ideal.
	Unnecessary waiting outside the room must be avoided.
Visiting children	Children should be allowed to visit and be told the truth about the patient's condition.
	Nurses should talk with the children before the first visit.
	The ICU should have places where the children can play.
Family needs	Apart from information, the family may need emotional, spiritual, and practical support.
Preparing the family	For some family members, being with a dying person is a new and potentially frightening experience, and they need information about symptoms and about what may happen.
	Generally, it is not possible to precisely predict how long the dying process will be for the individual patient.
	Families should be assured that patients' symptoms will be assessed and treated continuously.
Staff presence	Asking about the family's preferences regarding staff presence at the bedside is necessary.
	If the family prefers to be alone with the patient, the nurse should still go into the room frequently.
When the patient dies	After death of the patient, the family needs time to say goodbye.
	Family members can be involved in taking care of the dead patient.
After-death care of family	Some ICUs give mementoes such as handprints, locks of hair, and letters of condolence to give to the family.
	Follow-up practices such as telephone calls, a visit in the ICU, and follow-up cafés may improve outcomes for bereaved family members.
Caring for staff	It is helpful to talk with colleagues about one's experiences and ask others how they are and how they are coping after the death of a patient.
	EOL situations that have not been handled well may lead to burnout.

Abbreviations: EOL, end of life; ICU, intensive care unit.

Reproduced with permission from Jensen HI, Halvorsen K, Jerpseth H, et al: Practice Recommendations for End-of-Life Care in the Intensive Care Unit. Crit Care Nurse. 2020;40(3):14-22.

planning for the transition in that it is a sign that the patient is improving and making progress.

If the patient is transferring to another institution, such as an acute or subacute rehabilitation facility, suggest that the family visit the facility prior to transfer. This gives them an opportunity to meet the new caregivers, ask any questions they may have, and alleviate the patient's anxiety about the transfer. If the transfer is internal to another patient care unit and the patient's care is complex, consider working with the receiving unit staff in advance to inform them of the anticipated plan of care and any patient preferences. Identify a nurse in advance from the receiving unit, who may be able to take the time to meet the patient before the transfer. Clinical nurse specialists or nurse managers may also be able to meet the patient and family, describe the receiving unit, and act as a resource after the transfer, again giving a sense of control to the patient and family.

SUPPORTING PATIENTS AND FAMILIES DURING THE DYING PROCESS

Transitioning of care also includes planning care for the patient who is dying. Caring for the dying patient and their family can be a most rewarding challenge. The use of advance directives and Orders for Life-Sustaining Treatment provide a means for the acutely or critically ill patient to communicate wishes regarding end-of-life care. A dialogue with the patient and family about end-of-life care is an appropriate avenue for discussing values and beliefs associated with dying and living and understanding their goals of care. If advanced directives are in place, then the plan of care is designed to align with the preferences it describes. In the absence of an advanced directive, a person close to the patient may serve as a surrogate decision-maker. Further discussion about end-of-life decision making is in Chapter 8. Practice recommendations for end-of-life care are listed in Table 2-17.

An awareness of personal feelings about death is essential when caring for dying persons. Be genuine in providing care, touch, and presence, and do not feel compelled to talk. Take cues from the patient. Crying or laughing with the patient and family is an acknowledgment of humanness, an existential relationship, and a rare gift in a unique encounter.

PRINCIPLES OF MANAGEMENT

1. Use of interprofessional plans of care improves communication and collaboration in achieving optimal patient outcomes.
2. Optimal care of acutely and critically ill patients includes preventing complications common in the ICU setting such as VTEs, HAI, pressure injury, and sleep disturbances.
3. Prevention and prompt treatment of delirium, depression, and anxiety may prevent or ameliorate the negative long-term consequences of ICU stays for both patients and families.
4. Meeting patient and family needs through patient and family-centered care and education includes providing vital information regarding the patient's condition and care to allay their fears and concerns.
5. Careful planning and organization can minimize risks of transport in critically ill patients.

SELECTED BIBLIOGRAPHY

Patient and Family Needs

American Association of Critical-Care Nurses. AACN Practice Alert. Family visitation in the adult intensive care unit. *Crit Care Nurse.* 2017;37(4):88.

Chapman DK, Collingridge DS, Mitchell LA, et al. Satisfaction with elimination of all visitation restrictions in a mixed-profile intensive care unit. *Am J Crit Care.* 2016;25(1):46-50.

Coombs M, Puntillo KA, Franck LS, et al. Implementing the SCCM family-centered guidelines in critical care nursing practice. *AACN Adv Crit Care.* 2017;28(2):138-147.

Davidson J, Aslakson R, Long A, et al. Guidelines for family-centered care in the neonatal, pediatric, and adult ICU. *Crit Care Med.* 2017;45(1):103-128.

Miller J. Animal-assisted interventions. *Nursing Manage.* 2020; 51(4):16-23. doi:10.1097/01.NUMA.0000657240.17744.1b

Hardin SR, Kaplow R. *Synergy for Clinical Excellence: The AACN Synergy Model for Patient Care.* 2nd ed. Burlington, MA: Jones & Bartlett; 2017.

Høghaug G, Fagermoen MS, Lerdal A. The visitor's regard of their need for support, comfort, information, proximity, and assurance in the intensive care unit. *Intensive Crit Care Nurs.* 2012;28(5):263-268.

Huynh TG, Covalesky M, Sinclair S, et al. Measuring outcomes of an intensive care unit family diary program. *AACN Adv Crit Care.* 2017;28(2):179-190.

Jacob M, Horton C, Rance-Ashley S, et al. Needs of patients' family members in an intensive care unit with continuous visitation. *Am J Crit Care.* 2016;25(2):118-125.

Jensen H, Halvorsen K, Jerpseth H, Fridh I, Lind R. Practice recommendations for end-of-life care in the intensive care unit. *Crit Care Nurse.* 2020;40(3):14-22.

Kean L, Milner K. Implementation of open visitation in an adult intensive care unit: an evidence-based practice quality improvement project. *Crit Care Nurse.* 2020;40(2):76–79.

Kozub E, Scheler S, Necoechea G, O'Byrne N. Improving nurse satisfaction with open visitation in an adult intensive care unit. *Crit Care Nurs Q.* 2017;40(2):144-154.

Nikayin S, Rabiee A, Hashem M, et al. Anxiety symptoms in survivors of critical illness: a systematic review and meta-analysis. *Gen Hosp Psychiatry.* 2016;43:23-29.

Nydahl P, Egerod I, Hosey MM, Needham DM, Jones C, Bienvenu OJJ. Report on the Third International Intensive Care Unit Diary Conference. *Crit Care Nurse.* 2020;40(5):e18-e25. doi:10.4037/ ccn2020958

Obringer K, Hilgenberg C, Booker K. Needs of adult family members of intensive care unit patients. *J Clin Nurs.* 2012;21(11-12): 1651-1658.

Parker A, Sricharoenchai T, Raparla S, Schneck K, Bienvenu O, Needham D. Posttraumatic stress disorder in critical illness survivors: a metaanalysis. *Crit Care Med.* 2015;43(5):1121-1129.

Rabiee A, Nikayin S, Hashem M, et al. Depressive symptoms after critical illness: a systematic review and meta-analysis. *Crit Care Med.* 2016;44(9):1744-1753.

Rogan J, Zielke M, Drumright K, Boehm L. Institutional challenges and solutions to evidence-based, patient-centered practice: implementing ICU diaries. *Crit Care Nurse.* 2020;40(5):47-45.

Infection Prevention and Control

Centers for Disease Control and Prevention. Interim infection prevention and control recommendations for healthcare personnel during the coronavirus disease 2019 (COVID-19) pandemic. 2022. https://www.cdc.gov/coronavirus/2019-ncov/hcp/infection-control-recommendations.html.

Centers for Disease Control and Prevention. Transmission based precautions. 2022. https://www.cdc.gov/infectioncontrol/basics/transmission-based-precautions.html.

Kalil A, Metersky ML, Klompas M, et al. Management of adults with hospital-acquired and ventilator-associated pneumonia: 2016 clinical practice guidelines by the Infectious Diseases Society of America and the American Thoracic Society. *Clin Infect Dis.* 2016;63:e61.

McDonald C, Gerding DN, Johnson S, et al. Clinical practice guidelines for *Clostridium difficile* infection in adults and children: 2017 update by the Infectious Diseases Society of America (IDSA) and Society for Healthcare Epidemiology of America (SHEA). *Clin Infect Dis.* 2018;66(7):e1-e48.

National Health Safety Network. Bloodstream infection event (central line-associated bloodstream infection and non-central line associated bloodstream infection) 2021. https://www.cdc.gov/nhsn/pdfs/pscmanual/4psc_clabscurrent.pdf. Accessed June 28, 2021.

National Health Safety Network. Multidrug-resistant organism & *Clostridioides difficile* infection (MDRO/CDI) module. 2021. https://www.cdc.gov/nhsn/pdfs/pscmanual/12pscmdro_cdadcurrent.pdf. Accessed June 28, 2021.

National Health Safety Network. Urinary tract infection (catheter-associated urinary tract infection [CAUTI] and non-catheter-associated urinary tract infection [UTI]) events. 2021. https://www.cdc.gov/nhsn/pdfs/pscmanual/7psccauticurrent.pdf. Accessed June 28, 2021.

National Health Safety Network. Pneumonia (ventilator-associated [VAP] and non-ventilator-associated pneumonia [PNEU]) event. 2021. https://www.cdc.gov/nhsn/pdfs/pscmanual/6pscvapcurrent.pdf. Accessed June 28, 2021.

Occupational Safety and Health Administration. June 2021 regulations https://www.osha.gov/coronavirus/standards. Accessed July 18, 2021.

Patient and Family Education

Always Use Teach-Back! Welcome to the Always Use Teach-Back! Training toolkit, 2017. www.teachbacktraining.org. Accessed June 15, 2017.

Centrella-Nigro AM, Alexander C. Using the teach-back method in patient education to improve patient satisfaction. *J Contin Educ Nurs.* 2017;48(1):47-52.

Gillam SW, Gillam AR, Casier TL, Curcio K. Education for medications and side effects: a two part mechanism for improving the patient experience. *Appl Nurs Res.* 2016;31:72-78.

Psychosocial Support

Bell, L. Prevent post-intensive care syndrome (PICS) during COVID-19. May 4, 2020. https://www.aacn.org/blog/prevent-post-intensive-care-syndrome-pics-during-covid-19. Accessed June 28, 2021.

Critical Illness, Brain Dysfunction and Survivorship (CIBS) Center. ABCDEF (A2F) bundle overview. https://www.icudelirium.org/medical-professionals/overview. Accessed July 18, 2021.

Davidson JE, Harvey MA. Patient and family post-intensive care syndrome. *AACN Adv Crit Care.* 2016;27(2):184-186.

Kotfis K, Roberson SW, Wilson JE, Dabrowski W, Pun BT, Ely EW. COVID-19: ICU delirium management during SARS-CoV-2 pandemic. *Crit Care.* 2020;24:176.

Planetree International. *Family Presence Policy: Decision-Making Toolkit for Nurse Leaders.* May 2021. https://planetree.org/wp-content/uploads/2021/05/Family-Presence-Policy-Decision-Making-Toolkit.pdf.

Selim AA, Ely EW. Delirium the under-recognised syndrome: survey of healthcare professionals' awareness and practice in the intensive care units. *J Clin Nurs.* 2017;26(5-6):813-824.

Slooter AJ, Van de Leur RR, Zaal IJ. Delirium in critically ill patients. *Handb Clin Neurol.* 2017;141:449-466.

Sleep Deprivation

Blissitt PA. Sleep and mechanical ventilation. *Crit Care Nurs Clin North Am.* 2016;28:195-203.

Engwall M, Fridh I, Johansson L, Bergbom I, Lindahl B. Lighting, sleep and circadian rhythm: an intervention study in the intensive care unit. *Intensive Crit Care Nurs.* 2015;31(6):325-335.

Grimm J. Sleep deprivation in the intensive care patient. *Crit Care Nurse.* 2020;40(2):16-24.

Owens RL, Huynh TG, Netzer G. Sleep in the intensive care unit in a model of family-centered care. *AACN Adv Crit Care.* 2017;28(2):171-178.

Shaw R. Using music to promote sleep for hospitalized adults. *Am J Crit Care.* 2018;25(2):181-184.

Transport of Critically Ill Patients

Comeau, OY. Intrafacility transport of critically ill adult patients. *Crit Care Nurse.* 2020;40(2):70-72.

Comeau OY, Armendariz-Batiste J, Woodby SA. Safety first! Using a checklist for intrafacility transport of adult intensive care patients. *Crit Care Nurse.* 2015;35(5):16-25.

Evidence-Based Practice

AACN Scope and Standards for Progressive and Critical Care Nursing Practice. https://www.aacn.org/nursing-excellence/standards/aacn-scope-and-standards-for-progressive-and-critical-care-nursing-practice.

American Association of Critical-Care Nurses. AACN Practice Alert. Assessment and management of delirium across the life span. *Crit Care Nurse.* 2016;36(5):e14-e19.

American Association of Critical-Care Nurses. AACN Practice Alert. Prevention of aspiration in adults. *Crit Care Nurse.* 2017;37(3):88.

American Association of Critical-Care Nurses. AACN Practice Alert. Prevention of catheter-associated urinary tract infections in adults. *Crit Care Nurse.* 2018;38(1):84.

American Association of Critical-Care Nurses. AACN Practice Alert. Preventing venous thromboembolism in adults. *Crit Care Nurse.* 2018;38(3):88.

American Association of Critical-Care Nurses. Guideline update: bundle up for pain, agitation, and delirium. *Crit Care Nurse.* 2021;41(3):80.

Barnes G, Burnett A, Allen A, et al. Thromboembolism and anticoagulant therapy during the COVID-19 pandemic: interim clinical guidance from the anticoagulation forum. *J Thromb Thrombolysis.* 2020;50:72-81.

Centers for Disease Control and Prevention. Hand hygiene in healthcare settings. https://www.cdc.gov/handhygiene/index.html. Accessed June 28, 2021.

Devlin JW, Skrobik Y, Gélinas C, et al. Clinical practice guidelines for the prevention and management of pain, agitation/sedation, delirium, immobility, and sleep disruption in adult patients in the ICU. *Crit Care Med.* 2018;46(9):e825-e873.

Kearon C, Aki E, Ornelas J, et al. Antithrombic guidelines for VTE disease. *Chest.* 2016;149(2):315-352.

Klompas M, Branson R, Cawcut K, et al. Strategies to prevent ventilator-associated pneumonia, ventilator-associated events, and nonventilator hospital-acquired pneumonia in acute-care hospitals: 2022 update. *Infect Control Hosp Epidemiol.* 2022;43(6):687-713. doi:10.1017/ice.2022.88

National Pressure Ulcer Advisory Panel, European Pressure Ulcer Advisory Panel, Pan Pacific Pressure Ulcer Injury Alliance. Prevention and treatment of pressure ulcers: quick reference guide. https://npiap.com/page/Guidelines

Sedwick MB, Lance-Smith M, Reeder SJ, Nardi J. Using evidence-based practice to prevent ventilator-associated pneumonia. *Crit Care Nurse.* 2012;32(4):41-50.

Shadle H, Sabol V, Smith A, Stafford H, Thompson JA, Bowers M. A bundle-based approach to prevent catheter-associated urinary tract infections in the intensive care unit. *Crit Care Nurse.* 2021;41(2):62-71.

INTERPRETATION AND MANAGEMENT OF BASIC CARDIAC RHYTHMS

Carol Jacobson

3

KNOWLEDGE COMPETENCIES

1. Correctly identify key elements of electrocardiogram (ECG) waveforms, complexes, and intervals:
   - P wave
   - QRS complex
   - T wave
   - ST segment
   - PR interval
   - QT interval
   - RR interval
   - Rate (atrial and ventricular)

2. Compare and contrast the etiology, ECG characteristics, and management of common cardiac rhythms and conduction abnormalities:
   - Sinus node rhythms
   - Atrial rhythms
   - Junctional rhythms
   - Ventricular rhythms
   - AV blocks

3. Describe the indications for, and use of, temporary pacemakers, defibrillation, and cardioversion for the treatment of serious cardiac dysrhythmias.[*]

While different professional organizations may prefer the use of the term arrhythmia versus dysrhythmia, they are synonymous. This chapter uses dysrhythmia, the exception being the use of arrhythmia in selected professional statements, protocols, and practice statements.

Continuous monitoring of cardiac rhythm in the critically or acutely ill patient is an important aspect of cardiovascular assessment. Frequent analysis of electrocardiogram (ECG) rate and rhythm provides for early identification and treatment of alterations in cardiac rhythm, as well as abnormal conditions in other body systems. This chapter presents a review of basic cardiac electrophysiology and information essential to the identification and treatment of common cardiac dysrhythmias. Advanced cardiac dysrhythmias, and 12-lead ECG interpretation, are described in Chapter 18, Advanced ECG Concepts.

BASIC ELECTROPHYSIOLOGY

The electrical impulse of the heart is the stimulus for cardiac contraction. The cardiac conduction system is responsible for the initiation of the electrical impulse and its sequential spread through the atria, atrioventricular (AV) junction, and ventricles. The conduction system of the heart consists of the following structures (Figure 3-1):

Sinus node: The sinus node is a small group of cells in the upper right atrium that functions as the normal pacemaker of the heart because it has the highest rate of automaticity of all potential pacemaker sites. The sinus node normally depolarizes at a regular rate of 60 to 100 times/min.

AV node: The AV node is a small group of cells in the low right atrium near the tricuspid valve. The AV node has three main functions:

1. Its major job is to slow conduction of the impulse from the atria to the ventricles to allow time for the atria to contract and empty their blood into the ventricles.

2. Its rate of automaticity is 40 to 60 beats/min and can function as a backup pacemaker if the sinus node fails.

3. It screens out rapid atrial impulses to protect the ventricles from dangerously fast rates when the atrial rate is very rapid.

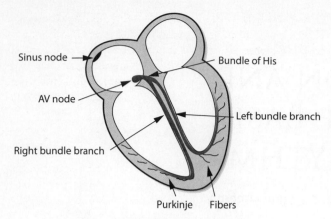

Figure 3-1. The conduction system of the heart.

Bundle of His: The bundle of His is a short bundle of fibers at the bottom of the AV node leading to the bundle branches. Conduction velocity accelerates in the bundle of His and the impulse is transmitted to both bundle branches.

Bundle branches: The bundle branches are bundles of fibers that rapidly conduct the impulse into the right and left ventricles. The *right bundle branch* travels along the right side of the interventricular septum and carries the impulse into the right ventricle. The *left bundle branch* has two main divisions: the anterior fascicle and

the posterior fascicle, which carry the impulse into the left ventricle.

Purkinje fibers: The Purkinje fibers are hairlike fibers that spread out from the bundle branches along the endocardial surface of both ventricles and rapidly conduct the impulse to the ventricular muscle cells. Cells in the Purkinje system have automaticity at a rate of 20 to 40 beats/min and can function as a backup pacemaker if all other pacemakers fail.

The electrical impulse normally begins in the sinus node and spreads through both atria in an inferior and leftward direction, resulting in depolarization of the atrial muscle. When the impulse reaches the AV node, its conduction velocity is slowed before it continues into the ventricles. When the impulse emerges from the AV node, it travels rapidly through the bundle of His and down the right and left bundle branches into the Purkinje network of both ventricles, and results in depolarization of the ventricular muscle. The spread of this wave of depolarization through the heart produces the classic surface ECG, which can be recorded by an electrocardiograph (ECG machine) or monitored continuously on a bedside cardiac monitor.

ECG WAVEFORMS, COMPLEXES, AND INTERVALS

The ECG waveforms, complexes, and intervals are illustrated in Figure 3-2.

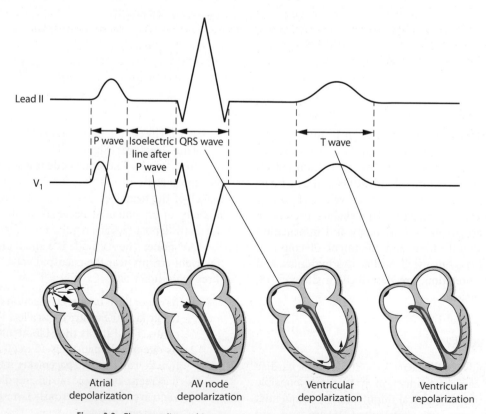

Figure 3-2. Electrocardiographic waves, complexes, and intervals in leads II and V_1.

P Wave

The P wave represents atrial muscle depolarization. It is normally 2.5 mm or less in height and 0.11 second or less in duration. P waves can be upright, inverted, or biphasic depending on how the electrical impulse conducts through the atria and on which lead it is being recorded.

QRS Complex

The QRS complex represents ventricular muscle depolarization. A Q wave is an initial negative deflection from baseline. An R wave is the first positive deflection from baseline. An S wave is a negative deflection that follows an R wave. The shape of the QRS complex depends on the lead being recorded and the ventricular activation sequence; not all leads record all waves of the QRS complex. Regardless of the shape of the complex, ventricular depolarization waves are called QRS complexes (Figure 3-3). The width of the QRS complex represents intraventricular conduction time and is measured from the point at which it first leaves the baseline to the point at which the last wave ends. Normal QRS width is 0.04 to 0.10 second in an adult. When describing the shape of the QRS complex in writing, a capital letter is used when the voltage of a wave is 5 mm or more, and a lowercase letter is used for smaller waves, as in Figure 3-3.

T Wave

The T wave represents ventricular muscle repolarization. It follows the QRS complex and is normally in the same direction as the QRS complex. T waves can be upright, flat, or inverted depending on many things, including the presence of myocardial ischemia, electrolyte levels, drug effect, myocardial disease, and the lead being recorded.

U Wave

The U wave is a small, rounded wave that sometimes follows the T wave and is thought to be due to repolarization of the M-cells (mid-myocardial cells) in the ventricles. U waves should be positive, especially when the T wave is positive. Large U waves can be seen when repolarization is abnormally prolonged; with electrolyte imbalances such as hypokalemia, hypocalcemia, hypomagnesemia; increased intracranial pressure; left ventricular hypertrophy; or with certain medications.

PR Interval

The PR interval is measured from the beginning of the P wave to the beginning of the QRS complex and represents the time required for the impulse to travel through the atria, AV junction, and to the Purkinje system. The normal PR interval in adults is 0.12 to 0.20 second. The PR segment extends from the end of the P wave to the beginning of the QRS complex.

ST Segment

The ST segment represents early ventricular repolarization. It begins at the end of the QRS complex (J point) and extends to the beginning of the T wave. The J point is where the QRS complex ends and the ST segment begins. The ST segment should be at the isoelectric line.

QT Interval

The QT interval measures the duration of ventricular depolarization and repolarization and varies with age, gender, and heart rate. The QT interval is measured from the beginning of the QRS complex to the end of the T wave. Because heart rate greatly affects the length of the QT interval, the QT interval must be corrected to a heart rate of 60 beats/min (corrected QT interval [QTc]). This correction is usually done using the Bazett formula:

QTc = measured QT interval divided by the square root of the RR interval (all measurements in seconds)

The QTc should not exceed 0.45 second in men and 0.46 second in women.

BASIC ELECTROCARDIOGRAPHY

The ECG is a graphic record of the electrical activity of the heart. The spread of the electrical impulse through the heart produces weak electrical currents that can be detected and amplified by the ECG machine and recorded on calibrated graph paper. These amplified signals form the ECG tracing which consists of the previously described waveforms and intervals inscribed onto grid paper. The grid on the paper consists of a series of small and large boxes, both horizontal and vertical; horizontal boxes measure time and vertical boxes measure voltage (Figure 3-4). On the horizontal axis, each small box is equal to 0.04 second, and each large box is equal to 0.20 second. On the vertical axis, each small box measures 1 mm and is equal to 0.1 mV; each large box

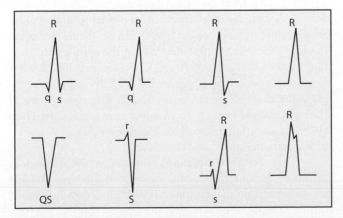

Figure 3-3. Examples of different configurations of QRS complexes. (*Reproduced with permission from Jacobson C, Marzlin K, Webner C. Cardiovascular Nursing Practice: A Comprehensive Resource Manual and Study Guide for Clinical Nurses. Burien, WA: Cardiovascular Nursing Education Associates; 2014.*)

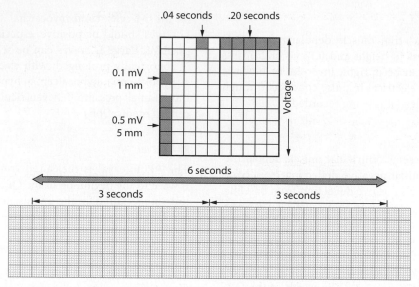

Figure 3-4. Time and voltage lines on ECG paper at standard paper speed of 25 mm/s. Horizontal axis measures time: each small box = 0.04 second, one large box = 0.20 *second. Vertical axis measures voltage and also represents mm of ST segment deviation: each small box = 0.1 mV or 1 mm, one large box = 0.5 mV or 5 mm.*

measures 5 mm and is equal to 0.5 mV. In addition to the grid, most ECG papers place a vertical line in the top margin at 3-second intervals or place a mark at 1-second intervals.

CARDIAC MONITORING

Cardiac monitoring provides continuous observation of the patient's heart rate and rhythm and is a routine nursing procedure in many types of acute and all critical care units as well as in emergency departments, postanesthesia recovery units, and many operating rooms. Cardiac monitoring has also become common in areas where patients receive treatments or procedures requiring moderate sedation or where the administration of certain medications could result in cardiac dysrhythmias. The goals of cardiac monitoring can range from simple heart rate and basic rhythm monitoring to sophisticated dysrhythmia diagnosis and ST-segment monitoring to detect cardiac ischemia. Cardiac monitoring can be done using a 3-wire, 5-wire, or 10-wire cable, which connects the patient to the cardiac monitor or portable telemetry box.

The choice of monitoring lead is based on the goals of monitoring in a particular patient population and by the patient's clinical situation. Because dysrhythmias are the most common complication of ischemic heart disease and myocardial infarction (MI), monitoring for dysrhythmia diagnosis is a priority in these patients. Although many dysrhythmias can be recognized in any lead, research consistently shows that leads V_1 and V_6, or their bipolar substitutes MCL_1 and MCL_6, are the best leads for differentiating wide QRS rhythms (Table 3-1). The QRS morphologies displayed in these leads are useful in differentiating ventricular tachycardia (VT) from supraventricular tachycardia (SVT) with aberrant intraventricular conduction and for recognizing right and left bundle branch block (see Chapter 18, Advanced ECG Concepts).

Correct placement of monitoring electrodes is critical for obtaining accurate information from any monitoring lead. Most currently available bedside monitors utilize either a 3-wire or a 5-wire monitoring cable. A 5-wire system offers several advantages over the 3-wire system (Table 3-2). With a 5-wire system, it is possible to monitor more than one lead at a time and it is possible to monitor a true unipolar V_1 lead, which is superior to its bipolar substitute MCL_1 in differentiating wide QRS rhythms. With a 5-wire system, all 12 standard ECG leads can be obtained by selecting the desired lead on the bedside monitor and moving the one chest lead to the appropriate spot on the thorax to record the precordial leads V_1 through V_6 (see Chapter 18, Advanced ECG Concepts). Figure 3-5 illustrates correct lead placement for a 5-wire system. Arm electrodes are placed on the shoulders as close as possible to where the arms join the torso. Placing the arm electrodes on the posterior shoulder keeps the anterior chest area clear for defibrillation paddles if needed and avoid irritating the skin in the subclavicular area where an intravenous (IV) catheter might need to be placed. Leg electrodes are placed at the level of the lowest ribs on the thorax or on the hips. Placing the chest electrode at the appropriate location on the chest and selecting "V" on the bedside monitor obtains the desired V or precordial lead. To monitor in V_1, place the chest electrode in the fourth intercostal space at the right sternal border. To monitor in V_6, place the chest electrode at the left midaxillary line at the V_4 level (V_4 level is fifth intercostal space, midclavicular line).

When using a 3-wire monitoring system with electrodes placed in their conventional locations on the right and left shoulders and on the left hip or low thorax, leads I, II, or III can be monitored by selecting the desired lead on the bedside monitor. It is not possible to obtain a true unipolar V_1 or V_6 lead with a 3-wire system. In this case, the bipolar substitutes MCL_1 and MCL_6 can be used but to obtain them requires

TABLE 3-1. EVIDENCE-BASED PRACTICE: BEDSIDE CARDIAC MONITORING FOR DYSRHYTHMIA DETECTION

Electrode Application
• Make sure skin is clean and dry before applying monitoring electrodes.
• Place arm electrodes on shoulder (front, top, or back) as close as possible to where arm joins torso.
• Place leg electrodes below the rib cage or on hips.
• Place V_1 electrode at the fourth intercostal space at right sternal border.
• Place V_6 electrode at the left midaxillary line at the V_4 level.
• Replace electrodes daily.
• Mark electrode position with indelible ink to ensure consistent lead placement.

Lead Selection
• Use lead V_1 as the primary dysrhythmia monitoring lead whenever possible.
• Use lead V_6 if lead V_1 is not available.
• Display at least two leads whenever possible.
• Use lead II to identify atrial activity if unclear in other leads and for R wave visualization during synchronized cardioversion.
• If using a 3-wire system, use MCL_1 as the primary lead and MCL_6 as the second choice lead.

Alarm Limits
• Set heart rate alarms as appropriate for patient's current heart rate and clinical condition.
• Never turn heart rate alarms off while patient's rhythm is being monitored.
• Set alarm limits on other parameters based on goals of patient care if using a computerized dysrhythmia monitoring system.

Documentation and Reporting
• Document the monitoring lead on every rhythm strip.
• Document heart rate, PR interval, QRS width, and QT interval every shift and with any significant rhythm change.
• Document rhythm strip with every significant rhythm change:
– Onset and termination of tachycardias.
– Symptomatic bradycardias or tachycardias.
– Conversion into or out of atrial flutter or atrial fibrillation.
– All rhythms requiring immediate treatment.
• Place rhythm strips flat on page (avoid folding or winding strips into chart).
• Report episodes of atrial fibrillation if no documented history of atrial fibrillation.
• Report rhythms with a short PR interval of <0.12 seconds (may indicate presence of accessory pathway).
• Report episodes of life-threatening dysrhythmias and rhythms requiring treatment.
• Document patient's tolerance of dysrhythmia and any symptoms.
• Document patient's response to treatment

Transporting Monitored Patients
• Continue cardiac monitoring using a portable, battery-operated monitor-defibrillator if patient is required to leave a monitored unit for diagnostic or therapeutic procedures.
• Monitored patients must be accompanied by a healthcare provider skilled in ECG interpretation and defibrillation during transport.
• Whenever possible, avoid transporting patients off the unit who have a corrected QT interval (QTc) of 0.50 seconds or greater until the prolonged QTc has been addressed.

AACN Practice Alert: Accurate dysrhythmia monitoring in adults. 2016.
Data from Sandau, Funk, Auerbach, et al. 2017.

placing electrodes in unconventional sites. Figure 3-5 shows electrode placement for a 3-wire system that allows the user to monitor either MCL_1 or MCL_6. Place the right arm electrode on the left shoulder, the left arm electrode at the

TABLE 3-2. ADVANTAGES OF COMMON MONITORING LEADS

Lead	Advantages
Preferred Monitoring Leads	
V_1 and V_6 (or MCL_1 and MCL_6 if using a 3-wire system)	Differentiate between right and left bundle branch block
	Morphology clues to differentiate between ventricular beats and supraventricular beats with aberrant conduction
	Differentiate between right and left ventricular ectopy
	Differentiate between right and left ventricular pacing
	Usually shows well-formed P waves
	Placement of electrodes keeps apex clear for auscultation or defibrillation
Other Monitoring Leads	
Lead II	Usually shows well-formed P waves
	Often best lead for identification of atrial flutter waves
	Usually has tall, upright QRS complex on which to synchronize machine for cardioversion
	Allows identification of retrograde P waves
Lead III or aVF	Assists in diagnosis of hemiblock
	Allows identification of retrograde P waves
	Allows identification of atrial flutter waves
	Best limb leads for ST-segment monitoring when 12-lead ECG showing ischemic fingerprint not available
Lewis lead (negative electrode at second right intercostal space, positive electrode at fourth right intercostal space)	Good lead to identify atrial activity when unclear in other leads
Atrial electrogram (recorded from atrial epicardial pacing wire)	Good lead to identify atrial activity when unclear in other leads

V_1 position (fourth intercostal space at the right sternal border), and the left leg electrode in the V_6 position (fifth intercostal space at the left midaxillary line). With electrodes in this position, select "lead I" on the monitor to obtain MCL_1 and switch to lead II on the monitor to record MCL_6.

The electrode sites on the skin should be clean, dry, and relatively flat. Remove excess hair, if present, and clean the skin with alcohol to remove any oils. Mildly abrade the skin with a gauze or abrading pad supplied on electrode packaging to improve transmission of the ECG signal. Apply the pregelled electrodes to the chest in the appropriate locations. Set the heart rate alarm limits based on the patient's clinical situation and current heart rate. Bedside monitoring systems have default alarms that adjust the high- and low-rate limits based on the learned heart rate. Electrodes are changed daily to prevent pressure injury and provide artifact-free tracings.

DETERMINATION OF THE HEART RATE

Heart rate can be obtained from the ECG strip by several methods. The first, and most accurate if the rhythm is regular, is to count the number of small boxes (one small

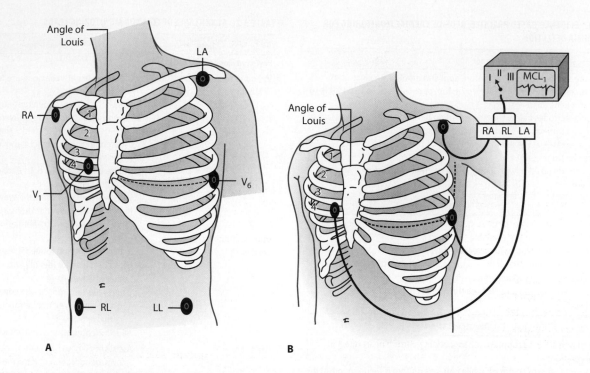

Figure 3-5. **(A)** Correct electrode placement for using a 5-wire monitoring cable. Right and left arm electrodes are placed on the shoulders and right and left leg electrodes are placed low on the thorax or on the hips. With the arm and leg electrodes placed as illustrated, leads I, II, III, aVR, aVL, and aVF can be obtained by selecting the desired lead on the bedside monitor. To obtain lead V_1, place the chest lead in the fourth intercostal space at the right sternal border and select "V" on the bedside monitor. To obtain lead V_6, place the chest lead at the level of V_4 in the left midaxillary line and select "V" on the bedside monitor. **(B)** Correct lead placement for obtaining MCL_1 and MCL_6 using a 3-wire lead system. Place the right arm electrode on the left shoulder; the left arm electrode in the fourth intercostal space at the right sternal border; and the left leg electrode at the level of V_4 in the left midaxillary line (V_6 position). To monitor in MCL_1, select lead I on the bedside monitor. To monitor in MCL_6, select lead II on the bedside monitor. (*Adapted with permission from Drew BJ. Bedside electrocardiogram monitoring.* AACN Clin Issues Crit Care Nurs. *1993;4(1):25-33.*)

box = 0.04 second) between two R waves, and then divide that number into 1500. There are 1500 boxes of 0.04-second interval in a 1-minute strip (Figure 3-6A). Another method is to count the number of large boxes (one large box = 0.20 second)

between two R waves, and then divide that number into 300 or use a standardized table (Table 3-3).

The third method for computing heart rate, especially useful when the rhythm is irregular, is to count the number

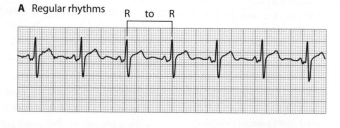

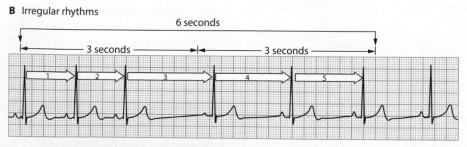

Figure 3-6. **(A)** Heart rate determination for a regular rhythm using little boxes between two R waves. One RR interval is marked at the top of the ECG paper. There are 18 little boxes between these two R waves. There are 1500 little boxes in a 60-second strip. By dividing 1500 by 18, one calculates a heart rate of 83 beats/min. Heart rate can also be determined for a regular rhythm counting large boxes between R waves. There are approximately four large boxes between R waves. There are 300 large boxes in a 60-second strip. By dividing 300 by 4, one calculates a heart rate of about 75 beats/min. **(B)** Heart rate determination for a regular or irregular rhythm using the number of RR intervals in a 6-second strip and multiplying by 10. There are five RR intervals in this example. Multiplying by 10 gives a heart rate of about 50 beats/min.

TABLE 3-3. HEART RATE DETERMINATION USING THE ELECTROCARDIOGRAM LARGE BOXES

Number of Large Boxes Between R Waves	Heart Rate (beats/min)
1	300
2	150
3	100
4	75
5	60
6	50
7	43
8	38
9	33
10	30

of RR intervals in 6 seconds and multiply that number by 10. The ECG paper is usually marked at 3-second intervals (15 large boxes horizontally) by a vertical line at the top of the paper (Figures 3-4 and 3-6B). The RR intervals are counted, not the QRS complexes, to avoid overestimating the heart rate.

The atrial rate can be calculated by using any of these three methods with P waves instead of R waves.

DETERMINATION OF CARDIAC RHYTHM

Correct determination of the cardiac rhythm requires a systematic evaluation of the ECG. The following steps are used to determine the cardiac rhythm:

1. Calculate the atrial (P wave) rate.
2. Calculate the ventricular (QRS complex) rate.
3. Determine the regularity and shape of the P waves.
4. Determine the regularity, shape, and width of the QRS complexes.
5. Measure the PR interval.
6. Interpret the dysrhythmia as described later.

COMMON DYSRHYTHMIAS

A *dysrhythmia* is any cardiac rhythm that is not normal sinus rhythm. The term dysrhythmia is synonymous with the term arrhythmia. A dysrhythmia may result from altered impulse formation or altered impulse conduction. The term *ectopic* refers to any beat or rhythm that arises from a location other than the sinus node. Ectopic beats can arise in the atria, AV junction, or ventricles. Dysrhythmias are named by the place where they originate and by their rate. Dysrhythmias are grouped as rhythms originating:

1. in the sinus node.
2. in the atria.
3. in the AV junction.
4. in the ventricle.
5. AV blocks.

The etiology, ECG characteristics, and treatment of the basic cardiac dysrhythmias are presented here and summarized in Chapter 25, Cardiac Rhythms, ECG Characteristics, and Treatment Guide.

RHYTHMS ORIGINATING IN THE SINUS NODE

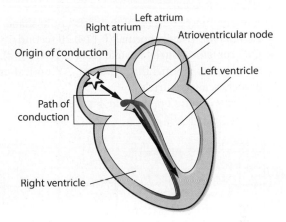

Figure 3-7. Demonstrates the path of conduction for rhythms originating in the sinus node.

Normal Sinus Rhythm

ECG Characteristics

- *Rate:* 60 to 100 beats/min.
- *Rhythm:* Regular.
- *P waves:* Precede every QRS complex; consistent in shape.
- *PR interval:* 0.12 to 0.20 second.
- *QRS complex:* 0.04 to 0.10 second.
- *Conduction:* Normal through atria, AV node, bundle branches, and ventricles.
- *Example of normal sinus rhythm:* Figure 3-8.

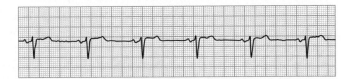

Figure 3-8. Normal sinus rhythm.

Sinus Bradycardia

All aspects of sinus bradycardia are the same as normal sinus rhythm except the rate is slower. It can be a normal finding in athletes and during sleep. Sinus bradycardia may be a response to vagal stimulation, such as carotid sinus massage, ocular pressure, or vomiting. Other causes of sinus bradycardia include inferior MI, obstructive sleep apnea, increased intracranial pressure and other central nervous system conditions (eg, stroke), anorexia nervosa, hypothyroidism, hypothermia, and some infectious diseases. Sinus bradycardia can be a response to several medications, including digitalis, beta-blockers, some calcium channel blockers, ivabradine, antiarrhythmics, and others.

ECG Characteristics

- *Rate:* traditionally defined as a rate less than 60 beats/min, but increasingly, research and practice guidelines define bradycardia as a rate <50 beats/min
- *Rhythm:* Regular.
- *P waves:* Precede every QRS; consistent in shape.
- *PR interval:* Usually normal (0.12-0.20 second).
- *QRS complex:* Usually normal (0.04-0.10 second).
- *Conduction:* Normal through atria, AV node, bundle branches, and ventricles.
- *Example of sinus bradycardia:* Figure 3-9.

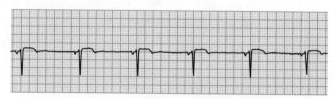

Figure 3-9. Sinus bradycardia, rate 42 beats/min.

Treatment

Treatment of sinus bradycardia in adults is not required unless the patient is symptomatic. If the dysrhythmia is accompanied by hypotension, confusion, diaphoresis, chest pain, or other signs of hemodynamic compromise or by ventricular ectopy, 0.5 mg of atropine IV is the treatment of choice. Attempts are made to decrease vagal stimulation. If the dysrhythmia is due to medications, they are held until their need has been reevaluated. Temporary or permanent pacing may be necessary.

Sinus Tachycardia

Sinus tachycardia is a sinus rhythm at a rate greater than 100 beats/min. Sinus tachycardia is a normal response to exercise and emotion. Sinus tachycardia that persists at rest usually indicates some underlying problem, such as fever, acute blood loss, shock, pain, anxiety, heart failure (HF), hypermetabolic states, pulmonary disease, or anemia. Sinus tachycardia is a normal physiologic response to a decrease in cardiac output; cardiac output is the product of heart rate and stroke volume. The following medications also cause sinus tachycardia: atropine, isoproterenol, epinephrine, dopamine, dobutamine, norepinephrine, nitroprusside, and caffeine.

ECG Characteristics

- *Rate:* Greater than 100 beats/min.
- *Rhythm:* Regular.
- *P waves:* Precede every QRS; consistent in shape; may be buried in the preceding T wave.
- *PR interval:* Usually normal; may be difficult to measure if P waves are buried in T waves.

- *QRS complex:* Usually normal.
- *Conduction:* Normal through atria, AV node, bundle branches, and ventricles.
- *Example of sinus tachycardia:* Figure 3-10.

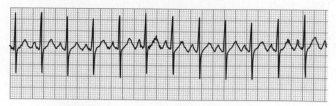

Figure 3-10. Sinus tachycardia, rate 125 beats/min.

Treatment

Treatment of sinus tachycardia is directed at the underlying cause. This dysrhythmia is a physiologic response to a decrease in cardiac output, and it should never be ignored, especially in the cardiac patient. Because the ventricles fill with blood and the coronary arteries perfuse during diastole, persistent tachycardia can cause decreased stroke volume, decreased cardiac output, and decreased coronary perfusion secondary to the decreased diastolic time that occurs with rapid heart rates. Carotid sinus pressure may slow the heart rate temporarily and thereby help in ruling out other dysrhythmias.

Sinus Dysrhythmia

Sinus dysrhythmia occurs when the sinus node discharges irregularly. It occurs frequently as a normal phenomenon, especially in younger people, and is commonly associated with the phases of respiration. During inspiration, the sinus node fires faster; during expiration, it slows. Digitalis toxicity may also cause this dysrhythmia. Sinus dysrhythmia looks like normal sinus rhythm except for the irregularity.

ECG Characteristics

- *Rate:* 60 to 100 beats/min.
- *Rhythm:* Irregular; phasic increase and decrease in rate, which may or may not be related to respiration.
- *P waves:* Precede every QRS complex; consistent in shape.
- *PR interval:* Usually normal.
- *QRS complex:* Usually normal.
- *Conduction:* Normal through atria, AV node, bundle branches, and ventricles.
- *Example of sinus dysrhythmia:* Figure 3-11.

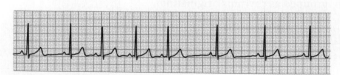

Figure 3-11. Sinus dysrhythmia.

Treatment

Treatment of sinus dysrhythmia usually is not necessary. If the dysrhythmia is thought to be because of digitalis toxicity, then digitalis is held. Atropine increases the rate and eliminates the irregularity.

Sinus Node Dysfunction

Sinus node dysfunction (SND), previously called sick sinus syndrome, consists of various abnormalities in sinus node impulse formation or conduction of the sinus impulse into the atrial myocardium. The 2018 guideline on the evaluation and management of patients with bradycardia and cardiac conduction delay lists the following conditions as components of the definition of SND:

- Sinus bradycardia: Sinus rate <50 beats/min.
- Ectopic atrial bradycardia: Sischarge of an atrial pacemaker outside the sinus node at a rate <50 beats/min.
- Sinoatrial exit block (also called sinus exit block): Evidence of failed conduction between the sinus node and surrounding atrial tissue.
- Sinus pause: Depolarization of the sinus node >3 seconds after the last atrial depolarization.
- Sinus arrest: No evidence of sinus node depolarization.
- Tachycardia-bradycardia ("tachy-brady") syndrome: Sinus bradycardia, ectopic atrial bradycardia, or sinus pause alternating with rapid atrial tachycardia (AT), atrial flutter, or atrial fibrillation (AF). Suppression of sinus node automaticity and sinus pauses can occur after termination of the atrial tachyarrhythmia.
- Chronotropic incompetence: Inability of the heart rate to increase appropriately with increased activity or demand. Some researchers define chronotropic incompetence as failure to reach 80% of expected heart rate reserve with exercise. Heart rate reserve is the difference between maximum predicted heart rate based on age (220 minus age) and the resting heart rate. For example, a 50 year old's maximum predicted heart rate is 170 beats/min (220 – 50). If the resting heart rate is 60 beats/min, the heart rate reserve is 110 beats/min (170 – 60). Failure of this person's heart rate to reach 88 beats/min during exercise (88 is 80% of 110) is chronotropic incompetence.

Patients with symptoms due to SND have a high risk of syncope, AF, and HF. The development of chronotropic incompetence with age is associated with increased risk of cardiovascular death and overall mortality.

Sinus Pause and Sinus Arrest (Failure of the Sinus Node to Fire)

ECG Characteristics

- *Rate:* Atrial—within normal range but may be in bradycardia range if several sinus impulses fail to form. Ventricular—within normal range but may be in bradycardia range if several sinus impulses fail to form and there are no junctional or ventricular escape beats. Ventricular rate may be faster than atrial rate if junctional or ventricular escape beats occur during periods of sinus arrest.
- *Rhythm:* Irregular due to transient absence of sinus node discharge.
- *P waves:* Present when sinus node fires and absent during periods of sinus arrest. When present, they precede every QRS complex and are consistent in shape. Because the sinus node occasionally fails to form impulses, the P-P interval is not an exact multiple of the sinus cycle. If junctional escape beats occur, P waves may be inverted either before or after the junctional QRS.
- *QRS complex:* Usually normal when sinus node is functioning and absent during periods of sinus arrest, unless escape beats occur. If ventricular escape beats occur, QRS is wide.
- *Conduction:* Normal through atria, AV node, bundle branches, and ventricles when sinus node fires. When sinus node fails to form impulses, there is no conduction through atria. If junctional escape beats occur, ventricular conduction is usually normal. If ventricular escape beats occur, ventricular conduction is abnormally slow.
- *Example of sinus arrest:* Figure 3-12

Treatment

Treat the cause, if known. SND rarely presents acutely, but if it does, atropine 0.5 mg IV may increase sinus rate temporarily. If SND is due to calcium channel blocker or beta-blocker overdose, IV glucagon, or high-dose insulin therapy may improve heart rate and symptoms. IV calcium can be used in calcium channel blocker toxicity. If SND is due to digoxin toxicity, digoxin Fab antibody fragment may be effective. Temporary or permanent pacemaker therapy may be necessary if other forms of therapy fail and in chronic SND.

Tachycardia-Bradycardia (Tachy-Brady) Syndrome

ECG Characteristics

- *Rate:* Atrial—varies from slow to normal to rapid as rhythm goes from sinus to atrial tachyarrhythmias. Ventricular—varies from slow to normal to rapid depending on atrial rate and rhythm.

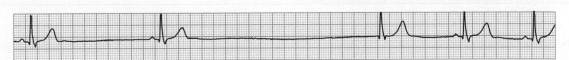

Figure 3-12. Sinus arrest.

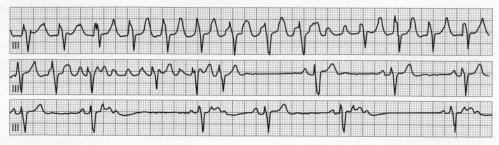

Figure 3-13. Bradycardia-tachycardia syndrome. Episodes of atrial tachycardia or atrial flutter alternating with episodes of sinus bradycardia.

- *Rhythm:* Irregular due to alternating bradycardia and tachycardia rhythms. Long pauses may occur following termination of tachyarrhythmias.
- *P waves:* Present during periods of sinus rhythm. When atrial flutter or fibrillation occurs, P waves are absent and atrial flutter or fibrillation waves are seen.
- *QRS complex:* Usually normal unless bundle branch block is present.
- *Conduction:* Sinus and atrial impulses conduct through the AV node, bundle branches, and ventricles. If junctional escape beats occur during pauses, ventricular conduction is usually normal. If ventricular escape beats occur, ventricular conduction is abnormally slow.
- *Example of tachycardia-bradycardia syndrome:* Figure 3-13.

DYSRHYTHMIAS ORIGINATING IN THE ATRIA

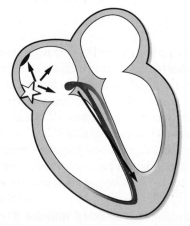

Figure 3-14. Dysrhythmias originating in the atria.

Premature Atrial Complexes

A premature atrial complex (PAC) occurs when an irritable focus in the atria fires before the next sinus node impulse is due to fire. PACs can be caused by caffeine, alcohol, nicotine, HF, pulmonary disease, interruptions in atrial blood supply by MI or infarction, anxiety, and hypermetabolic states. PACs can also occur in normal hearts.

ECG Characteristics
- *Rate:* Usually within normal range.
- *Rhythm:* Usually regular except when PACs occur, resulting in early beats. PACs usually have a noncompensatory pause (interval between the complex preceding and that following the PAC is less than two normal RR intervals) because premature depolarization of the atria by the PAC usually causes premature depolarization of the sinus node as well, thus causing the sinus node to "reset" itself.
- *P waves:* Precede every QRS complex. The configuration of the premature P wave differs from that of the sinus P waves because the premature impulse originates in a different part of the atria, with atrial depolarization occurring in a different pattern. Very early P waves may be buried in the preceding T wave.
- *PR interval:* May be normal or long depending on the prematurity of the beat; very early PACs may find the AV junction still partially refractory and unable to conduct at a normal rate, resulting in a prolonged PR interval.
- *QRS complex:* May be normal, aberrant (wide), or absent, depending on the prematurity of the beat. If the ventricles have repolarized completely, they will be able to conduct the early impulse normally, resulting in a normal QRS. If the PAC occurs during the relative refractory period of the AV node, bundle branches, or ventricles, the impulse will conduct aberrantly and the QRS will be wide. If the PAC occurs very early during the complete refractory period of the AV node, bundle branches, or ventricles, the impulse will not conduct to the ventricles and the QRS will be absent.
- *Conduction:* PACs travel through the atria differently from sinus impulses because they originate from a different spot; conduction through the AV node, bundle branches, and ventricles is usually normal unless the PAC is very early.
- *Example of PAC:* Figure 3-15A, B.

Treatment

Treatment of PACs usually is not necessary because they do not cause hemodynamic compromise. Patients with frequent or bothersome PACs are usually counseled to avoid smoking,

DYSRHYTHMIAS ORIGINATING IN THE ATRIA **47**

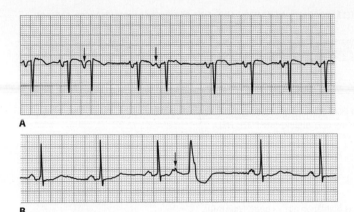

Figure 3-15. **(A)** PAC conducted normally in the ventricle. **(B)** PAC conducted aberrantly in the ventricle.

alcohol, and caffeine. Frequent PACs may precede more serious dysrhythmias such as AF. Treatment is directed at the cause. Medications such as beta-blockers, disopyramide, flecainide, and propafenone can be used to suppress atrial activity, but this is rarely necessary.

Wandering Atrial Pacemaker and Multifocal Atrial Tachycardia

Wandering atrial pacemaker (WAP) refers to rhythms that exhibit varying P-wave morphology as the site of impulse formation shifts from the sinus node to various sites in the atria or into the AV junction. This occurs when two (usually sinus and junctional) or more supraventricular pacemakers compete with each other for control of the heart. Because the rates of these competing pacemakers are almost identical, it is common to have atrial fusion occur as the atria are activated by more than one wave of depolarization at a time, resulting in varying P-wave morphology. WAP can be due to increased vagal tone that slows the sinus pacemaker or to enhanced automaticity in atrial or junctional pacemaker cells, causing them to compete with the sinus node for control. The term *multifocal atrial tachycardia (MAT)* is used when the rate is faster than 100 beats/min. MAT is commonly associated with chronic obstructive pulmonary disease (COPD) and other pulmonary diseases such as pneumonia and pulmonary embolism. It is also seen in HF and coronary, valvular, or hypertensive heart disease.

ECG Characteristics
- *Rate:* 60 to 100 beats/min. If the rate is faster than 100 beats/min, it is called MAT.
- *Rhythm:* May be slightly irregular.

- *P waves:* Varying shapes (upright, flat, inverted, notched) as impulses originate in different parts of the atria or junction. At least three different P-wave shapes should be seen.
- *PR interval:* May vary depending on proximity of the pacemaker to the AV node.
- *QRS complex:* Usually normal.
- *Conduction:* Conduction through the atria varies as they are depolarized from different spots. Conduction through the bundle branches and ventricles is usually normal.
- *Example of WAP:* Figure 3-16. *Example of MAT:* Figure 3-17.

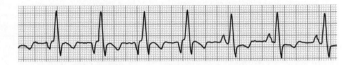

Figure 3-16. Wandering atrial pacemaker.

Treatment
Treatment of WAP usually is not necessary. If slow heart rates lead to symptoms, atropine can be given. Treatment of MAT is directed toward eliminating the underlying cause, including hypoxia, HF, and electrolyte imbalances. Maintaining normal magnesium and potassium levels is important in managing MAT. Antiarrhythmic drugs are not helpful in managing MAT. See Table 3-4 for recommendations for treating MAT.

Atrial Tachycardia

Atrial tachycardia (AT) is a rapid atrial rhythm occurring at a rate of 120 to 250 beats/min and can be due to abnormal automaticity or to reentry within the atrium (Figure 3-18). When the dysrhythmia abruptly starts and terminates, it is called *paroxysmal atrial tachycardia*. Rapid atrial rate can be caused by emotions, caffeine, tobacco, alcohol, fatigue, or sympathomimetic drugs. Whenever the atrial rate is rapid, the AV node begins to block some of the impulses attempting to travel through it to protect the ventricles from excessively rapid rates. In normal healthy hearts, the AV node can usually conduct each atrial impulse up to rates of about 180 to 200 beats/min. In patients with cardiac disease or who are on AV nodal blocking drugs such as digitalis, beta-blockers, or calcium channel blockers, the AV node may not be able to conduct each impulse and AT with block occurs. AT with block may indicate digitalis toxicity.

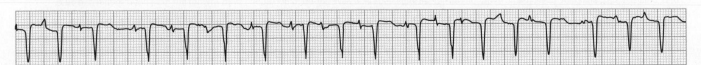

Figure 3-17. Multifocal atrial tachycardia.

TABLE 3-4. GUIDELINES FOR MANAGEMENT OF SUPRAVENTRICULAR ARRHYTHMIAS (CLASS OF RECOMMENDATION AND LEVEL OF EVIDENCE INDICATED [COR; LOE] FOR EACH RECOMMENDATION)

Treatment of SVT of Unknown Mechanism

Acute Treatment
1. Vagal maneuvers (Valsalva, CSM) for regular SVT (1; B-R)
2. Adenosine for regular SVT (1; B-R)
3. Synchronized cardioversion if hemodynamically unstable and vagal maneuvers or adenosine ineffective or not feasible (1; B-NR)
4. Synchronized cardioversion if hemodynamically stable and drug therapy ineffective or contraindicated (1; B-NR)
5. IV verapamil or diltiazem for acute treatment if hemodynamically stable (1Ia; B-R)
6. IV beta-blockers for acute treatment if hemodynamically stable (IIa; C-LD)

Ongoing Management
1. Oral beta-blockers, diltiazem, or verapamil if no pre-excitation (1; B-R)
2. EP study with option for ablation (I; B-NR)
3. Flecainide or propafenone if no structural heart disease or ischemic heart disease if ablation not an option (IIa; B-R)
4. Sotolol or dofetilide if ablation not an option and other drugs not effective (IIb; B-R)
5. Amiodarone or digoxin can be considered if ablation not an option and other drugs not effective (IIb; C-LD)

Treatment of Multifocal Atrial Tachycardia

Acute Treatment
1. IV metoprolol or verapamil if hemodynamically stable (IIa; C-LD)

Ongoing Management
1. Oral verapamil (IIa; B-NR) or metoprolol (IIa; C-LD) is reasonable for managing recurrent symptomatic MAT

Treatment of Suspected Focal Atrial Tachycardia

Acute Treatment
1. IV beta-blockers, diltiazem, or verapamil if hemodynamically stable (I; C-LD)
2. Synchronized cardioversion if hemodynamically unstable (I; C-LD)
3. Adenosine to restore sinus rhythm or diagnose tachycardia (IIa; B-NR)
4. IV amiodarone or ibutilide if hemodynamically stable (IIb; C-LD)

Ongoing Management
1. Catheter ablation as alternative to drug therapy (I; B-NR)
2. Oral beta-blockers, diltiazem, or verapamil (IIa; C-LD)
3. Flecainide or propafenone if no structural or ischemic heart disease (IIa; C-LD)
4. Sotalol or amiodarone (IIb; C-LD)

Treatment of AV Nodal Reentry Tachycardia (AVNRT)

Acute Treatment
1. Vagal maneuvers or adenosine (I; B-R)
2. Synchronized cardioversion for stable or unstable AVNRT when vagal maneuvers and adenosine ineffective (I; B-NR)
3. IV beta-blockers, diltiazem, or verapamil if hemodynamically stable (IIa; B-R)
4. Oral beta-blockers, diltiazem, or verapamil if hemodynamically stable (IIb; C-LD)
5. IV amiodarone if hemodynamically stable and other drugs ineffective (IIb; C-LD)

Ongoing Management
1. Catheter ablation (I; B-NR)—considered first-line therapy
2. Oral beta-blockers, verapamil, or diltiazem if ablation not an option (I; B-R)
3. Flecainide or propafenone if ablation not an option and other drugs ineffective and no structural or ischemic heart disease (IIa; B-R)
4. Clinical follow-up without other therapy reasonable if minimally symptomatic (IIa; B-NR)
5. Oral sotalol, dofetilide, digoxin, or amiodarone if ablation not an option (IIb; B-R)
6. Pill-in-the-pocket (verapamil, diltiazem, beta-blockers) if infrequent stable episodes (IIb; C-LD)

Treatment of Orthodromic AVRT or Circus Movement Tachycardia (CMT)

Acute Treatment
1. Vagal maneuvers or adenosine (I; B-R)
2. Synchronized cardioversion for stable or unstable AVRT when vagal maneuvers and adenosine ineffective (I; B-NR)
3. Synchronized cardioversion should be performed for hemodynamically unstable pre-excited AF (I; B-NR)
4. Ibutilide or IV procainamide beneficial for pre-excited AF if hemodynamically stable (I; C-LD)
5. IV diltiazem or verapamil (IIa; B-R) or beta-blockers (IIa; C-LD) if no pre-excitation during sinus rhythm
6. IV beta-blockers, diltiazem, or verapamil might be considered in patients who have pre-excitation during sinus rhythm but have not responded to other therapies (IIb; B-R)
7. IV digoxin, IV amiodarone, IV or oral beta-blockers, diltiazem, and verapamil are potentially harmful and contraindicated with pre-excited AF (III harm; C-LD)

(continued)

TABLE 3-4. GUIDELINES FOR MANAGEMENT OF SUPRAVENTRICULAR ARRHYTHMIAS (CLASS OF RECOMMENDATION AND LEVEL OF EVIDENCE INDICATED [COR; LOE] FOR EACH RECOMMENDATION) (CONTINUED)

Ongoing Management

1. Catheter ablation of accessory pathway for AVRT or pre-excited AF (I; B-NR)
2. Oral beta-blockers, verapamil, diltiazem if no pre-excitation on resting ECG (I; C-LD)
3. Oral flecainide or propafenone if no structural or ischemic heart disease for AVRT or pre-excited AF if ablation not an option (IIa; B-R)
4. Oral dofetilide or sotalol for AVRT or pre-excited AF if ablation not an option (IIb; B-R)
5. Oral beta-blockers, diltiazem, or verapamil in patients with pre-excitation on resting ECG and ablation not an option (IIb; C-LD)
6. Oral amiodarone for AVRT or pre-excited AF if ablation not an option and other drugs are ineffective (IIb; C-LD)
7. Oral digoxin if no pre-excitation on resting ECG and ablation not an option (IIb; C-LD)
8. Oral digoxin potentially harmful if AF with pre-excitation on resting ECG (III harm; C-LD)

Treatment of Atrial Flutter

Acute Treatment

1. Oral dofetilide or IV ibutilide for pharmacological cardioversion (I; A)
2. IV or oral beta-blockers, diltiazem, or verapamil for rate control if hemodynamically stable (I; B-R)
3. Synchronized cardioversion if hemodynamically unstable and drugs ineffective (I; B-NR)
4. Elective synchronized cardioversion if hemodynamically stable and rhythm control is goal (I; B-NR)
5. Rapid atrial pacing for conversion of atrial flutter if atrial pacing wires in place (I; C-LD)
6. Acute antithrombotic therapy same as for AF (Table 3-5) (I; B-NR)
7. IV amiodarone for rate control (if no pre-excitation) if systolic heart failure when beta-blockers contraindicated or ineffective (IIa; B-R)

Ongoing Management

1. Catheter ablation if symptomatic or refractory to rate control drugs (I; B-R)
2. Beta-blockers, diltiazem, or verapamil for rate control if hemodynamically stable (I; C-LD)
3. Catheter ablation for "atypical" flutter after failure of at least one antiarrhythmic drug (I; C-LD)
4. Ongoing antithrombotic therapy same as for AF (see Table 3-5) (I; B-R)
5. Amiodarone, dofetilide, or sotalol useful to maintain sinus rhythm with recurrent atrial flutter (IIa; B-R)
6. There are several COR IIa recommendations for catheter ablation of atrial flutter in various situations. See source below for more information.
7. Flecainide or propafenone to maintain sinus rhythm if no structural or ischemic heart disease (IIb; B-R)
8. Catheter ablation may be reasonable for asymptomatic patients with recurrent atrial flutter (IIb; C-LD)

Treatment of Junctional Tachycardia

There are no Class I recommendations for treatment of junctional tachycardia.

Acute Treatment

1. IV beta-blockers, diltiazem, procainamide, or verapamil (IIa; C-LD)

Ongoing Management

1. Oral beta-blockers, diltiazem, or verapamil (IIa; C-LD)
2. Flecainide or propafenone if no structural or ischemic heart disease (IIb; C-LD)
3. Catheter ablation when medical therapy ineffective or contraindicated (IIb; C-LD)

Class of Recommendation (COR)

Class I: Strong; benefit >>> risk

Class IIa: Moderate; benefit >> risk

Class IIb: Weak; benefit > risk

Class III no benefit: benefit = risk, not indicated, useful, or effective

Class III harm: risk > benefit; potentially harmful, contraindicated

Level of Evidence (LOE) Definitions

Level A: High-quality evidence from multiple randomized clinical trials (RCTs) or meta-analyses of high-quality RCTs.

Level B-R (randomized): Moderate-quality evidence from one or more RCTs or meta-analysis of moderate-quality RCTs.

Level B-NR (nonrandomized): Moderate-quality evidence from one or more nonrandomized studies, observational studies, or registry studies or meta-analyses of such studies.

Level C-LD (limited data): Randomized or nonrandomized observational or registry studies with limitations of design or execution; meta-analyses of such studies.

Level C-EO (expert opinion): Consensus of expert opinion based on clinical experience.

Abbreviations: AF: atrial fibrillation; AT: atrial tachycardia; AVNRT: atrioventricular nodal reentry tachycardia; BBB: bundle branch block; CMT: circus movement tachycardia; COR: class of recommendation; CSM: carotid sinus massage; EP: electrophysiology; LOE: level of evidence; LV: left ventricular; SVT: supraventricular tachycardia.

Data from Page RL, Joglar JA, Caldwell MA, et al. 2015 ACC/AHA/HRS Guideline for the Management of Adult Patients With Supraventricular Tachycardia: A Report of the American College of Cardiology/American Heart Association Task Force on Clinical Practice Guidelines and the Heart Rhythm Society. Circulation. 2016;133(14):e506-e574.

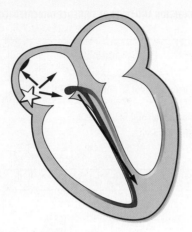

Figure 3-18. Atrial tachycardia.

ECG Characteristics

- *Rate:* Atrial rate is 120 to 250 beats/min.
- *Rhythm:* Regular unless there is variable block at the AV node.
- *P waves:* Differ in shape from sinus P waves because they are ectopic. Precede each QRS complex but may be hidden in preceding T wave. When block is present, more than one P wave will appear before each QRS complex.
- *PR interval:* May be shorter than normal but often difficult to measure because of hidden P waves.
- *QRS complex:* Usually normal but may be wide if aberrant conduction is present.
- *Conduction:* Usually normal through the AV node and into the ventricles. In AT with block, some atrial impulses do not conduct into the ventricles. Aberrant ventricular conduction may occur if atrial impulses are conducted into the ventricles while the bundle branches or ventricles are still partially refractory.
- *Example of AT:* Figure 3-19.

Treatment

Treatment of AT is directed at eliminating the cause, if possible, controlling the ventricular rate, and reestablishing sinus rhythm. If the patient is hemodynamically unstable due to a rapid AT, cardioversion can be attempted, although automatic ATs usually do not respond to cardioversion. Some ATs may terminate with IV adenosine, but more often IV verapamil or diltiazem, or an IV beta-blocker, is used for acute therapy to slow the ventricular rate, and they may occasionally terminate the AT. Other medications that can be used for management of recurrent AT are flecainide, propafenone, amiodarone, or sotalol. Catheter ablation is a class I recommendation for preventing recurrent AT. See Table 3-4 for recommendations for management of AT.

Atrial Flutter

In atrial flutter (Figure 3-20), the atria are depolarized at rates of 250 to 350 times/min. Classic or typical atrial flutter is due to a fixed reentry circuit in the right atrium around which the impulse circulates in a counterclockwise direction, resulting in negative flutter waves in leads II and III and an atrial rate between 250 and 350 beats/min (most commonly 300 beats/min). At such rapid atrial rates, the AV node usually blocks at least half of the impulses to protect the ventricles from excessive rates. Causes of atrial flutter include rheumatic heart disease, atherosclerotic heart disease, thyrotoxicosis, HF, and MI or infarction. Because the ventricular rate in atrial flutter can be quite fast, symptoms associated with decreased cardiac output can occur. Mural thrombi may form in the atria due to the fact that there is no strong atrial contraction, and blood stasis occurs, leading to a risk of systemic or pulmonary emboli.

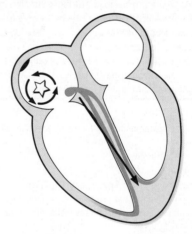

Figure 3-20. Atrial flutter.

ECG Characteristics

- *Rate:* Atrial rate varies between 250 and 350 beats/min, most commonly 300. Ventricular rate varies depending on the amount of block at the AV node. New onset atrial flutter usually has a ventricular rate around 150 beats/min, and rarely 300 beats/min if 1:1 conduction occurs to the ventricles. With medications that block AV node conduction, the ventricular rate is usually in the normal range, commonly around 75 beats/min.
- *Rhythm:* Atrial rhythm is regular. Ventricular rhythm may be regular or irregular because of varying AV block.

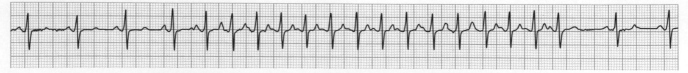

Figure 3-19. Sinus rhythm with an 18-beat run of atrial tachycardia at a rate of 167 beats/min.

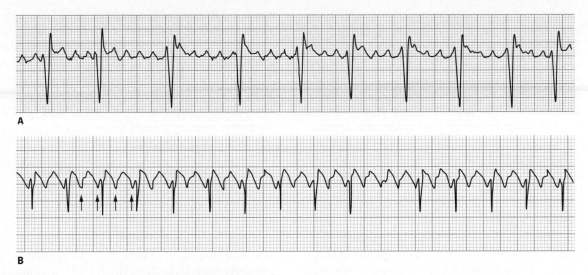

A

B

Figure 3-21. (A) Atrial flutter with 4:1 and 5:1 conduction. **(B)** Atrial flutter with 2:1 conduction.

- *F waves:* F waves (flutter waves) are seen, characterized by a very regular, "sawtooth" pattern. One F wave is usually hidden in the QRS complex, and when 2:1 conduction occurs, F waves may not be readily apparent.
- *FR interval (flutter wave to the beginning of the QRS complex):* May be consistent or may vary.
- *QRS complex:* Usually normal; aberration can occur.
- *Conduction:* Usually normal through the AV node and ventricles.
- *Example of atrial flutter:* Figure 3-21A, B.

Treatment

The immediate goal of treatment depends on the hemodynamic consequences of the dysrhythmia. Ventricular rate control is the priority if cardiac output is markedly compromised due to rapid ventricular rates. Electrical (direct current) cardioversion may be necessary as an immediate treatment, especially if 1:1 conduction occurs. IV calcium channel blockers (verapamil or diltiazem) or beta-blockers can be used for acute ventricular rate control. Conversion to sinus rhythm can be accomplished by electrical cardioversion, drug therapy, or overdrive atrial pacing. Oral dofetilide or IV ibutilide are useful for pharmacological cardioversion.

Medications that slow the atrial rate, like flecainide or propafenone, should not be used unless the ventricular rate has been controlled with an AV nodal blocking agent (a calcium channel blocker, beta-blocker, or digitalis). The danger of giving these medications alone is that the atrial rate may decrease from 300 beats/min to a slower rate, making it possible for the AV node to conduct each impulse and resulting in even faster ventricular rates. See Table 3-4 for treatment of atrial flutter.

Atrial Fibrillation

AF is an extremely rapid and disorganized pattern of depolarization in the atria, and is the most common dysrhythmia seen in clinical practice (Figure 3-22). AF commonly occurs in the presence of atherosclerotic or rheumatic heart disease, thyroid disease, HF, cardiomyopathy, valve disease,

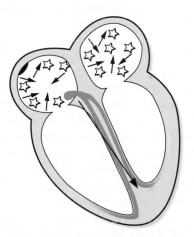

Figure 3-22. Atrial fibrillation.

pulmonary disease, MI, congenital heart disease, and after cardiac surgery. The following classification system is used when defining AF: *paroxysmal,* episodes that terminate spontaneously or with intervention within 7 days of onset; *persistent,* episodes that last more than 7 days; *long-standing persistent,* continuous AF lasting more than 12 months; and *permanent,* continuous AF lasting more than 12 months and decision has been made to stop attempts to restore and/or maintain sinus rhythm. The term *recurrent* is used when the patient has two or more episodes of AF, and the term *lone AF* is used when AF occurs in the absence of cardiac disease or any other known cause (usually in people <60 years of age). Nonvalvular AF occurs in patients without mitral valve disease, prosthetic valve, or history of valve surgery.

AF has several adverse consequences that require prompt recognition and treatment in order to prevent complications:

1. Decreased cardiac output due to loss of atrial kick, rapid ventricular rate, and irregular ventricular rhythm. Cardiac output is dependent on adequate ventricular filling, and the loss of atrial contraction

and the rapid ventricular rate that commonly occurs in AF contribute to reduced ventricular filling.

2. Tachycardia-induced cardiomyopathy can occur whenever the ventricular rate is rapid for a prolonged period of time. This is more common in asymptomatic patients who are unaware that they are in AF.

3. Thromboembolism because of formation of clots in the fibrillating atria, usually in the left atrial appendage (LAA). Stroke is the most common and potentially devastating embolic event, but pulmonary embolus and embolization to any other part of the body can also occur.

ECG Characteristics

- *Rate:* Atrial rate is 400 to 600 beats/min or faster. Ventricular rate varies depending on the amount of block at the AV node. In new AF, the ventricular response is usually quite rapid, 160 to 200 beats/min; in treated AF, the ventricular rate is controlled in the normal range of 60 to 100 beats/min.
- *Rhythm:* Irregular; one of the distinguishing features of AF is the marked irregularity of the ventricular response.
- *F waves:* Not present; atrial activity is chaotic with no formed atrial impulses visible; irregular F waves are often seen, and vary in size from coarse to very fine.
- *PR interval:* Not measurable; there are no P waves.
- *QRS complex:* Usually normal; aberration is common.
- *Conduction:* Conduction within the atria is disorganized and follows a very irregular pattern. Most of the atrial impulses are blocked within the AV junction. Those impulses that are conducted through the AV junction are usually conducted normally through the ventricles. If an atrial impulse reaches the bundle branch system during its refractory period, aberrant intraventricular conduction can occur.
- *Example of atrial fibrillation:* Figure 3-23A, B.

Pharmacological Treatment of Atrial Fibrillation

Treatment of AF is directed toward eliminating the cause, controlling ventricular rate, restoring and maintaining sinus rhythm, and preventing thromboembolism. The American College of Cardiology, American Heart Association, and the Heart Rhythm Society have collaborated to publish guidelines for the management of AF. See Table 3-5 for the guidelines for management of AF.

Ventricular rate control is aimed at improving hemodynamics and relieving symptoms. New onset AF often results in a very rapid ventricular rate that can be mildly to moderately symptomatic or cause extreme hemodynamic instability. Patients with Wolff-Parkinson-White (WPW) syndrome have an accessory pathway that can conduct AF impulses directly into the ventricle via the accessory pathway, resulting in an extremely rapid ventricular rate that can cause ventricular fibrillation (VF) and sudden cardiac death (see Chapter 18, Advanced ECG Concepts). In the unstable patient, ventricular rate control is a priority, and electrical cardioversion may be necessary if the patient is hemodynamically unstable because of rapid ventricular rate. Intravenous calcium channel blockers (eg, diltiazem, verapamil) and beta-blockers are commonly used in the acute situation for ventricular rate control but should be used with caution in the presence of HF or hypotension and are contraindicated if WPW is present. Beta-blockers, calcium channel blockers, and digitalis can be used orally for long-term rate control.

Rhythm control is restoration of sinus rhythm using pharmacologic or electrical cardioversion and maintenance of sinus rhythm using antiarrhythmic medications. Antiarrhythmic medications with a class I recommendation for pharmacological cardioversion of AF are flecainide, dofetilide, propafenone, and ibutilide; amiodarone is a class IIa recommendation. Medications are most effective in restoring sinus rhythm when started within 7 days of AF onset. Several antiarrhythmics can be effective in maintaining

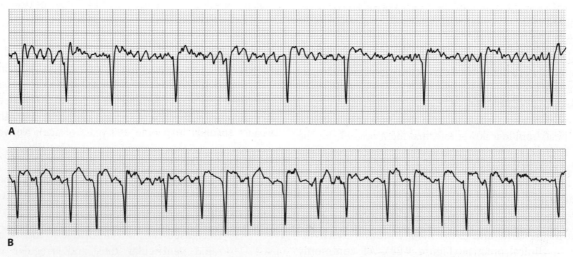

Figure 3-23. **(A)** Atrial fibrillation with a controlled ventricular response. **(B)** Atrial fibrillation with an uncontrolled ventricular response.

TABLE 3-5. GUIDELINES FOR MANAGEMENT OF ATRIAL FIBRILLATION (CLASS OF RECOMMENDATION AND LEVEL OF EVIDENCE [COR; LOE] INDICATED FOR EACH RECOMMENDATION)

Rate Control (see Source for Complete Guidelines and More Detailed Information)
1. Beta-blocker, diltiazem, or verapamil for paroxysmal, persistent, or permanent AF (I; B)
2. IV beta-blocker, diltiazem, or verapamil for acute rate control if no pre-excitation (I; B)
3. Synchronized cardioversion recommended if hemodynamically unstable (I; B)
4. A resting heart rate < 80 is reasonable for symptomatic AF (IIa; B)
5. IV amiodarone in critically ill patients without pre-excitation (IIa; B)
6. AV node ablation with permanent ventricular pacemaker when drug therapy ineffective (IIa; B)
7. A resting heart rate < 110 is reasonable if asymptomatic and LV systolic function preserved (IIb; B)
8. Oral amiodarone if other measures ineffective (IIb; C)

Preventing Thromboembolism (see Source for Complete Guidelines and More Detailed Information)
1. For patients with AF and an elevated CHA_2DS_2-VASc score of 2 or greater in men or 3 or greater in women, oral anticoagulants are recommended. Options include: (I; A)

  - Warfarin
  - Dabigatran
  - Rivaroxaban
  - Apixaban
  - Edoxaban

2. NOACs (dabigatran, rivaroxaban, apixaban, and edoxaban) are recommended over warfarin in NOAC-eligible patients with AF (except with moderate-to-severe mitral stenosis or a mechanical heart valve) (I; A)
3. Among patients treated with warfarin, the international normalized ratio (INR) should be determined at least weekly during initiation of anticoagulant therapy and at least monthly when anticoagulation (INR in range) is stable (I; A)
4. In patients with AF (except with moderate-to-severe mitral stenosis or a mechanical heart valve), the CHA_2DS_2-VASc score is recommended for assessment of stroke risk (I; B)
5. For patients with AF who have mechanical heart valves, warfarin is recommended (I; B)
6. Selection of anticoagulant therapy should be based on the risk of thromboembolism, irrespective of whether the AF pattern is paroxysmal, persistent, or permanent (I; B)
7. Renal function and hepatic function should be evaluated before initiation of a NOAC and should be re-evaluated at least annually (I; B-NR)
8. For patients with AF (except with moderate-to-severe mitral stenosis or a mechanical heart valve) who are unable to maintain a therapeutic INR level with warfarin, use of a NOAC is recommended (I; C-EO)
9. For patients with AF (except with moderate-to-severe mitral stenosis or a mechanical heart valve) and a CHA_2DS_2-VASc score of 0 in men or 1 in women, it is reasonable to omit anticoagulant therapy (IIa; B)
10. For patients with AF (except with moderate-to-severe mitral stenosis or a mechanical heart valve) and a CHA_2DS_2-VASc score of 1 in men and 2 in women, prescribing an oral anticoagulant to reduce thromboembolic stroke risk may be considered (IIb; B-R)

Cardioversion of Atrial Fibrillation and Atrial Flutter

Direct-Current Cardioversion
1. Cardioversion is recommended to restore sinus rhythm. If unsuccessful, attempts can be repeated (I; B)
2. Cardioversion recommended for AF or flutter with rapid ventricular rate that does not respond to drugs (I; C)
3. Cardioversion recommended for AF or flutter with pre-excitation and hemodynamic instability (I; C)
4. It is reasonable to repeat cardioversion in persistent AF when sinus rhythm can be maintained for a clinically meaningful time period between procedures (IIb; C)

Pharmacological Cardioversion
1. Flecainide, dofetilide, propafenone, and IV ibutilide in absence of contraindications (I; A)
2. Amiodarone is reasonable (IIa; A)
3. Propafenone or flecainide ("pill-in-the-pocket") to terminate AF out of hospital is reasonable once observed to be safe in a monitored setting (IIa; B)
4. Dofetilide should not be initiated out of hospital (III; B)

Prevention of Thromboembolism
1. For patients with AF or atrial flutter of 48 hours duration or longer, or when the duration of AF is unknown, anticoagulation with warfarin (INR 2.0 to 3.0), a factor Xa inhibitor, or direct thrombin inhibitor is recommended for at least 3 weeks before and at least 4 weeks after cardioversion, regardless of the CHA_2DS_2-VASc score or the method (electrical or pharmacological) used to restore sinus rhythm (I; B-R)
2. For patients with AF or atrial flutter of more than 48 hours duration or unknown duration that requires immediate cardioversion for hemodynamic instability, anticoagulation should be initiated as soon as possible and continued for at least 4 weeks after cardioversion unless contraindicated (I; C)
3. After cardioversion for AF of any duration, the decision about long-term anticoagulation therapy should be based on the thromboembolic risk profile and bleeding risk profile (I; C-EO)
4. For patients with AF or atrial flutter of less than 48 hours duration with a CHA_2DS_2-VASc score of 2 or greater in men and 3 or greater in women, administration of heparin, a factor Xa inhibitor, or a direct thrombin inhibitor is reasonable as soon as possible before cardioversion, followed by long-term anticoagulation therapy (IIa; B-NR)

(continued)

TABLE 3-5. GUIDELINES FOR MANAGEMENT OF ATRIAL FIBRILLATION (CLASS OF RECOMMENDATION AND LEVEL OF EVIDENCE [COR; LOE] INDICATED FOR EACH RECOMMENDATION) (CONTINUED)

5. For patients with AF or atrial flutter of 48 hours' duration or longer or of unknown duration who have not been anticoagulated for the preceding 3 weeks, it is reasonable to perform transesophageal echocardiography before cardioversion and proceed with cardioversion if no left atrial thrombus is identified, including in the LAA, provided that anticoagulation is achieved before transesophageal echocardiography and maintained after cardioversion for at least 4 weeks (IIa; B)

6. For patients with AF or atrial flutter of less than 48 hours' duration with a CHA2 DS2-VASc score of 0 in men or 1 in women, administration of heparin, a factor Xa inhibitor, or a direct thrombin inhibitor versus no anticoagulant therapy, may be considered before cardioversion, without the need for postcardioversion oral anticoagulation (IIb; B-NR)

Maintenance of Sinus Rhythm

1. Amiodarone, dofetilide, dronedarone, flecainide, propafenone, or sotalol are recommended depending on underlying heart disease and comorbidities (I; A)
2. The risks of antiarrhythmic drugs should be considered before initiation (I; C)
3. Amiodarone should only be used after other agents have failed or are contraindicated (I; C)
4. A rhythm-control strategy with drug therapy can be useful for treatment of tachycardia-induced cardiomyopathy (IIa; C)
5. It may be reasonable to continue antiarrhythmic drug therapy in the setting of infrequent, well-tolerated recurrences of AF when the drug has reduced the frequency or symptoms (IIb; C)
6. Antiarrhythmic drugs should not be continued when AF becomes permanent and dronedarone should not be used for treatment of AF in patients with NYHA class III or IV heart failure or who have had decompensated heart failure in the past 4 weeks (III; B)
7. Dronedarone should not be used for treatment of AF in patients with NYHA class III and IV HF or patients who have had an episode of decompensated HF in the past 4 weeks (III; B)

Class of Recommendation (COR)

Class I: Strong; benefit >>> risk

Class IIa: Moderate; benefit >> risk

Class IIb: Weak; benefit > risk

Class III no benefit or may cause harm

Level of Evidence (LOE)

Level A: High-quality evidence from more than 1 RCT; meta-analyses of high-quality RCTs; one or more RCTs corroborated by high-quality registry studies.

Level B-R (randomized): Moderate-quality evidence from 1 or more RCTs; Meta-analyses of moderate-quality RCTs. Level B-NR (nonrandomized): Moderate-quality evidence from 1 or more well-designed, well-executed nonrandomized studies, observational studies, or registry studies; meta-analyses of such studies.

Level C-LD (limited data): Randomized or nonrandomized observational or registry studies with limitations of design or execution; meta-analyses of such studies; physiological or mechanistic studies in human subjects.

Level C-EO (expert opinion): Consensus of expert opinion based on clinical experience.

Abbreviations: AF: atrial fibrillation; HF: heart failure; INR: international normalized ratio; LAA: left atrial appendage; LMWH: low-molecular-weight heparin; LV: left ventricular; MI: myocardial infarction; NOAC: non-vitamin K oral anticoagulant; NYHA: New York Heart Association; RCT: randomized control trial, TIA: transient ischemic attack.

Data from January CT, Wann LS, Alpert JS, et al. 2014 AHA/ACC/HRS guideline for the management of patients with atrial fibrillation: a report of the American College of Cardiology/American Heart Association Task Force on practice guidelines and the Heart Rhythm Society. Circulation. 2014;130(23):e199-e267 and January CT, Wann LS, Calkins H, et al. 2019 AHA/ACC/HRS focused update of the 2014 AHA/ACC/HRS guideline for the management of patients with atrial fibrillation: a report of the American College of Cardiology/American Heart Association Task Force on practice guidelines and the Heart Rhythm Society. Circulation. 2019;140:e125-e151.

sinus rhythm after conversion, including amiodarone, dofetilide, dronedarone, flecainide, propafenone, and sotalol. Oral beta-blockers or amiodarone are often used to try to prevent postoperative AF in patients undergoing cardiac surgery. Refer to specific drug guidelines for patient selection criteria.

Preventing thromboembolism is a goal in all patients with AF regardless of rhythm or rate control strategy. Antithrombotic therapy is recommended for all patients with AF based on stroke risk. The risk of stroke must be weighed against the risk of bleeding when considering anticoagulation for thromboembolism prevention. The CHA_2DS_2VASc score is used to assess stroke risk in AF patients and assigns 1 point for each item unless otherwise indicated: C = congestive heart failure, H = hypertension, A_2 = age >75 years (2 points), D = diabetes, and S_2 = history of stroke, TIA, or thromboembolism (2 points), V = vascular disease (prior MI, peripheral artery disease, or aortic plaque), A = age 65 to 74, Sc = sex

category female. Oral anticoagulation with warfarin to maintain INR between 2.0 and 3.0 (target INR = 2.5) is recommended for patients with mechanical heart valves. Options for patients with a CHA_2DS_2VASc score of 2 or higher in men or 3 or higher in women include warfarin or a non-vitamin K oral anticoagulant (NOAC) dabigatran, rivaroxaban, apixaban or edoxaban. For patients with a CHA_2DS_2VASc score of 0 in men or 1 in women, no antithrombotic therapy or oral anticoagulant may be considered. See Table 3-5 for recommendations for thromboembolism prevention in patients with AF.

Nonpharmacological Management of Atrial Fibrillation

Radiofrequency (RF) catheter ablation and surgical management of AF include AV node ablation, pulmonary vein ablation, surgical or ablation Maze procedures, and occlusion or surgical removal of the LAA. These procedures are briefly described here.

ESSENTIAL CONTENT CASE

Atrial Dysrhythmia and Cardioversion

You are caring for a patient who was admitted for an elective cardioversion. She was seen in her physician's office this morning for complaints of SOB and palpitations that started around 7 AM. She has a history of hypertension and diabetes but no previous cardiac history. In the office, her ECG showed AF with a ventricular response between 120 and 130 beats/min. Previous ECGs had all shown normal sinus rhythm, and since her symptoms were new and time of onset was just a few hours ago, her physician elected to treat her with cardioversion. Her BP is 136/74 and she is breathing comfortably at this time. You place her on the bedside cardiac monitor in lead V_1.

Case Question 1. What are the diagnostic features of AF that you expect to see on the monitor?
Figure 3-24A shows her rhythm strip:

Case Question 2. Is her admitting diagnosis of AF correct?

Case Question 3. What other treatments besides electrical cardioversion would be appropriate for managing this rhythm?
You gather the equipment and supplies needed for the cardioversion. The cardiologist arrives and an anesthesiologist is present to sedate the patient. The cardiologist asks you to deliver a synchronized 100 J shock after the patient is asleep.

Case Question 4. What safety considerations are necessary before delivering the cardioversion shock?
The shock is delivered and Figure 3-24B shows the post-shock rhythm.

Case Question 5. What is the rhythm?

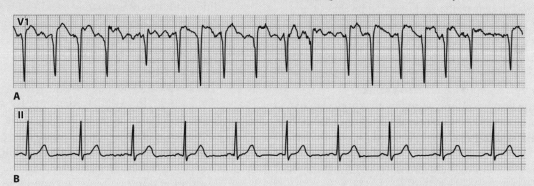

Figure 3-24. (A) Rhythm strip when monitoring is initiated. **(B)** Post-shock rhythm strip.

Answers
1. AF is characterized by the presence of "fibrillation" waves instead of organized P waves, and an irregularly irregular ventricular response.
2. Yes. This is a typical example of AF.
3. The first goal of treatment for AF is ventricular rate control. AV nodal blocking agents such as a beta-blocker or calcium channel blocker (ie, verapamil or diltiazem) are used for rate control. Antiarrhythmics such as flecainide, dofetilide, propafenone, ibutilide, or amiodarone can be used for pharmacological conversion of AF to sinus rhythm. Patients with persistent AF are on chronic therapy with a rate control drug and oral anticoagulation.
4. Every member of the team participating in the procedure should be involved in assuring patient safety. The patient should be monitored with noninvasive BP monitoring and pulse oximetry. Airway management supplies, emergency drugs, and sedation reversal agents should be present at the bedside. The patient should be adequately sedated prior to shock delivery. The defibrillator must be synchronized on the QRS complex to avoid delivering the shock on the T wave, which could cause VF. Prior to shock delivery, the operator should ensure that no one is touching the patient or the bed.
5. This is normal sinus rhythm, indicating a successful cardioversion.

RF AV node ablation is the most common nonpharmacologic method of rate control in AF and is usually done only when drug therapy for rate control is ineffective or not tolerated. RF energy is directed at the AV node to heat the tissue and destroy its ability to conduct impulses to the ventricle. This procedure results in complete AV block and requires a ventricular pacemaker implant to maintain an adequate ventricular rate. AV node ablation does not stop AF; therefore, patients must be chronically anticoagulated to prevent stroke.

RF ablation of AF trigger sites in the pulmonary veins or atria is the mainstay of ablation therapy for AF. The most common site of AF triggers is the first 2 to 4 cm inside the pulmonary veins leading into the left atrium, although triggers can be present in multiple sites within both atria. The most successful procedures are segmental ostial pulmonary vein isolation (PVI) and circumferential PVI. In segmental ostial PVI, specific sites of electrical conduction in the ostia of the pulmonary veins are ablated. In circumferential PVI, continuous ablation lesions encircle the ostia of all four pulmonary veins, usually in two pairs (ie, one circle of lesions around the left pulmonary veins and another circle around the right pulmonary veins). These ablation lesions completely isolate the pulmonary veins from the atrial myocardium and prevent conduction from trigger sites in to the atria.

The Cox-Maze III procedure involves creation of multiple incisions within both atria using the "cut and sew" technique during cardiac surgery. The incisions create scars in the atria that direct the impulse from the sinus node to the AV node through both atria in an orderly fashion and prevent reentry of impulses that could lead to AF. Because it is time consuming, requires cardiopulmonary bypass, and is technically difficult, the Cox-Maze III procedure is rarely done today and has been replaced with the Cox-Maze IV procedure, which is the current gold standard for surgical ablation. The Cox-Maze IV procedure can be done through a mini-thoracotomy or via median sternotomy and creates ablation lines by using bipolar RF and/or cryothermal energy devices. These ablation lines direct the sinus impulse through the atria, similar to the scars created by the cut and sew method. Catheter-based RF ablation procedures create the lesions from the endocardial approach and are done percutaneously in the electrophysiology laboratory rather than requiring surgery. Hybrid procedures using ablation catheters and the surgical approach are also available.

LAA amputation is done along with surgical Cox-Maze procedures as well as with mitral valve procedures to reduce the likelihood of thromboembolism, since most clots develop in the LAA during AF. LAA occlusion devices can be inserted via the right femoral vein and into the LAA through an atrial trans-septal approach and expanded within the LAA to seal it from the rest of the atrium, thus trapping clots and preventing them from embolizing.

Patients who have atrial tachyarrhythmias detected by implanted pacemakers or ICDs are at increased risk of stroke and other thromboembolic events. These devices store electrograms that can be reviewed for the presence of silent AF or other atrial tachyarrhythmias and provide information on frequency and duration of episodes that increase stroke risk. High-rate episodes recorded on implanted devices should be evaluated to document episodes of AF and guide appropriate treatment. In 20% to 40% of patients with ischemic stroke, the cause is unknown (referred to as cryptogenic stroke). Implantation of a cardiac monitor (loop recorder) may show episodes of silent AF that increase risk for stroke.

Supraventricular Tachycardia

A SVT by definition is any rhythm at a rate faster than 100 beats/min, which originates above the ventricle or utilizes the atria or AV junction as part of the circuit that maintains the tachycardia. Technically, SVT can include sinus tachycardia, AT, atrial flutter, AF, and junctional tachycardia. However, the term SVT is meant to be used to describe a regular, narrow QRS tachycardia in which the exact mechanism cannot be determined from the surface ECG. If P waves or atrial activity such a fibrillation or flutter waves can be clearly seen, then the mechanism can usually be identified. Occasionally in AT, the

P waves are hidden in preceding T waves and in that case use of the term SVT is appropriate.

The two most common dysrhythmias for which the term SVT is appropriate are AV nodal reentry tachycardia (AVNRT) and circus movement tachycardia (CMT) that occurs when an accessory pathway is present, such as in WPW. Another term used to describe CMT is AV reentry tachycardia (AVRT) but CMT is used here to prevent confusion between these two common dysrhythmias. The mechanisms of these SVTs are described in detail in Chapter 18, Advanced ECG Concepts. ECG characteristics of both SVTs are very similar and described here.

ECG Characteristics

- *Rate:* 140 to 250 beats/min.
- *Rhythm:* Regular.
- *P waves:* Usually not visible. In AVNRT, the P wave is hidden in the QRS or barely peeking out at the end of the QRS. In CMT, the P wave is usually present in the ST segment, but is often not visible.
- *PR interval:* Not measurable, since P waves are usually not visible.
- *QRS complex:* Usually normal.
- *Conduction:* In AVNRT, the impulse travels in a small circuit that includes the AV node as one limb of the circuit and a slower conducting pathway just outside the AV node as the second limb of the circuit. The impulse depolarizes the atria in a retrograde direction at the same time as it depolarizes the ventricles through the normal His-Purkinje system, resulting in a regular narrow QRS tachycardia. In CMT, the impulse follows a reentry circuit that includes the atria, AV node, ventricles, and accessory pathway. The most common type of CMT is called orthodromic CMT, in which the impulse travels from atria to ventricles through the normal AV node and His-Purkinje system, then back to the atria from the ventricles through the accessory pathway. This results in a regular, narrow QRS tachycardia because the ventricles are depolarized via the normal conduction system. If the circuit reverses direction and the ventricles depolarize through conduction down the accessory pathway, this is called antidromic CMT, and the resulting tachycardia has a wide QRS complex.
- *Example of SVT:* See Figure 3-25A, B.

Treatment

These SVTs are usually well tolerated and often paroxysmal in nature. If the ventricular rate is very rapid and sustained, symptoms such as palpitations, dizziness, or syncope can occur.

Vagal maneuvers such as carotid sinus massage, Valsalva's maneuver, gagging or coughing, drinking ice water, or putting the face in ice water may be effective in terminating the tachycardia. Adenosine (6 mg given rapidly IV, may repeat with 12 mg if necessary) is the most effective drug to

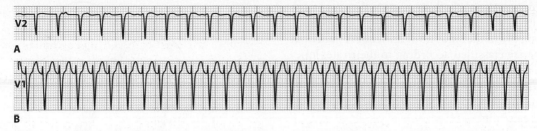

Figure 3-25. **(A)** SVT at a rate of 190 beats/min found to be AVNRT at electrophysiology study. **(B)** SVT at a rate of 214 found to be CMT at electrophysiology study.

terminate the tachycardia. Drugs that slow AV conduction, like calcium channel blockers (diltiazem, verapamil) or beta-blockers, can terminate tachycardia and can be used long term to prevent recurrences. Synchronized cardioversion can be used if drugs are contraindicated or fail to terminate tachycardia. RF ablation offers a cure for AVNRT and CMT. See Table 3-4 for recommendations for management of SVTs.

DYSRHYTHMIAS ORIGINATING IN THE ATRIOVENTRICULAR JUNCTION

Cells surrounding the AV node in the AV junction are capable of initiating impulses and controlling the heart rhythm (Figure 3-26). Junctional beats and junctional rhythms can appear in any of three ways on the ECG depending on the location of the junctional pacemaker and the speed of conduction of the impulse into the atria and ventricles:

- When a junctional focus fires, the wave of depolarization spreads backward (retrograde) into the atria as well as forward (antegrade) into the ventricles. If the impulse arrives in the atria before it arrives in the ventricles, the ECG shows a P wave (usually inverted because the atria are depolarizing from bottom to top) followed immediately by a QRS complex as the impulse reaches the ventricles. In this case, the PR interval is very short, usually 0.10 second or less.
- If the junctional impulse reaches both the atria and the ventricles at the same time, only a QRS is seen on the ECG because the ventricles are much larger than the atria and only ventricular depolarization will be seen, even though the atria are also depolarizing.

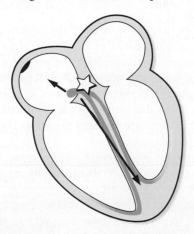

Figure 3-26. Dysrhythmias originating in the AV junction.

- If the junctional impulse reaches the ventricles before it reaches the atria, the QRS precedes the P wave on the ECG. Again, the P wave is usually inverted because of retrograde atrial depolarization, and the RP interval (distance from the beginning of the QRS to the beginning of the following P wave) is short.

Premature Junctional Complexes

Premature junctional complexes (PJCs) are due to an irritable focus in the AV junction. Irritability can be because of coronary heart disease or MI disrupting blood flow to the AV junction, nicotine, caffeine, emotions, or medications such as digitalis.

ECG Characteristics

- *Rate:* 60 to 100 beats/min or whatever the rate of the basic rhythm.
- *Rhythm:* Regular except for occurrence of premature beats.
- *P waves:* May occur before, during, or after the QRS complex of the premature beat and are usually inverted.
- *PR interval:* Short, usually 0.10 second or less when P waves precede the QRS.
- *QRS complex:* Usually normal but may be aberrant if the PJC occurs very early and conducts into the ventricles during the refractory period of a bundle branch.
- *Conduction:* Retrograde through the atria; usually normal through the ventricles.
- *Example of PJCs:* Figure 3-27.

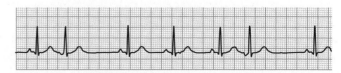

Figure 3-27. Premature junctional complexes.

Treatment

Treatment is not necessary for PJCs.

Junctional Rhythm, Accelerated Junctional Rhythm, and Junctional Tachycardia

Junctional rhythms can occur if the sinus node rate falls below the rate of the AV junctional pacemakers or when atrial conduction through the AV junction has been disrupted. Junctional rhythms commonly occur from digitalis toxicity or following inferior MI owing to disruption of blood supply to the sinus node and the AV junction. These rhythms are classified according to their rate. Junctional rhythm usually occurs at a rate of 40 to 60 beats/min, accelerated junctional rhythm occurs at a rate of 60 to 100 beats/min, and junctional tachycardia occurs at a rate of 100 to 250 beats/min.

ECG Characteristics

- *Rate:* Junctional rhythm, 40 to 60 beats/min; accelerated junctional rhythm, 60 to 100 beats/min; junctional tachycardia, 100 to 250 beats/min.
- *Rhythm:* Regular.
- *P waves:* May precede or follow QRS.
- *PR interval:* Short, 0.10 second or less.
- *QRS complex:* Usually normal.
- *Conduction:* Retrograde through the atria; normal through the ventricles.
- *Example of junctional rhythm and accelerated junctional rhythm:* Figure 3-28A, B.

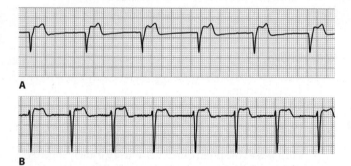

Figure 3-28. (A) Junctional rhythm, rate 52 beats/min. **(B)** Accelerated junctional rhythm, rate 70 beats/min.

Treatment

Treatment of junctional rhythm rarely is required unless the rate is too slow or too fast to maintain adequate cardiac output. If the rate is slow, atropine is given to increase the sinus rate and override the junctional focus or to increase the rate of firing of the junctional pacemaker. If the rate is fast, medications such as verapamil, propranolol, or beta-blockers may be effective in slowing the rate or terminating the dysrhythmia. Digitalis toxicity is a common cause of junctional rhythms, and so is held or avoided in patients with this dysrhythmia. See Table 3-4 for recommended treatment of junctional tachycardia.

DYSRHYTHMIAS ORIGINATING IN THE VENTRICLES

Ventricular dysrhythmias originate in the ventricular muscle or Purkinje system and are considered to be more dangerous than other dysrhythmias because of their potential to initiate VT and severely decrease cardiac output (Figure 3-29). However, as with any dysrhythmia, ventricular rate is a key determinant of how well a patient can tolerate a ventricular

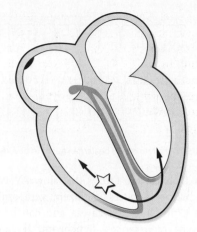

Figure 3-29. Dysrhythmias originating in the ventricles.

rhythm. Ventricular rhythms can range in severity from mild, well-tolerated rhythms to pulseless rhythms leading to sudden cardiac death.

Premature Ventricular Complexes

Premature ventricular complexes (PVCs) are caused by premature depolarization of cells in the ventricular myocardium or Purkinje system or to reentry in the ventricles. PVCs can be caused by hypoxia, MI, hypokalemia, acidosis, exercise, increased levels of circulating catecholamines, digitalis toxicity, caffeine, and alcohol, among other causes. PVCs increase with aging and are more common in people with coronary disease, valve disease, hypertension, cardiomyopathy, and other forms of heart disease. PVCs are not dangerous in people with normal hearts but are associated with higher mortality rates in patients with structural heart disease or acute MI, especially if left ventricular function is reduced. PVCs are considered potentially malignant when they occur more frequently than 10 per hour or are repetitive (occur in pairs, triplets, or more than three in a row) in patients with coronary disease, previous MI, cardiomyopathy, and reduced ejection fraction.

ECG Characteristics

- *Rate:* 60 to 100 beats/min or the rate of the basic rhythm.
- *Rhythm:* Irregular because of the early beats.
- *P waves:* Not related to the PVCs. Sinus rhythm is usually not interrupted by the premature beats, so sinus P waves can often be seen occurring regularly throughout the rhythm. P waves may occasionally follow PVCs due to retrograde conduction from the ventricle backward through the atria. These P waves are inverted.
- *PR interval:* Not present before most PVCs. If a P wave happens, by coincidence, to precede a PVC, the PR interval is short.
- *QRS complex:* Wide and bizarre; greater than 0.10 second in duration. These may vary in morphology (size, shape), if they originate from more than one focus in the ventricles (multifocal PVCs).

- *Conduction:* Impulses originating in the ventricles conduct through the ventricles from muscle cell to muscle cell rather than through Purkinje fibers, resulting in wide QRS complexes. Some PVCs may conduct retrograde into the atria, resulting in inverted P waves following the PVC. When the sinus rhythm is undisturbed by PVCs, the atria depolarize normally.
- *Example of PVCs:* Figure 3-30A, B.

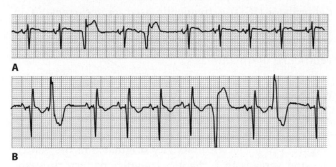

Figure 3-30. Premature ventricular complexes **(A)** Unifocal PVCs. **(B)** Multifocal PVCs.

Treatment

The significance of PVCs depends on the clinical setting in which they occur. Many people have chronic PVCs that do not need to be treated, and most of these people are asymptomatic. There is no evidence that suppression of PVCs reduces mortality, especially in patients with no structural heart disease. If PVCs cause bothersome palpitations, patients are told to avoid caffeine, tobacco, other stimulants, and try stress reduction techniques. Low-dose beta-blockers may reduce PVC frequency and the perception of palpitations and can be used for symptom relief.

In the setting of an acute MI, PVCs may be precursors of more dangerous ventricular dysrhythmias, especially when they occur near the apex of the T wave (R on T PVCs). Unless PVCs result in hemodynamic instability or symptomatic VT, treatment is not recommended. Beta-blockers are often effective in suppressing repetitive PVCs and have become the drugs of choice for treating post-MI PVCs that are symptomatic. Several antiarrhythmic medications are effective in reducing the frequency of PVCs but are not recommended due to the risk of prodysrhythmia and their association with sudden cardiac death in patients with structural heart disease. Amiodarone and sotalol can be used for PVC suppression in symptomatic patients but they do not improve mortality. Catheter ablation is an option in patients with left ventricular dysfunction associated with PVCs.

Idioventricular Rhythm and Accelerated Idioventricular Rhythm

Idioventricular rhythm occurs when an ectopic focus in the ventricle fires at a rate less than 50 beats/min, commonly 20 to 40 beats/min. This rhythm occurs as an escape rhythm when the sinus node and junctional tissue fail to fire or fail to conduct their impulses to the ventricle. Accelerated

idioventricular rhythm (AIVR) occurs when an ectopic focus in the ventricles fires at a rate of 50 to 100 beats/min. AIVR commonly occurs in patients with acute MI, especially inferior wall MI, and is a common dysrhythmia after thrombolytic therapy, when reperfusion of the damaged myocardium occurs. However, AIVR is not a sensitive or specific marker for successful reperfusion.

ECG Characteristics

- *Rate:* Less than 50 beats/min and commonly 20 to 40 beats/min for ventricular rhythm and 50 to 100 beats/min for accelerated ventricular rhythm.
- *Rhythm:* Usually regular.
- *P waves:* May be seen but at a slower rate than the ventricular focus, with dissociation from the QRS complex.
- *PR interval:* Not measured.
- *QRS complex:* Wide and bizarre.
- *Conduction:* If sinus rhythm is the basic rhythm, atrial conduction is normal. Impulses originating in the ventricles conduct via muscle cell-to-cell conduction, resulting in the wide QRS complex.
- *Example of escape ventricular rhythm and accelerated ventricular rhythm:* Figure 3-31A, B.

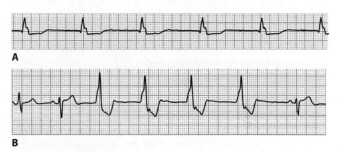

Figure 3-31. (A) Ventricular escape rhythm, rate 45 bpm. **(B)** Sinus rhythm with 4 beats of accelerated ventricular rhythm, rate 65 bpm.

Treatment

The treatment of AIVR depends on its cause and how well the patient is able to tolerate it. This dysrhythmia is usually transient and not harmful because the ventricular rate is within normal limits. Suppressive therapy is not indicated because abolishing the ventricular rhythm may leave an even less desirable heart rate. If the patient is symptomatic because of the loss of atrial kick, atropine can be used to increase the rate of the sinus node and overdrive the ventricular rhythm. If the ventricular rhythm is an escape rhythm, then treatment is directed toward increasing the rate of the escape rhythm or pacing the heart temporarily. Usually, accelerated ventricular rhythm is transient and benign and does not require treatment.

Ventricular Tachycardia

VT is a rapid ventricular rhythm at a rate greater than 100 beats/min. VT can be classified according to: (1) duration, *nonsustained* (lasts less than 30 seconds), *sustained* (lasts longer than 30 seconds), or *incessant* (VT present most of the time); and (2) morphology (ECG appearance of QRS complexes), *monomorphic* (QRS complexes have the same shape during tachycardia), *polymorphic* (QRS complexes vary randomly in shape), or *bidirectional* (alternating upright and negative QRS complexes during tachycardia). Polymorphic VT that occurs in the presence of a long QT interval is called *torsades de pointes* (meaning "twisting of the points"). The most common cause of VT is coronary artery disease, including acute ischemia, acute MI, and prior MI. Other causes include HF, cardiomyopathy, valvular heart disease, congenital heart disease, arrhythmogenic right ventricular dysplasia, cardiac tumors, cardiac surgery, and the proarrhythmic effects of many drugs. See Chapter 18 (Advanced ECG Concepts) for more information on VTs and the differential diagnosis of wide QRS tachycardias.

ECG Characteristics

- *Rate:* Ventricular rate is faster than 100 beats/min.
- *Rhythm:* Monomorphic VT is usually regular; polymorphic VT can be irregular.
- *P waves:* Dissociated from QRS complexes. If sinus rhythm is the underlying basic rhythm, they are regular. P waves may be seen but are not related to QRS complexes. P waves are often buried within QRS complexes.
- *PR interval:* Not measurable because of dissociation of P waves from QRS complexes.
- *QRS complex:* Usually 0.12 second or more in duration.
- *Conduction:* Impulse originates in one ventricle and spreads via muscle cell-to-cell conduction through both ventricles. There may be retrograde conduction through the atria, but more often the sinus node continues to fire regularly and depolarize the atria normally.
- *Example of VT:* Figure 3-32.

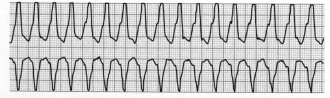

Figure 3-32. Monomorphic ventricular tachycardia.

Treatment

Immediate treatment of VT depends on how well the rhythm is tolerated by the patient. The two main determinants of patient tolerance of any tachycardia are ventricular rate and underlying left ventricular function. VT can be an emergency if cardiac output is severely decreased because of a very rapid rate or poor left ventricular function.

Hemodynamically unstable VT is treated with synchronized cardioversion. If VT is pulseless, then immediate defibrillation is required. VT that is hemodynamically stable can be treated with pharmacologic therapy. Amiodarone is often the drug of choice but lidocaine or procainamide can also be used. Medications used to treat VT on a long-term basis include amiodarone, sotalol, and beta-blockers. Some VTs can be treated with RF catheter ablation to abolish the ectopic focus. The implantable cardioverter defibrillator (ICD) is frequently used for recurrent VT in patients with reduced ejection fractions or drug refractory VT. See Table 3-6 for recommendations for management of ventricular dysrhythmias.

Ventricular Fibrillation

Ventricular fibrillation (VF) is rapid, ineffective quivering of the ventricles and is fatal without immediate treatment (Figure 3-33). Electrical activity originates in the ventricles and spreads in a chaotic, irregular pattern throughout both ventricles. There is no cardiac output or palpable pulse with VF.

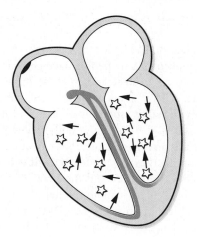

Figure 3-33. Ventricular fibrillation.

ECG Characteristics

- *Rate:* Rapid, uncoordinated, ineffective.
- *Rhythm:* Chaotic, irregular.
- *P waves:* None seen.
- *PR interval:* None.
- *QRS complex:* No formed QRS complexes seen; rapid, irregular undulations without any specific pattern.
- *Conduction:* Multiple ectopic foci firing simultaneously in ventricles and depolarizing them irregularly and without any organized pattern. Ventricles are not contracting.
- *Example of ventricular fibrillation:* Figure 3-34.

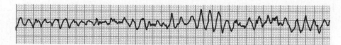

Figure 3-34. Ventricular fibrillation.

TABLE 3-6. TREATMENT OF VENTRICULAR ARRHYTHMIAS

Ventricular Tachycardia

Acute Treatment
1. Patients with a wide-QRS tachycardia should be presumed to have VT if the diagnosis is unclear. (I; C-EO)
2. Patients presenting with ventricular arrhythmias (VA) with hemodynamic instability should undergo direct current cardioversion (I; A)
3. In patients with hemodynamically stable VT, administration of intravenous procainamide can be useful to attempt to terminate VT (I; A)
4. In patients with hemodynamically stable VT, administration of intravenous amiodarone or sotalol may be considered to attempt to terminate VT (IIb; BR)
5. In patients with a recent MI who have VT/VF that repeatedly recurs despite direct current cardioversion and antiarrhythmic medications (VT/VF storm), an intravenous beta-blocker can be useful (IIa; B-NR)
6. In patients with suspected AMI, prophylactic administration of lidocaine or high-dose amiodarone for the prevention of VT is potentially harmful (III; B-R)
7. In patients with a wide QRS complex tachycardia of unknown origin, calcium channel blockers (eg, verapamil and diltiazem) are potentially harmful (III; C-LD)

Ongoing Management
1. In patients with ischemic heart disease, who either survive sudden cardiac arrest due to VT/VF or experience hemodynamically unstable VT (I; B-R) or stable VT (I; B-NR) not due to reversible causes, an ICD is recommended if meaningful survival greater than 1 year is expected.
2. In patients with ischemic heart disease and unexplained syncope who have inducible sustained monomorphic VT on electrophysiological study, an ICD is recommended if meaningful survival of greater than 1 year is expected (I; B-NR)
3. In patients with ischemic heart disease and recurrent VA, with significant symptoms or ICD shocks despite optimal device programming and ongoing treatment with a beta-blocker, amiodarone or sotalol is useful to suppress recurrent VA (I; B-R)
4. In patients with prior MI and recurrent episodes of symptomatic sustained VT or who present with VT or VF storm and have failed or are intolerant of amiodarone (I; B-R) or other antiarrhythmic medications (I; B-NR), catheter ablation is recommended.
5. In patients with ischemic heart disease and ICD shocks for sustained monomorphic VT or symptomatic sustained monomorphic VT that is recurrent or hemodynamically tolerated, catheter ablation as first-line therapy may be considered to reduce recurrent VA (IIb; C-LD)
6. In patients with prior MI, class IC antiarrhythmic medications (eg, flecainide and propafenone) should not be used (III; B-R)
7. In patients with ischemic heart disease and sustained monomorphic VT, coronary revascularization alone is an ineffective therapy to prevent recurrent VT (III; C-LD)
8. In patients with incessant VT or VF, an ICD should not be implanted until sufficient control of the arrhythmia is achieved to prevent repeated ICD shocks (III; C-LD)

Polymorphic Ventricular Tachycardia

Acute Treatment
1. In patients with polymorphic VT or VF with ST-elevation MI, angiography with emergency revascularization is recommended (I; B-NR)
2. In patients with polymorphic VT due to myocardial ischemia, intravenous beta-blockers can be useful (IIa; B-R)

Torsades de Pointes

Acute Treatment
1. For patients with QT prolongation due to a medication, hypokalemia, hypomagnesemia, or other acquired factor and recurrent torsades de pointes, administration of intravenous magnesium sulfate is recommended to suppress the arrhythmia (I; C-LD)
2. In patients with recurrent torsades de pointes associated with acquired QT prolongation and bradycardia that cannot be suppressed with intravenous magnesium administration, increasing the heart rate with atrial or ventricular pacing or isoproterenol are recommended to suppress the arrhythmia (I; B-NR)
3. For patients with torsades de pointes associated with acquired QT prolongation, potassium repletion to 4.0 mmol/L or more and magnesium repletion to normal values are beneficial (I; C-LD)
4. In patients with congenital or acquired long QT syndrome, QT-prolonging medications are potentially harmful (III; B-NR)

Class of Recommendation (COR)
Class I: Strong; benefit >>> risk
Class IIa: Moderate; benefit >> risk
Class IIb: Weak; benefit > risk
Class III: No benefit or may cause harm

Level of Evidence (LOE)
Level A: High-quality evidence from more than 1 RCT; meta-analyses of high-quality RCTs; one or more RCTs corroborated by high-quality registry studies.
Level B-R (randomized): Moderate-quality evidence from 1 or more RCTs; Meta-analyses of moderate-quality RCTs. Level B-NR (nonrandomized): Moderate-quality evidence from 1 or more well-designed, well-executed nonrandomized studies, observational studies, or registry studies; meta-analyses of such studies.
Level C-LD (limited data): Randomized or nonrandomized observational or registry studies with limitations of design or execution; meta-analyses of such studies; physiological or mechanistic studies in human subjects.
Level C-EO (expert opinion): Consensus of expert opinion based on clinical experience.

Data from Al-Khatib SM, Stevenson WG, Ackerman MJ, et al: 2017 AHA/ACC/HRS Guideline for Management of Patients With Ventricular Arrhythmias and the Prevention of Sudden Cardiac Death: A Report of the American College of Cardiology/American Heart Association Task Force on Clinical Practice Guidelines and the Heart Rhythm Society. Circulation. 2017 Oct 30.

Treatment

VF requires immediate defibrillation. Synchronized cardioversion is not possible because there are no formed QRS complexes on which to synchronize the shock. Cardiopulmonary resuscitation (CPR) must be performed until a defibrillator is available, and then defibrillation at 200 J (biphasic defibrillation) or 360 J (monophasic defibrillation) is recommended followed by CPR and pharmacologic therapy. IV amiodarone is the recommended antiarrhythmic during the resuscitation effort and as maintenance therapy for 24 to 48 hours following return of spontaneous circulation. Beta-blockers, amiodarone, and sotalol are most often used for long-term drug therapy. The ICD has become the standard of care for survivors of VF that occurs in the absence of acute ischemia.

Ventricular Asystole

Ventricular asystole is the absence of any ventricular rhythm: no QRS complex, no pulse, and no cardiac output (Figure 3-35). Ventricular asystole is always fatal unless the cause can be identified and treated immediately. If atrial activity is still present, the term "ventricular standstill" is used.

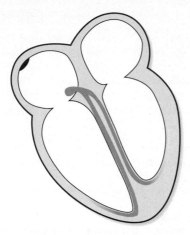

Figure 3-35. Ventricular asystole.

ECG Characteristics

- *Rate:* None.
- *Rhythm:* None.
- *P waves:* May be present if the sinus node is functioning.
- *PR interval:* None.
- *QRS complex:* None.
- *Conduction:* Atrial conduction may be normal, if the sinus node is functioning. There is no conduction into the ventricles.
- *Example of ventricular asystole:* Figure 3-36.

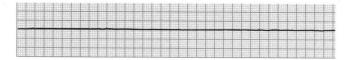

Figure 3-36. Ventricular asystole.

Treatment

CPR must be initiated immediately if the patient is to survive. IV epinephrine is the only drug currently recommended for treating asystole. The cause of asystole should be determined and treated as rapidly as possible to improve the chance of survival. Asystole has a very poor prognosis despite the best resuscitation efforts because it usually represents extensive MI or severe underlying metabolic problems. Pacing and atropine are no longer recommended for treatment for asystole.

ATRIOVENTRICULAR BLOCKS

The term *atrioventricular block* is used to describe dysrhythmias in which there is delayed or failed conduction of supraventricular impulses into the ventricles. AV blocks have been classified according to location of the block and severity of the conduction abnormality.

First-Degree Atrioventricular Block

First-degree AV block is defined as prolonged AV conduction time of supraventricular impulses into the ventricles (Figure 3-37). This delay usually occurs in the AV node, and all impulses are conducted to the ventricles, but with delayed conduction times. First-degree AV block can be due to coronary heart disease, rheumatic heart disease, or administration of digitalis, beta-blockers, or calcium channel blockers. First-degree AV block can be normal in people with slow heart rates or high vagal tone.

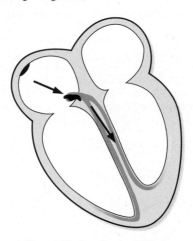

Figure 3-37. First-degree AV block.

ECG Characteristics

- *Rate:* Can occur at any sinus rate, usually 60 to 100 beats/min.
- *Rhythm:* Regular.
- *P waves:* Normal; precede every QRS complex.
- *PR interval:* Prolonged above 0.20 second.
- *QRS complex:* Usually normal.
- *Conduction:* Normal through the atria, delayed through the AV node, and normal through the ventricles.
- *Example of first-degree AV block:* Figure 3-38.

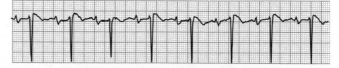

Figure 3-38. First-degree AV block, PR interval is 0.28 second.

Treatment

Treatment of first-degree AV block is usually not required, but the rhythm should be observed for progression to more severe block.

Second-Degree Atrioventricular Block

Second-degree AV block occurs when one atrial impulse at a time fails to be conducted to the ventricles. Second-degree

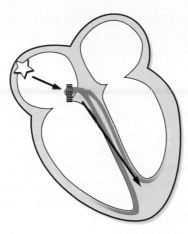

Figure 3-39. Type I second-degree AV block.

AV block can be divided into two distinct categories: type I block, occurring in the AV node (Figure 3-39), and type II block, occurring below the AV node in the bundle of His or bundle-branch system (Figure 3-40).

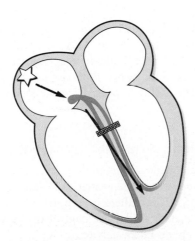

Figure 3-40. Type II second-degree AV block.

Type I Second-Degree Atrioventricular Block

Type I second-degree AV block, often referred to as *Wenckebach block,* is a progressive increase in conduction times of consecutive atrial impulses into the ventricles until one impulse fails to conduct, or is "dropped." The PR intervals gradually lengthen until one P wave fails to conduct and is not followed by a QRS complex, resulting in a pause, after which the cycle repeats itself. This type of block is commonly associated with inferior MI, coronary heart disease, aortic valve disease, mitral valve prolapse, atrial septal defects, and administration of digitalis, beta-blockers, or calcium channel blockers.

ECG Characteristics

- *Rate:* Can occur at any sinus or atrial rate.
- *Rhythm:* Irregular. Overall appearance of the rhythm demonstrates "group beating."

- *P waves:* Normal. Some P waves are not conducted to the ventricles, but only one at a time fails to conduct to the ventricle.
- *PR interval:* Gradually lengthens on consecutive beats. The PR interval preceding the pause is longer than that following the pause (unless 2:1 conduction is present).
- *QRS complex:* Usually normal unless there is associated bundle branch block.
- *Conduction:* Normal through the atria; progressively delayed through the AV node until an impulse fails to conduct. Ventricular conduction is normal. Conduction ratios can vary, with ratios as low as 2:1 (every other P wave is blocked) up to high ratios such as 15:14 (every 15th P wave is blocked).
- *Example of second-degree AV block type I:* Figure 3-41.

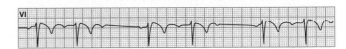

Figure 3-41. Second-degree AV block, type I. PR intervals progressively prolong before the blocked P waves.

Treatment

Treatment of type I second-degree AV block depends on the conduction ratio, the resulting ventricular rate, and the patient's tolerance for the rhythm. If ventricular rates are slow enough to decrease cardiac output, the treatment is atropine to increase the sinus rate and speed conduction through the AV node. At higher conduction ratios where the ventricular rate is within a normal range, no treatment is necessary. If the block is due to digitalis, calcium channel blockers, or beta-blockers, those medications are held. This type of block is usually temporary and benign, and seldom requires pacing, although temporary pacing may be needed when the ventricular rate is slow.

Type II Second-Degree Atrioventricular Block

Type II second-degree AV block is sudden failure of conduction of an atrial impulse to the ventricles without progressive increases in conduction time of consecutive P waves (Figure 3-40). Type II block occurs below the AV node and is usually associated with bundle branch block; therefore, the dropped beats are usually a manifestation of bilateral bundle branch block. This form of block appears on the ECG much the same as type I block except that there is no progressive increase in PR intervals before the blocked beats and the QRS is almost always wide. Type II block is less common than type I block, but is a more serious form of block. It occurs in rheumatic heart disease, coronary heart disease, primary disease of the conduction system, and in the presence of acute anterior MI. Type II block is more dangerous than type I because of a higher incidence of associated symptoms and progression to complete AV block.

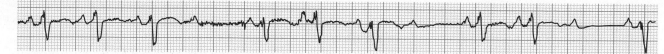

Figure 3-42. Second-degree AV block, type II. All PR intervals are constant.

ECG Characteristics

- *Rate:* Can occur at any basic rate.
- *Rhythm:* Irregular due to blocked beats.
- *P waves:* Usually regular and precede each QRS. Periodically a P wave is not followed by a QRS complex.
- *PR interval:* Constant before conducted beats. The PR interval preceding the pause is the same as that following the pause.
- *QRS complex:* Usually wide because of associated bundle branch block.
- *Conduction:* Normal through the atria and through the AV node but intermittently blocked in the bundle branch system and fails to reach the ventricles. Conduction through the ventricles is abnormally slow due to associated bundle branch block. Conduction ratios can vary from 2:1 to only occasional blocked beats.
- *Example of second-degree AV block type II:* Figure 3-42.

Treatment

Treatment usually includes pacemaker therapy because this type of block is often permanent and progresses to complete block. External pacing can be used for treatment of symptomatic type II block until transvenous pacing can be initiated. Atropine is not recommended because increasing the number of impulses conducting through the AV node may bombard the diseased bundles with more impulses than they can handle, resulting in further conduction failure and a slower ventricular rate.

High-Grade Atrioventricular Block

High-grade (or advanced) AV block is present when two or more consecutive atrial impulses are blocked when the atrial rate is reasonable (<135 beats/min) and conduction fails because of the block itself and not because of interference from an escape pacemaker. High-grade AV block may be type I, occurring in the AV node, or type II, occurring below the AV node. The importance of high-grade block depends on the conduction ratio and the resulting ventricular rate. Because ventricular rates tend to be slow, this dysrhythmia is frequently symptomatic and requires treatment.

ECG Characteristics

- *Rate:* Atrial rate less than 135 beats/min.
- *Rhythm:* Regular or irregular, depending on conduction pattern.
- *P waves:* Normal. Present before every conducted QRS, but several P waves appear without subsequent QRS complexes.
- *PR interval:* Constant before conducted beats. May be normal or prolonged.

- *QRS complex:* Usually normal in type I block and wide in type II block.
- *Conduction:* Normal through the atria. Two or more consecutive atrial impulses fail to conduct to the ventricles. Ventricular conduction is normal in type I block and abnormally slow in type II block.
- *Example of high-grade AV block:* Figure 3-43.

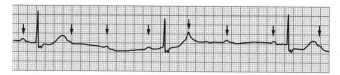

Figure 3-43. High-grade AV block. Two P waves in a row are blocked.

Treatment

Treatment of high-grade block is necessary, if the patient is symptomatic. Atropine can be given and is generally more effective in type I block. An external pacemaker may be required until transvenous pacing can be initiated, and permanent pacing is often necessary in type II high-grade block.

Third-Degree Atrioventricular Block (Complete Block)

Third-degree AV block is complete failure of conduction of all atrial impulses to the ventricles (Figure 3-44A, B). In third-degree AV block, there is complete AV dissociation; the atria are usually under the control of the sinus node, although complete block can occur with any atrial dysrhythmia; and either a junctional or ventricular pacemaker controls the ventricles. The ventricular rate is usually less than 45 beats/min; a faster rate could indicate an accelerated junctional or ventricular rhythm that interferes with conduction from the atria into the ventricles by causing physiologic refractoriness in the conduction system, thus causing a physiologic failure of conduction that must be differentiated from the abnormal conduction system function of complete AV block. Causes of complete AV block include coronary heart disease, MI, Lev disease, Lenègre disease, cardiac surgery, congenital heart disease, and medications that slow AV conduction such as digitalis, beta-blockers, and calcium channel blockers.

ECG Characteristics

- *Rate:* Atrial rate is usually normal. Ventricular rate is less than 45 beats/min.
- *Rhythm:* Regular.
- *P waves:* Normal but dissociated from QRS complexes.
- *PR interval:* No consistent PR intervals because there is no relationship between P waves and QRS complexes.

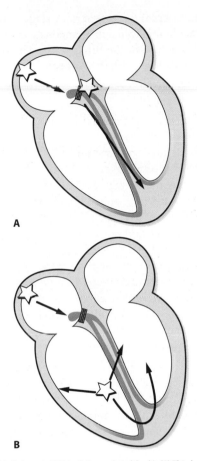

Figure 3-44. Third-degree AV block (complete block). **(A)** Third-degree AV block with junctional escape pacemaker. **(B)** Third-degree AV block with ventricular escape pacemaker. (*Reproduced with permission from Woods SL, Froelicher ES, Motzer SU. Cardiac Nursing, 3rd ed. Philadelphia, PA: JB Lippincott; 1995.*)

- *QRS complex:* Normal if ventricles are controlled by a junctional pacemaker. Wide if controlled by a ventricular pacemaker.
- *Conduction:* Normal through the atria. All impulses are blocked at the AV node or in the bundle branches, so there is no conduction to the ventricles. Conduction through the ventricles is normal if a junctional escape rhythm occurs, and abnormally slow if a ventricular escape rhythm occurs.
- *Examples of third-degree AV block:* Figure 3-45A, B.

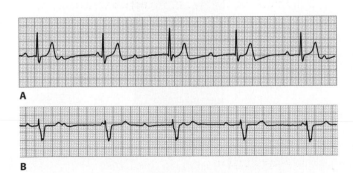

Figure 3-45. (A) Third-degree AV block with a junctional escape pacemaker at a rate of about 36 beats/min. **(B)** Third-degree AV block with a ventricular escape pacemaker at a rate of about 40 beats/min.

Treatment

Third-degree AV block can occur without significant symptoms if it occurs gradually and the heart has time to compensate for the slow ventricular rate. If it occurs suddenly in the presence of acute MI, its significance depends on the resulting ventricular rate and the patient's tolerance. Treatment of complete heart block with symptoms of decreased cardiac output includes external pacing until transvenous pacing can be initiated. Atropine can be given but is not usually effective in restoring conduction.

TEMPORARY PACING

Indications

If the heart fails to generate or conduct impulses to the ventricle, the myocardium can be electrically stimulated using a cardiac pacemaker. A cardiac pacemaker has two components: a pulse generator and a pacing electrode or lead. Temporary cardiac pacing is indicated in any situation in which bradycardia results in symptoms of decreased cerebral perfusion or hemodynamic compromise and does not respond to pharmacologic therapy. Signs and symptoms of hemodynamic instability are hypotension, change in mental status, angina, or pulmonary edema. Temporary pacing is also used to terminate some rapid reentrant tachycardias by briefly pacing the heart at a faster rate than the existing rate. When pacing is stopped, the sinus node may resume control of the rhythm if the tachycardia has been terminated. This type of pacing is termed *overdrive pacing* to distinguish it from pacing for bradycardic conditions.

Temporary cardiac pacing is accomplished by transvenous, epicardial, or external pacing methods. If continued cardiac pacing is required, insertion of permanent pacemakers is done electively. The following section presents an overview of temporary ventricular pacing principles. A more detailed explanation of pacemaker functions is covered in Chapter 18, Advanced ECG Concepts.

Transvenous Pacing

Transvenous pacing is usually done by percutaneous puncture of the internal jugular, subclavian, antecubital, or femoral vein and advancing a pacing lead into the apex of the right ventricle so that the tip of the pacing lead contacts the wall of the ventricle (Figure 3-46A). The transvenous pacing lead is attached to an external pulse generator that is kept either on the patient or at the bedside. Transvenous pacing is usually necessary only for a few days until the rhythm returns to normal or a permanent pacemaker is inserted.

Epicardial Pacing

Epicardial pacing is done through electrodes placed on the atria or ventricles during cardiac surgery. The pacing electrode end of the lead is looped through or loosely sutured to the epicardial surface of the atria or ventricles and the other end is pulled through the chest wall, sutured to the skin, and

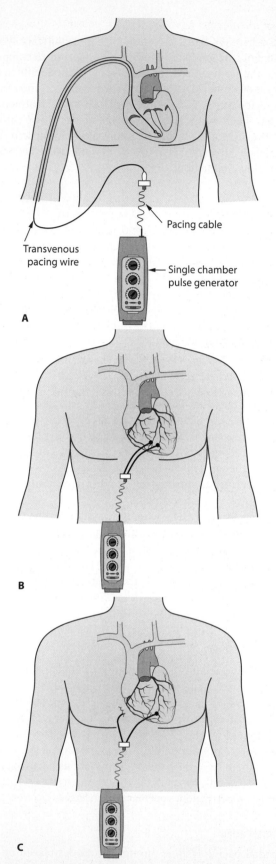

A

Transvenous
pacing wire

Pacing cable

Single chamber
pulse generator

B

C

Figure 3-46. Temporary single chamber ventricular pacing. **(A)** Transvenous pacing with pacing lead in apex of right ventricle. **(B)** Bipolar epicardial pacing with two epicardial wires on ventricle. **(C)** Unipolar epicardial pacing with one wire on ventricle and one ground wire in mediastinum.

attached to an external pulse generator (Figure 3-46B, C). A ground wire is often placed subcutaneously in the chest wall and pulled through with the other leads. The number and placement of leads vary with the surgeon.

Components of a Pacing System

The basic components of a cardiac pacing system are the pulse generator and the pacing lead. The *pulse generator* contains the power source (battery) and all of the electronic circuitry that controls pacemaker function. A temporary pulse generator is a box that is kept at the bedside and is usually powered by a regular 9-V battery. It has controls on the front that allow the operator to set pacing rate, strength of the pacing stimulus (output), and sensitivity settings (Figure 3-47).

The *pacing lead* is an insulated wire used to transmit the electrical current from the pulse generator to the myocardium. A unipolar lead contains a single wire and a bipolar lead contains two wires that are insulated from each other. In a unipolar lead, the electrode is an exposed metal tip at the end of the lead that contacts the myocardium and serves as the negative pole of the pacing circuit. In a bipolar lead, the end of the lead is a metal tip that contacts myocardium and serves as the negative pole, and the positive pole is an exposed metal ring located a few millimeters proximal to the distal tip.

Basics of Pacemaker Operation

Electrical current flows in a closed-loop circuit between two pieces of metal (poles). For current to flow, there must be conductive material (ie, a lead, muscle, or conductive solution) between the two poles. In the heart, the pacing lead,

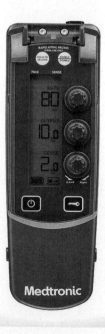

Figure 3-47. Temporary pacemaker pulse generator. ©2018 Medtronic. All rights reserved. (*Used with the permission of Medtronic.*)

cardiac muscle, and body tissues serve as conducting material for the flow of electrical current in the pacing system. The pacing circuit consists of the pacemaker pulse generator (the power source), the conducting lead (pacing lead), and the myocardium. The electrical stimulus travels from the pulse generator through the pacing lead to the myocardium, through the myocardium, and back to the pulse generator, thus completing the circuit.

Temporary transvenous pacing is done using a bipolar pacing lead with its tip in the apex of the RV (see Figure 3-46A). Epicardial pacing can be done with either bipolar or unipolar leads. The term *bipolar* means that both of the poles in the pacing system are in or on the heart (see Figure 3-46A, B). In a bipolar system, the pulse generator initiates the electrical impulse and delivers it out the negative terminal of the pacemaker to the pacing lead. The impulse travels down the lead to the distal electrode (negative pole or cathode) that is in contact with myocardium. As the impulse reaches the tip, it travels through the myocardium and returns to the positive pole (or anode) of the system, completing the circuit. In a transvenous bipolar system, the positive pole is the proximal ring located a few millimeters proximal to the distal tip. The circuit over which the electrical impulse travels in a bipolar system is small because the two poles are located close together on the lead. This results in a small pacing spike on the ECG as the pacing stimulus travels between the two poles. If the stimulus is strong enough to depolarize the myocardium, the pacing spike is immediately followed by a P wave if the lead is in the atrium or a wide QRS complex if the lead is in the ventricle.

A unipolar system has only one of the two poles in or on the heart (see Figure 3-46C). In a temporary unipolar epicardial pacing system, a ground lead placed in the subcutaneous tissue in the mediastinum serves as the second pole. Unipolar pacemakers work the same way as bipolar systems, but the circuit over which the impulse travels is larger because of the greater distance between the two poles. This results in a large pacing spike on the ECG as the impulse travels between the two poles.

Capture and Sensing

The two main functions of a pacing system are capture and sensing. *Capture* means that a pacing stimulus results in depolarization of the chamber being paced (Figure 3-48A). Capture is determined by the strength of the stimulus, which is measured in milliamperes (mA), the amount of time the stimulus is applied to the heart (pulse width), and by contact of the pacing electrode with the myocardium. Capture cannot occur unless the distal tip of the pacing lead is in contact with healthy myocardium that is capable of responding to the stimulus. Pacing in infarcted tissue usually prevents capture. Similarly, if the catheter is floating in the cavity of the ventricle and not in direct contact with myocardium, capture will not occur. In temporary pacing, the output dial on the face of the pulse generator controls stimulus strength, and can be set and changed easily by the operator. Temporary pulse generators usually are capable of delivering a stimulus of 0.1 to 20 mA.

Sensing means that the pacemaker is able to detect the presence of intrinsic cardiac activity (Figure 3-48B). The sensing circuit controls how sensitive the pacemaker is to intrinsic cardiac depolarizations. Intrinsic activity is measured in millivolts (mV), and the higher the number, the larger the intrinsic signal; for example, a 10-mV QRS complex is larger than a 2-mV QRS. When pacemaker sensitivity needs to be increased to make the pacemaker "see" smaller signals, the sensitivity number must be decreased; for example, a sensitivity of 2 mV is more sensitive than one of 5 mV.

A fence analogy may help to explain sensitivity. Think of sensitivity as a fence standing between the pacemaker and what it wants to see, the ventricle; for example, if there is a 10-ft-high fence (or a 10-mV sensitivity) between the two, the pacemaker may not see what the ventricle is doing.

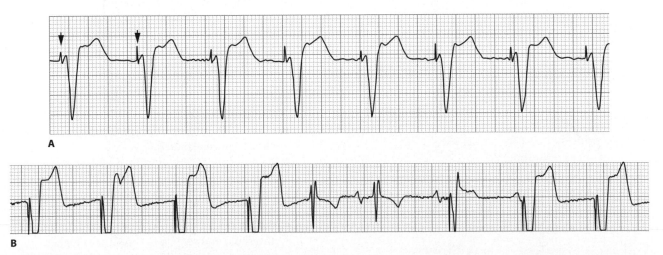

Figure 3-48. (A) Ventricular pacing with 100% capture. Arrows show pacing spikes, each one followed by a wide QRS complex indicating ventricular capture. **(B)** Rhythm strip of a ventricular pacemaker in the demand mode. There is appropriate sensing of intrinsic QRS complexes and appropriate pacing with ventricular capture when the intrinsic QRS complexes fall below the preset rate of the pacemaker. The seventh beat is fusion between the intrinsic QRS and the paced beat, a normal phenomenon in ventricular pacing.

To make the pacemaker able to see, the fence needs to be lowered. Lowering the fence to 2 ft would probably enable the pacemaker to see the ventricle. Changing the sensitivity from 10 to 2 mV is like lowering the fence—the pacemaker becomes more sensitive and is able to "see" intrinsic activity more easily. Thus, to increase the sensitivity of a pacemaker, the millivolt number (fence) must be decreased.

Asynchronous (Fixed-Rate) Pacing Mode

A pacemaker programmed to an asynchronous mode paces at the programmed rate regardless of intrinsic cardiac activity. This can result in competition between the pacemaker and the heart's own electrical activity. Asynchronous pacing in the ventricle is unsafe because of the potential for pacing stimuli to fall in the vulnerable period of repolarization and cause VF.

Demand Mode

The term *demand* means that the pacemaker paces only when the heart fails to depolarize on its own, that is, the pacemaker fires only "on demand." In demand mode, the pacemaker's sensing circuit is capable of sensing intrinsic cardiac activity and inhibiting pacer output when intrinsic activity is present. Sensing takes place between the two poles of the pacemaker. A bipolar system senses over a small area because the poles are close together, and this can result in "undersensing" of intrinsic signals. A unipolar system senses over a large area because the poles are far apart, and this can result in "oversensing." A unipolar system is more likely to sense myopotentials caused by muscle movement and inappropriately inhibit pacemaker output, potentially resulting in periods of asystole if the patient has no underlying cardiac rhythm. The demand mode should always be used for ventricular pacing to avoid the possibility of VF.

A paced ventricular beat begins with a pacing spike, which indicates that the pacemaker released an electrical stimulus (Figure 3-49). If the pacing stimulus is strong enough to depolarize the ventricle, the spike is followed by a wide QRS complex and a T wave that is oriented in the opposite direction of the QRS complex. Figure 3-48A illustrates ventricular pacing with consistent capture.

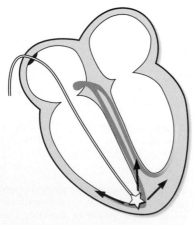

Figure 3-49. Temporary pacing lead in RV apex.

Figure 3-48B is the ECG of a ventricular pacemaker that is functioning correctly in the demand mode. The pacemaker generates an impulse when it senses that the heart rate has decreased below the set pacing rate. Therefore, the pacemaker senses the intrinsic cardiac rhythm of the patient and only generates an impulse when the rate falls below the preset pacing rate. Refer to Chapter 18, Advanced ECG Concepts, for more detailed information on single and dual-chamber pacing.

Initiating Transvenous Ventricular Pacing

Temporary transvenous pacing leads are bipolar and have two tails, one marked "positive" or "proximal" and the other marked "negative" or "distal," which are connected to the pulse generator. To initiate ventricular pacing using a transvenous lead (see Figure 3-46A):

1. Connect the negative terminal of the pulse generator to the distal end of the pacing lead.
2. Connect the positive terminal of the pulse generator to the proximal end of the pacing lead.
3. Set the rate at 70 to 80 beats/min or as ordered by physician.
4. Set the output at 5 mA, then determine stimulation threshold and set two to three times higher.
5. Set the sensitivity at 2 mV and adjust according to sensitivity threshold.

Initiating Epicardial Pacing

To initiate bipolar ventricular pacing (two leads on the ventricle; see Figure 3-46B):

1. Connect the negative terminal of the pulse generator to one of the ventricular leads.
2. Connect the positive terminal of the pulse generator to the other ventricular lead.
3. Set the rate at 70 to 80 beats/min or as ordered.
4. Set the output at 5 mA, then determine stimulation threshold and set two to three times higher.
5. Set the sensitivity at 2 mV and adjust according to sensitivity threshold.

To initiate unipolar ventricular pacing (one lead on the ventricle; see Figure 3-46C):

1. Connect the negative terminal of the pulse generator to the ventricular lead.
2. Connect the positive terminal of the pulse generator to the ground lead.
3. Set the rate at 70 to 80 beats/min or as ordered by physician.
4. Set the output at 5 mA, then determine stimulation threshold and set two to three times higher.
5. Set the sensitivity at 2 mV and adjust according to sensitivity threshold. See Chapter 18, Advanced ECG Concepts, for information on how to obtain capture and sensing thresholds.

External (Transcutaneous) Pacemakers

The emergent nature of many bradycardic rhythms requires immediate temporary pacing. Because transvenous catheter placement is difficult to accomplish quickly, external pacing is the preferred method for rapid, easy initiation of cardiac pacing in emergent situations until a transvenous pacemaker can be inserted. External pacing is done through large-surface adhesive electrodes attached to the anterior and posterior chest wall and connected to an external pacing unit (Figure 3-50). The pacing current passes through skin and chest wall structures to reach the heart; therefore, large energies are required to achieve capture. Sedation and analgesia are usually needed to minimize the discomfort felt by the patient during pacing. Transcutaneous pacing spikes are usually very large, often distorting the QRS complex. The presence of a pulse with every pacing spike confirms ventricular capture.

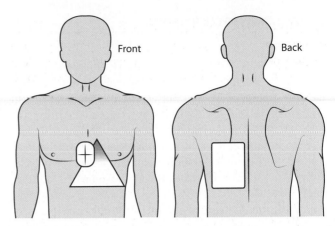

Figure 3-50. External pacemaker with pacing electrode pads on anterior and posterior chest and back.

ESSENTIAL CONTENT CASE

Heart Block and Epicardial Pacemaker

A patient underwent an aortic valve replacement yesterday. He has been extubated, he has a mediastinal chest tube, and two ventricular epicardial pacing leads are in place and coiled under a dressing. He is in sinus rhythm at a rate in the 80s, BP is 146/80, RR is 16, and he is breathing comfortably. The monitor alarm sounds and when you enter the room, he is pale and complaining of dizziness but no chest pain. The monitor shows the following rhythm:

Figure 3-51A

Case Question 1. What is his rhythm?
He is dizzy and his BP is 92/60.

Case Question 2. What can you do to treat this dysrhythmia?

Case Question 3. Describe how to initiate epicardial ventricular pacing.
You connect the pacing leads to a temporary pulse generator and set the rate at 70 beats/min.
This is the rhythm:

Figure 3-51B

Case Question 4. What is this rhythm?

Case Question 5. Evaluate pacemaker function in terms of ventricular capture and ventricular sensing.

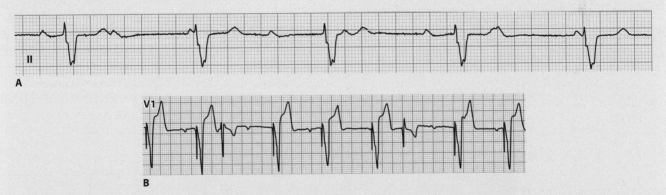

Figure 3-51. (A) Rhythm before treatment. (B) Rhythm after treatment.

Answers
1. This rhythm is third-degree AV block with a ventricular pacemaker at a rate of about 40 beats/min.
2. Third-degree AV block is best treated with pacing. Atropine may speed up the rate of the sinus rhythm but it does not improve conduction in complete heart block. Since this patient has ventricular epicardial pacing leads in place, the best treatment is to initiate temporary ventricular pacing.
3. To initiate ventricular epicardial pacing with two ventricular leads present, connect one epicardial lead to the negative terminal of the temporary pacemaker pulse generator and connect the other lead to the positive terminal of the pacemaker. Set the desired rate, output, and sensitivity and turn the pacemaker on.
4. Ventricular paced rhythm at a rate of 70 beats/min. Sinus P waves are present and two of them are conducted to the ventricles.
5. Capture is good: every ventricular pacing spike is followed by a wide QRS complex. Sensing is also good: the two conducted beats are sensed and the pacemaker inhibits its output appropriately.

DEFIBRILLATION AND CARDIOVERSION

Defibrillation

Defibrillation is the therapeutic delivery of electrical energy to the myocardium to terminate life-threatening ventricular dysrhythmias (VF and pulseless VT). The defibrillating shock depolarizes all cells in the heart simultaneously, stopping all electrical activity and allowing the sinus node to resume its function as the normal pacemaker of the heart. Early defibrillation is the only treatment for VF or pulseless VT and should not be delayed for any reason when a defibrillator is available. If a defibrillator is not immediately available, CPR should be started until a defibrillator arrives.

Defibrillation is done externally using two paddles or adhesive pads applied to the skin in the anterolateral position (Figure 3-52A). One paddle or pad is placed under the right clavicle to the right of the sternum and the other paddle or pad is placed to the left of the cardiac apex. If paddles are used, place conductive gel pads on the patient's skin, then place paddles on the gel pads using 25 lb of pressure to decrease transthoracic impedance and protect the skin from burns. Avoid placing paddles over medication patches or over pacemaker or ICD pulse generators.

Advanced Cardiac Life Support (ACLS) guidelines recommend an initial energy of 360 J with a monophasic defibrillator and the manufacturer's recommended energy level for biphasic defibrillators. If the manufacturer's suggested energy level is not known, a 200-J shock is recommended. Make sure no one is touching the patient, the bed, or anything attached to the patient when the shock is delivered; call "all clear" and visually verify before delivering the shock. Depress the discharge button to release the energy. If using paddles, depress both discharge buttons (one on each paddle) simultaneously. The shock is delivered immediately when buttons are pushed (Figure 3-53A). Immediately resume CPR for 2 minutes before rhythm and pulse check (this may be modified in a monitored situation where ECG and hemodynamic monitoring is available).

Automatic External Defibrillators

An automatic external defibrillator (AED) is a device that incorporates a rhythm-analysis system and a shock advisory system for use by trained laypeople or medical personnel in treating victims of sudden cardiac death. The American Heart Association recommends that AEDs should be available in selected areas where large gatherings of people occur and where immediate access to emergency care may be limited, such as on airplanes, in airports, sports stadiums, health and fitness facilities, and so on. It is well known that early defibrillation is the key to survival in patients experiencing VF or pulseless VT. Any delay in the delivery of the first shock, including delays related to waiting for the arrival of trained medical personnel and equipment, can decrease the chance of survival. The availability of an AED in public areas can prevent unnecessary delays in treatment and improve survival in victims of sudden cardiac death.

Operation of an AED is quite simple and can be performed by laypeople. Instructions for use are printed on the machines and voice commands also guide the operator in using the AED. Adhesive pads are placed in the standard defibrillation position on the chest (see Figure 3-52A), the machine is turned on, and the rhythm analysis system analyzes the patient's rhythm. If the rhythm analysis system detects a shockable rhythm, such as VF or rapid VT, a voice advises the operator to shock the patient. Delivery of the shock is a simple maneuver that only involves pushing a button. The operator is advised to "stand clear" prior to delivering the shock. After a shock is delivered, the system prompts the operator to resume CPR. After 2 minutes of CPR, it prompts the operator to stop CPR while it reanalyzes the rhythm.

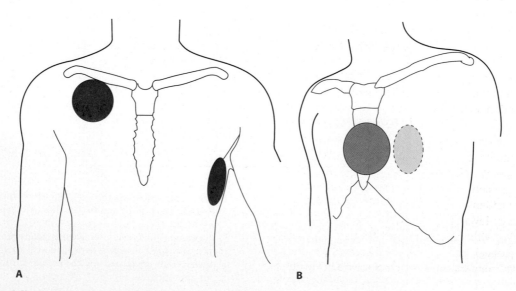

A   **B**

Figure 3-52. Paddle or adhesive pad placement for external defibrillation via **(A)** anterolateral position and **(B)** anteroposterior position.

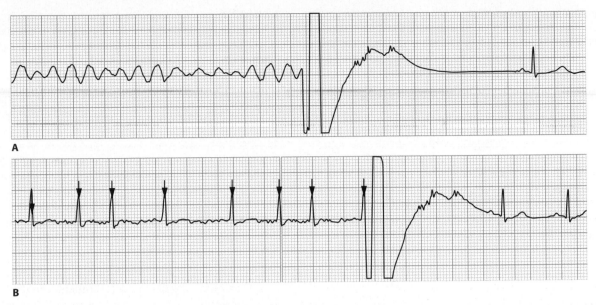

Figure 3-53. **(A)** Defibrillation of VF to sinus rhythm. **(B)** Cardioversion of atrial fibrillation to sinus rhythm. Note the synchronization mark on the QRS.

Cardioversion

Cardioversion is the delivery of electrical energy that is synchronized to the QRS complex so that the energy is delivered during ventricular depolarization in order to avoid the T wave and the vulnerable period of ventricular repolarization. The delivery of electrical energy near the T wave can lead to VF. Synchronized cardioversion is used to terminate both SVT and VTs and is usually an elective procedure, although it should be performed urgently if the patient is hemodynamically unstable. Cardioversion can be performed via anterolateral electrode placement (see Figure 3-52A) or via anteroposterior (AP) electrode placement (see Figure 3-52B). AP placement is preferred because less energy is required and the success rate is higher when energy travels through the short axis of the chest. Either paddles or hands-free adhesive pads can be used.

Sedation is required for cardioversion since the patient is usually awake and alert and able to feel the pain caused by the procedure. The selection of medications to accomplish sedation depends on physician discretion and hospital policy, or an anesthesiologist may be called to place the patient under deep sedation. Because sedation is used, an emergency cart equipped with emergency medications (lidocaine, epinephrine, amiodarone, atropine), sedation-reversal agents, O_2-delivery equipment, and suction equipment should be immediately available. The patient's blood pressure and oxygen saturation are continuously monitored during the procedure until the patient is completely awake and recovered.

Initial energy level for cardioversion is typically 50 to 100 J and varies with different dysrhythmias. If the first shock is unsuccessful, energy level is increased for subsequent shocks. The machine must be synchronized to the QRS complex for cardioversion. Most machines put a bright dot or similar marker on the QRS complex when in the "synch" mode (Figure 3-53B). The machine will not discharge its energy until it sees the synch marker. Make sure to visually verify that the synch marker is actually on the QRS complex and not on a tall T wave. When delivering energy during cardioversion, push and hold the discharge button until the energy is delivered; the synchronized machine will not discharge until it sees a QRS complex. When the energy is released, the machine automatically returns to the asynchronous mode, so if subsequent shocks are needed, the machine must be resynchronized.

SELECTED BIBLIOGRAPHY

Bradfield JS, Boyle NG, Shivkumar K. Ventricular arrhythmias. In: Fuster V, Harrington RA, Narula J, Eapen ZJ, eds. *Hurst's the Heart.* 14th ed. New York, NY: McGraw Hill; 2017.

Calkins H. Supraventricular tachycardia: atrial tachycardia, atrioventricular nodal reentry, and Wolff-Parkinson-White syndrome. In: Fuster V, Harrington RA, Narula J, Eapen ZJ, eds. *Hurst's the Heart.* 14th ed. New York, NY: McGraw Hill; 2017.

Jacobson C, Marzlin K, Webner C. *Cardiovascular Nursing Practice 3rd ed: Cardiac Arrhythmias & 12 Lead ECG Interpretation.* Burien, WA: Cardiovascular Nursing Education Associates; 2021.

Evidence-Based Practice

AACN Practice Alert: Accurate dysrhythmia monitoring in adults. *Crit Care Nurs.* 2016;36(6):e26-e34. https://www.aacn.org/clinical-resources/practice-alerts/dysrhythmia-monitoring

Al-Khatib SM, Stevenson WG, Ackerman MJ, et al. 2017 AHA/ACC/HRS guideline for management of patients with ventricular arrhythmias and the prevention of sudden cardiac death: a report of the American College of Cardiology/American Heart Association Task Force on Practice Guidelines and the Heart Rhythm Society. *Heart Rhythm.* 2018;15:e73-e189.

Drew BJ, Ackerman MJ, Funk M. Prevention of Torsade de Pointes in hospital settings. *J Am Coll Cardiol.* 2010;55:934-947.

January CT, Wann LS, Alpert JS, et al. 2014 AHA/ACC/HRS guideline for the management of patients with atrial fibrillation: a report of the American College of Cardiology/American Heart Association Task Force on Practice Guidelines and the Heart Rhythm Society. *Circulation*. 2014;130:e199-e267.

January, CT, Wann, LS, Calkins, H, et al. 2019 AHA/ACC/HRS focused update of the 2014 AHA/ACC/HRS guideline for the management of patients with atrial fibrillation: a report of the American College of Cardiology/American Heart Association Task Force on Practice Guidelines and the Heart Rhythm Society. *Circulation*. 2019;140:e125-e151.

Kusumoto, F.M., Schoenfeld. M.H., Barrett, C., et al. 2018 ACC/AHA/HRS guideline on the evaluation and management of patients with bradycardia and cardiac conduction delay: a report of the American College of Cardiology/American Heart Association Task Force on Clinical Practice Guidelines and the Heart Rhythm Society. *Circulation*. 2019;140:e382-e482.

Link MS, Berkow LC, Kudenchuk PJ, et al. Part 7: adult advanced cardiovascular life support: 2015 American Heart Association guidelines update for cardiopulmonary resuscitation and emergency cardiovascular care. *Circulation*. 2015;132:S444.

Page RL, Joglar JA, Caldwell MA, et al. ACC/AHA/HRS guideline for the management of adult patients with supraventricular tachycardia: a report of the American College of Cardiology/American Heart Association Task Force on Practice Guidelines and the Heart Rhythm Society. *Circulation*. 2016;133:e506-e574.

Priori SG, Blomstrom-Lundqvist C, Mazzanti A, et al. 2015 ESC guidelines for the management of patients with ventricular arrhythmias and the prevention of sudden cardiac death. *Eur Heart J*. 2015;36:2793-2867.

Sandau K, Funk M, Auerbach A, et al. Update to practice standards for electrocardiographic monitoring in hospital settings: a scientific statement from the American Heart Association. *Circulation*. 2017;136:e273-e344.

HEMODYNAMIC MONITORING

4

Mary Jo Kelly and Elizabeth J. Bridges

KNOWLEDGE COMPETENCIES

1. Identify the characteristics of normal and abnormal waveform pressures for the following hemodynamic monitoring parameters:
   - Central venous pressure
   - Pulmonary artery pressure
   - Arterial blood pressure

2. Describe the basic elements of hemodynamic pressure-monitoring equipment and methods used to ensure accurate pressure measurements.

3. Discuss the indications, contraindications, and general management principles for the following common hemodynamic monitoring parameters:
   - Central venous pressure
   - Pulmonary artery pressure
   - Mixed venous oxygenation

   - Arterial blood pressure
   - Cardiac output

4. Describe the use of SvO_2/$ScvO_2$ monitoring in the critically ill patient.

5. Describe the use of functional hemodynamic measures, including analysis of pulse pressure and stroke volume variation during positive pressure ventilation, and the passive leg raising maneuver.

6. Describe the use of peripheral perfusion indicators, including of capillary refill time and skin mottling in critically ill patients.

7. Compare and contrast the clinical implications and management approaches to abnormal hemodynamic values.

OVERVIEW

The term *hemodynamics* refers to the interrelationship of blood pressure (BP), blood flow, vascular volumes, heart rate (HR), ventricular function, and the physical properties of the blood. Monitoring the hemodynamic status of the critically ill patient is an integral part of critical care nursing. It is essential that critical care nurses have a working knowledge of how to obtain accurate data, analyze waveforms, and interpret and integrate the data.

Clinical examination findings such as mental status, urine output, edema, jugular venous distention, capillary refill time, skin mottling, skin temperature, and skin color provide some data about a patient's fluid balance,

oxygenation, and perfusion. Additional data can be obtained through noninvasive and invasive hemodynamic monitoring and functional hemodynamic assessment. Parameters such as arterial BP, cardiac output (CO), pulmonary arterial pressure (PAP), and intracardiac pressures can be directly measured and monitored with special indwelling catheters. Less invasive evaluations include the passive leg raise (PLR) maneuver and cardiovascular ultrasound. Analysis of changes in the arterial waveforms in patients on positive pressure mechanical ventilation can also provide information about the patient's fluid responsiveness that guides management. Understanding how to gather hemodynamic data and interpret it is an essential function of the critical care nurse.

Adapted from Leanna R. Miller

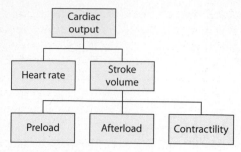

Figure 4-1. Factors affecting CO.

ANATOMY AND PHYSIOLOGY

Cardiac Output

CO is the amount of blood pumped by the ventricles each minute. It is the product of the HR and the stroke volume (SV) which is the amount of blood ejected by the ventricle with each contraction. See Figure 4-1.

$$CO = HR \times SV$$

The normal value of cardiac output is 4.0 to 8.0 L/min (Table 4-1). It is important to note that CO values are relative to size. Values within the normal range for a person 5-ft tall weighing 100 lb, may be totally inadequate for a 6-ft, 200-lb individual. Cardiac index (CI) is the CO that has been adjusted to individual body size. It is determined by dividing the CO by the individual's body surface area (BSA), which may be obtained from the DuBois body surface area chart. The conversion to CI has been automated into monitors. The normal value for CI is 2.5 to 4.3 L/min/m^2 (see Table 4-1).

$$CI = CO/BSA$$

CO measurements are used to assess the patient's perfusion status, response to therapy, and hemodynamic status.

$$CO = \text{Stroke Volume} \times \text{Heart Rate}$$

The stroke volume is the difference between the volume of blood in the ventricle just before contraction (end-diastolic volume) and the volume of blood left in the ventricle after contraction (end-systolic volume).

TABLE 4-1.   NORMAL HEMODYNAMIC AND BLOOD FLOW PARAMETERS

Parameter	Abbreviation	Formula	Normal Range
Cardiac output	CO	Stroke volume (SV) × heart rate (HR)	4-8 L/min
Cardiac index	CI	CO/BSA ÷ 1000	2.5-4.3 L/min/m^2
Cardiac Output (Fick)	CO	VO$_2$ × BSA/[(SaO$_2$ – SvO$_2$) × Hgb × 13.4 \newline *VO$_2$ = 125	
Mean arterial pressure	MAP	2(DBP) + SBP ÷ 3	70-105 mm Hg
Right atrial pressure	RAP	cm H$_2$O = mm Hg × 1.34	2-8 mm Hg
Pulmonary artery occlusion pressure	PAOP		8-12 mm Hg
Pulmonary artery systolic	PAS		15-35 mm Hg
Pulmonary artery diastolic	PAD		10-15 mm Hg
Pulmonary vascular resistance	PVR	PAM – PAOP × 80 ÷ CO	100-250 dynes/s/cm^{-5}
Pulmonary vascular resistance index	PVRI	PAM – PAOP × 80 ÷ CI	255-285 dynes/s/cm^{-5}/m^2
Pulmonary artery mean	PAM		15-20 mm Hg
Systemic vascular resistance	SVR	MAP – RAP × 80 ÷ CO	800-1200 dynes/s/cm^{-5}
Systemic vascular resistance index	SVRI	MAP – RAP × 80 ÷ CI	1970-2390 dynes/s/cm^{-5}/m^2
Right ventricular stroke work index	RVSWI	(PAM – RAP) SVI × 0.0138	7-12 g/m/m^2/beat
Left ventricular stroke work index	LVSWI	(MAP – PAOP) SVI × 0.0138	35-85 g/m/m^2/beat
Oxygen delivery	DO$_2$	CaO$_2$ × CO × 10 \newline (Hgb × 1.34 × SaO$_2$) × (HR × SV) × 10	900-1100 mL/min
Oxygen delivery index	DO$_2$I	CaO$_2$ × CI × 10	360-600 mL/min/m^2
Oxygen consumption	VO$_2$	C(a – v)O$_2$ × CO × 10	200-250 mL/min
Oxygen consumption index	VO$_2$I	C(a – v)O$_2$ × CI × 10	108-165 mL/min/m^2
Stroke volume	SV	CO/HR × 1000	50-100 mL/beat
Stroke volume index	SVI	CI/HR × 1000	35-60 mL/beat/m^2
Ejection fraction	EF		>60%
Right ventricular end-diastolic volume	RVEDV	SV/EF	100-160 mL
Right ventricular end-diastolic volume index	RVEDVI	EDV/BSA	600-100 mL/m^2
Right ventricular end-systolic volume	RVESV	EDV – SV	50-100 mL
Right ventricular end-systolic volume index	RVESVI	ESV/BSA	30-60 mL/m^2
Right ventricular ejection fraction	RVEF	SV/EDV	40%-60%
Mixed venous saturation	SvO$_2$		60%-80%
Oxygen extraction ratio	O$_2$ER	(CaO$_2$ – CvO$_2$)/CaO$_2$ × 100	22%-30%

Normal SV range is 50 to 100 mL/beat (see Table 4-1). SV depends on preload, afterload, and contractility. Therefore, CO is determined by:

1. Heart rate (and rhythm)
2. Preload
3. Afterload
4. Contractility

Low Cardiac Output/Cardiac Index

Because the SV of the left ventricle is a component used in the determination of CO, any condition or disease process that impairs the pumping (ejection) or filling of the ventricle may contribute to a decreased CO. Alterations that lead to diminished CO can be divided into two general categories: inadequate ventricular filling and inadequate ventricular emptying.

Factors that lead to inadequate ventricular filling include arrhythmias, hypovolemia, cardiac tamponade, mitral or tricuspid stenosis, diastolic dysfunction, constrictive pericarditis, and restrictive cardiomyopathy. Each of these abnormalities leads to a decrease in preload (the amount of volume in the ventricle at end diastole), which results in a decrease in SV and CO.

Factors that lead to inadequate ventricular emptying include mitral/tricuspid insufficiency, myocardial infarction, increased afterload (hypertension, aortic/pulmonic stenosis), myocardial diseases (myocarditis, cardiomyopathies), metabolic disorders (hypoglycemia, hypoxia, severe acidosis), and use of negative inotropic drugs (beta-blockers, calcium channel blockers).

High Cardiac Output/Index

In theory, in the normal, healthy individual, factors that increase heart rate and contractility and decrease afterload within normal compensatory limits, can contribute to an increase in venous return and preload, which increase the CO. Hyperdynamic states, such as in sepsis, anemia, pregnancy, and hyperthyroid crisis, may cause CO values to be increased. Increased heart rate is a major component in hyperdynamic states; however, in sepsis a profound decrease in afterload also contributes to an increased CO.

Components of Cardiac Output/Cardiac Index

Heart Rate

Normal heart rate is 60 to 100 beats/min. In a healthy individual, an increase in heart rate can lead to an increase in CO. In a person with cardiac dysfunction, increases in heart rate can lead to a decreased CO and may cause myocardial ischemia. An increase in heart rate to 130 beats/min or greater decreases the ventricular filling time causing a drop in preload and SV and subsequent decrease in CO. An increase in heart rate also decreases diastolic time, which results in a decrease in coronary artery perfusion.

A lower heart rate does not necessarily result in a decrease in CO. For example, athletes may have a decreased heart rate with a normal CO. Their training and conditioning strengthen the myocardium such that each cardiac contraction produces an increased SV. In individuals with left ventricular (LV) dysfunction, a slow heart rate can produce a decrease in CO. This is caused by decreased contractility, as well as fewer cardiac contractions each minute.

Because CO is a product of SV times heart rate, any change in SV normally produces a change in the heart rate. Bradycardias and tachycardias are potentially dangerous because they may result in a decrease in CO if adequate stroke volume is not maintained. Sudden-onset bradycardia may cause a decrease in CO. The cause of tachycardia, on the other hand, must be determined because it may not reflect a low output state but rather a normal physiologic response (eg, tachycardia secondary to fever). Heart rate varies between individuals and is related to many factors. Some are described here.

DECREASED HEART RATE

- Parasympathetic stimulation (vagus nerve stimulation) is a common occurrence in the critical care setting. It can occur with a Valsalva maneuver, such as excessive bearing down during a bowel movement, vomiting, coughing, and suctioning.
- Conduction abnormalities, especially second- and third-degree blocks, are often seen in patients with cardiovascular diseases. Many drugs used in the critical care setting may lead to a decreased heart rate, including digitalis, beta-blockers, calcium channel blockers, and reflex bradycardia may occur with phenylephrine (Neosynephrine).
- Athletes often have resting heart rates below 60 beats/min without compromising CO.
- The actual heart rate is not as important as the systemic effect of the heart rate. If the patient's heart rate leads to diminished perfusion (manifested as decreased level of consciousness, decreased urinary output, hypotension, prolonged capillary refill time, new-onset chest pain, etc.), treatment is initiated to increase the heart rate as appropriate.

INCREASED HEART RATE

- Stress, anxiety, pain, and conditions resulting in compensatory release of endogenous catecholamines such as hypovolemia (eg, hemorrhage, severe diarrhea), fever, anemia, and hypotension may all produce tachycardia.
- Drugs with a direct positive chronotropic effect include epinephrine, dopamine, and norepinephrine.

Tachycardia is common in critically ill patients. When evaluating a rapid heart rate, each of the main sources for the tachycardia is evaluated; for example, if a patient has a heart rate of 120 beats/min, the clinician considers such factors as fever, pain, and anxiety before assuming that the tachycardia is due to a reduced SV. The two most common reasons for a low SV are hypovolemia and LV dysfunction. Both causes of low SV can produce an increased heart rate if no abnormality exists in regulation of the heart rate (such as autonomic nervous system dysfunction or use of drugs that interfere with the sympathetic or parasympathetic nervous system such as beta-blockers).

An increased heart rate can compensate for a decrease in SV, although this compensation is limited. The faster the heart rate, the less time exists for ventricular filling. As an increased heart rate reduces diastolic filling time, the potential exists to eventually reduce the SV. There is no specific heart rate where diastolic filling is reduced so severely that SV decreases. However, as the heart rate increases, it is important to remember that SV may be negatively affected.

Increased heart rate also has the potential to increase myocardial oxygen demand (MVO_2). The higher the heart rate, the more likely it is that the heart consumes more oxygen. Some patients are more sensitive to elevated MVO_2 than others; for example, a young person may tolerate a sinus tachycardia as high as 160 beats/min for several days, whereas a patient with coronary artery disease may decompensate and develop pulmonary edema with a heart rate in the 130s. Controlling heart rate, particularly in patients with altered myocardial blood flow, is one way of protecting myocardial function.

Heart Rhythm

Supraventricular tachycardia, or a change from normal sinus rhythm to atrial fibrillation or flutter may cause clinical decompensation. Loss of "atrial kick" may contribute to decreased CO. Normally, atrial contraction contributes 20% to 40% of the ventricular filling volume. With tachycardia, that atrial contribution to SV may diminish significantly. Although those with normal cardiac function are unlikely to experience compromise, it is more likely in those with impaired cardiac function.

Stroke Volume and Stroke Volume Index

Stroke volume is the amount of blood ejected from each ventricle with each heartbeat. The right and left ventricles eject nearly the same amount, which is normally from 50 to 100 mL per heartbeat (see Table 4-1).

$$SV = CO/HR \times 1000$$

Just as CI indexes CO to patient BSA, stroke volume index (SVI) indexes SV to BSA. The BSA calculation is generally built into technology (based on body weight and height), but online calculators can also be used. A pharmacist can also assist with the calculation of BSA as it is frequently used to determine medication dosing. Indexing helps to compare values regardless of the patient's size. This is calculated by most monitors. Normal SVI is 35 to 60 mL/beat/m^2 (see Table 4-1). Common causes of decreased stroke volume/stroke volume index (SV/SVI) are inadequate blood volume (preload), impaired ventricular contractility (strength), increased systemic vascular resistance (SVR; afterload), and cardiac valve dysfunction. High SV/SVI occurs when the vascular resistance is low (as in

distributive shock states such as sepsis, use of vasodilators, neurogenic shock, and anaphylaxis).

Ejection Fraction

The *ejection fraction* (EF) is defined as a measurement, expressed as a percentage, of how much blood the ventricle pumps out with each contraction in relation to the volume of available blood. For example, assume the LV end-diastolic volume (LVEDV is the amount of blood left in the heart just before contraction) is 100 mL. If the SV is 80 mL the EF is 80%; 80 mL of the possible 100 mL in the ventricle was ejected. Right ventricular (RV) volumes are roughly equal to those of the left ventricle (see Table 4-1). A normal value for EF is greater than 60%.

The EF may change before the SV in certain conditions, such as LV failure and sepsis. For example, the left ventricle may dilate in response to LV dysfunction from coronary artery disease, and LVEDV increases. If the heart can contract effectively with this larger end-diastolic volume, the EF may remain the same. In heart failure, if the EF is <40%, this is referred to as Heart Failure with Reduced Ejection Fraction (HFrEF). It is important to remember that approximately 50% of the patients with heart failure (HF) have a normal EF (Heart Failure Preserved EF [HFpEF] > 40%), which will influence monitoring and volume resuscitation. Unfortunately, EF and LVEDV are not routinely available. The SV and SVI are measures to assess left and right ventricular dysfunction. The SV is very important because it typically decreases with hypovolemia or with left ventricular dysfunction (ie, the left ventricle is too weak to eject blood).

Factors Affecting Stroke Volume/Stroke Volume Index

Preload

Preload is the distending force that stretches the ventricular myocardium during diastole. Clinically, it is described as the filling pressure of the ventricles at the end of diastole; for example, right-ventricular end-diastolic pressure (estimated by RAP) is right-ventricular preload and left-ventricular end-diastolic pressure (estimated by the PAOP) is left-ventricular preload.

According to the Frank-Starling principle, the force of contraction is related to myocardial fiber stretch prior to contraction. As the fibers are stretched, the contractile force increases up to a certain point. Beyond this point, the contractile force decreases and is referred to as *ventricular failure* (Figure 4-2). Increased preload reflects an increase in end-diastolic blood volume, which stretches the myocardium, resulting in a more forceful ventricular contraction. This forceful ventricular contraction yields an increase in SV, and therefore, CO. Too much preload causes the ventricular contraction to be less effective (flat portion of the ventricular function curve).

Determinants of Preload

Preload is determined primarily by the amount of venous return to the heart. Venous constriction, venous dilation,

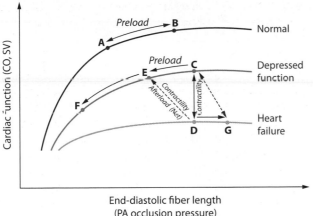

Figure 4-2. Family of ventricular function curves. Family of ventricular function curves representing normal, depressed, and severely depressed function. A change in preload is represented by a move up or down a single curve (Frank-Starling principle). Point A to point B and point B to point A reflect an increase and decrease, respectively, in preload. The response to volume loading is dependent on the position on the ventricular function curve and the shape of the curve. If both ventricles are on the steep portion of the curve the SV will increase in response to volume (responder). In contrast if the heart is on the flat portion of the curve the SV will not increase (nonresponder). A change in afterload results in a shift in the curve that appears similar to that caused by contractility, although the mechanism is different. Point D to E reflects the net effect of a decrease in afterload on a failing heart. This upward and lateral shift is the result of two actions. Point D to C reflects an increase in force of contraction and point C to E a decrease in preload due to increased systolic ejection. A change in contractility is represented by an upward or downward shift of the curve, that is, for any given preload and afterload, the CO is increased or decreased. In a failing heart, an additional effect of decreased contractility is an increase in preload due to decreased systolic ejection; thus, the net effect of a decrease in contractility is to shift the curve down and to the left (Point C to G). (*Reproduced with permission from Woods SL, Sivarajan-Froelicher ES, Motzer S, et al: Cardiac Nursing, 6th ed. Philadelphia, PA: Lippincott; 2010. Figure 21-8.*)

and alterations in the total blood volume all affect preload. Preload decreases with volume change. This can occur in hemorrhage (traumatic, surgical, gastrointestinal [GI], postpartum), diuresis (excessive use of diuretics, diabetic ketoacidosis, diabetes insipidus), vomiting and diarrhea, third spacing (ascites, severe burns, severe sepsis, HF), redistribution of blood flow (use of vasodilators, neurogenic shock, distributive shock states including severe sepsis), and profound diaphoresis. Venous dilatation also results in diminished preload. Etiologies that increase venous pooling and result in decreased venous return to the heart include hyperthermia, septic shock, anaphylactic shock, and medication administration (nitroglycerin, nitroprusside) (Table 4-2).

Factors leading to increased preload include excessive administration of crystalloids, colloids, or blood products, renal failure (oliguric phase and/or anuria), and venous constriction that results in the shunting of peripheral blood to the central organs (heart and brain). The increased venous return results in an increased preload. This may occur in hypothermia, some forms of shock (cardiogenic and

obstructive), and with administration of drugs that stimulate the alpha receptors (epinephrine, dopamine at doses >10 mcg/kg/min, norepinephrine) (see Table 4-2).

Clinical Indicators of Preload

The right ventricle (RV) ejects blood into the pulmonary circulation and the left ventricle ejects blood into the systemic circulation. Both circulatory systems are affected by preload, afterload, and contractility.

Right Ventricular Preload

Normal right ventricular (RV) pressure is 2 to 8 mm Hg or 2 to 10 cm H_2O (see Table 4-1) Right atrial pressure (RAP) is measured to assess right ventricular function, and the response to fluid and drug administration. While the central venous pressure (CVP) is often used in clinical practice as an indicator of intravascular volume, this is only one factor that affects the CVP/RAP. In general, there are three etiologies of RV failure:

1. Intrinsic disease such as RV infarct or cardiomyopathies;
2. Secondary to factors that increase pulmonary vascular resistance (PVR) such as pulmonary arterial hypertension, pulmonary embolism, hypoxemia, chronic obstructive pulmonary disease (COPD), cor pulmonale, acute respiratory distress syndrome (ARDS), acidosis and sepsis; and
3. Severe LV dysfunction as seen in mitral stenosis/insufficiency or LV failure.

The only clinically significant reason for a decreased CVP/RAP is hypovolemia (absolute or relative due to vasodilation). Note that an individual may have a relatively low CVP without hypovolemia. Thus a low CVP, without other indications of hypoperfusion, is not a reason for volume resuscitation. The CVP/RAP may be increased with volume resuscitation, right heart failure, concomitant left ventricular failure, hypoxia, and the application of positive end-expiratory pressure (PEEP) in mechanically ventilated patients. The CVP/RAP may also be increased by cardiac tamponade (effusion, blood, etc.) and restrictive cardiomyopathies. CVP/RAP is a late indicator of alterations in LV function therefore limiting its value in clinical decision making. In general, the CVP and RAP are not accurate predictors of whether a patient will respond to a fluid challenge.

Left Ventricular Preload

Normal LV preload is 8 to 12 mm Hg (PAEDP = pulmonary artery end-diastolic pressure; PAOP = pulmonary artery occlusion pressure; LAP = left atrial pressure). The most commonly used term is PAOP (see Table 4-1). With the insertion of 1.25 to 1.50 mL of air into the balloon port of the pulmonary artery (PA) catheter, the balloon becomes lodged in a portion of the PA that is smaller than the balloon, which occludes blood flow distal to the catheter tip. The pressure in the left atrium is then sensed at the catheter tip. When the

TABLE 4-2. HEMODYNAMIC EFFECTS OF CARDIOVASCULAR AGENTS

Drug	CO	PAOP	SVR	MAP	HR	CVP	PVR
Norepinephrine (Levophed)	↑ (slight)	↑	↑	↑	↔, ↑	↑	↑
Phenylephrine (Neosynephrine)	↔,↓	↑	↑	↑	↔,↓	↑	↑
Epinephrine (Asthmahaler)	↑	↑	↑	↑	↑	↑	↑
Dobutamine	↑	↓	↓	↑	↔, ↑	↓	↓
(Dobutrex)				(with ↑ CO)	(slight)		↑
Dopamine (Intropin)	↑	↑	↑	↑			↔
<5 mcg/kg/min	↑	↑↑	(slight)	(slight)	↑	↑↑	↑
>5 mcg/kg/min			↑↑	↑↑			
Digoxin (Lanoxin)	↑	↔	↔	↔	↓	↔	↔
Isoproterenol (Isuprel)	↑	↓	↓	↓	↑	↓	↓
Vasopressin	↔, ↓ (related to ↑ SVR)	↑	↑	↑	↔, ↓	↑	↑
Milrinone (Primacor)	↑	↓	↓	↔ (↓ in preload-sensitive patient)	↔ (↑ in preload-sensitive patient)	↓	↓
Nitroglycerin (Tridil)							
20-40 mcg/min	↔	↓	↔	↔	↔	↓	↔
50-250 mcg/min (max dose)	↑	↓	↓	↓	↑	↓	↓
Nitroprusside (Nipride)	↑	↓	↓	↓	↑	↓	↓

mitral valve is open during ventricular diastole, the pressure that is sensed is that of the left ventricle, the left ventricular end-diastolic pressure (LVEDP), or LV preload (Figure 4-3). PAOP thus estimates LVEDP.

PAOP increases because of conditions such as intravascular volume overload, cardiac tamponade (blood, effusion, etc.), impaired ventricular relaxation (diastolic dysfunction, restrictive cardiomyopathy, and constrictive pericarditis), and LV dysfunction. Common etiologies of LV dysfunction include mitral stenosis/insufficiency, aortic stenosis/insufficiency, and diminished LV compliance (ischemia, fibrosis, hypertrophy). Clinically significant reasons for a decreased PAOP

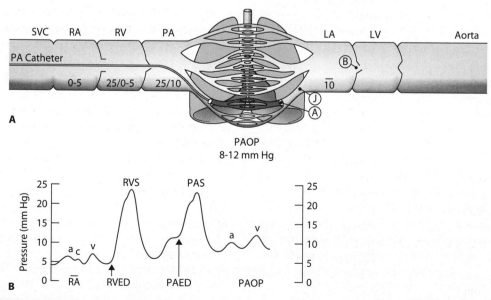

Figure 4-3. Schema of the cardiopulmonary circuit and the principle underlying the use of the PAOP as an indicator of LV preload. **(A)** When the inflated balloon on the catheter obstructs arterial flow, the catheter records the pressure at the junction of the static column of fluid and flowing venous channels (J-point). The J-point occurs in the venous system, approximately 1.5 cm from the left atria. **(B)** Characteristic waveforms observed as the PA catheter is "floated" from the RA through the right ventricle (RV) and into the PA where it occludes flow (pulmonary artery occlusion pressure [PAOP]). Note that the mean RA pressure is similar to the RV end-diastolic pressure (RVEDP), the RV systolic (RVS) and PA systolic (PAS) pressures are similar, and that there is a step-up in pressure as the catheter crosses the pulmonic valve and enters the PA. In a correctly positioned catheter, the PAOP is lower than the mean PA pressure and has a waveform that is relatively similar to the RAP (although slightly delayed relative to the ECG). (*Reproduced with permission from Woods SL, Sivarajan-Froelicher ES, Motzer S, et al: Cardiac Nursing, 6th ed. Philadelphia, PA: Lippincott; 2010. Figure 21-12.*)

are hypovolemia (absolute) and relative hypovolemia due to profound vasodilation.

There are some conditions in which PAOP and LVEDP do not correlate. LV failure with PAOP greater than 15 to 20 mm Hg and conditions with diminished LV compliance result in a PAOP less than the true LVEDP. Patients on PEEP (continuous positive airway pressure), zone 1 or 2 catheter tip placement, tachycardia (>130 beats/min), mitral stenosis/insufficiency, COPD, or pulmonary veno-occlusive disease have a measured PAOP that is greater than the true LVEDP. These factors must be considered prior to therapeutic management.

The PAEDP is normally 1 to 4 mm Hg higher than the PAOP due to resistance of blood flow into the pulmonary vessels. However, when the PA catheter is "wedged," there is no flow or resistance to flow, and the measured value reflects left atrial pressure (and left ventricular end-diastolic pressure when the mitral valve is open) transmitted across the static column of blood. In the presence of increased PVR, the PAEDP and PAOP no longer agree and cannot be used interchangeably. If the PAEDP and PAOP closely agree, the PAEDP can be used to trend the LVEDP without inflating the balloon. This allows prolonged balloon life, and reduces the risk for pulmonary ischemia, PA damage, and rupture that can occur with repeated PAOP measurements. Institutional policy guides the frequency of measuring PAOP.

Afterload

Afterload is the resistance to ventricular emptying during systole. It is the pressure or resistance that the ventricles must overcome to open the aortic and pulmonic valves and to pump blood into the systemic and pulmonary vasculature.

Vascular resistance is determined by the length of a vessel, its diameter or radius, and the viscosity of the blood. The length of the vessel is considered constant. The viscosity of the blood is relatively constant except when gross volume changes occur (eg, hemorrhage) or in polycythemia. Therefore, conditions that alter the diameter of the vessels, or the outflow tract, have a primary effect on the afterload of the ventricles.

As afterload increases, due to vasoconstriction or obstruction of the ventricular outflow tract, the heart must work harder to eject the volume. Afterload affects the isovolumetric contraction phase of the cardiac cycle. During this phase, the ventricular pressure rises so the ventricles are able to overcome the existing vascular resistance, open the semilunar valves, and eject the contents. Once the pressure within the ventricle is higher than the pressure in the aorta/pulmonary system, the valves open and the blood is ejected from the heart. With increased afterload the heart works harder to eject the contents, leading to increased myocardial oxygen consumption (MVO_2). This increased workload is a crucial period of myocardial susceptibility to ischemic injury and is a major reason to consider afterload reduction therapies.

Common causes of increased afterload include aortic/pulmonic stenosis, hypothermia, hypertension, compensatory responses to hypotension and decreased CO, classic shock states (hypovolemic, cardiogenic, and obstructive), and response to drugs that stimulate the alpha receptors (epinephrine, norepinephrine, dopamine, and phenylephrine) (see Table 4-2). Decreased afterload is seen in hyperthermia, the distributive shocks (septic, anaphylactic, and neurogenic), and after administration of vasodilating drugs (nitroprusside, nitroglycerin at higher doses, calcium channel blockers, betablockers, etc.) (see Table 4-2).

Clinical Indicators of Afterload

Unlike preload, afterload cannot be directly measured. Several hemodynamic parameters are calculated based on other measured variables. These parameters are usually referred to as *derived values*. Formulas for some common derived variables are listed in Table 4-1. Most bedside monitors perform the calculations necessary to determine these values. However, critical care nurses need to know which variables are included in the calculations. This knowledge is essential to understand how hemodynamic parameters interact, how derived variables are interpreted, and how they guide the selection of appropriate therapy.

Systemic Vascular Resistance

Normal SVR is 800 to 1200 dynes-s/cm^{-5} (see Table 4-1). If the SVR is elevated, the left ventricle faces an increased resistance to the ejection of blood. The SVR commonly elevates as a compensatory response in hypotension or a low CO, such as would occur in classic shock states. It is important for the clinician to know why the SVR is elevated; for example, if the SVR is elevated because of systemic hypertension, afterload-reducing agents are a critical part of the therapy. However, if the SVR is elevated secondary to a compensation for low CO, therapy is directed toward the primary goal of improving CO to reduce the SVR.

If the SVR is low, the left ventricle faces a lower resistance to the ejection of blood. Generally, the SVR only decreases as a pathologic response to inflammatory conditions that cause vasodilation (eg, systemic inflammatory response [SIRS], sepsis, fever). The SVR can also be reduced in hepatic disease due to increased collateral circulation or from neurogenic-induced central vasodilation. Generally, if the SVR is reduced, administration of fluid and/or vasopressor drugs is considered. More important, treating the underlying condition is essential. If the underlying condition leading to reduced SVR is not treated, the use of vasopressors provides only short-term improvement.

Pulmonary Vascular Resistance

PVR is lower in comparison to SVR. Normal PVR is about 100 to 250 dynes-s/cm^{-5} (see Table 4-1). Generally, only an elevated PVR is considered a problem, because it produces a strain on the RV. If this strain is unrelieved, the RV may eventually fail. Failure of the RV results in decreased RV stroke volume, which subsequently decreases left ventricular preload and stroke volume. Systemic hypotension may occur due to RV dysfunction. As noted previously, the most common causes of an increase in PVR include pulmonary arterial hypertension, pulmonary embolism, hypoxemia, COPD, cor pulmonale, ARDS, acidosis, and sepsis.

ESSENTIAL CONTENT CASE

High SVR

A 73-year-old woman is in the critical care unit with the diagnosis of acute decompensated HF. She presently is alert and oriented but complains of severe shortness of breath. Her pulse oximeter reveals a value of 89% on a fraction of inspired oxygen content (Fio_2) of 50% via a high-humidity face mask. She has crackles throughout both lung fields and has 3+ pitting edema of both lower legs, and jugular venous distention. She has a PA catheter inserted to aid in the interpretation of the situation. The following data are available:

BP	202/114 mm Hg	SVR	2674
P	74/min	PVR	191
RR	34 breaths/min		
T	37.6°C		
CO	3.9 L/min		
CI	1.9 L/min/m²		
SI	24		
PA	43/24		
PAOP	21 mm Hg		
CVP	13 mm Hg		
Svo_2	52%		

Case Question 1. What are signs and symptoms of heart failure in this patient?

Case Question 2. Which hemodynamic parameters are abnormal?

Case Question 3. What are the priorities of treatment in this patient?

Answers
1. This patient is presenting with severe shortness of breath on 50% FiO_2 with a SaO_2 of 89%. She has bilateral crackles and 3+ pitting edema. These signs validate biventricular failure.
2. BP 202/114 mm Hg; CI 1.9 L/min/m²; SI 24; PA 43/24; PAOP 21 mm Hg; CVP 13 mm Hg; SvO_2 52%; SVR 2674.
3. Based on this information the patient is in hypertensive urgency (systolic BP > 180 without end-organ damage, based on the information given). The goal is to gradually reduce BP by 20%, to less than 160/100 over several hours and have near normal control within 24 hours. Caution should be used when lowering the SVR and BP to avoid a rapid decrease resulting in decreased perfusion pressure. Patients with sustained elevated BPs can have a decrease in organ perfusion at higher pressures than the clinician might normally expect. This is especially common in the older adult. See Chapter 9 for a discussion of the management of hypertensive crisis.

Contractility

Contractility is the strength of the myocardial contraction, or the degree of myocardial fiber shortening with contraction independent of preload and afterload. Contractility contributes significantly to CO. If the other determinants of CO are constant, then a heart with a greater contractile force will produce a greater CO. However, contractility, while a separate property from preload and afterload, may be affected by both, based on the Frank-Starling law of the heart (Figure 4-2).

Electrolyte levels also have a major impact on the contractility of the heart. Monitoring and treating abnormal calcium, sodium, magnesium, potassium, and phosphorus levels is essential to ensure optimal contractility. Other factors that affect contractility include myocardial oxygenation (ischemia), amount of functional myocardium (infarction, cardiomyopathy), and administration of positive and negative inotropic drugs.

Clinical Indicators of Contractility

Myocardial contractility is reflected indirectly in the SVI, which is the SV adjusted according to body size, and the right and left ventricular stroke work index (RVSWI and LVSWI). The normal value for SVI is 35 to 60 mL/beat/m², RVSWI is 7 to 12 g-m/M², and LVSWI is 35 to 85 g-m/M² (see Table 4-1). These are not direct indicators of contractility, but trends can be used to identify patients at risk for poor contractility and to monitor the effects of therapeutic management.

BLOOD PRESSURE

Cardiac output is determined by heart rate and stroke volume. Anything impacting either element will impact the cardiac output. Blood pressure is determined by cardiac output and resistance. Measuring blood pressure provides dynamic information on cardiac output.

Blood pressure measures the force of the blood hitting the walls of the arteries with each cardiac cycle. As the heart beats, blood is ejected into the arteries, systolic blood pressure (SBP) is the peak pressure created in this cardiac cycle. In the period between heart beats, ventricular relaxation occurs. This is when the heart refills with blood and when diastolic pressure is measured.

Mean arterial pressure (MAP) is the average pressure exerted during one cardiac cycle. MAP is influenced by both SVR and CO. To perfuse vital organs a MAP of 60 mm Hg is needed. If the MAP is persistently <60, multiorgan failure may occur. Blood pressure including MAP changes dynamically with each heartbeat, this dynamic response provides valuable information on hemodynamic status.

Pulse pressure is the difference between systolic and diastolic blood pressure. If the systolic pressure =120 and the diastolic pressure = 70, the pulse pressure would be = 50 mm Hg.

A normal pulse pressure is approximately 40 mm Hg (eg, BP = 120/80 mm Hg). A widened pulse pressure ≥ 50 mm Hg is normal in the healthy, active person such as a runner. But in the less active person, a widened pulse pressure may indicate the heart is working harder or a decrease in arterial compliance. A low (narrow) pulse pressure is defined as a pulse pressure ≤ 1/4 of systolic pressure (generally <40 mm Hg) and is commonly present in heart failure, heart valve disease states, and injury with a loss of blood. Low pulse pressure, particularly in conjunction with a low SBP, may indicate the heart is not able to pump enough blood. Example: SBP = 90 mm Hg; DBP = 60 mm Hg; pulse pressure = 30 mm Hg.

Diastolic Blood Pressure

The major factor that affects diastolic blood pressure is vascular tone, although there are other factors such as the duration of the cardiac cycle, stroke volume, and arterial compliance. Under conditions where there is no acute change in intravascular volume or stroke volume and the arterial compliance is not changing, an increase in HR will decrease diastolic time, resulting in an increased diastolic blood pressure. With bradycardia, the diastolic period is longer, and the diastolic blood pressure may be lower. If a patient who is tachycardic has a low diastolic blood pressure (defined as less than 40 or 50 mm Hg) that is abnormal, and it indicates significant vasodilation. In addition to serving as an indicator of vascular tone, a low diastolic blood pressure also represents a marked risk to the heart as coronary artery filling is driven by the diastolic pressure and coronary perfusion occurs only during diastole.

Diastolic Shock Index

It is important to evaluate the diastolic blood pressure relative to the heart rate. Recently a new indicator has been introduced—diastolic shock index (DSI = HR/DBP). A study was conducted in over 700 patients with septic shock to determine if the DSI before the initiation of vasopressors was associated with clinical outcomes. Patients were divided into groups based on the DSI. For example, in a patient with an HR of 78 and a diastolic BP of 52, the DSI is equal to 78/52 = 1.5, which reflects adequate vascular tone. In contrast, the DSI is 3.3 for a heart rate of 128 and a diastolic blood pressure of 38, which indicates profound vasodilation. These data are consistent with the previous discussion related to diastolic blood pressure. Tachycardia in conjunction with a diastolic blood pressure < 50 mm Hg is indicative of severe vasodilation (this would be a DSI between 2 and 2.5). In this study, the patients with a higher DSI before the start of vasopressors (indicating more severe vasoplegia) had a higher mortality, needed more renal replacement therapy, had a higher lactate, received more fluids, and a higher vasopressor dose. A persistently elevated DSI, indicating failure to resolve the vasoplegia, was also associated with increased mortality. Although the use of the DSI is still experimental, it demonstrates the importance of interpreting the diastolic blood pressure relative to the heart rate.

Arterial Catheters

Blood pressure measurement with the indirect method (sphygmomanometer or oscillometric method) may not be as accurate as direct BP measurement, during conditions of abnormal blood flow (high or low CO states), and extremes of SVR. The prevalence of these conditions in critically ill patients may necessitate insertion of an arterial catheter to directly measure BP.

Insertion

Arterial catheters are short (<4 in) catheters that can be inserted into radial, brachial, axillary, femoral, or pedal arteries. The most common site is the radial artery. Arterial catheters can be placed by cut down or with percutaneous insertion techniques, the latter being the most common insertion method.

General insertion steps for percutaneous insertion are similar to IV catheter insertion. Prior to insertion of a radial artery catheter, however, an Allen test is performed to identify any neurovascular or circulatory impairment that may lead to potential complications (see Figure 4-4). The Allen test is performed by completely obstructing blood flow to the hand by compressing the radial and ulnar arteries for a minute or two. If adequate collateral blood flow exists, there will be rapid return of color, within 7 seconds, to the hand upon release of the ulnar artery.

During insertion, care is exercised not to damage the arterial vessel by excessive probing or movement of the needle. Bleeding into the tissues occurs quite easily if the vessel is damaged, causing obstruction to distal blood flow and nerve pressure. Following artery cannulation, the catheter is connected to the pressure transducer and a high-pressure infusion system to prevent blood from backing up into the tubing and fluid container. The AACN Procedure Manual provides a detailed chapter on arterial catheter insertion assistance, care, and removal that may provide additional guidance.

Removal

The removal of the arterial catheter is warranted when an accurate BP can be obtained via noninvasive methods, the BP is no longer labile, or when frequent arterial blood samples are no longer indicated. Removal of arterial catheters is commonly performed by the nurse using procedures similar to IV catheter removal, but because the catheter was in an artery, greater attention to achieving hemostasis is required. Following catheter removal, firm direct pressure is maintained at the site and 1 to 2 fingers width above the site for 5 minutes or longer until hemostasis occurs. This prevents bleeding and hematoma formation. For patients with coagulation abnormalities, manual pressure may need to be applied for 10 minutes or longer. Pressure dressings, rather

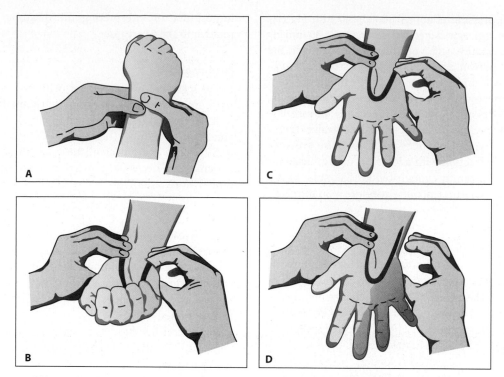

Figure 4-4. The Allen test. **(A)** locate the radial and ulner pulses **(B)** apply compression to both arteries **(C)** maintain compression and observe the color of the palm **(D)** watch for rapid return of color when only the ulner artery is released. (*Reproduced with permission from Bucher L, Melander SD: Critical care nursing. Philadelplhia, PA: WB Saunders; 1999. Figure 6-9.*)

than manual pressure, at the site are not recommended as a means to achieve hemostasis. Once hemostasis is achieved, a pressure dressing is applied to prevent rebleeding.

Frequent assessment of the site after catheter removal is recommended to identify rebleeding and thrombosis of the artery. Checking the extremity for the presence of pulses, circulation, and bleeding is recommended for a few hours after catheter removal.

Complications

A variety of complications are associated with arterial catheters (Table 4-3). The most serious are related to bleeding from the arterial catheter system or site and loss of arterial flow to the extremity from thrombus formation, which can lead to ischemia and loss of limb. Loose connections in the arterial system can lead to rapid and massive blood loss. The morbidity and mortality associated with these complications require stringent safeguards (Luer-Lock connections, minimum number of stopcocks, pressure alarm system activated at all times) to prevent bleeding and to rapidly identify disruptions in the arterial system. The catheters are removed as early as possible to prevent the potential for thrombus formation and reduce the risk of infection.

BASIC COMPONENTS OF HEMODYNAMIC MONITORING SYSTEMS

The basic components of a hemodynamic monitoring system include an indwelling catheter connected to a pressure transducer and flush system and a bedside monitor. All components that come in contact with the vascular system must be sterile, with meticulous attention paid to maintaining a closed sterile system during use.

Pressure Tubing

The pressure tubing is a key component of any hemodynamic monitoring system. It is designed to be a stiff (noncompliant) tubing to ensure accurate transfer of intravascular pressures to the transducer. The pressure tubing connects the intravascular catheter to the transducer. The pressure tubing may have stopcocks in line to facilitate blood sampling and zeroing and referencing the transducer (described later). Normally, the pressure tubing is kept as short as possible (no more than 3-4 ft), with a minimal number of stopcocks, to increase the accuracy of pressure measurements. Inclusion of a blood-conserving device in the existing monitoring circuit may affect its dynamic response characteristics.

Pressure Transducer

The pressure transducer is a small electronic sensor that converts the mechanical pressure (vascular pressure) into an electrical signal. This electrical signal can then be displayed on the pressure amplifier.

Pressure Amplifier

The pressure amplifier, or "bedside monitor," augments the signal from the transducer and displays the converted

TABLE 4-3. **PROBLEMS ENCOUNTERED WITH ARTERIAL CATHETERS**

Problem	Cause	Prevention	Treatment[a]
Hematoma after withdrawal of needle	Bleeding or oozing at puncture site.	Maintain firm pressure on site during withdrawal of catheter and for 5-15 min (as necessary) after withdrawal. Apply elastic tape (Elastoplast) firmly over puncture site. For femoral arterial puncture sites, leave a sandbag on site for 1-2 hours to prevent oozing. If patient is receiving unfractionated heparin, discontinue 2 hours before catheter removal.	Continue to hold pressure to puncture site until oozing stops. Apply sandbag to femoral puncture site for 1-2 hours after removal of catheter.
Decreased or absent pulse distal to puncture site	Spasm of artery. Thrombosis of artery.	Introduce arterial needle cleanly, nontraumatically. Use 1 U unfractionated heparin to 1 mL IV fluid.	Inject lidocaine locally at insertion site and 10 mg into arterial catheter. Arteriotomy and Fogarty catheterization both distally and proximally from the puncture site result in return of pulse in >90% of cases if brachial or femoral artery is used.
Bleedback into tubing, dome, or transducer	Insufficient pressure on IV bag. Loose connections.	Maintain 300 mm Hg pressure on IV bag. Use Luer-Lock stopcocks; tighten periodically.	Replace transducer. "Fast-flush" through system. Tighten all connections.
Hemorrhage	Loose connections.	Keep all connecting sites visible. Observe connecting sites frequently. Use built-in alarm system. Use Luer-Lock stopcocks.	Tighten all connections.
Emboli	Clot from catheter tip into bloodstream.	Always aspirate and discard before flushing. Use continuous flush device. Use 1 U unfractionated heparin to 1 mL IV fluid. Gently flush < 2-4 mL.	Remove catheter.
Local infection	Forward movement of contaminated catheter. Break in sterile technique. Prolonged catheter use.	Carefully secure catheter at insertion site. Always use aseptic technique. Remove catheter as early as possible. Inspect and care for insertion site daily.	Remove catheter.
Bloodstream infection	Break in sterile technique. Prolonged catheter use. Bacterial growth in IV fluid.	Use percutaneous insertion. Always use aseptic technique. Remove catheters as early as possible. Change transducer, stopcocks, and tubing every 72 hours. Do not use IV fluid containing glucose. Use a closed-system flush system rather than an open system. Carefully flush remaining blood from stopcocks after blood sampling.	Remove catheter.

[a]*For some of the treatment options noted in this table, the critical care provider should be contacted to rectify problem. Please refer to specific procedures and policies in your institution.*
Data from Lough ME. Hemodynamic Monitoring Emerging Technologies and Clinical Practice. *St Louis, MO: Elsevier; 2016 and Wiegand, DL.* Procedure Manual for High Acuity, Progressive and Critical Care. *St Louis, MO: Elsevier; 2017.*

vascular pressure as an electrical signal. This signal is used to display a continuous waveform on the oscilloscope of the monitor and to provide a numerical display of the pressure measurement. Most bedside monitors also have a graphic recorder to print out the pressure waveform.

Pressure Bag and Flush Device

In addition to being attached to the pressure amplifier, the transducer is connected to an intravenous (IV) solution, which is placed in a pressure bag. The IV solution is normally 500 to 1000 mL of normal saline (NS, 0.9% sodium chloride). Solutions with dextrose should be avoided as the dextrose will increase the risk for infection. After the initial line setup, the IV solution is placed under 300 mm Hg of pressure to prevent backflow of blood into the system from the vascular catheter. The IV solution is placed under pressure for another reason. Included in most pressure systems is a flush device. The flush device regulates fluid flow through the pressure tubing at a slow, continuous rate to prevent occlusion of the vascular catheter. Normally, the flush device restricts fluid flow to approximately 1 to 4 mL/h. If the flush device is activated, by squeezing or pulling the flush device, a rapid flow of fluid enters the pressure tubing. Flush devices are activated for two reasons: to rapidly clear the tubing of air (never into the patient) or blood and to check the accuracy of the tubing/catheter system with a dynamic response assessment (square wave test). Measuring the fluid in the IV solution is done on every shift to determine the amount of fluid infused from the pressure bag.

Studies comparing heparin intermittent flushing with 0.9% NS flushing for central venous/PA/arterial catheter maintenance found no conclusive evidence of differences in efficacy or safety. Due to the increased expense and the potential for complications (thrombocytopenia) with the use of a heparin flush, it is generally not recommended. Hospital policy or individual patient circumstances must also be considered in the decision to use heparin in the flush system.

Alarms

Bedside monitors have alarms for each of the hemodynamic pressures being monitored. Normally, every parameter that is being monitored has high and low alarms, which can be set to detect variations from the current value. Alarm limits are generally set to detect significant decreases or increases in pressures or rates, typically ±10% of the current values. When alarm limits are too narrow, the frequency of monitor alarms will increase. Studies show that when alarms are frequent and do not accurately indicate a change in a patient's condition, response times increase, placing patients at risk. Setting alarm limits at liberal levels also creates a risk to patient safety, as the monitor may not alarm when in fact, there is a change in condition that warrants intervention. Tailoring alarm limits for the individual patient may increase patient safety and reduce nuisance alarms. Refer to the AACN Procedure Alert: Managing Alarms in Acute Care Across the Life Span: Electrocardiography and Pulse Oximetry for additional evidence-based recommendations.

OBTAINING ACCURATE HEMODYNAMIC VALUES

The information obtained from hemodynamic monitoring technology must be verified for accuracy by the bedside clinician.

Leveling the Transducer

Leveling (or referencing) is the process of aligning the air-fluid interface on the transducer with the anatomical reference that represents the position of the atrium, known as the phlebostatic axis. Leveling minimizes the effect of hydrostatic pressure on the transducer, improving the accuracy of the readings. If the transducer is positioned too low, it will cause an erroneous increase in pressure. If the transducer is positioned too high, the fluid within the tubing above the transducer exerts a lower pressure and results in an abnormally low-pressure value. The reference point is the phlebostatic axis and is found at the intersection between the fourth intercostal space (ICS) and half the AP diameter of the chest (Figure 4-5).

When the transducer and stopcocks are mounted on a pole close to the bed, the pole height is adjusted to have the stopcock opening horizontal to the external reference. To ensure horizontal positioning, a carpenter's level (or similar device) is usually necessary. Each time the bed height or patient position is altered, this leveling procedure must be repeated. Leveling must be performed when obtaining the first set of hemodynamic information and any time the patient position changes relative to the transducer location. When obtaining the first set of readings, zeroing, and leveling are frequently performed simultaneously.

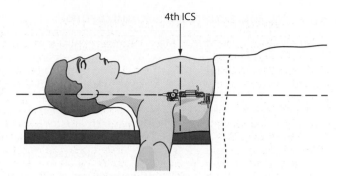

Figure 4-5. The phlebostatic axis is determined by drawing an imaginary vertical line from the fourth ICS on the sternal border to the right side of the chest and a second imaginary line is drawn horizontally at the level of the midpoint between the anterior and posterior surface of the chest. The phlebostatic axis is located at the intersection of the two lines. Note, this may be different than the midaxillary line. The transducer is leveled at the phlebostatic axis.

Zeroing the Transducer

A fundamental step in obtaining accurate hemodynamic values is to zero the transducer amplifier system. *Zeroing* is the act of electronically compensating for any offset (distortion) in the transducer. This is normally done by exposing the transducer to air and pushing an automatic zero button on the bedside monitor. Zeroing is done for each pressure line attached to the PA catheter or the arterial catheter. This step is performed at least once before obtaining the first hemodynamic reading after catheter insertion. Zeroing should be repeated when accuracy of waveform values is in question, following disconnection of the transducer cable, and per institutional policy.

Ensuring Accurate Waveform Transmission

For hemodynamic monitoring to provide accurate information, the vascular pressure must be transmitted back to the transducer unaltered. For this waveform to be transmitted unaltered, no obstructions or distortions to the signal should be present along the transmission route. A variety of factors can cause distortions to the waveform, including catheter obstructions (eg, clots, catheter bending, blood or air in tubing), excessive tubing or connectors, and transducer damage. Verification of an accurate transmission of the waveform to the transducer is checked by the bedside nurse by performing a dynamic response test (square wave test), at the beginning of each shift and any time the waveform configuration changes (see Table 4-4).

Dynamic Response Test

The dynamic response test (square wave test) is performed on all hemodynamic pressure systems before assuming the waveforms and pressures obtained are accurate. The square wave test is performed by assessing the pressure waveform after fast flushing the catheter (Table 4-5A). The fast-flush valve is pulled or squeezed, depending on the model, and then rapidly released. The tracing should show a rapid rise

TABLE 4-4. EVIDENCED-BASED PRACTICE: PULMONARY ARTERY PRESSURE MEASUREMENT

- Verify the accuracy of the transducer-patient interface by performing a square waveform test (dynamic response) at the beginning of each shift and any time the system has been disturbed.
- PAP/PAOP/CVP measurements should be made with the patient supine (HOB elevated between 0° and 60°), in lateral position (20°, 30°, or 90°), or prone.
- Level the transducer air-fluid interface to the phlebostatic axis (4th ICS/½ AP diameter of the chest) with the patient in a supine position prior to PAP/RAP/PAOP measurements.
- Obtain PAP/RAP/PAOP measurements from a graphic (analog) tracing at end-expiration.
- Use a simultaneous ECG tracing to assist with proper PAP/RAP/PAOP waveform identification.
- PA catheters can be safely withdrawn and removed by competent registered nurses (see AACN Procedure Manual).
- With airway pressure release ventilation (APRV), patients breathe spontaneously around the upper pressure limit; thus, the airway pressure tracing is used to identify spontaneous end-expiration, which occurs immediately before the release of airway pressure and the initiation of inspiration.
- Accurate alternatives to measuring CVP include measuring peripheral venous pressure (PVP); PVP measurements are obtained from a catheter in the dorsum of the hand or forearm, or from a peripherally inserted central catheter (PICC).[a]
- Continuity from the peripheral venous catheter tip to the central circulation should be verified by checking for an increase in the PVP in response to circumferential occlusion of the arm or leg proximal to the catheter or in response to a sustained inspiratory breath or Valsalva maneuver.

[a]Data from American Association of Critical-Care Nurses, 2016.

TABLE 4-5. ASSESSING DAMPING CONCEPTS FROM SQUARE WAVE TEST

Square Wave Test	Clinical Effect	Corrective Action
A: Optimally damped system. When the fast flush of the continuous flush system is activated and quickly released, a sharp upstroke terminates in a flat line at the maximal indicator on the monitor and hard copy. This is followed by an immediate and rapid downstroke extending below the baseline with just 1 or 2 oscillations within 0.12 seconds (minimal ringing) and a quick return to baseline. The patient's pressure waveform is also clearly defined with all components of the waveform, such as the dicrotic notch on an arterial waveform, clearly visible. Intervention: There is no adjustment in the monitoring system required. Optimally damped Observed waveform	Produces accurate waveform and pressure.	None required.
B: Overdamped system. The upstroke of the square wave appears somewhat slurred, the waveform does not extend below the baseline after the fast flush, and there is no ringing after the flush. The patient's waveform displays a falsely decreased systolic pressure and a falsely high diastolic pressure, as well as poorly defined components of the pressure tracing, such as a diminished or absent dicrotic notch on arterial waveforms. Interventions: To correct the problem—(1) check for the presence of blood clots, blood left in the catheter following blood sampling, or air bubbles at any point from the catheter tip to the transducer and eliminate them as necessary; (2) use low compliance (rigid), short (<3-4 ft) monitoring tubing; (3) ensure there are no loose connections; and (4) check for kinks in the line. Overdamped Observed waveform	Produces a falsely low systolic and high diastolic value.	Check the system for air, blood, loose connections, or kinks in the tubing or catheter. Verify extension tubing has not been added.
C: Underdamped system. The waveform is characterized by numerous amplified oscillations above and below the baseline following the fast flush. The monitored pressure wave displays falsely high systolic pressure (overshoot), possibly falsely low diastolic pressures, and "ringing" artifacts on the waveform. Intervention: To correct the problem, remove all air bubbles in the fluid system. Use large bore, shorter tubing Underdamped Observed waveform	Produces a falsely high systolic and low diastolic value.	Remove unnecessary tubing and stopcocks.

Reproduced with permission from Darovic GO. Hemodynamic Monitoring: Invasive and Noninvasive Clinical Application, 2nd ed. Philadelphia, PA: WB Saunders Co; 1995. Table 6-2.

in the waveform to the top of the graph paper, with a square pattern. Release of the flush device should show a rapid decrease in pressure below the baseline of the pressure waveform (undershoot), followed immediately by a small increase above the baseline (overshoot) prior to resumption of the normal pressure waveform. While it is common to look at the oscillations from the activation of the fast flush to assess if the system is optimally damped, the most important information is how far apart the oscillations are rather than how many oscillations there are. Optimally damped systems have 1 to 1.5 little boxes (on the ECG paper) between them. In general, there will be one to two oscillations. An optimally damped system will faithfully reproduce most complex waveforms. If there are more than two boxes between the oscillations the system is most likely underdamped (usually evidenced by ringing with multiple oscillations in response to the fast flush) and the system requires further optimization. The most common cause of underdamping is air bubbles (including microbubbles and air in the stopcock). If there are more than 2.5 little boxes between the oscillations, the system is inadequate and cannot be used without correction. In general, there will be damping of the waveforms. There is no evidence to support the practice of comparing the arterial line to the oscillometric blood pressure measurement as an indicator of the accuracy of the arterial line. These two methods are measuring different phenomena (pressure vs flow) at different locations on the body.

Two problems may exist with waveform transmissions, and these are referred to as *overdamping* and *underdamping* (Table 4-5B, C).

Overdamping

If something absorbs the pressure wave (like large air bubbles, blood in the tubing, loose stopcocks/connections, or low fluid level in the flush bag), it is said to be *overdamped*. Overdamping decreases systolic pressures and increases diastolic pressures. An overdamped square wave test reflects the obstruction in waveform transmission. Characteristics of overdamping include a loss of the undershoot and overshoot waves after release of the flush valve and a slurring of the downstroke (Table 4-5B).

Underdamping

If something accentuates the pressure wave (like excessive tubing or small air bubbles), it is said to be *underdamped*. Underdamping increases systolic pressures and decreases diastolic pressures (Table 4-5C). An underdamped square wave test reflects the amplification of pressure waves and includes large undershoot and overshoot waves after the release of the flush valve. Table 4-6 summarizes the methods of assessing and ensuring the accuracy of hemodynamic monitoring systems.

Care of the Tubing/Catheter System

Nosocomial infections related to the tubing/catheter system are usually caused by the entry of organisms through

TABLE 4-6. SUMMARY OF METHODS FOR ASSESSING AND ENSURING ACCURACY OF HEMODYNAMIC MONITORING SYSTEMS[a]

Method	When Performed
Zero transducer	Performed at set up and once per shift. If the transducer zeros properly, a waveform should be visible on the monitor. (Note: the zero is also activated as a part of leveling.)
Level the transducer	Leveling should be confirmed at the start of every shift, prior to each pressure reading, after any position change and with any substantive change in pressures.
Square wave test	Should be performed prior to every reading and after blood has been withdrawn from the catheter.

[a]If a transducer has been zeroed, leveled, and has an optimally damped square wave test, the monitor display is accurate.

stopcocks. Stopcocks are opened for blood sampling and zeroing the transducer only when necessary. Closed, needleless systems are used whenever feasible to decrease the risks to the patient and clinician.

The Centers for Disease Control (CDC) and Infusion Nurses Society recommend tubing changes, including flush device, transducer, and flush solution, be done every 96 hours. There are widespread variations in site care techniques and materials used across hospitals, but the procedure for changing the dressing is always a sterile one. Current CDC recommendations state that central lines should be removed as soon as their exclusive use is no longer required.

Pulmonary Artery Catheters

The PA catheter is a multilumen catheter inserted into the PA (Figure 4-6). Each lumen or "port" has specific functions (Table 4-7). The PA catheter typically is inserted through an introducer sheath (large-diameter, short catheter with a diaphragm) placed in a major vein. Veins used for PA catheter insertion include the internal jugular, subclavian, and femoral.

Pulmonary artery catheters are used less frequently than 10 years ago, but the PA catheter is still considered the gold standard to assess hemodynamics and guide therapy. Many critically ill patients are now monitored with less invasive hemodynamic technology. Today, the PA catheter is used when advanced hemodynamic monitoring is required to guide medical management most commonly for heart dysfunction, respiratory failure, and post-cardiac surgery care. Studies have shown no clear mortality benefit from the use of the PA catheter alone. See the AACN Practice Alert "Pulmonary Artery/Central Venous Pressure Monitoring in Adults."

Insertion

Pulmonary artery catheters can be inserted into most large-diameter veins, with the internal jugular vein being the most common insertion site. Typically, the PA catheter is placed into a percutaneously inserted introducer sheath with a sterile sleeve to maintain the sterility of the PA catheter after insertion (Figure 4-7). As the catheter is advanced into the

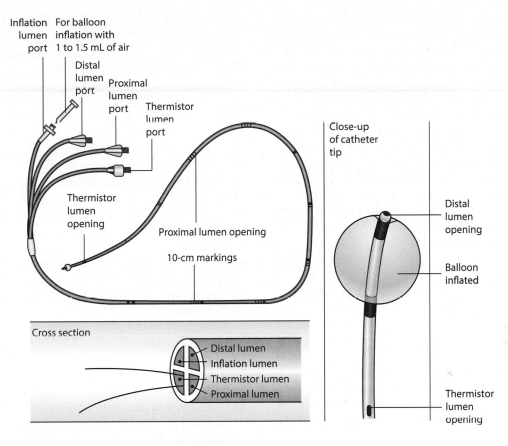

Figure 4-6. Flow-directed PA catheter.

RA, the balloon at the tip of the catheter is inflated with 1.25 to 1.50 mL of air. Inflation of the balloon during insertion allows blood flow through the heart to direct the catheter and it floats up into the PA. Following proper placement of the catheter within the PA, the balloon is deflated, and the waveform should be observed for a return to a PA waveform to confirm that the catheter is not wedged.

Pressure at the tip of the PA catheter is monitored continuously as the catheter is advanced through the right heart and into the PA (Figure 4-8). Changes in pressure and waveform configurations allow clinicians to identify the location of the PA catheter as it is directed into the RA, through the tricuspid valve into the RV, through the pulmonic valve, and into the PA (Figure 4-9 and Table 4-8). Normal pressures for each of the chambers are summarized in Tables 4-1 and 4-7. Occasionally, bedside fluoroscopy also is needed to assist with proper insertion of the catheter.

TABLE 4-7. PULMONARY ARTERY PORT FUNCTIONS

Type of Port	Functions
Distal tip port	Measures pressure at the tip of the catheter in the PA. With proper inflation of the balloon, measures the PAOP. Used to sample SvO_2 levels and for other blood sampling needs.
Proximal lumen port	Measures pressure 30 cm from the distal tip, usually in the right atrium (RA). CVP and RAP are synonymous terms. Injection site for CO determinations. Used to draw blood samples for laboratory tests requiring venous blood. If coagulation studies are drawn, completely remove unfractionated heparin from line prior to obtaining sample. Used for IV fluids and drug administration, if necessary.
Balloon inflation port	Inflated periodically with <1.5 mL of air to obtain PAOP tracing.
Ventricular port (on selected models of PA catheters)	Measures RV pressure. Used for insertion of a temporary pacemaker electrode in the RV.
Ventricular infusion port (on selected models of PA catheters)	An additional lumen for IV fluid or drug administration. Located close to the proximal lumen exit area. May be used for CO determinations or CVP measurements, if necessary.
CO port (thermistor lumen)	Measures blood temperature near the distal tip when connected to the CO computer. May be used to monitor body (core) temperature continuously.

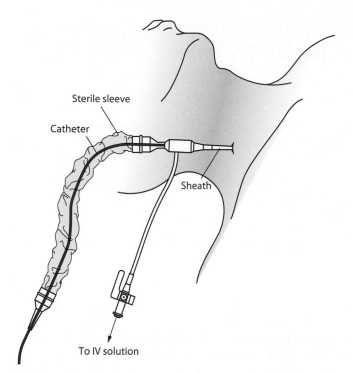

Figure 4-7. PA catheter inserted through an introducer sheath in the right internal jugular vein. The sterile sleeve of the introducer allows advancement of the PA catheter after insertion, if necessary. The side port of the sheath is connected to an IV to reduce clotting around the sheath and permit fluid administration. (*Reproduced with permission from Daily E, Schroeder J*. Techniques in Bedside Hemodynamic Monitoring, *3rd ed. St Louis, MO: CV Mosby; 1985.*)

Following insertion, the PA pressure waveform is monitored continuously to identify migration of the catheter tip either into a small branch of the PA, obstructing blood flow to distal lung tissue or backward into the RV. A chest x-ray is obtained after insertion to verify proper location and rule out pneumothorax, kinking of the catheter, or other complications.

Removal

Removing the PA catheter is a clinical decision based on the assessment that the data from the catheter are no longer contributing to decisions about the care of the patient. This decision may be made anywhere from a few hours to several days after insertion. The removal of the PA catheter is normally performed by a provider, although at some institutions nurses perform this task (see Table 4-4). Refer to the AACN Procedure Manual for High Acuity, Progressive, and Critical Care for the procedure. Nursing advocacy and the use of checklists can help ensure prompt removal of invasive lines.

After discontinuing infusions through the catheter, all stopcocks to the patient are turned off to avoid air entry into the venous system during catheter removal, and the balloon port is checked to ensure that the balloon is deflated. The patient is placed in a supine position with the head of the bed flat. While the catheter is being gently withdrawn, the patient is instructed to exhale or hold his or her breath to further decrease the chance of air embolus. Resistance during catheter withdrawal may indicate catheter knotting and/or entrapment in a valve leaflet or chordae tendineae. A chest x-ray is then necessary to confirm the problem and special removal procedures are performed to avoid structural damage to the heart.

Complications

Complications associated with PA catheters include those associated with insertion, maintenance, and removal of the device (Table 4-9). During insertion, the most common complication is ventricular ectopy (premature ventricular contractions [PVCs], ventricular tachycardia, or fibrillation) from catheter irritation of the ventricular wall. Similar to complications associated with central venous catheters, pneumothorax or air emboli may occur during insertion or removal of a PA catheter. Introduction of microorganisms and subsequent infection are always a risk. A rare but serious complication is damage to the tricuspid or pulmonic valves. Pulmonary hemorrhage or infarct may also occur during inadvertent migration of the PA catheter into small-diameter branches of the PA or from balloon rupture. Prevention and treatment strategies are summarized in Table 4-9 for each of these complications.

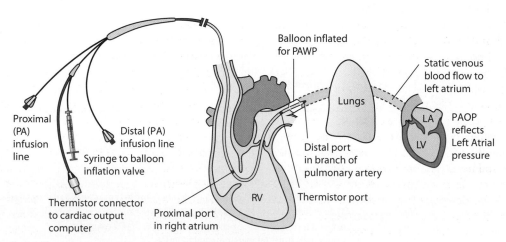

Figure 4-8. PA catheter inserted into the PA.

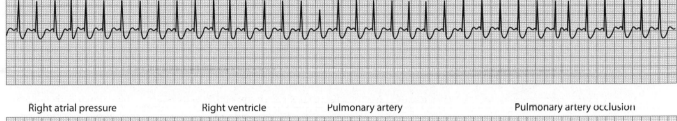

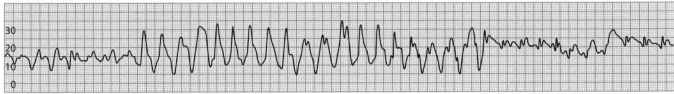

Right atrial pressure   Right ventricle   Pulmonary artery   Pulmonary artery occlusion

Figure 4-9. Change in waveforms as the PA catheter is "floated" from the right atrium (RA), through the right ventricle (RV) into the pulmonary artery (PA) and out to an occluded position in the pulmonary artery (PAOP). In this example, the patient is breathing spontaneously.

OBTAINING AND INTERPRETING HEMODYNAMIC WAVEFORMS

To obtain hemodynamic values, interpretation of hemodynamic waveforms is necessary. A multichannel strip recorder, which provides both an electrocardiographic (ECG) and pressure tracing, is a required element. Many institutions also use respiratory pressure waveforms, graphed simultaneously with the ECG and hemodynamic waveforms, to ensure accurate identification of end expiration. Each tracing also has calibration markings to aid in pressure identification, particularly if using a hard copy of the tracing (Figure 4-10).

A hard copy of the waveforms can be obtained by activating the record function of the bedside monitor. When obtaining waveforms for interpretation, make sure the calibration scales on the left side of the paper are properly aligned with the paper grid. Improperly aligned calibration marks increase the difficulty in reading the waveform and increase potential errors in interpretation.

Patient Positioning

The patient is placed in the supine position, with the backrest elevated anywhere from 0° to 60° (see Figure 4-11).

Accurate readings can also be achieved when the patient is in a 20°, 30°, or 90° lateral position with the head of bed (HOB) flat and in the prone position. When using prone position, it is important to allow adequate stabilization time after changing position (30-60 minutes) to ensure that CVP, PAP, and CO readings are accurate. Improper leveling affects accurate atrial and venous pressure readings. When using prone position, the phlebostatic axis remains the reference point. The reference point for leveling when patients are in the right lateral position is the intersection of the 4th intercoastal space and midsternum. If lying in the left lateral position the reference point for leveling is the 4th ICS and the left parasternal border. When the patient is in the 30° lateral position (right or left) the left atrial reference point is located one-half the vertical distance between the surface of the bed and the left sternal border.

It is important to remember that patient comfort is a key issue when obtaining hemodynamic waveform readings. Do not position a spontaneously breathing patient with dyspnea flat for the sole reason of obtaining hemodynamic readings. It is best to obtain values in the position in which the patient is most comfortable. If a patient demonstrates position-related changes, it is important to always measure in that position and to document the position to ensure consistency.

Interpretation

Correct interpretation of hemodynamic waveforms involves careful assessment of venous and arterial pressure waveforms. Normal values for each of the hemodynamic pressures are listed in Table 4-1. In addition, Chapter 24, Hemodynamic Monitoring Troubleshooting Guide, lists common problems and approaches to hemodynamic monitoring systems. The ability to recognize the characteristic waveforms associated with each chamber and the PA pressures is essential during insertion of the PA catheter as well as monitoring for incorrect positioning (Figure 4-9).

Atrial and Venous Waveforms

Pressures in the atrial and venous systems are significantly lower than in the ventricular and arterial systems. CVP (also called RAP) and PAOP are the atrial/venous pressures that are measured in critically ill patients. These pressures can be used to estimate ventricular pressures because, at the time of ventricular end diastole, the mitral and tricuspid valves are open (see Figure 4-3). This allows a clear communication between the ventricles and the atrium, with equilibration of pressures in the two chambers. Ideally, ventricular pressures are better measures of ventricular function than atrial estimates; however, direct ventricular pressure measurement is not always available. Atrial pressures are then used as a substitute. If ventricular waveforms are available, they are used in place of atrial pressures. CVP and PAOP are clinical

TABLE 4-8. PRESSURE WAVEFORMS OBSERVED DURING PULMONARY ARTERY CATHETER INSERTION

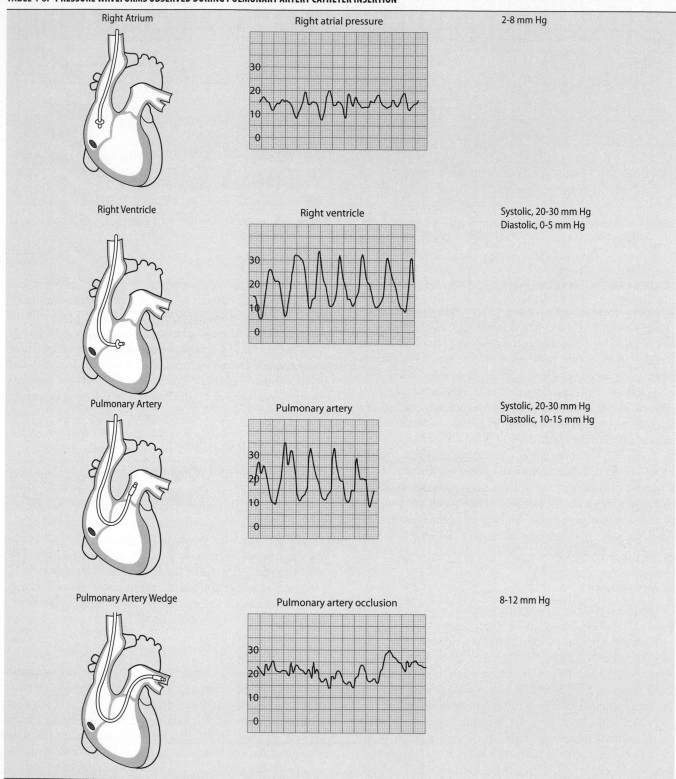

Right Atrium — Right atrial pressure — 2-8 mm Hg

Right Ventricle — Right ventricle — Systolic, 20-30 mm Hg / Diastolic, 0-5 mm Hg

Pulmonary Artery — Pulmonary artery — Systolic, 20-30 mm Hg / Diastolic, 10-15 mm Hg

Pulmonary Artery Wedge — Pulmonary artery occlusion — 8-12 mm Hg

Reproduced with permission from Boggs R, Woolridge-King M. AACN Procedure Manual, 3rd ed. Philadelphia, PA: WB Saunders; 1993.

TABLE 4-9. PROBLEMS ENCOUNTERED WITH PULMONARY ARTERY CATHETERS

Problem	Cause	Prevention	Treatment[a]
Phlebitis or local infection at insertion site	Mechanical irritation or contamination.	Prepare skin properly before insertion. Use sterile technique during insertion and dressing change. Insert smoothly and rapidly. Use Teflon-coated introducer. Attach silver-impregnated cuff to introducer. Change dressings, IV fluid bag, transducer, stopcocks, and connecting tubing every 96 hours. Remove catheter or change insertion site when no longer needed.	Remove catheter. Apply warm compresses. Give pain medication as necessary.
Ventricular irritability	Looping of excess catheter in RV. Migration of catheter from PA to RV. Irritation of the endocardium during catheter passage.	Carefully secure catheter at insertion site; check chest film. Position catheter tip in main right or left PA. Keep balloon inflated during advancement; advance gently.	Reposition catheter; remove loop. Inflate balloon to encourage catheter flotation out to PA. Advance rapidly out to PA. (Sometimes turning the patient may move catheter tip and stop the irritation.)
Apparent wedging of catheter with balloon deflated	Forward migration of catheter tip caused by blood flow, excessive loop in RV, or inadequate suturing of catheter at insertion site.	Check catheter tip by fluoroscopy; position in main right or left PA after insertion. Check catheter position after insertion on x-ray film if fluoroscopy is not used. Carefully secure catheter in place at insertion site.	Aspirate blood from catheter; if catheter is wedged, sample will be arterialized and obtained with difficulty. If wedged, slowly pull back catheter until PA waveform appears. If not wedged, gently aspirate and flush catheter with saline; catheter tip can partially clot, causing damping that resembles damped PAOP waveform.
Pulmonary hemorrhage or infarction, or both	Distal migration of catheter tip. Continuous or prolonged wedging of catheter. Overinflation of balloon while catheter is wedged. Failure of balloon to deflate.	Check chest film immediately after insertion and 12-24 hours later; remove any catheter loop in RA or RV. Leave balloon deflated. Carefully secure catheter at skin to prevent inadvertent advancement. Position catheter in main right or left PA. Pull catheter back to pulmonary artery if it spontaneously wedges. Do not flush catheter when in wedge position. Inflate balloon slowly with only enough air to obtain a PAOP waveform. Do not inflate 7-Fr catheter with more than 1.25-1.5 mL of air. Do not inflate if resistance is met.	Deflate balloon. Place patient on side (catheter tip down). Stop anticoagulation. Consider "wedge" angiogram. Intubate with double-lumen ET. Recommend surgery, if severe hemorrhage.
"Overwedging" or damped PAOP	Overinflation of balloon. Frequent inflation of balloon.	Watch waveform during inflation; inject only enough air to obtain PAOP. Check inflated balloon shape before insertion.	Deflate balloon; reinflate slowly with only enough air to obtain PAOP pressure. Deflate balloon; reposition and slowly reinflate.
PA balloon rupture	Overinflation of balloon. Frequent inflations of balloon. Syringe deflation, damaging wall of balloon.	Inflate slowly with only enough air to obtain a PAOP. Monitor PAD pressure as reflection of PAOP and LVEDP. Allow passive deflation of balloon. Remove syringe after inflation.	Remove syringe to prevent further air injection. Monitor PAD pressure.
Infection	Nonsterile insertion techniques. Contamination via skin. Contamination through stopcock ports or catheter hub. Fluid contamination from transducer through cracked membrane of disposable dome. Prolonged catheter placement.	Use sterile techniques. Use sterile catheter sleeve. Prepare skin with effective antiseptic (chlorhexidine). Use sterile CDC approved dressing (change gauze dressing every 2 days and transparent dressing every 7 days). Inspect site daily. Reassess need for catheter after 3 days. Avoid internal jugular approach. Use a closed system flush system rather than an open system. Use sterile dead-end caps on all stopcock ports. Change IV tubing, flush device, and solution every 72 to 96 hours. Do not use IV solution that contains glucose. Check transducer domes for cracks. Change transducers every 72 to 96 hours. Change catheter and/or insertion site with any local signs of infection and for infections without obvious source (should obtain cultures).	Remove catheter. Use antibiotics. Use temporary pacemaker or flotation catheter with pacing wire.

(continued)

TABLE 4-9. PROBLEMS ENCOUNTERED WITH PULMONARY ARTERY CATHETERS (CONTINUED)

Problem	Cause	Prevention	Treatment[a]
Heart block during insertion of catheter	Mechanical irritation of His bundle in patients with preexisting left bundle branch block.	Remove catheter as soon as clinically possible. Insert catheter expeditiously with balloon inflated. Insert transvenous pacing catheter before PA catheter insertion.	

Abbreviations: PA, pulmonary artery; PAOP, pulmonary artery occlusion pressure; RV, right ventricle.

[a]For some of the treatment options noted in this table, the provider should be contacted STAT to rectify problem. In some medical centers, the critical care nurse is allowed to perform these interventions. Please refer to specific procedures in your institution.

Adapted with permission from Lough ME. Hemodynamic Monitoring Emerging Technologies and Clinical Practice. St Louis, MO: Elsevier; 2016 and Wiegand, DL. Procedure Manual for High Acuity, Progressive and Critical Care. St Louis, MO: Elsevier; 2017.

measurements that assess "preload" of the right and left ventricles, respectively.

The traditional approach to fluid resuscitation consisted of measuring a pressure parameter such as the CVP or PAOP together with a CO determination. A "fluid challenge" and reassessment of the parameter(s) were then done. This approach has been largely discredited by the data indicating that the CVP and PAOP do not reliably predict volume responsiveness.

Central Venous Pressure

A normal CVP is between 2- and 8 mm Hg and provides information about right ventricular preload. Low CVP values may reflect hypovolemia or decreased venous return. High CVP values may reflect overhydration, increased venous return, or right-sided cardiac failure. The CVP is not evaluated in isolation but is one piece of data that is considered along with the SV, CO, and the results of functional hemodynamic measurements. If the CVP and SV are low and functional hemodynamics indicate fluid responsiveness, hypovolemia is assumed. If the CVP is high and the SV is low and functional hemodynamics indicate that the patient is not fluid responsive, RV dysfunction is more likely to be the cause.

CVP is obtained from the proximal port of the PA catheter or the tip of a central venous catheter. There are three waves on atrial waveforms (a, c, and v waves). Measurement of CVP is done simultaneously with the ECG. The "a" wave

of the CVP waveform starts just after the P wave on the ECG is observed and represents atrial contraction. The peak of the "a" wave usually follows the P wave of the ECG by 80 msec (0.08 seconds) (Figure 4-12). There are several ways proposed to read the CVP pressure. The first is to bisect the a, c, and v waves, so there is an equal area above and below. Other strategies include using the mean (average) of the "a" wave of the CVP waveform. The mean of the "a" wave most closely approximates ventricular end-diastolic pressure. Average the highest and lowest points on the "a" wave, to calculate the mean CVP reading.

Another method, the Z-point technique, also can be used to estimate ventricular end-diastolic pressures (Figure 4-12). The Z-point is taken just before the closure of the tricuspid valve. This point is located on a CVP tracing in the mid to late QRS complex area (0.08 seconds after the onset of the QRS complex). The Z-point technique is especially useful when an "a" wave does not exist, for example, in atrial fibrillation when atrial contraction is absent.

By isolating the "a" wave or using the Z-point technique, atrial pressures can reasonably estimate ventricular end-diastolic pressure. It is helpful to read these values off a multichannel strip recorder and not the digital display on the bedside monitor. The stop-cursor function or the hard copy method may be used to improve the accuracy of digital numbers, particularly when there is variation or abnormal waveforms.

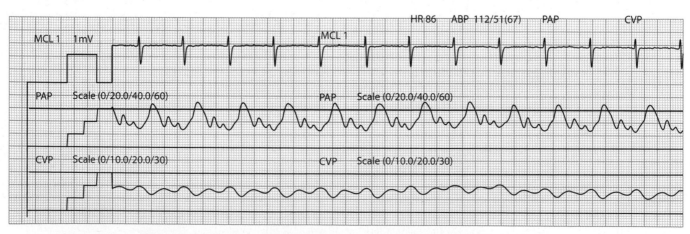

Figure 4-10. Sample printout for interpretation of CVP and PAP waveforms that includes ECG tracing.

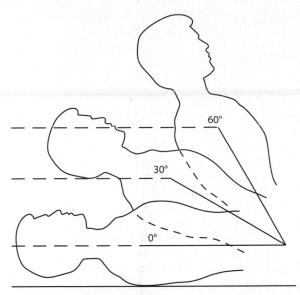

Figure 4-11. The level of the phlebostatic axis as the patient moves flat to a higher level of backrest. The level of the axis for referencing and zeroing the air-fluid interface rotates on the axis and remains horizontal as the patient moves from flat to increasingly higher backrest positions. For accurate hemodynamic pressure readings at different backrest elevations, the air-fluid interface must be at the level of the phlebostatic axis. (*Reproduced with permission from Bridges EJ, Woods SL. Pulmonary artery pressure measurement: state of the art. Heart Lung. 1993;22(2):99-111.*)

Central Venous Pressure: Abnormal Venous Waveforms

Two types of abnormal CVP waveforms are common. Large A waves (also called *cannon A waves*) occur when the atrium contracts against a closed tricuspid value). This occurs most commonly with arrhythmias like PVCs or third-degree heart block. Giant V waves are common in conditions such as tricuspid insufficiency or ventricular failure. Using the Z-point for CVP readings prevents incorrect interpretations associated with the use of large A or V waves.

PA Waveforms

Pulmonary artery pressures are obtained from a flow-directed PA catheter (see Figure 4-3). The PA pressure is a ventricular waveform that reflects RV SV and the PVR. A ventricular waveform has three characteristics, that are also observed in a systemic arterial waveform: rapid upstroke, rapid drop in pressure, and terminal diastolic rise. Systole and diastole are read in the same manner as for an arterial waveform. Normally, RV waveforms are only observed during insertion of the PA catheter or if an extra lumen on the catheter is positioned in the RV (see Table 4-8). If an RV waveform is present during monitoring, it is important to verify the location of the catheter (Figure 4-9). The catheter may have migrated out of the PA and into the RV. If the catheter tip is in the RV, there is an increased risk of ventricular ectopy due to irritation. LA and LV waveforms are not available in the clinical area but can be obtained during cardiac catheterization.

The PA pressure, which is obtained from the distal port of the PA catheter after it has passed through the pulmonic valve and is positioned in the pulmonary artery, is typically low in comparison to the systemic pressure. PA systolic pressure is generally 20 to 30 mm Hg, and the PA end-diastolic pressure is 10 to 15 mm Hg. (Figure 4-13).

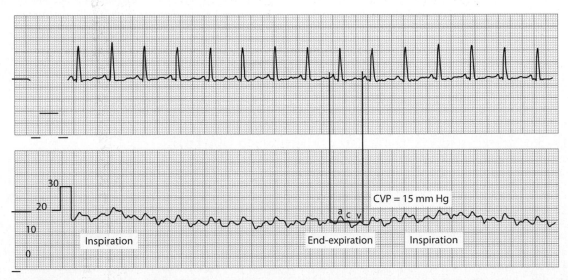

Figure 4-12. CVP tracing from a ventilated patient. The CVP is read at end-expiration. There are five mechanical components of the CVP, "a" wave, "c" wave and "v" wave and the "x descent" (downslope of the "a" wave) and the "y" descent (downslope of the "v" wave). The mean CVP, is determined by bisecting the a, c, and v waves so that there is an equal area above and below. Other options include measuring at the leading edge of the c wave (also known as the "z" point) or bisecting the "a" wave. Because the "c" wave represents closure of the tricuspid valve, the onset of the "c" wave reflects right ventricular end-diastolic pressure just before systole. To identify the "a" wave, draw a line down from the start of the P wave on the ECG. This electrical activity (atrial depolarization) will precede atrial contraction (a wave). The peak of the "a" wave typically follows the P wave by about 80 msec. The "c" wave, which reflects tricuspid valve closure, follows the "a" wave by a time interval approximately equivalent to the PR interval. The v wave, with reflects right atrial filling against the closed tricuspid valve, generally occurs at the peak of the T wave. In the absence of a P wave, there will not be an "a" wave. In this case, to identify the mean pressure, draw a straight line through the center of the Q wave (0.08 sec after onset) to locate the "Z" point. In this tracing, the CVP is elevated (15 mm Hg). (*Reproduced with permission from Bridges EJ. Monitoring pulmonary artery pressures: just the facts. Crit Care Nurse. 2000;20(6):59-78.*)

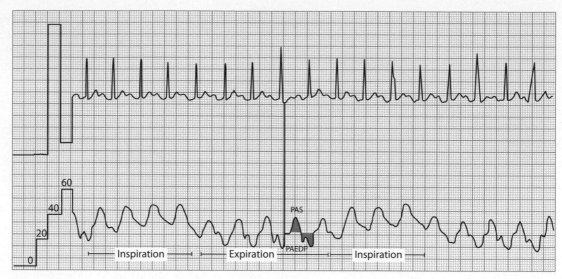

Figure 4-13. PA pressure waveform in ventilated patient. The PA pressure is measured at end expiration. The PA end-diastolic pressure is read 0.08 second after the onset of the QRS, followed by the peak systolic pressure. The PA mean is determined by bisecting the waveform. PA pressure 38/20/26. (*Reproduced with permission from Elizabeth J. Bridges.*)

With inflation of the balloon, the catheter floats forward and wedges in the pulmonary artery (pulmonary artery occlusion pressure—PAOP also sometimes called pulmonary artery wedge pressure (PAWP)) (Figures 4-14 and 4-15).

The PAOP looks similar to the CVP, but is damped and phase delayed (ie, occurs later relative to the ECG) (Figure 4-16).

The low-pressure pulmonary system is critical to adequate gas exchange in the lungs. If the pressure in the pulmonary vasculature is high, the capillary hydrostatic pressure exceeds capillary osmotic pressure and forces fluid out of

the vessels. If the pulmonary lymphatic drainage capability is exceeded, interstitial and alveolar flooding occurs, interfering with oxygen and carbon dioxide exchange.

Normally, the PA pressure is high enough to ensure blood flow through the lungs to the left atrium. Subsequently, pressure in the pulmonary arteries only needs to be high enough to overcome the resistance in the left atrium. The mean PA pressure must always be higher than LA pressure or blood flow through the lungs is not possible. As a practical guideline, the PAEDP is higher than the mean LA pressure (the mean LA pressure is generally estimated by PAOP).

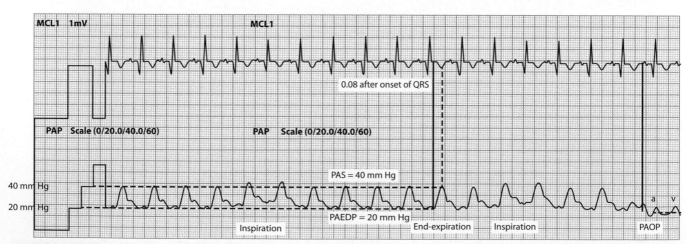

Figure 4-14. Pulmonary artery pressure transitioning into a PAOP on a 0/20/40/60 mm Hg scale. The PA pressure is read at end-expiration. Three PA pressures are measured: PA end-diastolic (PAEDP), PA systolic (PAS), and PA mean (PAM). The PAEDP is measured 0.08 seconds after the onset of the QRS. The PAS usually occurs after the QRS complex or near the T wave on the ECG. The PA mean is determined by bisecting the PA waveform so there is an equal area above and below the bisection. This PA pressure is slightly elevated 40/20 mm Hg. The waveform characteristics change at the end of the tracing as the balloon is inflated and the catheter floats forward into the wedge position. The PAOP has two positive waveforms ("a" and "v" waves). To locate the "a" wave (reflecting atrial contraction), draw a line straight down from the ECG (before the P wave). The a and v waves are shifted to the right compared to the CVP; due to the time it takes for the pressure waveform to be transmitted through the pulmonary vasculature to the distal port of the PA catheter. The "v" wave on the PAOP tracing generally occurs after the T wave. The PAOP is measured by bisecting the a and v waves, so there is an equal area above and below the bisection. In this tracing the PAOP is approximately 18 mm Hg.

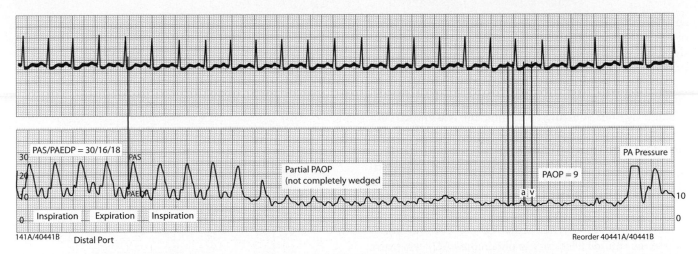

Figure 4-15. PA waveform progressing to PAOP and returning to PA waveform with balloon deflation. The waveform demonstrates an incomplete wedge (note how the waveform continues to change in the wedge position. The alignment of the a and v waves with the ECG is shifted compared to the CVP tracing. To find the "a" wave, locate the P wave. The "a" wave is usually 200 to 240 msec after the P wave (approximately five to six small boxes on the ECG paper). The v wave aligns with the T-P interval. (*Reproduced with permission from Elizabeth J. Bridges.*)

If the PAEDP value is less than the left atrial or wedge pressure, either a very low pulmonary blood flow state exists, or the waveforms have been misinterpreted.

While placement of a pulmonary artery catheter carries a risk of complications, measurement of PA pressures can be helpful in certain circumstances such as in assessing patients with pulmonary hypertension or cardiogenic shock to determine an optimal treatment plan. Elevated PA pressures also occur in chronic pulmonary disease, mitral valve disease, aortic valve disease, LV failure, hypoxia, and pulmonary emboli. Below-normal PA pressures occur primarily in conditions that produce hypovolemia. If blood volume or intravascular volume is reduced, less resistance to ventricular ejection occurs, resulting in a drop in arterial pressures. In this situation, the PAED pressure is also close to the LA pressure.

Pulmonary Artery Occlusion Pressure

Although the CVP is useful in assessing RV function, the assessment of LV function is generally more important. In LV dysfunction (eg, with myocardial infarction or cardiomyopathies), low CO impairs tissue oxygenation. The PAOP is used to assess LV function and determine appropriate therapy. Interpreting the PAOP is very similar to interpreting a CVP waveform with the obvious exception that the PAOP assesses LVEDP, not RVEDP. The LVEDP is used to assess LV function and systemic fluid status.

A normal PAOP is 8 to 12 mm Hg and rises to 15 to 18 mm Hg in patients with LV failure. PAOP greater than 18 mm Hg generally contributes to pulmonary edema in patients who have not adapted to these higher pressures. Low values reflect hypovolemia, with high values indicating hypervolemia and/or LV failure. However, the PAOP is

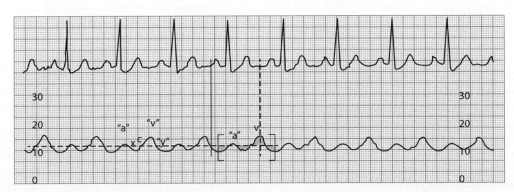

Figure 4-16. The PAOP has two primary waveforms (a and v waves) and the x (downslope of the "a" wave—left atrial relaxation) and y descent (downslope of the "v" wave—passive emptying of the left atria into the left ventricle after the mitral valve opens). The "c" wave, which reflects closure of the mitral valve and onset of left ventricular systole, may not be visible. To locate the "a" wave (reflecting atrial contraction), draw a line straight down from the ECG (before the P wave). The electrical activity (atrial depolarization) precedes mechanical activity (atrial contraction) followed by the v wave (venous outflow into the left atrium against a closed mitral valve). The "a" and "v" waves are shifted to the right compared to the CVP; due to the time it takes for the pressure wave to be transmitted back through the pulmonary vasculature to the distal port of the PA catheter. The "v" wave on the PAOP tracing generally occurs in the T-P interval. The PAOP is measured by bisecting the "a" and "v" waves, so there is an equal area above and below the bisection. In this tracing the PAOP is approximately 13 mm Hg. There is minimal respiratory variation in this strip. (*Reproduced with permission from Elizabeth J. Bridges.*)

an indirect indicator of volume, it is not an indicator of the heart's ability to respond to a fluid challenge (eg, fluid responsiveness). Mitral valve abnormalities also cause elevations in PAOP. When PAOP and SV are normal, normovolemia and acceptable LV function is assumed. If the PAOP and SV are both low, hypovolemia is likely. When PAOP is high (usually >18 mm Hg), but SV is low, LV dysfunction is assumed. Thus the use of bedside echocardiography combined with PA data may aid in a definitive diagnosis.

A PAOP waveform is obtained from the distal port of the PA catheter when the balloon on the catheter is inflated. Inflation of the balloon is performed for only a few seconds (8-15 seconds) to avoid a disruption in pulmonary blood flow. When inflating the balloon, inflate only to the volume necessary to obtain the PAOP waveform (1.25-1.50 mL). Record how much air it takes to inflate the balloon. If it takes less air to obtain a PAOP value than at a previous inflation, the catheter may have migrated further into the pulmonary artery. If it takes more air to obtain a PAOP, the catheter may have moved back. If no resistance is felt when the balloon is inflated and no PAOP tracing occurs, notify the physician or provider of a possible balloon rupture. When deflating the balloon, allow air to leave the balloon passively. Actively aspirating the air out of the balloon damages the balloon and is not necessary for complete emptying.

The characteristics and interpretation of PAOP and CVP waveforms are similar. The difference between interpreting a CVP and a PAOP waveform mainly centers on the delay in waveform correlation with the ECG (Figure 4-16). On a PAOP waveform, the "a" wave begins near the end of the QRS complex. The PAOP is measured by bisecting the a and v waves, so there is an equal area above and below the bisection. Averaging the "a" wave's highest and lowest values, is another method for obtaining the PAOP. If the Z-point is to be used for a PAOP reading, this point is 0.08 to 0.12 sec after the QRS complex (Figure 4-17). The PAOP is read at end-expiration (Figure 4-18).

Indirect assessment of LV pressures is commonly measured with the PAOP. The use of the PAOP to estimate LVEDP assumes that a measurement from an obstructed pulmonary capillary reflects an uninterrupted flow of blood to the left atrium because no valves exist in the PA system. A second assumption is that when the mitral valve is open, left atrial pressures reflect LVEDP. As long as these assumptions are accurate, the use of the PAOP to estimate LVEDP is acceptable.

Pulmonary Artery Occlusion Pressure: Abnormal Waveforms

Similar abnormal PAOP waveforms occur as with CVP measurements. Large A waves (Cannon A wave) are observed when the left atrium contracts against a closed mitral valve, which may occur with cardiac dysrhythmias (eg, wide-complex tachycardia). Large V waves (10 mm Hg greater than the "a" wave) are observed during mitral valve insufficiency and left heart failure. In the presence

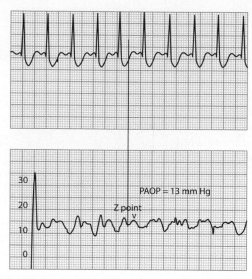

Figure 4-17. In cases where there is not a clear P wave (SVT, atrial fibrillation), the PAOP should be read at the (Z point), which is located 80–120 msec (0.08–0.12 sec) after the QRS on the ECG. In atrial fibrillation, because of the variation in cardiac cycle length, the PAOP should be measured on at least three cardiac cycles and averaged. (Reproduced with permission from Elizabeth J. Bridges.)

of a large V wave, the LVEDP is best correlated with the trough (nadir) of the x descent (downslope of the "a" wave). Regardless of the cause of the large V wave, there is an increase in pulmonary capillary pressure, which increases the risk for pulmonary edema.

Systemic Arterial Pressures

An arterial waveform, such as seen in systemic and PA tracings, has three common characteristics: rapid upstroke, dicrotic notch, and progressive diastolic runoff (Figure 4-19). Diastole is read near the end of the QRS complex with systole read before the peak of the T wave. The mean arterial pressure can be calculated (see Table 4-1) or obtained from the digital display on the bedside monitor.

Direct measurement of systemic arterial pressures is obtained when the transducer for the arterial line is leveled to the phlebostatic axis (see Figure 4-5), with pressure waveforms interpreted as described. Normal pressures are generally in the region of 100 to 120 mm Hg systolic, 60 to 80 mm Hg diastolic, and 70 to 105 mm Hg mean (see Table 4-1).

Systemic arterial pressures are not interpreted without other clinical information. In general, however, hypotension is assumed if the mean arterial pressure drops below 65 mm Hg. Hypertension is assumed if the systolic blood pressure (SBP) is greater than 140 to 160 mm Hg or the diastolic pressure exceeds 90 mm Hg.

The arterial pressure is one of the most commonly used parameters for assessing the adequacy of tissues. BP is determined by two factors: CO and SVR. Changes in BP do not necessarily reflect early clinical changes in hemodynamics because of the interaction with CO and SVR.

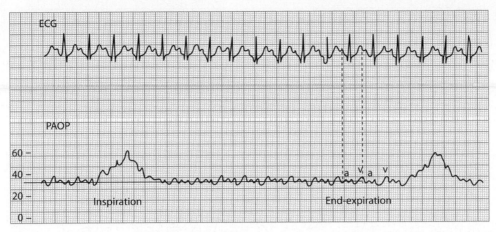

Figure 4-18. PAOP in ventilated patient. There is artifact, or possibly a c wave. The PAOP is very high (~36 mm Hg). Note the effects of mechanical ventilation. The pressure is read at end-expiration.

In addition, the CO consists of heart rate and SV. These two interact to maintain a normal CO. Subsequently, if the SV begins to fall due to loss of volume (hypovolemia) or dysfunction (LV failure), the heart rate increases to offset the decrease in SV. The net effect is to maintain the CO at near normal levels. If the CO does not change, then the drop in SV does not affect the BP.

The key point for the nurse to consider is that because of compensatory mechanisms, BP may not signal early clinical changes in hemodynamic status. If a patient begins to bleed postoperatively, the BP generally does not reflect this change until compensation is no longer possible. In addition, hypotension is sometimes difficult to evaluate. It is possible that true hypotension exists only when tissue hypoxia is present and end organs are affected. Although tradition dictates that we identify hypotension using predefined levels of BP, other measures such as mixed venous saturation of hemoglobin (Svo_2) and lactate levels may be better indicators of tissue perfusion. Svo_2 monitoring is described later in the section Continuous Mixed and Central Venous Oxygen Monitoring (Svo_2/$Scvo_2$).

Although studies identify the role of hypertension in circulatory damage, the specific level of hypertension that results in damage is unclear. Therefore, any SBP over 140 mm Hg is considered potentially injurious to the vasculature.

Artifacts in Hemodynamic Waveforms: Respiratory Influence

Respiration can physiologically change hemodynamic pressures. Spontaneous breathing augments venous return and slightly increases resistance to left ventricle filling. Mechanical ventilation does the opposite, potentially reducing venous return and reducing the resistance on the heart. The effect of respiration on waveforms is noted in Figures 4-20 and 4-21.

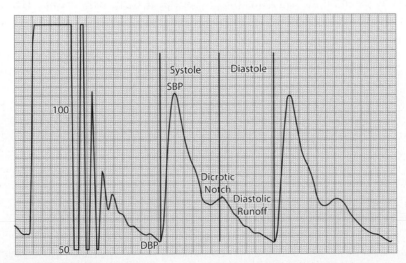

Figure 4-19. Arterial waveform tracing (105/52) from the radial artery in a patient with a heart rate of 73 bpm. The waveform is adequately damped. The upstroke of the arterial waveform begins approximately 0.2 seconds after the onset of the QRS. The dicrotic notch reflects the closure of the aortic valve and the onset of diastole. With tachycardia, the diastolic phase shortens and the diastolic BP usually increases due to the shortened diastolic runoff time (except if there is profound vasodilation).

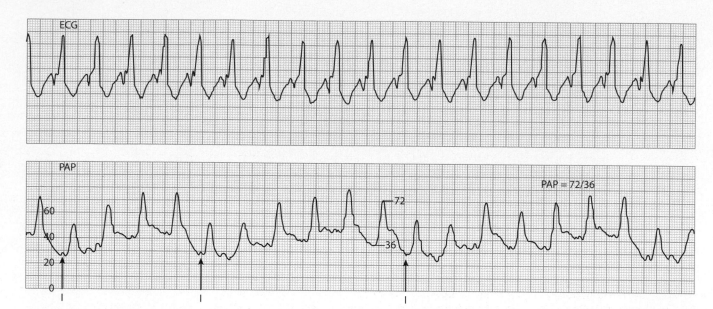

Figure 4-20. Respiratory fluctuations of pulmonary artery pressure (PAP) waveform in a spontaneously breathing patient. The location of the inspiration (I) is marked on the waveform. The points just before inspiration are end expiration, where the readings are taken. (*Reproduced with permission from AACN Procedure Manual or High Acuity, Progressive and Critical Care, 7th ed. St. Louis, MO: Elsevier; 2017.*)

A spontaneous breath or a triggered ventilator breath produces a drop in the waveform because of the decrease in pleural pressure. A ventilator breath produces an upward distortion of the baseline, due to an increase in pleural and intrathoracic pressure (Figure 4-22). The key to reading the waveform correctly is to isolate the point where pleural pressure is closest to atmospheric pressure. This point is usually at end expiration, just prior to inspiration.

Invasive Cardiac Output Monitoring

The PA catheter provides information on the measurement of blood flow parameters (CO and SV). Understanding these flow parameters is essential to assessing the adequacy of cardiac function. Flow parameters CO and SV are the first parameters assessed when monitoring hemodynamic data.

If flow parameters are adequate, tissue oxygenation is generally maintained. It is important to remember that when the CO and BP are normal, there may still be alterations in the microcirculation that affect tissue oxygenation. In the presence of abnormal flow parameters, the clinician must suspect a threat to tissue oxygenation and consider interventions to improve cardiac function. Other signs of altered blood flow present later and are less specific, including changes in level of consciousness, decreased urine output, and loss of pulse. Blood flow is essential in assuring adequate tissue oxygenation. Hemodynamic monitoring is

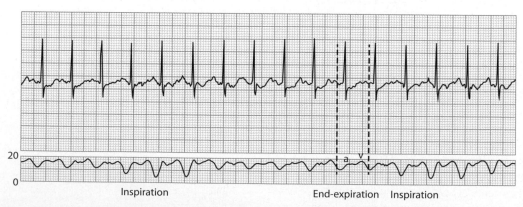

Figure 4-21. Reading the right atrial (RAP) from the paper printout at end expiration in a spontaneously breathing patient. While observing the patient, identify inspiration (see decrease in pressure). The point just before inspiration is end expiration. Locate the a wave by drawing a line down from the P wave on the ECG. The next waveform reflects atrial contraction. The v wave occurs in the T-P section of the ECG. By bisecting the a and v wave, the mean CVP is approximately 16 mm Hg. (*Reproduced with permission from AACN Procedure Manual or High Acuity, Progressive and Critical Care, 7th ed. St. Louis, MO: Elsevier; 2017.*)

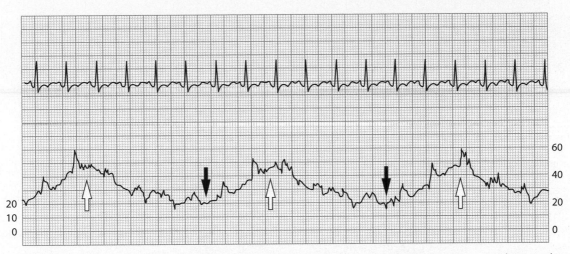

Figure 4-22. Right atrial waveform, from a PA catheter with simultaneously recorded ECG from a head-injured patient with neurogenic pulmonary edema. The patient is being maintained on controlled mechanical ventilation with 30 cm H_2O PEEP. Peak inspiratory pressure is 100 cm H_2O. The open arrows indicate the positive-pressure (ventilator) breaths and the solid arrows indicate end expiration. It is at this point that the RAP is recorded. Note that the end-expiratory pressure measurement is approximately 20 mm Hg. This grossly elevated value should not be considered to be a "true" indication of intravascular volume or RV function. Rather, the pressure measurement is spuriously elevated as a result of the excessively high intrathoracic pressure surrounding the heart and blood vessels. (*Reproduced with permission from Darovic GO.* Hemodynamic Monitoring: Invasive and Noninvasive Clinical Application, *2nd ed. Philadelphia, PA: WB Saunders Co; 1995.*)

a means of assessing the adequacy of blood flow and, tissue oxygen delivery.

Measurement of Cardiac Output

CO measurements using a PA catheter are obtained using the intermittent thermodilution technique (TDCO) or the continuous CO (CCO) technique. Both types of measures rely on measuring changes in blood temperatures. Most centers now use the CCO measurement technique using a modified pulmonary artery catheter with a heated filament. Both methods are reliable. The CCO is a closed system that reduces infection risk by avoiding multiple entries into the system. The AACN procedure manual provides detailed directions to obtain invasive cardiac output measurements.

Key Concepts in Measuring Cardiac Output

To correctly measure the CO, the nurse needs to program the bedside CO computer with the patient's height and weight or BSA if known. The CI is the CO adjusted for BSA, making it a more precise measurement. The CO computer device uses a proprietary computation constant that is pre-programmed into the monitor to ensure accuracy of values.

Factors Affecting Accuracy

The TDCO measures right ventricular outflow. A functioning tricuspid and pulmonic valve, no ventricular septal defect, and a stable cardiac rhythm are needed to ensure accuracy. The CCO displays an update of data every 30 to 60 seconds with an average of data over the last 3 to 6 minutes. If a patient has an acute change it may take up to 10 minutes for this change to be displayed on the monitor. Chapter 24, Hemodynamic Monitoring Troubleshooting Guide and the AACN procedure manual identify common problems associated with measurement of CO.

Interpreting Cardiac Output and Cardiac Index

Changes in HR or SV will impact CO and CI, with clinically significant changes indicating a change in blood flow and potentially an alteration in oxygen delivery. The CI is best tracked by trending CI values rather than a single value. A CI less than 2.5 $L/min/m^2$ is considered a circulatory compromise, and further assessment is warranted. If the CI drops to less than 2.2 $L/min/m^2$, the need for intervention becomes urgent. However, some patients tolerate low CI without clinical problems. Having a shared understanding with the care team on what CI value requires intervention and notification of the provider may reduce treatment delays and increase patient safety. Using both CI and tissue oxygenation parameters, such as $Svo_2/Scvo_2$ and lactate, may enhance the identification of a clinically significant event (Table 4-10). If you doubt the accuracy of the CO/CI, the Fick equation, which uses Sao_2 and Svo_2 (Table 4-1) may be a useful alternative. The use of the Fick equation is more reliable in specific conditions such as tricuspid regurgitation and low output states.

TABLE 4-10. ARTERIAL BLOOD GAS/TISSUE OXYGENATION PARAMETERS

Parameters	Normal Range
PaO_2	80-105 mm Hg
$PaCO_2$	35-45 mm Hg
pH	7.35-7.45
HCO3	22-26 mEq/L
Base excess, deficit	0 ± 2.3 mEq/L
SaO_2	≥94%
SvO_2	60%-80%
$ScVO_2$	70%-75%
Lactate	1-2 mEq/L
Pyruvate	0.1-0.1 mEq/L

ESSENTIAL CONTENT CASE

Svo₂

A 35-year-old woman with pancreatitis and acute respiratory distress syndrome (ARDS) experiences a progressively worsening oxygenation status. The care team decides to replace her PA catheter with a Svo_2 catheter to better monitor and manage her care. Once the Svo_2 catheter is in place and calibrated, it is noted that her Svo_2 is only 55%. A quick assessment of oxygen supply variables yields the following:

Hct	20%
CO	6 L/min
PAOP	18 mm Hg
Sao₂	91% on an Fio₂ of 0.6, PEEP of 15 cm H₂O

Given the high level of ventilator support already in place, the team felt that augmentation of oxygen-carrying capacity with transfusions of packed red blood cells (PRBCs) would provide the greatest boost to oxygenation. Following the infusion of 2 U of PRBC, the Svo_2 increased to 70%. Over the course of the next few days, decreases in ventilator support were evaluated by monitoring changes in Svo_2 in conjunction with other supply-side variables.

On day 6, she became increasingly agitated and her Svo_2 decreased to 60%. She was febrile and her sputum was noted to be purulent appearing. Sputum cultures were obtained and other reasons for the agitation were also considered. A STAT chest radiograph was obtained which ruled out pneumothorax, and an arterial blood gas revealed a $Paco_2$ of 45 mm Hg, a Pao_2 of 55 mm Hg, and a Sao_2 of 88%. Her ventilator settings were SIMV of 12/min (spontaneous rate was 10 above the ventilation), Fio_2 of 0.45, PEEP of 5 cm H₂O, Hct of 29%, and CO of 6 L/min.

The team recognized that both supply and demand needed to be addressed to optimize her oxygenation. Thus, ventilator settings were increased as follows:

Fio₂	0.60
PEEP	10 cm H₂O
SIMV	20/min

Case Question 1. What factors contributed to the low SvO₂ when the monitor was first placed?

Case Question 2. What factors contributed to the change in SvO₂ on day 6?

Answers

1. Parameters that determine Svo_2 are CO, hemoglobin (measured here as hematocrit), Sao_2, and oxygen consumption. Normal value is 60% to 80%. Alarms should be set at 60%, so the patient's monitor will alarm when the level drops. In the first part of the case, the patient's hematocrit was low, suggesting that inadequate oxygen-carrying capacity may be affecting the supply of oxygen, leading to a drop in Svo_2. The Svo_2 normalized after transfusion and the patient was able to wean from ventilator support.

2. On day 6, when the patient's Svo_2 dropped again, the CO and hematocrit are stable, so the parameters causing a drop in Svo_2 are most likely Sao_2 and oxygen consumption. The patient was noted to be agitated and febrile and this may be contributing to her increased oxygen consumption. The changes to the ventilator setting, increasing the PEEP and Fio_2 will increase the supply of oxygen, while increasing the respiratory rate may lower her demand for oxygen. Additional strategies that might benefit this patient by reducing her oxygen consumption include antipyretics to treat her fever, antibiotics for infection, and pain management if an assessment reveals that pain is contributing to her agitation.

CONTINUOUS MIXED AND CENTRAL VENOUS OXYGEN MONITORING

Monitoring Principles (Technical)

In addition to monitoring CO/CI, the PA catheter provides monitoring of mixed venous oxygenation. Svo_2 catheters are different from other PA catheters; they have two special fiber-optic bundles within the catheter that determine the oxygen saturation of hemoglobin by measuring the wavelength (color) of reflected light. Light is transmitted down one bundle and is reflected off the oxygen-saturated hemoglobin, returning up the other bundle. This information is quantified by the bedside computer and continuously displayed as the percentage of saturation of the mixed venous blood. Spot checking of SVO₂ is still possible with PA catheters without the SVO₂ fiberoptic; the mixed venous sample is drawn from the PA port and sent to the lab.

The measurement of central venous oxygen saturation (Scvo₂) requires the insertion of a central venous catheter with a fiberoptic chip for continuous monitoring.

Spot checking of Scvo₂ is possible; the sample is drawn from the distal tip of a triple-lumen catheter or PICC line. Theoretically, the Scvo₂ measures the degree of oxygen extraction from the brain and upper body and trends well with Svo₂. The Scvo₂ is usually less than the Svo₂ except in shock states due to redistribution of blood flow in classic shock states.

Continuous Svo₂ or Scvo₂ monitoring is used as a diagnostic tool. It provides early warning of alterations in hemodynamic status and a continuous measure of oxygen delivery and consumption. In addition, continuous Svo₂/Scvo₂ monitoring augments other patient data allowing for a more precise understanding of the impact of clinical changes on patient perfusion. Continuous Svo₂ and Scvo₂ monitoring demonstrate how well the body's demand for oxygen is being met under different clinical conditions. Blood leaves the left heart 100% saturated with oxygen and is transported to the tissues for cellular use based on the amount of perfusion (CO). Under normal conditions, only about 25% to 30% of the oxygen available on the hemoglobin is extracted by the tissues, with blood returning to the right heart with approximately 70% to 75% of the hemoglobin saturated with oxygen (Figure 4-23). Normal values for mixed venous oxygen saturation (Svo_2) are 60% to 75%. Normal values for $Scvo_2$ >70%.

In situations where tissue demands for oxygen increase, oxygen saturation of blood returning to the right heart may be lower than 60%. Clinical conditions of increased tissue demand (consumption) for oxygen include shivering, fever, pain, anxiety, infection, seizures, and some "routine" nursing activities like turning and suctioning. In contrast, hypothermia dramatically decreases oxygen consumption by the tissues.

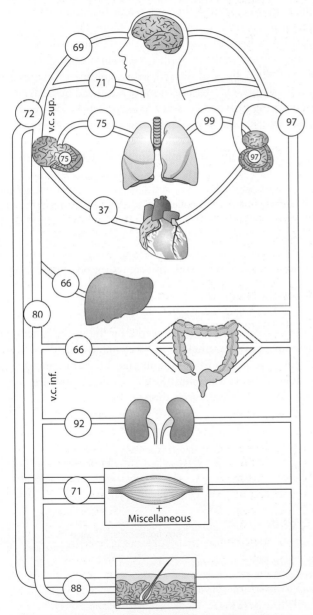

Arterial oxygen saturation are shown on the right, and venous ones on the left. The numbers shown are percentages. v.c. inf, inferior vena cava; v.c. sup, superior vena cava.

Figure 4-23. Arterial and venous oxygen saturations in various vascular regions. (*Reproduced with permission from Marx G, Reinhart K. Venous oximetry. Curr Opin Crit Care. 2006;12(3):263-268.*)

Continuous Svo_2 and $Scvo_2$ monitoring thus allow the healthcare team to identify the need for specific interventions that will bring oxygen supply (delivery) and oxygen demand (consumption) into balance.

The concept of oxygen utilization is often referred to as supply and demand (or consumption) and is the essential concept inherent in Svo_2 monitoring. Because tissue oxygenation depends on hemoglobin level, saturation of hemoglobin, oxygen consumption, and CO, the saturation of blood returning to the PA tells us much about the interaction of these four variables and can be used to assess the adequacy of interventions.

Selected Examples of Clinical Applications

Svo_2 and Low Cardiac Output

In low output states, hemoglobin is moved more slowly through the body, so there is a decrease in oxygen delivery (supply). There also is more time for oxygen extraction at the tissue level. Svo_2 levels in someone with cardiogenic shock are typically low (<60%) due to slow perfusion and high tissue extraction of oxygen. Adding an inotropic agent such as dobutamine may increase the CO and thus increase the Svo_2. Conversely, decreases in Svo_2 may be observed as inotropic agents are weaned, indicating decreases in CO. Svo_2 values between 30% and 49% have been associated with disruptions in the ability to produce adenosine triphosphate. This appreciably increases the rate of anaerobic metabolism and can contribute to an elevated lactate level.

Svo_2 and High Output States

In sepsis, CO is often very high (>10 L/min). In this hypermetabolic, hyperdynamic output state, there is microcirculatory obstruction and diminished blood flow to the tissues. Svo_2 levels are frequently above normal (>80%), indicating that oxygen extraction at the tissue level is low. Despite oxygen availability, tissue hypoxia exists and is confirmed with lactate measurements (although this is a late sign of tissue hypoxia). Because sepsis involves a dysregulated response to infection, the elevated CO seen in patients with sepsis does not improve morbidity or mortality. Effective treatment includes early intervention with fluid resuscitation and antimicrobial therapy. If a patient with sepsis is persistently hypotensive or has an elevated lactate after initial fluid replacement, the volume status and tissue perfusion are reassessed. Volume status can be reassessed by measuring CVP, or $Scvo_2$, performing a bedside cardiovascular ultrasound, or dynamic assessment of fluid responsiveness with PLR or fluid challenge. A repeat focused examination reassesses tissue perfusion. See Chapter 11 for a full discussion of sepsis and septic shock.

Svo_2 and Blood Loss

In acute blood loss, hemoglobin decreases, and the body extracts more from the available hemoglobin. Svo_2 levels decrease and are an early indication of acute blood loss. Transfusions (providing they are adequate in number and rate) increase Svo_2.

To enhance oxygen delivery and decrease consumption, the supply and demand components are considered. Oxygen supply may be increased by improving CO (fluids followed by inotropes), increasing oxygen saturation (Fio_2 level and PEEP for patients on mechanical ventilation), and by increasing hemoglobin (transfusion of red cells). Due to significant complications associated with blood transfusions, infections, and pulmonary complications (TRALI and fluid overload), a "restrictive" strategy of RBC transfusion is recommended. Replacement is considered with an Hgb of 7.0 g/dL except in acute hemorrhage, or 8.0 g/dL in patients with acute myocardial ischemia. Examples of how oxygen demand may be lowered include decreasing activity, controlling patient-ventilator dyssynchrony, preventing agitation and thrashing, and avoiding shivering. The Svo_2 catheter may be used to rapidly calculate and assess oxygen supply and consumption (Table 4-1) and direct therapies.

Troubleshooting the SvO2 Catheter

The instructions for calibration of the Svo_2 catheter must be followed if readings are to be accurate. The measurements are compared periodically with co-oximeter measurements of Svo_2 drawn slowly from the distal port of the PA. The Svo_2 monitor can be recalibrated if saturations vary. This is referred to as an in vivo calibration.

To provide accurate data, the Svo_2 catheters must be free-floating in the PA and not have fibrin or clots attached to the end, which might affect the fiber-optic measurement of saturation. A guide for this is called light intensity and refers to the amount of transmitted light required to obtain a suitable reflected signal back to the monitor. Guidelines for the levels of light intensity help the clinician to assess the accuracy of the Svo_2 readings. The size and position of the light intensity signal (called signal quality index, or SQI, on many monitors) help the nurse detect such complications as a catheter in wedge position or clot formation.

Svo_2 catheters can be helpful in the assessment of oxygenation in critically ill patients. An additional benefit may be a reduction in the need for frequent CO measurements, arterial blood gas parameters, and hemoglobin levels. However, as with any tool, the successful application of Svo_2 monitoring depends on user familiarity and comprehensive knowledge of essential concepts.

LESS INVASIVE HEMODYNAMIC MONITORING

Noninvasive Hemodynamic Technology

Pulmonary artery catheter use has decreased over the past 10 years in part due to limited evidence of benefit and the advancing technology. The goal of hemodynamic monitoring remains to identify hemodynamic instability and to correct it prior to the onset of organ failure. Often critically ill patients may be managed by physical exam, monitoring of urine output, capillary refill time, skin mottling, and vital signs. When signs of altered stroke volume or changes in heart rate present, the use of more advanced hemodynamic monitoring may be necessary to accurately guide treatment that optimize cardiac output and perfusion. Noninvasive hemodynamic monitoring may be used to assess cardiovascular function and determine appropriate therapies including fluid administration, vasopressors, or inotropes.

Noninvasive hemodynamic monitoring technology has advanced, but each device and method have strengths and limitations. Table 4-11 highlights some of the current noninvasive technology available and the application of these devices. As with all products, it is good to approach them with curiosity and consider your clinical setting and population.

Noninvasive Assessment

Functional Hemodynamic Monitoring

There are over 20 years of research on the use of functional hemodynamic parameters in perioperative and critically ill patients. The most commonly used dynamic indicators, systolic pressure variation (SPV) and pulse pressure variation (PPV), are measured directly from the arterial blood

TABLE 4-11. NONINVASIVE HEMODYNAMIC MONITORING TECHNOLOGY

Technology	Description	Considerations
Capnography-End Tidal CO_2	Paired with the passive leg raise. A increase in $ETCO_2$ of 5% or more indicates an increase in CI- patient is a fluid responder. If <5% increase, suggests patient is a fluid non-responder and may require other therapies.	Only validated in mechanically ventilated patients. Excellent predictor of need for fluid resuscitation.
Non-Invasive Pulse Contour Systems (Finger cuff technology)	Uses pulse contour analysis applied to blood pressure waveform to derive estimated SV, SVI, CO, CI, and SVV	Non-Calibrated May not be reliable if patient is vasoconstricted or has significant edema
Bioreactance Evaluates the change in SV and SV Index.	Two sets of electrodes are applied to anterior chest. The device measures over two phases, the time it takes for a small electrical current to travel across the thorax. Measures: HR, SV, SVI, CO, CI, and an estimate of afterload using total peripheral resistance (TPR). Can be used for PLR.	Non-Calibrated
Ultrasound Cardiac Output Measurement (USCOM)	Uses a noninvasive transcutaneous doppler device to measure continuous transaortic or transpulmonary doppler waveforms to determine CO, CI, SV, SVI, SVR, and DO_2	Non-Calibrated
Ultrasound – (POCUS)	Point of Care Ultrasound is used to evaluate the inferior vena cava for collapsibility in non-ventilated patients and the diameter in vented patients.	
Esophageal Doppler	Doppler	Velocity-time integral (VTi), SV, CO

Frank–Starling Curve

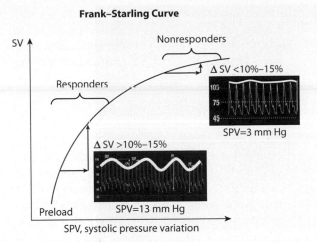

Figure 4-24. Frank-Starling ventricular function curve demonstrating the effects of the shape of the curve (steep vs flat) on the corresponding ventilator-induced changes in arterial pressure waveforms. Similar effects would also be observed on the SV. (*Reproduced with permission from Bridges E. Using functional hemodynamic indicators to guide fluid therapy. Am J Nurs. 2013;113(5):42-50.*)

pressure tracing or indirectly using noninvasive technology (eg, bioreactance or finger cuff technology). The stroke volume variation (SVV), as well as SV and CO, can be derived from technologies using the arterial waveform, noninvasive bioreactance, or finger cuff technology. Each of these dynamic parameters reflects the interaction between the heart and lungs during mechanical ventilation.

Functional hemodynamic parameters, which help answer the question—is the patient a fluid responder—are based on an understanding of the physiology of the heart as described by the Frank-Starling curve or the ventricular function curve (Figure 4-24).

If preload is increased with a fluid bolus, how much the SV increases depends on the shape and position of the ventricular function curve. If both ventricles are on the ascending portion of the curve, the increase in preload should cause a clinically significant increase in SV (fluid responders). For the same increase in preload in a patient who is on the flat portion of the ventricular function curve, there will be a smaller change in SV (fluid nonresponders).

In practice, determination of the patient's fluid response status can be made by observing the ventilator-induced changes in arterial BP (SBP and PP), which are due to positive pressure ventilation. During inspiration the intrathoracic pressure increases, which decreases preload to the heart. The decreased preload results in a decrease in SV for right and left ventricles, which subsequently causes a decrease in BP. By looking at the arterial BP tracing we can observe the ventilator-induced change in BP. A large variation in systolic BP (SPV), pulse pressure (PPV), or a derived SV waveform (SVV) suggests the heart is on the steep portion of the ventricular function curve and the administration of a fluid bolus would likely increase the SV. However, if the arterial BP tracing or derived SV has minimal variation, this suggests the heart is on the flat portion of the

ventricular function curve. If the patient is a fluid nonresponder the administration of a fluid challenge would not increase SV or CO and another treatment, such as addition of a vasopressor may be needed. Figure 4-25 is an example of arterial blood pressure tracings (sweep speed = 6.25 mm/sec) demonstrating the effects of progressive blood volume replacement on the PPV in a model of hemorrhagic shock resuscitation. These changes reflect moving up the ventricular function curve.

The original studies and fluid responsiveness thresholds come from research in mechanically ventilated patients receiving >8 mL/kg tidal volume, with PPV and SVV demonstrating the greatest diagnostic accuracy (Table 4-12). There are parameters from ultrasonography that can also be used to assess fluid responsiveness including inferior and superior vena cava variation during controlled ventilation and aortic velocity time integral (VTI) after passive leg raising.

It is important to note that there are also limitations to the use of these parameters (Table 4-13). Additionally, in fluid responders the effect of a fluid challenge may be transient. The CO may decrease within 30 minutes indicating the need for continued monitoring of perfusion state (eg, capillary refill time, knee mottling).

Performance of Functional Hemodynamic Measurements. There is proprietary technology available to continuously monitor functional hemodynamic indices using both invasive (arterial line) and noninvasive methods (bioimpedance, finger cuff). All of these technologies directly or indirectly measure SPV, PPV and derive SVV, SV, and CO. The SPV and the PPV can also be accurately measured intermittently using the arterial blood pressure tracing and the bedside monitor (Figure 4-26).

Passive Leg Raise Maneuver

The passive leg raising (PLR) maneuver involves moving the patient from a head-of-bed elevated position to torso flat with the legs elevated 30° to 45° (see Figure 4-27). This shift in body position causes a transfer of approximately 300 mL of blood from the lower extremities and splanchnic bed into the central circulation and heart and mimics a fluid challenge. The benefit of the PLRM is that it is reversible as soon as the legs are lowered. Additionally, it can be used in patients who are breathing spontaneously, have arrhythmias, or are receiving low tidal volume ventilation. The primary outcome is a change in SV or CO and there is limited evidence supporting the use of changes in end-tidal CO_2. It is important to note that there are contraindications and limitations to the PLR maneuver (Table 4-14).

The PLR maneuver may be useful in assessing fluid responsiveness in patients with ARDS on lung protective ventilation if the arterial-based measurements (eg, PPV, SVV) are uncertain. In this case, these indicators may be below threshold due to the small change in intrathoracic pressure that may be insufficient to cause sufficient changes in preload.

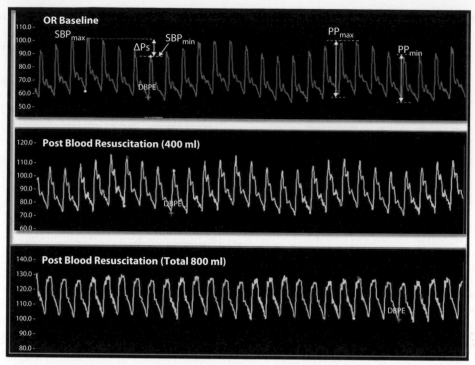

Figure 4-25. Arterial tracing from a model of hemorrhagic shock. **(A)** At baseline, there was marked ventilator-induced variation in the arterial waveform, with a PPV of 18% (fluid responder). **(B)** Following the administration of one unit of whole blood, the PPV decreased to 15% (fluid responder). One additional unit of whole blood was administered. **(C)** Post-resuscitation there was minimal variation in arterial waveform, with a PPV of 11.7% (nonresponder). Further administration of fluids would not increase the SV but would risk volume overload. (*Reproduced with permission from Elizabeth J. Bridges.*)

TABLE 4-12. FUNCTIONAL HEMODYNAMIC PARAMETERS

Formulas		
Variable	**Equation**	**Threshold for Responders**
SPV (Systolic pressure variation)	$SBP_{max} - SBP_{min}$	>10 mm Hg
SPV % (percent variation in SPV)	$([SBP_{max} - SBP_{min}]/[SBP_{max} + SBP_{min}/2]) \times 100$	>10%
*****PPV %** (pulse pressure variation)	$([PP_{max} - PP_{min}]/[PP_{max} + PP_{min}/2]) \times 100$	>12.5%
*****SVV %** (stroke volume variation)	$([SV_{max} - SV_{min}]/[SV_{max} + SV_{min}/2]) \times 100$	>12%
PVI (pleth variability index)	Derived from oximeter perfusion index	12%-16%
ΔSV (Change in SV)	(Post SV – Baseline SV)/ Baseline SV × 100	>10-15%
ΔCO (Change in SV)	(Post CO – Baseline CO)/ Baseline CO × 100	>10-15%
Inferior Vena Cava (IVC) Variation (ventilated)	Ultrasonography measurement	>10%
IVC Variation (spontaneous breathing)	Ultrasonography measurement	>40%
VTi (Velocity Time integral - ventilated)	Echocardiographic measurement	>10%
VTi (spontaneous breathing)	Echocardiographic measurement	>12.5%

The PPV and SVV remain accurate predictors of fluid response status when the patient is receiving <8 mL/kg tidal volume, but the threshold is lower. Use of passive leg raising maneuver should also be considered for patients receiving low tidal volume ventilation.
Data from Headley JM. The goldilocks principle: using functional hemodynamics for fluid optimization. Nurs Crit Care. 2016;11(3):23-27.

Example: Patient with ARDS on lung protective ventilation (Vt < 8 mL/kg PBW)*

- Functional indicator (eg, PPV, SVV) > threshold = Fluid Responder
- Functional indicator < threshold = Uncertain
- Perform PLR maneuver
  - ΔCO > 10% = Fluid Responder
  - Δ CO < 10% = Fluid Nonresponder (do not administer fluids)

Functional hemodynamic indicators may also provide insight into the tolerance of procedures or therapeutic

TABLE 4-13. LIMITATIONS FOR FUNCTIONAL HEMODYNAMICS

- Cannot be measured in spontaneously breathing patients including those receiving mechanical ventilation
- Cannot be reliably performed in patients on biphasic noninvasive ventilation
- Cannot be used with sustained arrhythmias
- Cannot be used with open chest
- Magnitude of the indicator (PPV, SVV) depends on the tidal volume
- Requires a functional arterial line
- Limited studies in patients with decreased ejection fraction
- Low tidal volume (<8 ml/kg) affects threshold (may not see as large a ΔCO)—consider PLRM
- Very high respiratory rate (HR/RR < 3.6) may cause a false negative
- Right heart failure may cause a false positive (limited evidence and has not been seen with ARDS)

*Assumes no right heart dysfunction

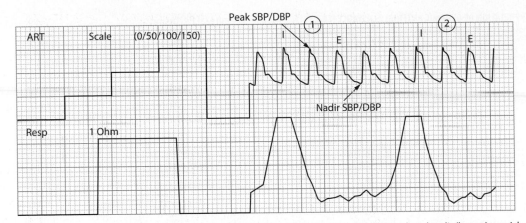

Figure 4-26. Example of a frozen screen used during the manual estimation of SPV and PPV, demonstrating the peak and nadir (lowest) arterial waveforms. Use the ventilatory waveform to identify one ventilator cycle. Within a single ventilator cycle, identify the arterial waveform with the highest systolic blood pressure (SBP); this is the waveform used to measure the peak SBP and DBP. Additionally, this waveform most likely has the largest pulse pressure (PP). Next identify the nadir SBP (this should be during the expiratory phase of the ventilator cycle. Use this waveform for the nadir SBP, DBP, and PP. Identify the exact pressures using the horizontal cursor, which traces along the waveform and provides direct measurements, in contrast to the vertical cursor, which requires estimation of the correct cursor position. Obtain BP values from a single ventilator breath and average over three ventilator cycles. E = expiration; I = inspiration. (*Reproduced with permission from Tyler L, Greco S, Bridges E, et al: Accuracy of stop-cursor method for determining systolic and pulse pressure variation. Am J Crit Care. 2013;22(4):298-305.*)

maneuvers that alter intrathoracic pressure. It is important that the technology used to assess the response to the PLR provide a real-time assessment of the change in SV/CO (eg, bioreactance, echocardiography, pulse contour). The change in BP and the use of the "stat" mode on a continuous cardiac output monitor cannot be used.

Hemodynamic Response to Changes in PEEP. Functional indicators can be used to predict the hemodynamic effects of PEEP. The higher the PPV on zero PEEP (indicating that the patient is on the steep portion of the ventricular function curve) the greater the decrease in CO in response to increased PEEP.

Prediction of Intradialytic Hemodynamic Instability. A combination of hemodynamic indicators reflecting macro-hemodynamics (eg, BP) and perfusion can be used to predict intradialytic hemodynamic instability (IHI). For example, a three-point scale was evaluated in patients undergoing the first run of dialysis, with one point assigned to each of the following parameters obtained immediately before initiation of dialysis: Cardiovascular SOFA score > 1; index finger capillary refill time > 3 seconds; and lactate > 2 mmol/L. The incidence of IHI during the first dialysis run increased with higher scores (0 = 10%; 1 = 33%, 2 = 55%; 3 = 80%), with most of the instability during the first hour. Other studies have found that indications of fluid responsiveness (decreased

pulse pressure index, IVC collapse) and vascular tone (low DBP) are also associated with increased likelihood of IHI.

Pressure Responders

Fluids are administered to patients with acute circulatory failure to increase mean systemic pressure and cardiac output, and ultimately to increase tissue perfusion. As noted above, only approximately half of critically ill patients with indications for a fluid challenge are fluid responders and among

TABLE 4-14. PLR PROCEDURE

- Shift patient from HOB 45° to legs elevated 45°
- Avoid inducing pain, coughing, awakening, which may cause adrenergic stimulation. Sympathetic stimulation may be suspected with a significant increase in HR.
- Shift causes an auto-transfusion of 300-500 mL blood (volume decreased if start from HOB 0°)
- Maximal ΔCO or ΔSV occurs within 1-2 minutes after leg elevation (must use technology that allows for real-time assessment of changes in SV/CO (eg, pulse contour, bioreactance, TEE)
- ΔBP is not a sensitive indicator of fluid responsiveness (direct or noninvasive)
- Fluid Responder: Increase in CO or SV > 10%-15%
- Fluid Nonresponder: Increase in CO or SV < 10% (indication to stop fluid infusion and consider other therapies (eg, vasopressor or inotrope)
- Time to perform maneuver ~ 2-3 minutes

Example of ΔCO Calculation:
Baseline CO = 3.2 L/min; Post CO = 3.6 L/min.
(Increase/Baseline) × 100 = (0.4/3.2) × 100 = ↑12.5%

Contraindications
- Unstable spine fracture
- Orthopedic—transtibial leg fracture
- Increased intracranial pressure
- Suspected or confirmed pulmonary edema
- Intraabdominal hypertension may cause a false negative test

Limitations
- Risk of aspiration
- Compression stockings (eg, TEDs) may decrease the volume of venous return and intermitting sequential compression devices may cause variation in CO

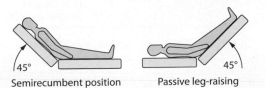

45°   45°

Semirecumbent position   Passive leg-raising

Figure 4-27. Passive leg raising (PLR) maneuver. The PLR is performed by raising the patient's legs to a 45° elevation while simultaneously lowering the patient's head and upper torso from a semi-recumbent (head of bed elevated 45° to a supine (flat) position. This maneuver tests for fluid responsiveness. (*Reproduced with permission from Marik PE, Monnet X, Teboul JL. Hemodynamic parameters to guide fluid therapy. Ann Intensive Care. 2011;1(1):1.*)

TABLE 4-15. INTERPRETATION OF DYNAMIC ARTERIAL ELASTANCE (Ea$_{dyn}$)*

Ea$_{dyn}$ (PPV/SVV)	Interpretation
1.2-2	Normal range indicating patient is likely to be a pressure responder. Example PPV = 14/SVV = 12; Eadyn = 1.2
0.9-1.2	Gray zone – not conclusive
<0.9	Profound vasodilat ion. A low Ea$_{dyn}$ does not preclude the administration of fluids, but the patient may also require a vasopressor. Example PPV = 12/SVV = 16; Eadyn = 0.75

Patient must be considered a fluid responder to apply the Ea$_{dyn}$. If they are not a fluid responder, a fluid challenge would not be expected to increase the CO or BP.

those who are fluid responders only half will also respond with an increase in MAP > 10% (pressure responder). Reasons for the failed pressure response may be because the fluid challenge and increased CO did not adequately increase venous return or there are alterations in arterial tone.

Dynamic arterial elastance (Eadyn). Dynamic arterial elastance is a newer hemodynamic parameter that can be used to predict if a patient who is a fluid responder will also be a pressure responder (Table 4-15). This parameter is based on the assumption that, all things being equal, an increase in the SV will cause an increase in the pulse pressure. How much the pulse pressure increases is dependent on the arterial tone. Under conditions of vasoconstriction, an increase in the SV will be associated with a larger increase in pulse pressure. Conversely, under conditions of vasodilation, an increase in SV may not cause a large increase in pulse pressure. Using the functional hemodynamic measures of PPV and SVV a continuous, dynamic parameter can be calculated (Eadyn = PPV/SVV). The Eadyn is different from systemic vascular resistance; it is a functional measure of arterial stiffness, which is partially determined by vascular tone. The Eadyn allows for the prediction of pressure response (ie, will a fluid responder also be a pressure responder).

Peripheral Perfusion

The assessment of peripheral perfusion is based on the physiological response to shock, which is the redistribution of blood to vital organs and away from less vital vasculature beds, such as the skin. Peripheral perfusion can be assessed using several noninvasive methods including skin mottling and capillary refill time (CRT). The 2021 Surviving Sepsis Campaign international guidelines suggest using CRT as an adjunct to other perfusion measures. Similarly, the National Institutes of Health COVID-19 Guidelines for the Care of Critically Ill Adults with COVID-19 specifically recommends "the use of dynamic parameters, skin temperature, capillary refilling time, and or lactate over static parameters to assess fluid responsiveness."

Skin Mottling

Knee mottling is the patchy purplish skin discoloration that usually starts at the knee due to heterogenic small vessel vasoconstriction, reflecting abnormal skin microperfusion. While skin mottling may be seen on other areas of the body, it can only be reliably assessed on the anterior aspect of the legs. The mottling reflects small vessel vasoconstriction and indicates abnormal skin microperfusion. The skin lacks autoregulation (it is primarily involved with thermal control); thus, the mottling reflects sympathetic activation. Changes in skin mottling occur independent of macrohemodynamics (ie, BP and CO). A limitation of knee mottling is that the research has been primarily done on individuals with a lighter skin tone, which limits its use. Ait Oufella et al. created a scoring system to standardize the evaluation of skin mottling, with scores ranging from 0 to 5 (Figure 4-28). Further research is urgently needed to ensure accurate measurement in all skin tones.

When assessing darker skin tone for pallor or mottling use natural light or halogen light rather than fluorescent light,

ESSENTIAL CONTENT CASE

Pressure Responder (Dynamic Arterial Elastance)

Case 1. A patient is hemodynamically unstable. Consideration is being given to administering a fluid challenge. The patient is a fluid responder and is not at risk for fluid overload. The next question is whether they are also a pressure responder.

HR	SBP/DBP/MAP	DSI	PPV	SVV	Eadyn	Interpretation
115	102/43/63	2.7	12	17	0.7	Fluid responder + Pressure responder –

In Case 1, the patient is a fluid responder but not a pressure responder. The DSI suggests profound vasodilation, which is supported by the Eadyn < 0.9. In this case, fluids may still be appropriate, but a vasopressor may also be needed.

Case 2. A patient has indications of hypoperfusion (elevated lactate, prolonged CRT) despite a normal BP. Consideration is being given to administering a fluid challenge.

The patient is a fluid responder and is not at risk for fluid overload. The next question is whether they are also a pressure responder.

HR	SBP/DBP/MAP	DSI	PPV	SVV	Eadyn	Interpretation
91	112/58/76	1.9	22	15	1.5	Fluid responder + Pressure responder +

In Case 2, the patient is both a fluid responder and a pressure responder as indicated by the Eadyn. Additionally, while the DBP is low, the DSI does not suggest profound vasodilation. The initial and the fluid challenge would be appropriate treatment. This case also demonstrates the integration of indicators of peripheral perfusion along with macrohemodynamics (eg, BP, HR) to detect indications of hypoperfusion.

Mottling score

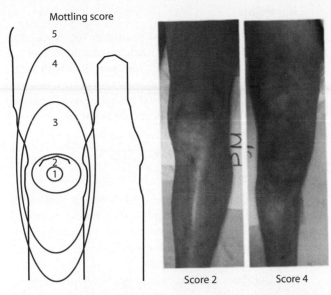

Score 2   Score 4

Figure 4-28. The skin mottling score is based on the extension of the mottling on the leg. Score 0 indicates no mottling; score 1, modest mottling area (coin size) localized to the center of the knee; score 2, moderate mottling area that does not exceed the superior edge of the kneecap; score 3, mild mottling area that does not exceed the middle thigh; score 4, severe mottling area that does not exceed the fold of the groin; score 5, extremely severe mottling area that exceeds the fold of the groin. (*Reproduced with permission from Ait-Oufella H, Lemoinne S, Boelle PY, et al: Mottling score predicts survival in septic shock.* Intensive Care Med. *2011;37(5):801-807.*)

which may alter the skin's true color. In individuals with light skin tone, cyanosis or increased unoxygenated blood generally appears bluish/purple. In contrast in individuals with darker skin tone the unoxygenated blood may cause a gray or whitish coloration and in individuals with yellow skin tones, unoxygenated blood may cause a grayish-greenish tone. If skin mottling on the anterior legs cannot be seen, consider a more general exam of other body areas for pallor (eg, buccal mucosa, conjunctiva, palms). Also consider other methods to assess perfusion, such as capillary refill time.

Capillary Refill Time (CRT)

The CRT refers to the time required for blood flow (thus color) to return to the distal capillaries after the release of compression sufficient to cause blanching of the fingertip, knee, or sternum. CRT reflects peripheral perfusion, with a longer CRT denoting reduced capillary perfusion. To allow for comparison across time, it is critical that all care providers perform the CRT using the same location and technique. Although there are no standard recommendations, Table 4-16 summarizes key aspects of performance, including where on the body the CRT can be reliably measured, how long and how hard to compress.

What do the knee mottling and CRT tell us? Most of the recent research related to skin mottling and CRT has been done in patients undergoing septic shock resuscitation. Studies found that patients with worse knee mottling and longer CRT after 6-hours of resuscitation had a higher risk of death. For example, in a study of patients with septic shock,

TABLE 4-16. PERFORMANCE OF CAPILLARY REFILL TIME EVALUATION

Location	There are three areas on the adult that can be used for reliable CRT measurements: Distal phalanx of the fingers (optimally the middle finger with observation of the nailbed or the pulp), kneecap, sternum. For the hand the arm must be supported at heart level.
Compression time	5-15 seconds, with no significant difference between the two compression periods. The key is standardization across personnel as different compression time will cause a different response.
Compression depth	Moderate pressure, which can be visualized as enough pressure to create a crescent on the tip of examiners nail bed.

after six hours of resuscitation, the CRT in the survivors was 2.3 ± 1.8 seconds versus 5.6 ± 3.5 seconds in nonsurvivors. The CRT on the kneecap was longer overall than the finger (2.3 ± 1.8 seconds vs 4.7 ± 3.8 seconds), with a normal value (2.9 ± 1.7 seconds) in survivors and prolonged value (7.6 ± 4.6 seconds) in nonsurvivors. The thresholds for normal and abnormal vary depending on the location on the body where the measurement is performed. For the most common locations (the index finger) a CRT < 3 seconds is considered normal and a CRT > 4 seconds is abnormal. The CRT on the knee is slightly longer, with a normal time < 3 seconds and a CRT > 5 seconds indicative of impaired perfusion. A recent study found that the risk of death was 4.6 times higher in patients with a CRT > 3.5 seconds at the end of resuscitation compared to those with a normal CRT.

Normalization of the knee mottling and CRT during resuscitation are associated with improved outcomes. Patients who fail to demonstrate an improvement in peripheral perfusion during resuscitation, even if their macrohemo-dynamics (eg, HR, BP, CO) improve, have worse outcomes. In post-cardiac arrest patients, the CRT is prolonged during hypothermia. After rewarming, failure to normalize the CRT is associated with poor survival. In 95 patients with sepsis and elevated lactate present on admission to the ED, 65 had a normal CRT (defined as a CRT < 3 seconds on the distal phalanx after 10 seconds compression) and 30 had an abnormal CRT. After resuscitation 87 patients had a normal CRT. The eight patients with an abnormal CRT, had a higher risk of adverse events (88% vs 20%) and hospital mortality (63% vs 9%). Patients with a normal CRT after resuscitation required less mechanical ventilation and ICU admission. The CRT at the time of a rapid response activation may also be a predictor of adverse events. At the time of activation of a rapid response, an abnormal CRT (>3 seconds) predicted the need to transfer to a higher level of care and mortality. Other risk factors for adverse events present at rapid response activation included the presence of hypoxemia (Spo$_2$ < 92% or increasing O$_2$ requirements), hypotension, or oliguria.

Caution must be used when interpreting the Spo$_2$. Several studies have demonstrated that in individuals with darker skin tone, there is a positive bias in the reported Spo$_2$

measures (ie, the Spo_2 is greater than the Sao_2). This positive bias (~2%) may cause hidden (occult) hypoxemia and also delay the initiation of therapies. At the time of this writing, there is not a specific clinical practice recommendation on how to correct for this disparity; thus a high index of suspicion is needed when a patient has signs of hypoxemia and a normal Spo_2.

Capillary refill time has also been used to guide treatment in the resuscitation of patients with septic shock. In the ANDROMEDA-SHOCK trial, resuscitation was guided by the evaluation of CRT (every 30 minutes until ≤3 seconds) compared to lactate (>20% decrease over 2 hours or normalize). There was lower mortality in the CRT group (34.9% vs 43.4%; p = 0.06), although the difference was not statistically significant. Additionally in the CRT group there was less organ dysfunction, faster organ dysfunction resolution and these patients received less resuscitation fluids and required less vasopressor support. This study demonstrates the potential utility of integrating indicators of peripheral perfusion into treatment decisions. It does not indicate that CRT should be the sole indicator; rather it should be used in conjunction with other routinely monitored hemodynamic parameters, including lactate. A new study (ANDROMEDA-2), that is ongoing is integrating readily accessible hemodynamic parameters (PP and DBP), peripheral perfusion (CRT), fluid responsiveness, and assessment of cardiac dysfunction to guide decisions about fluid therapy and the use of vasopressors and inotropes.

Key Points

- Failure of the peripheral perfusion (eg, knee mottling, CRT) to improve with resuscitation (even if the HR and BP normalize) is associated with worse outcomes.
- Peripheral perfusion should be re-assessed frequently (eg, every 30 minutes during resuscitation.

APPLICATION OF HEMODYNAMIC PARAMETERS

Low Cardiac Output States

Hemodynamic disturbances present as either a high or low blood flow state. Initially, compensatory mechanisms may keep blood flow normal, but eventually the output becomes either too high or too low. The most common alteration is the development of a low CO state.

Low CO states fall into two categories: hypovolemia or LV dysfunction. Although many conditions can cause either hypovolemia or LV dysfunction, all produce a low CO state. Before the CO falls, however, the SV decreases. Therefore, the SV or SI is an earlier warning sign of impending low-flow states. As such, it should be examined before the CO or index. When a declining SV can no longer be compensated (by heart rate), the total blood flow (CO) decreases. From a tissue oxygenation perspective, the drop in SV does not harm oxygen delivery as long as the total blood flow (CO) is maintained. Parameters such as Svo_2 remain normal as long as

---

ESSENTIAL CONTENT CASE

Hypovolemia

A 67-year-old woman is admitted to the critical care unit with the diagnosis of hypotension of unknown origin. She is unresponsive and intubated for airway protection. Breath sounds are clear, urine output is 15 mL in 8 hours, and her skin is cool. Findings from the Focused Assessment with Sonography in Trauma (FAST) examination are inconclusive, so a PA catheter is inserted to aid in the interpretation of the situation. The following data are available:

BP	86/54 mm Hg	SI	16 mL/m²
P	118/min	PA	24/10
RR	30 breaths/min	PAOP	6 mm Hg
T	37.3°C	CVP	3 mm Hg
CI	1.9 L/min/m²	SvO₂	50%

Case Question 1. Which hemodynamic parameters are abnormal?

Case Question 2. What is the significance of the abnormal findings?

Case Question 3. What strategies can be used to determine if the patient will respond to fluid resuscitation?

Answers
1. BP, SI, PAOP, CVP, CI, and SvO_2 are all low. HR is elevated (compensatory response to decrease in BP and CI).

2. Note the low blood flow (CI and SI below normal) and low intracardiac pressures (PAOP). This combination of low flow and intracardiac pressures is consistent with hypovolemia. In addition, the SvO_2 is low, indicating that a threat to tissue oxygenation is likely. The exact cause of the hypovolemia cannot be discerned from the hemodynamics. Further investigation to isolate the exact problem, such as GI bleeding, dehydration, or other forms of blood or fluid loss, is necessary to diagnose the underlying cause of the hypovolemia.

3. Fluid challenges are considered the cornerstone of resuscitation in critically ill patients. However, clinical studies have demonstrated that only about 50% of hemodynamically unstable patients are volume responsive. Increasing evidence suggests that excess fluid resuscitation is associated with increased mortality. It is vital to assess a patient's fluid responsiveness prior to embarking on fluid loading. Static pressure (CVP, PAOP) and echocardiographic (IVC diameter) parameters are not reliable predictors of volume responsiveness. Dynamic parameters (SPV, PPV, SVV) are reliable predictors of fluid response and are measured based on evaluating arterial pressure data as it changes over the course of the respiratory cycle in a patient on positive pressure mechanical ventilation. In spontaneously breathing patients, the passive leg raise test is highly predictive of volume responsiveness.

total blood flow is unchanged. Because SV and SVI decrease in both hypovolemia and LV dysfunction, without necessarily changing CO or Svo_2 levels, it is important to assess SV and SVI first when examining hemodynamic parameters.

Identifying the cause of the low-flow state (eg, hypovolemia or LV dysfunction) is based on a combination of clinical and hemodynamic information. For example, the patient's physical assessment and history might reveal the presence of a pathologic clinical condition such as LV failure. From a hemodynamic monitoring perspective, the use of intracardiac pressures (PAOP, CVP) is the most common method of differentiating the cause of the low blood flow state. Management of low CO states begins by treating problems of either LV dysfunction or hypovolemia.

Left Ventricular Dysfunction

Low CO states that are caused by LV dysfunction are managed with interventions that decrease LV work and improve performance: increase contractility and reduce preload and afterload. Generally, pharmacologic therapies are used to treat the dysfunctional left ventricle. However, a few physical interventions are available, such as allowing the patient to sit up, attempting to reduce anxiety, as well as mechanical supports, such as intra-aortic balloon pumping and ventricular assist devices (see Chapter 19, Advanced Cardiovascular Concepts). Improvement of LV function, however, relies heavily on pharmacologic support (see Table 4-2).

It is possible to perform ambulatory PA pressure and heart rate monitoring using the CardioMEMS™ in patients with preserved or reduced ejection heart failure with NYHA Class III symptoms who have been hospitalized in the past year (see Figure 4-29). A transcatheter is implanted into the left pulmonary artery. The device trends PA pressures and waveforms and transmits this information to a care provider. The data from the CardioMEMS™ precedes clinical deterioration and allows for early intervention. The CHAMPION trial showed a 28% reduction of HF hospitalization in 6 months and 37% reduction in 15 months.

Improvement of Contractility

If a patient presents with symptoms of LV dysfunction, relief is obtained by improving LV function. Inotropic therapy is commonly employed during an acute episode of LV dysfunction. Inotropic therapy increases the strength of the cardiac contraction, thereby increasing EF, SV, CO, and tissue oxygenation.

Two common inotropic drugs are used in critical care to improve ventricular contractility: dobutamine (Dobutrex) and milrinone (Primacor) (Table 4-17). Dobutamine acts as a sympathetic stimulant, increasing the stimulation of beta cells of the sympathetic nervous system. This stimulation produces a positive inotropic (contractile) response, as well as a positive chronotropic (heart rate) response. Heart rate response will be minimal unless the patient has a diminished preload. Dobutamine also has a slight vasodilator effect due to B_2 stimulation, causing a slight reduction in preload and afterload. Based on these effects, dobutamine is an ideal first choice to pharmacologically increase the CO and SV.

If dobutamine is not effective, milrinone may be used because its action is different from dobutamine. Dobutamine may not be effective in cases where sympathetic stimulation has already achieved its maximal impact. Milrinone is a phosphodiesterase inhibitor, increasing the availability of intracellular calcium. Milrinone reduces both the preload and afterload and must be used carefully in patients with acute decompensated congestive heart failure.

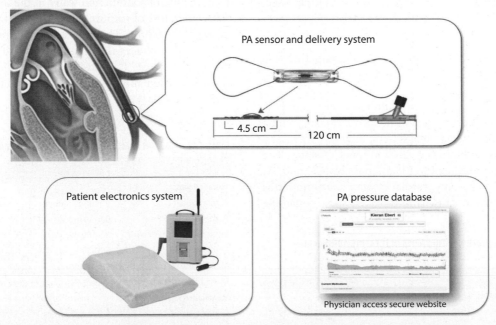

Figure 4-29. CardioMEMS HF system including pressure sensor and external measurement unit. CardioMEMS™. (*CardioMEMS, Champion and St. Jude Medical are trademarks of St. Jude Medical, LLC or its related companies. Reproduced with permission of St. Jude Medical, ©2018. All rights reserved.*)

Ambulatory PA Pressure Monitoring

A 75-year-old male diagnosed with heart failure with reduced EF (hFrEF) has been admitted to hospital three times in the past 6 months with progressively worsening heart failure. He is admitted for the placement of a CardioMEMS PA pressure monitoring device. Other comorbidities include diabetes, atrial fibrillation, CAD, COPD, and gout.

Medications included valsartan, carvedilol CR, spironolactone, furosemide, insulin, allopurinol, digoxin, warfarin, and metformin. Initial hemodynamic findings are:

EF	25%
CO	3.2 L/min
PA	65/32 mm Hg

Following implantation of the device, he has no further hospitalization for a period of 1 year and 6 months. Adjustment of medication is made remotely.

Case Question 1. What is a normal PA systolic, diastolic, and mean?

Case Question 2. What is the benefit of ambulatory PA pressure monitoring?

Answers

1. A normal PA systolic is 15 to 35 mm Hg; PA diastolic is 10 to 15 mm Hg; PA mean is 15 to 20 mm Hg.
2. Ambulatory PA pressure monitoring allows the HCP to identify periods of clinical deterioration remotely. It allows for same-day or next-day medication adjustments to prevent decompensation. It greatly reduces readmission of patients for heart failure decompensation providing a more proactive approach to medical management.

Although milrinone is associated with coagulopathic side effects (decreases platelet count), it is a logical alternative to dobutamine or dopamine.

Dopamine also can be used to improve the contractile state of the heart. Because dopamine also stimulates alpha cells of the sympathetic nervous system, afterload increases, a situation that is not always desired in low CO states. The net effect is an improvement in BP and possibly CO and SV, but the cost in terms of myocardial oxygen consumption is higher than with the other two inotropes. As such, dopamine

TABLE 4-17. COMMON INOTROPIC THERAPIES IN TREATING ABNORMAL HEMODYNAMICS

Drug	Dosage	Onset of Action	Route
Dobutamine (Dobutrex)	1-20 mcg/kg/min	1-2 min	IV
Dopamine (Intropin)	2-10 mcg/kg/min	1-2 min	IV
Milrinone (Primacor)	Loading 0.75 mg/kg, then 5-10 mcg/kg/min	<5 min	IV

is not a first-line drug to treat acute LV dysfunction unless hypotension is present.

The potential negative effect of inotropic therapy is the increase in myocardial oxygen consumption that accompanies the increased contractile state. Unfortunately, it is not easy to measure myocardial oxygenation. Because of this potential problem, many clinicians prefer to use agents that either reduce preload or afterload, because these agents do not increase myocardial oxygen consumption.

Preload Reduction

Reduction of preload is thought to be beneficial in the patient with LV dysfunction by decreasing the distention of overstretched myocardial muscle fibers. Many therapies have been designed for preload reduction, although they generally fall into one of two groups: drugs that reduce blood volume (diuretics) and those that promote venous vasodilation (nitrates, calcium channel blockers, beta-blockers, and morphine sulfate) (Table 4-18).

The most common approach to reduce preload is diuretic therapy. Diuretics are preferred because they eliminate excess fluid. As the left ventricle begins to fail, blood flow is decreased to the kidneys. This reduced blood flow is interpreted by the kidneys as insufficient blood volume. The kidneys then increase the reabsorption of water, producing an increase in intravascular volume. This increase contributes to venous engorgement and dependent edema in HF. Remember the use of preload reduction in patients with a systolic pressure less than 90 mm Hg can lead to worsening clinical presentation.

The most common diuretics used to reduce preload are the loop diuretics. Loop diuretics work by blocking the reabsorption of sodium and water in the loop of Henle. The subsequent loss of sodium and water allows for a reduction in vascular volume. The reduction in intravascular volume theoretically reduces the amount of blood returning to the heart and reduces the tension on myocardial muscle. The reduced tension allows the heart to return to a more normal contractile state.

TABLE 4-18. COMMON PRELOAD REDUCERS FOR ABNORMAL HEMODYNAMICS

Drug	Dosage	Onset of Action	Route
Diuretic Agents			
Furosemide (Lasix)	20 mg or higher	<5 min	IV/PO
Bumetanide (Bumex)	0.5-10 mg/day	<5 min	IV/PO
Ethacrynic Acid (Edecrin)	50-100 mg/day	<5 min	IV/PO
Chlorothiazide (Diuril)	500-2000 mg/day	1-2 h	IV/PO
Metolazone (Zaroxolyn)	2.5-20 mg/day	1 h	PO
Mannitol (Osmitrol)	12.5-200 g/day	<5 min	IV
Vasodilating Agents			
Dopamine (Intropin)	1-2 mcg/kg/min	5 min	IV
Nitroglycerin (Tridil, Nitrostat IV)	5-400 mcg	1-2 min	IV

ESSENTIAL CONTENT CASE

Left Ventricular Dysfunction

A 76-year-old man is admitted to the critical care unit with the diagnosis of acute inferior wall myocardial infarction and a history of COPD. During the shift he begins to complain of shortness of breath. He has crackles one-third of the way up his posterior lobes along with expiratory wheezing. He has an S_3 (gallop) and an II/VI systolic murmur. The following hemodynamic information is obtained on admission:

BP	100/58 mm Hg	PA	38/23
P	112/min	PAOP	21 mm Hg
CI	2.1 L/min/m²	CVP	13 mm Hg
CO	4.6 L/min	SvO_2	49%
SI	19		

Case Question 1. Which hemodynamic parameters are abnormal?

Case Question 2. What is the significance of these findings?

Case Question 3. What are the treatment priorities for this patient?

Answers
1. PA pressures, PAOP, CVP elevated; SI, CI, and SvO_2 decreased.
2. This patient presents with low blood flow (CI and SI) and high intracardiac pressures (PAOP, CVP). The combination of low blood flow and high filling pressures suggests LV and RV dysfunction. The low SvO_2 level suggests a serious disturbance in tissue oxygenation (alteration between oxygen delivery and oxygen consumption).
3. Interventions to support CI are required. Monitor heart rate and stroke volume. Reduce preload, assess afterload and contractility. The CI is not profoundly low so further investigation into the reason for the extremely low SvO_2 is needed. Further investigation to isolate the cause of LV dysfunction, such as HF, myocardial infarction, or cardiomyopathy, is necessary.

ESSENTIAL CONTENT CASE

Inotropic Therapy

A 71-year-old man is admitted to the ICU with hypotension of unknown origin. He presently has a fiber-optic PA catheter in place to determine the origin of the hypotension. He is unresponsive with a Glasgow Coma Scale of 4. His vital signs and PA catheter reveal the following information:

BP	102/68 mm Hg
P	101/min
CO	3.9 L/min
CI	2.3 L/min/m²
SI	23
PA	42/22
PAOP	18 mm Hg
CVP	12 mm Hg
SvO_2	51%

Case Question 1. Which hemodynamic parameters are abnormal?

Case Question 2. What are the treatment priorities for this patient?

Answers
1. CI, SI, and SvO_2 are low. HR, PA pressures, PAOP, and CVP are elevated.
2. Dobutamine is added to the patient's management regime. One hour after the dobutamine, a repeat set of hemodynamics reveals the following:

BP	104/66 mm Hg
P	106/min
CO	4.4 L/min
CI	2.6 L/min/m²
SI	25
PA	40/20
PAOP	14 mm Hg
CVP	13 mm Hg
SvO_2	57%

Based on the slight improvement in SI, CI, and SvO_2, as well as the decrease in PAOP, there has been a mild improvement in the hemodynamic parameters. Further titration of dobutamine should be considered because SvO_2 is not within normal limits. Milrinone is another option that could improve this patient's presentation. Remember the importance of following trends. Results are usually not immediate, so close monitoring of trends will allow improved outcomes. Consideration may also be given to the careful administration of vasodilators (although dobutamine also causes vasodilation) and diuresis.

Other preload reducers, such as nitroglycerin, act by promoting vasodilation. The result of vasodilation is to reduce the amount of blood returning to the heart. The net effect is to reduce preload and improve the LV contractile state. In clinical practice, it is common to use either form of preload reduction or both. Preload reducers such as nitroglycerin have the added benefit of improving myocardial blood flow. However, they do not contribute to diuresis. Morphine sulfate is also used as a preload reducer in patients with congestive heart failure and works as a peripheral vasodilator resulting in venous pooling.

Afterload Reduction

The cornerstone of long-term LV dysfunction management is the use of drugs to reduce afterload (resistance to ejection of blood). Short-term reduction of afterload, such as one sees in the acutely ill patient with LV dysfunction, is important, but is used only after ensuring the presence of an adequate SV. When afterload reduction should be used in acute care

TABLE 4-19. COMMON AFTERLOAD-REDUCING AGENTS

Drug	Dose	Onset of Action	Route
Smooth Muscle Relaxants and Alpha Inhibitors			
Nitroprusside (Nipride)	0.5-10 mcg/kg/min	1-2 min	IV
Nitroglycerin (Tridil, Nitrostat IV)	5-400 mcg	1-2 min	IV
Hydralazine (Apresoline)	10-40 mg	10-20 min	IV/IM
Phentolamine (Regitine)	0.1-2 mg/min	<1 min	IV
Angiotension-Converting Enzyme Inhibitors			
Captopril (Capoten)	25-400 mg/day in 2-3 doses	15-30 min	PO
Enalapril/Enalaprilat (Vasotec/ Vasotec IV)	2.5-4.0 mg/day	15 min	PO/IV
Lisinopril (Zestril)	10-40 mg/day	1 h	PO

is not universally agreed upon. However, it may be beneficial to lower BP or SVR to decrease afterload because doing so reduces LV work, improves LV contractility, and reduces myocardial oxygen consumption.

In an acutely ill patient with LV dysfunction, afterload reduction is employed when the patient is hypertensive or has a high SVR. Generally, afterload reducers are used initially only if the BP or high SVR is considered to be the cause of the LV dysfunction. Otherwise, afterload reducers are added after inotropic therapy and preload reduction.

In acute management of an increased afterload, the most common afterload reducer is nitroprusside (Nipride) (Table 4-19). This arterial dilating agent works very fast (within 2 minutes) and has only a short-acting half-life (about 2 minutes). The disadvantage of nitroprusside is that it breaks down into thiocyanate, a precursor to cyanide. Toxic levels of thiocyanate can accumulate within 2 days of administration at higher doses, particularly in patients with renal impairment. The antidote for thiocyanate poisoning is sodium thiosulfate. The sodium thiosulfate can be added to the nitroprusside infusion to reduce the likelihood of thiocyanate toxicity.

Other rapid afterload-reducing agents are available, including newer calcium channel and beta-blocking agents. Keep in mind that these agents might act as negative inotropes and actually weaken heart contractility. Their use in acute management of LV dysfunction is controversial, although their long-term use in managing HF is well established.

Other common agents to reduce afterload are the angiotensin-converting enzyme inhibitors. Generally, these drugs are used for the chronic management of afterload in an oral form, although some IV forms are available (enalapril). See Chapter 7, Pharmacology, for additional information on drug therapy.

Hypovolemia

If the underlying cause of the low CO state is hypovolemia, two key approaches are used: preload augmentation and

---

ESSENTIAL CONTENT CASE

Preload Reduction

A 77-year-old woman is in the intensive care unit following an episode of angina that precipitated an exacerbation of HF. She has a PA catheter in place, which was used to measure initial hemodynamics. A repeat evaluation was done following the initiation of nitroglycerin.

	Initial Values	Post-Nitroglycerin Values
BP	114/76 mm Hg	112/72 mm Hg
P	106/min	92/min
CI	2.4 L/min/m^2	2.6 L/min/m^2
SI	23	28
PA	40/23	35/20
PAOP	22 mm Hg	17 mm Hg
CVP	12 mm Hg	9 mm Hg
SvO$_2$	53%	58%

Case Question 1. Based on these data, was the nitroglycerin effective in improving her hemodynamics?

Case Question 2. Is the patient stabilized?

Answers
1. Based on the increase in SI and SvO$_2$, as well as a decrease in PAOP, this therapy appears to have been effective. Even though the CO did not change markedly, the increase was enough to improve tissue oxygenation. This example illustrates the need to evaluate more than one parameter (such as PAOP, SvO$_2$, etc.).
2. No. The patient is stabilized when the SvO$_2$ is between 60% and 80%. Consider titrating the nitroglycerin up, re-evaluating the hemodynamic values, and monitoring signs of tissue perfusion such as lactate level. Further diagnostic workup for the cause of her angina is also needed.

---

identification of the optimal type of preload agent. Identifying when to treat a patient who is potentially hypovolemic is greatly enhanced with hemodynamic monitoring. It is critical to use the guidelines outlined to avoid common errors in interpretation of hemodynamic monitoring data. For example, in the patient who is hypovolemic, the SV or SVI changes when vascular volume has been significantly altered. This change in SV is frequently accompanied by reduced cardiac pressures (eg, PAOP, CVP). However, the key parameter to monitor is SV. Keep in mind that cardiac pressures do not necessarily reflect changes in volume, due to ventricular compliance. To avoid errors in interpreting hypovolemia, always examine if a low SV is present before examining the cardiac pressures and consider functional (eg, SPV, PPV, or SVV) instead of static parameters (eg, CVP or PAOP).

Perhaps one of the most controversial areas in the treatment of hypovolemia is the choice of the agent to use to increase vascular volume. There are three major categories of agents to be considered: blood, crystalloids, and colloids.

ESSENTIAL CONTENT CASE

Hypovolemia

A 62-year-old man is in the critical care unit due to a ruptured diverticula. He presently is unresponsive and is being prepared for surgery. Breath sounds are clear, urine output is 20 mL in 9 hours, and his skin is cool and dry. A PA catheter is inserted to aid in the interpretation of the situation. The following data are available:

BP	82/58 mm Hg
P	111/min
RR	33/min
T	38.4°C
CI	1.7 L/min/m^2
SI	15
PA	23/11
PAOP	7 mm Hg
CVP	2 mm Hg
SvO$_2$	53%

After administration of fluid, PLR test is performed. The change in SV is less than 10%.

Case Question 1. Which hemodynamic parameters are abnormal?

Case Question 2. What is the treatment priority for this patient?

Case Question 3. What is the significance of the PLR test result?

Answers

1. BP, CI, SI, PAOP, CVP, and Svo$_2$ are all low. HR and temperature are elevated.
2. The most important parameters to treat are the low SI, CI, and Svo$_2$. A threat to tissue oxygenation clearly exists based on these parameters. Immediate supportive therapy includes a fluid bolus of NS or lactated Ringer solution. Infusing LR may contribute to an elevated lactate level. Lactate levels are important to monitor if the patient is in shock. Blood products (whole blood, albumin) may also be considered until the patient is taken to surgery. The other factor affecting tissue oxygenation in this patient is probable sepsis. Fluid administration, blood cultures, and administration of antibiotics are a high priority. If he is persistently hypotensive or has an elevated lactate level after initial fluid replacement, reassess volume status and tissue perfusion. Volume status can be reassessed by measuring CVP, or Scvo$_2$, performing a bedside cardiovascular ultrasound, or dynamic assessment of fluid responsiveness with passive leg raise or fluid challenge. Tissue perfusion is reassessed by a repeat focused examination.
3. Based on initial hemodynamic measurements (BP, CI, SI, PAOP, CVP, and Svo$_2$) treatment with intravenous fluids is the priority. However, only approximately 50% of the hemodynamically unstable patients improve their perfusion with administration of IV fluids. Since assessment with PLR after initial fluid resuscitation showed a change in SV of less than 10%, this patient would probably not benefit from further fluid administration. A vasopressor should be considered to provide hemodynamic stability. PLR is a useful test for predicting fluid responsiveness in hemodynamically unstable patients. In intubated patients, assessing SVV or PPV over the course of the respiratory cycle is also a noninvasive way to assess the fluid responsiveness.

Blood transfusion as described above is indicated in acute blood loss and when the hemoglobin reaches a specific threshold. Crystalloids are solutions such as NS and lactated Ringer solution. They obtain their benefit primarily through the sodium in the solution. The electrolyte levels in crystalloid solutions may vary from plasma levels. For example, in 0.9% NS, the Na+ and Cl− are both 154 mEq/L and there is no potassium or calcium. In Lactated Ringers, the Na+ is 130 mEq/L, K+ is 4.0 mEq/L, Cl− is 10.9 mEq/L, and calcium is 2.7 mmol/L. Colloids are solutions such as blood products (albumin) or synthetic solutions (hetastarch, a glucose polymer). Hetastarch use is very limited in practice due to its adverse renal and coagulation effects. Their fluid-retaining effect is because of the large molecules (protein or glucose polymers) in the solution.

There are several advantages of crystalloid solutions. They are inexpensive and produce limited immunologic responses. The key clinical advantage is that they expand into all fluid compartments (vascular, interstitial, and intracellular) because most of the solution does not remain in just the vascular bed; for example, if 1000 mL of a crystalloid such as (0.9% sodium chloride, is given, less than 200 mL stays in the vascular bed. The rest diffuses into the other fluid compartments. This makes crystalloids ideal for treating patients who have chronic hypovolemia or dehydration. This advantage is also a limitation in some cases. If a rapid vascular expansion is required, it takes large volumes of crystalloids because most of the solution is not staying in the vascular system. An additional disadvantage is that the acidity of NS, and the administration of large volumes may cause hyperchloremic metabolic acidosis.

Colloids have one key advantage over crystalloids in that they rapidly expand the vascular volume. Virtually all the colloid solution infused remains in the vascular bed, at least initially. This allows for much more rapid treatment of hypovolemia, frequently necessary in conditions such as trauma and postoperative bleeding. One disadvantage to colloids is their expense. Controversy does exist, however, about whether colloids are any more effective than crystalloids. Concerns have been raised that colloids may potentially cause harm in conditions with capillary leak syndromes (eg, sepsis and ARDS). In these conditions, the leakage of fluid through damaged capillaries is exacerbated if large proteins (or glucose polymers) leak through the capillaries because they pull large amounts of fluid along with them.

Further research is needed to determine the best fluid to use in different clinical situations. Each has its own benefits and limitations. Regardless of which is to be used, its effect should be measured on how well it improves tissue oxygenation, SV, SVI, and intracardiac pressures.

High Cardiac Output States

Though less common, elevations in CO also occur in critically ill patients. In healthy people, CO is increased when the demand for oxygen increases, such as during physical activity or psychological stimulation (fear, anxiety). In critical care, high CO states occur in response to a systemic inflammation, hepatic disease, or neurogenic-mediated vasodilation (Table 4-20). The most common reason for the CO to elevate is systemic inflammation, which is part of the dysregulated response to sepsis, and leads to a drop in SVR. This decrease in resistance produces a compensatory increase in CO. The increase in CO might be minimal or marked. The key point to remember is that an elevation in CO is a sign of a problem and not a problem in and of itself. If the problem is treated, the CO will return to normal.

When a patient has high COs in sepsis, it does not mean the heart is functioning normally. Because of the release of myocardial depressant factors, the EF normally is depressed in sepsis. The method by which the SV is maintained is through an increase in EDV. This increase in EDV allows SV to be maintained even though the EF is reduced.

If the hemodynamic problem in a high CO state is a low SVR, initial treatment centers on increasing afterload (SVR), augmenting preload, and administration of inotropic therapy. None of these therapies for managing low SVR states is curative, and the underlying cause of the low SVR (such as infection) must be corrected. Fluid administration with crystalloids (or colloids) is common because the vasodilation in low SVR produces a pseudohypovolemia. As described in the Essential Content Case, Hypovolemia, administration of

fluid resuscitation is followed by an assessment, such as PLR, to determine if the patient will benefit from further fluid administration.

An additional intervention for patients with low SVR is administration of an alpha-stimulating medication. Three common IV agents used for this purpose are norepinephrine (Levophed), dopamine (Intropin), and phenylephrine (Neosynephrine). Norepinephrine and dopamine have a combination of alpha and beta stimulation, producing both vasoconstriction and increased cardiac stimulation (inotropic and chronotropic responses). This makes the heart contract more forcefully and faster. These two agents have a greater likelihood of increasing BP and SVR due to this combined cardiac and vascular effect. Phenylephrine is only an alpha stimulant, which has some advantages; however, it is generally a third-line drug of choice. Because it only causes alpha stimulation, there is less direct effect on the heart. Although the SVR and BP might not be increased as quickly with phenylephrine, it does avoid some of the direct increase of myocardial oxygen consumption that is seen with norepinephrine and dopamine. Clinically, any of these agents may be used to increase the SVR. Because they are strong alpha stimulants, their use should be considered with a degree of caution.

Direct alpha stimulants can cause severe vasoconstriction. These agents are so strong that if they infiltrate into tissue, the resulting vasoconstriction might cause local tissue death. As a precaution, most institutions have policies that require vasopressors to be administered via large, central veins, or if necessary, for a short duration through a peripheral line while central access is obtained. The incidence of complications associated with peripheral vasopressors is relatively low (<2%–4%). If peripheral vasopressors are required, the IV catheter should be proximal to the antecubital fossa, the lowest concentration of vasopressor possible, should be used, and transition to central venous administration as occur as soon as possible.

From an assessment perspective, if these drugs are effective, the SVR should increase as well as the BP. However, it is critical to remember that when these drugs are used, tissue oxygenation as well as SVR and BP must be assessed. If the SVR or BP increases, parameters such as Svo_2

TABLE 4-20. HEMODYNAMIC PROFILES IN SHOCK

Parameters	Hypovolemic Shock	Cardiogenic Shock	Neurogenic Shock	Anaphylactic Shock	Septic Shock Early	Septic Shock Late	Obstructive Shock
RAP	↓	↑	↓	↓	↓	↑	↑
PAOP	↓	↑	↓	↓	↓	↑	↑
CO/CI	↓	↓	N↓	↓	N↑	↓	↓
BP	↓	↓	↓	↓	↓	↓	↓
PAP	N↓↑	↑	N↓	N↓↑	N↓	↑	↑
SVR	↑	↑	↓	↓	↓	↑	↑

Abbreviation: N, normal.

ESSENTIAL CONTENT CASE

Low SVR

A 65-year-old man is in the critical care unit after developing hypotension on the floor. He had femoral-popliteal bypass surgery 4 days earlier and was doing well until yesterday. He began to complain of generalized malaise with the following vital signs:

BP	102/58 mm Hg	RR	27 breaths/min
P	110/min	T	38.1°C

His wound site is reddened but has no drainage. This morning, he was disoriented and hypotensive (BP 88/54, P 114/min), prompting the transfer to the intensive care unit. A lactate level was obtained and was 3.2 mmol/L. He does not complain of any discomfort or shortness of breath. His lung sounds are clear, and he has a pulse oximeter value of 99%. A flow-directed PA catheter is inserted to assist in the assessment of the cause of hypotension. The following data are available from the PA catheter:

CO	10.5 L/min	SVR	475
CI	6.0 L/min/m^2	PVR	51
PA	22/11	CVP	2 mm Hg
PAOP	8 mm Hg	SvO$_2$	84%

Case Question 1. Which hemodynamic parameters are abnormal?

Case Question 2. What is the treatment required for this patient?

Answers

1. CI, HR, and SvO$_2$ are elevated. BP, SVR, PAOP, and CVP are decreased.
2. Based on this information, the patient is in septic shock as evidenced by a MAP < 65 mm Hg and a lactate level > 2 mmol/L. In addition, the vasodilation is also producing low cardiac pressures. The current recommendation is fluid resuscitation of up to 30 mg/kg. If after fluid resuscitation the BP remains low, further evaluation to determine fluid responsiveness is needed. If the patient is not fluid responsive a vasopressor such as norepinephrine is initiated. The 2021 Sepsis Guideline recommends the addition of vasopressin with norepinephrine in the setting of septic shock. Definitive therapy to treat the underlying cause of his septic shock must begin as soon as possible and includes appropriate antibiotic therapy and cultures.

also increase. SVR and BP do not always directly correlate with blood flow, which makes the addition of tissue oxygenation parameters (like SvO$_2$) an essential part of assessing the effect of vasopressors like norepinephrine, dopamine, and phenylephrine.

In some cases, patients with low SVR may benefit from inotropic therapy to improve oxygen delivery.

Administration of inotropic therapy might seem unusual in a patient with a normal or high CO. However, the rationale for this therapy is to provide supranormal oxygenation to address the microcapillary shunting and diminished cellular oxygenation that occurs in sepsis and other low SVR states (Figure 4-30). In such patients, the SvO$_2$ levels are high, reflecting the regional maldistribution of blood flow and

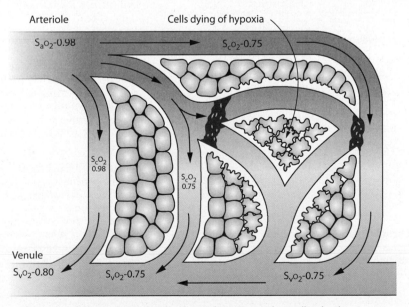

Figure 4-30. Microcirculatory shunting due to obstruction at the capillary level.

diminished oxygen consumption. Because of a lack of blood flow to some regions, oxygen delivery may be increased in an attempt to increase oxygen to threatened areas. Whether this therapy is effective is still being investigated. If the problem is simply microcapillary shunting, increasing oxygen delivery might be sufficient. However, if the problem is diminished cellular oxygenation or an inability to effectively use oxygen, then increased oxygen delivery alone is unlikely to be helpful.

Current management guidelines focus on the need to restore microcirculatory oxygenation, pressure, and flow variables. Despite normalization of global parameters (BP, CI, lactate, base excess, etc.), microcirculatory and regional perfusion alterations may still occur. Persistence of these alterations has been associated with worsened prognosis. The use of near-infrared spectroscopy (NIRS), which measures tissue oxygenation (Sto_2) and provides a method to monitor regional circulation shows great promise in assessing brain microcirculation and oxygenation. However, widespread use of the technology to assess shock states has not yet occurred. Future studies may provide insight into how best the technology may be used (Figure 4-31).

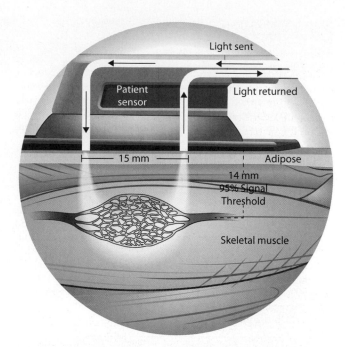

Figure 4-31. StO_2 is derived from measurement of the near-infrared spectra of the tissue bed sampled. A near-infrared light source shines light into the tissue bed. It is used to measure the percentage of hemoglobin saturation. The normal value is 0.75 to 0.90.

ESSENTIAL CASE STUDY

Initial Assessment Using Routine Vital Signs

Case: 52-year-old male s/p emergent colectomy (ruptured diverticulum with peritonitis). PMH: Hypertension, mild LV hypertrophy with diastolic dysfunction; EF 56%. Intraoperative: EBL 300 mL (replaced with 1 u PRBCs) plus 750 mL crystalloid (3-250 mL boluses). Fio_2 50%.

Parameter	Value	Interpretation
HR (bpm)	108	• HR 108, DBP 54; DSI = 2 (vasodilation not profound)
SBP/DBP/MAP (mm Hg)	92/54/66	• Hypotension
Pulse pressure (mm Hg)	38	• MAP = 66 (concern in patient with HTN)
RR	22	• ↑Lactate 3.6 mmol/L suggesting hypoperfusion
Temp (°C)	38.1	• ↓Pulse pressure (normal 40-60 mm Hg). PP < 40 suggests SV is low
Spo_2 (%)	100	
Lactate	3.6	• ↑Shock index (HR/SBP = 1.17; abnormal > 0.9)
Hgb (g/dL)	10.2	
Knee mottling score	3	• ↓peripheral perfusion (knee mottling and prolonged CRT)
CRT (sec)	4	

Q. Is the patient hemodynamically unstable?
Yes – the patient is tachycardic and hypotensive (of greater concern in a patient with a history of hypertension) and his shock index (HR/SBP) is greater than 0.9. He is tachypneic and febrile, and despite a MAP greater than 65 mmHg.

Q. What are the indications of hypoperfusion?
He has a lactate of 3.6 mmol/L, his CRT =4 (above the normal threshold of 3) and his skin mottling score is elevated at 3. Given these findings indicating hypoperfusion and his risk for infection – he has probable diagnosis of septic shock.

Q. Is this a cardiac output problem?
The most likely cause of the hypotension is a CO problem as indicated by the decreased SBP and narrow PP. A bedside echo could be performed to assess cardiac function if needed. Although vasodilation is a primary finding in distributive shock staes such as sepsis, for this patient it does not appear to be profound. The patient is tachycardic (HR 108) with a DBP of 58 and a diastolic shock index of 2.

Q. What is the initial treatment for this patient?
In this patient, hypoperfusion and an increased risk for infection should trigger a sepsis alert. The initial treatment would be aimed at optimizing cardiac output with fluids. The integration of functional hemodynamic parameters would further refine treatment decisions. This case demonstrates and example of using less-invasive methods of assessment to guide therapy in a patient.

SELECTED BIBLIOGRAPHY

Hemodynamic Monitoring—General

Bakker J, Kattan E, Annane D, et al. Current practice and evolving concepts in septic shock resuscitation. *Intensive Care Med.* 2022;48:148-163.

Cecconi M, Hernandez G, Dunser M, et al. Fluid administration for acute circulatory dysfunction using basic monitoring: narrative review and expert panel recommendations from an ESICM task force. *Intensive Care Med.* 2019;45:21–32.

Cinel I, Kasapoglu US, Gul F, Dellinger RP. The initial resuscitation of septic shock. *J Crit Care.* 2020;57:108-117.

De Backer D. Detailing the cardiovascular profile in shock patients. *Crit Care.* 2017;21(Suppl 3):311.

De Backer D, Foulon P. Minimizing catecholamines and optimizing perfusion. *Crit Care.* 2019;23(Suppl 1):149.

Knapp, R, ed. *Hemodynamic Monitoring Made Incredibly Visual.* 4th ed., Wolters Kluwer, 2020. Philadelphia, PA.

Kupchik N. Principles of resuscitation. *Crit Care Nurse Clin N Am.* 2021;33:225-244.

Ltaief Z, Schneider AG, Liaudet L. Pathophysiology and clinical implications of the veno-arterial PCO_2 gap. *Crit Care.* 2021;25:318.

Maheshwari K, Nathanson BH, Munson SH, et al. Abnormal shock index exposure and clinical outcomes among critically ill patients: a retrospective cohort analysis. *J Crit Care.* 2020;57:5-12.

Messina A, Collino F, Cecconi M. Fluid administration for acute circulatory dysfunction using basic monitoring. *Ann Trans Med.* 2020;8(12):788.

Messmer AS, Zingg C, Müller M, Gerber JL, Schefold JC, Pfortmueller CA. Fluid overload and mortality in adult critical care patients—a systematic review and meta-analysis of observational studies [published online October 1, 2020]. *Crit Care Med.* doi:10.1097/ccm.0000000000004617

Osman M, Balla S, Dupont A, O'Neill WW, Babar Basir M. Reviving invasive hemodynamic monitoring in cardiogenic shock. Invasive hemodynamic monitoring in cardiogenic shock. *Am J Cardiol.* 2021;150:128-129.

Pinsky, M, Teboul, J, Vincent, J, ed. *Hemodynamic Monitoring Lessons from the ICU.* Springer, 2019. Switzerland.

Sanfilippo F, Messina A, Cecconi M, Astuto M. Ten answers to key questions for fluid management in intensive care. *Medicina Intensiva.* 2021;45:552-562.

Saxena A, Garan AR, Kapur NK, et al. Value of hemodynamic monitoring in patients with cardiogenic shock undergoing mechanical circulatory support. *Circulation.* 2020;141(14):1184-1197.

Scheeren TWL, Bakker J, Kaufmann T, et al. Current use of inotropes in circulatory shock. *Ann. Intensive Care.* 2021;11:21. https://doi.org/10.1186/s13613-021-00806-8

van der Ven WH, Terwindt LE, Risvanoglu N, et al. Performance of a machine-learning algorithm to predict hypotension in mechanically ventilated patients with COVID-19 admitted to the intensive care unit: a cohort study. *J Clin Monit Comput.* 2021;13:1-9.

VanDyck TJ, Pinsky MR. Hemodynamic monitoring in cardiogenic shock. *Curr Opin Crit Care.* 2021 Aug 1;27(4):454-459.

Vincent JL. The fluid challenge. *Crit Care.* 2020;24:703.

Vincent JL. Bakker J. Blood lactate levels in sepsis: in 8 questions. *Curr Opin Crit Care.* 2021;27(3):298-302.

Vincent JL, Joosten A, Saugel B. Hemodynamic monitoring and support. *Crit Care Med.* 2021;49(10):1638-1650.

Wiegand D, ed. *AACN Procedure Manual for High Acuity, Progressive and Critical Care. Section 9: Hemodynamic Monitoring.* 7th ed. Elsevier; 2017.

Blood Pressure Monitoring

Bridges E, Middleton R. Direct arterial vs oscillometric monitoring of blood pressure: stop comparing and pick one (a decision-making algorithm). *Crit Care Nurse.* 1997;17(3):58-66, 68-72. https://www.ncbi.nlm.nih.gov/pubmed/9313412

Kim SH, Lilot M, Sidhu KS, et al. Accuracy and precision of continuous noninvasive arterial pressure monitoring compared with invasive arterial pressure: a systematic review and meta-analysis. *Anesthesiology.* 2014;120(5):1080-1097.

McGhee BH, Bridges EJ. Monitoring arterial blood pressure: what you may not know. *Crit Care Nurse.* 2002;22(2):60-64, 66-70, 73 passim. http://www.ncbi.nlm.nih.gov/pubmed/11961944

PA Catheter

Bootsma IT, Boerma EC, de Lange F, Scheeren TWL. The contemporary pulmonary artery catheter. Part 1: placement and waveform analysis. *J Clin Monit Comput.* 2022;36:5 15.

Bootsma IT, Boerma EC, Scheeren TWL, de Lange F. The contemporary pulmonary artery catheter. Part 2: measurements, limitations, and clinical applications. *J Clin Monit Comput.* 2022;36(1):17-31.

Cronhjort M, Wall O, Nyberg E, et al. Impact of hemodynamic goal-directed resuscitation on mortality in adult critically ill patients: a systematic review and meta-analysis. *J Clin Monit Comput.* 2018;32(3):403-414.

De Backer D, Bakker J, Cecconi M, et al. Alternatives to the Swan–Ganz catheter. *Intensive Care Med.* 2018;44:730-741.

Headley JM, Ahrens T. Narrative history of the Swan-Ganz catheter: development, education, controversies, and clinician acumen. *AACN Adv Crit Care.* 2020;31(1):25-33.

Thurman P. Mixed shock states: a case for the pulmonary artery catheter. *AACN Adv Crit Care.* 2020;31(1):67-74.

Von Rueden KT. Bridging the gap between clinical practice and the AACN practice alert on pulmonary artery/central venous pressure monitoring in adults. *AACN Adv Crit Care.* 2020;31(1):34-40.

CVP

Marik PE, Cavallazzi R. Does the central venous pressure predict fluid responsiveness? An updated meta-analysis and a plea for some common sense. *Crit Care Med.* 2013;41:1774-1781.

Sanfilippo F, Noto A, Martucci G, Farbo M, Burgio G, Biasucci DG. Central venous pressure monitoring via peripherally or centrally inserted central catheters: a systematic review and meta-analysis. *J Vasc Access.* 2017;18(4):273-278.

SpO$_2$

Bickler P, Tremper KK. The pulse oximeter is amazing, but not perfect. *Anesthesiology.* 2022;136(5):670-671.

Garrett W Burnett 1, Blaine Stannard 1, David B Wax 1, Hung-Mo Lin 2, Chantal Pyram-Vincent 1, Samuel DeMaria 1, Matthew A Levin 3 et al. Self-reported race/ethnicity and intraoperative occult hypoxemia: a retrospective cohort study. *Anesthesiology.* 2022;136:688–696.

Fawzy A, Wu TD, Wang K, et al. Racial and ethnic discrepancy in pulse oximetry and delayed identification of treatment eligibility among patients with COVID-19. *JAMA Intern Med.* 2022;182(7):730–738. doi:10.1001/jamainternmed.2022.1906.

Gottlieb ER, Ziiegler J, Morley K. Assessment of racial and ethnic differences in oxygen supplementation among patients in the intensive care unit. *JAMA Internal Med.* 2022;59(4):2103246.

Henry NR. Disparities in hypoxemia detection by pulse oximetry across self-identified racial groups and associations with clinical outcomes. *Crit Care Med.* 2022;50:204–211.

Okunlola O, Lipnick MS, Batchelder P, Bernstein M, Feiner J, Bickler P. Pulse oximeter performance, racial inequity, and the work ahead. *Respir Care.* 2022;67:252-257.

Sjoding MW, Dickson RP, Iwashyna TJ, Gay SE, Valley TS. Racial Bias in Pulse Oximetry Measurement. *N Engl J Med.* 2020 Dec 17;383(25):2477-2478. doi: 10.1056/NEJMc2029240. Erratum in: *N Engl J Med.* 2021 Dec 23;385(26):2496. PMID: 33326721; PMCID: PMC7808260.

Wong A-KI, Charpignon M, Kim H, Josef C, de Hond AAH, Fojas JJ, Tabaie A, Liu X, Mireles-Cabodevila E, Carvalho L, Kamaleswaran R, Madushani RWMA, Adhikari L, Holder AL, Steyerberg EW, Buchman TG, Lough ME, Celi LA. Analysis of discrepancies between pulse oximetry and arterial oxygen saturation measurements by race and ethnicity and association with organ dysfunction and mortality. *JAMA Netw Open.* 2021 Nov 1;4(11):e2131674. doi: 10.1001/jamanetworkopen.2021.31674. Erratum in: JAMA Netw Open. 2022 Feb 1;5(2):e221210. PMID: 34730820; PMCID: PMC9178439.

SvO$_2$/ScvO$_2$

Messina A, Greco M, Cecconi, M. What should I use next if clinical evaluation and echocardiographic haemodynamic assessment is not enough? *Curr Opin Crit Care.* 2019;25(3):259-265.

ETCO$_2$/Pa-vCO$_2$

Al Duhailib Z, Hegazy AF, Lalli R, et al. The use of central venous to arterial carbon dioxide tension gap for outcome prediction in critically ill patients: a systematic review and meta-analysis. *Crit Care Med.* 2020;48(12):1855-1861.

Gavelli F, Teboul JL, Monnet X. How can CO$_2$-derived indices guide resuscitation in critically ill patients? *J Thorac Dis.* 2019;11(Suppl 11):S1528-S1537.

Helmy TA, El-reweny EM, Ghazy FG. Prognostic value of venous to arterial carbon dioxide difference during early resuscitation in critically ill patients with septic shock. *Indian J Crit Care Med.* 2017;21(9):589-593.

Huang H, Wu C, Shen Q, Fang Y, Xu H. Value of variation of end-tidal carbon dioxide for predicting fluid responsiveness during the passive leg raising test in patients with mechanical ventilation: a systematic review and meta-analysis. *Crit Care.* 2022;26(1):20.

Naumann DN, Midwinter MJ, Hutchings S. Venous-to-arterial CO$_2$ differences and the quest for bedside point-of-care monitoring to assess the microcirculation during shock. *Ann Transl Med.* 2016;4(2):37.

Wireless/Remote Monitoring

Abraham WT, Adamson PB, Bourge RC, et al. Wireless pulmonary artery haemodynamic monitoring in chronic heart failure: a randomised controlled trial. *Lancet.* 2011;377(9766):658-666.

Abraham WT, Stevenson LW, Bourge RC, et al. Sustained efficacy of pulmonary artery pressure to guide adjustment of chronic heart failure therapy: complete follow-up results from the CHAMPION randomised trial. *Lancet.* 2016;387:453–461.

Joshi R, Nair A. The utility of CardioMEMS, a wireless hemodynamic monitoring system in reducing heart failure related hospital readmissions. *J Nurse Pract.* 2021;17(3):267-272.

Kanat N, Nichols M. CardioMEMS for effective management of heart failure: reducing healthcare utilization and 30 day readmissions. *Heart Lung.* 2017;46(2017):211-214.

Kotalczyk A, Imberti JF, Lip GYH, Wright DJ. Telemedical monitoring based on implantable devices-the evolution beyond the CardioMEMS^{TM} technology. *Curr Heart Fail Rep.* 2022;19(1):7-14.

Lander MM, Aldweib N, Abraham WT. Wireless hemodynamic monitoring in patients with heart failure. *Curr Heart Failure Rep.* 2021 epub, https://doi.org/10.1007/s11897-020-00498-4

Preister S, Case L, Deibert J. Pulmonary artery sensor (CardioMEMS) effect on hospital admissions and emergency department visits. *Heart Lung.* 2017;46:215-219.

Sauld C, Pedersen R, Sulemanjee N. Remote hemodynamic monitoring program: a single center experience in reducing heart failure admissions. *Heart Lung.* 2017;46:215-219.

Less-Invasive CO Monitoring

Ameloot K, Palmers PJ, Malbrain M. The accuracy of noninvasive cardiac output and pressure measurements with finger cuff: a concise review. *Curr Opin Crit Care.* 2015;21:232-239.

Asamoto M, Orli R, Otsuji M, Bougaki M, Imai Y, Yamada Y. Reliability of cardiac output measurements using LiDCOrapid^{TM} and FloTrac/Vigileo^{TM} across broad ranges of cardiac output values. *J Clin Monit Comput.* 2017;31(4):709-716.

Cemaj S, Visenio MR, Sheppard OO, Johnson DW, Bauman ZM. Ultrasound and other advanced hemodynamic monitoring techniques in the intensive care unit. *Surg Clin North Am.* 2022 Feb;102(1):37-52.

De Backer D, Vincent, R. Noninvasive monitoring in the ICU. *Semin Respir Crit Care Med.* 2021;42(1):40-46.

Hodgson LE, Venn R, Forni LG, Samuels TL, Wakeling HG. Measuring the cardiac output in acute emergency admissions: use of the noninvasive ultrasonic cardiac output monitor (USCOM) with determination of the learning curve and inter-rater reliability. *J Intensive Care Soc.* 2016;17(2):122-128.

Huygh J, Peeters Y, Bernards J. Hemodynamic monitoring in the critically ill: an overview of current cardiac output monitoring methods. *F1000Res.* 2016;5(F1000 Faculty Rev):2855.

Johnson A, Stevenson J, Gu H, Huml J. Stroke volume optimization: utilization of the newest cardiac vital sign: considerations in recovery from cardiac surgery. *Crit Care Nurs Clin North Am.* 2019;31(3):329-348.

Messina A, Greco M, Cecconi M. What should I use next if clinical evaluation and echocardiographic haemodynamic assessment is not enough? *Curr Opin Crit Care.* 2019;25(3):259-265.

Peeters Y, Bernards J, Mekeirele M, et al. Hemodynamic monitoring: to calibrate or not to calibrate? Part 1—Calibrated techniques. *Anaesthesiol Intensive Ther.* 2015;47(5):487-500.

Rogge DE, Nicklas JY, Haas SA, Reuter DA, Saugel B. Continuous noninvasive arterial pressure monitoring using the vascular unloading technique (CNAP system) in obese patients during laparoscopic bariatric operations. *Anesth Analg.* 2018;126(2):454-463.

Tanios M, Epstein S, Sauser S, Chi A. Noninvasive monitoring of cardiac output during weaning from mechanical ventilation: a pilot study. *Am J Crit Care.* 2016;25(3):257-265.

NIRS/StO$_2$

Green MS, Sehgal S, Tariq R. Near-infrared spectroscopy: the new must have tool in the intensive care unit? *Semin Cardiothorac Vasc Anesth.* 2016 Sep,20(3).213-224.

Macdonald SPJ, Kinnear FB, Arendts G, Ho KM, Fatovich DM. Near-infrared spectroscopy to predict organ failure and outcome in sepsis: the Assessing Risk in Sepsis using a Tissue Oxygen Saturation (ARISTOS) study. *Eur J Emerg Med.* 2019 Jun;26(3):174-179.

Varis E, Pettilä V, Walkman E. Near-infrared spectroscopy in adult circulatory shock: a systematic review. *J Intensive Care Med.* 2020 Oct;35(10):943-962.

Functional Hemodynamics

Bakker J, Kattan E, Annane D, Castro R, Cecconi M, De Backer D, Dubin A, Evans L, Gong MN, Hamzaoui O, Ince C, Levy B, Monnet X, Ospina Tascón GA, Ostermann M, Pinsky MR, Russell JA, Saugel B, Scheeren TWL, Teboul JL, Vieillard Baron A, Vincent JL, Zampieri FG, Hernandez G. Current practice and evolving concepts in septic shock resuscitation. *Intensive Care Med.* 2022 Feb;48(2):148–163. doi: 10.1007/s00134-021-06595-9. Epub 2021 Dec 15. PMID: 34910228.

Bigé N, Lavillegrand JR, Dang J, et al. Bedside prediction of intra-dialytic hemodynamic instability in critically ill patients: the SOCRATE study. *Ann Intensive Care.* 2020;10:47.

Cecconi M, Monge Garcia MI, Gracia Romero M, et al. The use of pulse pressure variation and stroke volume variation in spontaneously breathing patients to assess dynamic arterial elastance and to predict arterial pressure response to fluid administration. *Anesth Analg.* 2015;120(1):76-84.

De Backer D, Vincent JL. Should we measure the central venous pressure to guide fluid management? Ten answers to 10 questions. *Crit Care.* 2018;22:43.

Douglas IS, Alapat PM, Corl KA, et al. Fluid response evaluation in sepsis, hypotension and shock: a randomized clinical trial. *Chest.* 2020;158(4):1431-1445. doi:10.1016/j.chest.2020.04.025

Eskesen TG, Wetterslev M, Perner A. Systematic review including re-analyses of 1148 individual data sets of central venous pressure as a predictor of fluid responsiveness. *Intensive Care Med.* 2016 Mar;42(3):324-332. doi:10.1007/s00134-015-4168-4. Epub 2015 Dec 9.

Georges D, de Courson H, Lanchon R, Sesay M, Nouette-Gaulain K, Bials M. End-expiratory occlusion maneuver to fluid responsiveness in the intensive care unit: an echocardiographic study. *Crit Care.* 2018;22(32):1-8.

Headley, J. Applying functional hemodynamics: a goal directed therapy (Webinar). American Association of Critical Care Nurses. 2020 Nov 19. https://www.aacn.org/education/webinar-series/wb0062/applying-functional-hemodynamics-a-goaldirected-strategy

Marik PE, Cavallazzi R. Does the central venous pressure predict fluid responsiveness? An updated meta-analysis and a plea for some common sense. *Crit Care Med.* 2013;41:1774-1781. 10.1097/CCM.0b013e31828a25fd

Messina A, Dell'Anna A, Baggiani M, et al. Functional hemodynamic tests: a systematic review and a metanalysis on the reliability of the end-expiratory occlusion test and of the mini-fluid challenge in predicting fluid responsiveness. *Crit Care.* 2019;23:264.

Monnet X, Marik PE, Teboul JL. Prediction of fluid responsiveness: an update. *Ann Intensive Care.* 2016;6:111. 10.1186/s13613-016-0216-7

Monnet X, Teboul JL. My patient has received fluid. How to assess its efficacy and side effects? *Ann Intensive Care.* 2018 Apr 24;8(1):54.

Pinsky MR. Functional hemodynamic monitoring. *Crit Care Clin.* 2015;31(1):89-111.

Shi R, Monnet X, Teboul JL. Parameters of fluid responsiveness. *Curr Opin Crit Care.* 2020;26:319-326.

Teboul JL, Monnet X, Chemla D, et al. Arterial pulse pressure variation with mechanical ventilation. *Am J Respir Crit Care Med.* 2019;199:22-31. 10.1164/rccm.201801-0088CI

Toscani L, Aya HD, Antonakaki D, et al. What is the impact of the fluid challenge technique on diagnosis of fluid responsiveness? A systematic review and meta-analysis. *Crit Care.* 2017;21(1):207. doi: 10.1186/s13054-017-1796-9

Tyler L, Greco S, Bridges E, et al. Accuracy of stop-cursor method for determining systolic and pulse pressure variation. *Am J Crit Care.* 2013;22(4):298-305. https://doi.org/22/4/298 [pii] 10.4037/ajcc2013295

van der Ven WH, Terwindt LE, Risvanoglu N, et al. Performance of a machine-learning algorithm to predict hypotension in mechanically ventilated patients with COVID-19 admitted to the intensive care unit: a cohort study. *J Clin Monit Comput.* 2021, epub.

Vincent J-L, Cecconi M, De Backer D. The fluid challenge. *Crit Care.* 2020;24(1):703.

PLR

Beurton, JL, Teboul V, Girotto L, et al. Intra-abdominal hypertension is responsible for false negatives to the passive leg raising test. *Crit Care Med.* 2019;47(8):e639-e647.

Beurton A, Teboul JL, Monnet X. Passive leg raising test in patients with intra-abdominal hypertension: do not throw it out. *Ann Transl Med.* 2020;8(12):806.

Cherpanath TG, Hirsch A, Geerts BF, et al. Predicting fluid responsiveness of passive leg raising: a systematic review and meta-analysis of 23 clinical trials. *Crit Care Med.* 2016;44(5):981-991.

Hamzaoui O, Gouëzel C, Jozwiak M, et al. Increase in central venous pressure during passive leg raising cannot detect fluid unresponsiveness. *Crit Care Med.* 2020;48:e684-e689.

Honore PM, Spapen HD. Passive leg raising test with minimally invasive monitoring: the way forward for guiding septic shock resuscitation? *J Intensive Care.* 2017;5(36):1-3.

Mesquida J, Gruatmoner G, Ferrer, R. Passive leg raising for assessment of volume responsiveness: a review. *Curr Opin Crit Care.* 2017;23(3):237-243.

Monnet X, Teboul JL. Passive leg raising: five rules, not a drop of fluid! *Crit Care.* 2015;19(18):1-3.

Monnet X, Marik P, Teboul J-L. Passive leg raising for predicting fluid responsiveness: a systematic review and meta-analysis. *Intensive Care Med.* 2016;42:1935-1947.

Monnet X, Teboul JL. Prediction of fluid responsiveness in spontaneously breathing patients. *Ann Transl Med.* 2020;8(12):790.

Pickett JD, Bridges E, Kritek PA. Passive leg-raising and prediction of fluid responsiveness: systematic review. *Crit Care Nurse.* 2017;37(2):32-48.

Pickett JD, Bridges E, Kritek PA, Whitney JD. Noninvasive blood pressure monitoring and prediction of fluid responsiveness to passive leg raising. *Am J Crit Care.* 2018;27(3):228-237.

Diastolic Shock Index

Benchekroune S, Karpati PC, Berton C, et al. Diastolic arterial blood pressure: a reliable early predictor of survival in human septic shock. *J Trauma.* 2008;64(5):1188-1195. https://doi.org/10.1097/TA.0b013e31811f3a45

Cinel I, Kasapoglu US, Gul F, Dellinger RP. The initial resuscitation of septic shock. *J Crit Care.* 2020;57:108-117. https://doi.org/10.1016/j.jcrc.2020.02.004

Dalmau, R. The diastolic shock index works ... but, what is it? *Ann Intensive Care.* 2020;10(1):103. https://doi.org/10.1186/s13613-020-00720-5

Hamzaoui O, Teboul JL. Importance of diastolic arterial pressure in septic shock rebuttal to comments of Dr. Magder. *J Crit Care.* 2019a;51:244. https://doi.org/10.1016/j.jcrc.2019.01.014

Hamzaoui O, Teboul JL. Importance of diastolic arterial pressure in septic shock: PRO. *J Crit Care.* 2019b;51:238-240. https://doi.org/10.1016/j.jcrc.2018.10.032

Magder, Sheldon. Importance of diastolic pressure in septic shock: Con–Response. *J Crit Care.* 2019;51:245-246. doi:10.1016/j.jcrc.2019.02.021

Ospina-Tascon GA, Hernandez G, Bakker J. Diastolic shock index (DSI) works ... and it could be a quite useful tool. *Ann Intensive Care.* 2020;10(1):109. https://doi.org/10.1186/s13613-020-00728-x

Ospina-Tascon GA, Teboul JL, Hernandez G, et al. Diastolic shock index and clinical outcomes in patients with septic shock. *Ann Intensive Care.* 2020;10(1):41. https://doi.org/10.1186/s13613-020-00658-8

Dynamic Elastance (Pressure Responders)

Bentzer P, Griesdale DE, Boyd J, et al. Will this hemodynamically unstable patient respond to a bolus of intravenous fluids? *JAMA.* 2016;316(12):1298-1309.

Cecconi M, Monge García MI, Gracia Romero, M, Mellinghoff J, Caliandro F, Grounds RM, & Rhodes A. The use of pulse pressure variation and stroke volume variation in spontaneously breathing patients to assess dynamic arterial elastance and to predict arterial pressure response to fluid administration. *Anesth Analg.* 2015;120(1):76-84. https://doi.org/10.1213/ANE.0000000000000442

Maheshwari K, Saugel B. Defining fluid responsiveness: Flow response vs. pressure response. *J Clin Anesth.* 2022;79:110667.

Monge García MI, Romero MG, Cano AG, Aya HD, Rhodes A, Grounds RM, & Cecconi M. Dynamic arterial elastance as a predictor of arterial pressure response to fluid administration: a validation study. *Crit Care* (London, England). 2014;18(6):626. https://doi.org/10.1186/s13054-014-0626-6

Monge García MI, Pinsky MR, & Cecconi M. Predicting vasopressor needs using dynamic parameters. *Intensive Care Med.* 2017;43(12):1841-1843. https://doi.org/10.1007/s00134-017-4752-x

Monge García MI & Barrasa González H. Why did arterial pressure not increase after fluid administration? *Med Intensiva.* 2017;41(9):546-549. https://doi.org/10.1016/j.medin.2017.03.005

Peripheral Perfusion

Ait-Oufella H, et al. Mottling score predicts survival in septic shock. *Intensive Care Med.* 2011;37:801-807.

Ait-Oufella H, Bakker J. Understanding clinical signs of poor tissue perfusion during septic shock. *Intensive Care Med.* 2016 (Epub—Feb 2016).

Ait-Oufella H, Bige N, Boelle PY, et al. Capillary refill time exploration during septic shock. *Intensive Care Med.* 2014;40:958–964.

Anderson B, Kelly AM, Kerr D, Clooney M, & Jolley D.. Impact of patient and environmental factors on capillary refill time in adults. *Am J Emerg Med.* 2008;26(1):62-65. https://doi.org/10.1016/j.ajem.2007.06.026

Angus D. How best to resuscitate patients with septic shock. *JAMA.* 2019;321(7):647-648.

Bakker J. Clinical use of peripheral perfusion parameters in septic shock. *Curr Opin Crit Care.* 2021;27(3):269-273.

Bakker J, Hernández G. Can peripheral skin perfusion be used to assess organ perfusion and guide resuscitation interventions? *Front Med.* 2020;7(291)1-4.

Bigé N, Lavillegrand JR, Dang J, Attias P, Deryckere S, Joffre J, Dubée V, Preda G, Dumas G, Hariri G, Pichereau C, Baudel JL, Guidet B, Maury E, Boelle PY, Ait-Oufella H. Bedside prediction of intradialytic hemodynamic instability in critically ill patients: the SOCRATE study. *Ann Intensive Care.* 2020 Apr 22;10(1):47. doi: 10.1186/s13613-020-00663-x. PMID: 32323060; PMCID: PMC7176798.

Bridges E. Assessing patients during septic shock resuscitation. *AJN.* 2017;117(10):34-40.

Castro R, et al. Effects of capillary refill time—vs. lactate-targeted fluid resuscitation on regional, microcirculatory and hypoxia-related perfusion parameters in septic shock: a randomized controlled trial. *Ann Intensive Care.* 2020;10:150.

Coudroy R, Jamet A, Frat JP, Veinstein A, Chatellier D, Goudet V, Cabasson S, Thille AW, & Robert R. Incidence and impact of skin mottling over the knee and its duration on outcome in critically ill patients. *Intensive Care Med.* 2015;41(3):452-459. https://doi.org/10.1007/s00134-014-3600-5

Dumas G, Lavillegrand JR, Joffre J, Bigé N, de-Moura EB, Baudel JL, Chevret S, Guidet B, Maury E, Amorim F, & Ait-Oufella H.. Mottling score is a strong predictor of 14-day mortality in septic patients whatever vasopressor doses and other tissue perfusion parameters. *Crit Care* (London, England). 2019;23(1):211. https://doi.org/10.1186/s13054-019-2496-4

Falotico JM, et al. Advances in the approaches using peripheral perfusion for monitoring hemodynamic status. *Front Med.* 2020;7:Article614326.

Hariri G, Joffre J, Leblanc G, et al. Narrative review: clinical assessment of peripheral tissue perfusion in septic shock. *Ann Intensive Care.* 2019;9(1):37.

Hernández G, Ospina-Tascón GA, Damiani LP, et al. Effect of a resuscitation strategy targeting peripheral perfusion status vs serum lactate levels on 28-day mortality among patients with septic shock: the ANDROMEDA-SHOCK randomized clinical trial. *JAMA.* 2019;321(7):654-664. doi:10.1001/jama.2019.0071

Hernández G, Kattan E, Ospina-Tascón G. et al. Capillary refill time status could identify different clinical phenotypes among septic shock patients fulfilling Sepsis-3 criteria: a post hoc analysis of ANDROMEDA-SHOCK trial. *Intensive Care Med.* 2020;46:816-818. https://doi.org/10.1007/s00134-020-05960-4

Hernández G, Castro R, & Bakker J. Capillary refill time: the missing link between macrocirculation and microcirculation in septic shock? *J Thorac Dis.* 2020;12(3):1127-1129. https://doi.org/10.21037/jtd.2019.12.102

Kanoore Edul VS, Caminos Eguillor JF, Ferrara G, Estenssoro E, Siles DSP, Cesio CE, & Dubin A. Microcirculation alterations in severe COVID-19 pneumonia. *J Crit Care*. 2021;61:73-75. https://doi.org/10.1016/j.jcrc.2020.10.002

Kattan E, Hernández G, Ospina-Tascón G, Valenzuela ED, Bakker J, Castro R, & ANDROMEDA-SHOCK Study Investigators and the Latin America Intensive Care Network (LIVEN). A lactate-targeted resuscitation strategy may be associated with higher mortality in patients with septic shock and normal capillary refill time: a post hoc analysis of the ANDROMEDA-SHOCK study. *Ann Intensive Care*. 2020;10(1):114. https://doi.org/10.1186/s13613-020-00732-1

Lara B, Enberg L, Ortega M, et al. Capillary refill time during fluid resuscitation in patients with sepsis-related hyperlactatemia at the emergency department is related to mortality. *PLoS One*. 2017;12:e0188548 75.

Latham H, Bengtson C, Satterwhite L, et al. Sepsis resuscitation based on stroke volume optimization improves outcome and reduces cost of care. *Crit Care Med*. 2018;46:709. doi:10.1097/01.ccm.0000529453.26993.69

Makic MBF, Bridges E. CE: Managing sepsis and septic shock: current guidelines and definitions. *Am J Nurs*. 2018;118(2): 34-39.

Morocho JP, Martínez AF, Cevallos MM, Vasconez-Gonzalez J, Ortiz-Prado E, Barreto-Grimaldos A, & Vélez-Páez JL. (2022). Prolonged capillary refilling as a predictor of mortality in patients with septic shock. *J Intensive Care Med*. 2021;37(3):423-429. https://doi.org/10.1177/08850666211003507

Schriger DL. Defining normal capillary refill: variation with age, sex, and temperature. *Ann Emerg Med*. 1988;17(9):932-935.

Schriger DL. Capillary refill—is it a useful predictor of hypovolemic states? *Ann Emerg Med*. 1991;20:601-605.

Sebat C, Vandegrift MA, Oldroyd S, Kramer A, & Sebat F. Capillary refill time as part of an early warning score for rapid response team activation is an independent predictor of outcomes. *Resuscitation*. 2020;153:105-110. https://doi.org/10.1016/j.resuscitation.2020.05.044

van Genderen ME, van Bommel J, & Lima A. Monitoring peripheral perfusion in critically ill patients at the bedside. *Curr Opin Crit Care*. 2012;18(3):273-279. https://doi.org/10.1097/MCC.0b013e3283533924

van Genderen ME, Lima A, Akkerhuis M, et al. Persistent peripheral and microcirculatory perfusion alterations after out-of-hospital cardiac arrest are associated with poor survival. *Crit Care Med*. 2012;40(8):2287-2294.

van Genderen ME, Paauwe J, de Jonge J, et al. Clinical assessment of peripheral perfusion to predict postoperative complications after major abdominal surgery early: a prospective observational study in adults. *Crit Care*. 2014;18:R114 77.

Van Genderen ME, Engels N, van der Valk, RJ, Lima A, Klijn E, Bakker J, & van Bommel J. Early peripheral perfusion-guided fluid therapy in patients with septic shock. *Am J Resp Crit Care Med*. 2015;191(4):477-480. https://doi.org/10.1164/rccm.201408-1575LE

Vera M, Kattan E, Castro R, & Hernández G. The seven T's of capillary refill time: more than a clinical sign for septic shock patients. *Eur J Emerg Med*: official journal of the European Society for Emergency Medicine. 2020;27(3):169-171. https://doi.org/10.1097/MEJ.0000000000000705

Peripheral Vasopressors

Delaney A, Finnis M, Bellomo R, Udy A, Jones D, Keijzers G, MacDonald S, & Peake S. Initiation of vasopressor infusions via peripheral versus central access in patients with early septic shock: A retrospective cohort study. *Emerg Med Australasia*: EMA. 2020;32(2):210-219. https://doi.org/10.1111/1742-6723.13394

Lewis T, Merchan C, Altshuler D, & Papadopoulos J, (2019). Safety of the Peripheral Administration of Vasopressor Agents. *J Intens Care Med*. 2019;34(1):26-33. https://doi.org/10.1177/0885066616686035

Loubani OM, & Green RS, (2015). A systematic review of extravasation and local tissue injury from administration of vasopressors through peripheral intravenous catheters and central venous catheters. *J Crit Care*. 2015;30(3),653.e9-653.e6.53E17. https://doi.org/10.1016/j.jcrc.2015.01.014

Nickel B. Peripheral intravenous administration of high-risk infusions in critical care: a risk-benefit analysis. *Crit Care Nurse*. 2019;39(6):16-28.

Nguyen TT, Surrey A, Barmaan B, Miller S, Oswalt A, Evans D, & Dhindsa H. (2021). Utilization and extravasation of peripheral norepinephrine in the emergency department. *The American journal of emergency medicine*, 39, 55–59. https://doi.org/10.1016/j.ajem.2020.01.014.

Owen VS, Rosgen BK, Cherak SJ, et al. Adverse events associated with administration of vasopressor medications through a peripheral intravenous catheter: a systematic review and meta-analysis. *Crit Care*. 2021;25:146.

Pancaro C, Shah N, Pasma W, Saager L, Cassidy R, van Klei W, Kooij F, Vittali D, Hollmann MW, Kheterpal S, & Lirk P. Risk of major complications after perioperative norepinephrine infusion through peripheral intravenous lines in a multicenter study. *Anesth Analg*. 2020;131(4):1060-1065. https://doi.org/10.1213/ANE.0000000000004445

Tian DH, Smyth C, Keijzers G, Macdonald S P, Peake S, Udy A, & Delaney A. Safety of peripheral administration of vasopressor medications: A systematic review. *Emerg Med Australasia*: EMA. 2020;32(2):220-227. https://doi.org/10.1111/1742-6723.13406

Udy AA, Finnis M, Jones D, Delaney A, Macdonald S, Bellomo R, Peake S, & ARISE Investigators. Incidence, patient characteristics, mode of drug delivery, and outcomes of septic shock patients treated with vasopressors in the arise trial. *Shock*. (Augusta, Ga.), 2019;52(4):400-407. https://doi.org/10.1097/SHK.0000000000001281

Evidence-Based Practice Guidelines (Update)

AACN. Practice alert: obtaining accurate non-invasive blood pressure measurements in adults (Last reviewed May 2021) https://www.aacn.org/clinical-resources/practice-alerts/obtaining-accurate-noninvasive-blood-pressure-measurements-in-adults (Accessed 28 Mar 2022).

AACN. Practice alert: pulmonary artery/central venous pressure monitoring in adults (Last reviewed 2021). https://www.aacn.org/clinical-resources/practice-alerts/pulmonary-artery-pressure-measurement (Accessed 28 Mar 2022).

AACN. Practice alert: managing alarms in acute care across the life span: electrocardiography and pulse oximetry. 2018. https://www.aacn.org/clinical-resources/practice-alerts/managing-alarms-in-acute-care-across-the-life-span (Accessed 29 Mar 2022).

Airway and Ventilatory Management

5

Robert E. St. John and Maureen A. Seckel

KNOWLEDGE COMPETENCIES

1. Interpret normal and abnormal arterial blood gas (ABG) results and determine common management strategies for treatment.

2. Identify indications, complications, and management strategies for artificial airways, oxygen delivery, and monitoring devices.

3. Identify indications, principles of operation, complications, and management strategies for mechanical ventilation.

4. Explain the concepts of respiratory muscle fatigue, rest, and conditioning as they relate to the mechanically ventilated weaning patient.

5. Discuss essential components for successful weaning from short- and long-term ventilation, and multidisciplinary institutional approaches to the care of prolonged mechanically ventilated patients.

DIAGNOSTIC TESTS, MONITORING SYSTEMS, AND RESPIRATORY ASSESSMENT TECHNIQUES

Arterial Blood Gas Monitoring

Arterial blood gas (ABG) monitoring is frequently performed in critically ill patients to assess acid-base balance, ventilation, and oxygenation. An arterial blood sample is analyzed for oxygen tension (Pao_2), carbon dioxide tension ($Paco_2$), and pH using a blood gas analyzer. From these measurements, several other parameters are calculated by the blood gas analyzer, including base excess (BE), bicarbonate (HCO_3^-), and oxygen saturation (Sao_2). Fractional arterial Sao_2 can be directly measured, if a co-oximeter is available. Normal ABG values are listed in Table 5-1.

ABG samples are obtained by direct puncture of an artery, usually the radial artery, or by withdrawing blood through an indwelling arterial catheter system. A heparinized syringe is used to collect the sample to prevent clotting of the blood prior to analysis. Blood gas samples are kept on ice unless there is the ability to immediately analyze to prevent the continued transfer of CO_2 and O_2 in and out of the red blood cells. ABG analysis equipment is often kept in or near the critical care unit to maximize accuracy and decrease the time for reporting of results. Additionally, portable point-of-care devices are available at many hospitals, which allow measurement at the bedside. Regardless of the method used to obtain the ABG sample, practitioners should wear gloves and follow standard precautions to prevent exposure to blood during the sampling procedure.

Techniques
Indwelling Arterial Catheters
Pressure monitoring systems used with indwelling arterial catheters have sites where samples of arterial blood can be withdrawn for ABG analysis or other laboratory testing (Figure 5-1). Using the stopcock closest to the catheter insertion site, or the indwelling syringe or reservoir of the needleless systems, a 3- to 5-mL sample of blood is withdrawn to clear the catheter system of any flush system fluid. A 1-mL sample for ABG analysis is then obtained in a heparinized syringe. Any air remaining in the syringe is then removed, an airtight cap is placed on the end of the syringe, and the sample is placed on ice to ensure accuracy of the measurement. The arterial catheter system is then flushed

TABLE 5-1. LABORATORY AND CALCULATED RESPIRATORY VALUES

Parameter	Value
Arterial Blood Gases	
• pH	7.35-7.45
• $Paco_2$	35-45 mm Hg
• HCO_3^-	21-28 mEq/L
• Base	−2 to +2 mEq/L
• Pao_2	80-100 mm Hg (normals vary with age and altitude)
• Sao_2	>95% (normals vary with age and altitude)
Mixed Venous Blood Gases	
• pH	7.31-7.41
• $Pmvco_2$	40-50 mm Hg
• $Pmvo_2$	35-45 mm Hg
• Svo_2	60%-80%
Respiratory Parameters	
• Tidal volume (V_T)	6-8 mL/kg
• Respiratory rate	8-16/min
• Respiratory static compliance	70-100 mL/cm H_2O
• Negative inspiratory force (NIF)	≤−20 cm H_2O
• Alveolar gas equation (PAo_2)	100 mm Hg at sea level on room air
• Minute volume (MV)	5-6 L/min
Respiratory Calculations	
• Alveolar gas equation (PAo_2)	$PAo_2 = Fio_2(PATM − PH_2O)$
• Static compliance	V_T/(Plateau pressure − PEEP)

to clear the line of any residual blood. Management of pressure monitoring via indwelling arterial catheters is guided by institutional policy and procedures.

Complications associated with this technique for obtaining ABG samples include infection and hemorrhage. Any time an invasive system is used, the potential exists for contamination of the sterile system. The use of needleless systems on indwelling catheter systems decreases patients' risk for infection, and reduces the risk for accidental needlestick injuries and so should be used whenever feasible. Hemorrhage is a rare complication, occurring when stopcocks are inadvertently left in the wrong position after blood withdrawal or when the tubing is disconnected. These complications can be avoided by carefully following the proper technique during blood sampling, limiting sample withdrawal to experienced practitioners, and keeping the pressure alarm system of the bedside monitoring system activated at all times.

Arterial Puncture
When indwelling arterial catheters are not in place, ABG samples are obtained by directly puncturing the artery with a needle and syringe. The most common sites for arterial puncture are the radial, brachial, and femoral arteries. Similar to venipuncture, the technique for obtaining an ABG sample is relatively simple, but success in obtaining the sample requires experience.

An Allen test is performed prior to obtaining an ABG by percutaneous puncture and prior to the insertion of an arterial line into the radial artery. The Allen test requires that both the ulnar and radial pulses be manually occluded for a brief period of time with the forearm held upward to facilitate blood emptying from the hand. Once blanching of the hand is observed, the forearm is placed in a downward position, the ulnar artery is released, and the hand is observed for flushing. If the hand flushes, it is an indication that the ulnar artery is capable of supplying blood to the fingers should the radial artery be damaged. Documentation of the Allen test is included in the record of the procedure.

Following location of the pulsating artery and antiseptic preparation of the skin, the needle is inserted into the artery at a 45° angle with the bevel facing upward. The needle is slowly advanced until arterial blood appears in the syringe barrel, or the insertion depth is below the artery location. If blood is not obtained, the needle is pulled back to just below the skin and relocation of the pulsating artery is verified prior to advancing the needle again.

As soon as the 1-mL sample of arterial blood is obtained, the syringe is withdrawn, and firm pressure quickly applied to the insertion site with a sterile gauze pad. Handheld pressure is maintained for at least 5 minutes and the site inspected for bleeding or oozing. If present, pressure is reapplied until all evidence of oozing has stopped. In patients who have a coagulopathy or are on anticoagulation therapy, it may be necessary to apply local pressure for greater than 5 minutes. Pressure dressings are not applied until hemostasis has been achieved.

As described, all air must be removed from the ABG syringe, and an airtight cap applied to the end (remove the needle first). Given the importance of maintaining pressure at the puncture site, it is helpful to have another provider assisting during arterial puncture to ensure appropriate handling of the blood sample.

Complications associated with arterial puncture include arterial vessel tear, air embolism, hemorrhage, arterial obstruction, loss of extremity, and infection. Using a proper technique during sampling can dramatically decrease the incidence of these complications. Damage to the artery may be decreased by using a small diameter needle (21-23 gauge in adults) and by avoiding multiple puncture attempts at the same site. After one or two failed attempts at entering the artery, a different site is selected, or another experienced practitioner enlisted to attempt the ABG sampling. All facilities have specific policies and procedures providing guidance on sample acquisition and handling of ABGs, and the reader is encouraged to follow their institutional guidelines.

Hemorrhage can occur easily into the surrounding tissues if adequate hemostasis is not achieved with direct pressure following the puncture. Bleeding into the tissue can range from small blood loss with minimal local damage to large blood loss with loss of distal circulation and even exsanguination. Large blood loss is more commonly seen with femoral punctures and is often the result of inadequate pressure on the artery following needle removal. Bleeding from the femoral artery is difficult to visualize, so significant blood loss can occur before practitioners are alerted to the problem. For this reason, the femoral site is the least preferred site for ABG sampling and is used only when other sites are not accessible.

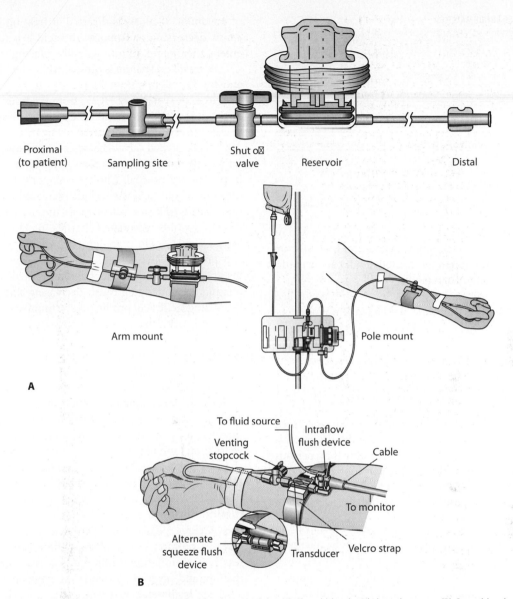

Proximal
(to patient)   Sampling site   Shut off
valve   Reservoir   Distal

Arm mount   Pole mount

A

To fluid source
Intraflow
flush device
Venting
stopcock   Cable

To monitor

Alternate
squeeze flush
device   Transducer   Velcro strap

B

Figure 5-1. Examples of indwelling arterial catheter systems for blood gas analysis. **(A)** Closed blood withdrawal system. **(B)** Open blood withdrawal system. (*Reproduced with permission from Edwards Lifesciences LLC, Irvine, CA.*)

The need for frequent ABG sampling for ventilation and oxygenation assessment and management may require the insertion of an arterial catheter and monitoring system to decrease the risks associated with repetitive arterial punctures.

Analysis

The best approach to analyzing the results of ABGs is a systematic one. Analysis is accomplished by evaluating acid-base and oxygenation status. Upon receipt of ABG results, the practitioner first identifies any abnormal values (see Table 5-1). Then a systematic evaluation of acid-base and oxygenation status is done.

Acid-Base Analysis

Optimal cellular functioning occurs when the pH of the blood is between 7.35 and 7.45. Decreases in pH below 7.35 are termed *acidemia,* and increases in pH above 7.45 are termed *alkalemia.* When the amount of acids or bases in the body

increases or decreases, the pH changes if the ratio of acids to bases is altered; for example, if acid production increases, and there is no change in the amount of base production, pH decreases. If the base production were to increase as well, as a response to increased acid production, then no change in pH would occur because the ratio of acids to bases would be maintained. Because the body functions best at a pH in the 7.35 to 7.45 range, there are strong homeostatic mechanisms in place to maintain the balance between acids and bases, even if one of those components is functioning abnormally. Although a variety of regulatory systems are involved in acid-base balance, the bicarbonate (HCO_3^-) and carbon dioxide (CO_2) levels are the primary regulators.

- *Metabolic component:* HCO_3^- levels are controlled primarily by the kidneys and are called the *metabolic component* of the acid-base system. By increasing or decreasing the amount of HCO_3^- excreted in

TABLE 5-2. ACID-BASE ABNORMALITIES

Acid-Base Abnormality	Primary ABG Abnormalities			ABG Changes With Compensation (If Present)	
	pH	Paco$_2$	HCO$_3^-$	Respiratory (Paco$_2$)	Metabolic (HCO$_3^-$)
Alkalemia					
Metabolic	↑		↑	↑	
Respiratory	↑	↓			↓
Acidemia					
Metabolic	↓		↓	↓	
Respiratory	↓	↑			↑

the kidneys, the pH of the blood can be increased or decreased. Changes in HCO$_3^-$ excretion may take up to 24 hours or longer to accomplish but can be maintained for prolonged periods.

- *Respiratory component:* CO$_2$ levels are controlled primarily by the lungs and are called the *respiratory component* of the acid-base system. By increasing or decreasing the amount of CO$_2$ excreted by the lungs, the pH of the blood can be increased or decreased. Changes in CO$_2$ excretion can occur rapidly, within a minute, by increasing or decreasing the respiratory rate (RR) and/or the depth of ventilation or tidal volume (Vt) with each breath resulting in an increased minute volume (MV). Compensation by the respiratory system is difficult to maintain over long periods of time (24 hours) due to respiratory muscle fatigue.
- *Acid-base abnormalities:* A variety of conditions may result in acid-base abnormalities (Tables 5-2 and 5-3).

Metabolic alkalemia is present when the pH is above 7.45 and the HCO$_3^-$ more than 26 mEq/L. In metabolic alkalosis, there is either a primary increase in hydrogen ion (H$^+$) loss or HCO$_3^-$ gain. The respiratory system attempts to compensate for the increased pH by decreasing the amount of CO$_2$ eliminated from the body (alveolar hypoventilation). This compensatory attempt by the respiratory system results in a change in pH, but rarely to a normal value. Clinical situations or conditions that cause metabolic alkalemia include loss of body acids (nasogastric suction of HCl, vomiting, excessive diuretic therapy, steroids, hypokalemia) and ingestion of exogenous bicarbonate or citrate substances. Management

of metabolic alkalosis is directed at treating the underlying cause, decreasing or stopping the acid loss (eg, use of anti-emetic therapy for vomiting), and replacing electrolytes.

Metabolic acidemia is present when the pH is below 7.35 and the HCO$_3^-$ less than 21 mEq/L. In metabolic acidosis, there is excessive loss of HCO$_3^-$ from the body by the kidneys or the accumulation of acid. The respiratory system attempts to compensate for the decreased pH by increasing the amount of CO$_2$ eliminated (alveolar hyperventilation). This compensatory attempt by the respiratory system results in a change in pH toward normal. Clinical situations or conditions that cause metabolic acidosis include increased metabolic formation of acids (diabetic ketoacidosis, uremic acidosis, lactic acidosis), loss of bicarbonate (diarrhea, renal tubular acidosis), hyperkalemia, toxin ingestion (salicylates overdose, ethylene and propylene glycol, methanol, paraldehyde), and adrenal insufficiency. Management of metabolic acidosis is directed at treating the underlying cause, decreasing acid formation (eg, decreasing lactic acid production by improving cardiac output [CO] in shock), decreasing bicarbonate losses (eg, treatment of diarrhea), or removal of toxins through dialysis or cathartics. When metabolic acidosis is severe and the underlying cause is not amenable to rapid correction, administration of sodium bicarbonate (NaHCO$_3$) may be considered.

Respiratory alkalemia occurs when the pH is above 7.45 and the Paco$_2$ is below 35 mm Hg. In respiratory alkalosis, there is an excessive amount of ventilation (alveolar hyperventilation) and removal of CO$_2$ from the body. If these ABG changes persist for 24 hours or more, the kidneys attempt to compensate for the elevated pH by increasing the excretion of HCO$_3^-$ until normal or near-normal pH levels occur. Clinical situations or conditions that cause respiratory alkalosis include neurogenic hyperventilation, interstitial lung diseases, pulmonary embolism, asthma, acute anxiety/stress/fear, hyperventilation syndromes, excessive mechanical ventilation, and severe hypoxemia. Management of respiratory alkalosis is directed at treating the underlying cause and decreasing excessive ventilation if possible.

Respiratory acidemia occurs when the pH is below 7.35 and the Paco$_2$ is above 45 mm Hg. In respiratory acidosis, there is an inadequate amount of ventilation (alveolar hypoventilation) and removal of CO$_2$ from the body. If these changes persist for 24 hours or more, the kidneys attempt to compensate for the decreased pH by increasing the amount of HCO$_3^-$ in the

TABLE 5-3. EXAMPLES OF ARTERIAL BLOOD GAS RESULTS

ABG Analysis	pH	Paco$_2$ (mm Hg)	HCO$_3^-$ (mEq/L)	Base Excess	Pao$_2$ (mm Hg)	Sao$_2$ (%)
Normal ABG	7.37	38	24	−1	85	96
Respiratory acidosis, no compensation, with hypoxemia	7.28	51	25	−1	63	89
Metabolic acidosis, no compensation, without hypoxemia	7.23	35	14	−12	92	97
Metabolic alkalosis, partial compensation, without hypoxemia	7.49	48	37	+11	84	95
Respiratory acidosis, full compensation, with hypoxemia	7.35	59	33	+6	55	86
Respiratory alkalosis, no compensation, with hypoxemia	7.52	31	24	0	60	88
Metabolic acidosis, partial compensation, with hypoxemia	7.30	29	16	−9	54	85
Laboratory error	7.31	32	28	0	92	96

body (decreased excretion of HCO_3^- in the urine) until normal or near-normal pH levels occur. Clinical situations or conditions that cause respiratory acidosis include hypoventilation associated with respiratory failure (eg, acute respiratory distress syndrome [ARDS], severe asthma, pneumonia, chronic obstructive pulmonary diseases [COPDs], sleep apnea), pulmonary embolism, pulmonary edema, pneumothorax, respiratory center depression, neuromuscular disturbances in the presence of normal lungs, and inadequate mechanical ventilation. Management of respiratory acidosis is directed at treating the underlying cause and improving ventilation.

Mixed (combined) disturbance is the simultaneous development of a primary respiratory and metabolic acid-base disturbance; for example, metabolic acidosis may occur from diabetic ketoacidosis, with respiratory acidosis occurring from respiratory failure associated with aspiration pneumonia. Mixed acid-base disturbances create a more complex picture, beyond the scope of this chapter, and suggest multisystem dysfunction.

Oxygenation

After determining the acid-base status from the ABG, the adequacy of oxygenation is assessed. Normal values for Pao_2 depend on age and altitude. Lower levels of Pao_2 are acceptable as normal with increasing age and altitude levels. In general, Pao_2 levels between 80 and 100 mm Hg are considered normal on room air.

Sao_2 levels are also affected by age and altitude, with values above 95% considered normal. Hemoglobin saturation with oxygen is primarily influenced by the amount of available oxygen in the plasma (Figure 5-2). The S shape to the normal oxyhemoglobin disassociation curve emphasizes that as long as Pao_2 levels are above 60 mm Hg with an arterial blood pH above 7.35, 90% or more of the available hemoglobin is bound or saturated with O_2. Factors that can shift the oxyhemoglobin curve to the right and left include temperature, pH, $Paco_2$, and abnormal hemoglobin conditions. In general, shifting the curve to the right (reducing the pH) decreases the affinity of oxygen for hemoglobin, resulting in an increase in the amount of oxygen released to the tissues. Shifting of the curve to the left (increasing the pH) increases the affinity of oxygen for hemoglobin, resulting in a decreased amount of oxygen released to the tissues.

A decrease in Pao_2 below normal values is *hypoxemia*. A variety of conditions cause hypoxemia:

- *Low inspired oxygen:* Usually, the fraction of inspired oxygen concentration (Fio_2) is reduced at high altitudes or when toxic gases are inhaled. Inadequate or inappropriately low Fio_2 administration may contribute to hypoxic respiratory failure in patients with other cardiopulmonary diseases.
- *Overall hypoventilation:* Decreases in tidal volume (V_T), respiratory rate, or both reduce minute ventilation and cause hypoventilation. Alveoli are underventilated, leading to a fall in arterial oxygen tension (Pao_2) and increased $Paco_2$ levels. Causes of hypoventilation include respiratory center depression from drug overdose, anesthesia, excessive analgesic administration, neuromuscular disturbances, and respiratory muscle fatigue.
- *Ventilation-perfusion (V/Q) mismatch:* When the balance between adequately ventilated and perfused alveoli is altered, hypoxemia develops. Perfusion past under ventilated alveoli leads to poorly oxygenated blood in the pulmonary vasculature and a right to left intrapulmonary shunt. V/Q mismatch also occurs when ventilated alveoli are poorly perfused, a situation referred to as dead space, such as when there is pulmonary emboli or severe hypotension.
- *Shunt:* When blood bypasses or shunts past the alveoli, gas exchange cannot occur and blood returns to the left side of the heart without being oxygenated. Shunts caused anatomically include pulmonary arteriovenous fistulas or congenital cardiac anomalies of the heart and great vessels, such as tetralogy of Fallot. Physiologic shunts are caused by a variety of conditions that result in closed, nonventilated alveoli such as seen in ARDS, and severe forms of COVID-19.
- *Diffusion defect:* Thickening of the alveolar-capillary membrane decreases oxygen diffusion and leads to hypoxemia. Causes of diffusion defects are chronic disease states such as pulmonary fibrosis and sarcoidosis. Hypoxemia usually responds to supplemental oxygen in conditions of diffusion impairment (eg, interstitial lung disease).
- *Low mixed venous oxygenation:* Under normal conditions, the lungs fully oxygenate the pulmonary arterial blood and mixed venous oxygen tension ($Pmvo_2$) does not affect Pao_2 significantly. However, a reduced $Pmvo_2$ can lower the Pao_2 significantly when either ventilation-perfusion mismatch or right-to-left

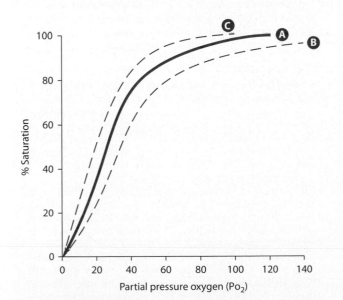

Figure 5-2. Oxyhemoglobin dissociation curve. **(A)** Normal. **(B)** Shift to the right. **(C)** Shift to the left.

intrapulmonary shunting is present. Conditions that can contribute to low mixed venous oxygenation include low CO, anemia, hypoxemia, and increased oxygen consumption. Improving tissue oxygen delivery by increasing CO or hemoglobin usually improves mixed venous oxygen saturation.

Venous Blood Gas Monitoring

Analysis of oxygen and carbon dioxide levels in the venous blood provides additional information about the adequacy of perfusion and oxygen use by the tissues. Venous blood gas analysis, also referred to as a *mixed venous blood gas sample*, is obtained from the distal tip of a pulmonary artery (PA) catheter or from a central venous pressure (CVP) catheter. If the distal tip of the PA catheter is used, withdrawal of the blood should be done slowly over a 20-second period to avoid arterialization of the PA blood. This approach is not important when sampling through a CVP catheter. Normal values for venous blood gas are listed in Table 5-1. Central venous saturation ($Scvo_2$) can be obtained from any central venous catheter with the tip positioned in the superior vena cava. Svo_2 can only be obtained from a PA or specialized catheter. More information on Svo_2 and $Scvo_2$ monitoring is found in Chapter 4, Hemodynamic Monitoring.

ESSENTIAL CONTENT CASE

Respiratory Failure: Asthma

A 35-year-old woman with a history of asthma is admitted to the emergency department with an asthma exacerbation secondary to viral pneumonia. Vital signs and laboratory tests on admission were:

Temperature:	38.1°C (oral)
Heart rate:	110/min, slightly labored
BP:	148/90 mm Hg

Lung sounds: pronounced wheezing noted in all lung fields. ABG on room air was:

pH:	7.45
$Paco_2$:	35 mm Hg
HCO_3^-:	23 mEq/L
BE:	0 mEq/L
Pao_2:	53 mm Hg

She is started on oxygen therapy via a non-rebreather mask at 100% O_2. IV fluids, steroids, and albuterol continuous nebulizers are also initiated along with empiric antibiotics. Within 30 minutes, her BP, heart rate, and respiratory rate have decreased to normal values, with improvement in her Pao_2 level (81 mm Hg). She is transferred to the progressive care unit 3 hours later. The patient is stable until approximately 6 hours following her admission to the hospital. At that time, she becomes increasingly lethargic, with quiet lung sounds, and has an increased heart rate, BP, and respiratory rate. ABGs during a Rapid Response Team assessment show a respiratory acidosis with partial compensation and hypoxemia despite 4 L of O_2 by nasal cannula:

pH:	7.28
$Paco_2$:	55 mm Hg
HCO_3^-:	26.8 mEq/L
BE:	0.9 mEq/L
Pao_2:	48 mm Hg

The patient is intubated with a 7.5-mm oral endotracheal tube (ET) tube without difficulty and placed on a ventilator (mode, AC; rate, 15/min; V_T, 600 mL; Fio_2, 1.0; positive end-expiratory pressure [PEEP], 5 cm H_2O). Immediately after intubation and initiation of mechanical ventilation, her BP drops to 88/64 mm Hg. Following a 500-mL bolus of IV fluids, her BP is 118/70. ABG 15 minutes after intubation is as follows:

pH:	7.36
$Paco_2$:	47 mm Hg
HCO_3^-:	27.3 mEq/L
BE:	2.1 mEq/L
Pao_2:	165 mm Hg

Case Question 1. Why do you think the patient's BP decreased after intubation?

Case Question 2. What ventilator changes if any would you anticipate?

Answers

1. Hypotension post-intubation is multifactorial. The increased intrathoracic pressure caused by PEEP and positive pressure ventilation can cause a decrease in venous return to the heart along with a decrease in CO, which may be exaggerated in patients with hypovolemia. For this patient with severe asthma, hemodynamic stability is further compromised by lung hyperinflation and auto-PEEP. Other potential causes of post-intubation hypotension include hemothorax, pneumothorax, or the sequelae of medications used to intubate.

2. (A) Decrease Fio_2: Initial Ventilator setting recommendations for intubation include FiO_2 of 100%. The patient is on 100% O_2 and her Pao_2 is 165 post-intubation. Anticipate orders to titrate Fio_2 down incrementally. Her hypoxia has improved with intubation and treatment of her hypercarbic respiratory failure.

3. (B) Initiate interventions to decrease auto-PEEP and dynamic hyperinflation. A likely cause of hypotension in this patient is hyperinflation and auto-PEEP associated with her history of asthma. There are several strategies to prevent further complications. Auto-PEEP and plateau pressure measurements should be performed. Low tidal volumes, low ventilator rates, short inspiratory times, and long expiratory times may help to prevent hyperinflation. Ensure adequate exhalation time to minimize hyperinflation and auto-PEEP if present.

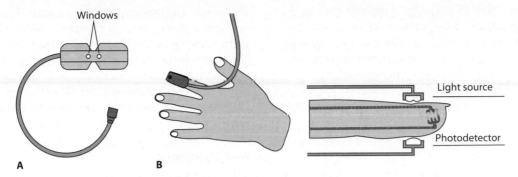

Figure 5-3. Pulse oximeter. **(A)** Sensor. **(B)** Schematic of sensor operation on finger.

Pulse Oximetry

Pulse oximetry is a common method for the continuous, non-invasive monitoring of Sao_2. A reusable multi-patient sensor or disposable single patient use adhesive sensor is applied to skin over areas with strong arterial pulsatile blood flow, typically a finger or toe (Figure 5-3). Alternative sites include the bridge of the nose or nostril, ear, and forehead (Figure 5-4). The forehead sensor is a reflectance sensor and provides a central monitoring site location. Sensors are typically sized according to body weight and intended sensor placement location. It is critical to place sensors only on the manufacturer-approved anatomic locations for which they were designed and Food and Drug Administration (FDA) approved. For example, a pulse oximeter sensor designed and intended to be placed on a finger should not be used on the ear or forehead. While the monitor may display an apparently normal Sao_2 value and

pulse waveform, the accuracy of this value is highly questionable. Additionally when using adhesive sensors, additional tape or other adhesive material should never be applied to the sensor as this may result in circulation constriction of the monitoring site as well as measurement error. The pulse oximeter sensor (Spo_2) is connected to a pulse oximeter monitor unit via a cable. Light-emitting diodes (LEDs) on one side of the sensor transmit light of two different wavelengths (infrared [IR] and red [R]) through arterial blood flowing under the sensor. Depending on the level of Sao_2 of hemoglobin in the arterial blood, different amounts of IR and R light are absorbed and detected on the other side of the sensor (transmission) or via scattered light on the same side of the light emitters (reflectance). The sensor uses photodetection to transmit the ratio of IR and R light information during the pulsatile and non-pulsatile intervals of the cardiac cycle to the microprocessor within the monitor, which then uses various internal software algorithms and sensor calibration curve information for calculation and digital display of the Sao_2 and pulse rate.

When blood perfusion is adequate and Sao_2 levels are greater than 70%, depending on the type of sensor being used and monitoring site, there is generally a close correlation between the saturation reading from the pulse oximeter (Spo_2) and Sao_2 directly measured from ABGs. In situations where perfusion or pulse signal strength to the sensor is markedly diminished (eg, peripheral vasoconstriction due to disease, drugs, or hypothermia), the ability of the pulse oximeter to detect a signal may be less than under normal perfusion conditions. Newer generation hospital grade-pulse oximeters have the ability to adequately detect signals during most poor perfusion conditions as well as sources of signal interference, such as motion or other conditions, which create the potential for artifact. As a result of the world-wide COVID-19 pandemic, the use of small non–hospital-grade finger-based pulse oximeter devices have dramatically increased. Some of these devices have variable accuracy and performance. Clinicians should exercise great caution surrounding use of these products. Only FDA-approved, hospital-grade pulse oximeter monitors and sensors should be used for patient clinical assessment and management to ensure accurate and reliable performance.

Pulse oximetry has several advantages for respiratory monitoring. The ability to have continuous information on

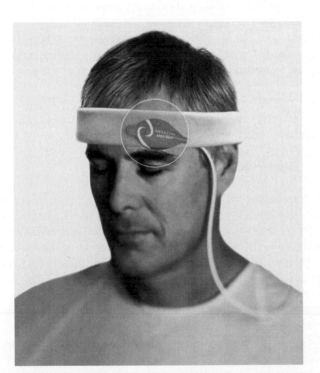

Figure 5-4. Forehead reflectance pulse oximeter sensor. (*©2018 Medtronic. All rights reserved. Used with the permission of Medtronic.*)

the estimated SaO_2 level of critically ill patients without the need for an invasive arterial punctures decreases infection risks and blood loss from frequent ABG analysis. In addition, these monitors are easy to use, well tolerated by most patients, and portable enough to use during transport.

The major disadvantage of pulse oximeters for assessing oxygen status is that their accuracy depends in large part on the ability to acquire an adequate arterial pulsatile signal. Clinical situations that decrease the accuracy of the device include:

- Hypotension
- Low CO states
- Vasoconstriction or vasoactive drugs
- Hypothermia
- Peripheral arterial disease
- Movement of the sensor and/or poor skin adherence

Research shows that SpO_2 readings may be less accurate in patients with darkly pigmented skin, representing a disparity in clinical data. Establishing a higher target range for pulse oximeter readings such as 94% to 98% for all patients may be helpful in ensuring oxygen saturations above 88%. Other sources of potential interference may include venous pulsation, bone and tendon, sensor movement, skin pigmentation, use of certain intravascular dyes, direct exposure to bright ambient light, and certain nail polish applications and treatments. Because these conditions are commonly encountered in any patient connected to a pulse oximeter, including those in a critical care setting, caution is exercised when using pulse oximetry in critical care units. Proper use (Table 5-4) and periodic validation of the accuracy of the devices with ABG analysis utilizing a co-oximeter instrument is essential to avoid erroneous patient assessment. Routinely used pulse oximeters measure light absorbance at only two wavelengths of light. As such, dyshemoglobinemias such as methemoglobinemia

(Met-Hgb) and carboxyhemoglobinemia (CO-Hgb) cannot be measured. Further, the presence of such elevations may cause errors in interpretation of pulse oximetry. Although there are noninvasive devices available for detecting such dyshemoglobinemias, the most widely used and recognized "gold standard" technique for determining the presence of dyshemoglobinemias is co-oximetry via invasive ABG analysis.

Assessing Pulmonary Function

A variety of measurements in addition to ABG analysis can be used to further evaluate the critically ill patient's respiratory system.

Measurement of selected lung volumes can be easily accomplished at the bedside. V_T, exhaled minute ventilation (V_E), and negative inspiratory force (NIF) are measured with portable, handheld equipment (spirometer and NIF meter, respectively). Lung compliance and alveolar oxygen content can be calculated with standard formulas (see Table 5-1). Frequent trend monitoring of these parameters provides an objective evaluation of the patient's response to interventions.

ABG analysis for arterial partial pressure of carbon dioxide ($PaCO_2$) is an important parameter in critically ill patients for assessment of ventilation. To limit invasive procedures or for more continuous monitoring or $PaCO_2$, clinicians may sometimes rely on venous blood gases or capnography. Each of these techniques for assessing ventilation status has certain advantages and limitations. Central venous PCO_2 allows accurate estimation of $PaCO_2$, so long as CO_2 is relatively normal. PCO_2 measured from a central vein is normally approximately 4 mm Hg higher than $PaCO_2$. However, peripheral venous PCO_2 is a poor predictor of $PaCO_2$. Measurement of exhaled carbon dioxide or capnography offers measurement of the partial pressure of end-tidal PCO_2 ($PetCO_2$), a value that is close to $PaCO_2$ when the lung is healthy. It has the advantages of being noninvasive and can be monitored continuously on a breath-by-breath basis.

End-Tidal Carbon Dioxide Monitoring

Carbon dioxide is a by-product of cellular metabolism and is transported via the venous blood to the lungs where it is eliminated by the lungs during exhalation. End-tidal CO_2 (also referred to as partial pressure of end-tidal CO_2: $PetCO_2$) is the concentration of CO_2 present at the end of exhalation and is expressed either as a percentage ($PetCO_2$%) or partial pressure ($PetCO_2$ mm Hg). The normal range for $PetCO_2$ is typically 35 to 45 mm Hg and 2 to 5 mm Hg less than the arterial carbon dioxide tension or $PaCO_2$. For this reason, clinicians have sought to use this noninvasive monitoring method for assessing ventilation status over time. Under conditions of normal $\dot{V}/\dot{Q}$ matching, the relationship between $PetCO_2$ and $PaCO_2$ is relatively close. In critical illness where $\dot{V}/\dot{Q}$ relationships are frequently abnormal, this

TABLE 5-4. TIPS TO MAXIMIZE SAFETY AND ACCURACY OF PULSE OXIMETRY

- Apply sensor to dry finger of nondominant hand according to manufacturer's directions and observe for adequate cardiac-based arterial pulse wave generation or signal on pulse oximeter unit.
- Avoid tension on the sensor cable.
- Rotate application sites and change sensors according to manufacturer's directions whenever adherence is poor.
- In children and elderly patients, assess application sites more often and carefully assess skin integrity when using adhesive sensors.
- Never use pulse oximeter sensors on non-approved monitoring site locations, such as finger or digit sensor use on the ear or forehead.
- If pulse wave generation is inadequate or a signal alert message is displayed check for proper adherence to skin and position. Apply a new sensor to another site if necessary.
- Compare pulse oximeter displayed SaO_2 values with arterial blood gases periodically when changes in the clinical condition may decrease accuracy and/or when values do not fit the clinical situation.
- Be aware of factors that affect pulse oximetry accuracy including skin pigmentation, poor circulation, skin thickness, skin temperature, and the use of nail polish.

gradient or difference may be as high as 20 mm Hg or more, which limits the use of this technology to accurately reflect $Paco_2$. However, in most clinical circumstances, an increase in $PetCO_2$ can be interpreted as a sign of hypoventilation. Assessing the arterial to end-tidal CO_2 gradient as a trend also may be useful. An increasing gradient over time reflects a worsening condition and a narrowing gradient may reflect improved ventilation/perfusion matching.

Currently available end-tidal CO_2 monitoring devices fall into one of several categories: colorimetric, capnometric (numeric display only), or capnographic (numeric and graphical display). Colorimetric devices are pH-sensitive colored paper strips that change color in response to different concentrations of carbon dioxide (Figure 5-5). They are typically used for either initial or intermittent monitoring purposes such as verifying ET placement in the trachea following intubation or in some cases, to rule out inadvertent pulmonary placement of enteral feeding tubes following insertion. A capnometer provides a visual analog or digital display of the concentration of the $PetCO_2$. Capnography includes both capnometry plus the addition of a calibrated graphic waveform recording of the exhaled CO_2 on a breath-by-breath basis, and it is perhaps the most common instrument used for continuous monitoring. Figure 5-6 demonstrates the various phases of a normal carbon dioxide waveform during exhalation.

Capnography devices measure exhaled carbon dioxide using one of several different techniques: infrared spectrography, Raman spectrography, mass spectrometry, or a laser-based technology called molecular correlation spectroscopy as the infrared emission source. The laser creates an infrared emission precisely matching the absorption rate spectrum of CO_2 and eliminates the need for moving parts. A capnography

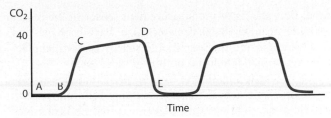

Figure 5-6. Capnogram waveform phases. Phase A to B: Early exhalation. This represents anatomic dead space and contains little carbon dioxide. Phase B to C: Combination of dead space and alveolar gas. Phase C to D: Exhalation of mostly alveolar gas (alveolar plateau). D: End-tidal point, that is, exhalation of carbon dioxide at maximum point. Phase D to E: Inspiration begins and carbon dioxide concentration rapidly falls to baseline or zero. (©2018 Medtronic. All rights reserved. Used with the permission of Medtronic.)

device using this technology is shown in Figure 5-7. All capnographs sample and measure expired gases either directly at the patient-ventilator interface (mainstream analysis) or are collected and transported via moisture and bacteria-filtered

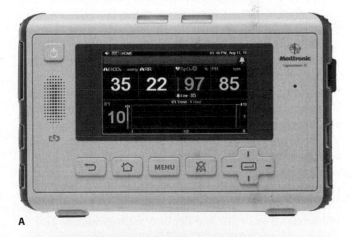

A

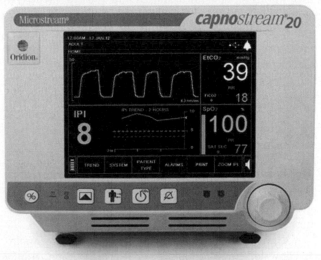

B

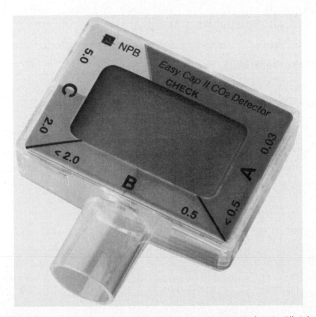

Figure 5-5. Colorimetric carbon dioxide detector. (©2018 Medtronic. All rights reserved. Used with the permission of Medtronic.)

Figure 5-7. Handheld **(A)** and Bedside **(B)** combined capnography (sidestream) and pulse oximetry instruments. (©2018 Medtronic. All rights reserved. Used with the permission of Medtronic.)

small-bore tubing to the measurement sensor in the monitor (sidestream analysis). Each technique has advantages and disadvantages and the user should strictly follow manufacturer recommendations for optimal performance.

Clinical application of capnography includes assessment of endotracheal or tracheostomy tube placement, gastric or small bowel tube placement, pulmonary blood flow, and alveolar ventilation, provided $\dot{V}/\dot{Q}$ relationships are normal. The AHA Guidelines for ACLS recommend using quantitative waveform capnography in intubated patients during CPR. Waveform capnography allows nurses and other caregivers to monitor CPR quality, optimize chest compressions, and detect return of spontaneous circulation (ROSC) during chest compressions. High-quality chest compressions are achieved when the end-tidal CO_2 value is at least 10 to 20 mm Hg. During CPR, an abrupt increase in the $PetCO_2$ to 35 to 40 mm Hg is reasonable to consider as an indication of ROSC. In intubated patients, failure to achieve a $PetCO_2$ of greater than 10 mm Hg, and ideally greater than or equal to 20 mm Hg by waveform capnography may be a useful marker for CPR quality and one component of a multimodal approach to decide when to end resuscitative efforts. An ideal target has not been identified.

When using end-tidal CO_2 adapters in-line for intubated patients (cuffed ETT or tracheostomy tube), it is important to position the sampling line (sidestream) or measurement head adapter (mainstream) in the ventilator circuit as close as possible to the artificial airway for the best fidelity in readings. Care should be taken to not block the ability to pass a suction catheter.

Assessment of the capnographic waveform alone can yield useful information in assessment of ventilator malfunction, patient response to changes in ventilator settings and weaning attempts, and depth of neuromuscular blockade in intubated patients. Capnography can also be used to monitor nonintubated patients via a nasal/oral sampling cannula. Patients with known or suspected obstructive sleep apnea, severe pneumonia, acute exacerbation of asthma or COPD, and in particular, patients receiving opioids or other related respiratory depressant medications, all face a risk for impaired ventilation. While pulse oximetry is a very useful tool for assessing oxygenation status, it is a poor ventilation monitor, especially in patients receiving supplemental oxygen. Whenever clinicians use capnography in the clinical setting, it is important to follow manufacturer recommendations regarding set-up, maintenance, and troubleshooting of equipment. Institutional policies and protocols regarding clinical management for patient care should also be followed.

Advances in noninvasive patient monitoring technologies allow for combined pulse oximetry and capnography monitoring which may have the capability to remotely monitor either at the bedside, a central station, or via PC, smart tablet or phone and virtually connect to the hospital EMR for automatic charting and alarm notification (Figure 5-8).

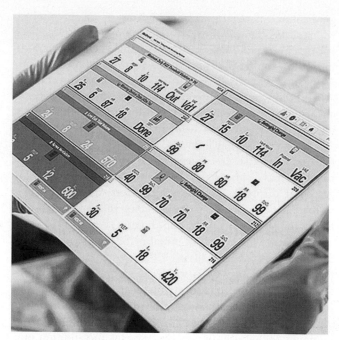

Figure 5-8. Remote monitoring system for continuous display of noninvasive respiratory monitoring instruments (© *2021 Medtronic. All rights reserved. Used with permission of Medtronic.*)

It is becoming increasingly common in progressive care and medical/surgical patient care units.

AIRWAY MANAGEMENT

Maintaining an open and patent airway is an important aspect of critical care management. Patency can be ensured through conservative techniques such as coughing, head and neck positioning, and alignment. If conservative techniques fail, insertion of an oral or nasal airway or endotracheal intubation may be required.

Oropharyngeal Airway

The oropharyngeal airway, or oral bite block, is an airway adjunct used to relieve upper airway obstruction caused by tongue relaxation (eg, postanesthesia or during unconsciousness), secretions, seizures, or biting down on oral ETs (Figure 5-9A). Oral airways are made of rigid plastic or rubber material, semicircular in shape, and available in sizes ranging from infants to adults. The airway is inserted with the concave curve of the airway facing up into the roof of the mouth. The oral airway is then rotated down 180° during insertion to fit the curvature of the tongue and ensure the tongue is not obstructing the airway. The tip of the oropharyngeal airway rests near the posterior pharyngeal wall. For this reason, oral airways are not recommended for use in alert patients because they may trigger the gag reflex and cause vomiting. Oropharyngeal airways are temporary devices for achieving airway patency.

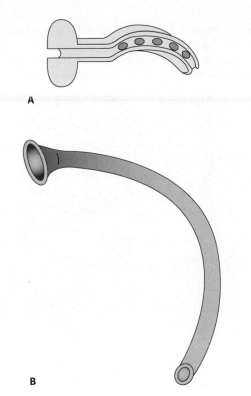

Figure 5-9. **(A)** Oropharyngeal and **(B)** Nasopharyngeal airways.

Management of oropharyngeal airways includes assessment of the lips and tongue to identify pressure injuries. At least every 24 hours, the airway is removed, and the lips and tongue are assessed and oral hygiene is provided.

Nasopharyngeal Airway

The nasopharyngeal airway, or nasal trumpet, is another type of airway adjunct device used to help maintain airway patency, especially in the semiconscious patient (Figure 5-9B). The nasopharyngeal airway is also used to facilitate nasotracheal suctioning. Made of soft malleable rubber or soft plastic, the nasal airway ranges in sizes from 26 to 35 Fr. Depending on hospital policy, a topical anesthetic (such as viscous lidocaine) may be applied to the nares prior to insertion of the airway. The nasopharyngeal airway, lubricated with a water-soluble gel, is gently inserted into one of the nares. To assess the patency of the airway, listen for or feel for air movement during expiration. The airway is secured using a chevron taping technique to the nose with a small piece of tape to prevent displacement. Complications of these airways include bleeding, sinusitis, and erosion of the mucous membranes.

Care of the patient with a nasal airway includes frequent assessment for pressure injuries and occlusion of the airway with dried secretions. Sinusitis has been documented as a complication. The continued need for the nasal airway is assessed daily and rotation of the airway from nostril to nostril is done on a daily basis. When performing nasotracheal suctioning through the nasal airway, the suction catheter is

lubricated with a water-soluble gel to ease passage. Refer to the following discussion on suctioning for additional standards of care.

Laryngeal Mask Airway

The laryngeal mask airway (LMA) is an ET with a small mask on one end that can be passed orally over the larynx to provide ventilatory assistance and prevent aspiration. Placement of the LMA is easier than intubation using a standard ET. Commonly used as the primary airway device in the operating room for certain types of surgical procedures, it is to be considered only a temporary airway for patients who require prolonged ventilatory support. LMA is often used in the management of the difficult airway; primarily in the "cannot intubate" or "cannot ventilate" clinical scenarios.

Artificial Airways

Artificial airways (oral and nasal ETs, tracheostomy tubes) are used when a patent airway cannot be maintained with an adjunct airway device, when patients require mechanical ventilation, or to manage severe airway obstruction. The artificial airway also provides some protection for the lower airway from aspiration of oral or gastric secretions and allows for easier secretion removal.

Types of Artificial Airways and Insertion

Endotracheal and tracheostomy tubes are made of either polyvinyl chloride or silicone and are available in a variety of sizes and lengths (Figure 5-10). Standard features include a 15-mm adapter at the end of the tube for connection to life-support equipment such as mechanical ventilation circuits, closed-suction catheter systems, swivel adapters, or a manual resuscitation bag (MRB). Tubes may be cuffed or uncuffed. For cuffed tubes, air is manually injected into the cuff located near the distal tip of the ET tube through a small one-way pilot valve and inflation lumen. Distance markers are located along the side of the tube for identification of tube position. A radiopaque line is also located on all tubes so as to aid in determining proper position radiographically.

ETs are inserted into the patient's trachea either through the mouth or nose (Figures 5-11 and 5-12). Orally inserted ET tubes are more common than the nasal route because nasal intubation is associated with sinus infections and is considered an independent risk factor for developing ventilator-associated pneumonia (VAP). With use of the laryngoscope, the upper airway is visualized and the tube is inserted through the vocal cords into the trachea, 2 to 4 cm above the carina. The presence of bilateral breath sounds, along with equal chest excursion during inspiration and the absence of breath sounds over the stomach, preliminarily confirms proper tube placement. An end-tidal CO_2 with waveform verification monitor is used as an immediate assessment for determining tracheal placement. If not available, a colorimetric CO_2 detector may be used. A portable chest x-ray

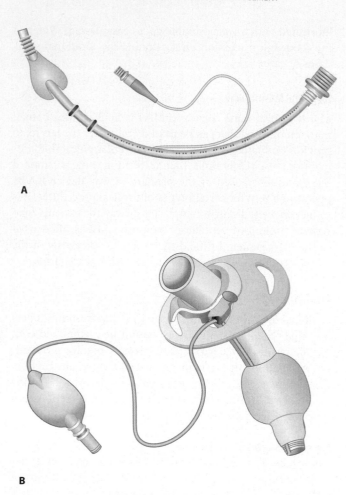

A

B

Figure 5-10. Artificial airways. **(A)** Cuffed endotracheal tube. **(B)** Cuffed tracheostomy tube. (©2018 Medtronic. All rights reserved. Used with the permission of Medtronic.)

verifies proper tube placement. Once proper placement is confirmed, the tube is anchored with either tape or a special ET fixation device to prevent movement (Figure 5-13). The centimeter marking of the ET tube at the lip is documented and checked during each shift to monitor proper tube placement. Documentation of the procedure in accordance with institutional policy, includes the assessments that confirmed tube placement.

ET sizes are typically identified by the tube's internal diameter in millimeters (mm ID). The size of the tube is printed on the tube and generally also on the outside packaging. Knowledge of the tube ID is critical; the smaller the mm ID, the higher the resistance to breathing through the tube, thus increasing the work of breathing (WOB). The most common ET sizes used in adults are 7.0 to 8.0 mm ID.

Complications of ET intubation are numerous and include laryngeal and tracheal damage, laryngospasm, aspiration, infection, discomfort, sinusitis, and subglottic injury. ETs can, in some situations, be safely left in place for up to 2 to 3 weeks, but tracheostomy is often considered following 10 to 14 days of intubation or less if a prolonged recovery is anticipated. The decision to place a tracheostomy ideally also

takes into account the patient's goals of care and the disease prognosis.

The majority of tracheostomy tubes used in critically ill patients is made of medical-grade plastic or silicone and

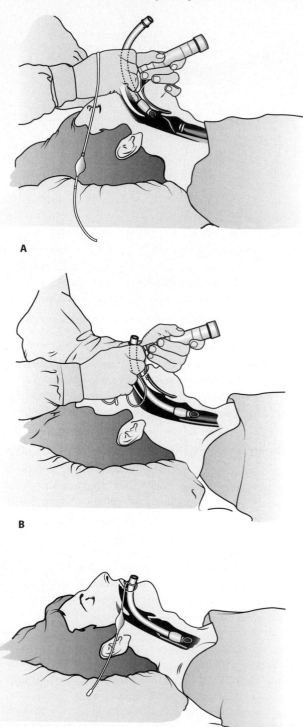

A

B

C

Figure 5-11. Oral intubation with an endotracheal (ET) tube. **(A)** Insertion of ET tube through the mouth with the aid of a laryngoscope. **(B)** ET tube advanced through the vocal cords into the trachea. **(C)** ET tube positioned with the cuff below the vocal cords. (*Reproduced with permission from Boggs R, Wooldridge-King M. AACN Procedure Manual for Critical Care, 3rd ed. Philadelphia, PA: WB Saunders; 1993.*)

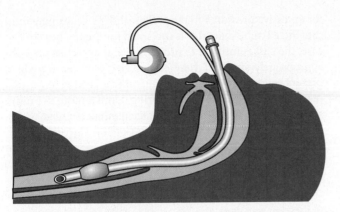

Figure 5-12. Nasal endotracheal tube. *(©2018 Medtronic. All rights reserved. Used with the permission of Medtronic.)*

come in a variety of sizes (Figure 5-10B). Tracheostomy tubes may be cuffed or uncuffed. As with ET tubes, a standard 15-mm adapter at the proximal end ensures universal connection to MRBs and ventilator circuits. Tracheostomy tubes may be inserted as an elective procedure using a standard open surgical technique in the operating room or at the bedside via a percutaneous insertion. This technique involves a procedure in which a small incision is made in the neck and a series of dilators are manually passed into the trachea over a guide wire, creating a stoma opening through which the tracheostomy tube is inserted. Bedside placement obviates the need for general anesthesia and for patient transport outside the intensive care unit (ICU) with its associated risks.

Tracheostomies are secured with cotton twill tape or latex-free Velcro tube holders attached to openings on the neck flange or plate of the tube. Many tracheostomy tubes have inner cannula that can be easily removed for periodic cleaning (reusable) or replacement (disposable). Some tracheostomy tubes incorporate an additional opening along the outer tube cannula referred to as a fenestration. A fenestrated tracheostomy tube is sometimes used as an aid for facilitating vocalization by allowing airflow upward and through the vocal cords. A fenestration is not necessary to be able to talk with a tracheostomy tube. Patients generally tolerate tracheostomy tubes and find them more comfortable than oral or nasal ET tubes. Further, there are more nutrition and communication options available to patients with tracheostomy tubes than with ETs.

Complications of tracheostomies include hemorrhage from erosion of the innominate artery; tracheal stenosis, malacia, or perforation; laryngeal nerve injury; aspiration; infection; air leak; device-related pressure injury; and mechanical problems. Most of these complications can be prevented with proper management.

Cuff Inflation

Following insertion of an endotracheal or tracheostomy tube, the cuff of the tube is inflated with just enough air to create an effective seal. The cuff is typically inflated with the lowest possible pressure that prevents air leak during mechanical ventilation and decreases the risk of pulmonary aspiration.

Cuff pressure is maintained at less than 25 mm Hg (30 cm H_2O). Excessive cuff pressure causes tracheal ischemia, necrosis, and erosion, as well as overinflation-related obstruction of the distal airway from cuff herniation. It is important to recognize that even a properly inflated cuffed artificial airway does not completely protect the patient from aspiration.

There are two common techniques to ensure proper cuff inflation without overinflation: the minimal leak and minimal occlusive volume techniques (MLT and MOV,

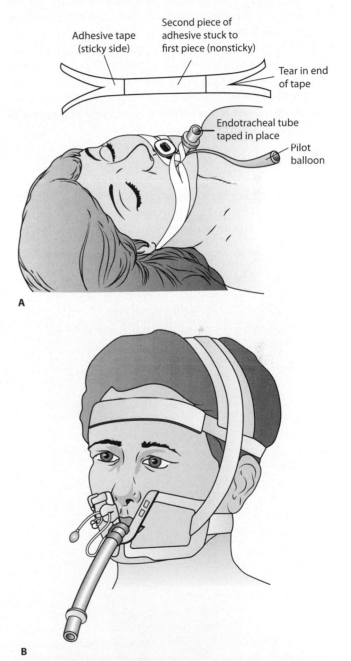

Figure 5-13. Methods for anchoring an endotracheal tube to prevent movement. **(A)** Taping of an oral ET tube. *(Reproduced with permission from Boggs R, Wooldridge-King M. AACN Procedure Manual for Critical Care, 3rd ed. Philadelphia, PA: WB Saunders; 1993.)* **(B)** Use of a special fixation device. *(Reproduced with permission from Kaplow R, Bookbinder M. A comparison of four endotracheal tube holders. Heart Lung. 1994;23(1):59-66.)*

respectively). The minimal leak technique involves listening over the larynx during positive pressure breaths with a stethoscope while slowly inflating the tube cuff in 1- to 2-mL increments. Inflation continues until only a small air leak, or rush of air, is heard over the larynx during peak inspiration. The minimal leak technique should result in no more than a 50- to 100-mL air loss per breath during mechanical ventilation. The cuff pressure and amount of air instilled into the cuff are recorded following the maneuver.

The MOV cuff inflation technique is similar to the minimal leak technique. Cuff inflation continues, however, until the air leak completely disappears. The amount of air instilled and the cuff pressure are recorded during cuff inflation and periodically to ensure an intracuff pressure of less than 25 mm Hg (30 cm H_2O). Manual palpation of the tube pilot balloon does not ensure optimal inflation. An additional device that is less common is available and measures continuous cuff pressures.

Cuff Pressure Measurement

The connection of the ET tube pilot balloon to an intracuff measuring manometer device, such as a manual handheld cuff inflator, allows for the simultaneous measurement of pressure during inflation or periodic checking (Figure 5-14). The need

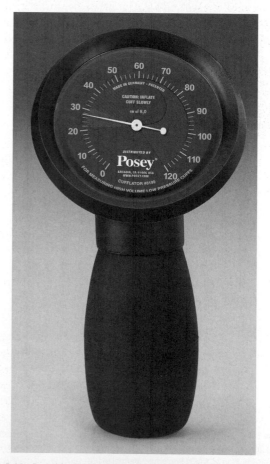

Figure 5-14. Portable endotracheal tube cuff inflator and manometer. (*Reproduced with permission from Posey Company, Arcadia, CA.*)

for excessive pressures to properly seal the trachea may indicate the ET tube diameter is too small for the trachea. In this case, the cuff is inflated to properly seal the trachea until the appropriately sized ET tube can be electively reinserted. At present, evidence of long-term outcomes is lacking to warrant mandatory cuff pressure monitoring. Until a more definitive statement may be made, the clinician is encouraged to follow tube manufacturer and hospital policy. Currently available clinical and laboratory testing evidence does suggest that intracuff pressure may be an important contributing factor to the development of complications related to cuffed endotracheal and tracheostomy tubes; however, morbidity secondary to these airway devices is invariably multifactorial.

Endotracheal and Tracheostomy Suctioning

Pulmonary secretion removal is normally accomplished by coughing. An effective cough requires a closed epiglottis so that intrathoracic pressure can be increased prior to sudden opening of the epiglottis and secretion expulsion. The presence of an artificial airway may prevent glottic closure and effective coughing, necessitating the use of periodic endotracheal suctioning to remove secretions.

Currently, two methods are commonly used for ET or tracheostomy tube suctioning while the patient is mechanically ventilated: the closed and open methods. *Closed suctioning* means the ventilator circuit remains closed while suctioning is performed, whereas *open suctioning* means the ventilator circuit is opened, or removed, during suctioning. The open method requires disconnection of the ET or tracheostomy tube from the mechanical ventilator or oxygen therapy source and insertion of a suction catheter each time the patient requires suctioning and is less commonly used today. The closed method refers to an in-line suction catheter device that remains attached to the ventilator circuit, allowing periodic insertion of the suction catheter through a diaphragm to suction without removing the patient from the ventilator. Following suctioning, the catheter is withdrawn into a plastic sleeve where it is stored until the next suctioning procedure. Closed systems offer an advantage in reducing the risk of infection.

Indications

The need for suctioning is determined by a variety of clinical signs and symptoms, such as visible or audible secretions in the airway, respiratory distress with increased respiratory rate and/or coughing, increased inspiratory pressures on the ventilator, and the presence of adventitious sounds (rhonchi, gurgling) during chest auscultation. Suctioning may also be performed when airway patency is questioned. Suctioning is only done when there is a clinical indication and never on a routine schedule.

Procedure

Hyperoxygenation with 100% O_2 for a minimum of 30 seconds is provided prior to each suctioning episode, whether using an open or closed technique (Table 5-5). Hyperoxygenation helps prevent decreases in arterial oxygen levels after suctioning. Hyperoxygenation can be achieved by increasing the FiO_2 setting on the mechanical ventilator or by using the "suction" button or temporary oxygen-enrichment function available on most microprocessor ventilators. Manual ventilation of the patient using an MRB is not recommended as the best choice and has been shown to be ineffective for providing delivered FiO_2 of 1.0. If no other alternative is available to hyperoxygenate, then an MRB can be used. At least 30 seconds of manual breaths with 100% FiO_2 are provided before and after each pass of the suction catheter. In spontaneously breathing patients, encourage several deep breaths of 100% O_2 before and after each suction pass. Usually two or three suction passes are sufficient to clear the airway. The mechanical act of inserting the

suction catheter into the trachea can stimulate the vagus nerve and result in bradycardia or asystole. Because of this risk, suctioning passes stop once the airway is clear and each pass of the suction catheter is 10 seconds or less.

The instillation of 5 to 10 mL of normal saline during ET or tracheostomy tube suctioning has risks and no documented benefits and therefore is not recommended. This practice was previously thought to decrease secretion viscosity and increase secretion removal during suctioning. However, bolus saline instillation has not been shown to be beneficial and is associated with SaO_2 decreases, patient discomfort, and bronchospasm.

Complications

A variety of complications are associated with ET or tracheostomy tube suctioning. Decreases in PaO_2 are well documented when no hyperoxygenation therapy is provided prior to suctioning. Serious cardiac arrhythmias can occur with suctioning, including bradycardia, asystole, ventricular tachycardia, and heart block. Less severe arrhythmias frequently occur with suctioning and include premature ventricular contractions, atrial contractions, and supraventricular tachycardia. Other complications associated with suctioning include increases in arterial pressure and intracranial pressure, bronchospasm, hypoxemia, and tracheal wall damage including bleeding, pain, and anxiety. Many of these complications can be minimized by using sterile technique, vigilant monitoring during and after suctioning, and hyperoxygenation before and after each suction pass.

Extubation

Extubation refers to the removal of an ET tube. The reversal or significant improvement of the underlying condition(s) that led to the use of ET tube usually signals the readiness for removal of the airway. Common indicators of readiness for ET tube removal include the patient's ability to:

- maintain spontaneous breathing and adequate ABG values with minimal to moderate amounts of O_2 administration ($FiO_2 < 0.50$),
- protect their airway by being alert and able to maintain airway alignment, and
- clear pulmonary secretions.

Removal of an artificial airway usually occurs following weaning from mechanical ventilatory support (see the discussion on weaning later). Preparations for extubation include an explanation to the patient and family of what to expect, the need to cough, medication for pain as needed, setting up the appropriate method for delivering O_2 therapy (eg, face mask, high flow nasal cannula), and positioning the patient with the head of the bed elevated at 30° to 45° to improve diaphragmatic function. Suctioning of the artificial airway and oral cavity is usually performed prior to extubation.

TABLE 5-5. STEPS FOR SUCTIONING THROUGH AN ARTIFICIAL AIRWAY

1. Assess for clinical indications:
   - Secretions visible or audible in the airway
   - Suspected aspiration
   - Decreased breath sounds, inspiratory wheezes, or expiratory crackles
   - Increase in peak airway pressures or decreased tidal volume
   - Restlessness or decreased level of consciousness
   - Ineffective or frequent cough
   - Tachypnea, shallow, or decreased respirations
   - Gradual or sudden decrease in PaO_2, SaO_2, or SpO_2
   - Sudden onset of respiratory distress
2. Hyperoxygenate with 100% oxygen for minimum of 30 s with one of the following:
   - Press the suction hyperoxygenation button to increase the FiO_2 to 1.0 (100%) on the ventilator (preferred),
   - Manually increase the FiO_2 to 1.0 (100%), or
   - Disconnect from the ventilator and manually ventilate with MRB (also called bag valve mask)
3. Insert catheter (closed or open system) gently until resistance is met, then pull back 1-2 cm
4. Place the nondominant thumb over the control vent of the suction catheter to apply continuous or intermittent suction as the catheter is completely withdrawn
   NOTE: Suction should be applied only as needed and for as short a time as possible
5. Hyperoxygenate for 30 s as described in step 2
6. Repeat steps 3, 4, and 5 as needed if secretions remain and patient is tolerating the procedure
7. Monitor cardiopulmonary status before, during, and after suctioning for the following:
   - Decreased oxygen saturation (SpO_2, arterial or mixed venous)
   - Cardiac dysrhythmias
   - Bronchospasm
   - Respiratory distress or coughing
   - Diminished breath sounds
   - Cardiac arrest
   - Hypertension or hypotension
   - Increased ICP
   - Decreased SvO_2
   - Anxiety, agitation, pain, or change in level of consciousness
   - Increased peak airway pressure
   - Pulmonary hemorrhage or bleeding
   - Increased work of breathing

Data from Wiegand DL. AACN Procedure Manual for Critical Care. 7th ed. St. Louis, MO: Elsevier Saunders; 2016.

Obtaining a baseline cardiopulmonary assessment also is important for later evaluation of the response to extubation. Extubation is best performed when the interdisciplinary team is available to assist if reintubation is required.

Hyperoxygenation with 100% O_2 is provided for 30 to 60 seconds prior to extubation in case respiratory distress occurs immediately after extubation and reintubation is necessary. The patient is asked to take a deep breath in and the artificial airway is then removed following complete deflation of the ET cuff, if present. Immediately apply the oxygen delivery method and encourage the patient to cough and take deep breaths.

Monitor the patient's response to the extubation. Changes in heart rate, respiratory rate, and/or blood pressure of more than 10% of baseline values may indicate respiratory compromise, necessitating more extensive assessment and possible reintubation. Pulmonary auscultation is also performed.

Complications associated with extubation include aspiration, bronchospasm, and tracheal damage. Monitor the patients' vital signs and upper airway for stridor, and encourage coughing and deep breathing. Inspiratory stridor occurs from glottic and subglottic edema and may develop immediately or take several hours. If the patient's clinical status permits, 2.5% racemic epinephrine (0.5 mL in 3 mL of normal saline) is administered via an aerosol delivery device. If the upper airway obstruction persists or worsens, reintubation is generally required along with a short course of intravenous steroids. A reattempt at extubation is usually delayed for 24 to 72 hours following reintubation for upper airway obstruction to allow further assessment and treatment of any swelling.

DECANNULATION

Decannulation refers to the removal of a tracheostomy tube. The reversal or significant improvement of the underlying condition(s) that led to the insertion of the tracheostomy tube usually signals the readiness for removal of the airway. Common indicators of readiness for tracheostomy tube removal include the patient's ability to:

- maintain spontaneous breathing and adequate Spo_2 without mechanical ventilation,
- maintain a patent upper airway without stridor or labored breathing, and
- clear pulmonary secretions with minimal secretions and effective cough.

Patients with compromised airway patency manifested by tracheal stenosis, granulation tissue, or abnormal vocal cords require additional assessment prior to decannulation. Additional assessments and protocols vary per facility but may include tracheostomy downsizing and capping trials to assess tolerance prior to removal.

Preparations for decannulation include an explanation to the patient and family of what to expect, the need to cough, setting up the appropriate method for delivering O_2 therapy (eg, face mask, nasal cannula), and positioning the patient with the head of the bed elevated at 30° to 45° to improve diaphragmatic function. Hyperoxygenation and suctioning of the artificial airway and oral cavity is usually performed prior to decannulation. Obtaining a baseline neurological and cardiopulmonary assessment also is important for later evaluation of the response to decannulation. Decannulation is best performed when the interdisciplinary team is available to assist if reinsertion of the tracheostomy tube is required.

The patient is asked to take a deep breath in and the artificial airway is then removed following removal of securement device. Place a dry sterile 4×4 dressing over stoma. Immediately apply the oxygen delivery method and encourage the patient to cough and take deep breaths.

Monitor the patient's response to decannulation. Changes in heart rate, respiratory rate, and/or blood pressure of more than 10% of baseline values may indicate respiratory compromise, Pulmonary auscultation is also performed. Encourage the gentle application of 1 to 2 fingers over the stoma while coughing or vocalizing to minimize leak.

The tracheostomy stoma closes generally within 2 to 7 days. Complications associated with decannulation include tracheomalacia (abnormal collapse of the tracheal walls) and aspiration. Decannulation failure has been reported to range from 2% to 5% and may require reinsertion.

OXYGEN THERAPY

Oxygen is used for any number of clinical problems (Table 5-6). The goals for oxygen use include increasing alveolar O_2 tension (Pao_2) to treat hypoxemia, decreasing the WOB, and maximizing myocardial and tissue oxygen supply.

TABLE 5-6. COMMON INDICATIONS FOR OXYGEN THERAPY

- Decreased cardiac performance
- Increased metabolic need for O_2 (fever, burns)
- Acute changes in level of consciousness (restlessness, confusion)
- Acute shortness of breath
- Decreased O_2 saturation
- $Pao_2 < 60$ mm Hg or $Sao_2 < 90\%$
- Normal Pao_2 or Sao_2 with signs and symptoms of significant hypoxia
- Acute myocardial infarction with $Spo_2 < 90\%$, respiratory distress, or signs of hypoxemia
- Carbon monoxide (CO) poisoning
- Methemoglobinemia (a form of hemoglobin where ferrous iron is oxidized to ferric form, causing a high affinity for O_2 with decreased O_2 release at tissue level)
- Acute anemia
- Cardiopulmonary arrest
- Reduced cardiac output
- In the presence of hypotension, tachycardia, cyanosis, chest pain, dyspnea, and acute neurologic dysfunction
- During stressful procedures and situations, especially in high-risk patients (eg, endotracheal suctioning, bronchoscopy, thoracentesis, pulmonary artery [PA] catheterization, travel at high altitudes)

Complications

As with any drug, oxygen is used cautiously. The hazards of oxygen misuse include alveolar hypoventilation, absorption atelectasis, and oxygen toxicity and can be life threatening.

Alveolar Hypoventilation

Alveolar hypoventilation is under ventilation of alveoli, and it is a side effect of great concern in patients with COPD with carbon dioxide retention. It was once thought that because the patient with COPD adjusts to chronically high levels of $Paco_2$, the chemoreceptors in the medulla of the brain lose responsiveness to high $Paco_2$ levels and hypoxemia becomes the primary stimulus for ventilation. However, there are several other physiologic mechanisms in the patient with COPD that contribute to increased $Paco_2$ levels including inability to increase minute ventilation and lack of hypoxic vasoconstriction, which leads to increased dead space ventilation. Correction of hypoxemia in the patient with COPD remains important with a target Pao_2 of 55 to 60 mm Hg ($Sao_2 \geq 90\%$), despite the presence of hypercapnia (see Chapter 10, Respiratory System).

Absorption Atelectasis

Absorption atelectasis results when high concentrations of O_2 (>90%) are given for long periods of time and nitrogen is washed out of the lungs. The nitrogen in inspired gas is approximately 79% of the total atmospheric gases. The large partial pressure of nitrogen in the alveoli helps keep the alveoli open because it is not absorbed. When the inspired gas is 90% to 100% oxygen, alveolar closure occurs because oxygen readily diffuses into the pulmonary capillary.

Oxygen Toxicity (Hyperoxia)

The toxic effects of oxygen are targeted primarily to the pulmonary and central nervous systems (CNS). CNS toxicity usually occurs with hyperbaric oxygen treatment. Signs and symptoms include nausea, anxiety, numbness, visual disturbances, muscular twitching, and grand mal seizures. The physiologic mechanism is not understood fully but is probably related to subtle neural and biochemical changes that alter the electric activity of the CNS.

Hyperoxia may lead to ARDS or bronchopulmonary dysplasia. Two phases of lung injury occur with prolonged exposure to high Fio_2 levels. The first phase occurs after 1 to 4 days of exposure to higher O_2 levels and is manifested by decreased tracheal mucosal blood flow and tracheobronchitis. Vital capacity decreases due to poor lung expansion and progressive atelectasis persists. The alveolar-capillary membrane becomes progressively impaired, decreasing gas exchange. The second phase occurs after 12 days of high exposure. The alveolar septa thicken and ARDS develops, with associated high mortality (see Chapter 10, Respiratory System).

Caring for the patient who requires high levels of oxygen requires astute monitoring and titration by the critical care nurse to maintain the lowest concentration of oxygen that promotes oxygen delivery and reduces oxygen demand. Monitor those patients at risk for absorption atelectasis and oxygen toxicity. Signs and symptoms include nonproductive cough, substernal chest pain, general malaise, fatigue, nausea, and vomiting. Newer therapies that have developed during the COVID-19 pandemic include encouraging patients to awake self-prone position for patients on HFNC along with traditional prone positioning (refer to Chapter 10, Respiratory System).

An oxygen concentration of 100% ($Fio_2 = 1.0$) is regarded as safe for short periods of time (<24 hours). Oxygen concentrations greater than 60% for more than 24 to 48 hours may damage the lungs and worsen respiratory problems. Fio_2 levels are decreased as soon as Pao_2 levels reach clinically acceptable levels (>60 mm Hg or higher).

Oxygen Delivery

Noninvasive Devices

Face masks and nasal cannulas are standard oxygen delivery devices for the spontaneously breathing patient (Figure 5-15). Oxygen can be delivered with a high- or low-flow device, with the concentration of O_2 delivered ranging from 21% to approximately 100% (Table 5-7). An example of a high-flow device is the Venturi mask system that can deliver precise concentrations of oxygen (Figure 5-16). The usual Fio_2 values delivered with this type of mask are 24%, 28%, 31%, 35%, 40%, and 50%. Often, Venturi masks are useful in patients with COPD and hypercapnia because the clinician can titrate the Pao_2 to minimize carbon dioxide retention.

An example of a low-flow system is the nasal cannula or prongs. Nasal prongs flow rate ranges are limited to 6 L/min. Flow rates less than 4 L/min need not be humidified. The main advantage of nasal prongs is that the patient can drink, eat, and speak during oxygen administration. Their disadvantage is that the exact Fio_2 delivered is unknown, because it is influenced by the patient's peak inspiratory flow demand and breathing pattern. As a general guide, 1 L/min of O_2 flow is an approximate equivalent to Fio_2 of 24%, and each additional liter of oxygen flow increases the Fio_2 by approximately 4%.

Simple oxygen face masks can provide an Fio_2 of 34% to 50% depending on fit, at flow rates from 5 to 10 L/min. Flow rates should be maintained at 5 L/min or more in order to avoid rebreathing exhaled CO_2 that can be retained in the mask. Limitations of using a simple face mask include difficulty in delivering accurate delivery of low concentrations of oxygen and long-term use can lead to skin irritation and potential pressure breakdown.

Non-rebreathing masks can achieve high oxygen concentrations of between 60% and 80% with a minimum flow

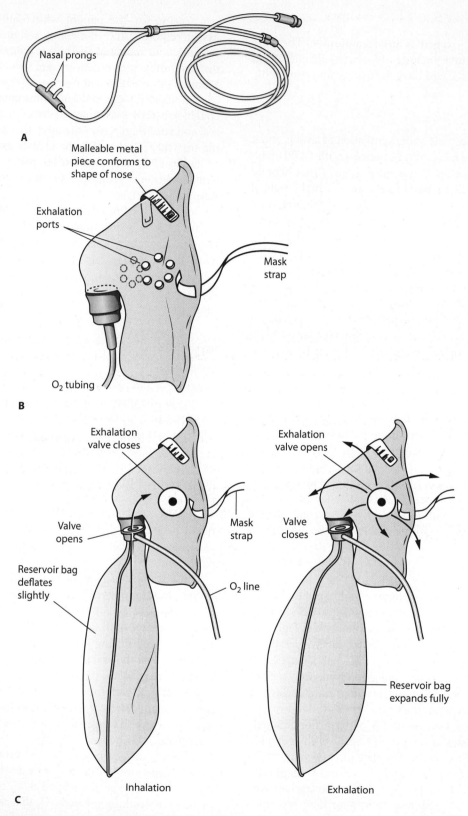

Figure 5-15. Noninvasive and invasive methods for O$_2$ delivery. **(A)** Nasal prongs. **(B)** Face mask. **(C)** Non-rebreathing mask. (*Reproduced with permission from Kersten L. Comprehensive Respiratory Nursing. Philadelphia, PA: WB Saunders; 1989.*)

TABLE 5-7. APPROXIMATE OXYGEN DELIVERY WITH COMMON NONINVASIVE AND INVASIVE OXYGEN DEVICES[a]

Device	% O$_2$
Nasal Prongs/Cannula	
• 2 L/min	28
• 4 L/min	36
• 5 L/min	40
High-Flow Nasal Cannula	
• 1-60 L/min	21-100[b]
Face Mask	
• 5 L/min	30
• 10 L/min	50
Non-rebreathing mask 10 L/min	60-80
Partial Rebreathing Mask 6-10 L/min	40-70
Venturi Mask	
• 24%	24
• 28%	28
• 35%	35
Manual Resuscitation Bag (MRB) or Bag-Mask-Valve	
• Disposable MRB	Dependent on model

[a]Actual delivery dependent on minute ventilation rates except for Venturi mask.
[b]Actual oxygen concentration dependent on oxygen blender setting.

rate of 10 L/min. A one-way valve placed between the mask and the reservoir bag with a non-rebreathing system prevents exhaled gases from entering the bag, thus maximizing the delivered Fio$_2$.

A variation of the non-rebreathing mask without the one-way valves is called a partial rebreathing mask. Oxygen is always supplied to maintain the reservoir bag at least one-third to one-half inflated on inspiration. At a flow of 6 to 10 L/min, the system can provide 40% to 70% oxygen. High-flow delivery devices such as aerosol masks or face tents, tracheostomy collars, and t-tube adapters can be used with supplemental oxygen systems. A continuous aerosol generator or large-volume reservoir humidifier can humidify the gas flow. Some aerosol generators cannot provide adequate flows at high oxygen concentrations.

Unlike conventional low-flow nasal cannulas and oxygen masks, which are constrained by flow, humidity, and accuracy of delivered inspired oxygen, high-flow nasal cannula (HFNC) oxygen devices are capable of delivering well-humidified, blended, and actively warmed oxygen (using vapor) across a wide range of oxygen concentrations. These devices (Figure 5-17) are useful in patients who require a higher flow of oxygen than can be delivered with traditional low-flow oxygen devices. HFNC can provide oxygen at very high flow rates, between 30 and 60 L/min and a moderate PEEP. Improved outcomes in patients placed on HFNC following a period of mechanical ventilation are due to a controlled oxygen concentration which may reduce transient hypoxemic episodes, and high flows which wash nasopharyngeal dead space, thus reducing CO$_2$ rebreathing, respiratory rate, and minute ventilation. Lastly, the small amount of PEEP generated with HFNC may help reduce lung collapse, enable improved gas exchange and reduce the WOB. Use of such high-flow oxygen delivery devices has dramatically increased during the COVID-19 pandemic as a result of the severe oxygenation challenges seen in some patients with hypoxemia and acute lung injury.

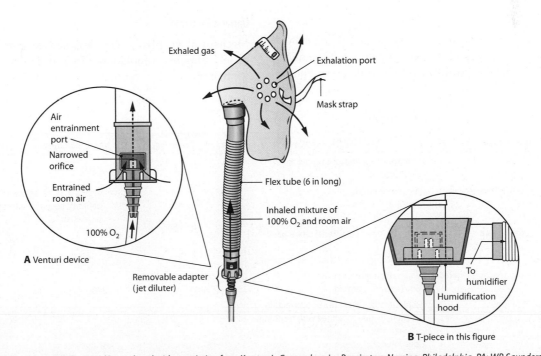

Figure 5-16. A. Venturi device **B.** T-piece. (*Reproduced with permission from Kersten L. Comprehensive Respiratory Nursing. Philadelphia, PA: WB Saunders; 1989.*)

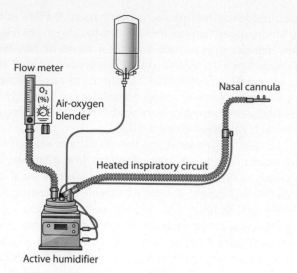

Figure 5-17. Diagram of high flow nasal cannula delivery system (*Reproduced with permission from Nishimura M. High-flow nasal cannula oxygen therapy in adults. J Intensive Care. 2015;3(1):15.*)

Invasive Devices

Manual Resuscitation Bags

MRBs (also called bag-valve mask) provide 40% to 100% O_2 at adult V_T and respiratory rates when attached to an ET or tracheostomy tube.

Mechanical Ventilators

The most common method for delivering oxygen invasively is with a mechanical ventilator. Oxygen can be accurately delivered from 21% to 100% O_2. Mechanical ventilation is discussed below in more detail.

T-Piece

Oxygen can also be provided directly to an ET or tracheostomy tube with a T-piece, or blow by, in spontaneously breathing patients who do not require ventilatory support.

The T-piece is connected directly to the ET tube or tracheostomy tube 15-mm adapter providing 21% to 80% O_2.

BASIC VENTILATORY MANAGEMENT

Indications

Mechanical ventilation is indicated when noninvasive management modalities fail to adequately support oxygenation and/or ventilation. The decision to initiate mechanical ventilation is based on the ability of the patient to support their oxygenation and/or ventilation needs. The inability of the patient to maintain clinically acceptable CO_2 levels and acid-base status or *hypercapnia* is recognized as one type of *respiratory failure* and is a common indicator for mechanical ventilation. *Refractory hypoxemia*, which is the inability to establish and maintain acceptable arterial oxygenation levels despite the administration of oxygen-enriched breathing environments, is another type of *respiratory failure* and also a common reason for mechanical ventilation. Table 5-8 presents a variety of physiologic indicators for initiating mechanical ventilation. By monitoring these indicators, it is possible to differentiate stable or improving values from continuing decompensation. The need for mechanical ventilation may then be anticipated to avoid emergent use of ventilatory support.

Depending on the underlying cause of the respiratory failure, different indicators may be assessed to determine the need for mechanical ventilation. Many of the causes of respiratory failure, however, are due to inadequate alveolar ventilation and/or hypoxemia, with abnormal ABG values and physical assessment as the primary indicators for ventilatory support.

General Principles

Mechanical ventilators are designed to partially or completely support ventilation. Two different categories of ventilators provide ventilatory support. Negative-pressure

TABLE 5-8. INDICATIONS FOR MECHANICAL VENTILATION

Basic Physiologic Impairment	Best Available Indicators	Approximate Normal Range	Values Indicating Need for Ventilatory Support
Apnea	Neuromuscular and/or cardiovascular collapse		
Acute ventilatory failure (hypercarbic respiratory failure)	$Paco_2 > 50$ mm Hg pH ≤ 7.25	35-45 7.35-7.45	Acute $Paco_2$ increase from normal or patient's baseline with decrease in pH (acidosis)
Impending ventilatory failure	Serial decrement of arterial blood gas values Symptoms of increased work of breathing		
Hypoxemia (acute oxygenation failure)	$Pao_2 < 50$ on room air Pao_2/Fio_2 ratio, mm Hg	80-100 mm Hg >300	<300
Respiratory muscle fatigue	Respiratory muscles are not contracting optimally due to fatigue with resulting hypercarbia Tidal volume, mL/kg Vital capacity, mL/kg Respiratory rate, breaths/min (adult)	5-7 65-75 10-20	<5 <10-12 <10 or >35

Data from Wiegand DL. AACN Procedure Manual for Critical Care. 7th ed. St. Louis, MO: Elsevier Saunders; 2016.

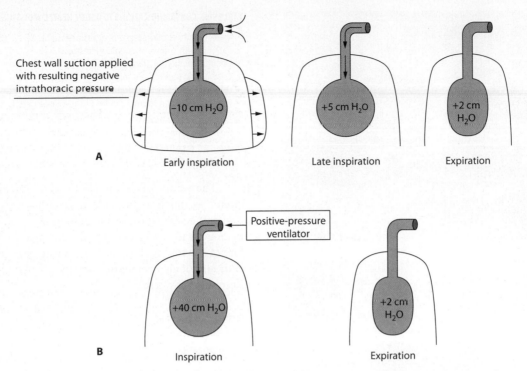

Figure 5-18. Principles of mechanical ventilation as provided by **(A)** negative-pressure and **(B)** positive-pressure ventilators.

ventilators (NPVs) decrease intrathoracic pressure by applying negative pressure to the chest wall, typically with a shell placed around the chest (Figure 5-18A). The decrease in intrathoracic pressure causes atmospheric gas to be drawn into the lungs. Positive-pressure ventilators deliver pressurized gases into the lung during inspiration (Figure 5-18B). Positive-pressure ventilators can dramatically increase intrathoracic pressures during inspiration, potentially decreasing venous return and CO.

NPVs are rarely used to manage acute respiratory problems in critical care and were first used during the polio pandemic. These devices are typically used for long-term noninvasive ventilatory support when respiratory muscle strength is inadequate to support unassisted, spontaneous breathing. Since the emergence of other noninvasive modes of positive-pressure (eg, bilevel positive airway pressure [BiPAP], BiLevel) ventilation and HFNC therapy, which are easier to apply and less cumbersome for patients, NPVs are infrequently selected (refer to Chapter 20, Advanced Respiratory Concepts: Modes of Ventilation). However, because of the rarity of this type of ventilator, and access to same, this chapter focuses only on the use of positive-pressure ventilators for ventilatory support.

Patient-Ventilator System

Positive-pressure ventilatory support can be accomplished invasively or noninvasively. Invasive mechanical ventilation is still widely used in most hospitals for supporting ventilation, although noninvasive technologies, which do not require the use of an artificial airway, are becoming more popular. To provide invasive positive-pressure ventilation, intubation of the trachea is required via an ET or tracheostomy tube. The ventilator is then connected to the artificial airway with a tubing circuit to maintain a closed delivery system (Figure 5-19). During the inspiratory cycle, gas from the ventilator is directed through a heated humidifier or a heat and moisture exchanger (HME) prior to entering the lungs through the ET tube or tracheostomy tube. Contraindications to HME use are listed in Table 5-9. At the completion of inspiration, gas is passively exhaled through the expiratory side of the tubing circuit.

Ventilator Tubing Circuit

The humidifier located on the inspiratory side of the circuit is necessary to overcome two primary problems. First, the presence of an artificial airway allows gas entering the lungs to bypass the normal upper airway humidification process. Second, the higher flows and larger volumes typically administered during mechanical ventilation require additional humidification to avoid excessive intrapulmonary membrane drying. The HME is generally placed between the breathing circuit and the Y-piece and some HME devices also serve as filters.

Pressure within the ventilator tubing circuit is continuously monitored to alert clinicians to excessively high or low airway pressures. Airway pressure is dynamically displayed on the front of the ventilator control panel.

Ventilator circuits with a heated humidifier contain wires that run through the inspiratory and expiratory limbs of the circuit. These wires maintain the temperature of the

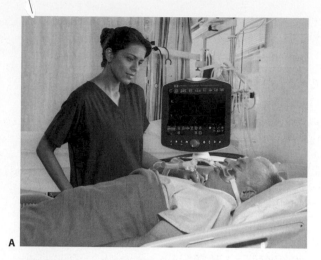

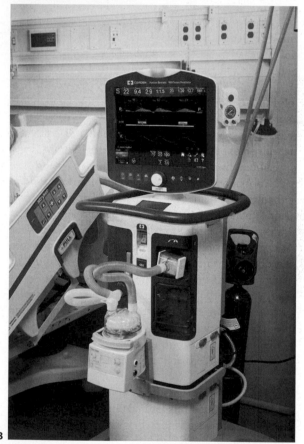

Figure 5-19. Typical setup of a ventilator with a closed system tubing circuit connected to an ET tube (**A**), and common ventilator components (**B**) including display panel, humidifier, and inspiratory gas filter. (*©2018 Medtronic. All rights reserved. Used with the permission of Medtronic.*)

TABLE 5-9. CONTRAINDICATIONS TO USE OF HEATED MOISTURE EXCHANGER (HME)

- Frank bloody or thick, copious secretions
- Patients with large bronchopleural fistulas
- Uncuffed or malfunctioning ET tube cuffs
- During lung protective strategies such as patients with ARDS
- Patients with body temperature < 32°C
- Patients with high spontaneous minute volume (>10 L/min)

Data from American Association for Respiratory Care: AARC clinical practice guideline: humidification during invasive and noninvasive mechanical ventilation: 2012. Resp Care. 2012;57:782-788.

The ventilator tubing circuit is maintained as a closed circuit as much as possible to avoid interrupting ventilation and oxygenation to the patient and potential spread of pathogens to caregivers as well as to decrease the potential for VAP. Avoiding frequent or routine changes of the ventilator circuit also decreases the risk of VAP (see Chapter 10, Respiratory System).

Ventilator Control Panel

The user interface or control panel of the ventilator usually incorporates three basic sections or areas:

1. Control settings for the type and amount of ventilation and oxygen delivery;
2. Alarm settings to specify desired high and low limits for key ventilatory measurements; and
3. Visual displays of monitored parameters (Figure 5-20).

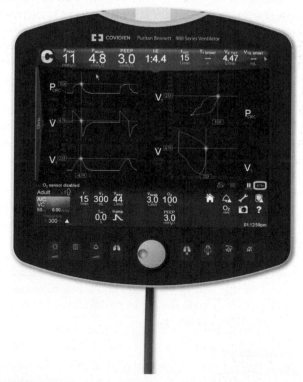

Figure 5-20. Ventilator visual display control panel for setting and adjusting ventilator parameters and alarms used in the assessment of patient-ventilator interaction and synchrony. (*©2018 Medtronic. All rights reserved. Used with the permission of Medtronic.*)

gas at or close to body temperature, significantly reducing the condensation and rainout of humidity in the gas and eliminating the need for in-line water traps. Certain medications, such as bronchodilators or steroids, can also be administered via a metered dose inhaler (MDI) or nebulized into the lungs through a low-volume aerosol-generating device located on the inspiratory side of the circuit.

TABLE 5-10. TRADITIONAL VENTILATOR ALARMS

Disconnect Alarms (Low-Pressure or Low-Volume Alarms)
- It is essential that when disconnection occurs, the clinician be immediately notified. Generally, this alarm is a continuous one and is triggered when a preselected inspiratory pressure level or minute ventilation is not sensed. With circuit leaks, this same alarm may be activated even though the patient may still be receiving a portion of the preset breath. Physical assessment, digital displays, and manometers are helpful in troubleshooting the cause of the alarms.

Pressure Alarms
- *High-pressure alarms* are set with volume modes of ventilation to ensure notification of pressures exceeding the selected threshold. These alarms are usually set 10-15 cm H_2O above the usual peak inspiratory pressure (PIP). Some causes for alarm activation (generally an intermittent alarm) include secretions, condensate in the tubing, biting on the endotracheal tubing, increased resistance (ie, bronchospasm), decreased compliance (eg, pulmonary edema, pneumothorax), and tubing compression.
- *Low-pressure alarms* are used to sense disconnection, circuit leaks, and changing compliance and resistance. They are generally set 5-10 cm H_2O below the usual PIP or 1-2 cm H_2O below the PEEP level or both.
- *Minute ventilation alarms* may be used to sense disconnection or changes in breathing patterns (rate and volume). Generally, low-minute ventilation and high-minute ventilation alarms are set (usually 5-10 L/min above and below usual minute ventilation). When stand-alone pressure support ventilation (PSV) is in use, this alarm may be the only audible alarm available on some ventilators.
- Fio_2 alarms: Most new ventilators provide Fio_2 above and below the selected Fio_2. Alarms are set 5% above and below the selected Fio_2.
- *Alarm silence or pause:* Because it is essential that alarms stay activated at all times, ventilator manufacturers have built-in silence or pause options so that clinicians can temporarily silence alarms for short periods (ie, 20 s). The ventilators "reset" the alarms automatically. Alarms provide important protection for ventilated patients. However, inappropriate threshold settings decrease usefulness. When threshold gradients are set too narrowly, alarms occur needlessly and frequently. Conversely, alarms that are set too loosely (wide gradients) do not allow for accurate and timely assessments.

Reproduced with permission from Kinney MR. AACN Clinical Reference for Critical Care Nursing. 4th ed. St Louis, MO: Mosby; 1998.

The number and configuration of these controls and displays vary from ventilator model to model, but their function and principles remain essentially the same.

Control Settings
The control settings area of the user interface allows the clinician to set the mode of ventilation, volume, pressure, respiratory rate, Fio_2, PEEP level, inspiratory trigger sensitivity or effort, and a variety of other breath delivery options (eg, inspiratory flow rate, inspiratory waveform pattern).

Alarm Settings
Alarms, which continuously monitor ventilator function, are essential to ensure safe and effective mechanical ventilation. Both high and low alarms are typically set to identify when critical parameters vary from the desired levels. Common alarms include low exhaled V_T, high or low exhaled minute volume, low Fio_2 delivery, high or low respiratory rate, and high or low airway pressures (Table 5-10).

Visual Displays
Airway pressures, respiratory rate, exhaled volumes, and the inspiratory to expiratory (I:E) ratio are among the most common visually displayed breath-to-breath values on the ventilator. Airway pressures are monitored during inspiration and exhalation and are often displayed as peak pressure, mean pressure, and end-expiratory pressure. A breath delivered by the ventilator produces higher airway pressures than an unassisted, spontaneous breath by the patient (Figure 5-21). The presence of PEEP is identified by a positive value at the end of expiration rather than 0 cm H_2O. Careful observation of the airway pressures provides the clinician with a great deal of information about the patient's respiratory effort, coordination with the ventilator, and changes in lung compliance.

The display of the patient's exhaled V_T reflects the amount of gas that is returned to the ventilator via the expiratory tubing with each respiratory cycle. Exhaled volumes are measured and displayed with each breath. The patient's total exhaled minute volume is also often displayed. Exhaled V_{TS} for ventilator-assisted mandatory breaths should be similar ($\pm 10\%$) to the desired V_T setting selected on the control panel. The V_T of spontaneous breaths, or partially ventilator-supported breaths, however, may be different from the V_T control setting.

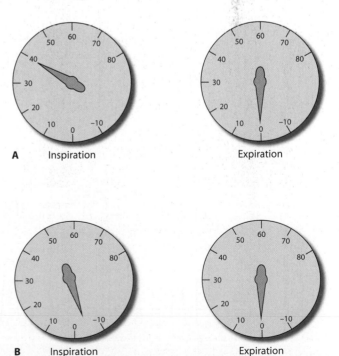

Figure 5-21. Typical airway pressure gauge changes during a **(A)** ventilator-assisted breath and a **(B)** spontaneous breath (cm H_2O).

Modes

The *mode* of ventilation refers to one of several different methods by which a ventilator supports ventilation. Modes are often classified as invasive (via an ET tube or tracheostomy tube) or noninvasive (via a face or nasal interface). These modes generate different levels of airway pressures, flow rates, volumes, and patterns of respiration and, therefore, different levels of support. The greater the level of ventilator support, the less muscle work is performed by the patient. This "work of breathing" varies considerably with each of the modes of ventilation (see Chapter 20, Advanced Respiratory Concepts: Modes of Ventilation).

The different modes of ventilation used to support ventilation depend on the underlying respiratory problem and clinical preferences. A brief description of the basic modes of mechanical ventilation follows. Applications of modes of ventilation and more complex modes are discussed in Chapter 20, Advanced Respiratory Concepts: Modes of Ventilation.

Control Ventilation

The control mode of ventilation ensures that patients receive a predetermined number and volume of breaths each minute. No deviations from the respiratory rate or V_T settings are delivered with this mode of ventilation. Generally, the patient is heavily sedated and possibly paralyzed with neuromuscular blocking agents to achieve the goal (see Chapter 6, Pain, Sedation, and Neuromuscular Blockade Management). The airway pressures, V_T delivery, and pattern of breathing typically observed with control ventilation are shown in Figure 5-22A. All the inspiratory waveforms appear in a regular pattern and appear the same in configuration. The lack of waveform deflections prior to inspiration indicates the breath was initiated by the ventilator and not by the patient.

Assist-Control Ventilation

In the assist-control or volume-controlled mode of ventilation (eg. A/C, VC, or AMV), the ventilator delivers a predetermined number and volume of breaths each minute, should the patient not initiate respirations at that rate or above. If the patient attempts to initiate breaths at a rate greater than the set minimum value, the ventilator delivers the spontaneously initiated breaths at a predetermined V_T. So in this mode, the patient may determine the total rate (Figure 5-22B). WOB with this mode is variable mainly due to the ventilator delivering a fixed inspiratory flow rate that may not meet the patient's demand. In these circumstances,

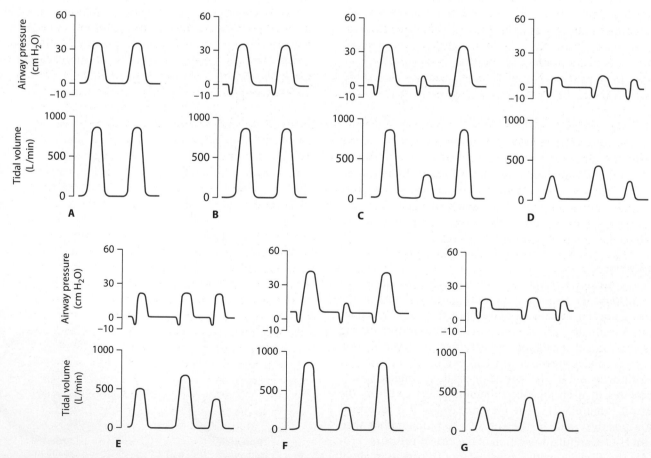

Figure 5-22. Airway pressures, tidal volumes (V_T), and patterns of breathing for different modes of mechanical ventilation. **(A)** Controlled ventilation. **(B)** Assist-control ventilation. **(C)** SIMV. **(D)** Spontaneous breathing. **(E)** Pressure support. **(F)** PEEP with SIMV. **(G)** Continuous positive airway pressure (CPAP). (*Reproduced with permission from Dossey B, Guzzetta C, Kenner C. Critical Care Nursing: Body-Mind-Spirit. Philadelphia, PA: JB Lippincott; 1992.*)

other modalities are now available which target a prescribed V_T but have the capability to generate a variable flowrate to better meet patient demand, thus reducing patient WOB (see Chapter 20, Advanced Respiratory Concepts: Modes of Ventilation).

Assist-control ventilation is often used when the patient is initially intubated (because minute ventilation requirements can be determined by both the patient and the ventilator), for short-term ventilatory support such as postanesthesia, and as a support mode when high levels of ventilatory support are required. Excessive ventilation can occur with this mode in situations where the patient's spontaneous respiratory rate increases for nonrespiratory reasons (eg, pain, CNS dysfunction). The increased minute volume may result in potentially dangerous respiratory alkalosis. Changing to a different mode of ventilation or addressing the underlying cause of the tachypnea may be necessary in these situations.

Synchronized Intermittent Mandatory Ventilation

The synchronized intermittent mandatory ventilation (SIMV) mode of ventilation ensures (or mandates) that a predetermined number of breaths at a selected V_T are delivered each minute. Any additional breaths initiated by the patient are allowed but, in contrast to the assist-control mode, the ventilator does not deliver these breaths. The patient is allowed to spontaneously breathe at the depth and rate desired until it is time for the next ventilator-assisted, or mandatory, breath. Mandatory breaths are synchronized with the patient's inspiratory effort, if present, to optimize patient-ventilator synchrony. The spontaneous breaths taken during SIMV are at the same Fio_2 as the mandatory breaths (Figure 5-22C).

Originally designated as a ventilator mode for the gradual weaning of patients from mechanical ventilation, the use of a high-rate setting of SIMV can provide total ventilatory support. Reduction of the number of mandatory breaths allows the patient to slowly resume greater responsibility for spontaneous breathing. SIMV can be used for similar indications as the assist-control mode, as well as for weaning the patient from mechanical ventilatory support.

The WOB with this mode of ventilation depends on the V_T and rate of the spontaneous breaths. When the mandatory, intermittent breaths provide the majority of minute volume, the WOB by the patient may be less than when spontaneous breathing constitutes a larger proportion of the patient's total minute volume.

Although strong clinician and institutional biases exist regarding whether to use SIMV or other modes for ventilatory support, little data exist to clarify which mode of ventilation is best. Close observation of the physiologic and psychological response to the ventilatory mode is required, and consideration is given to trials on alternative modes if warranted.

Spontaneous Breathing

Many ventilators have a mode that allows the patient to breathe spontaneously without ventilator support (Figure 5-22D).

This is similar to placing the patient on a T-piece or blow-by oxygen setup, except it does have the benefit of providing continuous monitoring of exhaled volumes, airway pressures, and other parameters along with maintaining a closed circuit. The patient performs all the WOB. Use of the ventilator rather than the T-piece during spontaneous breathing actually may slightly increase the WOB. This occurs because of the additional inspiratory muscle work that is required to trigger flow delivery for each spontaneous breath. The amount of additional work required varies with different ventilator models. In some situations, removing the patient from the ventilator for weaning may result in a decrease in the WOB.

This mode of ventilation is often identified as continuous positive airway pressure (CPAP), flow-by, or spontaneous (SPONT) on the ventilator. CPAP is a spontaneous breathing setting with the addition of PEEP during the breathing cycle (see the following text). If no PEEP has been applied, the CPAP setting is similar to spontaneous breathing.

Some ventilators have an additional adjunct that compensates for the resistance secondary to ET diameter. It is called automatic tube compensation (ATC). ATC can be used with ventilatory support or alone with spontaneous breathing.

Pressure Support

Pressure support (PS) is a spontaneous breath type, available in SIMV and SPONT modes, which maintains a set positive pressure during the spontaneous inspiration (Figure 5-22E). The volume of a gas delivered by the ventilator during each inspiration varies depending on the level of PS and the demand of the patient. The higher the PS level, the higher the amount of gas delivered with each breath. Higher levels of PS can augment the spontaneous V_T and decrease the WOB associated with spontaneous breathing. At low levels of support, PS is primarily used to overcome the airway resistance caused by breathing through the artificial airway and the breathing circuit. The airway pressure achieved during a PS breath is the result of the PS setting plus the set PEEP level.

Positive-End Expiratory Pressure/Continuous Positive Airway Pressure

PEEP is used in conjunction with any of the ventilator modes to help stabilize alveolar lung volume and improve oxygenation (Figure 5-22F, G). The application of positive pressure to the airways during expiration may keep alveoli open and prevent early closure during exhalation. Lung compliance and ventilation-perfusion matching are often improved by prevention of early alveolar closure. If alveolar "recruitment" is not needed and excessive PEEP/CPAP is applied, it may result in adverse hemodynamic or respiratory compromise.

PEEP/CPAP is indicated for hypoxemia, which is secondary to diffuse lung injury (eg, ARDS, interstitial pneumonitis). PEEP/CPAP levels of 5 cm Hg or less are often used to provide "physiologic PEEP." The presence of the artificial airway allows intrathoracic pressure to fall to zero, which is below the usual level of intrathoracic pressure at end expiration (2 or 3 cm H_2O).

Use of PEEP may increase the risk of barotrauma due to higher mean and peak airway pressures during ventilation, especially when peak pressures are greater than 40 cm H_2O. High intrathoracic pressures also decrease venous return and CO. If CO decreases with PEEP/CPAP initiation and oxygenation is improved, a fluid bolus to correct hypovolemia may be required to improve CO. Other complications from PEEP/CPAP are increases in intracranial pressure, decreased renal perfusion, hepatic congestion, and worsening of intracardiac shunts.

Bilevel Positive Airway Pressure

BiPAP is a noninvasive mode of ventilation that combines two levels of positive pressure (PSV and PEEP) by means of a full-face mask, nasal mask (most common), hood, or nasal pillows. BiPAP can be delivered through a traditional ventilator or a separate noninvasive machine. The ventilator mode is designed to compensate for leaks in the setup, and a snug fit is needed usually requiring a head or chin straps. This form of therapy can be very labor intensive, requiring frequent assessment of patient tolerance. Full face mask ventilation is cautiously used because the potential for aspiration is high. If full face mask ventilation is chosen, the patient should be able to remove the mask quickly if nausea occurs or vomiting is imminent. The patient must be able to protect their airway during the use of BiPAP. For this reason, BiPAP is not recommended for use in obtunded patients and those with excessive secretions.

A number of options are available with BiPAP and include a spontaneous mode where the patient initiates all the pressure-supported breaths; a spontaneous-timed option, similar to PSV with a backup rate (some vendors call this A/C); and a control mode. The control mode requires the selection of a control rate and inspiratory time. A newer BiPAP mode adjusts pressure-supported breaths to maintain a targeted V_T and is known as average volume assured pressure support (AVAPS).

BiPAP is used successfully in a wide variety of patients such as those with sleep apnea, some patients with chronic hypoventilation syndromes, and also to prevent intubation and reintubation following extubation. Use of BiPAP in patients with COPD and heart failure is associated with decreased mortality and need for intubation. These patients are often difficult to wean from conventional mechanical ventilation given their underlying disease processes. Study results also demonstrate that outcomes in immunocompromised patients may also be better with noninvasive ventilation.

Complications of Mechanical Ventilation

Significant complications can arise from the use of mechanical ventilation and can be categorized as those associated with the patient's response to mechanical ventilation or those arising from ventilator malfunctions. Although the approach to minimizing or treating the complications of mechanical ventilation relate to the underlying cause, it is critical that frequent assessment of the patient, ventilator equipment, and the patient's response to ventilatory management be accomplished. Many clinicians participate in activities to assess the patient and ventilator, but the ultimate responsibility for ensuring continuous ventilatory support of the patient falls to the critical care team, including the nurse and respiratory therapist. Newer team members include the use of Tele-ICU staff when integrated into the critical care environment. Critically evaluating clinical indicators such as pH, $Paco_2$, Pao_2, Spo_2, heart rate, BP, and so on, in conjunction with patient status and ventilatory parameters, is essential to decrease complications associated with this highly complex technology.

Patient Response

Hemodynamic Compromise

Normal intrathoracic pressure changes during spontaneous breathing are negative throughout the ventilatory cycle. Intrapleural pressure varies from about +5 cm H_2O during exhalation to −8 cm H_2O during inhalation. This decrease in intrapleural pressure during inhalation facilitates lung inflation and venous return. Thoracic pressure fluctuations during positive-pressure ventilation are opposite to those that occur during spontaneous breathing. The mean intrathoracic pressure is usually positive and increases during inhalation and decreases during exhalation. The use of positive pressure ventilation increases peak airway pressures during inspiration, which in turn, increases mean airway pressures. This increase in mean airway pressure can impede venous return to the right atrium, thus decreasing CO. In some patients, the decrease in CO can be clinically significant, leading to increased heart rate, decreased blood pressure, and impaired perfusion to vital organs.

Whenever mechanical ventilation is instituted, or when ventilator changes are made, it is important to assess the patient's cardiovascular response. Approaches to managing hemodynamic compromise include increasing the preload of the heart (eg, fluid administration), decreasing the airway pressures exerted during mechanical ventilation by ensuring appropriate airway management techniques (suctioning, positioning, etc.), and by judiciously applying setting ventilator parameters. Ventilation strategies employing different modes and breath types may be helpful in managing airway pressures and are discussed in Chapter 20, Advanced Respiratory Concepts: Modes of Ventilation.

Barotrauma and Volutrauma

Barotrauma describes damage to the pulmonary system due to alveolar rupture from excessive airway pressures or overdistention of alveoli. Alveolar gas enters the interstitial pulmonary structures causing pneumothorax, pneumomediastinum, pneumoperitoneum, or subcutaneous emphysema. Because pneumothorax can lead to cardiovascular collapse, prompt recognition and management is essential. Pneumothorax should be considered whenever airway pressure increases acutely, breath sounds are diminished unilaterally, or blood pressure falls abruptly.

Patients with obstructive airway diseases (eg, asthma, bronchospasm), unevenly distributed lung disease (eg, lobar pneumonia), or hyperinflated lungs (eg, emphysema) are at high risk for barotrauma. Techniques to decrease the incidence of barotrauma include the use of small VTs, cautious use of PEEP, the avoidance of high airway pressures, and development of auto-PEEP in high-risk patients.

Volutrauma describes alveolar damage that results from high pressures resulting from large-volume ventilation in patients with ARDS. A common technique to reduce this risk is the use of smaller VTs (4-6 mL/kg of ideal body weight) and sometimes this is described as the "low stretch" protocol or low V_T ventilation. Different from barotrauma, this damage results in alveolar fractures and flooding (see Chapter 20, Advanced Respiratory Concepts: Modes of Ventilation).

Auto-PEEP occurs when a delivered breath is incompletely exhaled before the onset of the next inspiration. This gas trapping increases overall lung volumes, inadvertently raising the end-expiratory pressure in the alveoli. The presence of auto-PEEP increases the risk for complications from PEEP. Ventilator patients with COPD (eg, asthma, emphysema) or high respiratory rates are at increased risk for the development of auto-PEEP.

Auto-PEEP, also termed *intrinsic PEEP*, is difficult to diagnose because it cannot be observed on the airway pressure display at end expiration. The technique for assessment for auto-PEEP varies with different ventilator models and modes, but typically involves measuring the airway pressure close to the artificial airway during occlusion of the expiratory ventilator circuit during end expiration. This method requires that the patient be completely passive and not trigger a breath; it is not possible to measure auto-PEEP by this method in actively breathing patients. Another technique of monitoring auto-PEEP in actively breathing patients is the use of the flow-time curve displayed by the ventilator. If flow does not return to baseline at the end of exhalation before the next breath starts, the patient has auto-PEEP. Auto-PEEP can be minimized by:

- Maximizing the length of time for expiration (eg, increasing inspiratory flow rates by shortening inspiratory times)
- Decreasing high minute volume by lowering tidal volume or respiratory rate
- Decreasing obstructions to expiratory flow (eg, using larger diameter ET or tracheosotomy tubes, eliminating bronchospasm and secretions)
- Avoiding overventilation

Ventilator-Associated Pneumonia

VAP is a hospital-acquired complication and is associated with increased patient morbidity and mortality. Prevention includes evidence-based practices to limit the use of invasive ventilation, promote patient safety while undergoing invasive ventilation, and effective protocols for ventilator liberation. Interventions during ventilation are aimed at avoiding colonization and subsequent aspiration of bacteria into the

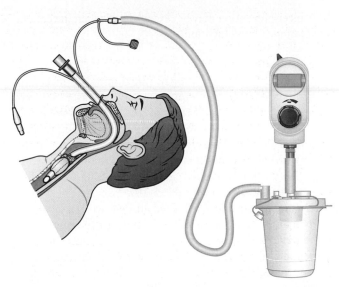

Figure 5-23. Cuffed endotracheal tube with dedicated lumen for continuous aspiration of subglottic secretions accumulated immediately above cuff. The dedicated lumen connector is attached to wall suction. (©2018 Medtronic. All rights reserved. Used with the permission of Medtronic.)

lower airway. Elevation of the head of the bed to 30° to 45° helps minimize aspiration of oral and gastric secretions. An ET tube with a subglottic suction port (Figure 5-23) incorporates a dedicated lumen above the ET cuff, which permits continuous low suction pressure (−20 mm Hg) or intermittent suctioning of subglottic secretions pooled above the cuff. Removal of the accumulated secretions may be particularly helpful before cuff deflation or manipulation. Studies have demonstrated that the application of continuous aspiration of subglottic secretions with ET tubes may prevent or delay the onset of VAP. Although subglottic suctioning is now available in some tracheostomy tubes, there are currently no recommendations for the use of subglottic suctioning in these tubes. In addition, oral care protocols including tooth brushing to remove plaque are important adjuncts to VAP prevention. See Chapter 10, Respiratory System for a complete discussion.

Positive Fluid Balance and Hyponatremia

Hyponatremia is a common occurrence following the institution of mechanical ventilation and develops from several factors, including applied PEEP, humidification of inspired gases, hypotonic fluid administration and diuretics, and increased levels of circulating antidiuretic hormone.

Upper Gastrointestinal Hemorrhage

Upper gastrointestinal (GI) bleeding may develop secondary to ulceration or gastritis. The prevention of stress ulcer bleeding requires ensuring hemodynamic stability and the administration of proton-pump inhibitors, H_2 receptor antagonists, antacids, or cytoprotective agents as appropriate in critically ill patients at high risk for GI bleeding (see Chapter 7, Pharmacology and Chapter 14, Gastrointestinal System for discussions of GI prophylaxis). Pharmacological therapy for stress ulcer prevention may be discontinued when the patient is tolerating enteral nutrition.

Ventilator Malfunction

Problems related to the proper functioning of mechanical ventilators, although rare, may have devastating consequences for patients. Many of the alarm systems on ventilators are designed to alert clinicians to improperly functioning ventilatory systems. These alarm systems must be activated at all times if ventilator malfunction problems are to be quickly identified and corrected, and untoward patient events avoided (see Table 5-10).

Many of the "problems" identified with ventilatory equipment are actually related to inappropriate setup or use of the devices. Examples of operator-related issues include ventilator circuits that are not properly connected, alarm systems that are set improperly, or inadequate ventilator settings for a particular clinical condition.

There are occasions, however, when ventilator systems do not operate properly. Examples of ventilator malfunctions include valve mechanisms sticking and obstructing gas flow, inadequate or excessive gas delivery, electronic circuit failures in microprocessing-based ventilators, failures with complete shutdown, and power failures or surges in the institution.

The most important approach to ventilator malfunction is to maintain a high level of vigilance to determine if ventilators are performing properly. Ensuring that alarm systems are set appropriately at all times, providing frequent routine assessment of ventilator functioning, and the use of experienced support personnel to maintain the ventilator systems are some of the most crucial activities necessary to avoid patient problems. In addition, whenever ventilator malfunction is suspected, the patient is immediately removed from the device and temporary ventilation and oxygenation provided with an MRB or another ventilator until the question of proper functioning is resolved. Any sudden change in the patient's respiratory or cardiovascular status alerts the clinician to consider potential ventilator malfunction as a cause.

Weaning from Short-Term Mechanical Ventilation

The process of transitioning the ventilator-dependent patient to unassisted spontaneous breathing is *weaning from mechanical ventilation*. This is a period of time where the level of ventilator support for oxygenation and ventilation is decreased, either gradually or abruptly, while monitoring the patient's response to the resumption of spontaneous breathing. A standardized approach along with weaning readiness criteria has been shown to reduce ventilator days and improve outcomes. Weaning, or "liberation," is considered to be complete, or successful, when the patient is extubated and does not require reintubation within 48 hours. The majority of patients intubated and ventilated for short periods of time (<72 hours) are successfully weaned with the first spontaneous breathing trial (SBT) or *Simple weaning*. Additionally, there is a subset of patients with long-term tracheostomy tubes, who may require short-term

mechanical ventilation, and are able to wean quickly once the clinical issue requiring mechanical ventilation is resolved. *Difficult weaning* may require multiple SBTs or up to 7 days to successfully achieve ventilator liberation with some patients requiring longer than 7 days or *Prolonged weaning*. Approximately 30% of patients require extended time periods for successful weaning, and some remain unable to breathe without partial or complete support from mechanical ventilation.

Weaning proceeds when the underlying cause of respiratory failure is addressed, and the patient is breathing spontaneously, maintaining adequate gas exchange, and protecting their own airway. Unnecessary delays in weaning from mechanical ventilation increase the likelihood of complications such as ventilator-induced lung injury, pneumonia, discomfort, and increases in hospitalization costs. Thus, the use of protocolized weaning including SBTs is encouraged both in ICU and PCU settings for *Simple weaning, Prolonged weaning,* and *Partial weaning.*

Steps in the Weaning Process

Assessment of Readiness

Readiness to wean from short-term mechanical ventilation may be assessed with a wide variety of criteria. However, in most institutions, for short-term ventilator patients, assessment of readiness to wean includes just three or four criteria. Along with assessing the patient's clinical stability, some examples are:

- ABGs within normal limits on minimal to moderate amounts of ventilatory support ($Fio_2 \leq 0.50$, minute ventilation ≤ 10 L/min, PEEP ≤ 5 cm H_2O, Pao_2/Fio_2 ratio > 200)
- NIF that is more negative than −20 cm H_2O
- Spontaneous V_T more than or equal to 4-6 mL/kg ideal body weight
- Vital capacity more than or equal to 10-15 mL/kg ideal body weight
- Respiratory rate less than 30 breaths/min
- Spontaneous rapid-shallow breathing index (RSBI) less than 105 breaths/min/L

An effective measure of weaning readiness should be incorporated into a bundled approach that includes both a daily safety screen and a collaborative weaning protocol. The "ABCDEF" bundle incorporates spontaneous awakening trials and SBTs (Figure 5-24), and other evidence-based practices for ICU management (Table 5-11). Bundles are a structured method of improving patient care processes and when collectively performed between nursing, providers and respiratory therapy have resulted in improved patient outcomes. Interventions such as minimizing sedation, assessing for delirium, promoting early mobility, and involving the family contribute to prompt ventilator liberation. Protocols that incorporate these important elements of care decrease practice variation and improve patient outcomes.

Following selection of the method for weaning (see the discussion later), the actual weaning trial can begin. It

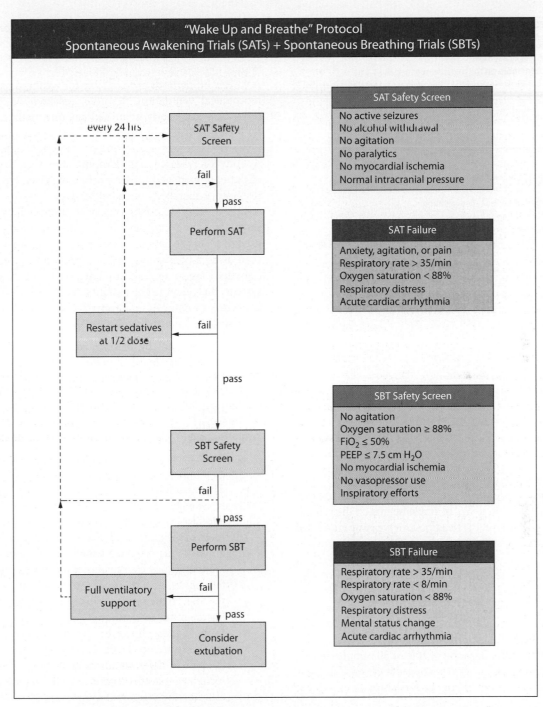

"Wake Up and Breathe" Protocol
Spontaneous Awakening Trials (SATs) + Spontaneous Breathing Trials (SBTs)

every 24 hrs

SAT Safety Screen

fail

pass

Perform SAT

Restart sedatives at 1/2 dose — fail

pass

SBT Safety Screen

fail

pass

Perform SBT

Full ventilatory support ← fail

pass

Consider extubation

SAT Safety Screen
No active seizures
No alcohol withdrawal
No agitation
No paralytics
No myocardial ischemia
Normal intracranial pressure

SAT Failure
Anxiety, agitation, or pain
Respiratory rate > 35/min
Oxygen saturation < 88%
Respiratory distress
Acute cardiac arrhythmia

SBT Safety Screen
No agitation
Oxygen saturation ≥ 88%
$FiO_2 \leq 50\%$
PEEP ≤ 7.5 cm H_2O
No myocardial ischemia
No vasopressor use
Inspiratory efforts

SBT Failure
Respiratory rate > 35/min
Respiratory rate < 8/min
Oxygen saturation < 88%
Respiratory distress
Mental status change
Acute cardiac arrhythmia

Figure 5-24. Spontaneous awakening trial—SAT (©2008 Vanderbilt University. All righs reserved.)

is important to prepare both the patient and the critical care environment properly to maximize the chances for weaning success (Table 5-12).

During an SBT, interventions include appropriate explanations of the process to the patient, positioning and medication to improve ventilatory efforts, and the avoidance of unnecessary activities. Continuous monitoring for signs and symptoms of respiratory distress or fatigue is essential. Many of these indicators are subtle, but careful monitoring of baseline levels before weaning progresses and throughout the trial provides objective indicators of the need to return the patient to previous levels of ventilator support.

The need to temporarily stop the weaning trial is not viewed as, or termed, a *failure*. Instead, it simply suggests that more time needs to be provided to ensure success. A full evaluation of the multiple reasons for inability to wean is necessary, however.

TABLE 5-11. ABCDEF BUNDLE AND COMPONENTS

Requires a coordinated effort between the healthcare team

A—Assess, Prevent, and Manage Pain
- See Chapter 6 for more on the management of pain

B—Both Spontaneous Awakening Trials (SAT) and Spontaneous Breathing Trials (SBT)
1. Spontaneous Awakening Trial
   - Daily assessment of SAT safety screen to turn off continuous sedation
   - Daily SAT (sedation interruption or light targeted level of sedation)
2. Spontaneous Breathing Trial
   - Daily assessment of SBT safety screen
   - Daily SBT

C—Choice of Analgesia and Sedation
Assessment of pain and sedation using validated tools (See Chapter 6 for more on management of pain and sedation
   - Sedation: Richmond Agitation Sedation Scale (RASS) or Sedation Agitation Scale (SAS)
   - Pain: Numeric Rating Scale (NRS), Behavioral Pain Scale (BPS), or Critical Care Pain Observation Tool (CPOT)

D—Delirium: Assess, Prevent, and Manage
Routine assessment of delirium using a validated tool
   - Confusion Assessment Method for the ICU (CAM-ICU)
   - Intensive Care Delirium Screening Checklist (ICDSC)

E—Early Mobility and Exercise
Daily assessment of mobility readiness and activity
   - Early Mobility Protocol
   - Mobility program

F—Family Engagement and Empowerment
Patient and family-centered care

Data from Society of Critical Care Medicine. ICU Liberation: ABCDEF Bundles. https://www.sccm.org/Clinical-Resources/ICULiberation-Home/ABCDEF-Bundles.

Weaning Trials

SBTs for patients undergoing STMV are usually done on T-piece or on the ventilator using CPAP or a low level of PS. Guidelines recommend that the initial SBT be implemented on the ventilator with CPAP or low level PS. Readiness for weaning is assessed daily using a "safety screen" which includes such factors as hemodynamic stability, oxygenation status, and improvement in the condition that necessitated the use of mechanical ventilation. Weaning protocols also include a daily trial of minimal to no continuous intravenous sedation, sometimes called a spontaneous awakening trial (SAT), which is done prior to or concurrently with the SBT. Once the patient is assessed as "ready," the SBT is initiated for a duration of at least 30 minutes but no more than 120 minutes. The trial is stopped if the patient shows signs of distress and/or deterioration. A decision to extubate if

TABLE 5-12. STRATEGIES TO FACILITATE WEANING

- Explain the weaning process to the patient/family and maintain open communication throughout weaning.
- Position to maximize ventilatory effort (sitting upright in bed or chair).
- Administer analgesics to relieve pain and sedatives to control anxiety, if appropriate.
- Remain with the patient during the weaning trial and/or provide a highly vigilant presence.
- Frequently assess the patient's response to the weaning trial.
- Avoid unnecessary physical exertion, painful procedures, and/or transports during the weaning trials.
- Maximize the physical environment to be conducive to weaning (eg, temperature, noise, distractions).

intubated or return to the ventilator or increase ventilator support is made with the conclusion of the trial.

Methods

A variety of methods are available for weaning patients from mechanical ventilation. To date, research on these techniques has not clearly identified any one method as optimal for weaning from short-term mechanical ventilation. Most institutions, however, use one or two approaches routinely. A body of research has demonstrated that the outcomes of patients managed under protocols driven by nurses and respiratory therapists were better than those managed with standard care. Most experts on weaning believe that, with short-term ventilator-dependent patients, the actual method used to wean the patient is less important to weaning success than using a consistently applied protocol strategy. In addition, there are some ventilators that have automated weaning systems that adapt to the patient's needs. Additional research is needed to determine automated ventilator weaning efficacy over clinician-driven protocols.

- *T-piece, blow by, or trach collar:* The T-piece method of weaning involves removing the patient from the mechanical ventilator and attaching an oxygen source to the artificial airway with a "T" piece for an SBT. A trach collar also provides oxygen but attaches by an elastic strap around the neck instead of directly to the artificial airway. No ventilatory support occurs with this device, with the patient completely breathing spontaneously the entire time this device is connected. The advantage of this method of weaning is that the resistance to breathing is low, because no special valves need to be opened to initiate gas flow. Rapid assessment of the patient's ability to spontaneously breathe is another purported advantage. Limitations of this SBT are that it may cause ventilatory muscle overload and fatigue. When this occurs, it usually appears early in the SBT, so the patient must be closely monitored during the initial few minutes. A PEEP valve can be added to the T-piece; however, similar to trach collar weaning, there are no alarms or backup systems to support the patient if ventilation is inadequate. It is critical to recognize that this technique relies on the clinician to monitor for signs and symptoms of respiratory difficulty and fatigue. Frequently, the Fio_2 is increased by at least 10% over the Fio_2 setting on the ventilator to prevent hypoxemia resulting from the lower V_T of spontaneous breaths. Patients who are unable to tolerate an SBT receive a stable, nonfatiguing, comfortable form of ventilatory support following the trial.

- *CPAP:* The use of the ventilator to allow spontaneous breathing periods without mandated breaths, similar to the T-piece, can be done with the CPAP mode. With this approach, ventilator alarm systems can be used to monitor spontaneous breathing rates and volumes, and a small amount of continuous pressure (5 cm H_2O) can be applied if needed. The disadvantage of this approach is that the WOB resulting from the need to open the demand valve to receive gas flow for the breath is higher than with the T-piece. For most patients, this slight additional WOB is not a critical factor to their weaning success or failure unless the trial is unduly long. To offset this workload, it is recommended that a low level of inspiratory PS (eg, 5-8 cm H_2O) be added during the SBT. In some ventilators, an additional feature, ATC can offset the additional workload imposed by the ventilator circuit and the ET.

- *Pressure support:* Another method for weaning from ventilation is the use of low-level PS ventilation. With this method, patients can spontaneously breathe on the ventilator with a small amount of ventilator *support* to augment their spontaneous breaths. This technique overcomes some of the resistance to breathing associated with ET tubes and demand valves. The lowest PS level that provides a respiratory rate of less than 20 breaths/min, no accessory muscle use, and a V_T of 6 to 10 mL/kg ideal body weight should be used. The main disadvantage with this approach is that clinicians may underestimate the degree of support that is provided and prematurely stop the weaning process.
- *SIMV:* One of the most popular methods of weaning patients in the past, this modality has been shown to prolong the duration of mechanical ventilation in comparison to weaning with daily SBTs or PS. By progressively decreasing the number of mandated breaths delivered by the ventilator, the patient performs more and more of the WOB by increasing spontaneous breathing. Advantages to the SIMV mode are the presence of built-in alarms to alert clinicians when ventilation problems occur and, in some modes, the guarantee of a minimum minute ventilation. The disadvantage of SIMV is that each spontaneous breath requires some additional WOB to open a valve, which allows gas flow to the patient for the spontaneous breath. SIMV is used either alone or in conjunction with PS (SIMV + PS).

Weaning From Prolonged Mechanical Ventilation

In contrast to patients who require short-term ventilation, those who require prolonged mechanical ventilation (PMV) may take days, weeks, or even months to liberate from the ventilator. This typically takes place outside of the ICU. In these PMV patients, the weaning process varies and consists of four stages. The first stage is marked by instability, high ventilatory support requirements, and either an inability to meet weaning criteria or failed SBTs. During the second stage, called the prewean stage, many physiologic factors continue to require optimization, and the patient's overall status may fluctuate. Ventilatory requirements are less and adjustments are made to maintain oxygenation and acid-base status as well as provide ventilatory muscle conditioning. The third, or weaning stage, is evident when the patient is stable, and rapid progress with weaning trials is possible. Finally, the last stage is called the outcome stage, which consists of successful extubation or provision of partial or full ventilatory support.

PMV is associated with high morbidity and mortality rates. Many patients are deconditioned due to prolonged illness and immobility and require a tracheostomy for long-term airway management. Strategies for these patients often include placement in long-term acute care settings (LTACs) or skilled nursing facilities (SNFs) for supportive care including rehabilitation. Research in PMV has suggested that the use of a standardized protocol is also important in this population. The following discussions of weaning patients from PMV address weaning readiness assessment, wean planning, and weaning modes and methods, including comprehensive institutional approaches.

Wean Assessment

Traditionally, the decision about when to begin the weaning process is determined once the condition that necessitates mechanical ventilation is improved or resolved. In the past, "traditional" weaning predictors were used to determine the optimal timing for extubation. More recently, investigators combined pulmonary assessments to improve predictive ability in PMV patients. One example is the rapid shallow breathing index (RSBI) (Table 5-13) which integrates rate and V_T. Unfortunately, these measures have not accurately predicted success in weaning. This is in part because they focus exclusively on pulmonary specific components to the exclusion of other important non-pulmonary factors that influence a patient's ability to breath spontaneously. Although standard weaning criteria are not predictive, the components are helpful for assessing the patient's overall condition and readiness for weaning.

As noted, assessment of weaning potential starts with an evaluation of the underlying reason for mechanical ventilation (sepsis, pneumonia, trauma, etc.). Resolution of the underlying cause is necessary before gains in the weaning process can be expected. However, it is important to remember that resolution alone is frequently not sufficient to ensure successful

TABLE 5-13. WEAN CLINICAL CRITERIA

SBT safety screen
• No agitation
• $Spo_2 \geq 88\%$
• Fraction of inspired oxygen (Fio_2) $\leq 50\%$
• PEEP ≤ 8 mm Hg
• No acute myocardial ischemia
• No vasopressor use
• Spontaneous inspiratory efforts
Traditional Weaning Criteria
• Spontaneous tidal volume (V_T) 4-6 mL/kg ideal body weight
• Vital capacity (VC) ≥ 10-15 mL/kg ideal body weight
• Minute volume (MV) ≤ 10 L/min (MV = Vt × RR)
• Negative inspiratory force (NIF) ≤ -20 cm H_2O
• Pao_2/Fio_2 ratio > 200 mm Hg
Integrated Weaning Criteria
• Rapid shallow breathing index (RSBI): frequency/tidal volume ratio (fx/V_T) ≤ 105 breaths/min/L

weaning. Patients who require PMV, sometimes referred to as the "chronically, critically ill," often suffer from a myriad of conditions that impede weaning. Even with resolution of the acute disease or condition that necessitated mechanical ventilation, the patient's overall status is often below baseline (frail, dehabilitated, malnourished, etc.). Therefore, a systematic, comprehensive approach to weaning is important.

Wean Planning

Once impediments to weaning are identified, plans that focus on improving the impediments are made in collaboration with an interdisciplinary team. A collaborative approach to assessment and planning greatly enhances positive outcomes in the PMV patient. However, for care planning to be successful, it must also be systematic. The wean process is dynamic and regular reassessment and adjustment of plans are necessary. Clinical pathways, protocols for weaning, and institution-wide approaches to managing and monitoring the patients are also effective strategies that ensure consistency in care and promote better outcomes.

Weaning Trials, Modes, and Methods

A wide variety of weaning modes and methods are available for weaning the patient ventilated short term as described earlier. To date, no data support the superiority of any one mode for weaning those requiring PMV; however, methods using protocols and other systematic, interdisciplinary approaches do appear to make a difference and are to be encouraged. These methods are described following a discussion of respiratory muscle fatigue, rest, and conditioning because these concepts are integrated into the section on protocols.

Respiratory Fatigue, Rest, and Conditioning

Respiratory muscle fatigue is common in ventilated weaning patients and occurs when the respiratory workload is excessive. When the workload exceeds metabolic stores, fatigue and hypercarbic respiratory failure ensue. Examples of those at risk include patients who are hypermetabolic, weak, or malnourished. Signs of encroaching fatigue include dyspnea,

---

ESSENTIAL CONTENT CASE

Long-Term Weaning

A 75-year-old man with COPD and oxygen dependence was admitted to the ED in respiratory distress. He was intubated and placed on the ventilator secondary to profound hypercarbia and acidosis and then transferred to the MICU for management of respiratory failure and right upper lobe pneumonia. On day 2, he meets criteria for his spontaneous awakening trial but does not meet criteria for an SBT. Weaning assessment parameters included:

NIF:	-10 cm H_2O
Fio_2:	0.55
RR:	37 breath/min
Spo_2:	92%

His sedation is at a minimal level with a sedation score of calm and comfortable, his delirium screen is negative, pain score is 0, and on day 3 he is lifted to the chair with a sling after failing his mobility egress test. Prolonged weaning is anticipated, and the patient and family agree to a tracheostomy tube. He receives a tracheostomy tube on day 5 and is transferred on day 6 to the respiratory progressive care unit for further management and weaning. Additional major impediments to weaning as assessed by the unit team include:

- Poor nutritional status (albumin 1.8 g/dL)
- Anxiety and agitation
- Debilitation and inability to ambulate
- Persistent upper lobe infiltrate
- Copious secretions
- NIF < 15 cm H_2O
- Minute ventilation: 15 L/min with a $Paco_2$ of 50 mm Hg
- RR 32 to 36 breaths/minutes

Case Question 1. What weaning modality could be used in this patient for long-term weaning and why?

Case Question 2. What components of the ABCDEF protocol were used for this patient?

Answers

1. As the research has not demonstrated any mode or method to be superior for a patient weaning with a tracheostomy, progressively longer SBTs may be used effectively. The modes can vary and include T-piece, trach collar, or low levels of PSV with intermittent rest periods on the ventilator (with support settings such as AC or a higher level of PSV). When the patient is able to sustain spontaneous breathing for a full 12 hours during the day, the nighttime ventilator support (at the "rest" level) may then be reduced, or if clinically appropriate, curtailed. The next steps would be to work on removal of the tracheostomy tube following downsizing and/or use of a talking trach to determine tolerance. This stepwise approach allows the patient to gradually transition to liberation from the ventilator.

2. The patient received daily spontaneous awakening and assessment for readiness to wean along with pain and sedation assessments (ABC). His delirium was addressed by using a modified sleep protocol and by using the family (F) to reorient the patient as well as encouraging the use of personal items when possible (D). Early exercise was implemented in the ICU and continued after transfer and integrated into his daily routine I. Family was an integral part of the plan of care and participated in his recovery on the unit (F).

tachypnea, chest-abdominal asynchrony, and elevated $Paco_2$ (a late sign). These signs and symptoms indicate a need for increased ventilatory support. Once fatigued, the muscles require 12 to 24 hours of rest to recover, which is accomplished through the selection of the appropriate mode of ventilation.

For the respiratory muscles to recover from fatigue, the inspiratory workload must be decreased. In the case of volume ventilation (eg, assist-control, intermittent mandatory ventilation), this means complete cessation of spontaneous effort, but in the case of pressure ventilation, a high level of PSV may accomplish the necessary "unloading." Generally, this means increasing the PSV level to attain a spontaneous respiratory rate of 20 breaths/min or less and the absence of accessory muscle use. However, in patients with obstructive diseases (eg, asthma and COPD), this higher level of support may result in further hyperinflation and adverse clinical outcomes. If the technique is used in these patients, it should be done cautiously.

Respiratory muscle conditioning employs concepts borrowed from exercise physiology. To condition muscles and attain an optimal training effect from exercise, the concepts of endurance and strength conditioning may be considered. With strength training, a large force is moved a short distance. The muscles are worked to fatigue (short duration intervals) and rested for long periods of time. SBTs on T-piece or CPAP both mimic this type of training because they employ high pressure and low-volume work.

Endurance conditioning, which requires that the workload be increased gradually, is easily accomplished with PSV because the level of support can be decreased over time. This kind of endurance training employs low pressure and high-volume work. Central to the application of both conditioning methods is the provision of adequate respiratory muscle rest between trials. Prolonging trials once the patient is fatigued serves no useful purpose and may be extremely detrimental physiologically and psychologically.

Wean Trial Protocols

Study results suggest that no mode of ventilation is superior for weaning, however, research does show that the process of weaning, specifically the use of protocols, decreases variations in care and improves outcomes. Protocols clearly delineate the actions caregivers take to promote successful weaning. The protocol components consist of weaning readiness criteria (wean screens), weaning trial method and duration (eg, CPAP, T-piece, or PSV), and parameters for assessing intolerance and providing respiratory muscle rest.

SBTs (described earlier), using CPAP or T-piece, are commonly used for weaning trials. The duration of such trials is generally between 30 minutes and 2 hours, although in those patients with tracheotomy tubes, the duration may be much longer. While CPAP or T-piece are most often used for weaning trials, other protocols may include the use of PSV (an endurance mode) and CPAP (a strengthening mode) and

providers may individualize to meet specific patient requirements. One example is that of patients with heart failure. In these patients, the sudden transition from ventilator support to the use of T-piece or CPAP for an SBT may result in an increased venous return that overwhelms the heart's ability to compensate. Until appropriate preload and after-load reduction is addressed in these patients, PSV may be a gentler method of weaning. Another example is that of patients with profound myopathies or extremely debilitated states that may benefit from more gradual increases in work such as those provided by PSV. Some new pressure modes, such as Proportional Assist Ventilation and Adaptive Support Ventilation, may potentially decrease the patient's workload during weaning. For more on this, see Chapter 20: Advanced Respiratory Concepts: Modes of Ventilation.

A popular and common-sense approach to wean trial progression is to attempt weaning trials during the daytime, allowing the patient to rest with increased ventilator support at night until the protocol threshold for extubation is reached. In the case of the patient with a tracheostomy, progressively longer episodes of spontaneous breathing, usually on tracheostomy collar or T-piece, are accomplished until tolerated for a specified amount of time. Then, decisions about discontinuation of ventilation and tracheostomy downsizing or decannulation may be made. Clearly communicating the wean plan to all members of the healthcare team, and especially the patient and family ensures team acceptance and consistent implementation. The aim is that the plan be sufficiently aggressive but safe and effective in meeting patient goals.

Other Protocols for Use

Patients who require PMV often face a variety of clinical conditions that not only prolong ventilator duration but also affect other outcomes, such as length of stay and mortality. Research has demonstrated that outcomes of critically ill patients are improved with protocol-directed management. The "ABCDEF" bundle, for instance, is effective evidence-based practice for patients who receive short-term mechanical ventilation. The principles of the bundle may also be useful in the PMV patient. More research is needed on protocol-directed management in the subset of patients who require PMV. See Table 5-14 for general guidelines on weaning patients on PMV.

Critical Pathways

Critical pathways are used to ensure that evidence-based care is provided and that variation in care delivery is reduced. Some pathways can be very directive such as those for patients undergoing hip replacements, where clinical progression can be anticipated by hours or days. However, such specificity is not possible in the ventilated patient. Instead, pathways for the PMV patient combine elements of care by specific time intervals (ie, begin deep vein thrombosis

TABLE 5-14. GENERAL WEANING GUIDELINES FOR PROLONGED MECHANICALLY VENTILATED PATIENTS

Active Weaning Should Occur

- When patient is stable and reason for mechanical ventilation is resolved or improving.
- When the "wean screen protocol criteria" are attained. A temporary hold and even an increase in support may be necessary when setbacks occur.
- During the daytime, not at night (to allow respiratory muscle rest).
- Include family in the patient wean plan.

Considerations for Temporary Hold

- With acute changes in condition.
- During procedures that require that the patient be flat or in the Trendelenburg position (ie, during line insertion).
- During or following "road trips" (consider increased ventilatory support to protect the patient while off the unit).
- If secretions are excessive requiring frequent suctioning (every half hour).
- Coordination of rehabilitation and mobility with weaning efforts will be patient dependent.

Rest and Sleep

- Rest is important for psychological and physiologic reasons. Complete rest in the mechanically ventilated patient is defined as that level of ventilatory support that offsets the work of breathing and decreases fatigue (refer to detailed description in text).
- A reasonable approach for the chronic or nonacute patient is to work on active weaning trials during the day until most of the daytime wean is accomplished (≥10 h). At night, the patient is allowed to sleep to help reduce delirium and ventilator support should be high enough to allow for relaxation and optimal resting. If pharmacological sleeping aids are used at night, administer them early in the night to enhance sleep and ventilatory synchronization so that the drugs can be metabolized before the daytime trials begin.

prophylaxis by day one) with those that are designated by the stage of illness (ie, patient up to the chair during the prewean stage). In addition to providing an evidence-based blueprint for a wide variety of care elements, the pathways encourage interdisciplinary input and collaboration. Ideally, they are incorporated into systematic institutional approaches to care of the PMV patient population.

Systematic Institutional Initiatives for the Management of the PMV Patient Population

Given the importance of systematic assessment and care planning, it is not surprising that many institutions have taken a comprehensive approach to the care of patient who requires PMV.

The healthcare environment is often chaotic and even more so since the start of the COVID-19 pandemic. Difficulty with accessing placement to LTACs or SNFs, and staffing shortages including increased use of agency personnel affect the continuity of care and contribute to gaps in practice and care planning. Given the complexity of the care of the PMV patient, a protocolized approach to care that decreases variation and promotes coordination may improve patient outcomes and are to be encouraged.

Troubleshooting Ventilators

The complexity of ventilators and the dynamic state of the patient's clinical condition, as well as the patient's response to ventilation, create a variety of common problems that may occur during mechanical ventilation. It is crucial that critical care clinicians be experts in the prevention, identification, and management of ventilator-associated problems in critically ill patients.

During mechanical ventilation, sudden changes in the clinical condition of the patient, particularly respiratory distress, and the occurrence of ventilator alarms or abnormal functioning of the ventilator, require immediate assessment and intervention. A systematic approach to each of these situations minimizes untoward ventilator events (Figure 5-25).

The first step is to determine the presence of respiratory distress or hemodynamic instability. If either is present, the patient is removed from the mechanical ventilator and manually ventilated with an MRB and 100% O_2 for a few minutes.

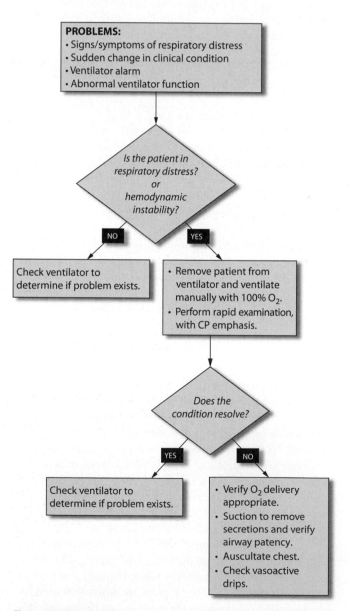

Figure 5-25. Algorithm for management of ventilator alarms and/or development of acute respiratory distress.

During manual ventilation, a quick assessment of the respiratory and cardiovascular systems is made, noting changes from previous status. Clinical improvement rapidly following removal from the ventilator suggests a ventilator problem. Manual ventilation is continued while another clinician corrects the ventilator problem (eg, tubing leaks or disconnections, inaccurate gas delivery) or replaces the ventilator. Continuation of respiratory distress after removal from the ventilator and during manual ventilation suggests a patient-related cause.

Nutrition

Patients with ET tubes are unable to eat orally and nutritional needs are usually met with feeding tubes (see Chapter 14, Gastrointestinal System). Recent studies have noted the importance of screening for postextubation dysphagia (PED) prior to oral feeding following extubation (Table 5-15). Studies have shown that up to 62% of patients intubated for greater than 48 hours can experience difficulty swallowing following extubation. "Swallow studies" such as fiberoptic evaluation of swallowing (FEES) or videofluoroscopic swallow studies (VFSS) are commonly done in these patients after failed PED screening and after consultation with speech language pathologist (SLP) and should also be considered in patients with a tracheostomy tube in place. Some chronic ventilator patients on stable ventilator settings may be able to tolerate an oral diet after evaluation by an SLP.

Communication

Mechanically ventilated patients are unable to speak and communicate verbally due to the presence of a cuffed ET or tracheostomy tube. The inability to speak is frustrating for the patient, nurse, and members of the healthcare team. Impaired communication results in patients experiencing anxiety and fear, symptoms that can have a deleterious effect on their physical and emotional conditions. Patients interviewed after extubation reveal how isolated and alone they felt because of their inability to speak.

Common Communication Problems

Patients' perceptions of communication difficulties related to mechanical ventilation include: (1) inability to communicate, (2) insufficient explanations, (3) inadequate understanding, (4) fears related to potential dangers associated with the inability to speak, and (5) difficulty with communication methods. Except for the problem of inability to vocalize, all of the problems cited by ventilated patients may be resolved by critical care nurses. For instance, "insufficient explanations" and "inadequate understanding" can be remedied by frequent repetition of all plans and procedures in language that is understandable to a nonmedical person and that takes into account that attention span and cognitive abilities, especially memory, are frequently diminished due to the underlying illness or injury, effects of medications and anesthesia, and the impact of the critical care environment.

TABLE 5-15. POSTEXTUBATION DYSPHAGIA SCREENING TOOL

Section A: Evaluation	
Patient has been evaluated by speech-language pathologist (SLP)	☐ Yes ☐ No If **Yes**, **stop** here and follow SLP recommendations.
Section B: Level of alertness	
Patient is awake and alert and able to follow commands	☐ Yes ☐ No If **No**, make patient NPO. Obtain order for SLP consult. If **Yes**, go to **Section C**
Level C: Respiratory status	
☐ Patient is able to remain off CPAP or BiPAP for more than 15 minutes ☐ Maintains SpO$_2$ without support of nonrebreather or Ventimask for more than 15 minutes ☐ RR is less than 30 breaths/minute	If **No** to any statement, stop here and reassess in 24 hours. If **Yes** to all statements, go to **Section D**
Level D: Symptoms and tubes	
☐ Patient has a feeding tube ☐ History of dysphagia ☐ Adverse changes in lung sounds ☐ Wet or gurgling vocal quality ☐ History of head/neck trauma ☐ No voice, nonverbal ☐ Poor voice volume ☐ Complaints of swallowing problems ☐ Cannot produce voluntary cough or clear throat ☐ Unexplained history of weight loss or dehydration ☐ History of head/neck cancer or surgery ☐ History of stroke, Parkinson disease, multiple sclerosis, or COPD	If **Yes** to any statement, **stop** here. Make patient NPO until SLP consult. If **No**, go to **Section E**
Section E: Verification to proceed for trial feedings	
Verify patient has diet orders and proceed to oral intake trial	

Adapted with permission from Johnson KL, Speirs L, Mitchell A, et al: Validation of a Postextubation Dysphagia Screening Tool for Patients After Prolonged Endotracheal Intubation. Am J Crit Care. 2018;27(2):89-96.

Although most messages the ventilated patient needs to communicate lie within a narrow range ("pain," "hunger," "water," and "sleep"), communicating these basic needs is often difficult. Most adults are accustomed to attending to their own basic needs, but in the critical care unit, not only are they unable to physically perform certain activities, they also may not be able to communicate their needs effectively. Basic needs include such activities as elimination, bathing, brushing teeth, combing hair, eating, drinking, and sleeping. Other examples include simple requests or statements such as "too hot," "too cold," "turn me," "up," "down," "straighten my legs," "my arm hurts," "I can't breathe," and "moisten my lips."

Patients have described difficulties with communication methods while being mechanically ventilated. This also can be avoided by assessing the patient's communication abilities. Is the patient alert and oriented? Can the patient answer or nod simple yes and no questions? Does the patient speak English? Can the patient use at least one hand to gesture? Does the patient have sufficient strength and dexterity to hold a pen and write, use a computer tablet, or point to a picture board? Are the patient's hearing and vision adequate? Knowledge of the patient's communication abilities assists the clinician to identify appropriate communication methods.

Once the most successful communication methods have been identified for a particular patient, they are written into the plan of care. Continuity among healthcare professionals in their approach to communication with nonvocal patients improves the quality of care and increases patient satisfaction.

Methods to Enhance Communication

A variety of methods for augmenting communication are available and can be classified into two categories: nonvocal treatments (gestures, lip reading, mouthing words, paper and pen, alphabet/numeric boards, flashcards, computers, tablets, etc.) and vocal treatments (talking tracheostomy tubes, speaking valves for tracheostomy tubes, and leak speech). The best way for the patient to communicate, who has an artificial airway or who is being mechanically ventilated, is still unknown so should be individualized to patient assessment and needs.

Nonvocal Treatments

Individual patient needs vary and it is recommended that the nurse use a variety of nonvocal treatments (eg, gestures, alphabet board, and paper and pen). Success with communication interventions varies with the diagnosis, age, type of injury or disease, type of respiratory assist devices, and psychosocial factors. For instance, lip reading can be successful in patients who have tracheostomies because the lips and mouth are visible, but in a patient with an ET tube, where tape and tube holders limit lip movement and visibility, lip reading may be less successful.

WRITING

Typically the easiest, most common method of communication readily available is the paper and pen. However, the supine position is not especially conducive to writing legibly.

In addition, the absence of proper eyeglasses, an injured or immobilized dominant writing hand, or lack of strength can make writing difficult for mechanically ventilated patients. Some patients prefer to use a pressure sensitive, inexpensive toy writing screen that is easy to use and easy to erase, allowing for privacy. Their low cost is an advantage, if isolation precludes re-use. Although costly, computer keyboards or touch screens may facilitate writing, especially in patients who are comfortable with "high-tech" solutions.

GESTURING

Another nonvocal method of communication that can be very effective is the deliberate use of gestures. Gestures are best suited for the short-term ventilated patient who is alert and can move at least one hand, even if only minimally. Generally, well-understood gestures are emblematic, have a low level of symbolism, and are easily interpreted by most people.

ALPHABET BOARD/PICTURE BOARD

For patients who face a language barrier, a picture board is sometimes useful along with well-understood gestures. Picture boards have images of common patient needs (eg, bedpan, glass of water, medications, family, doctor, nurse) that the patient can point to. Picture boards, although commercially available, can be made easily and laminated to more uniquely meet the needs of a specific critical care population.

Another approach is the use of flash cards that can be purchased or made. Language flash cards contain common words or phrases in the patient's preferred language.

Vocalization Techniques

If patients with tracheostomy tubes in place have intact organs of speech, they may benefit from vocal treatment strategies like pneumatic and electrical devices, fenestrated tracheostomy tubes, talking tracheostomy tubes, leak speech, and tracheostomy speaking valves. Several conditions preclude use of vocalization devices, such as neurologic conditions that impair vocalization (eg, Guillain-Barré syndrome), severe upper airway obstruction (eg, head/neck trauma), or vocal cord adduction (eg, presence of an ET tube).

A number of vocal treatments for patients with tracheostomies exist. Generally, they require that the cuff be completely deflated to allow for air to be breathed in and out through the mouth and nose as well as around the sides of the tracheostomy. On exhalation, the gases pass through the vocal cords allowing for speech. One method is known as leak speech which requires adjustment of the ventilator as the cuff is deflated to accommodate for tidal volume loss during mechanical ventilation. Some use one-way speaking valves (eg, Passy-Muir valve, shown in Figure 5-26) to allow for air to be inhaled through the valve but to close during exhalation to direct air up past the vocal cords. A fenestrated tracheostomy tube (Figure 5-27) also allows passage of air through the vocal cords. A cap, speaking valve, or intermittent digital occlusion may be used in conjunction with the fenestrated tube to ensure that all exhaled air moves through the vocal cords for vocalization. There are

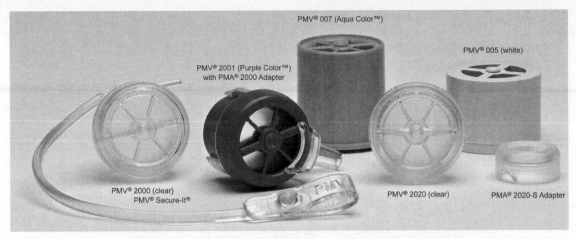

Figure 5-26. Examples of speaking valves for vocalization. (*Reproduced with permission from Passy-Muir, Inc., Irvine, CA.*)

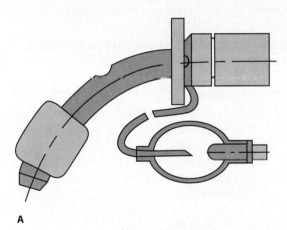

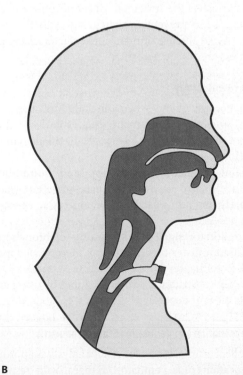

Figure 5-27. (A) Fenestrated tracheostomy tube. **(B)** Opening above the cuff site allowing gas, flow past the vocal cords during inspiration and expiration. (*©2018 Medtronic. All rights reserved. Used with the permission of Medtronic.*)

reports of granuloma tissue developing adjacent to the fenestration, which resolve after the removal of the tube. In addition, fenestrated ports often become clogged with secretions, again preventing the production of sound. It is imperative that if the tracheostomy tube is capped, the cuff of the tracheostomy be completely deflated.

Another vocal treatment is the talking tracheostomy tube, which is designed to provide a means of verbal communication for the ventilator-dependent patient. Patients who seemed unable to wean may take a renewed interest in the weaning process and successfully wean upon hearing their own voice. Currently there are two talking tracheostomy tubes available, which maintain a closed system with cuff inflation but differ in how they function.

1. *The Portex tracheostomy* operates by gas flowing (4-6 L/min) through an airflow line, which has a fenestration just above the tracheostomy tube cuff (Figure 5-28). The air flows through the glottis, thus supporting vocalization if the patient can form words with their mouth. However, an outside air source must be provided, which is usually not

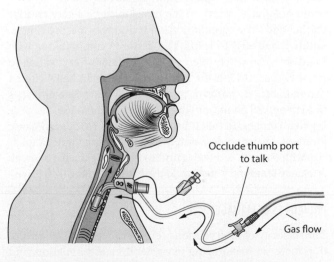

Figure 5-28. Tracheostomy tube with side port to facilitate speech (*Reproduced with permission from Smith Medical, Keen, NH.*)

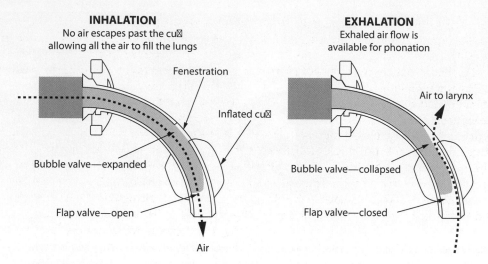

INHALATION
No air escapes past the cuff
allowing all the air to fill the lungs

Fenestration

Inflated cuff

Bubble valve—expanded

Flap valve—open

Air

EXHALATION
Exhaled air flow is
available for phonation

Air to larynx

Bubble valve—collapsed

Flap valve—closed

Figure 5-29. Tracheostomy tube with inner cannula for speaking (Blom tracheostomy tube system). (*Reproduced with permission from Pulmodyne, Indianapolis, IN.*)

humidified, and the trachea can become dry and irritated. The line for this air source requires diligent cleaning and flushing of the air port to prevent it from becoming clogged. The patient or staff must be able to manually divert air through the tube via a thumb port control.

2. *The Blom tracheostomy tube system* (Figure 5-29) uses a two-valve system in a specialized speech inner cannula that redirects air and does not require use of an air source. During inhalation the flap valve opens and the bubble valve seals the fenestration, preventing air leak to the upper airway. On exhalation, the flap valve closes, and the bubble valve collapses to unblock the fenestration to allow air to the vocal cords. An additional component is the exhaled volume reservoir, which is attached to the circuit and return volume to minimize false, low expiratory minute volume alarms.

Teaching Communication Methods

The critical care environment presents many teaching and learning challenges. Patients and families are under a considerable amount of stress, so the nurse must be a very creative teacher and offer communication techniques that are simple, effective, and easy to learn. The desire to communicate with loved ones, however, often makes the family very willing to learn. Frequently, it is the family who makes up large-lettered communication boards or purchases a writing slate or brings in a laptop, cell phone, or tablet for the patient to use. Suggesting that families do this is usually very well received, because loved ones want so desperately to help in some way. Emphasize with patients and their families that being unable to speak is usually temporary, just while the breathing tube is in place.

PRINCIPLES OF MANAGEMENT

The majority of interventions related to mechanical ventilation focus on maximizing oxygenation and ventilation, and preventing complications associated with artificial airways.

Maximizing Oxygenation, Ventilation, and Patient-Ventilator Synchrony

- Provide frequent explanations about the purpose of the ventilator.
- Monitor the patient's response to ventilator therapy and for signs that the patient is dyssynchronous with the ventilator respiratory pattern. The use of graphic displays, common on many ventilator systems, is often a helpful aid to patient assessment.
- Consider ventilator setting changes to maximize synchrony (eg, changes in flow rates, respiratory rates, sensitivities, and/or modes).
- Administer the minimal dose of sedative agents required to prevent dyssynchrony with the ventilator. Avoid the use of neuromuscular blocking agents unless absolutely necessary.

Maintain a Patent Airway

- Suction the airway when clinically indicated according to patient assessment (see Table 5-5). Routine suctioning that is not a response to the patient's condition is not recommended.
- Maintain adequate hydration and humidification of all inhaled gases to decrease secretion viscosity. Rarely, the administration of mucolytic agents may be necessary.
- Monitor for signs and symptoms of bronchospasm and administer bronchodilator therapy as appropriate (see Chapter 9, Cardiovascular System).
- Prevent obstruction of oral ET tubes by using an oral bite block if necessary.

Monitor Oxygenation and Ventilation Status Frequently

- Collect arterial blood for ABG analysis as appropriate (eg, after some ventilator changes, with respiratory distress or cardiovascular instability, or with significant changes in clinical condition).

- Use a noninvasive SpO_2 monitor continuously. Validate noninvasive measures with periodic ABG analysis (see Table 5-4).
- Observe for signs and symptoms of decreases in PaO_2, increases in $PaCO_2$, and respiratory distress. Development of respiratory distress requires immediate intervention (see Figure 5-25).
- Reposition the patient frequently to improve ventilation-perfusion relationships and prevent atelectasis.
- Aggressively manage pain, particularly chest and upper abdominal pain, to increase mobility, deep breathing, and coughing (see Chapter 6, Pain, Sedation, and Neuromuscular Blockade Management).

Physiotherapy and Monitoring

- Administer chest physiotherapy for selected clinical conditions (eg, large mucus production, lobar atelectasis).
- Closely monitor oxygenation status during chest physiotherapy for signs and symptoms of hypoxemia.

Maintain Oxygenation and Ventilatory Support at All Times

- Assess ventilator settings, alarm activation, and device function every 1 to 2 hours to ensure proper operation.
- During even brief periods of removal from mechanical ventilation, maintain ventilation and oxygenation with MRB. During intrahospital transport, verify adequacy of ventilatory support equipment, particularly the maintenance of PEEP (when >10 cm H_2O is required) and ensure adequate portable oxygen supply tank pressure. When possible, a portable mechanical ventilator should be used instead of an MRB.
- Keep emergency sources of portable oxygen readily available in the event of loss of wall oxygen capabilities.

Weaning From Mechanical Ventilation

- Systematically assess wean potential and address factors impeding weaning.
- Use a weaning protocol with a "wean screen." Ensure that the patient, family, and key caregivers are aware of weaning trials.
- Stop weaning trial if signs of intolerance or respiratory distress emerge.
- Promote the consistent use of an evidence-based intraprofessional approach to weaning.

Preventing Complications

- Maintain ET tube or tracheostomy cuff pressures less than 25 mm Hg (30 cm H_2O).
- Maintain artificial airway position by securing with a properly fitting holder device or selected tapes. Frequently verify proper ET position by noting ET marking at lip or nares placed after intubation.

- Ensure tape or devices used to secure the artificial airway are properly applied and are not causing pressure injury. Periodic repositioning of ET tubes may be required to prevent skin integrity problems.
- Use a bite block with oral ET tubes if necessary to prevent accidental biting of the tube.
- Provide frequent mouth care and assess for development of pressure areas from ET tubes. Move the ET from one side of the mouth to the other daily or more frequently depending on the device used.
- Assess for signs and symptoms of sinusitis with nasal ET tube use (eg, pain in sinus area with pressure, purulent drainage from nares, fever, increased white blood cell count).

Maximizing Communication

- Assess communication abilities and establish an approach for nonverbal communication. Assist family members in using that approach with the patient.
- Anticipate patient needs and concerns in the planning of care.
- Ensure that call lights, bells, or other methods for notifying unit personnel of patient needs are in place at all times.

Reducing Anxiety and Providing Psychosocial Support

- Maintain a calm, supportive environment to avoid unnecessary escalation of anxiety. Provide brief explanations of activities and procedures. The vigilance and presence of healthcare providers during periods of anxiety are crucial to avoid panic by patients and visiting family members.
- Teach the patient relaxation techniques to control anxiety.
- If needed, administer doses of anxiolytics that do not depress respiration (see Chapter 6, Pain, Sedation, and Neuromuscular Blockade; and Chapter 9, Cardiovascular System).
- Encourage the family to stay with the patient as much as desired and to participate in caregiver activities as appropriate. Presence of a family member provides comfort to the patient and assists the family member to better cope with the critical illness.
- Promote sleep at night by decreasing light, noise, and unnecessary interruptions.

SELECTED BIBLIOGRAPHY

General Critical Care

AACN. Pulmonary Management Pocket Reference. 2019.
AACN. Practice pointers: guideline update: bundle up for pain, agitation and delirium. *Crit Care Nurs*. 2021;41(3):80.

Alexander E, Allen J. Update on the prevention and treatment of intensive care delirium. *AACN Adv Crit Care*. 2021;32(1):5-10.

Balas MC, Devlin JW, Verceles AC, Morris P, Ely EW. Adapting the ABCDEF bundle to meet the needs of patients requiring prolonged mechanical ventilation in the long-term acute care hospital setting: historical perspectives and practical implications. *Semin Respir Crit Care Med*. 2016;37:119-135.

Balas MC, Pun BT, Pasero C, et al. Common challenges to effective ABCDEF bundle implementation: the ICU liberation campaign experience. *Crit Care Nurs*. 2019;39(1):46-60.

Bardwell J, Brimmer S, Davis W. Implementing the ABCDE bundle, Critical-Care Pain Observation Tool, and Richmond Agitation-Sedation Scale to reduce ventilator time. *AACN Adv Crit Care*. 2020;31(1):16-21.

Chesley CF, Lane-Fall MB, Panchanadam V, Harhay MO, Wani AA, Mikkelsen ME, Fuchs BD. Racial disparities in occult hypoxemia and clinically based mitigation strategies to apply in advance of technological advancements. *Respir Care*. 2022;10.4187/respcare.09769

Dexter AM, Scott JB. Airway management and ventilator-associated events. *Resp Care*. 2019;64(8):986-993.

El-Rabbany M, Zaghol N, Bhandari M, Azarpazhooh A. Prophylactic oral health procedures to prevent hospital-acquired and ventilator-associated pneumonia: a systemic review. *Int J Nurs Stud*. 2015;52:452-464.

Faust AC, Echevarria KL, Attridge RL, Shepherd L, Restrepo MI. Prophylactic acid-suppression therapy in hospitalized adults: indications, benefits, and infectious complications. *Crit Care Nurse*. 2017;37:18-29.

Fernandez R, Subira C, Frutos-Vivar F, et al. High-flow nasal cannula to prevent postextubation respiratory failure in high-risk non-hypercapnic patients: a randomized multicenter trial. *Ann Intensive Care*. 2017;7:47-52.

Gallagher JJ: Capnography monitoring during procedural sedation and analgesia. *AACN Adv Crit Care*. 2018;29(4):405–414.

Gershonovitch R, Yarom N, Findler M. Preventing ventilator-associated pneumonia in intensive care unit by improving oral care: a review of randomized control trials. *SN Comp Clin Med*. 2020;2:727-733.

Gonzalez S. Permissive hypoxmia versus normoxemia for critically ill patients receiving mechanical ventilation. *Crit Care Nurse*. 2015;35:80-81.

Good VS, Kirkwood PL, eds. *Advanced Critical Care Nursing*. 2nd ed. St. Louis, MO: Elsevier; 2018.

Grimm J. Sleep deprivation in the intensive care patient. *Crit Care Nurs*. 2020;40(2):e16-e24.

Hernandez G, Vaquero C, Colinas L. Effect of postextubation high-flow nasal cannula vs noninvasive ventilation on reintubation and postextubation respiratory failure in high-risk patients: a randomized clinical trial. *JAMA*. 2016;316:1565-1574.

Huang HB, Jiang W, Wang CY, et al. Stress ulcer prophylaxis in intensive care unit patients receiving enteral nutrition: a systematic review and meta-analysis. *Crit Care*. 2018;22:20.

Johnson KL, Speirs L, Mitchell A, et al. Validation of a postextubation dysphagia screening tool for patients after prolonged endotracheal intubation. *Am J Crit Care*. 2018;27(2):89-96.

Jongerden IP, Rovers MM, Grypdonck MH, Bonten MJ. Open and closed endotracheal suction systems in mechanically ventilated intensive care patients: a meta-analysis. *Crit Care Med*. 2007;35:260-270.

Kazmarek, RM, Stoller JK, Heur AJ. *Egan's Fundamentals of Respiratory Care*. 11th ed. St. Louis, MO: Mosby; 2016.

Klompas M, Anderson D, Trick W, et al. The preventability of ventilator-associated events. The CDC prevention epicenters wake-up and breathe collaborative. *Am J Resp Crit Care Med*. 2015;191:292-301.

Klompas M, Branson R, Eichenwald EC, et al. Strategies to prevent ventilator-associated pneumonia in acute care hospitals: 2014 update. *Inf Cont Hosp Epidemiol*. 2014;35:915-936.

Malinoski DJ, Todd SR, Slone S, Mullins RJ, Schreiber MA. Correlation of central venous and arterial blood gas measurements in mechanically ventilated trauma patients. *Arch Surg*. 2005;140:1122-1125.

Marra A, Kotfis K, Hosie A, et al. Delirium monitoring: yes or no? that is the question. *Am J Crit Care*. 2019;28(2):127-135.

Morris LL, Whitmer A, McIntosh E. Tracheostomy care and complications in the intensive care unit. *Crit Care Nurse*. 2013;33:18-30.

Munro N, Ruggiero M. Ventilator-associated pneumonia bundle. *AACN Adv Crit Care*. 2014;25:163-175.

Nassar BS, Schmidt GA. Estimating arterial partial pressure of carbon dioxide in ventilated patients: how valid are surrogate measures? *Ann Am Thorac Soc*. 2017;14:1005-1014.

Panchal AR, Bartos JA, Cabañas JG, et al. Part 3: adult basic and advanced life support; 2020 American Heart Association guidelines for cardiopulmonary resuscitation and emergency cardiovascular care. *Circulation*. 2020;142(suppl 2):S366-S468.

Rackley CR. Monitoring During Mechanical Ventilation. *Respir Care*. 2020;65(6):832-846.

Raoof S, Baumann MH. Ventilator-associated events: the new definition. *Am J Crit Care*. 2014;23:7-9.

Rose L, Burry L, Mallick R, et al. Prevalence, risk factors, and outcomes associated with physical restraint use in mechanically ventilated adults. *J Crit Care*. 2016;31:31-35.

Schallom L, Sona C, McSweeney M, et al. Comparison of forehead and digit oximetry in surgical/trauma patients at risk for decreased peripheral perfusion. *Heart Lung*. 2007;36:188-194.

Schmidt GA. Monitoring gas exchange. *Respir Care*. 2020 Jun;65(6):729-738.

Seckel MA. Ask the experts: does the use of a closed suction system help to prevent ventilator-associated pneumonia? *Crit Care Nurs*. 2008;28(1):65-66.

Seckel MA, Schulenburg K. Ask the experts: eating while receiving mechanical ventilation. *Crit Care Nurse*. 2011;31:95-97.

Seckel MA. Ask the experts: normal saline and mucous plugging. *Crit Care Nurse*. 2012;32:66-68.

Siobal MS. Monitoring exhaled carbon dioxide. *Respir Care*. 2016;61:1397-1416.

Smith SG. Ask the experts: best method for securing an endotracheal tube. *Crit Care Nurse*. 2016;36:78-80.

St John RE, Malen JF. Airway management. *Crit Care Nurs Clin N Am*. 2004;16:413-430.

Stolling JL, Barnes-Daly MA, Devlin JW, et al. Implementing the ABCDEF bundle: top 8 questions asked during the ICU liberation ABCDEF bundle improvement collaborative. *Crit Care Nurs*. 2019;39(10:36-45.

Stolling JL, Devlin JQ, Lin JC, Pun BT, Byrum D, Barr J. Best practices for conducting interprofessional team rounds to facilitate performance of the ICU liberation (ABCEDF) bundle. *Crit Care Med*. 2020;48(4):562-570.

Toftegaard M, Rees SE, Andreassen S. Correlation between acid–base parameters measured in arterial blood and venous blood sampled peripherally, from vena cavae superior, and from the pulmonary artery. *Eur J Emerg Med*. 2008;15:86-91.

Valdez-Lowe C, Ghareeb SA, Artinian NT. Pulse oximetry in adults. *AJN*. 2009;109(6):52-59.

Wang C, Tsai J, Chen S, et al. Normal saline instillation before suctioning: a meta-analysis of randomized controlled trials. *J Australian Crit Care*. 2016. http://dx.doi.org/10.1016/j.aucc.2016.11.001.

Zhao T, Wu X, Zhang Q, Li C, Worthington HV, Hua F. Oral hygiene care for critically ill patients to prevent ventilator-associated pneumonia. *Cochrane Database Syst Rev*. 2020;Issue 12. Art. No.: CD008367. doi: 10.1002/14651858.CD008367.pub4. Accessed July 09, 2021.

COVID-19

Alhazzani V., Evans L, Alshamsi F, et al. Surviving Sepsis Campaign guidelines on the management of adults with coronavirus disease 2019 (COVID-19) in the ICU: first update. *Crit Care Med*. January 28, 2021, Volume online first. doi: 10.1097/CCM.0000000000004899

COVID-19 Treatment Guidelines Panel. Coronavirus disease 2019 (COVID-19) treatment guidelines. National Institutes of Health. Available at https://www.covid19treatmentguidelines.nih.gov/. Accessed July 23, 2021.

Pandian V, Morris LL, Brodsky, et al. Critical care guidance for tracheostomy care during the COVID-19 pandemic: a global, multidisciplinary approach. *Am J Crit Care*. 2020;29(6):e116-e127.

Ventilator Management

Burns SM. Pressure modes of mechanical ventilation: the good, the bad, and the ugly. *AACN Adv Crit Care*. 2008;19:399-411.

Cvach MM, Stokes JE, Manzoor SH, et al. Ventilator alarms in intensive care units: frequency, duration, priority, and relationship to ventilator parameters. *Anesth Analg*. 2020;130:e9-e13.

Hess D, Kacmarek KM. *Essentials of Mechanical Ventilation*. 4th ed. New York, NY: McGraw-Hill Medical Publishing Division; 2019.

Kallett RH. Ventilator bundles in transition: from prevention of ventilator-associated pneumonia to prevention of ventilator-associated events. *Respir Care*. 2019;64(8):994-1006.

Restrepo RD, Walsh BK. Humidification during invasive and noninvasive mechanical ventilation: 2012. *Resp Care*. 2012;57:782-788.

Talbert S, Detrick CW, Emery K, et al. Intubation setting, aspiration, and ventilator-associated conditions. *Am J Crit Care*. 2020;29:371-378.

Vargas M, Chiumello D, Sutherasan Y, et al. Heat and moisture exchangers (HMEs) and heated humidifiers (HHs) in adult critically ill patients: a systematic review, meta-analysis and meta-regression of randomized controlled trials. *Crit Care*. 2017;221:123. doi: 10.1186/s13054-017-1710-5

Weaning From Mechanical Ventilation

Bell L. Safe weaning from mechanical ventilation. *Am J Crit Care*. 2015;24:130.

Burns SM, Fisher C, Tribble SS, et al. Multifactor clinical score and outcome of mechanical ventilation weaning trials: Burns Wean Assessment Program. *Am J Crit Care*. 2010;19(5):431-9. doi: 10.4037/ajcc2010273

Burns SM, Fisher C, Tribble SS, et al. The relationship of 26 clinical factors to weaning outcome. *Am J Crit Care*. 2012;21:52-58.

Girard TD, Kress JP, Fuchs BD, et al. Efficacy and safety of a paired sedation and ventilator weaning protocol for mechanically ventilated patients in intensive care (awakening and breathing controlled trial): a randomised controlled trial. *Lancet*. 2008;371:126-134.

Greenberg JA, Balk RA, Shah RC. Score for predicting ventilator weaning duration in patients with tracheostomies. *Am J Crit Care*. 2018;27(6):477-485.

Gupta P, Geihler K, Walters RW, Meyerink K, Modrykamien AM. The effect of mechanical ventilation discontinuation protocol in patients with simple and difficult weaning: impact on clinical outcomes. *Resp Care*. 2014;59:170-177.

Haas CF, Loik PS. Ventilator discontinuation protocols. *Resp Care*. 2012;57:1649-1662.

Jung B, Vaschetto R, Jaber S. Ten tips to optimize weaning and extubation success in the critically ill. *Intensive Care Med*. 2020;46:2461-2463.

MacIntyre NR. Evidence-based assessments in the ventilator discontinuation process. *Resp Care*. 2012;57:1611-1618.

Olff C, Clark-Wadkins C. Tele-ICU partners enhanced evidence-based practice: ventilator weaning initiative. *AACN Adv Crit Care*. 2012;23:312-322.

Rose L, Schultz MJ, Cardwell CR, et al. Automated versus non-automated weaning for reducing the duration of mechanical ventilation for critically ill adults and children: a Cochrane systematic review and meta-analysis. *Crit Care*. 2015;48. doi: 10.1186/s13054-015-0755-6

Schreiber AF, Ceriana P, Ambrosino N, Malovini A, Nava S. Physiotherapy and weaning from prolonged mechanical ventilation. *Respir Care*. 2019;64(1):17-25.

Seckel MA. Mechanical ventilation and weaning. In: Good VS, Kirkwood PL, eds. *Advanced Critical Care Nursing*. 2nd ed. St Louis, MO: Elsevier; 2018.

Surani S, Sharma M, Middagh K, et al. Weaning from mechanical ventilator in a long-term acute care hospital: a retrospective analysis. *Open Respir Med J*. 2020;14:62-66.

Villalba D, Rossetti GG, Scrigna M, et al. Prevalence of and risk factors for mechanical ventilation reinstitution in patients weaned from prolonged mechanical ventilation. *Respir Care*. 2020;65(2):210-216.

Communication

Grant M. Resolving communication challenges in the intensive care unit. *AACN Adv Crit Care*. 2015;26:123-130.

Grossbach I, Stranberg S, Chlan L. Promoting effective communication for patients receiving mechanical ventilation. *Crit Care Nurse*. 2011;31:46-61.

Hoorn S, Elbers PW, Girbes AR, Tuinman PR. Communicating with conscious and mechanically ventilated critically ill patients: a systematic review. *Crit Care*. 2016;30:33. doi: 10.1186/s13054-016-1483-2

Morris LL, Bedon AM, McIntosh E, Whitmer A. Restoring speech to tracheostomy patients. *Crit Care Nurse*. 2015;35:13-27.

Pandian V, Boisen S, Mathews S, Brenner MJ. Speech and safety in tracheostomy patients receiving mechanical ventilation: a systematic review. *Am J Crit Care*. 2019;28(6):441-450.

Rodriquez CS, Rowe M, Thomas L, et al. Enhancing the communication of suddenly speechless critical care patients. *Am J Crit Care*. 2016;25:e40-e47.

Evidence-Based Resources

American Association of Critical Care Nurses (AACN). *Practice Alert: Assessment and Management of Delirium Across the Lifespan.* Aliso Viejo, CA: AACN; 2018. www.aacn.org. Accessed July 8, 2021.

American Association of Critical Care Nurses (AACN). *Practice Alert: Managing Alarms in Acute Care Across the Life Span: Electrocardiography and Pulse Oximetry.* Aliso Viejo, CA: AACN; 2018. www.aacn.org. Accessed July 8, 2021.

American Association of Critical Care Nurses (AACN). *Practice Alert: Prevention of Aspiration in Adults.* Aliso Viejo, CA: AACN; 2018. www.aacn.org. Assessed June 8, 2021.

American Association of Respiratory Care. AARC clinical practice guideline: endotracheal suctioning of mechanically ventilated patients with artificial airways: 2010. *Resp Care.* 2010;55:758-764.

American Association of Respiratory Care. AARC clinical practice guideline: capnography/capnometry during mechanical ventilation: 2011. *Resp Care.* 2011;56:503-509.

American Association of Respiratory Care. AARC clinical practice guideline: effectiveness of nonpharmacologic airway clearance therapies in hospitalized patients. *Resp Care.* 2013;58:2187-2193.

American Association of Respiratory Care. AARC clinical practice guideline: effectiveness of pharmacologic airway clearance therapies in hospitalized patients. *Resp Care.* 2015;60(7):1071-1077.

American Association for Respiratory Care. AARC clinical practice guideline: care of the ventilator circuit and it relation to ventilator-associated pneumonia. *Resp Care.* 2003;48:869-879.

American Association for Respiratory Care. AARC clinical practice guideline: removal of the endotracheal tube-2007 revision and update. *Resp Care.* 2007;52;81-93.

Barden, C, Davis T, Seckel M, et al. AACN Tele-ICU Nursing Practice Guidelines. 2013. Available at http://www.aacn.org/wd/practice/docs/tele-icu-guidelines.pdf.

Centers for Disease Control and Prevention National Healthcare Safety Network. Ventilator-associated events. 2021. https://www.cdc.gov/nhsn/pdfs/pscmanual/10-vae_final.pdf. Accessed July 9, 2021.

Devlin JW, et al: Executive summary: clinical practice guidelines for the prevention and management of pain, agitation/sedation, delirium, immobility, and sleep disruption in adult patients in the ICU. *Crit Care Med.* 2018;46:1532-1548.

Fan E, Del Sorbo L, Goligher EC, et al. An Official American Thoracic Society/European Society of Intensive Care Medicine/Society of Critical Care Medicine Clinical Practice Guideline: mechanical ventilation in adult patients with acute respiratory distress syndrome. *Am J Respir Crit Care.* 2017;195:1253-1263.

Girard TD, Alhazzani W, Kress JP, et al. An official American Thoracic Society/American College of Chest Physicians clinical practice guideline: liberation from mechanical ventilation in critically ill adults: rehabilitation protocols. ventilator liberation protocols, and cuff leak tests. *Am J Resp Crit Care Med.* 2017;195:120-133.

Kalil AC, Metersky ML, Klompas M, et al. Management of adults with hospital-acquired and ventilator-associated pneumonia: 2016 clinical practice guidelines by the Infectious Diseases Society of America and the American Thoracic Society. *Clin Infect Dis.* 2016;63:e61-e111.

Klompas M, Branson R, Eichenwald EC, et al. Strategies to prevent ventilator-associated pneumonia in acute care hospitals: 2014 update. *Infect Control Hosp Epidemiol.* 2014;35(8);915-936.

Mitchell RB, Hussey HM, Setzen G, et al. Clinical consensus statement: tracheostomy care. *Otolaryngol Head Neck Surg.* 2013;148:6-20.

Mussa CC, Gomaa D, Rowley DD, et al. AARC clinical practice guideline: management of adult patients with tracheostomy in the acute care setting. *Resp Care.* 2021;6(1):156-169.

Ouellette DR, Patel S, Girard TD, et al. Liberation from mechanical ventilation in critically ill adults: an official American College of Chest Physicians/American Thoracic Society clinical practice guideline. Inspiratory pressure augmentation during spontaneous breathing trials, protocols minimizing sedation, and noninvasive ventilation immediately after extubation. *Chest.* 2017;151:166-180.

Qaseem A, Etzeandia-Ikobaltzeta I, Fitterman N, Williams JW, Kansagara D. Appropriate use of high-flow nasal oxygen in hospitalized patient for initial or postextubation management of acute respiratory failure: a clinical guideline from the American College of Physicians. *Ann Intern Med.* 2021;174(7):976-986.

Raimondi N, Vial MR, Calleja J, et al. Evidence-based guidelines for the use of tracheostomy in critically ill patients. *J Crit Care.* 2017;38:304-318.

Rochwerg B, Brochard L, Elliott MW, et al. Official ERS/ATS clinical practice guidelines: noninvasive ventilation for acute respiratory failure. *Eur Respir J.* 2017;50. https://doi.org/10.1183/13993003.02426-2016

Schmidt GA, Girard TD, Kress JP, et al. Official executive summary of the American Thoracic Society/American College of Chest Physicians clinical practice guideline: liberation from mechanical ventilation in critically ill adults. *Am J Respir Crit Care Med.* 2017;195:115-119.

Society of Critical Care Medicine. *ABCDEF bundle.* https://www.sccm.org/Clinical-Resources/ICULiberation-Home/ABCDEF-Bundles. Accessed July 23, 2021.

Society of Critical Care Medicine—Guidelines for the Prevention and Management of Pain, Agitation/Sedation, Delirium, Immobility, and Sleep Disruption in Adult Patients in the ICU. 2018. https://www.sccm.org/Clinical-Resources/Guidelines/Guidelines/Guidelines-for-the-Prevention-and-Management-of-Pa

Vanderbilt University Medical Center. Delirium prevention and safety: Starting with the ABCDEF's. http://www.icudelirium.org/medicalprofessionals.html. Accessed July 8, 2021.

Wiegand DL, ed. *AACN Procedure Manual for Critical Care.* 7th ed. St. Louis, MO: Elsevier Saunders; 2016.

PAIN, SEDATION, AND NEUROMUSCULAR BLOCKADE MANAGEMENT

6

Yvonne D'Arcy and Sara Knippa

KNOWLEDGE COMPETENCIES

1. Describe the elements of pain assessment in critically ill patients.

2. Describe how to use a behavioral pain scale to assess pain in patients who cannot self-report.

3. Compare and contrast pain-relieving modalities for the critically ill:
   • Nonsteroidal anti-inflammatory drugs
   • Opioids, including patient-controlled analgesia (PCA)
   • Epidural analgesia with opioids and/or local anesthetics (LAs)
   • Elastomeric pumps with local anesthetic (LA)
   • Nonpharmacologic modalities: distraction, cutaneous stimulation, imagery, and relaxation techniques

4. Identify the important elements of pain control for a patient who has a substance use disorder, is dependent on opioids for pain relief, on medication management for opioid addiction, or has a past history of substance abuse.

5. Describe special considerations for pain management in vulnerable populations such as older adults.

6. Identify the need for sedation, commonly used sedatives, and potential complications.

7. Discuss how to monitor and manage patients requiring sedation and interventions to address sedation-related issues.

8. Discuss different neuromuscular blocking agents used in critically ill ventilated patients, clinical indications, and monitoring.

Pain management is central to the care of the critically ill or injured patient. Often, critically ill patients are not able to self-report their pain management needs to their healthcare team. Patients identify physical care that promotes pain relief and comfort as an important element of their hospitalization and recovery, especially while in the critical care environment. Providing optimum pain relief for critically ill patients not only enhances their emotional well-being, but can also help avert additional physiologic injury for a patient who is already compromised. This chapter explores a multimodal approach to pain management in critically ill patients based on the physiologic mechanisms of pain transmission and human responses to pain. Specific pharmacologic and nonpharmacologic pain management techniques are described, including the integral relationships among relaxation, sedation, and

pain relief. Strategies also are presented that promote comfort and are easy to incorporate into a plan of care for critically ill patients. Finally, special considerations are delineated for vulnerable populations within the critical care setting.

PHYSIOLOGIC MECHANISMS OF PAIN

Peripheral Mechanisms

The pain response is elicited with tissue injuries, whether actual or potential. Undifferentiated free nerve endings, or *nociceptors*, are the major receptors signaling tissue injury (Figure 6-1). Nociceptors are polymodal and can be stimulated by thermal, mechanical, and chemical stimuli. Nociception refers to the transmission of impulses by sensory nerves, which signal tissue injury.

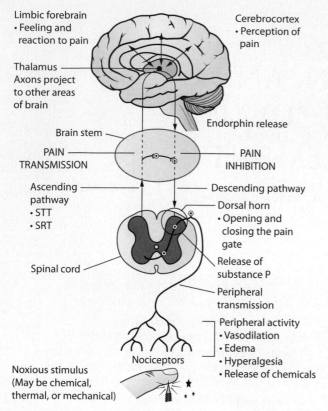

Figure 6-1. Physiologic pathway of pain transmission. (*Reproduced with permission from Copstead L. Perspectives on Pathophysiology. Philadelphia, PA: WB Saunders; 1995.*)

At the site of injury, the release of a variety of neurochemical substances potentiates the activation of peripheral nociceptors. Many of these substances are also mediators of the inflammatory response and they can facilitate or inhibit the pain impulse. These substances include histamine, kinins, prostaglandins, serotonin, and leukotrienes (Figure 6-2).

The nociceptive impulse travels to the spinal cord via specialized, afferent sensory fibers. Small, myelinated A-delta (δ) fibers conduct nociceptive signals rapidly to the spinal cord. The A-delta fibers transmit sensations that are generally localized and sharp in quality. In addition to A-delta fibers, smaller, unmyelinated C fibers also transmit nociceptive signals to the spinal cord. Because C fibers are unmyelinated, their conduction speed is much slower than their A-delta counterparts. The sensory quality of signals carried by C fibers tends to be dull and unlocalized (Figure 6-3).

Spinal Cord Integration

Sensory afferent fibers enter the spinal cord via the dorsal nerve, synapsing with cell bodies of spinal cord interneurons in the dorsal horn (see Figure 6-1). Most of the A-delta and C fibers synapse in laminae I through V in an area referred to as the *substantia gelatinosa*. Numerous neurotransmitters (eg, substance P, glutamate, and calcitonin gene-related peptide [CGRP]) and other receptor systems (eg, opiate, alpha-adrenergic, and serotonergic receptors) modulate the processing of nociceptive inputs in the spinal cord.

Stimulus	Representative receptor
NGF	TrkA
Bradykinin	BK$_2$
Seratonin	5-HT$_3$
ATP	P2X3
H+	ASIC3/VR1
Lipids	PGE$_2$/CB1/VR1
Heat	VR1/VRL-1
Pressure	DEG/ENaC

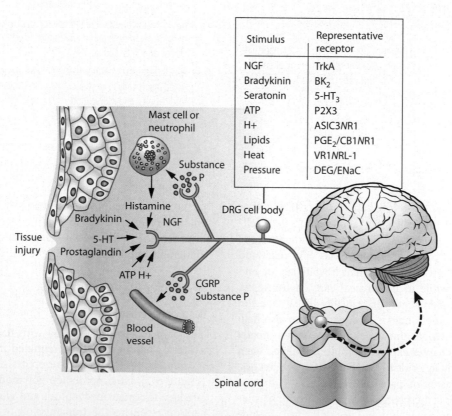

Figure 6-2. Peripheral nociceptors and the inflammatory response at the site of injury. (*Reproduced with permission from Julius D, Basbaum AI. Molecular mechanisms of nociception, Nature. 2001;413(6852):203-210.*)

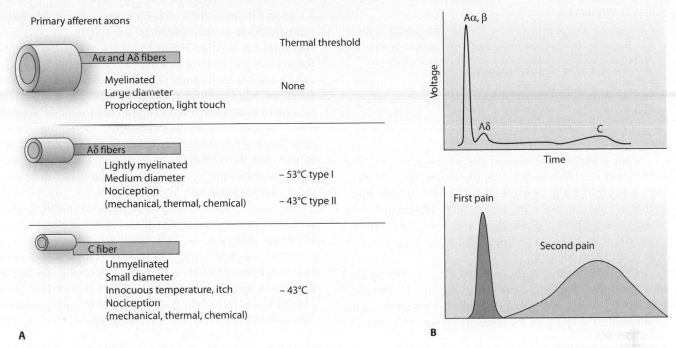

Figure 6-3. Different nociceptors detect different types of pain. **(A)** Peripheral nerves include small-diameter (Aδ) and medium- to large-diameter (Aα, β) myelinated afferent fibers, as well as small-diameter unmyelinated afferent fibers (C). **(B)** The fact that conduction velocity is directly related to fiber diameter is highlighted in the compound action potential recording from a peripheral nerve. Most nociceptors are either Aδ or C fibers, and their different conduction velocities (6-25 and ~1.0 m/s, respectively) account for the first (fast) and second (slow) pain responses to injury.

Central Processing

Following spinal cord integration, nociceptive impulses travel to the brain via specialized, ascending somatosensory pathways (see Figure 6-1). The spinothalamic tract conducts nociceptive signals directly from the spinal cord to the thalamus. The spinoreticulothalamic tract projects signals to the reticular formation and the mesencephalon in the midbrain, as well as to the thalamus. From the thalamus, axons project to somatosensory areas of the cerebrocortex and limbic forebrain. The unique physiologic, cognitive, and emotional responses to pain are determined and modulated by the specific areas to which the somatosensory pathways project. The stimulus to the cerebrocortex can also activate the patient's previous memories of the experience of pain; for example, the thalamus regulates the neurochemical response to pain, and the cortical and limbic projections are responsible for the perception of pain and aversive response to pain, respectively. Similarly, the reticular activating system regulates the heightened state of awareness that accompanies pain. The modulation of pain by activities in these specific areas of the brain is the basis of many of the analgesic modalities available to treat pain.

RESPONSES TO PAIN

Human responses to pain can be both physical and emotional. The physiologic responses to pain are the result of hypothalamic activation of the sympathetic nervous system associated with the stress response. Sympathetic activation leads to:

- A shift in circulation away from superficial vessels and toward striated muscle, the heart, the lungs, and the nervous system
- Dilation of the bronchioles to increase oxygenation
- Increased cardiac contractility
- Inhibition of gastric secretions and contraction
- Increases in circulating blood glucose for energy

Signs and symptoms of sympathetic activation that frequently accompany nociception and pain include:

- Increased heart rate
- Increased blood pressure
- Increased respiratory rate
- Pupil dilation
- Pallor and perspiration
- Nausea and vomiting

Although patients experiencing acute pain often exhibit signs and symptoms as noted above, it is critical to note that the absence or presence of any or all of these signs and symptoms does not negate or confirm the presence of pain. In fact, some patients, especially those who are critically ill and have little or no compensatory reserves, may exhibit a shock-like clinical picture in the presence of pain. Patients who are accustomed to underlying chronic pain may have a decreased physiologic response to it while the actual intensity of the pain remains high (Table 6-1).

TABLE 6-1. TYPES OF PAIN

Pain is defined as an unpleasant sensory and emotional experience associated with actual or potential tissue damage (APS, 2008). There are three main types of pain that can occur alone or in combination:
- Acute pain from which the patient expects to recover
- Chronic pain that lasts beyond the normal healing period
- Neuropathic pain is a special type of chronic pain that is the result of nerve damage

Pain is expressed both verbally and nonverbally. The expressions can take many forms, some of which are subtle cues that could easily be overlooked (Table 6-2). Any signs that may indicate pain warrant further exploration and assessment. Although physiologic and behavioral expressions of acute pain have been described, each person's response to pain is unique.

Critically ill patients who are receiving neuromuscular blocking agents (eg, mivacurium, vecuronium, atracurium, or cisatracurium) are unable to exhibit even subtle signs of discomfort because of the therapeutic paralysis. Neuromuscular blocking agents do not affect sensory nerves and have no analgesic qualities. Consequently, patients who are receiving blockade will require a continuous infusion of opioids to ensure pain relief.

PAIN ASSESSMENT

Pain assessment is a core element of ongoing surveillance of the critically ill patient. Self-report of pain intensity and distress is recommended whenever possible, especially for patients who can talk or communicate effectively and reliably. In those who cannot communicate, the use of a standardized assessment tool such as the Behavioral Pain Scale (BPS) or the Critical Care Pain Observation Tool (CPOT) is recommended in the 2018 Clinical Practice Guidelines for the Prevention and Management of Pain, Agitation/Sedation, Delirium, Immobility, and Sleep Disruption in Adult Patients in the ICU (PADIS guidelines). Unfortunately, these tools are under-used; studies show that up to a third of critical care nurses do not use pain assessment tools with their patients who are unable to communicate. Regular documentation of pain assessment not only helps monitor the efficacy of analgesic modalities, but also helps ensure consistency and communication among caregivers regarding patients' pain.

TABLE 6-2. EXAMPLES OF PAIN EXPRESSION IN CRITICALLY ILL PATIENTS

Verbal Cues	Facial Cues	Body Movements
Moaning	Grimacing	Splinting
Crying	Wincing	Rubbing
Screaming	Eye signals	Rocking
Silence		Rhythmic movement of extremity
		Shaking or tapping bed rails
		Grabbing the nurse's arm

Data from Herr K, Coyne P, Kry T, et al. Pain assessment in the nonverbal patient: position statement with clinical practice recommendations. Pain Manag Nurs. 2006;7(2):44-52.

For patients who can self-report, the numeric rating scale (NRS) is recommended in the PADIS guideline and uses numbers between 0 and 10 to describe pain intensity; the anchors are "no pain to worst pain imaginable." The NRS can be used with patients who are intubated or unable to speak for other medical reasons; for example, patients can be asked to use their fingers to indicate a number between 0 and 10; similarly, patients can be asked to indicate by nodding their head or pointing to a written chart. It is important to note that the NRS is the only currently validated way to assess intensity of pain. For example, a rating of 7 indicates a more intense pain than a rating of 2.

In some cases, critically ill patients are unable to indicate their pain intensity verbally or nonverbally. In these situations, nurses must often use other criteria to assess their patient's pain. Using a pain assessment scale based on behavioral cues provides a guide for identifying and assessing pain in nonverbal patients. There are two of these types of pain scales recommended by the PADIS guidelines: the BPS or the CPOT. They both have a set of behavior categories that are rated and when the score is summed, pain is considered present when the score is over a threshold (BPS > 3 and CPOT > 2). Neither of these scales are currently validated to indicate pain intensity. For example, a score of 6 on BPS is not considered greater pain than a score of 4; both scores simply indicate that pain is present. Tables 6-3 and 6-4 provide the criteria for two tools.

A MULTIMODAL APPROACH TO PAIN MANAGEMENT

Today there are numerous approaches and modalities available to treat acute pain. Pharmacologic techniques traditionally have been the mainstay of analgesia, other complementary or nonpharmacologic methods are growing in their acceptance and use in clinical practice. Most modalities used in the treatment of acute pain can be used effectively in the critically ill. Evidenced-based practice guidelines to maximize analgesia in critically ill patients are summarized in Table 6-5.

One of the central goals of pain management is to combine therapies or modalities that target as many of the processes involved in nociception and pain transmission as possible. Analgesic modalities, both pharmacologic and nonpharmacologic, exert their effects by altering nociception at specific structures within the peripheral or central nervous system (CNS); ie, the peripheral nociceptors, the spinal cord, or the brain or by altering the transmission of nociceptive impulses between these structures (Figure 6-4). By understanding the different sites where analgesic modalities work, nurses can select a combination of strategies to best treat the source or type of pain the patient is experiencing. A multimodal approach to pain control can achieve optimal analgesia with minimal side effects.

In response to the increasing number of patients diagnosed with a substance use disorder (SUD) the Centers for

TABLE 6-3. CRITICAL CARE PAIN OBSERVATION TOOL

Indicator	Description	Score	
Facial expressions	No muscle tension observed	Relaxed, neutral	0
	Presence of frowning, brow lowering, orbit tightening and levator contraction or any other change (e.g. opening eyes or tearing during nociceptive procedures)	Tense	1
		Grimacing	2
	All previous facial movements plus eyelid tightly closed (the patient may present with mouth open or biting the endotracheal tube)		
Body movements	Does not move at all (doesn't necessarily mean absence of pain) or normal position (movements not aimed toward the pain site or not made for the purpose of protection)	Absence of movements or normal position	0
			1
	Slow, cautious movements, touching or rubbing the pain site, seeking attention through movements	Protection	2
		Restlessness/Agitation	
	Pulling tube, attempting to sit up, moving limbs/thrashing, not Following commands, striking at staff, trying to climb out of bed		
Muscle tension	No resistance to passive movements	Relaxed	0
Evaluation by passive flexion and extension of upper limbs when patient is at rest or evaluation when patient is being turned	Resistance to passive movements	Tense, rigid	1
	Strong resistance to passive movements or incapacity to complete them	Very tense or rigid	2
Compliance with the ventilator (intubated patients)	Alarms not activated, easy ventilation	Tolerating ventilator or movement	0
	Coughing, alarms may be activated but stop spontaneously	Coughing but tolerating	1
OR	Asynchrony: blocking ventilation, alarms frequently activated	Fighting ventilator	2
Vocalization (extubated patients)	Talking in normal tone or no sound	Talking in normal tone or no sound	0
	Sighing, moaning	Sighing, moaning	1
	Crying out, sobbing	Crying out sobbing	2
Total			0-8

Reproduced with permission from Gélinas C, Fillion L, Puntillo KA, et al: Validation of the critical-care pain observation tool in adult patients. Am J Crit Care. 2006;15(4):420-427.

Disease Control and Prevention (CDC) drafted guidelines for using opioids in patients with chronic pain. These recommendations do not apply to cancer patients, or to patients who are receiving palliative care or end-of-life care. In addition, these guidelines do not specifically address the management of acute pain. However, understanding these guidelines is pertinent in critical care, as patients often have ongoing comorbidities such as fibromyalgia, arthritis, or painful neuropathic conditions that may complicate acute pain control. Patients may develop chronic pain as a result of trauma or surgical procedures such as amputations. Thus, the CDC guidelines may be useful to consider when caring for critically and acutely ill patients with chronic pain.

CDC 2018 Chronic pain guidelines

- Use nonpharmacologic and non-opioid medications as a first option
- If opioids are indicated, use short-acting opioids as the first opioid option
- Limit postoperative opioids prescriptions to 3 to 7 days
- Keep opioid equivalents to 50 morphine milligram equivalents (MME) with a maximum of 90 MME a day

TABLE 6-4. THE BEHAVIOR PAIN ASSESSMENT TOOLS

Item	Description	Score
Facial expression	Relaxed	1
	Partially tightened (e.g., brow lowering)	2
	Fully tightened (e.g., eyelid closing)	3
	Grimacing	4
Upper limbs	No movement	1
	Partially bent	2
	Fully bent with finger flexion	3
	Permanently retracted	4
Compliance with ventilation	Tolerating movement	1
	Coughing but tolerating ventilation for most of the time	2
	Fighting ventilator	3
	Unable to control ventilation	4

Reproduced with permission from Payen JF, Bru O, Bosson JL, et al: Assessing pain in critically ill sedated patients by using a behavioral pain scale. Crit Care Med. 2001;29(12):2258-2263.

TABLE 6-5. EVIDENCE-BASED GUIDELINES: PAIN MANAGEMENT

- Pain should be routinely monitored
- Use the behavioral pain scale BPS or critical-care pain observation tool (CPOT) for patients who cannot self-report pain
- Do not use vital signs alone for pain assessment in ICU patients
- Use preemptive analgesia prior to procedures
- Consider IV opioids as the first line to treat non-neuropathic pain
- Non-opioids and coanalgesics such as gabapentin or carbamazepine be considered for use with opioids
- Epidural analgesia is recommended for rib fractures and postoperative analgesia for abdominal aortic aneurysm

Data from Barr J, Fraser G, Puntillo K, et al. Clinical practice guidelines for the management of pain, agitation, and delirium in adult patients in the intensive care unit. Crit Care Med. 2013;41(1):263-306.

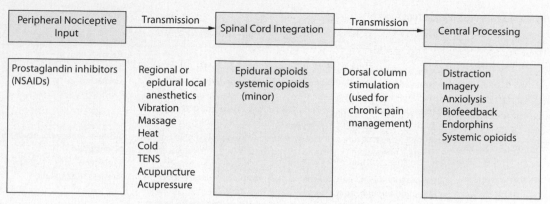

Figure 6-4. A multimodal approach to pain management.

Although these indications may not immediately apply to the critical care patient, awareness of the guidelines is helpful in considering appropriate medication use and pain management options during the recovery period.

To assist nurses in the selection and use of analgesic modalities, the following descriptions of each modality include where and how it works, clinical situations where it can be used most effectively, and strategies for titrating the modality. Finally, because few modalities exert a singular effect, a summary of commonly associated secondary or side effects and strategies to minimize their occurrence are also addressed.

NONSTEROIDAL ANTI-INFLAMMATORY DRUGS

Nonsteroidal anti-inflammatory drugs (NSAIDs) target the peripheral nociceptors. The NSAIDs exert their effect by modifying or reducing the amount of prostaglandin produced at the site of injury by inhibiting the formation of the enzyme cyclooxygenase, which is also responsible for the breakdown of arachidonic acid. By modifying and reducing the production of prostaglandin, the NSAIDs have been shown to have opioid-sparing effects and are very effective in managing pain associated with inflammation, trauma to peripheral tissues (e.g., soft tissue injuries), bone pain (e.g., fractures, metastatic disease), and pain associated with indwelling tubes and drains (e.g., chest tubes).

One of the NSAIDs commonly used in the critical care setting is ketorolac tromethamine (Toradol). Ketorolac is currently the only parenteral NSAID preparation available in the United States and can be administered safely via the intravenous (IV) route. Intramuscular administration is not recommended due to the potential for irregular and unpredictable absorption. Recommended dosing for ketorolac is a 30-mg loading dose followed by 15 mg every 6 hours. Like all NSAIDs, ketorolac has a ceiling effect where administration of higher doses offers no additional therapeutic benefit yet significantly increases the risk of toxicity. While not a NSAID, acetaminophen IV (Ofirmev) is another non-opioid alternative for patients who cannot tolerate ketorolac and do not have liver disease or other potential contraindications.

The PADIS Guidelines recommend the use of adjuvant analgesics such as NSAIDs to reduce opioid analgesic use and reduce opioid-related side effects.

Side Effects

The side effects associated with the use of NSAIDs relate to the function of prostaglandins in physiologic processes other than nociception; for example, gastrointestinal (GI) irritation, and bleeding may result from NSAID use because prostaglandins are necessary for maintaining the mucous lining of the stomach. Similarly, the enzyme cyclooxygenase is needed for the eventual production of thromboxane, a key substance involved in platelet function. As a result, when NSAIDs are used chronically or in high doses, platelet aggregation may be altered, leading to bleeding problems. Prostaglandin inhibition by NSAIDs can also cause vasoconstriction of the renal afferent arterioles, reducing glomerular blood flow and contributing to renal toxicity, particularly when NSAIDs are combined with other medications that affect kidney circulation. Cross-sensitivities with other NSAIDs have been documented (e.g., ibuprofen, naproxen, indomethacin, piroxicam, aspirin). For these reasons, ketorolac and other NSAIDs are avoided in patients who have a history of gastric ulceration, renal insufficiency, coagulopathies, or a documented sensitivity to aspirin or other NSAIDs. In addition, NSAID use is not recommended in patients with heart disease, recent heart bypass surgery, or patients with a history of ischemic attacks or strokes, or patients who have undergone spinal fusion surgery. An alternative to intravenous ketorolac for patients who are not good candidates for NSAIDs is intravenous acetaminophen, as noted above. The severity of all NSAID-related side effects increases with high doses or prolonged use. For this reason, ketorolac and other such medications are designed for short-term use only.

OPIOIDS

The primary medications for pain in the critical care setting continue to be opioids. The PADIS guidelines recommend that opioids be considered as first-line treatment for non-neuropathic pain. Traditionally referred to as *narcotics*, opioids produce their analgesic effects primarily by binding with specialized opiate receptors throughout the CNS and thereby altering the perception of pain. Opiate receptors are located in the brain, spinal cord, and GI tract. Although opioids work primarily within the CNS, they also have been shown to have some local or peripheral effects as well. There are at least 45 variations in opiate receptors that account for the varied responses in individual patients.

Opioids are well tolerated by most critically ill patients and can be administered by many routes including IV, oral, buccal, nasal, rectal, transdermal, and intraspinal. Morphine sulfate is still the most widely used opioid and serves as the gold standard against which others are compared. Other opioids commonly used in the care of the critically ill include hydromorphone (Dilaudid), fentanyl, and remifentanil. Opioid polymorphisms may cause opioids to affect patients differently, thus careful use and frequent assessment are necessary to determine optimal dosing. Opioids are further described in Chapter 7, Pharmacology.

For patients who have an SUD, are opioid dependent, on opioid medications to treat addiction or have a past history of addiction, opioid doses generally need to be higher than those not addicted. By identifying chronic opioid use on admission, it is possible to anticipate appropriate in-hospital opioid titration.

Side Effects

Patients' responses to opioids, both analgesic responses and side effects, are highly individualized. Just as all the opioid agents have similar pain-relieving potential, all opioids currently available share similar side effect profiles. When side effects do occur, it is important to remember that they are primarily the result of opioid pharmacology and patient response, as opposed to the route of administration.

Nausea and Vomiting

Nausea and vomiting are distressing side effects often related to opioids that, unfortunately, many patients experience. Generally, nausea and vomiting result from stimulation of the chemoreceptor trigger zone (CTZ) in the brain and/or from slowed GI peristalsis. Nausea and vomiting can often be managed effectively with antiemetic medications. Metoclopramide (Reglan), a procainamide derivative, works both centrally at the CTZ and at the GI level to increase gastric motility. However, there are significant risks with metoclopramide use, such as the potential for seizures and tardive dyskinesia. These conditions occur more commonly in older adults and with prolonged use.

The vestibular system also sends input to the CTZ. For this reason, movement frequently exacerbates opioid-related nausea. If patients complain of movement-related nausea, the application of a transdermal scopolamine patch can help prevent and treat opioid-induced nausea. The use of transdermal scopolamine is best avoided in patients older than 60 years because it has been reported to increase the incidence and severity of confusion in older patients.

The phenothiazines (ie, prochlorperazine [Compazine], and promethazine [Phenergan]) and the butyrophenones (droperidol [Inapsine]) treat nausea through the effects at the CTZ. The serotonin antagonist ondansetron (Zofran) is also effective for treatment of opioid-related nausea. The doses required for postoperative or opioid-related nausea are significantly smaller doses (4 mg IV) than those used with emetogenic chemotherapy.

Pruritus

Pruritus is another opioid-related side effect commonly reported by patients. The actual mechanisms producing opioid-related pruritus are unknown. Although antihistamines can provide symptomatic relief for some patients, the role of histamine in opioid-related pruritus is unclear. One of the drawbacks of using antihistamine agents, such as diphenhydramine (Benadryl), is the sedation associated with their use. In addition, the use of diphenhydramine has been shown to have a 70% increase in cognitive deterioration in older adult patients. Similar to other opioid side effects, the incidence and severity of pruritus is dose related and tends to diminish with ongoing use. Another option to treat opioid-induced pruritus is nalbuphine (Nubain), dosed at small doses of 2.5 to 5.0 mg IV every 6 hours as needed.

Constipation

Constipation, another common side effect, results from opioid binding at opiate receptors in the GI tract and decreased peristalsis. The incidence of constipation may be low or under-reported in some critically ill patients, but it is important to remember that it is likely to be a problem for many patients after the critical phase of their illness or injury. The best treatment for constipation is prevention by ensuring adequate hydration, as well as by administering stimulant laxatives and stool softeners as needed. For palliative care patients with opioid-induced constipation, methylnaltrexone (Relistor) can be given as a subcutaneous injection.

Urinary Retention

Urinary retention can result from increased smooth muscle tone caused by opioids, especially in the detrussor muscle of the bladder. Opioids have no effect on urine production and neither cause nor worsen oliguria. In the past urinary retention rarely occurred in critically ill patients because of indwelling urinary catheters. However, with the decreased use of indwelling urinary catheters in all hospitalized patients, this problem may occur in critical care patients as well.

Respiratory Depression

Respiratory depression, the most adverse side effect of opioids, occurs due to their impact on the respiratory centers in the brain stem. Both respiratory rate and the depth of breathing can decrease as a result of opioids, usually in a dose-dependent fashion. Patients at increased risk for respiratory depression include older adults, those with pre-existing cardiopulmonary diseases, patients receiving other respiratory depressive medications such as benzodiazepines, and those who receive high doses. Signs and symptoms of respiratory depression include altered level of consciousness, shallow breathing, decreased respiratory rate, pupil constriction, hypoxemia, and hypercarbia. The CDC discourages concomitant use of opioids and benzodiazepines related to the increased risk of oversedation.

Clinically significant respiratory depression resulting from opiate use is usually treated with IV naloxone (Narcan). Naloxone is an opioid antagonist; it binds with opiate receptors, temporarily displacing the opioid and suspending its pharmacologic effects. As with other medications, naloxone is administered in very small doses and titrated to the desired level of alertness since the abrupt, complete withdrawal of all opiate effect can cause an acute, severe, and frightening pain response (Table 6-6). The half-life of naloxone is short—approximately 30 to 45 minutes. Thus, ongoing assessment of the patient is essential as additional doses of naloxone may be required. A continuous infusion may be used in those who are profoundly sedated.

Naloxone is used with caution in patients with underlying cardiovascular disease. The acute onset of hypertension, pulmonary hypertension, and pulmonary edema with naloxone administration has been reported. Also, naloxone is avoided in patients who have developed a tolerance to opioids since opioid antagonists can precipitate withdrawal or acute abstinence syndrome.

Intravenous Opioids

Many critically ill patients are unable to use the oral route, thus the IV route is used most often. One of the advantages of IV opioids is their rapid onset of action, allowing for easy titration. The rapid onset is beneficial during most invasive procedures in critical care. Loading doses of IV opioids are administered to achieve an adequate blood level. Additional doses can then be administered intermittently to maintain analgesic levels.

Critically ill patients may benefit from the addition of a continuous IV opioid infusion. Pain control in patients

TABLE 6-6. ADMINISTRATION OF NALOXONE

1. Support ventilation.
2. Dilute 0.4 mg (400 mcg) ampule of naloxone with normal saline to constitute a 10-mL solution.
3. Administer in 1-mL increments, every 2-5 minutes, titrating to desired effect. Onset of action: approximately 2 minutes.
4. Continue to monitor patient; readminister naloxone as needed. Duration of action: approximately 45 minutes.
5. For patients requiring ongoing doses, consider naloxone infusion: Administer at 50-250 mcg/h, titrating to desired response.

who are not able to communicate their pain levels effectively, especially those receiving neuromuscular blocking agents, are provided with continuous infusions to assure comfort. The continuous infusion not only helps to achieve the appropriate blood levels, but also can be titrated as needed. Whenever appropriate, the maintenance dose for the infusion is based on patients' previous opioid requirements.

Patient-Controlled Analgesia

Patient-controlled analgesia (PCA) pumps can also be used effectively in the critical care setting with alert patients able to activate the PCA button. With PCA, patients self-administer small doses of an opioid infusion using a programmable pump. PCA prescriptions typically include a bolus dose of the selected medication, a lockout or delay interval, and either a 1- to 4-hour limit. The bolus dose refers to the amount of medication the patient receives following pump activation. The initial dose usually ranges between 0.5 and 2.0 mg of morphine, or its equivalent. The lockout or delay interval typically ranges between 5 and 10 minutes, which is enough time for the prescribed medication to circulate and take effect yet allows the patient to easily titrate the medication over time. The 1- to 4-hour limit serves as an additional safety feature by regulating the amount of medication the patient can receive over this period of time.

Assessing whether a critically ill patient is capable of using PCA is essential in order to assure success of this analgesic modality. PCA is not appropriate for patients unable to reliably self-administer pain medication (e.g., a patient with a decreased level of consciousness). However, a cognitively intact patient, who is unable to activate the PCA button due to lack of manual dexterity or strength, may use a PCA device that has been ergonomically adapted (eg, a pressure switch pad). Patients, family members, and visitors are educated to understand that the patient is the only person to activate the PCA device. Family members and friends may think they are helping by activating the PCA device for the patient and not realize that this can produce life-threatening sedation and respiratory depression.

Titrating PCA

Patients using PCAs usually find a dose and frequency that balances pain relief with other medication-related side effects such as sedation. It is best to start a PCA only after the patient has received loading doses to achieve adequate blood levels. For patients who continue to experience pain while using the PCA pump, the first step in titration is to give an additional loading dose and increase the bolus dose, usually by 25% to 50%, depending on the pain intensity. If patients continue to have pain despite the increased dose, the lockout interval or delay is then reduced, if possible.

Continuous PCA infusions are no longer recommended for the majority of patients as they increase sedation and do not provide additional pain relief. However, in patients who have preexisting opioid tolerance, a continuous infusion may maintain their baseline opioid requirements while the patient-controlled bolus doses are available to help manage any new pain they experience. The hourly dose of the continuous infusion is designed to be quianalgesic to the patient's preexisting opioid requirements.

Regional Analgesia

The combination of standard options such as opioids and regional analgesia is an additional method of reducing pain. This is commonly done with a nerve block performed during surgery. A regional block may last 6 to 8 hours using local anesthetics (LAs). An alternative is a continuous infusion using a small self-contained elastomeric pump. These pumps include the reservoir for the LA that resembles a filled softball and a preset flow control that allows the LA to infuse at a selected rate. The pump is attached to a catheter that can be placed along the surgical incision in a soaker hose configuration. It can also be placed along a nerve, such as the femoral nerve, for patients undergoing procedures such a total knee replacement where a continuous flow can be provided for a period of several days. The concentrations of regional analgesics do not cause motor blockade and are especially helpful to reduce pain associated with respiratory effort such as in thoracotomy patients.

Switching From IV to Oral Opioid Analgesia

Most often switching from IV to oral opioids is accomplished when acute pain subsides and the patient is able to tolerate

---

ESSENTIAL CONTENT CASE

Pain Management Using an Epidural Catheter

A 59-year-old man was admitted to the surgical ICU following a thoracotomy with wedge resection of the left lung for small-cell lung cancer. He was extubated on the morning of the first postoperative day. He had two left pleural chest tubes in place with moderate amounts of drainage and a continuing air leak. He was alert, responsive, and able to communicate his needs by writing notes and gesturing. He had a thoracic epidural catheter in place (T7-T8) with a bupivacaine (0.625 mg/mL) and fentanyl (4 mcg/mL) combination infusing at 6 mL/h. He also had an elastomeric infusion device that was providing a localized block at the incision site using LA only. When asked about his pain level, he wrote that it was 5 on a scale of 0 (no pain) to 10 (worst pain imaginable).

After he was extubated, his nurse noticed he was reluctant to cough and seemed to have some difficulty taking a deep breath. She also noticed his oxygen saturation was slowly drifting downward from 97% to 95%. His respiratory rate was increasing, as was his heart rate. When she listened to his breath sounds, they were bilateral and equal, but diminished throughout with scattered rhonchi. When she asked him about his pain, he said his pain was still a 5 as long as he did not move or cough. He also indicated that he tried to avoid taking a deep breath because it would make him cough and increase the pain level to an 8 or 10.

The nurse knew the patient needed to breathe deeply and cough to clear his lungs, but his pain and discomfort were limiting his ability to perform those maneuvers. He also refused to move from the bed to a chair. The nurse discussed strategies to help minimize the pain associated with this activity. First, she found an extra pillow for him to use as a splint to support his incision and chest wall, and to stabilize his chest tubes.

Then she called the anesthesiologist to confer about increasing the rate of the bupivacaine/fentanyl infusion to increase the pain relief. She also inquired about adding ketorolac or IV acetaminophen to his analgesic regimen to help with chest tube-associated pain.

Because the patient also had an elastomeric infusion pump with LA along the surgical incision, she checked to make sure the clamp was open and the medication was infusing. The addition of the pillows for splinting helped the patient to take deep breaths. The anesthesiologist prescribed a bolus of 3 mL of the epidural solution via the pump and increased the continuous rate to 8 mL/h and added ketorolac, 15 mg, IV every 6 hours and a dose of IV acetaminophen. Over the course of the next 2 hours, the patient was able to cough more effectively, with less pain. His oxygen saturation returned to 97% and he was also able to transfer to a chair for lunch.

Case Question 1: What are the advantages of using epidural analgesia?
(A) Local anesthetic blocks the entire surgical area
(B) Combining an opioid with LA improves pain relief, decreases opioid needs, and can increase respiratory efforts
(C) An epidural provides the patient with a method of continuous pain relief
(D) Patients like epidurals because they provide superior pain relief

Case Question 2: What is the value of adding ketorolac or acetaminophen to the pain regimen?
(A) IV medications work very quickly
(B) The two medications do not make the patient sedated
(C) Adding non-opioid medications can reduce opioid needs and decrease opioid-related side effects
(D) Patients have fewer allergies to non-opioid medications

Answers
1. B. Local anesthetics can have a short-term effect on pain relief and allow the patient to be more active and effectively cough and deep breathe. Combining the opioid and LA can have a synergistic effect increasing the overall pain relief more than using just a single medication.
2. C. Combining a non-opioid and opioid can also have a synergistic effect and decrease pain. The two different medications work on different areas of the pain mechanism. The combination can be used to help the patient become more active and if dosed at bedtime may help the patient to rest better.

oral or enteral nutrition. Patients who receive analgesics by mouth or via the enteral route may experience comparable pain relief to parenteral analgesia with less risk of infection and at a lower cost. Calculating the equianalgesic dose increases the likelihood that the transition to the oral route will be made without loss of pain control. A creative way to wean PCA is to substitute oral or enteral opioid (such as morphine or oxycodone) for one-half of the total dosage of PCA demand doses. Over the next 24 hours, reducing PCA consumption by increasing the lockout period or reducing the bolus size may help transition the patient and narrow the "analgesic gap" between different routes. To prevent opioid overdosage, controlled-release preparations of morphine and oxycodone, designed to be taken less frequently than their immediate-release counterparts, are not to be crushed, halved, or administered into enteral feeding tubes.

EPIDURAL ANALGESIA

Over the past decade the use of epidural analgesia has grown rapidly, especially in the critical care setting. The advantages of epidural analgesia include improved pain control with less sedation, lower overall opioid doses, and generally longer duration of pain management. Epidural analgesia has been associated with a lower morbidity and mortality in critically ill patients. Both opioids and LAs, either alone or in combination, are commonly administered via the epidural route. Epidural analgesia may be administered by several methods, including intermittent bolus dosing, continuous infusion or PCA technology. The mechanisms of action and the resultant clinical effects produced by epidurally administered opioids and LAs are distinct. For this reason, these agents are discussed separately and are important to distinguish in clinical practice.

Epidural Opioids

When opioids are administered epidurally, they diffuse into the cerebrospinal fluid and into the spinal cord (Figure 6-5).

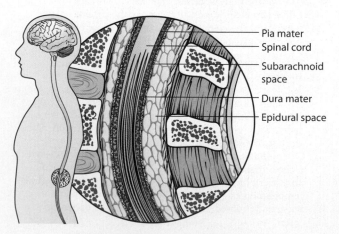

Figure 6-5. Epidural space for catheter placement.

There, the opioids bind with opiate receptors in the substantia gelatinosa, preventing the release of the neurotransmitter, substance P, and altering the transmission of nociceptive impulses from the spinal cord to the brain. Because the opioid is concentrated in the areas of high opiate receptor density where nociceptive impulses are entering the spinal cord, lower doses offer enhanced analgesia, with few supraspinal effects such as drowsiness.

A variety of opioids are commonly used for epidural analgesia including morphine, fentanyl, and hydromorphone. Preservative-free (PF) preparations are used because preservative agents can have neurotoxic effects. The opioids can be administered either by intermittent bolus or continuous infusion depending on the pharmacokinetic activity of the selected agent; for example, fentanyl is generally administered via continuous infusion due to its high lipid solubility, resulting in a short duration of action. In contrast, the low lipid solubility of PF morphine results in a delayed onset of action (30-60 minutes) and a prolonged duration of action (6-12 hours). Because of the delayed onset of action, PF morphine is recommended for use as a continuous infusion but not as a patient-controlled bolus dose.

Side Effects

The side effects associated with epidural opioids are the same as those described for oral and IV opioids. Side effects of opioids are determined primarily by the medication administered and not by the route of administration. For example, the incidence of nausea and vomiting with epidural morphine is similar to that associated with IV morphine. Although epidural opioids were once feared to be associated with a higher risk of respiratory depression, clinical studies and experience have not confirmed this risk. The incidence of respiratory depression has been reported as being no higher than 0.2%. Risk factors for respiratory depression are similar to those seen with IV opioids: increasing age, high doses, underlying cardiopulmonary dysfunction, obstructive sleep apnea, obesity, and the use of perioperative or the combination of epidural opioids with other agents that cause sedation such as benzodiazepines.

Epidural Local Anesthetics

Epidural opioids can also be combined with dilute concentrations of LAs. When administered in combination, these agents work synergistically, reducing the amount of each agent that is needed to produce analgesia. Whereas epidurally administered opioids work in the dorsal horn of the spinal cord, epidural LAs work primarily at the dorsal nerve root by blocking the conduction of afferent sensory fibers. The extent of the blockade is dose related. Higher LA concentrations block more afferent fibers within a given region, resulting in an increased density of the blockade. Higher infusion rates of LA-containing solutions increase the extent or spread of the blockade because more afferent fibers are blocked over a broader region.

ESSENTIAL CONTENT CASE

The Patient With a Substance Use Disorder

A 22-year-old woman was admitted to the cardiovascular ICU (CVICU) following a tricuspid valve replacement related to recurrent subacute bacterial endocarditis. She had a self-reported history of heroin use (approximately 2 g/day).

She was extubated within the first 24 hours after surgery, but remained in the CVICU for stabilization of fluid balance. During the change-of-shift report, the off-going nurse commented that: "She is a constant whiner. She refuses to do anything. All she wants is to go out for a smoke and more drugs. She had 10 mg of IV morphine so far this shift."

When the nurse came in to make her initial assessment, the patient said: "I can't take much more of this pain." The nurse probed further and asked her to use some numbers to describe her pain. She replied, "It's at 10!"

The nurse noticed that the patient was reluctant to move and refused to cough. Her vital signs were:

Heart rate	130 beats/min
BP	150/85 mm Hg
Temperature	38.5°C (orally)
Respiration rate	26 breaths/min, shallow

The nurse was concerned that due to the patient's preoperative use of heroin, she might not be receiving adequate doses of morphine to control her pain. She consulted the clinical nurse specialist for assistance in calculating an equivalent dose of morphine based on the usual heroin use. Using an estimated equivalence of heroin of 1 g = 10 to 15 mg morphine, the nurse calculated that the patient would need approximately 20 to 30 mg of morphine per day to account for her preexisting opioid tolerance. Consequently, analgesic dosing related to her surgery would also need to be relative to this baseline requirement. The patient's nurse approached the surgical team to discuss the potential benefits of using a PCA pump in addition to a continuous infusion of morphine. "By doing this," the nurse explained, "she will receive her baseline opioid requirements related to her drug tolerance." The continuous infusion will address her baseline opioid requirements while the patient-controlled boluses will allow her to treat the new surgical pain. "The PCA may also offer her some control during a time in her recovery when there are few options to do so." In addition to starting the PCA with a continuous infusion, the surgical team and the primary nurse also discussed using other non-opioid agents such as NSAIDs to augment her analgesia. The team also discussed adding morphine sulfate controlled-release (MS-Contin) to the patient's regimen once she was more comfortable on the PCA and titrating the oral medication doses up while decreasing the PCA. Once the MS-Contin was titrated to an effective dose, the PCA would be discontinued and short acting oral breakthrough medication used for additional pain relief. The nurse noted she would also need to monitor the patient for any signs or symptoms of withdrawal.

In addition to the changes in the medications, the primary nurse worked with the patient to use relaxation techniques. The nurse explained that relaxation techniques could be thought of as "boosters" to her pain medications and were something that she could do to help control the pain. They also agreed to try massage in the evening to promote sleep and relaxation.

Case Question 1: In order to maintain adequate pain control after surgery in a patient who is addicted to heroin or takes regular opioids, the nurse will need to:
(A) Provide a continuous rate on the PCA
(B) Provide a continuous rate on the PCA to account for her presurgical heroin usage and add additional pain medications for the surgical pain
(C) Try to limit the patient's opioid use because she has an SUD
(D) Substitute a non-opioid medication such as acetaminophen or ketorolac because the patients has an SUD

Case Question 2: The best way to control postoperative pain is to:
(A) Use opioids exclusively
(B) Use only medications
(C) Encourage the patient to cough and deep breathe
(D) Use a multimodal approach with medications and complementary techniques such as relaxation

Answers
1. B. It is essential to account for the presurgical heroin use when calculating the opioid doses so that additional medication may be added to reduce the pain to an acceptable level. Trying to limit opioids or substitute a non-opioid in a patient with an SUD with acute pain is not recommended and will have a negative effect on the pain relief.
2. D. Complementary techniques have been found to reduce anxiety and relax the patient. This in turn can help reduce the pain and help the patient cope with the pain.

Bupivacaine is the LA most commonly used for epidural analgesia and is usually administered in combination with either fentanyl or PF morphine as a continuous infusion. The concentration of bupivacaine used for epidural analgesia usually ranges between 1/16% (0.065 mg/mL) and 1/8% (1.25 mg/mL). These concentrations are significantly lower than those used for surgical anesthesia, which usually range between 1/4% and 1/2% bupivacaine. The type and concentration of opioid used in combination with bupivacaine vary by practitioner and organizational preferences, but usually range between 2 and 5 mcg/mL fentanyl or between 0.02 and 0.04 mg/mL PF morphine. Ropivacaine, an LA alternative to bupivacaine, has less potential for creating motor block. For older adults with rib fractures or flail chest, an epidural catheter with LA only may provide positive results with less respiratory compromise and reduced pain.

Side Effects

The side effects accompanying LAs are a direct result of the conduction blockade produced by the agents. Unfortunately, the LA agents are relatively nonspecific in their capacity to block nerve conduction. That is, LAs not only block sensory afferent fibers, but also can block the conduction of motor efferent and autonomic nerve fibers within the same dermatomal regions. Side effects associated with epidural LAs include hypotension—especially postural hypotension from sympathetic blockade—and functional motor deficits from varying degrees of efferent motor fiber blockade. Sensory deficits, including changes in proprioception in the joints of the lower extremities, can accompany epidural LA administration due to the blockade of non-nociceptive sensory afferents.

The extent and type of side effects that can be anticipated with epidural LAs depend on three primary factors: (1) the location of the epidural catheter, (2) the concentration of the LA administered, and (3) the volume or rate of infusion; for example, if a patient has an epidural catheter placed within the midthoracic region, one may anticipate signs of sympathetic nervous blockade, such as postural hypotension, because the sympathetic nerve fibers are concentrated in the thoracic region. In contrast, a patient with a lumbar catheter may experience a mild degree of motor weakness in the lower extremities because the motor efferent nerves exit the spine in the lumbar region. This usually presents clinically as either heaviness in a lower extremity or an inability to "lock" the knee in place when standing. Urinary retention may occur and in some cases, may be an indication for catheterization.

Both the concentration and infusion rate of the LA influence the severity and extent of side effects. The density of the blockade and intensity of observed side effects may be increased with high LA concentrations. With higher infusion volumes, greater spread of the LA can be anticipated which in turn may lead to a greater number or extent of side effects. If side effects occur, the dose of the LA often is reduced either by decreasing the concentration of the solution or by decreasing the rate. Additionally, low-dose vasopressors may be used to counteract hypotension caused by LA.

Titrating Epidural Analgesia

To maximize epidural analgesia, doses may need to be adjusted. With opioids alone, the dose needed to produce effective analgesia is best predicted by the patients' response as opposed to body size. Older adults typically require lower doses to achieve pain relief than those who are younger. Small bolus doses of fentanyl (eg, 50 mcg) may help safely titrate the epidural dose or infusion to treat pain. Similarly, a small bolus dose of fentanyl may also help treat breakthrough pain that occurs with increased patient activity or procedures. For patients receiving combinations of LAs and opioids, a small bolus dose of the prescribed infusate in conjunction with an increased rate can produce pain relief. Recall, that increasing the rate of the LA infusion increases the spread of the medication to additional dermatomes, whereas increasing the LA concentration increases the depth or intensity of the blockade and subsequent analgesia.

NON-PHARMACOLOGICAL PAIN MANAGEMENT

Cutaneous stimulation

One of the primary nonpharmacologic techniques for pain management used in the critical care setting is cutaneous stimulation. Cutaneous stimulation produces an analgesic effect by altering conduction of sensory impulses as they move from the periphery to the spinal cord through the stimulation of the largest sensory afferent fibers, known as the A-alpha (α) and A-beta (β) fibers. The sensory information transmitted by these large fibers is conducted more rapidly than that carried by their smaller counterparts (A-delta [δ] and C fibers) (see Figure 6-3). As a result, nociceptive input from the A-delta and C fibers can be preempted by the sensory input from the non-noxious cutaneous stimuli. Examples of cutaneous stimulation include the application of heat, cold, vibration, or massage. Transcutaneous electrical nerve stimulation (TENS) units produce similar effects by electrically stimulating large sensory fibers.

Cutaneous stimulation can produce analgesic effects whether used as a complementary modality with other pharmacologic treatments or as an independent treatment modality. Nurses can integrate these modalities easily and safely into analgesic treatment plans for the critically ill, especially for patients who are unable to tolerate higher opioid doses. To apply or administer cutaneous stimulation, one simply needs to stimulate sensory fibers anywhere between the site of injury and the spinal cord, but within the sensory dermatome (Figure 6-6). Massage, especially back massage, has additional analgesic benefits; it has been shown to promote relaxation and sleep, both of which can influence patients' responses to pain.

Distraction

Distraction techniques such as music, conversation, television viewing, laughter, and deep breathing for relaxation can be valuable adjuncts to pharmacologic modalities. These techniques produce their analgesic effects by sending intense stimuli through the thalamus, midbrain, and brain stem, which can increase the production of modulating substances such as endorphins. Also, because the brain can process only a limited number of incoming signals at any given time, the input provided by distraction techniques "competes" with nociceptive inputs. This is particularly true for the reticular activating system.

When planning for and using distraction techniques, keep in mind that they are most effective when activities are interesting to the patient (e.g., their favorite type of music, television program, or video) and when they involve multiple senses such as hearing, vision, touch, and movement. Flexible selection of activities that are consistent with patients' energy levels and changing requirements is essential for good outcomes.

Imagery

Imagery is another technique that can be used effectively with critically ill patients, particularly during planned

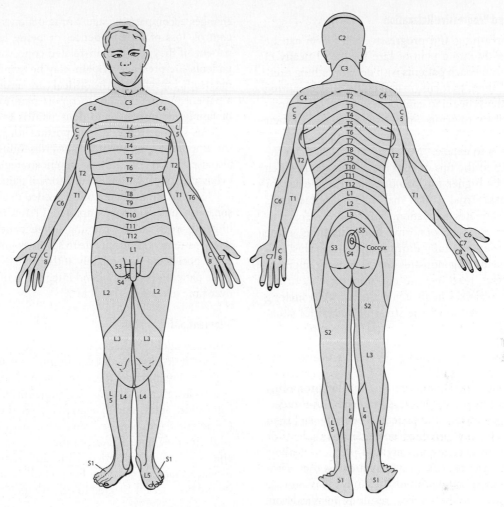

Figure 6-6. Sensory dermatomes.

procedures. Imagery alters the perception of pain stimuli, promotes relaxation, and increases the production of endorphins in the brain. Patients can use imagery independently or use guided imagery where a care provider, family member, or friend helps "guide" the patient in painting an imaginary picture. There are also audio recordings of guided imagery techniques that can be downloaded or played through a personal device. The more details pictured with the image, the more effective it can be. As with distraction techniques, tapping into multiple sensations is beneficial. Some patients prefer to involve the pain in their picture and imagine it melting or fading away. Other patients may prefer to paint a picture in their mind of a favorite place or activity. Strategies to help guide patients include the use of details to describe the imaginary scene (eg, "smell the fresh scent of the ocean air" or "see the intense red hue of the sun setting beyond the snow-capped mountains") and the use of relaxing sensory terms such as *floating, smooth, dissolving, lighter,* or *melting.* If patients can talk, it is helpful to have them describe the image they see using appropriate detail, although some patients will prefer not to talk and instead focus on their evolving image. Again, it is important to be flexible in the approach to imagery in order to maximize its benefits.

Relaxation techniques

Because critically ill patients experience numerous stressors and may have previously experienced tension or anxiety, many patients benefit from the inclusion of relaxation or anxiolytics. The use of relaxation techniques can help interrupt the vicious cycle involving pain, anxiety, and muscle tension that often develops when pain goes unrelieved. The physiologic response associated with relaxation includes decreased oxygen consumption, respiratory rate, heart rate, and muscle tension; blood pressure may either normalize or decrease.

A wide variety of pharmacologic and nonpharmacologic techniques can be used safely and effectively with critically ill patients to achieve relaxation and/or sedation. Relaxation techniques are simple to use and may be particularly useful in situations involving brief procedures such as turning or minor dressing changes, and following coughing or endotracheal suctioning or other stressful events.

Deep Breathing and Progressive Relaxation

Guided deep breathing and progressive relaxation can be incorporated easily into a plan of care for the critically ill patient. Nurses can coach patients with deep breathing exercises by helping them to focus on and guide their breathing patterns. As patients begin to control their breathing, nurses can work with them to begin progressive relaxation of their muscles. To do this, the nurse can say to the patient as he or she just begins to exhale, "Now begin to relax, from the top of your head to the tips of your toes." Change the pitch of the voice to be higher for "top of your head," lower for "tips of your toes." Time it such that the final phrase ends as the patient completes exhalation. This procedure capitalizes on the positive aspects of normal body functions, as the body tends to relax naturally during exhalation. This process is practiced during nonstressful periods to augment its efficacy. In fact, teaching and coaching patients to use deep breathing exercises helps equip them with a lifelong skill that may be used any time stressful or painful situations arise.

Presence

Probably the single most important aspect of promoting comfort in the critically ill or injured patient is the underlying relationship between the patient, the family, and their care providers. Family presence at the patient's bedside has been shown to decrease anxiety and promote healing. Including the people identified by the patient as their family support (with a broad definition of family) may provide enormous comfort for the patient, resulting in relaxation. *Presence* refers not only to physically "being there," but also to psychologically "being with" a patient. Although presence has not been well defined as an intervention to promote comfort, patients have described the importance of nurses simply "being there" and "being with" them.

SPECIAL CONSIDERATIONS FOR PAIN MANAGEMENT IN OLDER ADULTS

Misperceptions about older adult's experience of pain abound. Some believe that older adults have less pain because their extensive life experiences have equipped them to cope with discomfort more effectively. This may be true for some individuals but to accept this as fact for all older adults is short sighted and incorrect. In fact, the incidence of and morbidity associated with pain is higher in older adults than in the general population. Many older adults continue to experience chronic pain in addition to any acute pain associated with their critical illness or injury. Major sources of underlying pain in older adults include low back pain, arthritis, headache, chest pain, and neuropathies.

Assessment

Older adults often report pain very differently from younger patients due to physiologic, psychological, and cultural changes accompanying age. Some patients may fear loss of control, loss of independence, or being labeled as a "bad patient" if they report pain-related concerns. Also, for some patients the presence of pain may be symbolic of impending death, especially in the critical care setting. In such cases, a patient may be reticent to report pain to a care provider or family member as if to deny pain is to deny death. For reasons such as these, it is important for nurses to explain the importance of reporting any discomfort. Nurses may also use a variety of pain assessment strategies to incorporate behavioral or physiologic indicators of pain.

Similar strategies are often needed to assess pain in persons who are cognitively impaired. Preliminary reports from ongoing work among nursing home patients suggest that many patients with moderate to severe cognitive impairment can report acute pain reliably at the time they are asked. For these patients, pain recall and integration of pain experience over time may be less reliable.

Interventions

Critically ill older adults can benefit from any of the analgesic modalities discussed. Older adults may tolerate opioids if the doses are individualized, and the patient is monitored for effect. However, medication requirements may be reduced in some older adults due to age-related renal insufficiency and the potential for decreased renal clearance of medications. In addition, they have a reduced muscle-to-body fat ratio that affects the way that opioids bind and activate in the body. Analgesic requirements are highly individualized, and doses should be carefully titrated to achieve pain relief.

Principles of Pain Management

- Pain is a common occurrence in critically ill patients either from trauma, surgery, procedures, and/or painful comorbidity.
- It is important to assess and treat pain on a regular basis so that adequate pain relief may be provided.
- Pain can be effectively managed by using a combination of pain relief options including medications, interventional techniques, and nonpharmacologic methods.
- Older adults require special attention during pain assessment as they may misunderstand the goals of pain management and be reticent about reporting pain.

SEDATION

A holistic, patient-centered approach to sedation in the critical care environment recognizes that agitation and sedation are interrelated with clinical concerns such as pain, delirium, immobility, and sleep. This constellation of issues and consequences are so connected that in 2018, the Society of Critical Care Medicine updated previous guidelines addressing pain, agitation, and delirium to include recommendations that address immobility and sleep as well (the PADIS guidelines introduced in the previous section). The PADIS guidelines, as well as the accompanying ICU Liberation Bundle (ABCDEF Bundle—see Figure 6-7), represent best practices at the time of this publication, and further research is ongoing.

The critical care environment can be uncomfortable and anxiety provoking for patients. Once pain is addressed, anxiolysis may be appropriate to enhance comfort, decrease anxiety or agitation, and induce sleep. In some situations, the use of sedatives may be necessary to ensure tolerance of medical interventions, achieve clinical stability, or protect patients from inadvertent self-harm. While the treatment of anxiety is an important aspect of critical care, frequent dosing methods (infusions or IV boluses) intended to induce a depressed sensorium (ie, amnesia) are discouraged. Decisions about sedation must consider benefits and risks. For

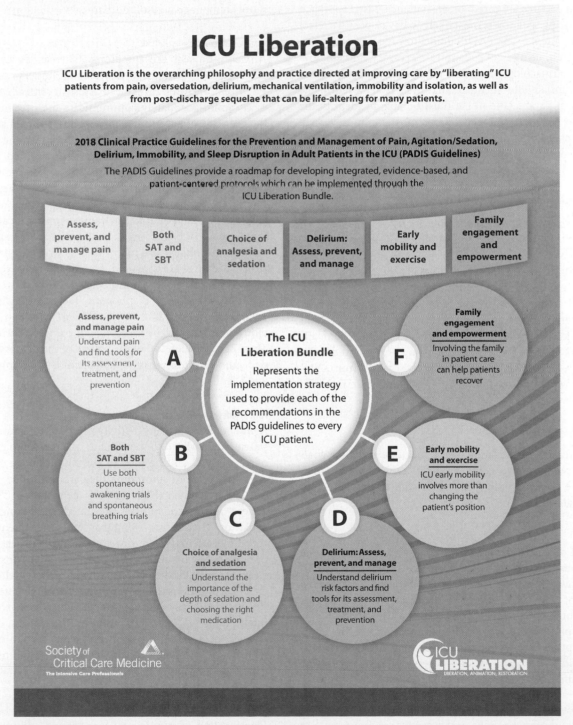

Figure 6-7. ABCEDF bundle from Liberation ICU. (© 2020 Society of Critical Care Medicine The Society of Critical Care Medicine and SCCM are registered trademarks of the Society of Critical Care Medicine.)

instance, sedation with benzodiazepines is associated with delirium, may be correlated with sleep disruption, and oversedation may prevent patients from mobilizing.

The use of sedation infusions in mechanically ventilated patients has been associated with negative outcomes such as prolonged mechanical ventilation, increased lengths of stay, and even death. Further, there is a strong association between benzodiazepine infusion use and delirium. As a result, in critical care and progressive care units where mechanically ventilated patients are cared for, an evidence-based approach of minimizing sedation is most likely to have a positive effect for these patients. The PADIS guidelines recommend treating pain first, using light sedation if necessary, and employing nonpharmacologic means of promoting sleep. To ensure that appropriate and adequate anxiolysis is achieved in the critically ill patient, the nurse must be able to identify the reason for sedation, the medications most commonly used, the level of sedation required, and how to monitor and manage the sedated patient. Clear identification of the reason for sedation is the first step in the process.

Analgosedation

Evidence-based patient care should focus on preventing or treating the cause of a patient's agitation, if possible, before using sedative medications. The previous sections of this chapter have emphasized the necessity of adequate pain management and a variety of options for pain relief. Since pain is a frequent cause for agitation, the PADIS guidelines recommend treating pain before a sedative agent is considered. Analgosedation is a strategy for mechanically ventilated patients that prioritizes pain control and analgesia use, reserving sedative agents for "rescue" from agitation that remains after the maximum opioid dose has been administered.

Reasons for Sedation

A clear reason for sedation helps to guide sedation goals and choice of sedative agent. As stated above, light sedation should be targeted unless there is a clinical indication for deep sedation.

Amnesia

The goal of attaining amnesia is appropriate in the case of procedures, surgery, and other invasive critical care interventions. However, when used to create amnesia for extended lengths of time (>24 hours), patients may experience the negative outcomes described previously. Amnesia may not be an appropriate reason for prolonged sedation use, the absolute exception being when neuromuscular blockade (NMB) is required. When paralytics are necessary, it is essential that both comfort (with analgesics) and sedation are ensured.

Ventilator Tolerance

Ineffective, dyssynchronous, and excessive respiratory efforts result in increased work of breathing and increased oxygen consumption. The reason for the dyssynchronous breathing should be quickly assessed and managed. Efforts are made to improve tolerance by first treating potential pain and adjusting the ventilator to optimize patient-ventilator interaction. Sedative use in the form of infusions or frequent IV bolus dosing in severe cases of patient/ventilator dyssynchrony may be necessary and in some cases lifesaving (see Chapter 5, Airway and Ventilatory Management and Chapter 20, Advanced Respiratory Concepts: Modes of Ventilation, for more on management of mechanical ventilation).

Anxiety and Fear

Anxiety and fear are symptoms that can be experienced by critically ill patients who are conscious. However, these symptoms are often difficult to assess in critically ill patients who cannot adequately communicate their feelings, due to the presence of an artificial airway, or a reduced sensorium. When the patient can identify anxiety or fear, the treatment goals are clear. Treatment of patient-identified anxiety is appropriate and rarely results in adverse effects. Generally, the sedatives are provided orally. The doses are adjusted to prevent excessive drowsiness or respiratory depression. However, in the patient who cannot communicate anxiety, the presence of behaviors and signs that are associated with anxiety and/or fear are often used as evidence and are the reason sedatives are provided. Manifestations of severe anxiety and/or fear include nonspecific signs of distress such as agitation, thrashing, diaphoresis, facial grimacing, blood pressure elevation, and increased heart rate. These nonspecific signs may also be indicative of pain or delirium. Thus, an in-depth evaluation of the source of the distress (eg, pain, delirium, etc) is essential if the patient is to be appropriately and adequately treated.

Patient Safety and Agitation

Agitation includes any activity that appears unhelpful or potentially harmful to the patient. The patient may be aware of the activity and be able to communicate the reason for the activity; more commonly they are not aware, making it difficult to identify the reason for the agitation. The patient appears distressed, and the associated activity includes episodic or continuous nonpurposeful movements, severe thrashing, attempts to remove tubes, efforts to get out of bed, or other behaviors which may threaten patient or staff safety. Reasons for agitation include pain and anxiety, delirium, preexisting conditions that require pharmacologic interventions (ie, preexisting psychiatric history), withdrawal from certain medications (eg, benzodiazepines), illicit drugs, or alcohol (see Chapter 11, Multisystem Problems, section on alcohol withdrawal). All potential reasons for the agitation should be explored so that appropriate therapy may be initiated.

Goals and Management of Sedation

Identification of a clear goal for sedation administration is important to determine the appropriate approach. The goal should include a target level of sedation. For example, in the patient who is anxious and unable to sleep, the goal is very different than for the patient who is unstable, on a ventilator, and suffering from profound hypoxemia.

Monitoring Sedation

Sedation scales have been developed to assist with the management of sedation and are helpful tools for the bedside clinician. Sedation scales allow the healthcare team to select a target level of sedation for the patient and assess the patient's response to a sedative. Descriptors of each level of sedation are provided so that the sedative may be adjusted appropriately. Sedation monitoring should be done routinely and frequently, and the level of sedation achieved should be recorded. Use of a valid and reliable sedation assessment scale is recommended (Table 6-7). The two scales endorsed by the PADIS guidelines are the Richmond Agitation Sedation Scale (RASS) and Sedation Agitation Scale (SAS). While not endorsed for all patients, objective sedation monitoring tools such as Bispectral index (BIS) monitoring may be helpful in sedative titration, especially when a sedative scale cannot be used (such as during NMB). It is important for the interdisciplinary team to determine the goal and level of sedation prior to beginning sedation and, in situations of ongoing sedation, readdress the goal at least daily.

Management of Short-Term Moderate Sedation

A technique referred to as "moderate sedation" (also known as conscious or procedural sedation) is commonly used to facilitate a non-intubated patient's tolerance of invasive procedures. In the critical care unit, procedures may occur at the bedside or in special procedural areas. Moderate sedation uses a combination of analgesics and sedatives to minimize discomfort during a procedure while assuring that the patient can communicate and maintain ventilation throughout the procedure. Amnesia is anticipated and often desired. The patient's ability to maintain a patent airway is central to the decision to use moderate sedation. Patients considered "lowest risk" are generally those who are recommended for the technique, although higher-risk individuals may also undergo moderate sedation based on consultation with the healthcare team. The American Society of Anesthesiology (ASA) Patient Classification Status is used to guide level of sedation (Table 6-8). Institutional guidelines for the use of moderate sedation vary somewhat, however, they generally follow ASA recommendations and include the use of continuous real-time monitoring such as respiratory rate and pattern, pulse oximetry, capnography, and heart rhythm in addition to very frequent (ie, every 5 minutes during the procedure) assessment of vital signs and evaluation of sedation level. Personnel on the team performing moderate sedation should be prepared to rescue the patient from a deeper-than-intended level of sedation.

Management of Continuous Sedation

In patients who require continuous sedation (eg, during mechanical ventilation for >24 hours), best practice recommends targeting light sedation as opposed to deep sedation. Light sedation is associated with improved outcomes such as shorter time to extubation and shorter ICU length of stay. Two recommended techniques for achieving light sedation goals are daily sedative interruption (DSI) and nurse-protocolized targeted sedation. A DSI, also known as a spontaneous awakening trial (SAT), is a planned period of time each day when sedative infusions are discontinued to allow the patient to become alert. Usually, the aim is to achieve a SAS score of 4 to 5 or a RASS score of −1 to 0 (see Table 6-7). DSI prompts the reevaluation of a patient's true sedation

TABLE 6-7. SEDATION ASSESSMENT SCALES WITH VALIDITY AND RELIABILITY IN ADULT PATIENTS

Sedation-Agitation Scale[a]	Richmond Agitation-Sedation Scale[b]
1 Unarousable (minimal or no response to noxious stimuli, does not communicate or follow commands)	− 5 Unresponsive (no response to voice or physical stimulation)
2 Very sedated (arouses to physical stimuli but does not communicate or follow commands; may move spontaneously)	− 4 Deep sedation (no response to voice, but any movement to physical stimulation)
3 Sedated (difficult to arouse, awakens to verbal stimuli or gentle shaking but drifts off again, follows simple commands)	− 3 Moderate sedation (any movement, but no eye contact to voice)
4 Calm and cooperative (calm, awakens easily, follows commands)	− 2 Light sedation (briefly, <10 seconds, awakening with eye contact to voice)
5 Agitated (anxious or mildly agitated, attempting to sit up, calms down to verbal instructions)	− 1 Drowsy (not fully alert, but has sustained, >10 seconds, awakening with eye contact to voice)
6 Very agitated (does not calm, despite frequent verbal reminding of limits; requires physical restraints, biting ET tube)	0 Alert and calm
7 Dangerous agitation (pulling at ET tube, trying to remove catheter, climbing over bed rail, striking at staff, thrashing side to side)	1 Restless (anxious or apprehensive but movements not aggressive or vigorous)
	2 Agitated (frequent nonpurposeful movement or patient-ventilator dyssynchrony)
	3 Very agitated (pulls on or removes tubes or catheters or has aggressive behavior toward staff)
	4 Combative (overly combative or violent; immediate danger to staff)

Data compiled from:
[a]Riker R, Picard J, Fraser G, et al (1994).
[b]Sessler C, Gosnet M, Grap MJ, et al (2002).

TABLE 6-8.   ASA CONTINUUM OF DEPTH OF SEDATION: DEFINITION OF GENERAL ANESTHESIA AND LEVELS OF SEDATION/ANALGESIA

	Minimal Sedation (Anxiolysis)	Moderate Sedation/Analgesia (Conscious Sedation)	Deep Sedation/Analgesia	General Anesthesia
Responsiveness	Normal response to verbal stimulation	Purposeful[a] response to verbal or tactile stimulation	Purposeful[a] response after repeated or painful stimulation	Unarousable, even with painful stimulus
Airway	Unaffected	No intervention required	Intervention may be required	Intervention often required
Spontaneous ventilation	Unaffected	Adequate	May be inadequate	Frequently inadequate
Cardiovascular function	Unaffected	Usually maintained	Usually maintained	May be impaired

Minimal Sedation (Anxiolysis) = a drug-induced state during which patients respond normally to verbal commands. Although cognitive function and coordination may be impaired, ventilatory and cardiovascular functions are unaffected.

Moderate Sedation/Analgesia (Conscious Sedation) = a drug-induced depression of consciousness during which patients respond purposefully[a] to verbal commands, either alone or accompanied by light tactile stimulation. No interventions are required to maintain a patent airway, and spontaneous ventilation is adequate. Cardiovascular function is usually maintained.

Deep Sedation/Analgesia = a drug-induced depression of consciousness during which patients cannot be easily aroused but respond purposefully[a] following repeated or painful stimulation. The ability to independently maintain ventilatory function may be impaired. Patients may require assistance in maintaining a patent airway, and spontaneous ventilation may be inadequate. Cardiovascular function is usually maintained.

General Anesthesia = a drug-induced loss of consciousness during which patients are not arousable, even by painful stimulation. The ability to independently maintain ventilatory function is often impaired. Patients often require assistance in maintaining a patent airway, and positive pressure ventilation may be required because of depressed spontaneous ventilation or drug-induced depression of neuromuscular function. Cardiovascular function may be impaired.

Since sedation is a continuum, it is not always possible to predict how an individual patient will respond. Hence, practitioners intending to produce a given level of sedation should be able to rescue patients whose level of sedation becomes deeper than initially intended. Individuals administering Moderate Sedation/Analgesia (Conscious Sedation) should be able to rescue patients who enter a state of Deep Sedation/Analgesia, while those administering Deep Sedation/Analgesia should be able to rescue patients who enter a state of general anesthesia.

[a]Reflex withdrawal from a painful stimulus is not considered a purposeful response.

Reproduced with permission from American Society of Anesthesiologists Task Force on Sedation and Analgesia by Non-Anesthesiologists: Practice guidelines for sedation and analgesia by non-anesthesiologists, Anesthesiology 2002;96(4):1004-1017.

needs, as sedation is restarted (usually at a lower dose such as half of previous rate) only if the patient demonstrates an indication for it. Nurse-protocolized sedation is the use of an established protocol by nurses at the bedside to determine sedative choices and titrate them to a prescribed target. Many protocols combine both nurse-protocolized sedation using targets and DSI.

In certain clinical situations, it may be appropriate to target continuous deep sedation for mechanically ventilated patients. Deep sedation may be necessary to help patients tolerate therapies such as targeted temperature management, prone positioning, or NMB, or to reduce a patient's respiratory drive and promote ventilator synchrony. However, deep sedation is associated with poor patient outcomes. Thus, the use of continuous deep sedation should be re-evaluated frequently to ensure it is only used for the shortest amount of time that is needed.

Sedative Medications

After ensuring that the presence of pain is either ruled out or addressed with the appropriate administration of analgesics, sedatives may be selected based on patient-specific factors such as the level and duration of sedation required. The choice of which sedative is used for an individual patient is so important that the "C" in the ABCDEF bundle is devoted to "Choice of Analgesia & Sedation." It is important for critical care nurses to understand the difference between various sedatives for appropriate patient monitoring and to support evidence-based sedative choices. Summaries of various sedative categories follow, and comprehensive descriptions of the medications are found in Chapter 7, Pharmacology.

Benzodiazepines

These sedatives are used to decrease anxiety and induce amnesia; they also have anticonvulsant properties (see Chapter 7). While there may be specific situations, such as alcohol withdrawal when benzodiazepines are indicated, the PADIS guidelines emphasize that propofol or dexmedetomidine are first-line agents and should be chosen over benzodiazepines for sedation for most critically ill patients. In general, the use of benzodiazepines in critical care patients should be avoided unless there is a specific indication or a circumstance in which no other alternative is available. Patients who do receive them require close monitoring for respiratory depression and oversedation.

- *Midazolam* is a popular benzodiazepine with a rapid onset of action and a short duration of effect. It can be administered intermittently in a bolus IV form or as a continuous infusion. Long-term infusions (>24 hours) of midazolam are discouraged because it has an active metabolite that may accumulate in the presence of other medications, renal disease, liver disease, or advanced age.
- *Lorazepam* has an intermediate onset of action and duration of effect when given orally or in a bolus intermittent form; however, when used as a continuous infusion (>24 hours) its effect is more long term (and it should be considered as such) because awakening may take hours to days to accomplish.
- *Diazepam*, a long-acting benzodiazepine, is not often used in critical care; however, it may be selected for treatment of alcohol withdrawal. It may be given orally or as an IV bolus.

Propofol

Propofol is an IV general anesthetic designed for use in the critical care unit as a continuous infusion. This medication is often preferred for short-term sedation use (ie, <24 hours) and when a very rapid onset of effect is desired. Propofol is lipid-based and serves as a source of calories. It is used cautiously in those with high triglycerides and is contraindicated in those with egg allergies. Frequent changes of the containers and tubing are required to prevent potential growth of microorganisms. Patients receiving propofol should be monitored for respiratory depression and hypotension (due to vasodilation). Propofol Infusion Syndrome (PRIS) is a rare but serious complication with various effects that include metabolic acidosis, hypotension, hypertriglyceridemia, and arrhythmias. The current evidence-based guidelines recommend the use of propofol or dexmedetomidine (discussed next) over sedation with benzodiazepines (either midazolam or lorazepam) to improve outcomes in mechanically ventilated patients, and propofol over benzodiazepines specifically in mechanically ventilated patients after cardiac surgery.

Dexmedetomidine

Dexmedetomidine is a centrally acting alpha-2 receptor agonist that has sedative and anesthetic properties. The major benefit of this agent is the fact that it does not produce respiratory depression when used as designed (ie, boluses are not recommended). Further, patients on dexmedetomidine are rapidly arousable and alert when stimulated. Bradycardia and hypotension may be dose-limiting side effects, and this medication alone will not provide adequate sedation when deep sedation is indicated (eg, during NMB). A study of mechanically ventilated ICU patients with sepsis showed that light sedation with dexmedetomidine offered equivalent patient outcomes to light sedation with propofol. Further study of sedation selection in critically ill patients is needed.

Ketamine

Ketamine is an IV general anesthetic that produces analgesia, anesthesia, and amnesia without loss of consciousness. It may be given intravenously, intranasally, or orally. Although contraindicated in patients with elevated intracranial pressure (ICP), its bronchodilatory properties make it a good choice in those with asthma. A well-known side effect of ketamine is hallucinations; however, these may be prevented with concurrent use of benzodiazepines. Ketamine can increase oral secretions. It is rarely a first-line sedative of choice but is commonly used as an opioid adjunct or for patients requiring painful, frequent procedures (eg, burn care). The nurse should be aware of hospital policy for use of this medication as some hospitals allow it only in specific circumstances.

Sedation Considerations During Drug Shortages

During the COVID-19 pandemic, intensive care units experience surges of high numbers of patients who require sedation, analgesia, and NMB. Some patients with severe ARDS require deep sedation and NMB to manage their respiratory drive even after ventilator settings were optimized. At the same time, the pandemic also creates uncertainty in the supply of medications, and shortages can be a common occurrence. Strategies to conserve medication supplies are needed and understanding of the various half-lives and properties of medications is crucial when patients are switched from one sedative or analgesic to another because of supply issues.

With propofol and dexmedetomidine being the preferred sedatives for mechanically ventilated patients to reduce delirium, a proposed strategy is to reserve propofol for patients requiring deep sedation, using dexmedetomidine for patients managed with light sedation. Other strategies include the use of alternative sedatives such as ketamine or benzodiazepines. Ketamine may also be used as an adjunct sedative to decrease the doses of other sedative infusions, and clonidine can be used as an adjunct to facilitate weaning from dexmedetomidine. Additional conservation strategies that are not currently well studied may include the use of enteral formulations to reduce intravenous sedative requirements, and use of sedative medications such as phenobarbital or inhaled anesthetic agents.

Issues Related to Sedation

Delirium

Delirium is said to be present in 50% to 80% of critically ill patients. Patients are especially at risk if they are older, have preexisting dementia, have a high severity of illness at admission, or have pre-ICU trauma or surgery. Modifiable risks include benzodiazepine use and blood transfusion. As noted earlier, the risk of worse outcomes, increased ICU length of stay, and long-term cognitive dysfunction is increased in patients who experience delirium. There are three types of presentations for delirium: hyperactive, hypoactive, and mixed presentation. In the past, delirium was commonly associated only with agitation. In fact, in medical ICUs the agitated presentation of delirium accounts for a minority of those who experience the condition. The remainder present with the hypoactive (calm, quiet) or mixed presentation of the condition. This hypoactive category is underdiagnosed and the associated outcomes are worse than for those with the agitated/active form of delirium. The hallmarks of the condition are disorientation and disorganized thinking.

Awareness of the potential for delirium and early recognition are essential for effective management and prevention of undesirable outcomes. Routine assessment for delirium should include the use of a valid and reliable tool such as Brief Confusion Assessment Method (bCAM) and Confusion Assessment Method for Intensive Care Units (CAM-ICU).

In the past, the most commonly used medication for the prevention and treatment of delirium in critical care units was haloperidol. Haloperidol provides sedation without significant respiratory depression and is not associated with potential development of tolerance or dependence. It, however, has potential adverse side effects that must be closely monitored. Extrapyramidal reactions such as dystonia and neuroleptic malignant syndrome are possible. Another adverse effect of haloperidol is prolonged QTc intervals; QTc interval monitoring is essential in patients receiving this medication. PADIS guidelines recommend against the routine use of haloperidol or HMG-CoA reductase inhibitors (ie, statins) to prevent or treat delirium. The guidelines do leave room for the use of a short-term atypical antipsychotic such as haloperidol for patients experiencing significant distress or agitation because of delirium. They should be used for behavioral control only and for the shortest duration at the lowest dose. The guidelines also suggest dexmedetomidine for delirium in patients whose agitation is preventing extubation (see Chapter 7, Pharmacology for more on these classes of medications).

Best practice related to delirium is to implement a bundle of nonpharmacologic interventions aimed to prevent delirium, such as the previously mentioned ABCDEF bundle. Examples of nonpharmacologic components of a bundle include early mobility, family involvement in care, cognitive stimulation such as reorientation, correction of sensory deficits with glasses and hearing aids, and ensuring adequate sleep and wakefulness. Further research on medication and nonpharmacologic interventions to reduce the incidence and severity of delirium is needed.

Sleep Disruption

Sleep disruption is common among critically ill patients (see Table 6-9). Although patients may appear restful, physiologically they may never experience stages of sleep that provide a restorative state (ie, rapid eye movement sleep, stage 3 slow wave sleep). These restorative stages of sleep are adversely affected by many factors, including a wide variety of medications. Sleep deprivation is also common among those with pain, discomfort, and anxiety. Additionally, sleep fragmentation may be a result of the increased auditory, tactile, and visual stimuli ubiquitous to the critical care environment. The PADIS guidelines recommend the use of nonpharmacologic interventions and environmental adjustment when possible. In some patients, pharmacologic sleep aids may be prescribed; however, the guidelines make no recommendation for a specific class or drug to be used and instead suggest that multicomponent sleep protocols to be used. Sleep promotion may be helpful in preventing or ameliorating Post-Intensive Care Syndrome (PICS).

NEUROMUSCULAR BLOCKADE

The use of NMB in the critical care unit is generally confined to severe situations where management with analgesics and sedatives is not enough to ensure desired outcomes.

TABLE 6-9. ADDRESSING SLEEP DISRUPTION

Type of Disruption	Examples	Strategies for addressing
Environmental factors: external features of the hospital room or unit that interfere with sleep	• Noise, light, bad odors, uncomfortable bed • Visitors, sound from hand hygiene	• Identify specific "quiet times" in which noise and light are reduced • Collaborate with family to prioritize patient sleep and schedule visits accordingly • Use pillows for positioning in bed
Physiological factors: elements of the patient's internal environment that interfere with sleep	• Discomfort (pain, nausea, trouble breathing, feeling too hot or too cold) • Coughing • Thirst and hunger • Needing to use bedpan or urinal	• Assess for discomfort, including pain, nausea, and shortness of breath before initiating quiet time for sleep • Assess patient's comfort with temperature and add or remove blankets • Provide oral care before "quiet time" starts • Offer urinal/bedpan before "quiet time"
Psychological factors: factors related to the patient's state of mind that interfere with sleep	• Worry, anxiety, stress, fear, loneliness • Unfamiliar environment • Disorientation to time • Lack of privacy • Missing bedtime routine • Not knowing nurses' names and not understanding medical terms	• Offer reassurance; reorient to time, place, plan of care, your name and role in care, and the plan for family presence, if applicable • Provide privacy when possible, using curtains, doors, and bed covers • Ask family about familiar routines that can be replicated or important items to place at bedside for reassurance
Patient care: activities by the healthcare team that can interfere with sleep	• Nursing care and medication administration • Procedures and diagnostic tests • Vital sign checks • Restricted mobility from lines/catheters/monitors • Respiratory devices: oxygen mask, endotracheal tube	• Cluster nursing care activities to reduce the number of night-time interruptions • Collaborate with the healthcare team to identify a safe frequency of patient assessment and vital-sign checks that respects patient's need for sleep and to plan procedures and tests for daytime hours when possible • Prior to quiet time initiation, position catheters, lines, and monitor wires to allow for movement in bed

Data from Devlin JW, Skrobik Y, Gélinas C, et al: Clinical Practice Guidelines for the Prevention and Management of Pain, Agitation/Sedation, Delirium, Immobility, and Sleep Disruption in Adult Patients in the ICU. Crit Care Med. 2018;46(9):e825-e873.

In these cases, the patient's muscular movements contribute to hemodynamic, pulmonary, and/or neurologic instability and NMB may be a lifesaving intervention. NMB may be indicated for treatment of ventilated patients with ARDS or acute severe asthma (ASA) if ventilator optimization strategies are not tolerated or fail to relieve refractory hypoxemia (see Chapter 20, Advanced Respiratory Concepts: Modes of Ventilation). NMB may prevent patient-ventilator dyssynchrony, improve oxygenation, and reduce the risk of barotrauma. Additional clinical indications for NMB include rapid sequence intubation, management of shivering during targeted temperature management (ie, for neurologic protection after cardiac arrest) and to control elevated intracranial or intra-abdominal pressure.

The decision to use NMB is individualized, weighing the benefits against the risks to the patient. For the purposes described, the use of NMB agents may be lifesaving and is an important part of care. However, risks of NMB include ICU-acquired neuropathies and myopathies (especially in patients who are also receiving glucocorticoids), increased duration of mechanical ventilation, awareness during paralysis, inability to assess neurologic status, and complications of immobility. Thus, NMB agents should be used sparingly and only in the most severe situations.

Neuromuscular Blocking Agents

The most common neuromuscular blocking agents used in critical care are the nondepolarizing agents (see Chapter 7, Pharmacology, for a comprehensive discussion of chemical paralytic agents). The agents block the transmission of nerve impulses by blocking cholinergic receptors, resulting in muscle paralysis. The degree of blockade varies depending on the dose and the amount of receptor blockade. Examples of short, intermediate, and long-acting NMB agents follow.

Short-Acting NMB

Mivacurium is rapid acting and has a short duration of action (15 minutes). It is a nondepolarizing neuromuscular-blocking medication. It may be given as an IV bolus initially but then is provided by infusion. Mivacurium is metabolized by pseudocholinesterase.

Succinylcholine, the lone depolarizing agent commonly used in critical care, has a very short duration of action (3-5 minutes) and is therefore used for short procedures such as endotracheal intubation. Adverse effects can include hyperkalemia and malignant hyperthermia; it should not be used in patients at risk for hyperkalemia or with underlying neuromuscular disease.

Intermediate-Acting NMB

These agents are rapidly metabolized over approximately 30 to 60 minutes. They may be administered via intravenous bolus as needed or by continuous infusion (it is recommended that an infusion, if used, last 48 hours or less). *Rocuronium*, a steroidal-like medication, may be used for

procedures as an alternative to succinylcholine since it has the shortest onset (45-60 seconds) and duration (30 minutes) of the intermediate-acting agents. It has the potential to exacerbate tachycardia due to inhibition of vagal activity. *Vecuronium*, another steroidal-like agent, is metabolized by the liver and excreted renally. The combination of steroids and vecuronium may contribute to myopathies. *Atracurium* and *cisatracurium* are metabolized in the plasma by Hoffmann elimination and unaffected by liver or kidney function, although hypothermia may slow the elimination process.

Long-Acting NMB

Pancuronium also has a steroidal-like molecular structure. It is generally given by intermittent IV bolus. Although labor intensive to use (the bolus is often required hourly), the intermittent dosing does allow for frequent reassessment. Pancuronium is vagolytic and can cause tachycardia; it may be contraindicated in patients with cardiovascular disease. Pancuronium is metabolized by the liver and is renally excreted.

Reversal Agents

Sugammadex is an NMB reversal agent approved for use in the United States in 2015. It provides rapid and predictable reversal of rocuronium and (to a lesser extent) vecuronium since it binds directly to the agent. *Neostigmine* is the more traditional reversal agent that increases the concentration of acetylcholine in the neuromuscular junction, allowing the acetylcholine to compete with the nondepolarizing NMB agent for receptor sites. An anticholinergic agent (eg, atropine, glycopyrrolate) may be given with neostigmine to prevent parasympathetic-induced bradycardia.

Monitoring and Management

Monitoring NMB is accomplished with clinical assessment along with the use of a peripheral nerve stimulator or by monitoring airway pressure waveforms. Monitoring should guide the titration of NMB infusion or the frequency of NMB bolus doses. The goal is to provide the least amount of medication required so that the patient meets clinical goals and can recover rapidly when NMB is no longer indicated. How these aspects of care and others are managed is essential to ensuring the best possible outcomes.

Peripheral Nerve Stimulation

Peripheral nerve stimulators are devices that deliver a series of electrical stimuli via electrodes to nerves under the skin (Figure 6-8). The electrical stimuli cause muscular contractions if the neuromuscular junction is functioning properly. Typically, peripheral nerve stimulation (PNS) is performed on the ulnar nerve at the wrist, with the temple area of the head as another potential site for nerve stimulation. When electrical stimuli are applied to the ulnar nerve, the thumb abducts and the fingers flex if the neuromuscular junction is intact.

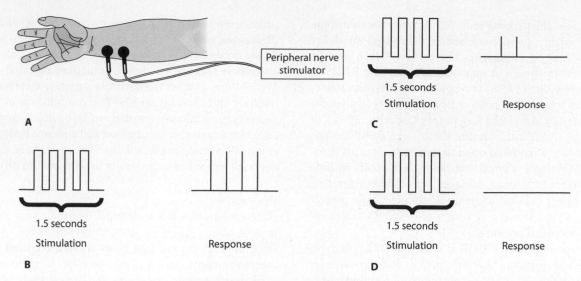

Figure 6-8 **(A)** PNS and graphic display of a train-of-four pattern for: **(B)** no NMB, **(C)** moderate block (80%), and **(D)** complete block.

The stimulator technique most commonly used to assess NMB is the train of four. With this technique, four small electrical stimuli are given every half second. The number of muscle twitches observed or palpated during the series of four electrical stimuli indicates the degree of NMB (see Figure 6-8). When no NMB is present, four twitches of similar intensity, or height, are noted. Following the administration of a nondepolarizing neuromuscular blocking agent, many of the neuromuscular junctions are blocked. This produces minimal response to the four delivered stimuli. As the level of NMB decreases over time, the number of twitches observed increases until four strong, equal twitches are observed, indicating that no NMB is present.

The degree of NMB is approximately 90% when one small twitch is palpated, 80% with two small twitches, and about 75% with three small twitches. Typically, in critical care patients, a moderate blockade level of 75% to 80% (two or three twitches in response to the train of four) indicates a reasonable level of NMB. At this level of blockade, stimulation of the nerve does not result in excessive muscular contraction but saturation (100% block) has not occurred. However, since various factors may influence the response to PNS, the achievement of clinical goals (ie, lack of muscle movements or intrinsic respiratory effort) guides dose titration.

Although PNS is helpful in the short term, it may be less reliable in patients requiring NMB for days. This is especially true when anasarca is present because the increase in edema decreases stimulus transmission. The presence of hypothermia may also influence the accuracy of PNS. It is important to remember that the technique is somewhat uncomfortable and frequent assessments using PNS are avoided if possible.

Airway Pressure Monitoring

Most ventilators provide respiratory waveform graphic displays. The simplest of the waveforms, airway pressure, may be used to monitor patient-generated respiratory activity (Figure 6-9). Regardless of the mode of ventilation, if chemical paralysis is adequate, there is an absence of spontaneous respiratory effort. If a spontaneous effort is noted on the waveform (a negative deflection), the NMB agents may need to be increased. The airway pressure monitoring technique is especially helpful when initiating NMB and to assess reducing or discontinuing it.

Management

Patients who are paralyzed may still experience pain, anxiety, and fear. To that end, it is essential that patients receiving NMB agents be provided with analgesics and sedatives. With

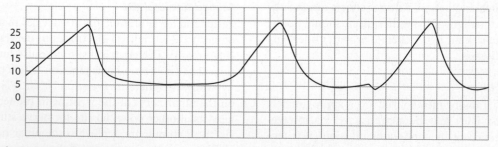

Figure 6-9. Example of spontaneous effort on assist-control volume ventilation. Note negative deflection prior to volume breath indicating inadequate level of NMB. (*Reproduced with permission from Suzanne M. Burns.*)

ESSENTIAL CONTENT CASE

Sedation and Neuromuscular Blockade

A 52-year-old woman with suspected pneumonia and sepsis is admitted to the ICU. She is confused, lethargic, and experiencing respiratory distress. Her pulse oximetry reading is 76%, heart rate 170 (sinus tachycardia), blood pressure 135/87 mm Hg, and respiratory rate 28/min and labored. The team quickly intubates her after induction with IV boluses of fentanyl, midazolam, and succinylcholine. She is ventilated on the assist-control mode: fraction of inspired oxygen (FiO_2) 80%, respiratory rate 15 breaths/min, tidal volume 400 mL, and PEEP 8 cm H_2O. The sepsis bundle and fluid resuscitation are initiated.

Following intubation, the patient's BP decreases to 60/30. Additional intravenous fluids are given, and a norepinephrine infusion is started, raising the BP to 110/60. The patient begins to awaken and appears agitated and dyssynchronous with the ventilator. The RASS score is +2 and the Behavioral Pain Scale (BPS) score is 10 despite additional IV boluses of fentanyl. After consultation with the team, the nurse starts a continuous infusion of fentanyl, and the BPS score decreases to 4. A continuous infusion of dexmedetomidine is started with a target goal of light sedation. When the RASS score is –1, patient-ventilator synchrony is achieved.

The following day the patient becomes increasingly dyssynchronous with the ventilator, demonstrates increased respiratory effort, and the pulse oximetry reading is 82% even after the FiO_2 is increased to 100% on the ventilator. The team decides to target deep sedation, so a propofol infusion replaces the dexmedetomidine and a RASS of –4 is achieved. Chest radiograph and arterial blood gas analysis indicate severe Acute Respiratory Distress Syndrome (ARDS). The respiratory therapist increases the inspiratory time and PEEP on the ventilator, then implements a trial of airway pressure release ventilation (APRV) mode. The patient remains dyssynchronous with the ventilator and hypoxemia is worsening. After ensuring deep sedation and adequate analgesia, a single bolus dose of cisatracurium is given, with improvement in hypoxemia. Assist control ventilation mode is resumed and the patient is placed in the prone position. When the patient begins to initiate breaths and becomes hypoxemic again, a cisatracurium infusion is started. The nurse monitors the airway pressure waveform to assure patient spontaneous breathing ceases and tests the train of four with the peripheral nerve stimulator.

The team's plan includes the daily reevaluation of the patient's need for prone positioning and NMB. Two days later, NMB is discontinued, PEEP and FiO_2 are reduced, and the patient maintains adequate oxygenation while lying supine. The team begins to consider the patient's eligibility for a daily sedation interruption (DSI). When the blood pressure is 110/60, respiratory rate is 16, and pulse oximetry is 95%, the propofol infusion is discontinued and fentanyl is used to continue to manage pain.

Case Question 1: Why did the patient's BP drop so precipitously following intubation and mechanical ventilation?
(A) Sedatives and narcotics potentiate the actions of each other and in some cases may result in hypotension.
(B) While experiencing severe shortness of breath, the patient is in a fight-or-flight mode and intrinsic stores of

epinephrine are released, constricting the peripheral vasculature and elevating BP. Once relaxed, the vessels dilate resulting in a lower BP.
(C) Septic shock results in vasodilation and capillary leak, contributing to hypotension and intravascular volume depletion.
(D) High PEEP can result in transmission of elevated intrathoracic pressure to the capillary bed (especially if the patient is dehydrated) causing decreased venous return and subsequent hypotension.
(E) All the above.

Case Question 2: When considering the choice of sedatives and monitoring for this patient, which of the following apply?
(A) Use a long-acting sedative since she will require sedation for a long time.
(B) If she is paralyzed, she will not feel any pain or remember anything, so analgesics and sedatives aren't necessary.
(C) Train of four is a helpful measurement when NMB is being used because it tests the depth of sedation.
(D) While NMB is maintained, sedatives are used for their amnesic properties in addition to concomitant analgesics for potential pain.

Case Question 3: Which of the following assessment findings during the DSI indicate that the nurse should restart the sedative infusion?
(A) The patient is grimacing and pointing at her throat.
(B) The respiratory rate is 35 and the pulse oximetry reading is 87%.
(C) The CAM-ICU screening is positive and the RASS score is 0.

Answers
1. E. All the above.
2. D. Neuromuscular blocking agents do not treat pain or induce amnesia, so it is important to achieve deep sedation and pain control before use of NMB to ensure amnesia. Their use without sedatives and narcotics (B) should never be done. Once clinical goals are achieved and the acute phase has passed, NMB should be discontinued. When awake and breathing spontaneously patients should be extubated as soon as possible. To that end short-acting sedatives are preferred (A). Train-of-four tests the degree of block attained by the paralytic agent, not sedation (C).
3. B. Signs of respiratory distress indicate that the patient is not ready to progress toward a spontaneous breathing trial and extubation. When a DSI is "failed," it has still been valuable because it confirms the ongoing need for sedation. The nurse should restart the sedative at a lower dose and titrate to effect to ensure that the patient receives only as much sedative as is truly needed. Indications of pain (A) should be treated with analgesics, not sedatives. Delirium without agitation (C) should not be treated with sedation.

virtually no exceptions, deep sedation and analgesia are used in combination for those receiving NMB agents. Amnesia is a desired outcome; no patient should experience a "trapped in body" state. It has been proposed that technology such as electroencephalogram-derived, depth-of-anesthesia monitoring systems may be helpful in ensuring adequate sedation during administration of NMB agents. To date, research has indicated high variability in the devices' ability to discriminate between levels of sedation and the benefit of using them is unclear.

In addition, because patients are unable to move or breathe on their own, the nurse must be vigilant in monitoring for safety. Situations that present a greater hazard to patients on NMB include accidental ventilator disconnections, unplanned extubations, harm from external forces, and complications of immobility including pressure injury and venous thromboembolism. Interventions to prevent complications are extremely important and include the use of eye lubricants, frequent turning, a physiotherapy regimen, and the use of prophylactic agents such as heparin to prevent deep vein thrombosis. Because the patient cannot communicate yet may hear, it is important to verbally reassure the patient and provide frequent explanations about what is happening throughout the course of the day and night.

The goal is to use NMB for the shortest time possible but determining when to discontinue this therapy may be difficult. One practical method is to stop the infusions of NMB agents daily to assess the need for continuation. Then, if signs of intolerance such as oxygen desaturation occur, the analgesic and sedative doses may be increased first. Tolerance to sedatives and analgesics is common and to be expected; increasing doses of the medications may be necessary. If intolerance is still noted, the NMB agents may be resumed. NMB agents are discontinued and given time to be metabolized prior to assessing a patient for brain death, as chemically induced paralysis would confound that examination. Decisions about starting, continuing, and stopping NMB require input from the interprofessional team to ensure their use is appropriate.

Principles of Management for the Use of Sedatives and Neuromuscular Blocking Agents

- Treat pain prior to providing sedation.
- Target the lightest level of sedation that will allow individualized treatment goals to be achieved. However, whenever using NMB the target should be a deep level of sedation.
- Assess sedation level with a valid and reliable scale, including during moderate sedation procedures.
- Routinely monitor for, prevent, and treat delirium.
- Provide sedation, analgesia, and meticulous physical care when NMB is administered.
- Use clinical assessment in conjunction with peripheral nerve stimulation and/or airway pressure monitoring to evaluate level of NMB.

SELECTED BIBLIOGRAPHY

Pain Management

AACN Scope and Standards for Progressive and Critical Care Nursing Practice. https://www.aacn.org/nursing-excellence/standards/aacn-scope-and-standards-for-progressive-and-critical-care-nursing-practice

American Association of Critical Care Nurses. Assessing pain in the critically ill adult. 2018. https://www.aacn.org/clinical-resources/practice-alerts/assessing-pain-in-critically-ill-adults. Accessed January 18, 2022.

American Society for Pain Management Nursing (ASPMN) Position Statements. http://www.aspmn.org/Pages/ASPMNPositionStatements.aspx

Barthélémy O, Limbourg T, Collet J, et al. Impact of non-steroidal anti-inflammatory drugs (NSAIDs) on cardiovascular outcomes in patients with stable atherothrombosis or multiple risk factors. *Int J Cardiol.* 2013;163(3):266-271.

Centers for Disease Control and Prevention Guidelines for prescribing opioids for chronic pain. 2018. Available at https://www.cdc.gov

D'Arcy Y. *A Compact Clinical Guide to Acute Pain Management.* New York, NY: Springer Publishing; 2011.

Delgado S. Managing pain in critically ill adults: A holistic approach. *Am J Nurs.* 2020;120(5):34-42.

Gelinas C, Joffe A, Szumita P, et al. A Psychometric Analysis Update of Behavioral Pain Assessment Tools for noncommunicative, critically ill adults. *AACN Crit Care.* 2019;30(4):365-387.

Gélinas C. Puntillo KA, Levin P, Azoulay E. The behavior pain assessment tool for critically ill adults: a validation study in 28 countries. *Pain.* 2017;158(5):811-821.

Julius D, Basbaum AI. Molecular mechanisms of nociception. *Nature.* 2001;413:203-210.

Marmo L, D'Arcy Y. *A Compact Clinical Guide to Critical Care, ER, and Trauma Pain Management.* New York, NY: Springer Publishing; 2013.

Martorella G. Characteristics of nonpharmacological interventions for pain management in the ICU: A scoping review. *AACN Adv Crit Care.* 2019;30(4):388-397.

Pain Management and the Opioid Epidemic: Balancing Societal and Individual Benefits and Risks of Prescription Opioid Use. National Academies Press; 2017. https://nap.nationalacademies.org/catalog/24781/pain-management-and-the-opioid-epidemic-balancing-societal-and-individual.

Pasero C, Quinlan-Colwell A, Rae D, et al. American Society for Pain Management Nursing position statement: prescribing and administering opioid doses based solely on pain intensity. *Pain Manag Nurs* 2016;17(3):170-180.

Pasternak GW. Molecular biology of opioid analgesia. *J Pain Symp Manage.* 2005;29(5S):S2-S9.

Rahu MA, Grap M, Ferguson P, Joseph P, Sherman S, Elswik R. Validity and Sensitivity of 6 Pain Scales in critically ill, intubated adults. *Am J Critical Care.* 2019;Nov;24(6):514-523.

Rose L, Smith O, Gélinas C, et al. Critical care nurses' pain assessment and management practices: a survey in Canada. *Am J Crit Care.* 2012;21(4):151-259.

Wu CL, Cohen SR, Richman JM, et al. Efficacy of postoperative patient-controlled and continuous infusion epidural analgesia versus intravenous patient-controlled analgesia with opioids: a meta-analysis. *Anesthesiology.* 2005;103(5):1079-1088.

Sedation and Neuromuscular Blockade

American Association of Critical Care Nurses. AACN Practice Alert: assessment and management of delirium across the life span. *Crit Care Nurse.* 2016;36(5):e14-e19.

Ammar MA, Sacha GL, Welch SC, et al. Sedation, analgesia, and paralysis in COVID-19 patients in the setting of drug shortages. *J Intensive Care Med.* 2021;36(2):157-174.

Balas MC, Vasilevskis EE, Olsen KM, et al. Effectiveness and safety of the awakening and breathing coordination, delirium monitoring/management, and early exercise/mobility bundle. *Crit Care Med.* 2014;42(5):1024-1036.

Chanques G, Constantin JM, Devlin JW, et al. Analgesia and sedation in patients with ARDS. *Intensive Care Med.* 2020;46: 2342-2356. https://doi.org/10.1007/s00134-020-06307-9

Cruickshank M, Henderson L, MacLennan G, et al. Alpha-2 agonists for sedation of mechanically ventilated adults in intensive care units: a systematic review. *Health Technol Assess.* 2016;20(25):v-xx.

Ely EW, Truman B, Shintani A, et al. Monitoring sedation status over time in ICU patients: reliability and validity of the Richmond Agitation-Sedation Scale (RASS). *JAMA.* 2003;289(22):2983-2991.

Hristovska AM, Duch P, Allingstrup M, Afshari A. Efficacy and safety of sugammadex versus neostigmine in reversing neuromuscular blockade in adults. *Cochrane Database of Syst Rev.* 2017;Issue 8. Art. No.: CD012763. DOI: 10.1002/14651858.CD012763

Hughes CG, Mailloux PT, Devlin JW, et al. Dexmedetomidine or propofol for sedation in mechanically ventilated adults with sepsis. *N Engl J Med.* 2021;384(15):1424-1436. https://doi.org/10.1056/NEJMoa2024922

Marra A, Ely WE, Pandharipande PP, Patel MB. The ABCDEF bundle in critical care. *Crit Care Clin.* 2017;33:225-243.

Pulak LM, Jensen L. Sleep in the intensive care unit: a review. *J Intensive Care Med.* 2016;31(1):14-23.

Rasheed AM, Amirah MF, Abdallah M, Parameaswari PJ, Issa M, Alharthy A. Ramsay Sedation Scale and Richmond Agitation Sedation Scale: a cross-sectional study. *Dimens Crit Care Nurs.* 2019;38(2):90-95.

Riker RR, Picard JT, Fraser GL. Prospective evaluation of the Sedation-Agitation Scale for adult critically ill patients. *Critical Care Medicine.* 1999;27(7):1325-1329.

Sessler C, Gosnet M, Grap MJ. The Richmond agitation-sedation scale: validity and reliability in adult intensive care unit patients. *Am J Respir Crit Care Med.* 2002;166:1338-1344.

Shetty RM, Bellini A, Wijayatilake DS, et al. BIS monitoring versus clinical assessment for sedation in mechanically ventilated adults in the intensive care unit and its impact on clinical outcomes and resource utilization. *Cochrane Database Syst Rev.* 2018;Issue 2. Art. No.: CD011240. DOI: 10.1002/14651858.CD011240.pub2

Tarazan N, Alshehri M, Sharif S, et al. Neuromuscular blocking agents in acute respiratory distress syndrome: updated systematic review and meta-analysis of randomized trials. *Intensive Care Med Exp.* 2020;8(61). https://doi.org/10.1186/s40635-020-00348-6

Wiatrowski R, Norton C, Giffen D. Analgosedation: Improving patient outcomes in ICU sedation and pain management. *Pain Manag Nurs.* 2016;17(3):204-217.

Zhang Z, Chen K, Ni H, Zhang X, Fan H. Sedation of mechanically ventilated adults in intensive care unit: a network meta-analysis. *Sci Rep.* 2017;7:44979. doi: 10.1038/srep44979

Evidence-Based Practice Guidelines

Alhazzani W, Belley-Cote E, Moller MH, et al. Neuromuscular blockade in patients with ARDS: a rapid practice guideline. *Intensive Care Med.* 2020;46:1977-1986. https://doi.org/10.1007/s00134-020-06227-8

American Geriatric Society (AGS). Pharmacological management of persistent pain in older persons. *J Am Geriatr Soc.* 2009;57(8):1331-1346.

American Society of Anesthesiologists Task Force on Acute Pain Management. Practice guidelines for acute pain management in the perioperative setting: an update report by the American Society of Anesthesiologist Task Force on Acute Pain Management. *Anesthesiology.* 2012;116:248-273.

Centers for Disease Control. Opioid Prescribing Guidelines for Chronic Pain, 2016. https://www.cdc.gov/drugoverdose/prescribing/guideline.html. Accessed June 30, 2018.

Chou R, Gordon DB, de Leon-Casasola OA, et al. Management of postoperative pain: a clinical practice guideline from the American Pain Society, the American Society of Regional Anesthesia and Pain Medicine, American Society of Anesthesiologists' Committee of Regional Anesthesia, Executive Committee and Administrative Council. *J Pain.* 2016;17(2):131-157.

Devlin JW, Skrobik Y, Gélinas C, et al. Clinical practice guidelines for the prevention and management of pain, agitation/sedation, delirium, immobility, and sleep disruption in adult patients in the ICU. *Crit Care Med.* 2018;46(9):e825-e873.

Herr K, Coyne P, Kry T, et al. Pain assessment in the nonverbal patient: position statement with clinical practice recommendations. *Pain Manag Nurs.* 2006;7(2):44-52.

Murray MJ, DeBlock H, Erstad B, et al. Clinical practice guidelines for sustained neuromuscular blockade in the adult critically ill patient. *Crit Care Med.* 2016;44(11):2079-2103.

Ouellette DR, Patel S, Girard TD, et al. Liberation from mechanical ventilation in critically ill adults: an Official American College of Chest Physicians/American Thoracic Society Clinical Practice Guideline. *Chest.* 2017;151(1):166-180.

PHARMACOLOGY

7

Earnest Alexander

KNOWLEDGE COMPETENCIES

1. Discuss advantages and disadvantages of various routes for medication delivery in critically ill patients.

2. Identify indications for use, mechanism of action, administration guidelines, side effects, and contraindications for drugs commonly administered in critical illness.

Critically ill adult patients often receive multiple medications during their admissions to an intensive care unit (ICU). These patients may be at risk for increased adverse effects from their medications because of altered metabolism and elimination that is commonly seen in the critically ill patient. Organ dysfunction or drug interactions may produce increased serum drug or active metabolite concentrations, resulting in enhanced or adverse pharmacologic effects. Therefore, it is important to be familiar with each patient's medications, including the drug's metabolic profile, drug interactions, and adverse effect profile. This chapter reviews medications commonly used in ICUs and discusses mechanisms of action, indications for use, common adverse effects, contraindications, and usual doses.

MEDICATION SAFETY

In the care of the critically ill, the medication-use process (which includes prescribing, preparation, dispensing, administration, and monitoring) is particularly complex. Each step in the process is fraught with the potential for breakdowns in medication safety (ie, adverse drug events [ADEs], medication errors). Improvement in medication safety requires interdisciplinary focus and attention. The Institute for Safe Medication Practices (ISMP) has highlighted the following

key elements that must be optimized in order to maintain patient safety in the medication use-process:

- *Patient information:* Having essential patient information at the time of medication prescribing, dispensing, and administration will result in a significant decrease in preventable ADEs.
- *Drug information:* Providing accurate and usable drug information to all healthcare practitioners involved in the medication-use process reduces the amount of preventable ADEs.
- *Communication of drug information:* Miscommunication between physicians, pharmacists, and nurses is a common cause of medication errors. To minimize medication errors caused by miscommunication, it is important to always verify drug information and eliminate communication barriers.
- *Drug labeling, packaging, and nomenclature:* Drug names that look alike or sound alike, as well as products that have confusing drug labeling and nondistinct drug packaging significantly contribute to medication errors. The incidence of medication errors is reduced with the use of proper labeling and the use of unit dose systems within hospitals.
- *Drug storage, stock, standardization, and distribution:* Standardizing drug administration times, drug

191

concentrations, and limiting the concentration of drugs available in patient care areas will reduce the risk of medication errors or minimize their consequences if an error occurs.

- *Drug device acquisition, use, and monitoring:* Appropriate safety assessment of drug delivery devices is made both prior to their purchase and during their use. Also, a system of independent double checks within the institution helps prevent device-related errors such as selecting the wrong drug or drug concentration, setting the rate improperly, or mixing the infusion line up with another.
- *Environmental factors:* A well-designed system offers the best chance of preventing errors; however, sometimes the ICU environment may contribute to medication errors. Environmental factors that can often contribute to medication errors include poor lighting, noise, interruptions, and a significant workload.
- *Staff competency and education:* Staff education is focused on priority topics, such as new medications being used in the hospital, high-alert medications, medication errors that have occurred both internally and externally, protocols, policies, and procedures related to medication use. Staff education can be an important error-prevention strategy when combined with the other key elements for medication safety.
- *Patient education:* Patients must receive ongoing education from physicians, pharmacists, and the nursing staff about the brand and generic names of medications they are receiving, their indications, usual and actual doses, expected and possible adverse effects, drug or food interactions, and how to protect themselves from errors. Patients can play a vital role in preventing medication errors when they are encouraged to ask questions and seek answers about their medications before drugs are dispensed at a pharmacy or administered in a hospital.
- *Quality processes and risk management:* The way to prevent errors is to redesign the systems and processes that lead to errors rather than focus on correcting the individuals who make errors. Effective strategies for reducing errors include making it difficult for staff to make an error and promoting the detection and correction of errors before they reach a patient and cause harm.

MEDICATION ADMINISTRATION METHODS

Intravenous

Intravenous administration is the preferred route for medications in critically ill patients because it permits complete and reliable delivery. Depending on the indication and the therapy, medications may be administered by IV push, intermittent infusion, or continuous infusion. Typically, *IV push* refers to administration of a drug over 3 to 5 minutes; *intermittent infusion* refers to 15-minute to 2-hour drug administration at set intervals throughout day, and *continuous infusion* administration occurs over a prolonged period of time.

Intramuscular or Subcutaneous

Intramuscular (IM) or subcutaneous (SC) administration of medications are rarely be used in critically ill patients. This is due to a number of factors including delayed onset of action, unreliable absorption because of decreased peripheral perfusion (particularly in patients who are hypotensive or hypovolemic), or inadequate muscle or decreased SC fat tissue. Furthermore, SC/IM administration may result in incomplete, unpredictable, or erratic drug absorption. If medication is not absorbed from the injection site, a depot of medication can develop. If this occurs, once perfusion is restored, absorption can potentially lead to supratherapeutic or toxic effects. Additionally, patients with thrombocytopenia or who are receiving thrombolytic agents or anticoagulants may develop hematomas and bleeding complications due to SC or IM administration. Finally, administering frequent IM injections may also be inconvenient and painful for patients.

Oral

Oral (PO) administration of medication in the critically ill patient can also result in incomplete, unpredictable, or erratic absorption. This may be caused by a number of factors including the presence of an ileus impairing drug absorption, or to diarrhea decreasing gastrointestinal (GI) tract transit time and time for drug absorption. Diarrhea may have a pronounced effect on the absorption of sustained-release preparations such as calcium channel–blocking agents, resulting in a suboptimal serum drug concentration or clinical response. Several medications such as fluconazole and the fluoroquinolones have been shown to exhibit excellent bioavailability when orally administered to critically ill patients. The availability of an oral suspension for some of these agents makes oral administration a reliable and cost-effective alternative for patients with limited IV access.

In patients unable to swallow, tablets are often crushed and capsules opened for administration through nasogastric or orogastric tubes. This practice is time consuming and can result in blockage of the tube, necessitating the removal of the clogged tube and insertion of a new tube. If enteral nutrition is being administered through the tube, it often has to be stopped for medication administration, resulting in inadequate nutrition for patients. Also, several medications (eg, phenytoin, carbamazepine, levothyroxine, and warfarin) have been shown to compete, or interact, with enteral nutrition solutions. This interaction results in decreased absorption of these agents, or complex formation with the nutrition solution leading to precipitation and clogging of the feeding tube. To avoid reduced medication absorption, enteral nutrition may be held before and after administration of these medications. In these instances, caloric intake will be reduced unless feeding rates are adjusted using volume-based strategies.

Liquid medications may circumvent the need to crush tablets or open capsules, but have their own limitations. An example is ciprofloxacin (Cipro) oral suspension, which is an oil-based preparation that is not given via feeding tube because of the high probability of clogs. Many liquid dosage forms contain sorbitol as a flavoring agent or as the primary delivery vehicle. Sorbitol's hyperosmolarity is a frequent cause of diarrhea in critically ill patients, especially in patients receiving enteral nutrition. Potassium chloride elixir is extremely hyperosmolar and requires dilution with 120 to 160 mL of water before administration. Administering undiluted potassium chloride elixir can result in osmotic diarrhea. Lastly, sustained-release or enteric-coated preparations are difficult to administer to critically ill patients. When sustained-release products are crushed, the patient absorbs the entire dose immediately as opposed to gradually over a period of 6, 8, 12, or 24 hours. This results in supratherapeutic or potentially toxic effects soon after the administration of the medication, with subtherapeutic effects at the end of the dosing interval. Sustained-release preparations must be converted to equivalent daily doses of immediate-release dosing forms and administered at more frequent dosing intervals. Enteric-coated dosage forms that are crushed may be inactivated by gastric juices or may cause stomach irritation. Enteric-coated tablets are specifically formulated to pass through the stomach intact so that they can enter the small intestine before they begin to dissolve.

Sublingual

Because of the high degree of vascularity of the sublingual mucosa, sublingual administration of medication often produces serum concentrations of medication that parallel IV administration, and an onset of action that is often faster than orally administered medications.

Traditionally, there are few medications administered sublingually (SL) to critically ill patients. Examples include nitroglycerin, and olanzapine sublingual formulations. Several oral and IV medications, however, have been shown to produce therapeutic effects after sublingual administration. Tacrolimus may be administered sublingually by opening the capsules and administering the contents sublingually in patients unable to swallow capsules. Captopril reliably and predictably lowers blood pressure in patients with hypertensive urgency. Oral lorazepam tablets can be administered SL to treat patients in status epilepticus; preparations of oral triazolam and IV midazolam have been shown to produce sedation after sublingual administration.

Intranasal

Intranasal administration is a way to effectively administer sedative and analgesic agents. The high degree of vascularity of the nasal mucosa results in rapid and complete absorption of medication. Agents that have been administered successfully intranasally include meperidine, fentanyl, sufentanil, butorphanol, ketamine, midazolam, and naloxone.

Transdermal

Transdermal administration of medication is of limited value in critically ill patients. Although nitroglycerin paste is extremely effective as a temporizing measure before IV access is established in the acute management of patients with angina, heart failure (HF), pulmonary edema, or hypertension, nitroglycerin transdermal patches are of limited benefit in this population because of their slow onset of activity and their inability for dose titration. Also, patients with decreased peripheral perfusion may not sufficiently absorb transdermally administered medications to produce the desired therapeutic effect. Transdermal preparations of clonidine, nitroglycerin, or fentanyl may be beneficial in patients who have been stabilized on IV or oral doses, but require chronic administration of these agents. Chronic use of nitroglycerin transdermal patches is further complicated by the development of tolerance. However, the development of tolerance can be avoided by removing the patch at bedtime, allowing for an 8- to 10-hour "nitrate-free" period.

A eutectic mixture of local anesthetic (EMLA) is a combination of lidocaine and prilocaine. This local anesthetic mixture can be used to anesthetize the skin before insertion of IV catheters or the injection of local anesthetics that may be required to produce deeper levels of topical anesthesia.

Although transdermal administration of medications is an infrequent method of drug administration in critically ill patients, its use is not overlooked as a potential cause of adverse effects in this patient population. Extensive application to burned, abraded, or denuded skin can result in significant systemic absorption of topically applied medications. Excessive use of viscous lidocaine products or mouthwashes containing lidocaine to provide local anesthesia for mucositis or esophagitis also can result in significant systemic absorption of lidocaine. Lidocaine administered topically to the oral mucosa has resulted in serum concentrations capable of producing seizures. The diffuse application of topical glucocorticosteroid preparations also can lead to absorption capable of producing adrenal suppression. This is especially true with the high-potency fluorinated steroid preparations such as betamethasone dipropionate, clobetasol propionate, desoximetasone, or fluocinonide.

CENTRAL NERVOUS SYSTEM PHARMACOLOGY

Sedatives

Sedatives can be divided into four main categories: benzodiazepines, barbiturates, neuroleptics, and miscellaneous agents. Benzodiazepines are appropriate for specific indications, such as alcohol withdrawal, but miscellaneous agents are preferred for sedation in critically ill patients due to the association of benzodiazepines with delirium. Barbiturates are reserved for patients with refractory status epilepticus, head injuries, and increased intracranial pressure. Neuroleptics have a limited use in patients who manifest a psychological or behavioral component to their sedative needs; indiscriminate use is discouraged. Propofol is a short-acting IV general anesthetic that is approved for use as a sedative for mechanically ventilated patients. Dexmedetomidine is another short-acting IV general anesthetic used for light sedation. Propofol and dexmedetomidine are the recommended choices for light sedation in critically ill patients in the 2018 Society of Critical Care Medicine guidelines. Dosing of sedatives is guided by frequent assessment of the level of sedation with a valid and reliable sedation assessment scale (see Chapter 6, Pain Management/Sedation).

Benzodiazepines

Benzodiazepines are frequently used agents in critically ill patients. These agents provide sedation, decrease anxiety, have anticonvulsant properties, possess indirect muscle-relaxant properties, and induce anterograde amnesia. Benzodiazepines bind to gamma-aminobutyric acid (GABA) receptors located in the central nervous system, modulating this inhibitory neurotransmitter. These agents have a wide margin of safety as well as flexibility in their routes of administration.

Benzodiazepines are often used to provide short-term sedation and amnesia during imaging procedures, other diagnostic procedures, and invasive procedures such as central venous catheter placement or bronchoscopy. Excessive sedation and confusion can occur with initial doses, and these effects may diminish as tolerance develops during therapy. Older adult and pediatric patients may exhibit a paradoxical effect manifested as irritability, agitation, hostility, hallucinations, and anxiety. Respiratory depression may be seen more commonly in patients receiving concurrent narcotics, as well as in elderly patients and patients with chronic obstructive pulmonary disease (COPD) or obstructive sleep apnea (OSA). Benzodiazepines have also been associated with the development of delirium, which has been linked with worse clinical outcomes. As a result, long-term use of benzodiazepines for sedation is not recommended. When used, there is a trend toward bolus dosing over continuous infusions. This trend is aimed at reducing the level of sedation and the duration of mechanical ventilation. Additional comparative trials are needed to demonstrate the best dosing strategy. Patients with histories of prior benzodiazepine or chronic alcohol use may require higher benzodiazepine doses to achieve the desired effect.

Monitoring Parameters

- Mental status, level of consciousness, respiratory rate, and level of comfort should be monitored in any patient receiving a benzodiazepine.
- Signs and symptoms of withdrawal reactions are monitored in patients receiving short-acting agents (ie, midazolam).
- Monitor level of sedation and use the lowest dose that produces the desired effect.

Midazolam

Midazolam is a short-acting, highly lipophilic (at physiologic pH) benzodiazepine that may be administered IV, IM, SL, PO, intranasally, or rectally. Clearance of midazolam has been shown to be extremely variable in critically ill patients. The elimination half-life can be increased by as much as 6 to 12 hours in patients with liver disease, shock, or concurrently receiving enzyme-inhibiting drugs such as erythromycin or fluconazole, and hypoalbuminemia. Midazolam's two primary metabolites, 1-hydroxymidazolam and 1-hydroxymidazolam glucuronide, have been shown to accumulate in critically ill patients, especially those with renal dysfunction, contributing additional pharmacologic effects. Older adult patients demonstrate prolonged half-lives secondary to age-related reduction in liver function.

Dose

- *IV bolus:* 0.025 to 0.05 mg/kg q 1-4h
- *Continuous infusion:* 0.02 to 0.1 mg/kg/h

Lorazepam

Lorazepam is an intermediate-acting benzodiazepine that offers the advantage of not having its metabolism affected by impaired hepatic function, age, or interacting drugs. Glucuronidation in the liver is the route of elimination of lorazepam. Because lorazepam is relatively water insoluble, it must be diluted in propylene glycol, and it is propylene glycol that is responsible for the hypotension that may be seen after bolus IV administration. Large volumes of fluid are required to maintain the drug in solution, so that only 20 to 40 mg can be safely dissolved in 250 mL of dextrose-5%-water (D_5W). In-line filters are recommended when administering lorazepam by continuous infusion because of the potential for the drug to precipitate. Finally, lorazepam's long elimination half-life of 10 to 20 hours limits its dosing flexibility by continuous infusion. Patients requiring high-dose infusions may be at risk for developing propylene glycol toxicity, which is manifested as a hyperosmolar state with a metabolic acidosis.

Dose

- *IV bolus:* 0.5 to 2 mg q1-4h
- *Continuous infusion:* 0.06 to 0.1 mg/kg/h

Diazepam

Diazepam is a long-acting benzodiazepine with a faster onset of action than lorazepam or midazolam. Although its duration of action is 1 to 2 hours after a single dose, it displays cumulative effects because its active metabolites contribute to its pharmacologic effect. Desmethyldiazepam has a half-life of approximately 150 to 200 hours, so it accumulates slowly and then is slowly eliminated from the body after diazepam is discontinued. Diazepam metabolism is reduced in patients with hepatic failure and in patients receiving drugs that inhibit hepatic microsomal enzymes. Diazepam may be used for one or two doses as a periprocedure anxiolytic and amnestic, but is not used for routine sedation of mechanically ventilated patients.

Dose

- *IV bolus:* 2.5 to 10 mg q2-4h
- *Continuous infusion:* Not recommended

Benzodiazepine Antagonist
Flumazenil
Flumazenil is a specific benzodiazepine antagonist indicated for the reversal of benzodiazepine-induced moderate sedation, recurrent sedation, and benzodiazepine overdose. It is used with caution in patients who have received benzodiazepines for an extended period of time to prevent the precipitation of withdrawal reactions.

Dose

- *Reversal of conscious sedation:* 0.2 mg IV over 15 seconds followed in 45 seconds by 0.2 mg repeated every minute as needed to a maximum dose of 1 mg. Reversal of recurrent sedation is the same as for conscious sedation, except doses may be repeated every 20 minutes as needed.
- *Benzodiazepine overdose:* 0.2 mg over 30 seconds followed by 0.3 mg over 30 seconds; repeated doses of 0.5 mg can be administered over 30 seconds at 1-minute intervals up to a cumulative dose of 3 mg. With a partial response after 3 mg, additional doses up to a total dose of 5 mg may be administered. In all of the above-mentioned scenarios, no more than 1 mg is administered at any one time, and no more than 3 mg in any 1 hour.
- *Continuous infusion:* 0.1 to 0.5 mg/h (for the reversal of long-acting benzodiazepines or massive overdoses).

Monitoring Parameters

- Level of consciousness and signs and symptoms of withdrawal reactions.

Neuroleptics
Haloperidol
Haloperidol is a major tranquilizer that has been used for the management of agitated or delirious patients who fail to respond to nonpharmacologic interventions or other sedatives. It is important to note that despite the common usage of this agent to treat delirium, there is no published evidence that haloperidol reduces the duration of delirium. The lack of supporting evidence is leading to the reconsideration of the role of haloperidol in this setting compared with other agents with fewer side effects (ie, atypical antipsychotics). Prolonged QTc is a significant adverse reaction and the risk for dysrhythmia must be carefully weighed against the potential benefit of haloperidol. Advantages of haloperidol are that it causes limited respiratory depression and has little potential for the development of tolerance or dependence. Although its exact mechanism of action is unknown, it probably involves dopaminergic receptor blockade in the central nervous system, resulting in central nervous system depression at the subcortical level of the brain.

Initial doses of 2 to 5 mg may be doubled every 15 to 20 minutes until the patient is adequately sedated. As soon as the patient's symptoms are controlled, the total dose required to calm the patient is divided into four equal doses and administered every 6 hours on a regularly scheduled basis. When the patient's symptoms are stable, the daily dose is rapidly tapered to the smallest dose that controls the patient's symptoms. Higher doses and IV administration of haloperidol may prolong the QTc interval in patients, especially those patients receiving haloperidol continuous infusions, or concomitant administration with other medications that prolong QTc. Monitoring the QTc interval is mandatory for all patients receiving haloperidol by IV injection or continuous infusion.

Another major side effect of haloperidol is its extrapyramidal reactions, such as akathisia and dystonia. These reactions usually occur early in therapy and may resolve with dose reduction or discontinuation of the drug. However, in more severe cases, diphenhydramine, 25 to 50 mg IV, or benztropine, 1 to 2 mg IV, may be required to relieve the symptoms. Extrapyramidal reactions appear to be more common after oral haloperidol than after IV haloperidol administration. Neuroleptic malignant syndrome may also be seen with this agent, manifested by hyperthermia, severe extrapyramidal reactions, severe muscle rigidity, altered mental status, and autonomic instability. Treatment involves supportive care and the administration of dantrolene. Cardiovascular side effects include hypotension.

Dose

- *IV or IM bolus:* 1 to 10 mg (titrated up as clinically indicated)
- *Continuous infusion:* 10 mg/h (not generally recommended)

Monitoring Parameters

- Mental status, blood pressure, electrocardiogram (ECG), bedside delirium monitoring, and electrolytes (especially with continuous infusions), signs of extrapyramidal reaction

Atypical Antipsychotics
Atypical antipsychotic agents such as quetiapine, olanzapine, risperidone, and ziprasidone have been suggested as possible alternatives to haloperidol, due to their similar mechanism of action and more favorable side effect profile, including reduced incidence of extrapyramidal reactions and QT prolongation. The use of atypical antipsychotics to manage ICU delirium has increased during recent years with reported usage as high as 40% in some studies. Despite these increases, additional well-controlled studies are warranted as their efficacy remains uncertain.

Monitoring Parameters

- Mental status, level of consciousness, ECG, bedside delirium monitoring

Quetiapine
Quetiapine is the most well studied of these agents to this point, with a randomized, placebo-controlled trial demonstrating a reduction in duration of delirium. Quetiapine can

be administered as scheduled dosing, with additional doses of haloperidol as needed. Dose escalation of the scheduled quetiapine may be required in 50 mg increments in patients still requiring breakthrough management with haloperidol. Sedation is the most commonly associated adverse effect. A limitation of quetiapine is that it is only available as an oral preparation.

Dose

- *PO or per tube:* 50 to 200 mg q12h

Monitoring Parameters

- Mental status, level of consciousness, ECG, bedside delirium monitoring

Barbiturates

Barbiturates are used to reduce intracranial pressure in head injury patients after conservative therapy has failed, and also in the setting of refractory status epilepticus. Barbiturates decrease cerebral oxygen consumption, decrease cerebral blood flow, and potentially scavenge free oxygen radicals.

The general central nervous system depression associated with the use of barbiturates may cause excessive sedation as well as respiratory depression. Barbiturates produce direct myocardial depression, reducing cardiac output and increasing venous capacitance. Rapid IV administration can result in arrhythmias and hypotension.

Pentobarbital

Pentobarbital continuous infusions are commonly used to induce barbiturate coma. The infusion is titrated to maintain intracranial pressure less than 20 mm Hg and cerebral perfusion pressure greater than 60 mm Hg. The mean arterial pressure (MAP) is maintained in a range that provides an adequate cerebral perfusion pressure. Therapeutic serum pentobarbital concentrations are 20 to 50 mg/L.

Dose

- *IV bolus:* 5 to 10 mg/kg infused over 2 hours
- *Continuous infusion:* 0.5 to 4 mg/kg/h

Monitoring Parameters

- Level of consciousness, intracranial pressure, cerebral perfusion pressure, blood pressure, and serum pentobarbital concentration

Miscellaneous Agents

Propofol

Propofol is an IV general anesthetic used for sedation of mechanically ventilated patients. The agent is often used as the primary sedative and is held or reduced during daily awakening protocols. The advantages of propofol are its rapid onset and short duration of action compared to the benzodiazepines. Propofol is associated with pain on injection, respiratory depression, and hypotension, especially in critically ill patients who are already hypotensive or hypovolemic. Hypotension can be avoided by limiting bolus doses to 0.25 to 0.5 mg/kg and the initial infusion rate to 5 mcg/kg/min. The fat-emulsion vehicle of propofol has been shown to support the growth of microorganisms. The manufacturer recommends changing the IV tubing of extemporaneously prepared infusions every 6 hours or every 12 hours, if the infusion bottles are used. Propofol is formulated in a fat-emulsion vehicle that provides 1.1 kcal/mL, and its infusion rate must be accounted for when determining a patient's nutrition support regimen because the fat-emulsion base can be considered as a calorie source. High infusion rates can be a cause of hypertriglyceridemia. This agent can also cause a rare but serious adverse effect known as propofol-related infusion syndrome (PRIS). PRIS is associated with the use of propofol for more than 48 hours and at doses greater than 75 mcg/kg/min. Hyperkalemia, tachyarrhythmia, bradycardia, rhabdomyolysis, and lactic acidosis combined with hypertriglyceridemia as previously described are common signs of PRIS. The bedside nurse monitors closely for these signs as discontinuance of therapy may avoid the serious outcomes of PRIS: myocardial failure, metabolic acidosis, rhabdomyolysis, dysrhythmias, and renal failure. Propofol is available in 50- and 100-mL infusion vials. To decrease waste, 50-mL vials may be used when changing vials in patients who are scheduled for IV line changes, extubation from mechanical ventilation, and low infusion rates.

Dose

- *IV bolus:* 0.25 to 0.5 mg/kg
- *Continuous infusion:* 5 to 50 mcg/kg/min

Monitoring Parameters

- Level of consciousness, blood pressure, lactic acid, creatinine kinase, and serum triglyceride level, especially at high infusion rates

Ketamine

Ketamine is an analog of phencyclidine that is commonly used as an IV general anesthetic. It is an agent that produces analgesia, anesthesia, and amnesia without the loss of consciousness. The sedation noted with this agent is dissociative and dose dependent. Doses of 0.1 to 0.5 mg/kg provide analgesia only with no sedation, while doses greater than 0.5 mg/kg provide some degree of sedation. The onset of anesthesia after a single 0.5- to 1.0-mg/kg bolus dose is within 1 to 2 minutes and lasts approximately 5 to 10 minutes. Ketamine causes sympathetic stimulation that normally increases blood pressure and heart rate while maintaining cardiac output. This may be important in patients with hypovolemia. Ketamine is useful in patients who require repeated painful procedures such as wound debridement. The bronchodilatory effects of ketamine may be beneficial in patients experiencing status asthmaticus. However, ketamine may increase intracranial pressure and is avoided or used with caution in patients with head injuries, space-occupying lesions, or any other conditions that may cause an increase in intracranial pressure. Emergence reactions or hallucinations, commonly seen after ketamine anesthesia, may be prevented with the concurrent use of benzodiazepines.

Dose

- *IV bolus:* 0.1 to 1 mg/kg
- *Continuous infusion:* 0.05 to 3 mg/kg/h
- *Oral:* 10 mg/kg diluted in 1 to 2 oz of juice
- *Intranasal:* 5 mg/kg

Monitoring Parameters

- Levels of sedation and analgesia, heart rate, blood pressure, and mental status

Dexmedetomidine

Dexmedetomidine is a relatively selective alpha-2-adrenergic agonist with sedative properties indicated for light sedation of intubated and mechanically ventilated patients. Dexmedetomidine is not associated with respiratory depression but has been associated with reductions in heart rate and blood pressure. Some patients may complain of increased awareness while receiving the drug in the ICU. Dexmedetomidine has minimal amnestic properties and most patients require breakthrough doses of sedatives and analgesics while receiving the drug. Additionally, hypotension is commonly encountered during the loading dose, thus loading doses should be avoided in hemodynamically unstable patients.

The agent has been evaluated for longer-term sedation, up to 28 days in a limited number of patients. In this setting, a reduction of the loading infusion or elimination altogether is advised to minimize cardiovascular depression. However, a higher maintenance infusion (up to 1.5 mcg/kg/h) may be required compared to short-term sedation, with bradycardia being the most common adverse effect limiting the patient's dose. Patients receiving prolonged infusions of dexmedetomidine may be at risk for withdrawal symptoms, reflex tachycardia, and neurologic manifestations (eg, agitation, irritability, speech abnormalities), following abrupt discontinuation. Patients are monitored for 12 to 24 hours following discontinuation. To prevent withdrawal, dexmedetomidine can be tapered in patients who have received therapy greater than 24 hours (eg, infusion reduced by 0.1 mcg/kg/h every 12-24 hours).

Dexmedetomidine is the preferred sedative compared with benzodiazepines for reducing the duration of delirium in adult ICU patients with delirium unrelated to alcohol or benzodiazepine withdrawal.

Dose

- *IV bolus:* 1 mcg/kg over 10 minutes
- *Continuous infusion:* 0.2 to 1.5 mcg/kg/h

Monitoring Parameters

- Levels of sedation and analgesia, heart rate, and blood pressure

Analgesics

Opioids

Opioids, also known as narcotics, produce their effects by reversibly binding to the mu, delta, kappa, and sigma opiate receptors located in the central nervous system. Mu-1 receptors are associated with analgesia, and mu-2 receptors are associated with respiratory depression, bradycardia, euphoria, and dependence. Delta receptors have no selective agonist and modulate mu-receptor activity. Kappa receptors function at the spinal and supraspinal levels and are associated with sedation. Sigma receptors are associated with dysphoria and psychotomimetic effects.

Monitoring Parameters

- Level of pain or comfort, blood pressure, renal function, hepatic function, and respiratory rate

Morphine

Morphine is a commonly used narcotic analgesic. Morphine is hepatically metabolized to several metabolites, including morphine-6-glucuronide (M6G), which is approximately 5 to 10 times more potent than morphine. M6G is renally eliminated and after repeated doses can accumulate in patients with renal dysfunction, producing enhanced pharmacologic effects. Morphine's clearance is reduced in critically ill patients due to increased protein binding, decreased hepatic blood flow, reduced renal function, or reduced hepatocellular function. Morphine possesses vasodilatory properties and can produce hypotension because of either direct effects on the vasculature or histamine release.

Dose

- *IV bolus:* 2 to 5 mg
- *Continuous infusion:* 2 to 30 mg/h

Patient-Controlled Analgesia (PCA)

- *IV bolus:* 0.5 to 3 mg
- *Lockout interval:* 5 to 20 minutes

Meperidine

Meperidine is a short-acting opioid that has one-seventh the potency of morphine. It is hepatically metabolized to normeperidine, which is eliminated through the kidneys, and is also a neurotoxin. Normeperidine can accumulate in patients with renal dysfunction, resulting in seizures. Meperidine is avoided in patients taking monoamine oxidase inhibitors because of the potential for development of a hypertensive crisis when these agents are administered concurrently. The role of this agent as an analgesic has been reduced dramatically due to seizure potential. In many institutions, the agent has been limited to serve as an adjunctive therapy to minimize shivering in hypothermic patients.

Dose

- *IV bolus:* 25 to 100 mg

Fentanyl

Fentanyl is an analog of meperidine that is 100 times more potent than morphine. After single doses, its duration of action is limited by its rapid distribution into fat tissue. However, after repeated dosing or continuous infusion administration, fat stores become saturated, thereby prolonging its terminal elimination half-life to more than 24 hours. Fentanyl does not have active metabolites, although accumulation can occur in hepatic dysfunction. Unlike morphine, fentanyl does not cause histamine release.

Dose

- *IV bolus:* 25 to 100 mcg q1-2h
- *Continuous infusion:* 50 to 300 mcg/h
- *Transdermal:* Patients not previously on opioids: 25 mcg/h
- *Opioid-tolerant patients:* 25 to 100 mcg/h

PCA

- *IV bolus:* 25 to 100 mcg
- *Lockout interval:* 5 to 10 minutes

Hydromorphone

Hydromorphone is a morphine derivative that is 5 to 7.5 times more potent than morphine with a similar duration of action. Because of the relative potency compared to morphine, caution must be used in dose conversions. Hydromorphone can accumulate and intensify pharmacologic effects in patients with hepatic and renal impairment. The agent primarily has a role in refractory pain management.

Dose

- *IV bolus:* 0.4 to 2 mg
- *Continuous infusion:* 0.2 to 3 mg/h

PCA

- *IV bolus:* 0.1 to 1 mg
- *Lockout interval:* 5 to 20 minutes

Opioid Antagonist
Naloxone

Naloxone is a pure opiate antagonist that displaces opioid agonists from the mu-, delta-, and kappa-receptor–binding sites. Naloxone reverses narcotic-induced respiratory depression, producing an increase in respiratory rate and minute ventilation, a decrease in arterial PCO_2, and normalization of blood pressure if reduced. Narcotic-induced sedation or sleep is also reversed by naloxone. Naloxone reverses analgesia, increases sympathetic nervous system activity, and may result in tachycardia, hypertension, pulmonary edema, and cardiac arrhythmias. Naloxone administration produces withdrawal symptoms in patients who have been taking narcotic analgesics chronically. In non-life-threatening situations (eg, postsurgical patient with respiratory depression, but not in cardiac or respiratory arrest), diluting and slowly administering naloxone in incremental doses can prevent the precipitation of acute withdrawal reactions as well as prevent the increase in sympathetic stimulation that may accompany the reversal of analgesia. One 0.4-mg ampule is diluted with 0.9% NaCl (saline) to 10 mL to produce a concentration of 0.04 mg/mL. Sequential doses of 0.04 to 0.08 mg are administered slowly until the desired response is obtained. A more aggressive dosing approach may be warranted in life-threatening situations. Because its duration of action is generally shorter than that of opiates, the effect of opiates may return after the effects of naloxone dissipate, approximately 30 to 120 minutes. To combat this, continuous infusions may be required in situations of overdose with extended-release opioid formulations.

Dose

- *Opiate depression:* Initial dose: 0.1 to 0.2 mg given at 2- to 3-minute intervals until the desired response is obtained. Additional doses may be necessary depending on the response of the patient and the dose and duration of the opiate administered.
- *Known or suspected opiate overdose:* Initial dose: 0.4 to 2.0 mg administered at 2- to 3-minute intervals if necessary. If no response is observed after a total of 10 mg has been administered, other causes of the depressive state should be determined.
- *Continuous infusion:* Initial infusion rates can be customized based on calculating 2/3 of the initial effective intermittent dosing, given hourly. Typical rates range 2.5 to 5 mcg/kg/h, titrated to the patient's response.

Monitoring Parameters

- Signs and symptoms of withdrawal reactions, respiratory rate, blood pressure, mental status, level of consciousness, and pupil size

Nonsteroidal Anti-Inflammatory Drugs
Ketorolac

Ketorolac is a nonsteroidal anti-inflammatory drug (NSAID) that is indicated for the short-term treatment of moderate to severe acute pain that requires analgesia at the opioid level. The drug exhibits anti-inflammatory, analgesic, and antipyretic properties. Its mechanism of action is thought to be due to inhibition of prostaglandin synthesis by inhibiting cyclooxygenase, an enzyme that catalyzes the formation of endoperoxidases from arachidonic acid. NSAIDs are more efficacious in the treatment of prostaglandin-mediated pain. Ketorolac is the only currently available NSAID approved for IM, IV, and oral administration, and it is often used in combination with other analgesics because pain often involves multiple mechanisms. Combination therapy may be more efficacious than single-drug regimens, and combinations with narcotics can decrease narcotic requirements, minimizing narcotic side effects.

Ketorolac is associated with the same adverse effects as orally administered NSAIDs, such as reversible platelet inhibition, GI bleeding, and reduced renal function. Ketorolac is contraindicated in patients with advanced renal failure and in patients at risk for renal failure because of volume depletion. Therefore, volume depletion is corrected before administering ketorolac. Dose reduction of 50% is recommended for mild and moderate renal impairment. Because of the potential for significant adverse effects, the maximum combined duration of parenteral and oral use is limited to 5 days.

Dose

- *Loading dose:* Less than 65 years: 30 to 60 mg; more than 65 years or less than 50 kg: 15 to 30 mg
- *Maintenance dose:* Less than 65 years: 30 mg q6h; more than 65 years or less than 50 kg: 15 mg q6h

Monitoring Parameters

- Renal function and volume status

Acetaminophen

Acetaminophen is an analgesic and antipyretic available in a number of dosage forms, including an IV formulation. IV acetaminophen is indicated for the management of mild to moderate pain, and management of moderate to severe pain with adjunctive opioid analgesics. The preferred route of administration for acetaminophen continues to be oral with comparable dosing (eg, 650 mg oral every 4 hours or 1 g oral every 6 hours), but the IV route has proven beneficial in the perioperative setting when oral therapy is not feasible. The IV form of this agent is not cost-effective as an antipyretic because equally effective and less expensive options exist (eg, acetaminophen rectal suppositories). Use of IV acetaminophen is restricted to postsurgical patients who are unable to take oral or rectal acetaminophen.

Dose

- *IV bolus:* 1 g IV every 6 hours for 24 to 48 hours postoperative (maximum of 4 g in 24 hours)

Monitoring Parameters

- Liver function test, pain control, blood pressure

Neuromuscular Blocking Agents

Neuromuscular blocking agents (NMBAs) are primarily used to obtain, protect, and maintain a safe secure airway and to assist with mechanical ventilation. These agents have no sedative, amnestic, anesthetic, or analgesic properties. The indications for using NMBA in critically ill patients can be divided into short- and long-term indications. Short-term indications include endotracheal intubation, stability during patient transport, hemodynamic monitoring, radiologic procedures, dressing changes, and minor surgical procedures. The primary long-term indications are optimizing mechanical ventilation, decreasing oxygen consumption, controlling increased intracranial pressure, treating refractory shivering associated with hypothermia, and managing muscle spasms associated with tetanus. NMBAs are categorized as either depolarizing or nondepolarizing agents.

Depolarizing Agents

Succinylcholine

Succinylcholine is the only depolarizing agent available for clinical use and is the agent of choice for rapid intubation of the trachea. Succinylcholine binds to acetylcholine receptors causing a persistent depolarization of the muscle endplate resulting in paralysis.

Succinylcholine may increase serum potassium approximately 0.5 mEq/L after a standard intubating dose of 1 to 2 mg/kg. Critically ill patients with burns, spinal cord injury, and trauma with extensive skeletal muscle damage, upper and lower motor neuron disease, and prolonged bed rest are predisposed to the development of hyperkalemia after a dose of succinylcholine because of the development of nonfunctional extrajunctional acetylcholine receptors. These receptors bind succinylcholine without causing paralysis, but depolarize the muscle cells, releasing potassium and increasing serum potassium concentrations into the supratherapeutic or toxic range. Although hyperkalemia can occur within the first 24 hours after injury, patients are most at risk during the period from 7 days after injury until 9 months later. Therefore, succinylcholine is contraindicated in these patients. As a depolarizing agent, succinylcholine alone or in combination with inhalational anesthetics may trigger malignant hyperthermia. The mechanism appears to be related to increases in intracellular concentration of calcium in normal muscle. Because of the clear association with malignant hyperthermia, the agent should be avoided in patients with a family history of malignant hyperthermia. In situations where succinylcholine is contraindicated, a short-acting or intermediate-acting nondepolarizing agent may be used. Succinylcholine is rapidly hydrolyzed by pseudocholinesterase; however, patients with atypical pseudocholinesterase may experience prolonged blockade. Other conditions associated with prolonged blockade resulting from reduced cholinesterase activity include pregnancy, liver disease, acute infections, carcinomas, uremia, and burns.

Dose

- *Intubation:* 1 to 2 mg/kg IV

Monitoring Parameters

- Renal function, electrolytes (especially potassium), acid-base status, and level of paralysis

Nondepolarizing Agents

Nondepolarizing agents are competitive antagonists of acetylcholine at the acetylcholine receptor. Nondepolarizing agents are subdivided according to chemical class either aminosteroid (pancuronium, rocuronium, vecuronium) or benzylisoquinolinium (atracurium, cisatracurium). These agents are further classified according to duration of action: intermediate (atracurium, cisatracurium, rocuronium, vecuronium) and long (pancuronium).

Nondepolarizing agents can be used for short- or long-term indications in critically ill patients. Short-term indications include intubation, stability during intrahospital transport, and immobility during procedures. Long-term indications include mechanical ventilation after optimal doses of sedatives and analgesics have not been able to prevent patient/ventilator dyssynchrony, as well as to reduce and control high intracranial pressures.

Selecting an Agent

Several factors are considered when selecting the most appropriate agent for a patient. The onset and duration of paralysis should match that required by the procedure. Short procedures (ie, endotracheal intubation) may require a short-acting agent with rapid onset, such as succinylcholine. Bolus doses of intermediate- or long-acting agents may be selected for longer procedures (ie, dressing changes, radiologic scans). Long-term indications such as mechanical ventilation may require intermittent doses of long-acting agents or continuous infusions of intermediate-acting agents. The patient's underlying pathophysiology also must be considered when selecting an NMBA. Succinylcholine is avoided in patients at risk for developing hyperkalemia. Pancuronium's vagolytic effect can increase heart rate and blood pressure and is used with caution in patients with unstable coronary artery disease. Vecuronium and pancuronium are metabolized to 3-hydroxy metabolites that have 50% of the activity of the parent compounds. These metabolites are renally eliminated and have been shown to accumulate in patients with renal dysfunction producing prolonged periods of paralysis. Monitoring patients and adjusting doses, dosing intervals, or continuous infusion rates with the aid of a peripheral nerve stimulator to maintain one or two twitches of a train-of-four (TOF) stimulation can usually prevent this adverse effect from occurring (see Chapter 6, Pain, Sedation, and Neuromuscular Blockade Management). Atracurium or cisatracurium are considered for patients in multisystem organ failure because of their independence on organ function for metabolism and elimination.

NMBAs are used for management of an adult ICU patient only when all other means to manage the patient have been tried without success. Agent selection is variable based on patient population and local practice. Patients receiving NMBAs are assessed both clinically and by TOF monitoring with a goal of adjusting the NMBA to achieve one to two twitches. Patients receiving NMBA therapy are also medicated to provide adequate sedation (ie, deep sedation as defined by validated sedation monitoring tools) and analgesia. This assessment is critical at baseline, before NMBA therapy is initiated, as neuromuscular blockade will alter sedation monitoring during therapy. It is also important to note that bispectral index (BIS) monitoring has demonstrated value in evaluating levels of sedation during NMBA therapy, and is preferred compared with validated sedation monitoring tools (see Chapter 6, Pain, Sedation, and Neuromuscular Blockade Management).

Side Effects

Although adverse effects are minimal, several can be significant. Atracurium can cause histamine release after rapid IV bolus injection, resulting in hypotension and flushing. Injecting each agent over at least 60 seconds can prevent this adverse effect. Laudanosine, atracurium's primary metabolite, has been shown to produce seizures in dogs after it achieves high concentrations in the cerebral spinal fluid. However, there are no reports of critically ill patients experiencing adverse central nervous system events from the accumulation of laudanosine.

The steroid-based agents, pancuronium and vecuronium are metabolized to 3-hydroxy metabolites that have 50% of the activity of the parent compounds. These metabolites are renally eliminated and have been shown to accumulate in patients with renal dysfunction, producing prolonged periods of paralysis. Monitoring patients and adjusting doses, dosing intervals, or continuous infusion rates with the aid of a peripheral nerve stimulator to maintain one or two twitches of a TOF stimulation can usually prevent this adverse effect from occurring (see Chapter 6, Pain, Sedation, and Neuromuscular Blockade Management).

A more serious complication associated with the use of nondepolarizing agents is the development of a prolonged disuse atrophy syndrome. This syndrome has been shown to occur after the extended administration of steroid-based and benzylisoquinolinium agents and cannot be prevented with peripheral nerve stimulation monitoring. Patients receiving steroids may be predisposed to developing this complication; however, this association remains to be conclusively proven.

Tolerance or the need to increase doses to maintain a stable level of paralysis is often encountered in patients receiving these agents for an extended duration. Tolerance may be attributed to the proliferation of nonfunctional extrajunctional receptors that bind drug but do not cause paralysis, increased volume of distribution resulting in lower serum concentrations at the neuromuscular junction, and binding to acute phase reactant proteins, decreasing the free, pharmacologically active fraction. An additional consideration for patients requiring NMBAs is care that prevents secondary injury. This includes meticulous skin care to prevent pressure injury, the use of prophylactic eye care to prevent corneal abrasions, venous thromboembolism prophylaxis and oral care to prevent ventilator-associated pneumonia. For patients receiving NMBA and corticosteroids, every effort is made to discontinue the NMBAs as soon as possible.

Dose
Intermediate-Acting

- *Atracurium:* Intubation: 0.5 mg/kg IV; maintenance: 0.08 to 0.10 mg/kg IV; continuous infusion: 5 to 20 mcg/kg/min
- *Cisatracurium:* Intubation: 0.15 to 0.2 mg/kg IV; maintenance dose: 0.03 mg/kg IV; continuous infusion: 1 to 3 mcg/kg/min

- Rocuronium: Intubation: 0.45 to 1.2 mg/kg IV; maintenance dose: 0.075 to 0.15 mg/kg IV; continuous infusion: 10 to 14 mcg/kg/min
- Vecuronium: Intubation: 0.1 to 0.15 mg/kg IV; maintenance dose: 0.01 to 0.15 mg/kg IV; continuous infusion: 0.8 to 1.7 mcg/kg/min

Long-Acting

- Pancuronium: Intubation: 0.06 to 0.1 mg/kg IV; maintenance dose: 0.01 to 0.015 mg/kg IV; continuous infusion: 1 mcg/kg/min (not generally recommended)

Monitoring Parameters

- Level of paralysis (peripheral nerve stimulation), renal function, and liver function

Anticonvulsants

Hydantoins

Phenytoin

Phenytoin is an anticonvulsant used for the acute control of generalized tonic-clonic (GTC) seizures, following the administration of benzodiazepines, and for maintenance therapy once the seizure has been controlled. Phenytoin stabilizes neuronal cell membranes and decreases the spread of seizure activity. Phenytoin may inhibit neuronal depolarizations by blocking sodium channels in excitatory pathways and prevent increases in intracellular potassium concentrations and decreases in intracellular calcium concentrations.

The bioavailability of oral phenytoin is approximately 90% to 100%. Dissolution is the rate-limiting step in phenytoin absorption with peak serum concentrations occurring 1.5 (eg, oral liquid and immediate release) to 12 hours (eg, Dilantin Kapseal capsules) after a dose. The rate of absorption is dose dependent, with increasing times to peak concentration with increasing doses. In addition, the dissolution and absorption rate depend on the phenytoin formulation administered. The Dilantin Kapseal brand of phenytoin capsules has the dissolution characteristics of an extended-release preparation, whereas generic phenytoin products possess rapid-release characteristics and are absorbed more quickly. Extended-release and rapid-release products are not interchangeable, and only extended-release products may be administered in a single daily dose.

Phenytoin is 90% to 95% bound to albumin. In critically ill patients, the pharmacologically free fraction is highly variable and ranges between 10% and 27% of the total serum concentration. The free fraction has been shown to increase by more than 100% from baseline during the first week of illness and is generally associated with a significant reduction in serum albumin concentration. Alterations in albumin binding also may be seen in hypoalbuminemia (<2.5 g/dL), major trauma, sepsis, burns, malnutrition, and surgery, as well as liver or renal disease, and may result in an increase in a free concentration with potentially toxic effects. Significant alterations in phenytoin metabolism usually do not occur until the serum albumin falls below 2.5 g/dL. Equations used to normalize the phenytoin concentration in patients with hypoalbuminemia are usually unreliable, and direct measurement of the free phenytoin concentration is used to adjust therapy.

Phenytoin is metabolized by the cytochrome P-450 enzyme system to its inactive primary metabolite 5-(p-hydroxyphenyl)-5-phenylhydantoin, which is glucuronidated and renally eliminated. Phenytoin undergoes dose-dependent metabolism such that proportional increases in the dose may result in greater than proportional increases in the serum concentration. It is difficult to predict the concentration at which a patient's metabolism will become saturated, so that any changes in dose above 400 to 500 mg/day need to be carefully monitored. Because phenytoin displays nonlinear metabolism, *half-life* is an inappropriate term to describe phenytoin elimination. Phenytoin metabolism is usually referred to as the time it takes to eliminate 50% (t_{50}) of a given daily dose. In normal patients taking 300 mg/day, the t_{50} is about 22 hours. As the dose is increased, the t_{50} increases, with the time to reach steady state becoming progressively longer. The time to steady state may vary from several days to several weeks depending on the dose and the patient's ability to metabolize the drug.

Other medications can affect phenytoin metabolism by inducing or inhibiting its metabolic pathway. The effects of enzyme induction can occur within 2 days to 2 weeks after starting an agent. Inhibition usually occurs within 1 to 2 days after a drug is started and its effects usually last until the inhibiting drug is eliminated from the body. Phenytoin clearance is increased in critically ill patients, resulting in subtherapeutic serum concentrations. The mechanism for the increase in clearance is unclear, but may be caused by changes in protein binding, induction in phenytoin metabolism, or a stress-related transient increase in hepatic metabolic function.

Phenytoin precipitates in dextrose-containing solutions and should only be mixed in 0.9% sodium chloride solutions. Because of its short-stability, it is administered within 4 hours of compounding. To prevent phlebitis, the maximum concentration for peripheral administration is 10 mg/mL; a final concentration of 20 mg/mL may be used if the dose is being administered through a central venous catheter. Phenytoin solution must be administered through an in-line 1.2- or 5.0-μ filter to prevent the administration of phenytoin crystals into the systemic circulation. Phenytoin doses should not be administered at a rate faster than 50 mg/min because hypotension and arrhythmias may occur, with hypotension likely related to propylene glycol diluent. The infusion rate is decreased by 50%, if hypotension or arrhythmias develop.

Oral administration is not usually recommended in critically ill patients because of the risk of erratic or incomplete absorption. Phenytoin oral suspension may adhere to the inside walls of oro- or nasogastric tubes, reducing the dose delivered to the patient. If phenytoin is administered through a feeding tube, the tube is flushed with 30 to 60 mL of 0.9% sodium chloride before and after administering the dose. After the dose is administered, the feeding tube is clamped for an hour before restarting the feeding solution. Oral absorption may be impaired by concomitant administration with enteral nutrition solutions, reducing its bioavailability and resulting in erratic serum concentrations with seizures occurring as a result of subtherapeutic serum concentrations. Phenytoin oral solution must be shaken prior to use to ensure uniformity in the distribution of the phenytoin particles throughout the suspension. If the suspension is not shaken before obtaining a dose, the phenytoin powder settles to the bottom of the bottle producing subtherapeutic doses when the bottle is first opened and toxic doses as the bottle is used.

The normal therapeutic range for the total phenytoin serum concentration is 10 to 20 mg/L with the free fraction therapeutic range of 1 to 2 mg/L. Serum concentration of 20 to 30 mg/L may be required in patients who are having seizures. Phenytoin serum concentrations can be obtained 30 to 60 minutes after the IV loading dose is infused to assess the adequacy of the dose. Trough concentrations are monitored 2 to 3 times a week, particularly after the first week of therapy. Measurement of free phenytoin concentrations may be indicated in critically ill patients, patients with serum albumin concentrations less than 2.5 g/dL, renal failure, or receiving drugs known to displace phenytoin from albumin-binding sites. Other monitoring parameters include the patient's seizure activity and medication profile for agents known to alter phenytoin's metabolism.

Hemodialysis and hemofiltration have no effect on phenytoin clearance. Early adverse effects that may be associated with increasing concentrations are nystagmus (>20 mg/L), ataxia (>30 mg/L), lethargy, confusion, and impaired cognitive function (>40 mg/L).

Dose

- *Loading dose:* 15 to 20 mg/kg IV (18-20 mg/kg for status epilepticus or 15-18 mg/kg for seizure prophylaxis). An additional IV loading dose of up to 10 mg/kg can be given to status epilepticus patients refractory to the initial loading dose.
- *Maintenance dose:* 5 to 7.5 mg/kg/day IV or PO (5-6 mg/kg/day in typical adults or 6-7.5 mg/kg/day may be required in acutely ill or neurotrauma). IV doses administered every 6 to 8 hours.

Monitoring Parameters

- Seizure activity, electroencephalogram (EEG), serum phenytoin concentration (free phenytoin concentration if applicable), albumin, liver function, infusion rate, blood pressure, ECG with IV administration, and IV injection site
- Note that serum phenytoin concentrations should be drawn 2 to 4 hours after a loading dose in status epilepticus

Fosphenytoin

Fosphenytoin is a phenytoin prodrug with good aqueous solubility that was developed to be a water-soluble alternative to phenytoin. In patients unable to tolerate oral phenytoin, equimolar doses of fosphenytoin have been shown to produce equal or greater plasma phenytoin concentrations. Although phenytoin sodium 50 mg is equal to fosphenytoin sodium 75 mg, fosphenytoin doses are converted to an equivalent phenytoin dose known as phenytoin equivalents (PE) on a milligram-per-milligram basis. Thus, a phenytoin 300 mg dose is equal to fosphenytoin 300 mg PE.

Fosphenytoin, administered IM or IV, is rapidly and completely converted to phenytoin in vivo, resulting in essentially 100% bioavailability. The conversion half-life to phenytoin is about 33 minutes following IM administration and about 15 minutes after IV infusion. After IM administration, peak plasma fosphenytoin concentrations occur approximately 30 minutes postdose, with peak phenytoin concentrations occurring in about 3 hours. Fosphenytoin's peak concentration following IV administration occurs at the end of the infusion, with peak phenytoin concentrations occurring in approximately 40 to 75 minutes. In patients with renal or hepatic dysfunction or hypoalbuminemia, there is enhanced conversion to phenytoin without an increase in clearance. Fosphenytoin is 90% to 95% bound to plasma proteins and is saturable with the percent of bound fosphenytoin decreasing as the fosphenytoin dose increases.

The maximum total phenytoin concentration increases with increasing fosphenytoin doses, but the total phenytoin concentration is less affected by increasing fosphenytoin infusion rates. Maximum free phenytoin concentrations are nearly constant at infusion rates up to 50 mg PE/min, whereas they increase with faster infusion rates secondary to phenytoin displacement from albumin-binding sites in the presence of high fosphenytoin concentrations.

For the treatment of status epilepticus, the recommended loading dose of IV fosphenytoin is 15 to 20 PE/kg, and it is not administered faster than 150 mg PE/min because of the risk of hypotension. Fosphenytoin 15 to 20 mg PE/kg infused at 100 to 150 mg PE/min yields plasma-free phenytoin concentrations over time that approximate those achieved when an equimolar dose of IV phenytoin is administered at 50 mg/min. In the treatment of status epilepticus, total phenytoin concentrations greater than 10 mg/L and free phenytoin concentrations greater than 1 mg/mL are achieved within 10 to 20 minutes after starting the infusion.

In nonemergent situations, loading doses of 10 to 20 PE/kg administered IV or IM are recommended. In nonemergent situations, IV administration of infusion rates of 50 to 100 mg PE/min may be acceptable, but results in slightly lower and delayed maximum free phenytoin concentrations as compared with administration at higher infusion rates. The initial daily maintenance dose is 4 to 6 mg PE/kg/day. Dosing adjustments are not required when IM fosphenytoin is substituted temporarily for oral phenytoin. However, patients switched from once-daily extended-release phenytoin capsules may require twice-daily or more frequent administration of fosphenytoin to maintain similar peak and trough phenytoin concentrations.

The incidence of adverse effects tends to increase as both dose and infusion rate are increased. At doses above 15 mg PE/kg and infusion rates higher than 150 mg PE/min, transient pruritus, tinnitus, nystagmus, somnolence, and ataxia occur more frequently than at lower doses or infusion rates. Severe burning, itching, and paresthesias of the groin are commonly associated with infusion rates greater than 150 mg PE/min. Slowing or temporarily stopping the infusion can minimize the frequency and severity of these reactions. Continuous cardiac rate and rhythm, blood pressure, and respiratory function are monitored throughout the fosphenytoin infusion and for 10 to 20 minutes after the end of the infusion.

Following fosphenytoin administration, phenytoin concentrations are not monitored until the conversion to phenytoin is complete. This occurs within 2 hours after the end of an IV infusion and 5 hours after an IM injection. Prior to complete conversion, commonly used immunoanalytic techniques such as fluorescence polarization and enzyme-mediated assays may significantly overestimate plasma phenytoin concentrations because of cross-reactivity with fosphenytoin. Blood samples collected before complete conversion to phenytoin are collected in tubes containing EDTA as an anticoagulant to minimize the ex vivo conversion of fosphenytoin to phenytoin. Monitoring is similar to phenytoin. In critically ill patients with renal failure receiving fosphenytoin, one or more metabolites of adducts of fosphenytoin accumulate and display significant cross-reactivity with several phenytoin immunoassay methods.

Pyrrolidine Derivatives

Levetiracetam

Levetiracetam is a second-generation antiepileptic drug with increasing usage in the critical care setting. The agent leads to selective prevention of burst firing and seizure activity. Levetiracetam is commonly prescribed for adjunctive treatment of partial onset seizures with or without secondary generalization. Other approved indications include monotherapy treatment of partial onset seizures with or without secondary generalization, and adjunctive treatment of myoclonic seizures associated with juvenile myoclonic epilepsy and primary GTC seizures associated with idiopathic generalized epilepsy. Seizure prophylaxis in posttraumatic brain injury patients is also an established role for levetiracetam. Additionally, levetiracetam is used in neurologic emergencies (eg, status epilepticus) and rapid IV administration of undiluted levetiracetam has been proven safe and tolerable in doses of up to 1500 mg. This option is often preferred compared with IVPB, because of ready access to the undiluted drug for administration.

Levetiracetam lacks cytochrome P450 isoenzyme-inducing potential and is not associated with clinically significant interactions with other drugs, including other antiepileptic drugs. Sedation is the most common adverse effect noted.

Dose

- *Maintenance dose:* 250 mg to 1000 mg q12 IV or PO
- *Status epilepticus loading dose:*
  - *IVPB:* 20 mg/kg IV over 15 minutes.
  - *IV Push:* 20 mg/kg IV push. Maximum of 1500 mg over 5 minutes.

Monitoring Parameters

- Seizure activity, EEG, sedation

Miscellaneous agents

Lacosamide

Lacosamide is a functionalized amino acid anticonvulsant indicated for the treatment of partial onset and primary GTC seizures. Usage of this agent within the ICU has increased, as this agent is well tolerated. Both oral and injectable forms are available; the injectable form can be used when oral administration is temporarily not feasible.

Dose

- *Maintenance dose:* 150 mg to 200mg q12 IV or PO

Monitoring Parameters

- Seizure activity, EEG

Valproic acid

Valproic acid, which includes divalprocx sodium is an antiepileptic drug indicated for monotherapy and adjunctive therapy of complex partial seizures and simple and complex absence seizures, adjunctive therapy in patients with multiple seizure types that include absence seizures. There are a number of dosage forms available ranging from delayed and extended-release oral dosage forms, oral liquid, and parenteral. As such, these agents are very commonly used in various patient care settings.

Dose

- *Maintenance dose:* 10 to 15 mg/kg/day IV or PO titrated in 5 to 10 mg/kg/day increments at weekly intervals to a maximum of 60 mg/kg/day

Monitoring Parameters

- Seizure activity, EEG, liver function tests

Barbiturates

Pentobarbital

Pentobarbital is a barbiturate mainly used to control intracranial pressure in patients with head injuries. Pentobarbital may also be used in patients with status epilepticus who are refractory to other anticonvulsants. The central nervous system protective effect of pentobarbital may be attributed to decreased cerebral oxygen consumption allowing a proportionate decrease in cerebral blood flow and potentially scavenging free oxygen radicals. Its anticonvulsant effects are similar to phenobarbital. Pentobarbital produces a dose-dependent depression of the central nervous system beginning with sedation and ending with coma and death. At high serum concentrations, pentobarbital suppresses the respiratory drive necessitating mechanical ventilation during therapeutic pentobarbital coma.

Pentobarbital has a greater affinity for adipose tissue than phenobarbital. Its lipophilicity causes it to cross the blood-brain barrier faster than phenobarbital to produce its central nervous system effects. Pentobarbital is hepatically metabolized with an average half-life of 22 hours. In head-injured patients, pentobarbital's clearance is faster with its half-life averaging 15 to 19 hours. Alterations in hepatic microsomal enzymes can be expected to alter its clearance and half-life.

The infusion may be discontinued after 72 hours of intracranial pressure control or if there is deterioration in the cardiovascular status of the patient. The infusion is tapered over 48 to 72 hours by decreasing the infusion rate by 25% every 12 hours. The patient is monitored during this time for increases in intracranial pressure or the development of seizures.

Serum concentrations are obtained 1 to 2 hours after the loading infusion and then daily. The serum concentration within 24 hours after starting therapy does not reflect steady-state conditions. If the 24-hour concentration has changed from the post-loading dose by 33% to 50% and is less than 20 mg/L or greater than 50 mg/L, the infusion is increased or decreased by 0.5 to 1.0 mg/kg/h. Serum concentrations are monitored in conjunction with the patient's physiologic parameters such as brain stem reflexes, intracranial pressure, systemic blood pressure, EEG, and hemodynamic parameters. Acceptable therapeutic endpoints include an MAP of 70 to 80 mm Hg, cerebral perfusion pressure of greater than 60 mm Hg, intracranial pressure of less than 20 mm Hg, EEG showing a 30- to 60-second burst suppression pattern, and an absence of muscular movement and brainstem reflexes on neurologic examination. However, deeper levels of sedation may not be needed if seizures are controlled, or intracranial pressure is less than 20 mm Hg.

Dose
- *IV bolus:* 5 to 10 mg/kg IV over 2 hours for coma or status epilepticus
- *Continuous infusion:* 0.5 to 4 mg/kg/h (start at 0.5-1 mg/kg/h and increase in increments of 0.5-1 mg/kg/h

Monitoring Parameters
- Seizure activity, intracranial pressure, blood pressure, heart rate, respiratory rate, EEG

Phenobarbital

Phenobarbital may be added for patients who have not responded to other IV antiepileptics. Phenobarbital depresses excitatory postsynaptic seizure discharge and increases the

convulsive threshold for electrical and chemical stimulation. This effect is due to the inhibiting effects of GABA.

Phenobarbital is 90% to 100% bioavailable with peak concentrations occurring in 0.5 to 4 hours after an oral or IM dose. Peak brain concentrations occur approximately 20 to 40 minutes after an administered dose. Phenobarbital is primarily hepatically metabolized by the cytochrome P-450 microsomal enzyme system with approximately 25% of a dose excreted unchanged in the urine. The half-life of phenobarbital is 96 hours with steady-state conditions being achieved in about 2 to 3 weeks.

The usual loading dose of phenobarbital is 20 mg/kg and achieves a serum concentration of about 20 mg/L. Each 1 mg/kg dose increment increases the serum concentration by about 1.5 mg/L. The loading dose has the potential to decrease respiratory drive in patients who have received other central nervous system depressants. The maximum IV infusion rate is 50 mg/min or less. Infusion rates above 50 mg/min may cause hypotension because of its propylene glycol diluent. Blood pressure is monitored during the loading infusion, and the infusion rate is decreased by 50% if hypotension develops.

The maintenance dose is started within 24 hours after the loading dose. The typical adult maintenance dose of 2 to 4 mg/kg/day produces serum concentrations in the range of 10 to 30 mg/L. Each 1 mg/kg/day increase in the maintenance dose increases the serum concentration about 10 mg/L. Lower doses are used in elderly patients, patients with renal failure, and patients with liver dysfunction because of their reduced abilities to eliminate the drug. The maintenance dose is administered as a single daily dose because of its long half-life, with this dose usually given at bedtime because of phenobarbital's sedative properties. In cases of excessive sedation, the daily dose may be administered as smaller doses 2 to 3 times per day. Tolerance usually develops to sedation with long-term administration.

Hemodialysis removes a significant amount of phenobarbital. Posthemodialysis serum concentrations are monitored and supplemented doses administered after hemodialysis to maintain the serum concentration within the therapeutic range.

Phenobarbital serum concentrations can be monitored 30 to 60 minutes after the end of the loading infusion to assess the adequacy of the dose. Maintenance doses are monitored every 3 to 4 days in patients with changing hemodynamic status, because the patients may have alterations in their ability to eliminate the drug, resulting in increased or decreased serum concentrations. If the serum concentrations are fluctuating, they are monitored daily to prevent excessive rises in the serum concentrations and toxicity or subtherapeutic serum concentrations and seizures. The serum concentration may be monitored once a week if stable. Trough concentrations are typically monitored, but because of its long half-life, there is minimal peak-to-trough variation in the serum concentration so that a drug level can be drawn anytime during the dosing interval. When patients regain consciousness, serum levels may not be needed if the patients are not having seizures.

Dose

- *Loading dose:* 20 mg/kg IV (1 mg/kg increases the serum concentration 1 mg/L)
- *Maintenance dose:* 3 to 5 mg/kg/day IV or PO

Monitoring Parameters

- Seizure activity, EEG, serum phenobarbital concentration, infusion rate, blood pressure, and ECG with IV administration

Benzodiazepines

Benzodiazepines are the primary agents in the management of status epilepticus. These agents suppress the spread of seizure activity but do not abolish the abnormal discharge from a seizure focus. Although IV diazepam has the fastest onset of action, lorazepam or midazolam are equally efficacious in controlling seizure activity. They are the agents of choice to temporarily control seizures and to gain time for the loading of fosphenytoin, levetiracetam, or valproic acid.

Monitoring Parameters

- Seizure activity, EEG, and respiratory rate and quality

CARDIOVASCULAR SYSTEM PHARMACOLOGY

Miscellaneous Agents

Fenoldopam

Fenoldopam is a benzapine derivative with selective dopamine-1 receptor agonist properties, similar to dopamine. This dopaminergic stimulation results in a decrease in systemic blood pressure with an increase in natriuresis and urine output. The primary use of fenoldopam is limited to the management of severe hypertension, particularly in patients with renal impairment.

Dose

- *Continuous infusion:* 0.1 to 1.6 mcg/kg/min

Monitoring Parameters

- Blood pressure, urine output, and hemodynamic parameters

Parenteral Vasodilators

Nitrates

Sodium Nitroprusside

Sodium nitroprusside is a balanced vasodilator affecting the arterial and venous systems. Blood pressure reduction occurs within seconds after an infusion is started, with a duration of action of less than 10 minutes once the infusion is discontinued. Sodium nitroprusside was previously considered the agent of choice in acute hypertensive conditions such as hypertensive encephalopathy, intracerebral infarction, subarachnoid

hemorrhage, carotid endarterectomy, malignant hypertension, microangiopathic anemia, and aortic dissection, and after general surgical procedures, major vascular procedures, or renal transplantation. However, use of this agent has been severely restricted due to significant cost increases compared with effective, safer, and less costly alternatives.

If sodium nitroprusside is used for longer than 48 hours, there is a risk of thiocyanate toxicity. However, this may only be a concern in patients with renal dysfunction. In this setting, thiocyanate serum concentrations are monitored to ensure that they remain below 10 mg/dL. Other potential side effects include methemoglobinemia and cyanide toxicity. Nitroprusside should be used with caution in the setting of increased intracranial pressure, such as head trauma or postcraniotomy, where it may cause an increase in cerebral blood flow. Nitroprusside's effects on intracranial pressure may be attenuated by a lowered $PaCO_2$ and raised PaO_2. In pregnant women, nitroprusside is reserved only for refractory hypertension associated with eclampsia because of the potential risk to the fetus.

Dose

- *Continuous infusion:* 0.5 to 10 mcg/kg/min

Monitoring Parameters

- Blood pressure, renal function, thiocyanate concentration (prolonged infusions), acid-base status, and hemodynamic parameters

Nitroglycerin

Nitroglycerin is a preferential venous dilator affecting the venous system at low doses, but relaxes arterial smooth muscle at higher doses. The onset of blood pressure reduction after starting a nitroglycerin infusion is similar to sodium nitroprusside, approximately 1 to 3 minutes, with duration of action of less than 10 minutes. Headaches are a common adverse effect that may occur with nitroglycerin therapy and can be treated with acetaminophen. Tachyphylaxis can be seen with the IV infusion, similar to what is seen after the chronic use of topical nitroglycerin preparations. Tachyphylaxis is very common and the patient should be transitioned to another agent to meet the goal endpoint if needed. In patients receiving unfractionated heparin in addition to nitroglycerin, increased doses of unfractionated heparin may be required to maintain a therapeutic partial thromboplastin time (PTT). The mechanism by which nitroglycerin causes unfractionated heparin resistance is unknown. However, the PTT is closely monitored in patients receiving nitroglycerin and unfractionated heparin concurrently.

Nitroglycerin is the preferred agent in the setting of hypertension associated with myocardial ischemia or infarction because its net effect is a reduction in oxygen consumption.

Dose

- *Continuous infusion:* 10 to 300 mcg/min

Monitoring Parameters

- Blood pressure, heart rate, signs and symptoms of ischemia, hemodynamic parameters (if applicable), and PTT (in patients receiving unfractionated heparin concurrently)

Arterial Vasodilating Agents
Hydralazine

Hydralazine reduces peripheral vascular resistance by directly relaxing arterial smooth muscle. Blood pressure reduction occurs within 5 to 20 minutes after an IV dose and lasts approximately 2 to 6 hours. Common adverse effects include headache, nausea, vomiting, palpitations, and tachycardia. Reflex tachycardia may precipitate anginal attacks. Co-administration of a beta-receptor antagonist can decrease the incidence of tachycardia.

Dose

- 10 to 25 mg IV q2-4h

Monitoring Parameters

- Blood pressure and heart rate

Alpha- and Beta-Adrenergic Blocking Agents
Labetalol

Labetalol is a combined alpha- and beta-adrenergic blocking agent with a specificity of beta receptors to alpha receptors of approximately 7:1. Labetalol may be administered parenterally by escalating bolus doses or by continuous infusion. The onset of action after the administration of labetalol is within 5 minutes with a duration of effect from 2 to 12 hours. Because labetalol possesses beta-blocking properties, it may produce bronchospasm in individuals with asthma or reactive airway disease. It also may produce conduction system disturbances or bradycardia in susceptible individuals, and its negative inotropic properties may exacerbate symptoms of HF.

Labetalol may be considered as an alternative to sodium nitroprusside in the setting of hypertension associated with head trauma or postcraniotomy, spinal cord syndromes, transverse lesions of the spinal cord, Guillain-Barré syndrome, or autonomic hyperreflexia, as well as hypertension associated with sympathomimetics (eg, cocaine, amphetamines, phencyclidine, nasal decongestants, or certain diet pills) or withdrawal of centrally acting antihypertensive agents (eg, beta-blockers, clonidine, or methyldopa). It also may be used as an alternative to phentolamine in the setting of pheochromocytoma because of its alpha- and beta-blocking properties.

Dose

- *IV bolus:* 10 to 20 mg over 2 minutes, then 40 to 80 mg IV q10min to a total of 300 mg
- *Continuous infusion:* 1 to 6 mg/min and titrate to effect

Monitoring Parameters

- Blood pressure, heart rate, ECG, and signs and symptoms of HF or bronchospasm (if applicable)

Alpha-Adrenergic Blocking Agents
Phentolamine

Phentolamine is an alpha-adrenergic blocking agent that may be administered parenterally by bolus injection or continuous infusion. Onset of action is within 1 to 2 minutes, with a duration of action of 3 to 10 minutes. Potential adverse effects that may occur with phentolamine include tachycardia, GI stimulation, and hypoglycemia.

Phentolamine is considered the drug of choice for the treatment of hypertension associated with pheochromocytoma because of its ability to block alpha-adrenergic receptors. Also, it is the primary agent used to treat acute hypertensive episodes in patients receiving monoamine oxidase inhibitors.

Dose

- *IV bolus:* 5 to 10 mg q5-15min
- *Continuous infusion:* 1 to 10 mg/min

Monitoring Parameters

- Blood pressure and heart rate

Beta-Adrenergic Blocking Agents

Beta-adrenergic blocking agents available for IV delivery include propranolol, atenolol, esmolol, and metoprolol. Propranolol, atenolol, and metoprolol are administered by bolus injection, and esmolol is administered by continuous infusion. A continuous infusion of esmolol may or may not be preceded by an initial bolus injection.

Esmolol has the fastest onset and shortest duration of action, approximately 1 to 3 minutes and 20 to 30 minutes, respectively. Propranolol and metoprolol have similar onset times, but durations of action vary between 1 and 6 hours. The duration of action after a bolus dose of atenolol is approximately 12 hours.

All agents may produce bronchospasm in individuals with asthma or reactive airway disease and may produce conduction system disturbances or bradycardia in susceptible individuals. Also, because of their negative inotropic properties, they may exacerbate symptoms of HF. Beta-blocking agents typically are used as adjuncts with other agents in the treatment of acute hypertension. They may be used with sodium nitroprusside in the treatment of acute aortic dissections. They are administered to patients with hypertension associated with pheochromocytoma only after phentolamine has been given. Also, they are the agents of choice in patients who have been maintained on beta-blocking agents for the chronic management of hypertension but who have abruptly stopped therapy.

Beta-blocking agents are avoided in patients with hypertensive encephalopathy, intracranial infarctions, or subarachnoid hemorrhages because of their central nervous system depressant effects. They also are avoided in patients with acute pulmonary edema because of their negative inotropic properties. Finally, beta-blocking agents are avoided in hypertension associated with eclampsia and renal vasculature disorders.

Dose

- *Esmolol:* IV bolus 500 mcg/kg; continuous infusion: 50 to 400 mcg/kg/min
- *Metoprolol:* IV bolus: 5 mg IV q2min; maintenance 1.25 to 5 mg q6-12h
- *Propranolol:* IV bolus: 0.5 to 1 mg q5-15min

Monitoring Parameters

- Blood pressure, heart rate, ECG, and signs and symptoms of HF or bronchospasm (if applicable)

Angiotensin-Converting Enzyme Inhibitors

Angiotensin-converting enzyme (ACE) inhibitors competitively inhibit ACE, which is responsible for the conversion of angiotensin I to angiotensin II (a potent vasoconstrictor). In addition, ACE inhibitors increase the availability of bradykinin and other vasodilatory prostaglandins, and reduce plasma aldosterone concentrations. The net effect is a reduction in blood pressure in hypertensive patients and a reduction in afterload in patients with HF.

ACE inhibitors are indicated in the management of hypertension and HF. ACE inhibitors currently available in oral formulations include quinapril, ramipril, benazepril, captopril, enalapril, fosinopril, and lisinopril. Enalaprilat is the only IV formulation available. Adverse effects associated with ACE inhibitors include rash, taste disturbances, and cough. Additionally, ACE inhibitors can cause drug-induced angioedema, which most often affects the lips, tongue, face, and upper airway, and more rarely is associated with abdominal symptoms (eg, pain with diarrhea). Initial-dose hypotension may occur in patients who are hypovolemic, hyponatremic, or who have been aggressively diuresed. Hypotension may be avoided or minimized by starting with low doses or withholding diuretics for 24 to 48 hours. Worsening of renal function may occur in patients with bilateral renal artery stenosis. Additionally, hyperkalemia is also a possible complication of ACE inhibitor therapy, especially in patients with chronic kidney disease and in combination with other potassium-sparing medications.

Enalapril

Enalapril is unique among ACE inhibitors, as it is a prodrug that is converted in the liver to its active moiety, enalaprilat, a long-acting ACE inhibitor. Enalapril is available in an oral dosage form, and enalaprilat is available in the IV form. Following an IV dose of enalaprilat, blood pressure lowering occurs within 15 minutes and lasts 4 to 6 hours.

Dose

- *Enalaprilat:* IV bolus: 0.625 to 1.25 mg over 5 minutes q6h; continuous infusion: not recommended
- *Enalapril:* oral: 2.5 to 40 mg qd

Monitoring Parameters

- Blood pressure, heart rate, renal function, and electrolytes

Angiotensin Receptor Blockers

Angiotensin receptor blockers (ARBs) selectively block the binding of angiotensin II (a powerful vasoconstrictor in vascular smooth muscle) to the receptors in tissues such as vascular smooth muscle and the adrenal gland. This receptor blockade results in vasodilation and decreased secretion of aldosterone, which leads to increased sodium excretion and potassium-sparing effects. ARBs are indicated for both hypertension and HF. ARBs currently available in oral formulations include valsartan, candesartan, irbesartan, azilsartan, eprosartan, losartan, telmisartan, and olmesartan. The most common adverse effects of ARBs are hypotension, dizziness, and headache. Although rare, cough can also be associated with ARBs. This cough can be reversed by discontinuance of therapy. Overall, these agents are relatively well tolerated and thus commonly used for the chronic management of hypertension. The role in the acute blood pressure lowering is limited due to the lack of a parenteral formulation.

Monitoring Parameters

- Blood pressure and heart rate, and electrolytes

Calcium Channel–Blocking Agents

Calcium channel–blocking agents may be used as alternative therapy in the treatment of hypertension resulting from hypertensive encephalopathy, myocardial ischemia, malignant hypertension, or eclampsia, or after renal transplantation.

Nicardipine

Nicardipine is an IV calcium channel–blocking agent that is primarily indicated for the treatment of hypertension. Onset is within 5 minutes with duration of approximately 30 minutes. Nicardipine also is available in an oral dosage form, however not commonly administered. Patients started on IV therapy are more commonly converted to convert to nifedipine extended-release oral therapy or amlodipine enterally per tube when indicated.

Dose

- *Continuous infusion:* 5 mg/h, increase every 15 minutes to a maximum of 15 mg/h

Monitoring Parameters

- Blood pressure and heart rate

Clevidipine

Clevidipine is an IV calcium channel–blocking agent that is also indicated for the treatment of hypertension. An onset of 2 minutes is faster than nicardipine with a shorter duration of 10 minutes. Clevidipine is delivered as an injectable lipid emulsion (20%), similar to intralipids, and is not available in an oral dosage form. Similar to propofol, vials of clevidipine and IV tubing must be changed every 12 hours during therapy because the phospholipids support microbial growth.

Dose

- *Continuous infusion:* 1 to 2 mg/h, increase by doubling dose every 90-second interval initially to achieve blood pressure reduction. As the blood pressure approaches goal, increase dose less aggressively every 5 to 10 minutes. Maximum recommended dose of 32 mg/h, with an average rate of 21 mg/h for a maximum duration of 72 hours.

Monitoring Parameters

- Blood pressure and heart rate

Central Sympatholytic Agents

Clonidine

Clonidine is an oral agent that stimulates alpha-2-adrenergic receptors in the medulla oblongata, causing inhibition of sympathetic vasomotor centers. Although clonidine typically is used as maintenance antihypertensive therapy, it can be used in the setting of hypertensive urgencies or emergencies. Its antihypertensive effects may be seen within 30 minutes and last 8 to 12 hours. Once blood pressure is controlled, oral maintenance clonidine therapy may be started.

Centrally acting sympatholytics rarely are indicated as first-line agents except when hypertension may be due to the abrupt withdrawal of one of these agents.

Dose

- *Hypertensive urgency:* 0.2 mg PO initially, then 0.1 mg/h PO (to a maximum of 0.8 mg)
- *Transdermal:* TTS-1 (0.1 mg/day) to TTS-3 (0.3 mg/day) topically q1wk

Monitoring Parameters

- Blood pressure, heart rate, and mental status. Monitor for syncope with first dose

Antiarrhythmics

Antiarrhythmic agents are divided into five classes. Dosage information for individual antiarrhythmic agents is not provided in this chapter.

Class I Agents

Class I agents are further divided into three subclasses: Ia (procainamide, quinidine, disopyramide), Ib (lidocaine, mexiletine), and Ic (flecainide, propafenone). All class I agents block sodium channels in the myocardium and inhibit potassium-repolarizing currents to prolong repolarization.

Class Ia Agents

Class Ia agents inhibit the fast sodium channel (phase 0 of the action potential), slow conduction at elevated serum drug concentrations, and prolong action potential duration and repolarization. Class Ia agents can cause proarrhythmic complications by prolonging the QT interval or by depressing conduction and promoting reentry.

Monitoring Parameters

- ECG (QRS complex, QT interval, arrhythmia frequency)

Class Ib Agents

Class Ib agents have little effect on phase 0 depolarization and conduction velocity, but shorten the action potential duration and repolarization. QT prolongation typically does not occur with class Ib agents. Class Ib agents act selectively on diseased or ischemic tissue where they block conduction and interrupt reentry circuits.

Monitoring Parameters

- ECG (QT interval, arrhythmia frequency), hepatic function

Class Ic Agents

Class Ic agents inhibit the fast sodium channel and cause a marked depression of phase 0 of the action potential and slow conduction profoundly but have minimal effects on repolarization. The dramatic effects of these agents on conduction may account for their significant proarrhythmic effects, which limit their use in patients with supraventricular arrhythmias and structural heart disease.

Monitoring Parameters

- ECG (PR interval and QRS complex, arrhythmia frequency)

Class II Agents

Beta-blocking agents (esmolol, metoprolol, and propranolol) inactivate sodium channels and depress phase 4 depolarization and increase the refractory period of the atrioventricular node. These agents have no effect on repolarization. Beta-blockers competitively antagonize catecholamine binding at beta-adrenergic receptors.

Beta-blocking agents can be classified as selective or nonselective agents. *Nonselective agents* bind to beta-1 receptors located on myocardial cells and beta-2 receptors located on bronchial and skeletal smooth muscle. Stimulation of beta-1 receptors causes an increase in heart rate and contractility, whereas stimulation of beta-2 receptors results in bronchodilation and vasodilation. Selective beta-blocking agents block beta-1 receptors in the heart at low or moderate doses, but they become less selective with increasing doses.

Class II agents are used for the prophylaxis and treatment of both supraventricular arrhythmias and arrhythmias associated with catecholamine excess or stimulation, slowing the ventricular response in atrial fibrillation, lowering blood pressure, decreasing heart rate, and decreasing ischemia. Esmolol is useful especially for the rapid, short-term control of ventricular response in atrial fibrillation or flutter.

Nonselective beta-blocking agents are avoided or used with caution in patients with HF, atrioventricular nodal blockade, asthma, COPD, peripheral vascular disease, Raynaud phenomenon, and diabetes. Beta-1 selective beta-blocking agents are used with caution in these populations.

Monitoring Parameters

- ECG (heart rate, PR interval, arrhythmia frequency)

Class III Agents

Class III agents (amiodarone, dofetilide, and sotalol) lengthen the action potential duration and effective refractory period and prolong repolarization. Additionally, amiodarone possesses alpha- and beta-blocking effects and calcium channel–blocking properties and inhibits the fast sodium channel. Sotalol possesses nonselective beta-blocking properties. Although torsades de pointes is relatively rare with amiodarone, precautions are taken to prevent hypokalemia- or digitalis-toxicity–induced arrhythmias. Sotalol may be associated with proarrhythmic effects in the setting of hypokalemia, bradycardia, high sotalol dose, and QT-interval prolongation, and in patients with preexisting HF. Sotalol is also contraindicated in patients with severe renal impairment.

Amiodarone

The antiarrhythmic effect of amiodarone is due to the prolongation of the action potential duration and refractory period, and secondarily through alpha-adrenergic and beta-adrenergic blockade. In patients with recent-onset (<48 hours) atrial fibrillation or atrial flutter, IV amiodarone has been shown to restore normal sinus rhythm within 8 hours in approximately 60% to 70% of treated patients. Although IV amiodarone has been associated with negative inotropic effects, minimal side effects are associated with its short-term administration.

Amiodarone is recommended as an option for the treatment of wide-complex tachycardia; stable, narrow-complex supraventricular tachycardia; stable, monomorphic, or polymorphic ventricular tachycardia; atrial fibrillation and flutter; ventricular fibrillation; and pulseless ventricular tachycardia.

Dose

- *Atrial fibrillation:* 150 mg IV over 10 minutes, followed by 1 mg/min continuous IV infusion for 6 hours, then 0.5 mg/min continuous IV infusion for 18 hours. After 24 hours, change to oral dosing or consider decreasing rate to 0.25 mg/min.
- *Pulseless ventricular tachycardia:* 300 mg IV, which may be followed by 150 mg IV.

Monitoring Parameters

- ECG (PR and QT intervals, QRS complex, arrhythmia frequency)
- Longer-term toxicities monitored by liver function tests, thyroid function tests, pulmonary function tests, that are taken at baseline and monitored through the course of therapy

Dofetilide

Dofetilide is a class III antiarrhythmic (potassium channel blocker) agent used for rhythm conversion in patients with atrial fibrillation. Prior to 2016, the agent was Food and Drug Administration (FDA) approved with substantial restrictions, as prescribers were required to undergo drug-specific training before being permitted to prescribe it. Initiation of drug therapy was also limited to hospitalized patients with continuous ECG monitoring and dosing based on a prespecified dosing algorithm. These restrictions were based on substantial adverse events associated with dofetilide administration including proarrhythmic events and sudden cardiac death. Since 2016, these restrictions have been lifted. The dose is now adjusted according to QT prolongation and creatinine clearance. If the QTc is greater than 440 milliseconds (or >500 milliseconds in the setting of ventricular conduction abnormality), dofetilide is contraindicated. Dofetilide is also contraindicated in patients with severe renal impairment.

Dose

- Modified based on creatinine clearance and QT or QTc interval. The usual recommended oral dose is 250 mcg bid.

Monitoring Parameters

- Renal function, QTc interval at baseline and 2 to 3 hours after administration

Ibutilide

Ibutilide is a class III antiarrhythmic agent indicated for the conversion of recent-onset atrial fibrillation and atrial flutter to normal sinus rhythm. Ibutilide prolongs the refractory period and action potential duration, with little or no effect on conduction velocity or automaticity. Its electrophysiologic effects are predominantly derived from activation of a slow sodium inward current. Ibutilide can cause slowing of the sinus rate and atrioventricular node conduction, but has no effect on heart rate, PR interval, or QRS interval. The drug is associated with minimal hemodynamic effects with no significant effect on cardiac output, mean pulmonary arterial pressure, or pulmonary capillary wedge pressure. Ibutilide has not been shown to lower blood pressure or worsen HF.

Ibutilide has been shown to be more effective than procainamide and sotalol in terminating atrial fibrillation and atrial flutter. In addition, ibutilide has been shown to decrease the amount of joules required to treat resistant atrial fibrillation and atrial flutter during cardioversion. Depending on the duration of atrial fibrillation or flutter, ibutilide has an efficacy rate of 22% to 43% and 37% to 76%, respectively, for terminating these arrhythmias. Ibutilide is only available as an IV dosage form and cannot be used for the long-term maintenance of normal sinus rhythm.

Sustained and nonsustained polymorphic ventricular tachycardia is the most significant adverse effect associated with ibutilide. The overall incidence of polymorphic ventricular tachycardia diagnosed as torsades de pointes was 4.3%, including 1.7% of patients in whom the arrhythmia was sustained and required cardioversion. Ibutilide administration should be avoided in patients receiving other agents that prolong the QTc interval, including class Ia or III antiarrhythmic agents, phenothiazines, antipsychotics, antidepressants, haloperidol, and some antihistamines. Before ibutilide administration, patients are screened carefully to exclude high-risk individuals, such as those with a QTc interval greater than 440 milliseconds or bradycardia. Serum potassium and magnesium levels are measured and corrected before the drug is administered. The ibutilide infusion is stopped in the event of nonsustained or sustained ventricular tachycardia or marked prolongation in the QTc interval. Patients are monitored for at least 4 hours after the infusion or until the QTc returns to baseline, with longer monitoring if nonsustained ventricular tachycardia develops.

Dose

- Greater than or equal to 60 kg: 1 mg over 10 minutes; wait 10 minutes; then prn
- Less than 60 kg: 0.01 mg/kg over 10 minutes; wait 10 minutes; then prn

Monitoring Parameters

- ECG (heart rate, PR interval, ST segment, T wave, arrhythmia frequency) for at least 4 hours following infusion or until QTc has returned to baselines

Class IV Agents

Calcium channel–blocking agents inhibit calcium channels within the atrioventricular node and sinoatrial node, prolong conduction through the atrioventricular and sinoatrial nodes, and prolong the functional refractory period of the nodes, as well as depress phase 4 depolarization. Class IV agents are used for the prophylaxis and treatment of supraventricular arrhythmias and to slow the ventricular response in atrial fibrillation, flutter, and multifocal atrial tachycardia. These agents include diltiazem and verapamil.

Monitoring Parameters

- ECG (PR interval, arrhythmia frequency)

Class V Agents

Adenosine, digoxin, and atropine possess different pharmacologic properties but ultimately affect the sinoatrial node or atrioventricular node.

Adenosine

Adenosine depresses sinus node automaticity and atrioventricular nodal conduction. Adenosine is indicated for the acute termination of atrioventricular nodal and reentrant tachycardia, and for supraventricular tachycardias, including Wolff-Parkinson-White syndrome. Some side effects of adenosine include flushing, chest tightness, and a brief asystole or bradycardia that can occur shortly after rapid administration.

Atropine

Atropine increases the sinus rate and decreases atrioventricular nodal conduction time and effective refractory period by decreasing vagal tone. The major indications for the use of atropine include symptomatic sinus bradycardia and type I second-degree atrioventricular block.

Digoxin

Digoxin slows the sinoatrial node rate of depolarization and conduction through the atrioventricular node primarily through vagal stimulating effects. Digoxin is indicated for the treatment of supraventricular tachycardia and for controlling ventricular response associated with supraventricular tachycardia.

Monitoring Parameters

- ECG (heart rate, PR interval, ST segment, T wave, arrhythmia frequency)

Vasodilators and Remodeling Agents

Idiopathic pulmonary arterial hypertension (IPAH), formerly called primary pulmonary hypertension, is characterized by elevations in pulmonary arterial pressure in the absence of a demonstrable cause. Vasoconstriction in the pulmonary vasculature is thought to play an important role in the pathogenesis of IPAH. This vasoconstriction occurs secondary to either impaired production of endogenous vasodilators (prostacyclin and nitric oxide), or from increased production of endothelin, an endogenous vasoconstrictor. Thus, treatment strategies target these three pathways (nitric oxide, prostacyclin, and endothelin) and fit into corresponding categories.

Nitric Oxide

Nitric oxide is an odorless and tasteless gas with vasodilator properties that is administered by respiratory therapists via continuous inhalation using a closed system for targeted pulmonary hypertensive patients (acute pulmonary hypertension in postoperative setting or prior to initiation of chronic therapies). The goal of inhaled nitric oxide is to improve oxygenation and reduce the need for extracorporeal membrane oxygenation (ECMO). This is a restricted therapy considering the high cost, and potential risk of occupational gas exposure to clinicians. Given these risks, there should be clear institutional policies, procedures, and guidelines in place to identify appropriate patients who meet the criteria to receive this therapy, and ensure a closely monitored system to eliminate unintended exposure to this gas.

Prostacyclin Analogues

Epoprostenol (Flolan, Veletri), treprostinil (Remodulin, Tyvaso), and iloprost (Ventavis) are potent vasodilators, which also inhibit platelet aggregation and smooth muscle proliferation and are the mainstay of IPAH therapy. Epoprostenol is delivered intravenously via continuous infusion and also via inhalation. In these instances, the presence of protocols and procedures to assure optimum administration of this agent are essential. For long-term therapy, a permanently implanted central venous catheter and portable infusion pump are used. Side effects include jaw pain, diarrhea, and arthralgias. The doses are typically titrated based on impact on systemic blood pressure; therefore, monitoring is recommended whenever therapy is initiated. Treprostinil has several routes of administration. This agent can be administered via continuous IV infusion. Also, treprostinil has an advantage of continuous SC delivery and a longer half-life (possibly less immediately life-threatening if interrupted). A major disadvantage of treprostinil is the high rate of significant infusion site discomfort if the SC route is used. Additionally, treprostinil is available as a solution for inhalation administered using the Tyvaso Inhalation System. Iloprost is an aerosolized preparation which is delivered via a specialized nebulizer device.

Endothelin Receptor Antagonist

Bosentan (Tracleer), ambrisentan (Letairis), and macitentan (Opsumit) work by blocking the vasoconstrictive properties of endothelin and are only available orally. The main adverse event associated with these therapies is elevations in liver enzymes; therefore, close monitoring of liver function tests is required. These agents are often combined with prostacyclin analogues to treat refractory cases of IPAH.

Phosphodiesterase 5 Inhibitors

Numerous studies of patients with IPAH have demonstrated improvements in pulmonary hemodynamics after treatment with sildenafil (Viagra, Revatio). Tadalafil (Cialis) and vardenafil (Levitra) have similar mechanisms of action; however, there appear to be some differences in the degree of phosphodiesterase inhibition, leading to questions of whether these agents are interchangeable. Sildenafil is the most widely studied and therefore the most commonly prescribed phosphodiesterase inhibitor. Similar to bosentan, sildenafil's most prominent role appears to be in combination with prostacyclin analogues.

Calcium Channel Blockers

Nifedipine (Procardia, Adalat), amlodipine (Norvasc), and diltiazem (Cardizem) all have proven beneficial in IPAH therapy due to vasodilatory properties. Relatively high doses are required to see responses, with systemic hypotension and edema being the most significant adverse effects in these patients. The historical role for these agents has been first-line management; however, many clinicians currently opt for prostacyclin therapy or phosphodiesterase therapy initially.

Soluble Guanylate Cyclase Stimulators

Riociguat (Adempas) is an oral soluble guanylate cyclase (sGC) stimulator and is indicated for the treatment of adults with IPAH, and patients with persistent/recurrent chronic thromboembolic pulmonary hypertension (CTEPH) after surgical treatment or inoperable CTEPH. Riociguat is the first FDA-approved agent, which shows efficacy for patients with CTEPH. Soluble guanylate cyclase stimulators relax arteries to increase blood flow thereby decreasing blood pressure. Riociguat is an FDA pregnancy category X drug and is therefore, only available to female patients through a special restricted distribution program called the Adempas Risk Evaluation Mitigation Strategies (REMS) program.

Vasopressor Agents

The 2021 Surviving Sepsis Campaign international guidelines for management of sepsis and septic shock continue to recommend norepinephrine as the first-choice vasopressor in this setting. It is recommended that vasopressor therapy initially target a MAP of 65 mm Hg. Norepinephrine is a direct-acting vasoactive agent. It possesses alpha- and beta-adrenergic agonist properties producing mixed vasopressor and inotropic effects.

Vasopressin has emerged as an important therapeutic agent for the hemodynamic support of septic and vasodilatory shock. The 2021 Surviving Sepsis Campaign international guidelines recommend the addition of vasopressin in patients with inadequate MAP on lower doses of norepinephrine, instead of maximally titrating norepinephrine. Vasopressin is a hormone that mediates vasoconstriction via V1-receptor activation on vascular smooth muscle. During septic shock, vasopressin levels are particularly low. Exogenous vasopressin administration is based on the theory of hormone replacement. Vasopressin (up to 0.03 unit/min) can be added to norepinephrine with the intent of raising MAP to target or decreasing norepinephrine dosage. Low-dose vasopressin is not recommended as the single initial vasopressor for treatment of sepsis-induced hypotension, and vasopressin doses higher than 0.03 to 0.04 units/min are reserved for salvage therapy (failure to achieve an adequate MAP with other vasopressor agents). It is important to note that harmful vasoconstriction of the GI vasculature will occur with dose escalation greater than 0.04 units/min.

The 2021 Surviving Sepsis Campaign international guidelines also highlight epinephrine as an option in patients whose hypotension is refractory to norepinephrine and vasopressin combination with adequate volume status. Epinephrine possesses alpha- and beta-adrenergic effects, increasing heart rate, contractility, and vasoconstriction with higher doses. Epinephrine's use is reserved for when other vasoconstrictors are inadequate. Adverse effects include tachyarrhythmias; myocardial, mesenteric, renal, and extremity ischemia; and hyperglycemia.

Dopamine has fallen out of favor for sepsis, with use limited by tachyarrhythmias. Dopamine is both an indirect-acting and a direct-acting agent. Dopamine works indirectly by causing the release of norepinephrine from nerve terminal storage vesicles as well as directly by stimulating alpha and beta receptors. Dopamine is unique in that it produces different pharmacologic responses based on the dose infused. Doses between 5 and 10 mcg/kg/min are typically associated with an increase in inotropy resulting from stimulation of beta receptors in the heart, and doses above 10 mcg/kg/min stimulate peripheral alpha-adrenergic receptors, producing vasoconstriction and an increase in blood pressure.

Phenylephrine is not recommended in the treatment of septic shock except in the following circumstances: (a) norepinephrine is associated with serious arrhythmias, (b) cardiac output is known to be high and blood pressure persistently low, or (c) as salvage therapy when combined inotrope/vasopressor drugs and low-dose vasopressin have failed to achieve the MAP target. Phenylephrine is a pure alpha-adrenergic agonist. It produces vasoconstriction without a direct effect on the heart, although it may cause a reflex bradycardia. Phenylephrine may be useful when dopamine, dobutamine, norepinephrine, or epinephrine cause tachyarrhythmias and when a vasoconstrictor is required.

Dose

- *Norepinephrine:* 2 to 33 mcg/min IV
- *Epinephrine:* 1 to 10mcg/min IV
- *Phenylephrine:* 30 to 400 mcg/min IV
- *Vasopressin:* 0.01 to 0.04 units/min IV

Monitoring Parameters

- Blood pressure, heart rate, ECG, urine output, and hemodynamic parameters

Inotropic Agents

Catecholamines

Dobutamine

Dobutamine produces pronounced beta-adrenergic effects such as increases in inotropy and chronotropy along with vasodilation. Dobutamine is useful especially for the acute management of low cardiac output states, as in cardiogenic shock. Adverse effects associated with the use of dobutamine include tachyarrhythmias and ischemia.

A trial of dobutamine infusion up to 20 mcg/kg/min may be administered or added to vasopressors (if in use) in the presence of: (a) myocardial dysfunction as suggested by elevated cardiac filling pressures and low cardiac output, or (b) ongoing signs of hypoperfusion, despite achieving adequate intravascular volume and adequate MAP. Norepinephrine and dobutamine can be titrated separately to maintain both blood pressure and cardiac output.

The 2021 Surviving Sepsis Campaign international guidelines provide a weak recommendation suggesting the addition of dobutamine to norepinephrine or epinephrine alone in septic shock and cardiac dysfunction with persistent hypoperfusion despite adequate volume status and arterial blood pressure. It is important to note that more evidence is needed in this area.

Dopamine

Dopamine in the range of 5 to 10 mcg/kg/min typically produces an increase in inotropy and chronotropy. Doses above 10 mcg/kg/min typically produce alpha-adrenergic effects.

Isoproterenol

Isoproterenol is a potent pure beta-receptor agonist. It has potent inotropic, chronotropic, and vasodilatory properties. Its use typically is reserved for temporizing life-threatening bradycardia. The restrictions on this agent are further enhanced by dramatic price increases, which negate clinical benefit compared with other agents and devices

(eg, pacemakers). Adverse effects associated with isoproterenol include tachyarrhythmias, myocardial ischemia, and hypotension.

Epinephrine

Epinephrine produces pronounced effects on heart rate and contractility and is used when other inotropic agents have not resulted in the desired response. Epinephrine is associated with tachyarrhythmias; myocardial, mesenteric, renal, and extremity ischemia; and hyperglycemia.

Dose

- *Dobutamine:* 2 to 20 mcg/kg/min IV
- *Dopamine:* 2 to 20 mcg/kg/min IV
- *Isoproterenol:* 2 to 10 mcg/kg/min IV
- *Epinephrine*: 0.01 to 0.05 mcg/kg/min IV

Monitoring Parameters

- Blood pressure, heart rate, ECG, urine output, and hemodynamic parameters

Phosphodiesterase Inhibitors

Milrinone

Milrinone increases contractility and heart rate, and produces vasodilation. The mechanism of action of this agent is thought to be due to the inhibition of myocardial cyclic adenosine monophosphate phosphodiesterase (AMP) activity, resulting in increased cellular concentrations of cyclic AMP. This agent is useful in the setting of low-output HF and can be combined with dobutamine to increase cardiac output. Milrinone can produce tachyarrhythmias, ischemia, and hypotension. Of note, loading doses are often omitted due to concerns of hypotension.

Dose

- *Milrinone:* loading dose: 50 mcg/kg; maintenance dose: 0.375 to 0.75 mcg/kg/min

Monitoring Parameters

- Blood pressure, heart rate, ECG, urine output, hemodynamic parameters, and platelet count

ANTIBIOTIC PHARMACOLOGY

There are a wide variety of antibiotic agents used in hospitalized patients. Commonly used antibiotic classes include beta lactams or penicillins (eg, penicillin G potassium, ampicillin ± sulbactam, oxacillin, nafcillin, ticarcillin ± clavulanic acid, and piperacillin ± tazobactam), carbapenems (eg, meropenem, doripenem, and imipenem/cilastatin), monobactams (eg, aztreonam), cephalosporins (eg, cefazolin, cefotetan, cefoxitin, cefotaxime, ceftazidime, ceftriaxone, and cefepime), fluoroquinolones (eg, levofloxacin, moxifloxacin, and ciprofloxacin), macrolides (eg, azithromycin, erythromycin), lincosamides (eg, clindamycin), nitroimidazoles (eg, metronidazole), lipopeptides (eg, daptomycin), oxazolidinones (eg, linezolid), glycopeptides (eg, vancomycin, telavancin), and aminoglycosides (eg, amikacin, tobramycin, and gentamicin). Since the development of the first antibiotic (penicillin) in 1944, microorganisms have continually evolved by developing resistance to these agents. This has led to the need for newer and more innovative classes of antibiotics with different targets and ways to avoid resistance. Selection of the correct agent(s) is based on correct identification of the site of infection, and knowledge of resistance patterns within the institution. In some instances, combinations of different antibiotic classes (eg, aminoglycoside + beta lactam, or fluoroquinolone + beta lactam) may be used as a strategy to address resistance patterns. This is used particularly with gram-negative organisms. Additionally, the antibiotic dose, frequency, and/or length of infusion can also be modified as well.

As noted, there are a number of factors related to optimal antibiotic therapy. A complete review of all antibiotic classes is beyond the scope of this text, and the focus of this section is on vancomycin due to the commonality of usage and the link to therapeutic drug monitoring (TDM).

Vancomycin

Vancomycin is a glycopeptide antibiotic active against gram-positive and certain anaerobic organisms. It exerts its antimicrobial effects by binding with peptidoglycan and inhibiting bacterial cell wall synthesis. In addition, the antibacterial effects of vancomycin also include alteration of bacterial cell wall permeability and selective inhibition of RNA synthesis.

Vancomycin is minimally absorbed after oral administration so oral use is indicated only for intestinal infections such as *Clostridium difficile*. After single or multiple IV doses, therapeutic vancomycin concentrations can be found in ascitic, pericardial, peritoneal, pleural, and synovial fluids. Vancomycin penetrates poorly into cerebrospinal fluid (CSF), with CSF penetration being directly proportional to vancomycin dose and degree of meningeal inflammation. Vancomycin is eliminated through the kidneys primarily via glomerular filtration with a limited degree of tubular secretion. Nonrenal elimination occurs through the liver and accounts for about 30% of total clearance. The elimination half-life of vancomycin is 3 to 13 hours in patients with normal renal function and increases in proportion to decreasing creatinine clearance. In acute renal failure, nonrenal clearance is maintained but eventually declines approaching the nonrenal clearance in chronic renal failure. In critically ill patients with reduced renal function, the increase in half-life may be due to a reduction in clearance as well as an increase in the volume of distribution.

Vancomycin is removed minimally during hemodialysis with cuprophane filter membranes, so that dosage supplementation after hemodialysis is not necessary. Vancomycin's half-life averages 150 hours in patients with chronic renal failure. With the newer high-flux polysulfone hemodialysis filters, vancomycin is removed to a greater degree, resulting in significant reductions in vancomycin serum concentrations. However, there is a significant redistribution period

that takes place over the 12-hour period after the high-flux hemodialysis procedure with postdialysis concentrations similar to predialysis concentrations. Therefore, dose supplementation is based on concentrations obtained at least 12 hours after dialysis, and often obtained just before the next dialysis session. Vancomycin is removed very effectively by continuous renal replacement therapy (CRRT) resulting in a reduction in half-life to 24 to 48 hours. The CRRT flow rate helps to determine the approximate drug clearance, with most patients requiring daily supplemental vancomycin dosing during CRRT.

The most common adverse effect of vancomycin is the "red-man syndrome," which is a histamine-like reaction associated with rapid vancomycin infusion and characterized by flushing, tingling, pruritus, erythema, and a macular papular rash. It typically begins 15 to 45 minutes after starting the infusion and abates 10 to 60 minutes after stopping the infusion. It may be avoided or minimized by infusing the dose over 2 hours or by pretreating the patient with diphenhydramine, 25 to 50 mg, 15 to 30 minutes before the vancomycin infusion. Other rare, but reported, adverse effects include rash, thrombophlebitis, chills, fever, and neutropenia.

PULMONARY PHARMACOLOGY
Albuterol

Albuterol is a selective beta-2 agonist, used to treat or prevent reversible bronchospasm. Adverse effects tend to be associated with inadvertent beta-1 stimulation leading to cardiovascular events including tachycardia, premature ventricular contractions, and palpitations.

Monitoring Parameters
- Heart rate and pulmonary function tests

Levalbuterol

Levalbuterol is the active enantiomer of racemic albuterol. Dose-ranging studies in stable ambulatory asthmatics and patients with COPD have documented that levalbuterol 0.63 mg and albuterol 2.5 mg produced equivalent increases in the magnitude of FEV_1 for a similar duration. There are no studies evaluating the efficacy of levalbuterol in hospitalized or critically ill patients. One study assessing the tachycardic effects of these agents in critically ill patients showed a clinically insignificant increase in heart rate following the administration of either agent. This has led to restrictions of levalbuterol within many institutions to patients intolerant to albuterol, or with histories of tachyarrhythmias.

Monitoring Parameters
- Heart rate and pulmonary function tests

Ipratropium

Ipratropium is an inhaled anticholinergic, used most commonly as a bronchodilator for cholinergic-mediated bronchospasm associated with asthma or COPD. Ipratropium is often combined with inhaled short-acting beta-2 agonists (eg, albuterol) for the management of asthma or COPD exacerbations.

Monitoring Parameters

- Pulmonary function tests

GASTROINTESTINAL PHARMACOLOGY

Stress Ulcer Prophylaxis

Stress ulcers are superficial lesions commonly involving the mucosal layer of the stomach that appear after stressful events such as trauma, surgery, burns, sepsis, or organ failure. Risk factors for the development of stress ulcers include coagulopathy, patients requiring mechanical ventilation for more than 48 hours, patients with a history of GI ulceration or bleeding within the past year, sepsis, an ICU stay longer than 1 week, occult bleeding lasting more than 6 days, and the use of high-dose steroids (>0.250 mg of hydrocortisone or the equivalent). Numerous studies support the use of antacids, H_2-receptor antagonists, and sucralfate to treat stress ulcers. There are limited prospective comparative studies supporting the use of proton pump inhibitors (PPIs) for preventing stress ulcer formation in critically ill patients. More studies are warranted to highlight the role of PPIs in this setting. The use of any therapy to prevent stress ulcer formation requires a careful assessment of individual patient risk and benefit, particularly in light of the increased risk for ventilator-associated pneumonia and *c. difficile* that is associated with increasing gastric pH.

H2 Antagonists

Ranitidine and famotidine essentially have replaced antacids as therapy for the prevention of stress gastritis. These agents have the benefit of requiring administration only every 6 to 12 hours or may be delivered by continuous infusion. When they are administered by continuous infusion, they may be added to parenteral nutrition solutions, decreasing the need for multiple daily doses. Each agent has been associated with thrombocytopenia and mental status changes. Mental status changes typically occur in older adults or in patients with reduced renal function when the dose is not appropriately adjusted. Also, similar to antacids, alkalinization of the GI tract with H_2 antagonists may predispose patients to pneumonias with gram-negative organisms that originate in the GI tract.

Dose

- *Ranitidine:* Intermittent IV: 50 mg q8h; continuous infusion: 6.25 mg/h
- *Famotidine:* Intermittent IV: 20 mg q12h; continuous infusion: not recommended

Monitoring Parameters

- Nasogastric aspirate pH, platelet count, hemoglobin, hematocrit, and nasogastric aspirate and stool guaiac

Other Agents

Sucralfate

Sucralfate is an aluminum disaccharide compound that has been shown to be safe and effective for the prophylaxis of stress gastritis. Sucralfate may work by increasing bicarbonate secretion, mucus secretion, or prostaglandin synthesis to prevent the formation of stress ulcers. Sucralfate has no effect on gastric pH. It can be administered either as a suspension or as a tablet that can be partially dissolved in 10 to 30 mL of water and administered orally or through a nasogastric tube. Although sucralfate is free from systemic side effects, it has been reported to cause hypophosphatemia, constipation, and the formation of bezoars. Because sucralfate does not increase gastric pH, it lacks the ability to alkalinize the gastric environment and may decrease the development of gram-negative nosocomial pneumonias. Sucralfate has a limited role as an alternative to H_2 antagonists in patients with thrombocytopenia or mental status changes.

Dose

- 1 g PO, NG q6h

Monitoring Parameters

- Hemoglobin, hematocrit, nasogastric aspirate, and stool guaiac

Acute Peptic Ulcer Bleeding

Proton Pump Inhibitors

Proton pump inhibitors have demonstrated efficacy in preventing rebleeding and reducing transfusion requirements in several randomized controlled trials. The rationale for adjunctive acid-suppressant therapy is based on in vitro data demonstrating clot stability and enhanced platelet aggregation at gastric pHs more than 6. High-dose IV PPI therapy is recommended to be given continuously or intermittently for 3 days in conjunction with therapeutic endoscopy. This is the most cost-effective approach for the management of hospitalized patients with acute peptic ulcer bleeding.

Pantoprazole and esomeprazole are available in oral and injectable forms, while lansoprazole and omeprazole are available in oral forms only. It is advisable to transition to oral/enteral PPI therapy, if possible, after 72 hours of IV therapy. High-risk patients with peptic ulcer bleeding who received endoscopic hemostatic therapy followed by short-term high-dose PPI therapy in hospital can be continued on twice-daily PPI therapy until 2 weeks after index endoscopy.

Dose

- *Pantoprazole and esomeprazole:* IV bolus dosing: 40 to 80 mg IV q12h for 72 hours; continuous infusion: 80 mg IV bolus; then 8 mg/h for 72 hours

Monitoring Parameters

- Hemoglobin, hematocrit, and stool guaiac

Variceal Hemorrhage

Upper GI bleeding is a common problem encountered in the ICU. Its mortality remains around 10%. Vasoactive drugs to control bleeding play an important role in the immediate treatment of acute upper GI bleeding associated with variceal hemorrhage.

Vasopressin

Vasopressin remains a commonly used agent for acute variceal bleeding. Vasopressin is a nonspecific vasoconstrictor that reduces portal pressure by constricting the splanchnic bed and reducing blood flow into the portal system. Vasopressin is successful in stopping bleeding in about 50% of patients. Many of the adverse effects of vasopressin are caused by its relative nonselective vasoconstrictor effect. Myocardial, mesenteric, and cutaneous ischemia have been reported in association with its use. Drug-related adverse effects have been reported in up to 25% of patients receiving vasopressin. Therefore, octreotide is a more favorable agent due to decreased adverse effects with better efficacy data. The use of transdermal or IV nitrates with vasopressin reduces the incidence of these adverse effects.

Dose

- 0.3 to 0.9 units/min

Monitoring Parameters

- Hemoglobin, hematocrit, nasogastric aspirate, stool guaiac, ECG, signs and symptoms of ischemia, blood pressure, and heart rate

Octreotide

Octreotide, the longer-acting synthetic analog of somatostatin, reduces splanchnic blood flow and has a modest effect on hepatic blood flow and wedged hepatic venous pressure with little systemic circulation effects. Although octreotide produces the same results as vasopressin in the control of bleeding and transfusion requirements, it produces significantly fewer adverse effects. Continuous infusion of octreotide has been shown to be as effective as injection sclerotherapy in control of variceal hemorrhage.

Dose

- *Initial bolus dose:* 100 mcg, followed by 50 mcg/h continuous infusion

Monitoring Parameters

- Hemoglobin, hematocrit, nasogastric aspirate, and stool guaiac

Propranolol

Propranolol has been shown to reduce portal pressure both acutely and chronically in patients with portal hypertension by reducing splanchnic blood flow. The primary use of propranolol has been in the prevention of variceal bleeding. Propranolol or other beta-blockers are avoided in patients experiencing acute GI bleeding, because beta-blocking agents may prevent the compensatory tachycardia needed to maintain cardiac output and blood pressure in the setting of hemorrhage.

Monitoring Parameters

- Hemoglobin, hematocrit, heart rate, and blood pressure

RENAL PHARMACOLOGY

Diuretics

Diuretics may be categorized in a number of ways, including site of action, chemical structure, and potency. Although many diuretics are available for oral and IV administration, intravenously administered agents typically are given to critically ill patients because of their guaranteed absorption and more predictable responses. Therefore, the primary agents used in ICUs are the intravenously administered loop diuretics, thiazide diuretics, and osmotic agents. However, the oral thiazide-like agent, metolazone, is used commonly in combination with loop diuretics to maintain urine output for patients with diuretic resistance.

Monitoring Parameters

- Urine output, blood pressure, renal function, electrolytes, weight, fluid balance, and hemodynamic parameters (if applicable)

Loop Diuretics

Loop diuretics (furosemide, bumetanide, torsemide) act by inhibiting active transport of chloride and possibly sodium in the thick ascending loop of Henle. Administration of loop diuretics results in enhanced excretion of sodium, chloride, potassium, hydrogen, magnesium, ammonium, and bicarbonate. Maximum electrolyte loss is greater with loop diuretics than with thiazide diuretics. Furosemide, bumetanide, and torsemide have some renal vasodilator properties that reduce renal vascular resistance and increase renal blood flow. Additionally, these three agents decrease peripheral vascular resistance and increase venous capacitance. These effects may account for the decrease in left ventricular filling pressure that occurs before the onset of diuresis in patients with HF.

Loop diuretics typically are used for the treatment of edema associated with HF or oliguric renal failure, the management of hypertension complicated by HF or renal failure, in combination with hypotensive agents in the treatment of hypertensive crisis, especially when associated with acute pulmonary edema or renal failure, and in combination with 0.9% sodium chloride to increase calcium excretion in patients with hypercalcemia.

Common adverse effects associated with loop diuretic administration include hypotension from excessive reduction in plasma volume, hypokalemia and hypochloremia resulting in metabolic alkalosis, and hypomagnesemia. Reduction in these electrolytes may predispose patients to the development of supraventricular and ventricular ectopy.

Tinnitus, with reversible or permanent hearing impairment, may occur with the rapid administration of large IV doses. Typically, IV bolus doses of furosemide are not administered faster than 40 mg/min.

Dose

- *Furosemide:* IV bolus: 10 to 100 mg q1-6h; continuous infusion: 10 to 40 mg/h
- *Bumetanide:* IV bolus: 0.5 to 1 mg q1-2h; continuous infusion: 0.5 to 2 mg/h
- *Torsemide:* IV bolus: 5 to 20 mg qd

Thiazide Diuretics

Thiazide (IV chlorothiazide) and thiazide-like (PO metolazone) diuretics enhance excretion of sodium, chloride, and water by inhibiting the transport of sodium across the renal tubular epithelium in the cortical diluting segment of the nephron. Thiazides also increase the excretion of potassium and bicarbonate.

Thiazide diuretics are used in the management of edema and hypertension as monotherapy or in combination with other agents. They have less potent diuretic and antihypertensive effects than loop diuretics. IV chlorothiazide and oral metolazone are often used in combination with loop diuretics in patients with diuretic resistance. By acting at a different site in the nephron, this combination of agents may restore diuretic responsiveness. Thiazide diuretics decrease glomerular filtration rate, and this effect may contribute to their decreased efficacy in patients with reduced renal function (glomerular filtration rate < 20 mL/min). Metolazone, unlike thiazide diuretics, does not substantially decrease glomerular filtration rate or renal plasma flow and often produces a diuretic effect even in patients with glomerular filtration rates less than 20 mL/min.

Adverse effects that may occur with the administration of thiazide diuretics include hyponatremia, hypovolemia, hypotension, hypochloremia, and hypokalemia resulting in a metabolic alkalosis, hypercalcemia, hyperuricemia, and the precipitation of acute gouty attacks.

Dose

- *Chlorothiazide:* 500 to 1000 mg IV q12h
- *Metolazone:* 2.5 to 20 mg PO qd

Osmotic Diuretics

Mannitol

Mannitol is an osmotic diuretic commonly used in patients with increased intracranial pressure. Mannitol produces a diuretic effect by increasing the osmotic pressure of the glomerular filtrate and preventing the tubular reabsorption of water and solutes. Mannitol increases the excretion of sodium, water, potassium, and chloride, as well as other electrolytes.

Mannitol is used to treat acute oliguric renal failure and reduce intracranial and intraocular pressures. The renal protective effects of mannitol may be due to its ability to prevent nephrotoxins from becoming concentrated in the tubular fluid. However, its ability to prevent or reverse acute renal failure may be because of restoring renal blood flow, glomerular filtration rate, urine flow, and sodium excretion. To be effective in preventing or reversing renal failure, mannitol must be administered before reductions in glomerular filtration rate or renal blood flow have resulted in acute tubular damage. Mannitol is useful in the treatment of cerebral edema, especially when there is evidence of herniation or the development of cord compression.

The most severe adverse effect of mannitol is overexpansion of extracellular fluid and circulatory overload, producing acute HF and pulmonary edema. This effect typically occurs in patients with severely impaired renal function. Therefore, mannitol is not administered to individuals in whom adequate renal function and urine flow have not been established.

Dose

- 0.25 to 1 g/kg, then 0.25 to 0.5 g/kg q4h

Monitoring Parameters

- Urine output, blood pressure, renal function, electrolytes, weight, fluid balance, hemodynamic parameters (if applicable), serum osmolarity, and intracranial pressure (if applicable)

HEMATOLOGIC PHARMACOLOGY

Anticoagulants

Unfractionated Heparin

Unfractionated heparin consists of a group of mucopolysaccharides derived from the mast cells of porcine intestinal tissues. It binds with antithrombin III, accelerating the rate at which antithrombin III neutralizes coagulation factors II, VII, IX, X, XI, and XII. Unfractionated heparin is used for prophylaxis and treatment of venous thrombosis and pulmonary embolism, atrial fibrillation with embolization, and treatment of acute disseminated intravascular coagulation.

Subcutaneously administered unfractionated heparin is absorbed slowly and completely over the dosing interval. The total amount of unfractionated heparin required to achieve the same degree of anticoagulation over the same time period does not appear to differ whether the unfractionated heparin is administered subcutaneously or intravenously. The apparent volume of distribution of unfractionated heparin is directly proportional to body weight, but this process is likely saturable to some extent in obese patients. Literature describing dosing recommendations in the obese population is variable, with some suggesting ideal body weight for dosing and others proposing total body weight.

The metabolism and elimination of unfractionated heparin involve the process of depolymerization and desulfation. Enzymes reported to be involved in unfractionated heparin metabolism include heparinase and desulfatase, which cleave unfractionated heparin into oligosaccharides. The half-life of unfractionated heparin ranges from 0.4 to 2.5 hours. Patients with underlying thromboembolic disease have been shown to have shorter elimination half-lives, faster clearance, and require larger doses to maintain adequate anti-thrombotic activity.

A weight-based nomogram is utilized with a loading dose followed by a continuous infusion. The infusion is traditionally titrated based on activated PTT monitoring. Recently some centers have used antifactor Xa monitoring based on the proposed benefit of a smoother dose-response curve. The main adverse effects may be attributed to excessive anticoagulation. Bleeding occurs in 3% to 20% of patients receiving short-term, high-dose therapy. Bleeding is increased threefold when the PTT is 2 to 2.9 times above control and eightfold when the PTT is more than 3 times the control value. Unfractionated heparin-induced thrombocytopenia may occur in 1% to 5% of patients receiving the drug.

The PTT is the most commonly used test to monitor and adjust unfractionated heparin doses. Although unfractionated heparin is typically administered as a continuous infusion, it is important that samples are collected as close to steady state as possible. After starting unfractionated heparin therapy or adjusting the dose, PTT values are drawn at least 6 to 8 hours after the change. Samples drawn too early are misleading and may result in inappropriate dose adjustments. Once the unfractionated heparin dose has been determined, daily monitoring of the PTT for minor adjustments in the unfractionated heparin dose is indicated. Large variations in subsequent coagulation tests should be investigated to ensure that the patient's condition has not changed or the patient is not developing thrombocytopenia. A similar approach is used if antifactor Xa levels are monitored in lieu of PTT.

Platelet counts are monitored every 2 to 3 days while a patient is receiving unfractionated heparin to assess for unfractionated heparin-induced thrombocytopenia, thrombosis, or hemorrhage. Hemoglobin and hematocrit are monitored every 2 to 3 days to assess for the presence of bleeding. Additionally, sputum, urine, and stool are examined for the presence of blood. Patients are examined for signs of bleeding at IV access sites and for the development of hematomas and ecchymosis. In addition, IM injections are avoided in patients receiving unfractionated heparin and elective invasive procedures are avoided or rescheduled.

Dose

- *Individualized dosing:* Bolus: 80 units/kg followed by a continuous infusion of 18 units/kg/h; for the treatment of deep venous thrombosis (DVT) or pulmonary embolism; for the treatment of arterial thromboembolism including cerebral thromboembolism, or for the treatment of mural thrombosis. Lower bolus doses and initial infusion rates recommended for ST-Elevation Myocardial Infarction (STEMI), Non-ST-Elevation Myocardial Infarction (NSTEMI), and other indications. Infusion rates are adjusted to maintain a PTT between 1.5 and 2.0 times the control value, or antifactor Xa within institution specific therapeutic range (eg, 0.3-0.7 IU/mL)

Monitoring Parameters

- PTT or antifactor Xa, hemoglobin, hematocrit, platelet count, and signs of active bleeding

Low-Molecular-Weight Heparins

Low-molecular-weight heparins have a role in the treatment of DVT, pulmonary embolism, and acute MI. Low-molecular-weight heparins are less time consuming for nurses and laboratories and more comfortable for patients by allowing them to be discharged earlier from the hospital. The use of a fixed-dose regimen avoids the need for serial monitoring of the PTT and follow-up dose adjustments. Enoxaparin is the most studied low-molecular-weight heparin. Its dose for the treatment of DVT, pulmonary embolism, and acute MI is 1 mg/kg q12h. Dalteparin is another agent that has been shown to be as effective as unfractionated heparin in the treatment of thromboembolic disease and acute MI. Dalteparin 200 units/kg once daily is the typical dose used for the treatment of thromboembolic disease; 120 units/kg followed by 120 units/kg 12 hours later has been used in patients with acute MI receiving streptokinase. Warfarin can be started with the first dose of enoxaparin or dalteparin. When used as a bridge to warfarin therapy, enoxaparin or dalteparin are continued until two consecutive therapeutic international normalized ratio (INR) values are achieved, typically in about 5 to 7 days.

Both dalteparin and enoxaparin are primarily renally eliminated with the potential for drug accumulation in patients with renal impairment. The approach for managing these patients differs between the two drugs. Because these agents work by inhibiting factor Xa activity, it is possible to monitor their anticoagulation by measuring antifactor Xa levels. This is a useful monitoring tool, particularly when compared with serum drug levels. Doses of either agent may be adjusted based on antifactor Xa levels in patients with significant renal impairment (ie, creatinine clearance < 30 mL/min). The dosing adjustment for enoxaparin in patients with creatinine clearances less than 30 mL/min is to extend the dosing interval from 12 to 24 hours in both prophylaxis and treatment of thrombosis. No such dosage adjustment guideline has been approved for dalteparin, thus antifactor Xa levels may be required.

Several studies have documented that critically ill patients have significantly lower anti-Xa levels in response to single daily doses when compared to patients on general medical wards. Factor Xa activity may need to be monitored in critically ill patients to adjust doses to ensure adequate anticoagulation and prevent deep venous clots from developing.

Dose

- *Enoxaparin:* 1 mg/kg SC q12h, for treatment of DVT, pulmonary embolism, and acute MI

Monitoring Parameters

- Hemoglobin, hematocrit, and signs of active bleeding, platelet count, antifactor Xa levels

Warfarin

Warfarin prevents the conversion of vitamin K back to its active form from the vitamin K epoxide, impairing the formation of vitamin K–dependent clotting factors II, VII, IX, X, protein C, and protein S. Warfarin is indicated in the treatment of venous thrombosis or pulmonary embolism following full-dose parenteral anticoagulant (eg, unfractionated or low-molecular-weight heparin) therapy. Warfarin is also used for chronic therapy to reduce the risk of thromboembolic episodes in patients with chronic atrial fibrillation.

Warfarin is rapidly and extensively absorbed from the GI tract. Peak plasma concentrations occur between 60 and 90 minutes after an oral dose with bioavailability ranging between 75% and 100%. Albumin is the principal binding protein with 97.5% to 99.9% of warfarin being bound.

Warfarin's metabolism is stereospecific. The R-isomer is oxidized to 6-hydroxywarfarin and further reduced to 9S, 11R-warfarin alcohols. The S-isomer is oxidized to 7-hydroxywarfarin and further reduced to 9S, 11R-warfarin alcohols. The stereospecific isomer alcohol metabolites have anticoagulant activity in humans. The warfarin alcohols are renally eliminated. The elimination half-lives of the two warfarin isomers differ substantially. The S-isomer half-life is approximately 33 hours and the R-isomer half-life is 45 hours.

Warfarin therapy may be started on the first day of unfractionated or low-molecular-weight heparin therapy. Traditionally, warfarin 5 mg daily is given for the first 2 to 3 days and then adjusted to maintain the desired prothrombin time (PT) or INR. The timing of INR measurements relative to changes in daily dose is important. After the administration of a warfarin dose, the peak depression of coagulation occurs in about 36 hours. It is important to select an appropriate time during a given dosing interval and perform coagulation tests consistently at that time. After the first four to five doses, the fluctuation in the INR over a 24-hour dosing interval is minimal. The timeframe for stabilization of warfarin plasma concentrations and coagulation response during continued administration of maintenance doses is less clear. A minimum of 10 days appears to be necessary before the dose-response curve shows interval-to-interval stability. During the first week of therapy, two INR measurements are determined to assess the impact of warfarin accumulation on INR. Several factors are assessed when evaluating an unexpected response to warfarin. Laboratory results are verified to exclude inaccurate or spurious results. The medication profile is reviewed to exclude drug-drug interactions including changes in warfarin product, and the patient is evaluated for disease-drug interactions, nutritional-drug interactions, and nonadherence.

Bleeding is the major complication associated with the use of warfarin, occurring in 6% to 29% of patients receiving the drug. Bleeding complications include ecchymoses, hemoptysis, and epistaxis, as well as fatal or life-threatening hemorrhage. The effects of warfarin can be reversed with oral doses of vitamin K and with transfusion of fresh frozen plasma (FFP) to replace vitamin K-dependent clotting factors in patients without major bleed. In patients with major life threatening bleeding, 4-factor prothrombin complex concentrate (KCentra) plus vitamin K may be preferred compared with FFP, according to the 2012 American College of Chest Physicians Practice Guidelines for Oral Anticoagulant Therapy: Antithrombotic Therapy and Prevention of Thrombosis.

Dose

- 5 mg PO qd × 3 days, then adjusted to maintain the INR between 2 and 3
- To prevent thromboembolism associated with prosthetic heart valves, the dose should be adjusted to maintain an INR between 2.5 and 3.5

Monitoring Parameters

- INR, hemoglobin, hematocrit, and signs of active bleeding

Factor Xa Inhibitors

Rivaroxaban, Apixaban, and Edoxaban

Rivaroxaban and apixaban are oral factor Xa inhibitors, indicated for venous thromboembolism (VTE) prophylaxis, or prophylaxis of embolism or cerebrovascular accident (CVA) in patients with nonvalvular atrial fibrillation. The agents are also indicated for PE and DVT treatment. Andexanet (Andexxa) is a recombinant modified human factor Xa protein indicated for reversal of apixaban or rivaroxaban anticoagulation in patients with life-threatening or uncontrolled bleeding. It is currently the only FDA-approved reversal agent for apixaban and rivaroxaban. Andexanet has been associated with serious and life-threatening adverse events including arterial and venous thromboembolism, myocardial infarction, ischemic stroke, cardiac arrest, and sudden death. Outcomes data with 4-factor prothrombin complex concentrate (KCentra) reversal in bleeding and non-bleeding factor Xa inhibitor patients are limited to case reports and case series. Although these small studies indicate there may be some benefit, more robust research is needed to evaluate if there is a clear role in this setting.

Dose

Rivaroxaban:

- *VTE prophylaxis postsurgery:* 10 mg PO qd
- *Atrial fibrillation, nonvalvular-CVA prophylaxis:* 20 mg PO qd
- *DVT or PE treatment, and secondary prophylaxis:* 15 mg PO bid × 21 days followed by 20 mg PO qd

Apixaban:

- *Atrial fibrillation, nonvalvular-CVA prophylaxis:* For most patients, 5 mg PO bid. In patients with any two of the following characteristics: age more than or equal to 80 years; body weight less than or equal to 60 kg; or serum creatinine more than or equal to 1.5 mg/dL, reduce the dose to 2.5 mg PO bid

- *DVT or PE treatment, and secondary prophylaxis:* 10 mg PO bid × 7 days followed by 5 mg PO bid
- *VTE prophylaxis:* 2.5 mg PO bid

Monitoring Parameters

- Hemoglobin, hematocrit, renal function, and signs of active bleeding

Direct Thrombin Inhibitors

Dabigatran

Dabigatran is an oral direct thrombin inhibitor, indicated for use for stroke prevention in patients with nonvalvular atrial fibrillation. In clinical trials, dabigatran was superior to warfarin in reducing the risk for stroke and systemic embolism with lower minor bleed risk comparatively. Dabigatran also has a developing role as VTE prophylaxis after total knee or hip arthroplasty, as well as the treatment of DVT and PE. It is important to note that dabigatran capsules cannot be opened for feeding tube or oral administration. Additionally, this medication should be avoided in renal failure due to accumulation and bleeding events. This agent can be reversed with idarucizumab (Praxbind), which works by binding to dabigatran, causing inactivation.

Dose

- 150 mg PO bid

Monitoring Parameters

- Hemoglobin, hematocrit, aPTT, ecarin clotting time (ECT), renal function, and signs of active bleeding

Bivalirudin

Bivalirudin is an anticoagulant with direct thrombin inhibitor properties. Bivalirudin, when given with aspirin, is indicated for use as an anticoagulant in patients with unstable angina undergoing coronary angioplasty. It has been used as a substitute for unfractionated heparin. Potential advantages over unfractionated heparin include activity against clot-bound thrombin, more predictable anticoagulation, and no inhibition by components of the platelet release reaction. Numerous studies have compared bivalirudin to unfractionated heparin with or without a glycoprotein IIb/IIIa inhibitor, with mixed results. A major clinical trial published in 2015, MATRIX, demonstrated that bivalirudin, compared to unfractionated heparin with or without glycoprotein IIb/IIIa inhibitor, reduced bleeding complications, but resulted in higher rates of ischemic events, including acute stent thrombosis. Thus, bivalirudin may be considered a reasonable alternative to UFH primarily in patients at high risk of bleeding, heparin allergy or heparin-induced thrombocytopenia, undergoing percutaneous coronary intervention (PCI), or ECMO. There is no FDA-approved reversal agent for bivalirudin. In the event of bleeding, discontinuation of infusion is recommended and coagulation returns to baseline in approximately 1 hour following discontinuation with normal renal function. Please note that renal dysfunction will further delay clearance in this setting.

Dose

- *PCI including HIT:* 0.75 mg/kg IV bolus followed by 1.75 mg/kg/h continuous IV infusion for the duration of the procedure
- *Cardiopulmonary bypass:* 1 mg/kg IV bolus followed by 2.5 mg/kg/h continuous IV infusion × 4 hours, if necessary 0.2 mg/kg/h for up to 20 hours

Monitoring Parameters

- Activated PTT, activated clotting time (ACT), hemoglobin, hematocrit, and signs of active bleeding

Argatroban

Argatroban is a selective thrombin inhibitor indicated for the prevention or treatment of thrombosis in unfractionated heparin-induced thrombocytopenia and for use in PCIs. It has also shown effectiveness in ischemic stroke and as an adjunct to thrombolysis in patients with acute MI. Further studies are needed to establish effectiveness for other indications. Argatroban is dosed as a continuous infusion that is titrated based on activated PTT, similar to unfractionated heparin. During PCI, the ACT may be used. A notable drug-laboratory value interaction is the increase in PT and INR values that occurs with argatroban therapy, which may complicate the monitoring of warfarin therapy once oral anticoagulation is initiated. There is no FDA-approved reversal agent for argatroban. If bleeding occurs, discontinuation of infusion is recommended and coagulation returns to baseline in approximately 4 to 6 hours following discontinuation. This may be prolonged in hepatic impairment or critically ill.

Dose

- *Percutaneous coronary intervention:* Bolus: 350 mcg/kg; continuous infusion: 25 mcg/kg/min
- *Heparin-induced thrombocytopenia with thrombosis:* continuous infusion: 2 mcg/kg/min in non-critically ill. Lowering initial doses to 0.5 to 1 mcg/kg/min in critically ill patients is recommended

Monitoring Parameters

- Activated PTT, ACT, PT, INR, hemoglobin, hematocrit, and signs of active bleeding

Glycoprotein IIb/IIIa Inhibitor

Glycoprotein IIb/IIIa inhibitors are recommended, in addition to aspirin and unfractionated heparin, in patients with acute coronary syndrome awaiting PCI. If the glycoprotein IIb/IIIa inhibitor is started in the catheterization laboratory just before PCI, abciximab is the agent of choice.

Dose

- *Abciximab:* Bolus: 0.25 mg/kg over 1 to 5 minutes; continuous infusion: 0.125 mcg/kg/min for 12 hours (maximum infusion of 10 mcg/kg/min)

- *Tirofiban:* Bolus infusion: 25 mcg/kg within 5 minutes; continuous infusion: 0.1 mcg/kg/min for 12 to 24 hours after angioplasty or atherectomy
- *Eptifibatide:* Bolus: 180 mcg/kg; continuous infusion: 2 mcg/kg/min until discharge or coronary artery bypass grafting (maximum of 72 hours)

Monitoring Parameters

- Platelet count, hemoglobin, hematocrit, and signs of active bleeding

Thrombolytic Agents

Thrombolytic agents may be beneficial as reperfusion therapy in STEMI. The 2013 American College of Cardiology Foundation/American Heart Association guidelines for the management of STEMI include the following recommendations in order from most supported by published literature (Class I) to least supported (Class III).

Class I Recommendations

- In the absence of contraindications, fibrinolytic therapy should be given to patients with STEMI and onset of ischemic symptoms within the previous 12 hours when it is anticipated that primary PCI cannot be performed within 120 minutes of first medical contact.

Class IIa Recommendations

- In the absence of contraindications and when PCI is not available, fibrinolytic therapy is reasonable for patients with STEMI if there is clinical and/or electrocardiographic evidence of ongoing ischemia within 12 to 24 hours of symptom onset and a large area of myocardium at risk or hemodynamic instability.

Class III Recommendations

- Fibrinolytic therapy should not be administered to patients with ST depression except when a true posterior (inferobasal) MI is suspected or when associated with ST elevation in lead aVR.

Absolute contraindications to the use of thrombolytic agents include any active or recent bleeding; suspected aortic dissection; intracranial or intraspinal neoplasm; arteriovenous malformation or aneurysms; neurosurgery or significant closed head injury within the previous 3 months; ischemic stroke within the previous 3 months (except acute ischemic stroke within 3 hours); or facial trauma in the preceding 3 months. Relative contraindications include acute or chronic severe uncontrolled hypertension; ischemic stroke more than 3 months prior; traumatic or prolonged cardiopulmonary resuscitation greater than 10 minutes in duration; major surgery within the previous 3 weeks; internal bleeding within 2 to 4 weeks; noncompressible vascular punctures; prior allergic reaction to thrombolytics; pregnancy; active peptic ulcer; and current anticoagulation (risk increasing with increasing INR).

Adverse effects include bleeding from the GI or genitourinary tracts, as well as gingival bleeding and epistaxis. Superficial bleeding may occur from trauma sites such as those for IV access or invasive procedures. IM injections, and noncompressible arterial punctures, are avoided during thrombolytic therapy.

Monitoring Parameters

- For short-term thrombolytic therapy of MI: ECG, signs and symptoms of ischemia, and signs and symptoms of bleeding at IV injection sites (laboratory monitoring is of little value)
- Continuous infusion therapy: Thrombin time, activated PTT, and fibrinogen, in addition to above-mentioned monitoring parameters

Alteplase

Alteplase (recombinant tissue-type plasminogen activator or TPA) has a high affinity for fibrin-bound plasminogen, allowing activation on the fibrin surface. Most plasmin formed remains bound to the fibrin clot, minimizing systemic effects. The risk of an intracerebral bleed is approximately 0.5%.

Dose

- Acute MI: Accelerated infusion: patients over 67 kg, total dose 100 mg IV (15 mg IV bolus, then 50 mg over 30 minutes, then 35 mg over 60 minutes)
- Acute MI: Accelerated infusion: patients 67 kg or less (15 mg IV bolus, then 0.75 mg/kg over 30 minutes, then 0.5 mg/kg over 60 minutes); total dose not to exceed 100 mg
- Acute MI: 3-hour infusion: weight 65 kg or more, 60 mg IV in the first hour (6-10 mg of which to be given as bolus), then 20 mg over the second hour, and 20 mg over the third hour
- Acute MI: 3-hour infusion: weight less than 65 kg, 1.25 mg/kg IV administered over 3 hours, give 60% in the first hour (10% of which to be given as bolus), give remaining 40% over the next 2 hours
- Pulmonary embolism: 100 mg IV over 2 hours
- Ischemic stroke: 0.9 mg/kg (not to exceed 90 mg); 10% of total dose as IV bolus over 1 minute; then remaining 90% as IV infusion over 60 minutes

Tenecteplase

Tenecteplase (recombinant TNK-tissue-type plasminogen activator) has a longer elimination half-life (20-24 minutes) and is more resistant to inactivation by plasminogen activator inhibitor-1 than alteplase. Tenecteplase appears more fibrin specific than alteplase, which may account for a lower rate of noncerebral bleeding comparatively. However, there have been reports of antibody development to tenecteplase. Tenecteplase and alteplase have similar clinical efficacy for thrombolysis after MI.

Dose

- Acute MI: 30 to 50 mg (based on weight) IV over 5 seconds

Reteplase

Reteplase is a recombinant plasminogen activator for use in acute MI and pulmonary embolism as a thrombolytic agent. Reteplase has a longer half-life (13-16 minutes) than that of alteplase, allowing for bolus administration. The dosing regimen requires double bolus doses.

Dose

- *Acute MI and pulmonary embolism:* Two 10-unit IV bolus doses infused over 2 minutes via a dedicated line. The second dose is administered 30 minutes after the initiation of the first injection

IMMUNOSUPPRESSIVE AGENTS

Cyclosporine

Cyclosporine is used to prevent allograft rejection after solid organ transplantation and graft-versus-host disease in bone marrow transplant patients. Unlike other immunosuppressive agents, cyclosporine does not suppress bone marrow function. Cyclosporine inhibits cytokine synthesis and receptor expression needed for T-lymphocyte activation by interrupting signal transduction. A lack of cytokine disrupts the activation and proliferation of the helper and cytotoxic T-cells that are essential for rejection.

Cyclosporine is poorly absorbed from the GI tract with bioavailability averaging 30%. Its absorption is influenced by the type of organ transplant, time from transplantation, presence of biliary drainage, liver function, intestinal dysfunction, and the use of drugs that alter intestinal function. Cyclosporine is metabolized by cytochrome P 450 isoenzyme 3a to numerous metabolites with more than 90% of the dose excreted into the bile and eliminated in the feces. The kidneys eliminate less than 1% of the dose. There is no evidence that the metabolites have significant immunosuppressive activity compared with cyclosporine and none of the metabolites are known to cause nephrotoxicity.

Because of poor oral absorption, the oral dose is three times the IV dose. When converting from IV to oral administration, it is important to increase the oral dose by a factor of three to maintain stable cyclosporine concentrations. The oral solution can be administered diluted with chocolate milk or juice and administered through a nasogastric tube. The tube is flushed before and after cyclosporine is administered to ensure complete drug delivery and optimal absorption.

The microemulsion formulation of cyclosporine capsules and solution has increased bioavailability compared to the original formulation of cyclosporine capsules and solution. These formulations are not bioequivalent and cannot be used interchangeably. Converting from cyclosporine capsules and solution for microemulsion to cyclosporine capsules and oral solution using as 1:1 mg/kg/day ratio may result in lower cyclosporine blood concentrations. Conversion between formulations should be made utilizing increased monitoring to avoid toxicity due to high concentrations or possible organ rejection owing to low concentrations.

Nephrotoxicity is cyclosporine's major adverse effect. Three types of nephrotoxicity have been shown to occur. The first is an acute reversible reduction in glomerular filtration; second, tubular toxicity with possible enzymuria and aminoaciduria; and third, irreversible interstitial fibrosis and arteriopathy. The exact mechanism of cyclosporine nephrotoxicity is unclear, but may involve alterations in the various vasoactive substances in the kidney. Other side effects include a dose-dependent increase in bilirubin that occurs within the first 3 months after transplantation. Hyperkalemia can develop secondary to cyclosporine nephrotoxicity. Cyclosporine-induced hypomagnesemia can cause seizures. Neurotoxic effects such as tremors and paresthesias may occur in up to 15% of treated patients. Hypertension occurs frequently and may be because of the nephrotoxic effects or renal vasoconstrictive effects of the drug. Cyclosporine is a narrow therapeutic index drug and thus levels are monitored and doses adjusted accordingly. The target levels are individualized based on type of transplant, time since transplant, and concurrent immunosuppressants.

Tacrolimus (FK506)

Tacrolimus is a macrolide antibiotic produced by the fermentation broth of *Streptomyces tsukubaensis*. Although it bears no structural similarity to cyclosporine, its mode of action parallels cyclosporine. Tacrolimus exhibits similar in vitro effects to cyclosporine, but at concentrations 100 times lower than those of cyclosporine.

Tacrolimus is primarily metabolized in the liver by the cytochrome P-450 isoenzyme 3A4 to at least 15 metabolites. There is also some evidence to suggest that tacrolimus may be metabolized in the gut. The 13-O-demethyl-tacrolimus appears to be the major metabolite in patient blood. Less than 1% of a dose is excreted unchanged in the urine of liver transplant patients. Renal clearance accounts for less than 1% of total body clearance. The mean terminal elimination half-life is 12 hours but ranges from 8 to 40 hours. Patients with liver impairment have a longer tacrolimus half-life, reduced clearance, and elevated tacrolimus concentrations. The elevated tacrolimus concentrations are associated with increased nephrotoxicity in these patients. Because tacrolimus is primarily metabolized by the cytochrome P-450 enzyme system, it is anticipated that drugs known to interact with this enzyme system may affect tacrolimus disposition.

In most cases, IV therapy can be switched to oral therapy within 2 to 4 days after starting therapy. There may be variability among centers relative to the timing of transition to oral therapy. The oral dose starts 8 to 12 hours after the IV infusion has been stopped. The usual initial oral dose is 0.075 to 0.2 mg/kg/day, administered in two divided doses every 12 hours.

Nephrotoxicity is the most common adverse effect associated with the use of tacrolimus. Nephrotoxicity occurs in up to 40% of transplant patients receiving tacrolimus. Other side effects observed during tacrolimus therapy include headache, tremor, insomnia, diarrhea, hypertension, hyperglycemia, and hyperkalemia. Tacrolimus is a narrow therapeutic index drug and thus levels are monitored and doses adjusted accordingly. The target levels are individualized based on type of transplant, time since transplant, and concurrent immunosuppressants.

Sirolimus (Rapamycin)

Sirolimus is an immunosuppressive agent used for prophylaxis of organ rejection in patients receiving renal transplants. It typically is used in regimens containing cyclosporine and corticosteroids. Sirolimus inhibits T-lymphocyte activation and proliferation that occurs in response to antigenic and cytokine stimulation. Sirolimus also inhibits antibody production.

Sirolimus is administered orally once daily. The initial dose of sirolimus is administered as soon as possible after transplantation. It is recommended that sirolimus be taken 4 hours after cyclosporine modified oral solution or capsules.

Routine therapeutic drug level monitoring is not required in most patients. Sirolimus levels are monitored in patients with hepatic impairment, during concurrent administration of cytochrome P-450 cyp3a4 inducers and inhibitors, or when cyclosporine dosing is reduced or discontinued. Mean sirolimus whole blood trough concentrations, as measured by immunoassay, are approximately 9 ng/mL for the 2-mg/day dose and 17 ng/mL for the 5-mg/day dose. Results from other assays may differ from those with an immunoassay. On average, chromatographic methods such as HPLC or mass spectroscopy yield results that are 20% lower than immunoassay whole blood determinations.

SPECIAL DOSING CONSIDERATIONS

Continuous Renal Replacement Therapy

The techniques used to provide renal support to critically ill patients have changed considerably during the last 20 years. CRRTs such as continuous venovenous hemodialysis (CVVHD) and continuous venonvenous hemodialfiltration (CVVHDF) are replacing conventional hemodialysis in critically ill patients. Recommendations for drug dosage adjustments in conventional intermittent dialysis cannot be applied to continuous techniques with lower clearance rates. Clinical studies on the influence of CRRT on drug elimination are limited.

Hemofiltration alone typically produces an effective glomerular filtration rate of approximately 20 mL/min, and the addition of dialysis increases the effective glomerular filtration rate to 30 to 40 mL/min. Increasing the dialysis flow rate from 1 to 2 L/h further increases the effective glomerular filtration rate. Several points are important to remember when selecting drug doses in patients receiving any of these CRRT modes. First, drugs that are less than 80% protein bound, have a volume of distribution less than 1 L/kg, and a renal clearance greater than 35% will be removed during CRRT. Secondly, the following approaches may be used for dosage adjustments during CRRT (which includes dialysis) in the absence of published recommendations. The manufacturer's dosage recommendations for creatinine clearances below 30 to 40 mL/min may be used. Third, serum concentration monitoring is used to adjust the doses of aminoglycoside antibiotics and vancomycin. Finally, drugs such as catecholamines, narcotics, and sedatives are minimally removed during CRRT. The doses of these drug classes are titrated based on the patient's clinical response.

Drug Disposition in Older adults

Older adults are the fastest-growing segment of the population in the United States. Older patients consume nearly three times as many prescription drugs as younger patients and therefore are at risk for experiencing significantly more drug-drug interactions and ADEs. The most common risk factors that contribute to adverse events include polypharmacy, low body mass, preexisting chronic disease, excessive length of therapy, organ dysfunction, and prior history of drug reaction. Often the clinical trials in which safe dosing ranges are established do not include subjects who are older adults so a usual dose in an older adult may have unintended effects. Special attention must be paid on the part of healthcare professionals when dosing medications in older adults with low body mass and potentially impaired metabolism and clearance of drug secondary to age-related organ dysfunction (eg, renal or hepatic impairment). Agents that are of particular concern include sedatives, antihypertensives, narrow therapeutic index drugs, and anti-infectives. These agents often require a decrease in dose or longer intervals between doses to facilitate drug clearance and minimize the likelihood of toxicity.

Therapeutic Drug Monitoring

Therapeutic drug monitoring is the process of using drug concentrations, pharmacokinetic principles, and pharmacodynamics to optimize drug therapy. The goal of TDM is to maximize the therapeutic effect while avoiding toxicity. Drugs that are toxic at serum concentrations close to those required for therapeutic effect are the drugs most commonly monitored. The indications for TDM include narrow therapeutic range, limited objective monitoring parameters, potential for poor patient response, the need for therapeutic confirmation, unpredictable dose-response relationship, suspected toxicity, serious consequences of toxicity or lack of efficacy, correlation between serum concentration and efficacy or toxicity, identification of drug interactions, determination of individual pharmacokinetic parameters, and changes in patient pathophysiology or disease state.

The specific indication for TDM is important, because it affects the timing of the sample. Timing of sample collection

ESSENTIAL CONTENT CASE

Tips for Calculating IV Medication Infusion Rates

Information Required to Calculate IV Infusion Rates to Deliver Specific Medication Doses

- Dose to be infused (eg, mg/kg/min, mg/min, mg/h)
- Concentration of IV solution (eg, dopamine 400 mg in D_5W 250 mL = 1.6 mg/mL; nitroglycerin 50 mg in D_5W 250 mL = 200 mcg/mL)
- Patient's weight

Case Question 1: Calculate the IV infusion rate in milliliters per hour for a 70-kg patient requiring dobutamine 5 mcg/kg/min using a dobutamine admixture of 500 mg in D_5W 250 mL.

- Dose to be infused: 5 mcg/kg/min
- Dobutamine concentration: 500 mg/250 mL = 2 mg/mL or 2000 mcg/mL
- Patient weight: 70 kg

Calculation:

5 mcg/kg/min × 70 kg = 350 mcg/min
350 mcg/min × 60 min/h = 21,000 mcg/h
21,000 mcg/h ÷ 2000 mcg/mL = 10.5 mL/h

Case Question 2: Calculate the IV infusion rate in milliliters per hour for a 70-kg patient requiring nitroglycerin 50 mcg/m using a nitroglycerin admixture of 50 mg in D_5W 250 mL.

- Dose to be infused: 50 mcg/min

- Nitroglycerin concentration: 50 mg/250 mL = 0.2 mg/mL or 200 mcg/mL
- Patient weight: 70 kg

Calculation:

50 mcg/min × 60 min/h = 3000 mcg/h
3000 mcg/h ÷ 200 mcg/mL = 15 mL/h

Case Question 3: Calculate the IV infusion rate in milliliters per hour for a 70-kg patient requiring heparin 18 units/kg/h using a heparin admixture of 25,000 units in D_5W 500 mL.

- Maintenance infusion: 18 units/kg/h
- Heparin concentration: 25,000 units/500 mL = 50 units/mL
- Patient weight: 70 kg

Calculation:

Infusion rate: Heparin 18 units/kg/h × 70 kg = 1260 units/h ÷ 50 units/mL = 25.2 mL/h

Answers

1. Setting the infusion pump at 10.5 mL/h will deliver dobutamine at a dose of 5 mcg/kg/min.
2. Setting the infusion pump at 15 mL/h will deliver nitroglycerin at a dose of 50 mcg/min.
3. Setting the infusion pump at 25 mL/h will infuse the heparin at a dose of 18 units/kg/h.

---

depends on the question being asked. The timing of serum drug concentrations is critical for the interpretation of the results. The timing of peak serum drug concentrations depends on the route of administration and the drug product. Peak serum drug concentrations occur soon after an IV bolus dose, whereas they are delayed after IM, SC, or oral doses. Oral medications can be administered as either liquid or rapid- or slow-release dosage forms (eg, theophylline). The absorption and distribution phases must be considered when obtaining a peak serum drug concentration. The peak serum concentration may be much higher and occur earlier after a liquid or rapid-release dosage form compared to a sustained-release dosage form. Trough concentrations usually are obtained just prior to the next dose. Drugs with long half-lives (eg, phenobarbital) or sustained-release dosage forms (eg, theophylline) have minimal variation between their peak and trough concentrations. The timing of the determination of serum concentrations may be less critical in patients taking these dosage forms. Serum drug concentrations may be drawn at any time after achieving a steady state in a patient who is receiving a drug by continuous IV infusion. However, in patients receiving a drug by continuous infusion, the serum specimen should be drawn from a site away from where the drug is infusing. If toxicity is suspected, serum drug concentrations can be obtained at any time during the dosing interval.

Appropriate interpretation of serum concentrations is the step that requires an understanding of relevant patient factors, pharmacokinetics of the drug, and dosing regimen.

Misinterpretation of serum drug concentrations can result in ineffective and, at worst, harmful dosage adjustments. Interpreting serum concentrations includes an assessment of whether the patient's dose is appropriate, if the patient is at a steady state, the timing of the blood samples, an assessment of whether the time of blood sampling is appropriate for the indication, and an evaluation of the method of delivery to assess the completeness of drug delivery. Serum drug concentrations are interpreted within the context of the individual patient's condition. Therapeutic ranges serve as guidelines for each patient. Doses are not adjusted on the basis of laboratory results alone. Individual dosage ranges are developed for each patient as various patients may experience therapeutic efficacy, failure, or toxicity within a given therapeutic range.

SELECTED BIBLIOGRAPHY

General

Clinical Pharmacology [database online]. Tampa, FL: Gold Standard, Inc. http://www.clinicalpharmacology.com. Accessed May 22, 2021.

Drug Information Handbook. 29th ed. Hudson, OH: Wolters Kluwer Clinical Drug Information, Inc; 2020.

Faust AC, Echevarria KL, Attridge RL, et al. Prophylactic acid-suppressive therapy in hospitalized adults: indications, benefits, and infectious complications. *Crit Care Nurse.* 2017;37:18-29.

Institute of Safe Medication Practices. nwww.ismp.org. Accessed May 27, 2021.

Martin SJ, Olsen KM, Susla GM. *The Injectable Drug Reference.* 2nd ed. Des Plaines, IL: Society of Critical Care Medicine; 2006.

Papadopoulos J. *Pocket Guide to Critical Care Pharmacotherapy.* 2nd ed. Philadelphia, PA: Springer; 2015.

Sulsa GM, Suffredini AF, McAreavey D, et al. *The Handbook of Critical Care Drug Therapy.* 3rd ed. Philadelphia, PA: Lippincott William and Wilkins; 2006.

Vincent J, Abraham E, Kochanek P, et al. *Textbook of Critical Care.* 7th ed. Philadelphia, PA: Elsevier; 2016.

Evidence-Based Practice Guidelines

Ageno WA, Gallus AS, Wittkowsky A, et al. Clinical practice guidelines for oral anticoagulant therapy: antithrombotic therapy and prevention of thrombosis. *Chest.* 2012;141:e44S-e88S.

Devlin JW, Skrobik Y, Gélinas C, et al. Clinical practice guidelines for the prevention and management of pain, agitation/sedation, delirium, immobility, and sleep disruption in adult patients in the ICU. *Crit Care Med.* 2018;46:e825-e873.

Evans LE, Rhodes A, Alhazzani W, et al. Surviving sepsis campaign: international guidelines for management of sepsis and septic shock 2021. *Crit Care Med.* 2021;49:e1063-e1143.

Murray MJ, DeBlock H, Erstad B, et al. Clinical practice guidelines for sustained neuromuscular blockade in the adult critically ill patient. *Crit Care Med.* 2016;44:2079-2103.

O'Gara PT, Kushner FG, Ascheim DD, et al. American College of Cardiology Foundation/American Heart Association guidelines for management of ST-elevation myocardial infarction. Executive summary. *Circulation.* 2013;127:529-555.

ETHICAL AND LEGAL CONSIDERATIONS

8

Laura Webster

Ethical issues are pervasive in acute and critical care settings. Serious illness and its treatment constrain patient autonomy. Countless ailments bring prognostic uncertainty for patient outcomes in critical care, which can result in the patients, their loved ones, and healthcare teams struggling to determine the best ethical course of action. The COVID-19 pandemic both illuminated and exacerbated the ethical issues that critical care teams face.

The first step to managing ethical issues is the recognition that they exist, referred to as ethical sensitivity. Because of the complexity of the healthcare environment, differentiating issues that require moral reasoning from other common problems such as poor communication, differences of clinical opinion, or compassion fatigue can be challenging. Resolution of ethical issues depends on the ability to apply ethical decision-making skills and arrive at a conclusion about the best course of action for the situation in hand, knowing that many ethical dilemmas involve picking from bad options. Whether or not that action is taken depends not only on the motivation of the individual clinician but also on the environment in which treatments are provided. This chapter introduces the elements that serve as a foundation for addressing ethical issues including exploring terms, an introduction to and application of ethical frameworks, an overview of common ethical issues, a process to engage in ethical analysis, and problems that commonly occur in critical care setting are discussed.

FOUNDATIONAL TERMS: DEFINING ETHICS AND MORALITY

Many use the terms morality and ethics interchangeably. In this chapter, we use the terms differently to highlight difference between making a judgment and engaging in an ethical analysis. Vaughn's definition classifies ethics as the application of a moral theory, or theories, to sustain an ethically permissible argument. Whereas morality focuses on beliefs and judgments about what is "right" and what is "wrong" or what is "good" or what is "bad." Morality often makes a judgment and does not require supporting evidence or rationale. Ethics requires building and framing a stance using supportive rationale, it is not about right or wrong, or good or bad—ethics is about why a course of action is permissible. The practice of healthcare ethics seeks to unpack values to help clinicians, patients, and their surrogates make ethically informed decisions.

TYPES OF ETHICAL ISSUES

The most often cited ethical issues in health care are ethical dilemmas, moral uncertainty, moral hazard, and moral distress. While the issues are discussed from the nurse's perspective, all members of the healthcare team face similar ethical challenges. An ethical dilemma occurs when the nurse identifies two (or more) ethically permissible courses of action and they are often in opposition to each other. Both options can be supported with ethical rationale, yet each has undesirable consequences. In cases of moral uncertainty, a nurse recognizes that an ethical issue exists but is unable to identify the correct course of action. An analysis that includes considering all the possible actions, beyond those in opposition, can be helpful in resolving ethical dilemmas and moral uncertainty.

Much of healthcare occurs within a place of moral hazard. A moral hazard occurs when those who are empowered to parse risk and fashion responses to it (decision makers) are not those who suffer its burdens (decision bearers). When a person is a decision bearer, they must participate in action under the directions of another person. Marshall and Epstein believe moral hazard is the "background condition" for moral distress. While most actions a nurse takes involve entering a place of moral hazard, only a few results into moral distress.

When a nurse experiences moral distress, on the other hand, there is little uncertainty about what course of action feels correct but there is an inability to take that action. Internal factors such as fear of retribution and self-doubt can serve as the barrier to action. External factors that can constrain the nurse from acting include hierarchies within the healthcare system that create power imbalances, lack of administrative support, inappropriate staffing, and the presence or absence of hospital policies. While an ethical dilemma can lead the nurse to feel trapped between opposing courses of action, moral distress threatens their personal and professional integrity. Repeated episodes of moral distress can lead to the phenomenon of moral residue, in which the negative

feelings engendered by an ethical problem are compounded by unresolved feelings from past similar experiences. It should be noted that moral distress as a concept remains widely described and understood with over 34 definitions in the literature since Jameton's classic definition in 1984. However, all definitions highlight a person's moral judgment during a moral experience. More research on moral residue and its effect on nurses in acute care settings are needed. Table 8-1 provides the definition and examples of other types of ethical issues encountered in healthcare settings.

THE FOUNDATIONS FOR ETHICAL DECISION MAKING

Common Ethical Theories

The study of healthcare ethics involves exploring and applying multiple ethical frameworks from a vast array of ethical theories. Commonly used ethical theories in western healthcare include: virtue ethics, rule-based, principalism, relationship focused, casuistry, and outcome-based. This chapter briefly highlights each of these theories with an example of their application in nursing practice. Then the philosophical concept of rights explores the working environments for nurses. This chapter offers the 30,000-foot view knowing a single concept within a theory could be studied over a lifetime. This information barely scratches the surface. Table 8-2 summarizes common ethical theories.

Virtue Ethics

Virtue ethics supports virtues, or characteristics, valued according to a goal or purpose. The characteristics guide

TABLE 8-1. ETHICAL PROBLEMS

Type of Problem	Definition	Example
Ethical dilemma	The moral agent identifies two opposing but ethically permissible courses of action.	A patient on high-flow nasal cannula asks to leave against medical advice. The patient has decisional capacity and the surrogate came to take the patient home. The nurse worries the patient will quickly decompensate if they leave before their oxygen status stabilizes. Patients with capacity are allowed to refuse even lifesaving interventions, and nurses are asked to prevent foreseen complications and rescue patients in need.
Moral uncertainty	The moral agent is unable to determine what the best action is.	The nurse witnesses one adult family member verbally abusing another adult during their visit to a patient's room. The altercation occurred when the nurse was in the hall charting and has not affected the patient's plan of care. Is there an obligation to protect the patient from this family member after discharge? What action if any should be taken to prevent this from happening again?
Moral distress	A moral agent knows the right action to take but is unable to take that action.	An older adult with dementia and recurrent aspiration is scheduled for placement of a percutaneous endoscopic gastrostomy (PEG) tube for enteral nutrition. The nurse knows this treatment is inconsistent with current evidence, which shows that feeding tubes do not improve outcomes in patients with advanced dementia. However, the family has signed a consent form, the surgery is scheduled, and the nurse feels obligated to prepare the patient for the procedure.
Allocation of resources	A decision is required as to how to distribute a finite supply of goods or services across a group of people.	The principle of justice is the basis for allocation of resource problems. For example, when a hospital unit that provides a specific level of monitoring has one available bed and two patients, one in the operating room and one in the emergency room, who both require that level of care. Determining which patient will be admitted to the unit is an allocation of resources decision.
Locus of authority	Two or more individuals have a claim to the role of decision maker but do not agree on the course of action.	The patient's durable power of attorney for healthcare form indicates that both her adult children should make her healthcare decisions. They support opposing courses of treatment and it is unclear which course of action to take.

ESSENTIAL CONTENT CASE

Diagnosing Moral Distress

In selecting a topic for a graduate school assignment, Karen chose idiopathic pulmonary fibrosis, inspired by a patient, Adeline, she cared for in the medical intensive care unit (ICU), in room 576. Adeline was 66 years old and on high flow nasal cannula oxygen when Karen first met her and learned that she was a retired nurse. They chatted briefly about Adeline's career and her family while the patient awaited transfer to the operating room (OR) for a lung biopsy. Following the procedure, Adeline was intubated and sedated and Karen, rounding with the pulmonary team a few days later, was told that the biopsy showed a rare and very aggressive form of the disease. Over the subsequent week, Adeline's hypoxia worsened, and she was unable to undergo spontaneous breathing trials or sedation interruption without her oxygen saturation dropping to the low 80s. In a family conference, Adeline's sons presented the team with an advanced directive, which stated that in the event of a poor prognosis, Adeline did not desire life-sustaining measures such as mechanical ventilation. After much discussion, the family elected to remove Adeline from the ventilator. Because she had a chance to know Adeline, even very briefly, and to relate to her, Karen feels distressed observing her adult children as they grieve their loss. "This doesn't seem right" she thinks, "it's just so sad." After tearfully describing the situation to a colleague who is kind and gives her a hug, Karen decides she wants to learn more about this disease process.

A month later, Karen is again assigned to room 576. The patient, Gabriel, is a 72 year old with multiple medical problems who was admitted earlier that day with sepsis, requiring mechanical ventilation and vasopressors despite adequate fluid resuscitation. The nurse from the prior shift reports that she placed a urinary catheter, but no urine is draining from it. "But" she tells Karen "I know it's in. He's a man, after all!" After the prior nurse leaves, Karen finds that one of the antibiotics prescribed STAT and documented as administered is still hanging on the IV pole. Furthermore, the catheter remains without any urine. When she moves the collection bag to a lower position to prompt drainage, the sedated man twitches, as if uncomfortable. Karen removes the catheter and a stream of blood and urine are released. Based on the patient's history, she theorizes that an enlarged prostate impeded passage of the catheter into the bladder, and the balloon was actually inflated in the urethra, causing trauma. Karen is deeply concerned by the treatment her patient received and consults the charge nurse for guidance. The charge nurse points out that the nurse on the prior shift had a really tough assignment and

asks that Karen not mention what happened. She advises "you know what's it like to have a bad day, don't you? You don't want her to get in trouble for that and leave and then we're short staffed!" Karen feels distressed and does not know where to go for support. She is certain that the patient's adverse event was due to negligence by the nurse on the prior shift, and she feels obligated to protect him and other patients from further harm, but she is compelled to remain silent based on the guidance she was given by the charge nurse.

Case Question 1: How is the distress Karen experienced in these two situations different?

Case Question 2: How does identifying the form of distress help Karen?

Answers

1. In both cases, Karen felt a sense of distress, but the source of her distress is profoundly different. In the first situation, Karen felt emotional distress witnessing the grief engendered by the untimely death of a patient whom she briefly related to through a shared profession. In acute and critical care settings, emotionally distressing situations of this kind happen often. In the second scenario, Karen's distress was due to her inability to act in the way she felt was right (ie, formally reporting the errors). Furthermore, because her silence about her colleague's negligence is inconsistent with her professional values, her integrity suffered and shame ensued, creating an additional barrier to discussing the problem and getting support.

2. Distinguishing between emotional distress and moral distress is essential for the same reason that making an accurate diagnosis of the cause of shock is essential. The strategies to address these problems and their outcomes are very different. In the first scenario, Karen's emotional distress was alleviated by support from a friend and her own determination to learn more about the disease. Adeline's death seemed "not right" but nothing in that situation compelled Karen to act in a manner that she felt was wrong. With Gabriel, Karen felt complicit in the harm he suffered because she did not speak up about her colleague's negligence. Her professional integrity is threatened when she cannot take the action she believes to be right. Ethical analysis would not help Karen manage the emotional distress of caring for Adeline, but perhaps it could help her to navigate the moral distress she experienced with Gabriel.

---

acts by evaluating the general aim or purpose of a role and weighing the virtues at stake to avoid excess or deficiency of any one virtue. While in healthcare, most roles embrace similar virtues, their aims can allow the virtues to be applied differently. For example, the professional goal of a nurse is to navigate a patient's illness or injury and seeks to minimize pain and anxiety. Whereas the professional goal of a physician is to diagnose, to treat, and to realize when a patient is overmastered by their disease. These professional purposes align to work synergistically to give the best care to patients. Yet, when one profession disregards the goal of the other,

the clinicians may enter a place of moral hazard. A professional code of ethics, blends many ethical theories together, but when they outline professional goals and call out virtues important to a specific role, they are leaning into a virtue-ethics approach.

Professional Codes and Standards for Nurses

The *Code of Ethics for Nurses* developed by the American Nurses Association (ANA) articulates the essential values, principles, and obligations that guide nursing actions. The

TABLE 8-2. A SUMMARY OF COMMON MORAL THEORIES

Moral Theory	Basic Framework	Examples
Virtue based: (*Aristotelian*)	Virtues, character, obligations, and well-chosen habits	Clinician's obligations to both their families and their patients during COVID.
Consequence based: (*Consequentialist*)	Actions are guided by the outcome	Patient safety focuses on the outcome of keeping the patient safe, like when staff use restraints as a last resort to prevent harm to the patient or staff.
Principle or rule based: (*Deontological*)	Rules, duties, and principles	Law, policies, and common expectations.
Case based: (*Casuistry*)	Paradigm cases used to justify decisions	Evidence-based practice, like providing post-discharge follow-up care for patients with heart failure based on a study showing reduced readmissions for a similar program.
Relationship/Collective Focus: (*Care/Indigenous*)	Consideration of a group or all people guide decisions	A person who makes their healthcare decisions based on what is best for their family.
Social Equity Focus: (*Feminist*)	Actions aim to counteract and ameliorate inequity	Providing food, clothing, and transportation to a shelter for unhoused individuals when they are discharged

nine provisions of the ANA *Code of Ethics for Nurses* identify the ethical obligations of nurses and are applicable across all nursing roles (American Nurses Association, Code of Ethics for Nurses with Interpretive Statements, 2015. http://nursingworld.org/DocumentVault/Ethics-1/Code-of-Ethics-for-Nurses.html). While these provisions do not address specific ethical issues, they do provide a framework for examining issues and understanding the nurse's role in resolving them. The nurse's primary obligation to the patient, their role in patient advocacy, their duty to themselves, and their contribution to the work environment and to social justice are among the provisions in the *Code of Ethics for Nurses*.

In addition to the ANA *Code of Ethics for Nurses*, nurses' function in accordance with particular standards of practice and regulatory requirements. Professional organizations and statutory bodies delineate the standards that govern the practice of nursing in various jurisdictions. Most regulations are derived from nursing's implicit social contract with society. In addition, professional nursing standards define the criteria for the assessment and evaluation of nursing practice. External bodies, such as state boards of nursing, can impose certain regulations for licensure, regulate the practice of nursing, and evaluate and monitor the actions of professional nurses.

Nurses must be aware of the laws and regulations that impact their practice and also understand that such standards are not always consistent with their ethical obligations. There are rare situations when regulatory standards or laws conflict with a nurse's professional ethical obligations, and external support may be needed. Many organizations also delineate standards of practice for registered nurses in a defined area of specialty. For example, the American Association of Critical-Care Nurses (AACN) establishes expectations of performance for nurses practicing in acute and critical care and documents these in *the Scope and Standards for Progressive and Critical Care Nursing Practice*.

Standards of practice outlined by statutory bodies and specialty organizations are not confined to clinical skills and knowledge. Nurses are expected to function within the profession's code of ethics and are held morally and legally accountable for dishonorable practice. When allegations of unsafe, illegal, or immoral practice arise, the regulatory body serves to protect the public by investigating and disciplining the culpable professional. Although specialty organizations do not have authority to retract professional licensure, issues of professional misconduct are reviewed and may result in revocation of certification and notification of external parties.

Rule-Based

Rule-based (deontological) approaches to ethics use rules to help guide or make decisions. The application of a rule-based theory means examining the situation at hand and carefully framing the question to invoke the appropriate rule(s). For example, the legal system carries rules through a set of laws, and in practice, prosecutors must evaluate the potential crime at stake to develop the best arguments for or against different penal codes, before bringing charges for a specific crime. In rule-based theories, it remains vital to carefully examine the situation, frame the question and identify a rule or rules at stake in the dilemma.

In everyday practice, clinicians use institutional policies and legal standards as a set of rules to invoke whenever they are appropriate to follow.

Institutional Policies

Because nurses practice within organizations, institutional policies and procedures also guide their practice. Institutional guidelines such as those for assessing decision-making capacity, caring for patients who lack capacity, or policies for the determination of brain death are intended to guide employees of a healthcare facility when they are faced with moral uncertainty. These policies usually reflect expectations congruent with the professional codes of ethics. However, in some circumstances, organizations may assume a particular position or value and therefore expect the employees to uphold this position. For example, some hospitals endorse religious values and may prohibit professional practices that violate these positions. Ideally, the nurse and institution have complementary values and beliefs about professional responsibilities and obligations.

Institutions often provide internal resources to help clinicians resolve difficult ethical issues. Professional ethicists and those who provide ethics consultations help clinicians, patients, and surrogates during challenging situations. The process includes identifying differing values and providing guidance and support to health care teams who are uncertain about the correct action to take. Other resources for critical care nurses include institutional policies, colleagues with additional training in ethics, physicians, nurse managers, and advanced practice nurses. While the ANA code states that nurses act as advocates for patients, obtaining assistance when needed is an essential step in that process.

Legal Standards

The Affordable Care Act (ACA) passed in 2010 requires hospitals to report quality indicators, such as the rate of hospital-acquired infections (CMS, 2010). This legislation ties these indicators to Medicare reimbursement. The ACA thus creates financial incentives for hospital systems to implement strategies to prevent infection as a complication of hospital admission. In this way, the ACA offers a legal manifestation of the ethical principle of nonmaleficence, discussed in the following text. The Health Information Portability and Accountability Act (HIPAA) Privacy Rules similarly create a legal mandate to honor the ethical obligation of confidentiality.

State legislation can also influence acute care nursing practice. For instance, if a patient does not designate, through an advance directive, a surrogate decision maker, state law guides the selection of a family member to serve in this role. States differ in their recognition of unmarried domestic partners and friends to serve as the medical decision maker when a patient is rendered incapable by illness or injury.

When faced with an ethical issue, the professional codes, institutional policies, or legal standards can assist, and sometimes resolve, the issue. Thus, it is imperative that nurses be familiar with these resources and how to access them. However, nurses also need to recognize that guidelines and policies and even the law do not always answer the question of what the ethical course of action is. In such situations, the nurse must be prepared to identify the ethical principles involved and follow a step-wise approach to addressing the problem.

Principles of Ethics

Beauchamp and Childress wrote about principalism in the 1970s, which became one of the most influential perspectives in biomedical ethics. Inherent in this viewpoint is the belief that some basic moral principles define the essence of ethical obligations in human society and specifically in healthcare. Four basic principles, and derivative imperatives or rules, are considered *prima facie* binding. In other words, to breach a principle is wrong unless there are prevailing and compelling reasons that outweigh the necessary infringement. The principles and rules are binding but not absolute.

Because many approaches to ethics integrate the rules and principles outlined by the principle-oriented approach, it is helpful for nurses to understand these fundamental concepts. The primary principles in bioethics are nonmaleficence, beneficence, justice, and respect for persons (or autonomy). The principles are not ordered in a particular hierarchy, but their application and interpretation are based on the specific features of the ethical problem and the values of the team members involved. Articulating the principles involved and recognizing the personal values of the health care team members, patients, and families are essential steps to resolving an ethical problem.

Nonmaleficence

The principle of nonmaleficence imposes the duty to do no harm. This principle suggests that the nurse should not knowingly inflict actions that merely bring harm. In general, a nurse upholds the principle of nonmaleficence by maintaining competence and practicing within accepted standards of care.

Beneficence

The ethical principle of beneficence affirms an obligation to promote good by actively helping others to advance and realize their interests. In health care, understanding the values and preferences of the patient and family is intrinsic to this principle. The duty to do good requires that the healthcare team understand and agree on what is "good." Nurses, because of their close relationships with patients and their families, are often in the best position to understand the patient's interpretation of what is "good" in their plan of care.

Respect for Autonomy

The principle of respect for autonomy affirms the freedom and right of an individual to make decisions and choose actions based on that individual's personal values and beliefs. In other words, an autonomous choice is an informed decision made without coercion that reflects the individual's underlying interests and values. To respect a patient's autonomy is to recognize that patients may make choices and take actions that are incongruent with the values of the healthcare providers. In some cases, this concept is difficult to accept and endorse, particularly when the patient's choice conflicts with the caregivers' view of what is best in this situation.

Justice

The principle of justice covers a vast array of concepts. Justice can be simply defined as treating patients alike. Justice examines fairness, consistency, inequity, power, and privilege. When resources are limited, justice demands that they be fairly allocated. While there are many interpretations of the justice principle, three common theories will be described here by the following example. Imagine a population of people who have a set of goods that must be shared fairly among them. (1) *Egalitarian justice* would demand that the goods be divided into equal portions and every member of the population given the same share. (2) *Humanitarian justice* would demand that the goods be divided according to the needs of each member, with the neediest members getting larger portions. (3) *Libertarian justice* would demand the goods be distributed according to the contributions made by each member of the population; those making the greatest contributions get the greater share.

On a day-to-day basis, nurses make decisions involving the allocation of nursing care—like which patient they assess first or how to assign patients on the unit to the staff on the next shift. The complex and competing demands for nursing resources can sometimes lead to chaotic and random decisions. Such decisions may unintentionally compromise other important aims and additional scrutiny is warranted to preserve patient safety. The principle of justice argues for more than the basic allocation of resources; it demands a comprehensive, thoughtful approach to address competing claims to resources.

Relationship-Focused

Many ethical theories consider that humans exist in partnerships with other humans through relationships. These relationships highlight special obligations to not only the people in the relationship but to serve the relationship itself. When a person asks, what does it mean to be a "good" child, parent, or caregiver, they are leaning into to the weight of the relationship in a different manner than a virtue ethics approach. The relationship, not the role, becomes the most important to value during a dilemma.

Ethic of Care

One framework for ethics that is viewed as an alternative to the principle-based approach. The ethic of care emphasizes the important relationships in a case and identifies the correct ethical action as the one that preserves those relationships. In 1987, Carol Gilligan described the phenomenon of using relationships to identify moral actions after observing how children make ethical decisions. While some children adhere to rules (eg, "do not steal," "do not lie"), others consider how an action will affect others (eg, hurt feelings, loss of trust or respect). These ways of thinking carry through to adulthood. While Carol Gilligan's observations of children noted a gender difference in the application of care-based ethics, in adulthood, most people can view a situation through both the rules lens and the relationship lens.

The ethic of care begins from an attached, involved, and interdependent position. From this standpoint, morality is viewed as caring about others, developing relationships, and maintaining connections. Moral problems result from disturbances in interpersonal relationships and disruptions in perceived responsibilities. The resolution of moral issues emerges as the involved parties examine the contextual features and embrace the relevance of the relationship and the related responsibilities.

In contrast, a principle-oriented approach typically originates from a position of detachment and individuality. This approach recognizes the concepts of fairness, rights, and equality as the core of morality. Therefore, dilemmas arise when these elements are compromised. From this perspective, the approach to moral resolution is a reliance on formal logic, deductive reasoning, and a hierarchy of principles.

For nursing, the ethic of care provides a useful approach to moral analysis. The professional values of nursing emphasize attachment, caring, attention to context, and the development of relationships. To maintain this position, nurses develop proficiency in forming and sustaining relationships with patients and within families. The importance of relationships is also suggested in provision 1 of the *Code of Ethics for Nurses*. The ethic of care legitimizes and values the emotional, intuitive, and informal interpretation of moral issues. This perspective expands the sphere of inquiry and promotes the understanding and resolution of moral issues.

Casuistry

Casuistry uses prior cases to help guide decisions. A paradigm case occurs when the best knowledge at the time was applied and used to guide a complex case or situation. These "paradigm cases" are used to guide the actions for all similar future cases. In healthcare, the use of evidence-based practice (EBP) is the best example of casuistry in action. EBP literally guides clinicians on how to manage a certain ailment or injury with the best information available.

Outcome-Based

Outcome-based theories use potential outcomes to guide actions. These consequentialist, often utilitarian, frameworks establish a metric to achieve and while they may consider aspects of the process—the outcome remains vital to making and evaluating decisions. One example of an outcome-based theory is the application of crisis standards of care. During different stages of surge, one desired outcome is fair distribution of scarce resources that saves the most number of lives and a variety of strategies are leveraged to meet that aim.

SURGE CAPACITY AND CRISIS STANDARDS OF CARE

Surge capacity refers to a hospital's process to accommodate a sudden increase in patients or sudden decrease in available resources, like staffing. It is broken into three elements to be used on a spectrum with a goal to evaluate frequently and return to normal, or conventional, as soon as possible (See figure 8-1). This new section provides a higher level of detail than other sections in this chapter. Given the high potential for nurses, and other clinicians, to experience moral distress during a crisis, we hope this foundational knowledge will help when a crisis state occurs.

Conventional	Contingency	Crisis
This is a hospital's **normal state** with responses to an increase of **up to 120% of normal volume.**	This is a hospital's response to a sudden or progressive increase of **up to 200% of normal volume.**	In *rare* situations, this is a hospital's response to a sudden or progressive increase of **up to 300% of normal volume.**
Strategies: Conserve and Substitute to **maintain** the standards of care	Strategies: Conserve and Substitute + Adapt and Re-Use to **preserve** the standards of care	Strategies: Conserve and Substitute + Adapt and Re-Use + Allocate or Reallocate to **save** lives (the standards of *disaster* care)

Figure 8-1. *Data from Hick JL, Einav S, Hanfling D, et al: Surge capacity principles: care of the critically ill and injured during pandemics and disasters: CHEST consensus statement. Chest. 2014;146(4 Suppl):e1S-e16S.*

Surges traditionally describe situations in which there is a sudden influx of patients from a national disaster or mass causality incident. However, we are learning that a sudden decrease in available resources, including staff, can also result in changes to a hospital's surge state. While individual elements of staff, space, or supplies, can become scarce, any missing element can jeopardize the ability to provide the intervention itself. Each state has different strategies to avoid a crisis state. The National Academy of Sciences, Engineering, and Medicine outlined the following ethical values that apply to disaster response standards:

- Fairness—Standards that are, to the highest degree possible, recognized as fair by those affected by them—including the members of affected communities, practitioners, and provider organizations—and are evidence-based and responsive to specific needs of individuals and the population.
- Duty to care—Standards are focused on the duty of healthcare professionals to care for patients in need of medical care.
- Duty to steward resources—Healthcare institutions and public health officials have a duty to steward scarce resources, reflecting the utilitarian goal of saving the greatest possible number of lives.
- Transparency—In development, decision making, and information sharing.
- Consistency—In application across populations and among individuals regardless of their human condition (eg, race, age, disability, ethnicity, ability to pay, socioeconomic status, preexisting health conditions, relative worth, perceived obstacles to treatment, past use of resources).
- Proportionality—Public and individual requirements must be commensurate with the scale of the emergency and degree of scarce resources.
- Accountability—we must be accountable for our individual and institutional actions.

Crisis standards of care refer to change in standards of practice from our normal focus on the individual patient to one that examines the community as a whole. Crisis state occurs as a means of last resort, after all contingency measures are leveraged and existing resources remain insufficient. Until a balance between the demand for resources and their availability is restored, a shift in the standard of care may be warranted. Ethically, this shift is deliberate, transparent, and collaborative; it considers all available strategies for increasing and stretching the number of resources before initiating crisis allocation. The application of crisis standards of care should involve initiating a clear and consistent process for triaging patients and allocating the available resources. Often, there are state-specific guidelines to follow.

In a crisis, organizations implement guidelines using a systematic process of assessing available resources, identifying contingency measures to maintain usual standards whenever feasible, and finally shifting to triage to determine the most beneficial use of scarce resources. Table 8-3 provides definitions of the six "A"s for contingency and crisis response as described by the National Academy of Medicine. The example of managing personal protective equipment supplies is used to illustrate the application of each step in the cycle. Every stage of this cycle must include transparency, with communication to everyone affected by the crisis response.

There are practical, legal, and ethical elements in crisis standards of care. On a practical level, health care teams and their leaders seek to avoid applying a crisis standard and to maintain normal, also called conventional, standards. Limiting nonessential care and redeploying those staff to areas that are experiencing a surge in admissions is an example of a strategy that can help avoid a crisis. Legally, when state or federal officials declare a state of emergency and crisis standards of care are invoked, the liability of health care providers and the requirements of their role may shift. Ethically, applying crisis standards of care poses a threat to a nurse's moral integrity, while not applying them when needed risks unfairness and inconsistency to all in need. Most crisis standards are based on a utilitarian approach—seeking to do the greatest good for the greatest number—whereas the nursing code of ethics is often interpreted as emphasizing the nurse's obligation to each individual patient and family. As described in the AACN position statement on Ethical Triage and End-of-Life Care, health care institutions facing a crisis should implement shared transparent and compassionate processes that result in fair and ethical triage decisions. The statement also emphasizes nurses' obligation to provide optimal end-of-life care, especially for patients who do not receive a scarce life-saving resource.

TABLE 8-3. CONVENTIONAL, CONTINGENCY, AND CRISIS RESPONSE CYCLE

Step	Definition	Example: Supplies of Personal Protective Equipment
Awareness	The team or individual who serves as incident commander is aware of an existing or impending mismatch between resources available and the demand for resources.	The incident command team is notified about limited supplies of personal protective equipment (PPE).
Assess	Technical experts are identified, and a clinical care team to respond to resource challenges.	The supply of PPE and the rate at which it is being used is calculated.
Advice/anticipate	Teams with relevant technical and clinical expertise advise incident command on strategies to employ while anticipating further changes in resource availability and demand for care.	Supply specialists identify alternative sources for obtaining PPE (such as from community, state, or Strategic National Stockpile). The incident command team maintains and publishes a dashboard of existing PPE supplies.
Adapt	Changes in procedures are identified, starting with those that do not change the level of care provided, such as canceling non-essential services that require the resource in demand. Further adaptions that change the standard of care are implemented only if necessary.	Team models such as the use of warm zone configurations reduce donning and doffing of PPE. Crisis measures such as reusing PPE are employed if shortages persist.
Allocate	Triage teams employ consistent standards to determine the best use of a resource that is scarce.	Preserving N95s or equivalent supplies for aerosol-generating procedures and using face masks for other care activities. This strategy is only employed when the level of N95s available is at a crisis level.
Analysis	Monitor for opportunities to improve the allocation and establish thresholds for returning to contingency measures and maintaining standard of care and for continuing crisis standards.	The dashboard of PPE supplies is updated on a daily basis and procedures shift from contingency to crisis when supplies fall below a specific threshold and back to contingency when more resources are available. This step circles back to "advise/anticipate."

Data from Crisis Standards of Care: A Systems Framework for Catastrophic Disaster Response: Volume 1: Introduction and CSC Framework. Washington, DC: The National Academies Press; 2012

In crisis response, changes in care delivery are described along a continuum from conventional care in which patients receive the usual standard of care in the usual way, to contingency care where a functionally equivalent standard of care is provided through different means, and finally to crisis circumstances in which the standard is altered. Frequent reassessment of available resources and the demand for them is needed to ensure that the appropriate strategies along that continuum are applied. Operating under crisis standards of care when, in fact, contingency measures could be applied violates our duty to care, proportionality, and fairness.

Because resource availability will not be uniform, health care teams may be applying different standards to their processes at the same time. For instance, if space is adequate, patients may occupy hospital rooms in a conventional, usual way, while lack of staff is managed through a contingency measure using a team model, and simultaneously, severe deficits of personal protective equipment require application of a crisis standard of care. The continuum of conventional, contingency, and crisis standards is further described in chapter 23.

Hospitals and health systems can prepare for crisis situations by establishing in advance the guidelines that will be applied when resources and the demand for them are out of balance. As noted in Figure 8-2, two-way communication between direct care teams, system leaders, and local and state officials is an essential aspect of applying appropriate care in a crisis. Hospitals and health systems may maintain contingency levels of care if patients are transferred to a facility with more resources or when resources are shared across facilities. Appropriate preparation for a crisis thus includes

relationships between proximate facilities and collaboration with county and state officials. In addition, nurses with direct care experience must be engaged in establishing and implementing guidelines for crisis response. Nurses have a unique understanding of patient needs and strategies for applying scarce resources effectively. Their input in preparation for and during crisis response is essential.

The protracted nature of the COVID-19 pandemic which includes recurrent surges of patient admissions creates a unique, and in some cases, excruciating challenge for health care teams. Providing a different standard of care with the knowledge that it is an interim step and normal procedures will resume is ethically tolerable, whereas applying an altered standard for a long interval or repeatedly threatens professional integrity and trust in our health systems. As a result, the pandemic increases moral distress and the related but distinct phenomenon of burnout and highlights the importance of supporting healthcare workforce wellbeing. AACN's position statement on Moral Distress in Times of Crisis lists some of the actions that health systems and individuals can take to mitigate moral distress. In addition, adequate preparation for future crises based on lessons learned in responding to COVID-19 may help preserve the ethical integrity of nurses and their colleagues.

Rights

Most patients receive notice of their "patient rights" upon admission, and clinicians receive information about their workplace protections upon hiring. The concept of rights stems from rule-based theories and outlines areas in society that people should have access to, like the standard of

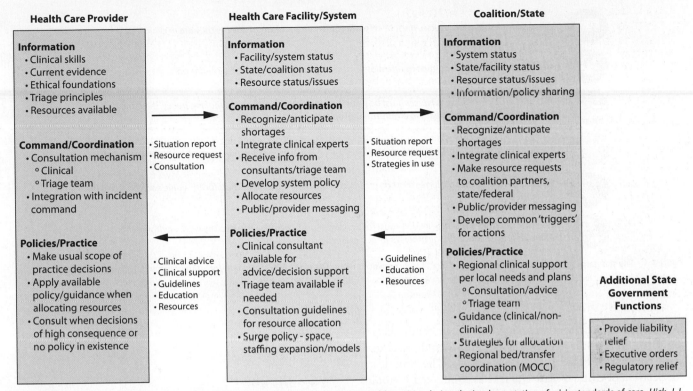

Figure 8-2. A model to demonstrate communication and collaboration among accountable entities during the implementation of crisis standards of care. *Hick, J. L., D. Hanfling, M. Wynia, and E. Toner. 2021. Crisis Standards of Care and COVID-19: What Did We Learn? How Do We Ensure Equity? What Should We Do? NAM Perspectives. Discussion, National Academy of Medicine, Washington, DC. https://doi.org/10.31478/202108e. Reproduced with permission from the National Academy of Sciences, courtesy of the National Academies Press.*

care, or should be free of like physical harm. Philosophically, rights are delineated into two types: negative rights and positive rights.

- A negative right states a person has the right to non-interference; for example, a patient's right to refuse medical treatment and a clinician's right to avoid threats to personal safety.
- A positive right states that someone is entitled to receive a good or service; for example, a patient's right to access the standard of care for a test or intervention.

Morally speaking, negative rights are generally much stronger than positive ones. We see this in all areas in society and in healthcare; we respect a patient's autonomy by not forcing them to participate in treatment they have declined. Positive rights, while important, often fluctuate in their availability in society and yet when tested, there is societal agreement that something is owed to someone else. In healthcare, clinicians began reviewing the workplace to explore the tension between a nurse's negative right to be free from harm and the positive services a nurse provides in the workplace.

BUILDING AN ETHICAL ENVIRONMENT

While the information in this chapter provides the basis for recognizing and analyzing ethical issues, evidence shows that that the environment has a profound effect on nurses'

ability to resolve ethical issues. A nurse may approach an ethical dilemma, such as the one described in the case "Applying the Process" below, with the intention of exploring all possible alternatives, using ethical creativity and motivated to take the action that ethical analysis supports. However, if factors within the environment such as incivility, lack of leadership, inadequate staffing, or hierarchical structures are barriers to action, preserving professional integrity requires additional navigation including identifying sources of support. When nurses feel unable to act because the work environment is not healthy, they are at risk for moral distress whenever an ethical concern arises. Furthermore, nurses who experience moral distress repeatedly are unlikely to meet their obligation to contribute to building a healthy work environment.

Healthy Work Environments

The AACN Standards for Establishing and Sustaining Healthy Work Environments provide a framework for identifying the elements of the environment that promote effective resolution of ethical issues. As shown in Figure 8-3, the six standards, skilled communication, true collaboration, authentic leadership, effective decisions making, meaningful recognition, and appropriate staffing, are not isolated characteristics but interdependent features that collectively contribute to an environment in which members of the healthcare team are able to make their optimal contribution

Skilled Communication: *Nurses must be as proficient in communication skills as they are in clinical skills*

 True Collaboration: *Nurses must be relentless in pursuing and fostering true collaboration*

 Effective Decision-Making: *Nurses must be valued and committed partners in making policy, directing and evaluating clinical care, and leading organizational operations*

 Appropriate Staffing: *Staffing must ensure the effective match between patient needs and nurse competencies*

 Meaningful Recognition: *Nurses must be recognized and must recognize others for the value each brings to the work of the organization*

 Authentic Leadership: *Nurse leaders must fully embrace the imperative of a healthy work environment, authentically live it, and engage others in its achievement*

Figure 8-3. The standards for establishing and sustaining healthy work environments. (*Data from ACN's Standards for Establishing and Sustaining a Healthy Work Environments. A Journey to Excellence, 2nd ed. Aliso Viejo, CA:* American Association of Critical-Care Nurses; 2016.)

to patient care. Environments in which these standards are practiced are not free of ethical issues but when those issues arise, there are mechanisms for responding. The American Association of Critical-Care Nurses has conducted periodic surveys of work environments since 2005. The results confirm a link between moral distress and perceptions of the work environment. Comparing results across the surveys, a concerning finding is that the number of respondents reporting moral distress has increased over time. Of note, these increases pre-date the COVID-19 pandemic which magnified existing sources of moral distress, such as inappropriate staffing and end-of-life care, and created new sources including inadequate personal protective equipment and restricted family visitation. The essential content case "The Impact of the Environment" describes how one situation is handled differently when it occurs in different environments.

Principles of Management

The attributes of a work environment are not static; they can change over time. Furthermore, the environment is not an entity in and of itself, it is a compilation of the attitudes and behaviors of the people who work there. Provision 6 of the *Code of Ethics for Nurses* describes the nurses' obligation to contribute to an ethical work environment. Ideally, novice nurses do this by learning from their preceptors, recognizing ethical issues, and seeking assistance appropriately. Experienced nurses can contribute as role models for skilled communication and true collaboration, expecting that members of the intraprofessional team will respond in kind and

---

ESSENTIAL CONTENT CASE

The Impact of the Environment

Henrietta is a 72-year-old woman who has been in the coronary care unit for 4 weeks following a large anterolateral myocardial infarction (MI). She has suffered from heart failure, pulmonary edema, and hypotension, and now has developed acute respiratory distress syndrome (ARDS) and renal failure. Currently, she requires pressure-controlled ventilator support, continuous renal replacement therapy (CRRT) and inotropic agents because of her low cardiac output. Her husband and her son visit often and seem to be supportive, but also overwhelmed by this sudden change in her health.

After 2 weeks without improvement and with episodes of worsening hemodynamic instability, the nurses are concerned that their care is prolonging Henrietta's inevitable death. Furthermore, during intervals when her sedation is weaned, the patient grimaces and reaches to remove tubes which the nurses interpret as an effort to communicate her discomfort with the current treatment modalities. Rhonda, the patient's primary nurse on dayshift, asks the physician, Dr. Smith, if a family conference should be planned. Dr. Smith responds that he has spoken to the family several times and "They just don't seem to get it. I think it's a waste of time to schedule another meeting. We'll just keep going until she codes, I guess." Rhonda is uncomfortable with this plan. Here are two possible outcomes of this situation that differ based on the work environment:

Healthy Work Environment

Rhonda uses skilled communication to engage the physician in further conversation. Using a professional tone, she states "I understand that you feel that a family meeting is a bad use of time, but I am concerned that we are not caring for our patient appropriately. Is this a good time for me to share my thoughts with you?" By restating what the physician has said, she demonstrates an understanding of his perspective. By referring to "we" and "our," she conveys her desire to collaborate in the management of this patient. Because Rhonda's communication is professional and clear, Dr. Smith agrees to talk further. "What are your thoughts?" he asks.

Rhonda recalls a workshop on palliative care communication skills that she attended, as part of the hospital's meaningful recognition program. She suggests "Maybe instead of trying to explain to them how sick she is, we should ask them what they think she feels about all this. I think we need to better understand what the patient would want." After a 5-minute conversation, Dr. Smith and Rhonda agree to plan a family conference for the following day.

When the time for the conference arrives, Rhonda asks her charge nurse to cover for her, so they can meet in the conference room. The charge nurse, Susan, replies that she cannot cover the patient on CRRT, as she is already covering for a nurse who has to take a patient to radiology. Recognizing that the meeting is important to Rhonda and her patient, Susan suggests that the doctor and Rhonda speak to the family in the patient's room. Rhonda agrees, and the charge nurse asks a nursing assistant to move extra chairs into the room so that Rhonda, the physician, and both family members can all sit.

Per the decision that Dr. Smith and Rhonda reached on the prior day, Rhonda starts the meeting with an open-ended question. She asks "Can you tell us a little more about Henrietta? We know about this illness but to make the right choices about her care we need to know more about her as a person." In prior interactions, neither man said more than a few words but with this invitation to talk about their wife and mother, they begin to speak with great affection. "You know, we've been married almost 50 years, and I've never seen her sit still for more than a few minutes. She is always on the go. You all must be giving her a lot of medicine to make her lie there so still." The physician sees an opening to provide information about Henrietta's disease and states "The medicine does keep her calm, but she is also very sick." "Will she get better soon?" the son asks. And Rhonda, recalling another palliative care communication skill from her past training, replies "We hope she will get better, but we are worried that she will never be as healthy as she was before the heart attack." The husband, tears in his eyes, asks, "So you're saying that all this." He gestures to the equipment in the room "may not be enough to get her back to who she was?" Rhonda instinctively takes his hand and nods "That is exactly what we are saying. And we need your help to understand what Henrietta would say about that."

Unhealthy Work Environment

Rhonda, having experienced moral distress when patients who clearly had a poor prognosis underwent CPR feels a surge of anxiety when the doctor suggests this will happen to Henrietta. Because other interactions between nurses and doctors in this unit have been characterized by incivility and mutual disrespect, she avoids further conversation with Dr. Smith. She continues to feel troubled by the care she is providing, however, and so decides that she will broach the issue with the family herself the following day. She wishes that she had been able to attend a conference on talking to patients about

end-of-life care, but her request was denied. The nurse manager is dealing with the unit's short staffing by limiting the number of schedule requests that staff can make.

The next day, Rhonda is in the patient's room when the spouse and son arrive and ask her for an update. She wants to answer honestly and begin a discussion that will allow her to help her patient but she is unsure how to do so. She explains the ventilator settings, the fluid balance, and the rate of the inotropic drip. The family nod but it is unclear how much of this information they take in. At that moment, Dr. Smith arrives and asks the family to wait in the waiting room while he examines the patient. Still troubled, Rhonda seeks the advice of the charge nurse but finds her totally overwhelmed and in need of support herself "We have a patient going to radiology today and a call out on the next shift and it's such pain that I'm in charge!" Just then the unit manager approaches to ask Rhonda why the family members are in the waiting room. "You know, we've already been written up for not adhering to the open visitation policy. You have to let the family stay in the room when they visit!" she tells Rhonda. Rhonda returns to Henrietta's room and completes her shift, mechanically providing the necessary nursing care.

Case Question 1: Which of the healthy work environment standards were evident in the first version of the case?

Case Question 2: Which of the healthy work environment standards were notably absent in the second version of the case?

Answers
1. Rhonda used skilled communication when she spoke to the doctor, the charge nurse, and the family. In addition, true collaboration took place in her work with the doctor and with the charge nurse. The charge nurse demonstrated authentic leadership in supporting Rhonda's desire for the family meeting and helping her to identify a strategy that worked around the staffing constraints. Rhonda experienced meaningful recognition when the hospital provided a professional development opportunity. Effective decision making occurred when the doctor invited Rhonda's input on approaching the family meeting and they decided, together on the flow of the meeting.

2. In the second case, there is evidence that poor communication is pervasive in the unit. Rhonda has experienced this in the past, and the charge nurse demonstrates this by venting openly about her role rather than seeking honest input into how she can manage the challenges she is facing. The manager's decision to limit staff access to professional development and her reprimand of Rhonda without hearing her side of the story are evidence that authentic leadership is lacking. Rhonda's anxiety and fear, a result of past experiences in the work environment, are barriers to developing a collaborative relationship with the doctor. Because she does not receive the support she seeks, effective decision making is also absent.

Additional Reflections
- Imagine you are Rhonda and reflect on how you would feel at the end of the shift in these two different versions of the story.
- Imagining that you are the patient's family, consider how the difference in work environment impacts your experience of Henrietta's illness.

include them in decisions that affect their work. Below are some actions that nurses can take to help address the health of their work environment:

- Engage in self-reflection to clarify values and better understand what guides personal and professional commitments. Help families and patients to clarify their values as well.
- Use open-ended questions to understand the perspectives of your colleagues, patients, and families. Recognize their use of different ethical frameworks and the principles they prioritize.
- Identify strategies such as journaling or talking to a friend or mentor for examining situations that lead to moral distress. There is no way to change past experiences but there may be opportunities to reframe them.
- Recognize the unique perspective that nursing brings to the healthcare team through their relationship with the patient and family and their understanding of the impact of serious illness. Expect other members of the healthcare team to value this as well.
- Use inclusive language—"we" instead of "I" or "you" and "our" instead of "my" or "your." Such language signals a desire for shared decision making and collaborative action.
- Review the literature, attend conferences, and use resources available from professional nursing organizations to develop communication skills.
- Provide meaningful recognition when colleagues demonstrate attention to the work environment. A simple statement such as "I appreciated working with you in the care of this patient" is a clear acknowledgment of a collaborative relationship.
- Consider forming a group with your colleagues to complete AACN's Healthy Work Environment Assessment, a tool that helps identify gaps in the work environment that can then be addressed with targeted interventions.
- Work with a manager or hospital administrators on projects for formal recognition such as Magnet status through the American Nurse Credentialing Center or the Beacon Award through the American Association of Critical-Care Nurses.

COMMON ETHICAL ISSUES

Nurses gain exposure to countless ethical issues, and these concepts stem from the ethical frameworks discussed earlier. A nurse's virtues of fidelity and veracity, the rules they follow, and the standards they embrace help navigate the ethical issues when they arise. This section includes descriptions of informed consent, end-of-life care, and evolving technology which are some of the contemporary issues that generate ethical issues for the healthcare team. This is by no means an all-inclusive list but rather is intended to provide examples of

how ethical analysis applies to situations that nurses working in critical care settings commonly encounter. Nursing interventions to respond to each issue are included.

Fidelity

Fidelity is the obligation to be faithful to commitments and promises and uphold implicit and explicit commitments to patients, colleagues, and employers. The concept of fidelity is particularly important in acute and critical care. The vulnerability of seriously ill patients increases their dependency on the relationship with the nurse, thus making the nurse's faithfulness to that relationship essential. Nurses demonstrate faithfulness by fulfilling the commitments of the relationship, which include the provision of competent care and advocacy on the patient's behalf. In addition, the nurse is obligated to demonstrate fidelity in relationships with colleagues and employers. In this way, the principle of fidelity can be difficult to uphold as institutions may have policies, such as those related to resource utilization, that the nurse finds conflict with the patient's best interests. When confronted with such situations, the nurse is wise to carefully weigh the ethical principles involved, to seek guidance if necessary, and to consider a role as an advocate for change if appropriate.

Privacy and Confidentiality

Privacy and confidentiality are associated, but distinct, concepts that are derived from the virtue of fidelity. Privacy refers to the right of an individual to be free from unjustified or unnecessary access by others. In acute care settings, the patient's privacy is sometimes disregarded. The design of many units includes easy visualization of patient rooms, and in their focus on addressing life-limiting illness, the healthcare team may assume that open access to the patient is for the best. The principle of privacy is honored when nurses request permission from the patient or family for any bodily intrusion or physical exposure. The casual infringement of an individual's privacy erodes trusting and caring nurse-patient relationships and contributes to the view of the patient as something other than an autonomous being.

Confidentiality refers to the protection of information. When the patient shares information with the nurse or any member of the healthcare team, the information should be treated as confidential and discussed only with those directly involved in the patient's care. Exceptions to confidentiality include quality improvement activities, mandatory disclosures to public health agencies, reporting abuse, or required disclosures in a judicial setting. Intentional disclosures of information obtained in a confidential manner take place only when strong and compelling reasons to do so exist such as when there is risk of harm to others. When possible, the patient is made aware of the impending disclosure, and ideally provides permission.

Violations of patient confidentiality may occur inadvertently. Casual conversations in hallways or elevators in which patient information is shared within earshot of strangers and unauthorized release of patient information to friends or family constitute a breach in confidentiality. The electronic health record (EHR) also introduces opportunities for violations of confidentiality, such as when a user does not log out of the system and patient information displayed on the computer screen can be viewed by anyone passing by. Social media created a new lens to evaluate a patient's privacy and confidentiality.

Veracity

The rule of veracity simply means that one should tell the truth and not lie or deceive others. Veracity is fundamental to relationships and society. The nurse-patient relationship is based on truthful communication and the expectation that each party will adhere to the rules of veracity. Deception, misrepresentation, or incomplete disclosure of information can undermine and erodes the patient's trust in healthcare providers.

Nearly every patient expects that information about their condition will be relayed in an open, honest, and sensitive manner. Without truthful communication, patients and/or their surrogates are unable to make fully informed decisions. However, the complex nature of acute illness does not always manifest as a single truth with clear boundaries. Uncertainty about the course of the illness, the appropriate treatment, or the plan of care is common in critical care and a single "truth" may not exist. In addition, some patients may have cultural beliefs around limiting information and the nurse should seek ethics guidance when such cases present. As emphasized in patient-centered care, patients or surrogate decision makers must be kept informed of the plan of care and areas of uncertainty should be openly acknowledged. Disclosure of uncertainty enables the patient or surrogate to realistically examine the proposed plan of care and stands as part of an informed consent process. Veracity asks nurses to not only be honest with what is known, but to identify the areas and be explicit about what remains unknown or unclear.

Informed Consent

The term "informed consent" is often interpreted as the task of ensuring that the appropriate form is completed and signed. From the standpoint of bioethics, informed consent is not a task but a process by which the healthcare team honors the autonomy of patients and their families. There are four elements that encompass informed consent: disclosure, comprehension, voluntariness, and competence.

Disclosure and Comprehension

The healthcare team is obligated to disclose information about specific treatments or treatment plans in a way the patient and family can understand. This can be challenging because healthcare treatments are complex, and their risks and benefits are not easily understood. Furthermore, patients and families who are facing serious illness may experience anxiety that impairs comprehension. Strategies such as rewording the same information, offering written information, and asking the patient or family member to restate information in their own words can improve comprehension. Without a confirmation that a patient desires limited information, deliberately omitting information about a treatment, minimizing its risks or benefits, or failing to address questions from a patient or family threatens the integrity of the informed consent process and represents dishonorable professional behavior.

Voluntariness

Decisions by the patient and family must be reached voluntarily. While any form of coercion, manipulation, or duress is not ethically supported, there are times when patients want to seek the guidance or even be influenced by their loved ones. In such cases, ethics assistance with an assessment of relational autonomy should be explored. The language used to describe treatment options is carefully chosen to avoid subtle forms of coercion that reflect personal views and do not constitute objective descriptions of the treatment involved. Consider a family member deciding about a do not resuscitate (DNR) order. If the provider describes cardiopulmonary resuscitation (CPR) as a potentially life-saving intervention without further details, the family member may feel compelled to refuse the DNR order. If instead, CPR is described as a painful intervention that prolongs the dying process and is not medically appropriate to offer, the family member's inclination will be very different. To the extent possible, balanced and objective descriptions of interventions are provided to ensure the element of voluntariness.

Principles of Management

Ideally, informed consent is comprised not only of documented conversations about specific treatments but also includes a series of interactions between the patient, family, and healthcare team to ensure a mutual understanding of the goals of care and strategies for achieving them. In this way, the healthcare team can disclose information at an appropriate pace, assessing the patient and family's comprehension and addressing questions as they arise.

Nursing interventions that uphold informed consent include:

- Providing and reinforcing information about disease, treatment options, risks, and benefits with patients and families.
- Honestly answering questions from patients and their families and consulting other members of the healthcare team for answers when needed.
- Using a teach back method in which decision makers are asked to restate in their own words the information they are given.

- Attending to environmental factors that impact disclosure and comprehension such as excess noise or inadequate seating. Seek private, quiet spaces for conversations about treatment options. When nurses and providers sit to talk to patients and families, they convey a willingness to listen and speak on an equal level.
- Taking time to consider and recognize personal views and opinions. If the family requests input in the form of "what would you do?" a nurse may want to first reframe the patient's values and that they are different than their own saying something like, "I would make that choice because of who I am. But this is about you (or about your loved one)" to redirect the discussion around the values of the patient and their family. If a response is still desired, it is permissible to share an honest answer as long as it is in the context of the nurse's own values.
- Choosing language carefully to increase comprehension and enhance voluntariness.
- Assuming that patients and families have capacity to make decisions and provide support for their decision-making skills.
- Increasing interaction between the healthcare team and the patient by using alternative methods of communication with intubated patients and asking for medical translators when needed.

Shared Decision Making

All decisions in health ought to be made through partnerships with the patients, their surrogates, and the healthcare team. Shared-decision making highlights the unique expertise each person brings. Clinicians are experts in identifying medically appropriate treatment options and patients, and/or their surrogates, are experts in their values and preferences of which of those options aligns with their values. The first part in making a shared decision outlines the obligation to understand who can make the decision at hand by assessing capacity.

Decision-Making Capacity

The final element of informed consent is capacity. Decision-making capacity is a healthcare assessment for decisions about the plan of care. Decision-making capacity reflects the ability of an individual to participate in the medical decision-making process based on four elements: (1) communicates a consistent choice, (2) understands the medical information, (3) appreciates the options and related benefits and consequences, and (4) engages in a process of reason. The assessment of capacity varies based on the amount of risk or harm possible and can be guided, in most (but not all states) by a profession's scope of practice. For example, a nurse can assess a patient's capacity to refuse to be turned in bed intermittently as it is a lower-risk refusal and nursing interventions fall within a nurses' scope of practice. Whereas a patient requesting to be removed from life-supportive treatments

may require multiple persons to assess their capacity because it is a high-stakes decision that requires a robust assessment. Capacity is not based on specific diagnoses or ailments or the ability to concur with healthcare providers or family members. It is a functional standard that focuses on the patient's ability as a decision maker. Some states outline specific guidelines about the assessment of decisional capacity, and many institutions have policies on determining capacity, and on the approach to patients who are unable to contribute to decision making.

Substitute Decision Making

When a patient lacks capacity due to illness or its treatment, a surrogate decision maker is usually assigned to provide informed consent. If the patient has assigned a friend or family member to the role of durable power of attorney for health care, that person is recognized as the surrogate decision maker. In the absence of documentation from the patient, state laws guide the designation of various legally related family members and, in some states, even close friends to the role of surrogate decision maker. If no surrogates are available, state guidelines may have a process to support decision making for unrepresented patients until a guardian can be appointed. The surrogate decision maker is not asked to make decisions based on their own values but rather to consider the values, goals, and preferences of the patient and how the patient would respond, if they could, to the information given by the healthcare team. Surrogates are often asked to use the Western framework to prioritize a patient's expressed wishes, a process called substituted judgment. If unable to arrive at a decision based on substituted judgment, surrogates may use the best interest standard.

The best interest standard can also be applied when patients who have never had capacity require care, such as infants and children who are unable to express their preferences at any time in their lives. The ethical analysis of the best interest standard includes considering the relief of suffering, restoration of function, and the acceptable quality of an extended life based on the patient's perspective when weighing options for treatment. Whenever a substitute decision maker is involved, it becomes important for clinicians to evaluate what it means to provide respectful care to humans in their presence.

Respect for Persons

When patients lack decisional capacity, clinicians move from the rule-based capacity assessment to a rule-based theory that focuses on patient autonomy, and voluntariness. Clinicians must provide respectful care to all patients whether they have decisional capacity or not. The Belmont report first established respect for persons and outlined that "individuals are [should be] treated as autonomous agents," and that "persons with diminished autonomy are entitled to protection."[1] It is because of respect for persons that patients are not restrained for chronic or routine care. Typically, bioethics only supports restraints to force treatments when specific situations are present:

1. Restraints are needed to maintain the physical safety of staff and the patient and discharge is not possible due to a patient's ongoing need for acute hospitalization.
2. An acute illness or injury that requires an emergent and immediate life-saving treatment or intervention when a patient's preferences are unknown.
   i. Example: a patient who needs emergent intubation without advance directives.
3. A limited time-trial to restore or improve a patient's decisional capacity.
   i. Example: an acutely psychotic patient on dialysis whose cognitive status may improve quickly.
4. A medically necessary procedure or limited treatment aligns with the patient's preferences according to the substituted decision maker and observed authentic statements. (For a Medical Intervention and the immediate post-intervention treatment only)
   i. Example: a substitute decision maker gives consent for a delirious patient for an emergent surgery, and later the still delirious patient refuses a post-operative intervention, like a wound check and dressing change, necessary to meet the patient's goals to discharge home.
5. A person who is an active danger to themselves or others. Many states carry specific laws about involuntary psychiatric treatment for patients with acute psychosis or active suicidality.

Respect for persons also asks clinicians to assess the patient's authentic statements. For patients who lack capacity, authentic statements can be assessed by reviewing a patient's statements and physical actions around a specific issue. When a person's communication and actions align and remain consistent and persistent over time, they can be identified as authentic. This principle highlights our desire to respect a person's bodily integrity and, whenever possible, to gain assent to provide treatments. Identifying authentic statements is highly nuanced assessment and ethics committees or ethics consult services can assist in this process. Once authentic statements are confirmed, clinicians should respect them.

End-of-Life Care

Providing end-of-life care is a common source of moral distress. When nurses participate in the use of life-sustaining

[1]https://www.hhs.gov/ohrp/regulations-and-policy/belmont-report/index.html

measures for patients whom they believe will derive little clinical benefit from it, they may feel that they are complicit in causing harm and unable to pursue what they believe is the right course of action. Conversely, patients and family members may decline treatment and generate similar distress among nurses who feel that such treatment would be of benefit to them. Ethical issues also arise when patients and families do not agree on the goals of care at end-of-life or when resources are not available to meet the needs of complex chronically ill patients as they approach end-of-life.

A wide range of circumstances contribute to the development of ethical issues during end-of-life care. This discussion reviews honoring patient preferences, decisions to forgo life-sustaining treatment, requests for potentially inappropriate care, decisions about resuscitation, and symptom management. Nursing management to promote ethical resolution is also described.

Honoring Patient Preferences

While nurses and the intraprofessional team seek to uphold the doctrine of informed consent in all situations involving patient decisions, discussions about end-of-life care have a unique complexity. Impending death is a source of duress for the patient, family, and healthcare team as they consider treatment options. When patients verbalize preferences about end-of-life care, they may identify specific circumstances such as who they want to be with and where they want to be, but they are not likely to speak of death itself as a desired outcome. Many times, preferences for end-of-life care are stated with the assumption that death will occur sometime in the distant future.

In addition, while some disease processes can be accurately predicted, many common chronic disorders such as heart failure, chronic obstructive pulmonary disease (COPD), and dementia impair quality of life but have an unpredictable impact on the duration of life. Healthcare teams may in fact provide end-of-life care, unwittingly, as they were not aware, until the patient's death, how near to dying the patient was. In such cases, even if the patient has established specific preferences regarding end-of-life care, the healthcare team may not recognize the appropriate point in time for initiating a treatment plan to meet those goals.

Advance Directives

In addition to conversations with the healthcare team, patients convey preferences regarding end-of-life care through written documents such as advanced directives. Advance directives are statements made by an individual with decision-making capacity that describe the care or treatment they wish to receive when no longer competent. Most states recognize two forms of advance directives, the treatment directive, or "living will," and documentation that identifies a surrogate decision maker. The treatment directive enables the individual to specify in advance his or her treatment choices and which interventions are desired. Usually treatment directives focus on CPR, mechanical ventilation, nutrition and hydration, and other life-sustaining technologies. In general, patients create treatment directives for one of three reasons, to direct the care they receive, to provide general guidance regarding their preferences, or to guide the decisions that families make on their behalf.

Documentation that identifies another decision maker if the patient cannot make their own decision is identified by different terms in different states. Some states use the term proxy directive, others refer to a durable power of attorney (DPOA) or a health care power of attorney (HCPA). The appointed individual is usually a relative or friend who assumes responsibility for healthcare decisions if the patient lacks the capacity to participate in the decision-making process. Treatment decisions by the appointed decision maker are based on an understanding of the patient's values and wishes regarding medical care. When a patient does not appoint a decision maker, most states have statutory provisions that recognize the legal authority of the healthcare substitute decision maker, and this individual is given authority to accept or refuse procedures or treatments on behalf of a patient based on their understanding of the patient's preferences.

Appointing a decision maker has some important advantages over a treatment directive. Many treatment directives are valid only under certain conditions. Terminal illness or an imminent death are common requirements before the treatment directive is enacted and prognostic uncertainty may render this condition difficult to meet. Such restrictions are not relevant in when documentation appoints a decision maker. The fact of the patient lacking decision-making capacity is sufficient to warrant the involvement of the assigned person. Furthermore, the process of authorizing a decision maker allows for consideration of the unique features of the specific situation before arriving at a decision. For example, a treatment directive may indicate refusal of mechanical ventilation, but the appointed decision maker speaking for the patient with a reversible acute respiratory process may consent to a trial of noninvasive ventilation when medically and ethically appropriate to offer. When the context of the medical ailment and the aim of directive are considered, it may highlight a clinical situation which the directive was intended to apply to. The appointed decision maker can make a more nuanced decision based on the benefits and burdens of proposed intervention and the knowledge and understanding of the patient's preferences and values. It is important to evaluate the laws in each state as some limit the authority of decision maker to alter a patient's written wishes, even when it is ethically appropriate to do so.

Decisions to Forego Life-Sustaining Treatments

Grounded in the principle of respect for patient autonomy, patients with capacity have the moral and legal right to forego life-sustaining treatments, including mechanical ventilation, medications, surgery, dialysis, nutrition, and hydration. The right of a capable patient to refuse treatment, even beneficial treatment, must be upheld if the elements of informed consent are met. Ongoing dialogue among the healthcare team, family, and patient is appropriate so that mutually satisfactory realistic goals are adopted. Patients must understand that refusal of treatment will not lead to inadequate care or abandonment by members of the healthcare team.

Conflicts regarding the discontinuation of life-sustaining treatments often reflect differences in values and beliefs. When patients or their surrogate decision makers choose to forego treatments that extend life, relinquishing the original goal of restoring health is sometimes difficult. Shifting to a paradigm that aligns treatments to a patient's values, which may advocate for a calm and peaceful death; this shift requires the nurse to change the treatment goals to promote comfort and support the grieving process.

Requests for Potentially Inappropriate Treatment

In some cases, surrogate decision makers request continued life-sustaining treatment which the healthcare team believes may not medically beneficial for the patient. In these cases, the clinical team needs to explore the supporting rationale (or lack of support) for the interventions in question. When clinicians are in consensus that a requested treatment is potentially inappropriate, an ethics consultation may help provide guidance on next steps. Justice, emotional, and social concerns can motivate individuals to request potentially inappropriate treatment. In such situations, nurses advocate for the medically appropriate treatment plan that best aligns with the patient's voice, based on their knowledge of the patient's prognosis, preferences, and the burdens and benefits that treatment options offer. Nurses should seek assistance from ethics when the plan of care is classified as not medically appropriate or does not reflect the patient's wishes, as this can be a source of moral distress.

A complicated array of factors including advances in healthcare technology, the aging of the population, and increased attention to burn-out syndrome in clinicians have intensified efforts to address the distress that members of the healthcare team experience when they participate in providing potentially inappropriate treatment. An official policy statement from five critical care professional organizations, including AACN, offers both system-level and clinician-level recommendations for mitigating and responding to requests for potentially inappropriate care. These include proactive, routine communication with the families of critically ill patients, early consultation with palliative care and/or ethics services, and institutional procedures for conflict resolution when disagreements in the plan of care persist. While this statement was created to address the issue of requests for inappropriate treatment in critical care settings, the recommendations are applicable to most acute care settings, including progressive care.

Informed Assent

In complex cases, it can be helpful for clinicians to provide recommendations. It can be very challenging to provide

TABLE 8-4. DEFINING CARE THAT IS NOT MEDICALLY APPROPRIATE

Defining Care That Is Not Medically Appropriate	
An intervention that meets one or more of the following: • It does not meet a patient's Goals of Care • It does not align clinically with the patient's treatment plan according to the standards of care • It is not clinically appropriate or indicated based on the illness, injury, or disease present	Critical Care Standards for determination of Not Medically Appropriate treatment include at least one of the following: • There is no reasonable expectation to restore a patient's cognitive function to allow the patient to perceive the benefit of treatment • There is no reasonable expectation that the patient will survive outside the acute care setting
Example: A patient with a new cancer who does not want any aggressive treatment and gives an informed refusal for resection and chemotherapy. Surgery and chemotherapy became not medically appropriate to continue to offer or recommend *based on the* patients goals of care.	Example: A patient who cannot be weaned from mechanical ventilation after maximum medical therapy and declines a tracheostomy will not survive outside of acute care setting. When treatment continues to be desired in cases like this, consider an ethics consultation.

Data from Bosslet GT, Pope TM, Rubenfeld GD, et al: An Official ATS/AACN/ACCP/ESICM/SCCM Policy Statement: Responding to Requests for Potentially Inappropriate Treatments in Intensive Care Units. Am J Respir Crit Care Med. 2015;191(11):1318-1330 and Kon AA, Shepard EK, Sederstrom NO, et al: Defining Futile and Potentially Inappropriate Interventions: A Policy Statement From the Society of Critical Care Medicine Ethics Committee. Crit Care Med. 2016;44(9):1769-1774.

recommendations to limit or to withdraw treatment. Clinicians should always elicit the patient's preferences and goals of care. When all clinicians agree a treatment is not medically appropriate to offer, then clinicians should give recommendations using an informed assent/nondissent format. Informed assent/nondissent means a clinician(s) provides medical recommendations in a statement form and the patient or surrogate assents (agrees) or nondissents (does not disagree) with the recommendations. Informed assent/nondissent does not require verbal agreement, it requires the patient or surrogate to understand the plan and does not disagree. The defining elements of treatment that is not medically appropriate are listed in Table 8-4.

Nurses use informed assent often without realizing it. When a patient covered in feces needs to be cleaned, a nurse usually arrives stating they are there to "freshen the patient up" they often do not ask questions and evaluate if the patient gives assent or communicates strong disagreement.

Resuscitation Decisions

Acute and critically ill patients are susceptible to sudden and unpredictable changes in cardiopulmonary status. The presumption exists that, unless stated otherwise, resuscitation efforts will be instituted immediately upon cardiopulmonary arrest. In-hospital resuscitation is moderately successful, and delay in efforts significantly reduces the chance of the patient's survival. The emergent nature, the questionable effectiveness, and the presumed consent for CPR contribute to the ethical dilemmas that surround this intervention.

Typically, "do not resuscitate" or "no code" are orders to withhold CPR only. Meaning, other medical or nursing interventions are not influenced by a DNR order. In other words, the decision to forego CPR is not a decision to forego any other interventions. Appropriate discussions with the patient or surrogate must occur before a resuscitation decision is made. Open communication and a shared understanding of the treatment plan are essential to understanding and responding to the patient's interests and preferences. When the issue of resuscitation status is not addressed with the patient or surrogate or the decision is not documented or communicated, then a code is initiated, risking the provision of unwanted care.

Most institutions have policies that address the process of writing and implementing a DNR order. In addition, many states have an approved process and forms to indicate a desire to forgo life support so that this wish can be conveyed across all healthcare settings. Examples of such forms include the Durable DNR form in Virginia and the Physician Order for Life-Sustaining Treatment or POLST form in California. These forms play an essential role in preventing the provision of undesired care as patients are never capable of verbally refusing in the moment when the need for resuscitation arises.

Symptom Management

When faced with a potentially life-limiting disease process, issues regarding symptom management also arise. Although palliation, the relief of troubling symptoms, is a priority in the care of all patients, once the decision to forego life-sustaining measures is made, palliation becomes the focus of care. In some circumstances, patients experience distressing symptoms despite the availability of pharmacologic agents to manage the uncomfortable effects of chronic and terminal illness. Whether due to a lack of knowledge, time, or a deliberate unwillingness to prescribe or administer the necessary medication, inadequate symptom management is not acceptable. In fact, a patient's right to pain relief carries state, national, and international support, and outside of rare exceptions, only the patient can decline interventions for pain relief. Nurses are obligated to ensure that patients receive care and treatments that are consistent with their choices. At the same time, provider colleagues are responsible for prescribing medications and ordering consults, such as for a palliative care service. A disagreement in which the nurse believes a particular order is justified and the provider does not agree can become an ethical problem, if effective communication between the two parties is absent.

Conflict can arise when patients require large doses of medications, such as narcotics, to effectively alleviate their symptoms. Legally and ethically, nurses must refrain from actions that hasten death and the side effect of respiratory depression may have an impact on the time of death. The essential element in this situation is the nurse's intent in providing the medication. When the intent is to relieve

ESSENTIAL CONTENT CASE

The Patient's Wishes

Medical Indications

A 20 year old with the deadname of Sue who is reported to self-identify as Scott, a transgender man, presented to the hospital intubated and sedated after a suicide attempt. (A deadname is a name, often the legal name assigned at birth, that a person asked to no longer be used.) The patient sustained multiple injuries from a jump from overpass including bilateral femur fractures, a left tibia fibula fracture, a left lung contusion, a right scapular laceration, and head lacerations. Shortly after the patient's first trip to the operating room, the patient developed a likely fat embolism syndrome with hypoxic respiratory failure, acute decrease in mental status, tachycardia, and fever with pulmonary embolism. After two weeks in the ICU, the patient is stable, with a tracheostomy and gastrostomy for tube feedings. When an ethics consultation was requested, the patient was comatose, ventilated, and unable to participate in an interview. When ethics arrive the bedside nurse reported the patient has begun to follow commands intermittently but remains unable to consistently answer yes/no questions.

The Patient Preferences

The patient is currently unable to confirm previously stated preferences; information was gathered second hand via family and friend's statements documented in chart notes. Clinicians and legal surrogates agree on all courses of clinical treatment and interventions. The patient's previously stated wishes about the gender the patient identifies with, and prefers, are in tension with the parents' concerns about the authenticity of their child's past statements.

The patient is reported to prefer the name of Scott and has recently started hormones as a transgender man. Multiple stakeholders have confirmed the patient prefers this chosen name. The patient's roommate confirmed the patient as Scott and only known as man. The patient's parent stated confirmed they learned about a year ago the patient told them they preferred the name Scott. About five months before the admission, the patient told his parents to use the name Scott and urged them to stop using his birth name. Since this time, the parents have been unable to use the name Scott and instead have used nicknames like "sport" instead. The parent told the bedside nurse they received a text message before the suicide attempt and also requested they no longer refer to him with the birth name.

Quality of Life

Currently, the patient is critically ill and the prognosis is unclear at this time. It is also unclear at this time what elements would be important to evaluate quality for the patient.

Case Narrative

There are many human rights movements inspiring education of clinicians and hospitals about the health disparities in the LGBTQAI+ community. This hospital was evaluated by the Healthcare Equality Index, a Human right movement, and recently became a leader in LBGTQ care. Clinicians in this case are acutely aware their patient is in a vulnerable state and want to be respectful to Scott and his parents, who are currently faced with the tragedy with their adult child's attempted suicide.

The patient's parent came from an authentic place and feels motivated to support an adult child. The parent is faced with both the tragic event of attempted suicide and the loss of identity of the child they have always known. The patient's parent calls the patient by their birth name and the bedside nurse reached out to ethics when the parent asked the nurse to use the patient's "legal name" and to stop calling the patient Scott.

The patient's parents identify as Christians who accept everyone regardless of who they are and choose to respectfully disagree with their choices. The patient's parents state they realize this may truly be their child's wish, and if they can talk in person, the parent voice that they are the ones who need to work on acceptance—not their child. They feel like during this critical time, they can't make this transition. The parents want clinicians to know they do not want to disrespect their child in any way and they are doing the best they can to cope during this difficult situation.

Case Question 1: Can a patient's parent make a decision about what name to call the patient?

Case Question 2: What options does the nurse have to find a path forward during the patient's recovery?

Answers
1. A patient's proxy or substitute decision maker makes healthcare decisions for their loved ones. While a patient's loved ones often give nurses a preferred name or nickname the patient responds to, this fall outside of a typical request. The parents request to use the birth name and birth pronouns, while the nurse knows this is not what the patient prefers and deadnaming is disrespectful. Since a patient's name is not a healthcare decision, it does not fall under the substituted decision-maker's authority. They cannot force clinicians to use the patient's birth name. The nurse's primary duty is to the patient first.
2. In this case, there is tension between the nurse's obligation to provide respect to their patient and to the patient's family. This is a very difficult situation and the nurse does have to provide care to both the patient and the family. Typically, this situation does not include a comatose patient who is unable to articulate their preferences. Most patients who have decisional capacity, examine care through "respect for autonomy"; whereas patients who lack decisional capacity, like Scott, embrace a broader focus of "respect for persons." Respect for persons in this case asks for clinicians to make their best effort to respect the human in front of them. This means respecting the patient's known wishes to called Scott and have male pronouns used. Respect for persons also asks clinicians to consider loved ones closest to the patient. To be respectful to both the patient and parents, clinicians can consider using gender-neutral terms around the patient's parents out of respect for them and while maintaining respect to the patient. Examples of this include stating, "our patient" or "your child" that allow conversations to occur during this critical recovery time. The nurse also, must align with the patient once the patient's communication is restored and seek to help the patient's parents find the resources and support they need to respect the patient.

pain and suffering, and not to deliberately hasten death, the action is morally justified. The concept that supports this reasoning is called the principle of double effect. This principle states that if an action has both a good and bad effect, a person is justified in taking that action if the intent was the good effect, the bad effect was a possible but not certain outcome of the action, and there was no additional course of action which could produce the good effect and avoid the bad one. The US Supreme Court cited the principle of double effect in a decision that distinguished palliative care from assisted suicide.

Principles of Management

The application of primary palliative care is one strategy that can help mitigate the moral distress and ethical conflicts that arise in end-of-life care. While hospice is a set of services that patients with a poor prognosis can enroll in if they meet specific criteria for insurance reimbursement, palliative care is an approach that applies to all seriously ill patients. Specialists in palliative care provide extra support to patients, families, and the healthcare team; however, in some cases, a palliative approach can be adopted by the team that is responsible for the patient's care without a specialist. Palliative care emphasizes symptom management, psychosocial support, and alignment of the patients' goals of care with the treatment plan. Skills in palliative care can be applied to patients even when the prognosis is uncertain, thus circumventing the issue of identifying an appropriate time for changing the goals of care. Below is a list of nursing interventions that can be used to implement a palliative care approach and may be helpful in preventing ethical issues in end-of-life care:

- Take advantage of the proximity that nurses have with the patient and family and seek to know the patient as a person
- Use open-ended questions and statements such as "tell me more" to clarify patient values and beliefs
- Share information about patients and families and goals of care with other members of the healthcare team
- Participate in family conferences to offer additional support to patients or their surrogate decision makers and to reinforce information about prognosis that is conveyed during the meeting
- Clarify personal preferences about the use of life-sustaining treatment and listen as other healthcare team members, patients, and families explain alternative preferences
- Use medications and nonpharmacologic strategies for a multimodal approach to symptom management (see Chapter 6, Pain Management/Sedation, for more on this)
- Be aware of patients' wishes regarding resuscitation efforts whether expressed verbally, through a surrogate decision maker, or in an advanced directive,

or other state-specific documentation such as an MOLST form (Medical Order for Life-Sustaining Treatment)
- Seek professional development opportunities for end-of-life management and palliative care

Evolving Technology

Technology not only affects the care that patients receive, but it also has implications for how that care is documented, and how healthcare team members communicate with each other and with patients. Because of the rapid pace of innovation, professional codes, state and federal laws, and institutional policies may not yet address all the issues that advance in technology introduce. While technology can improve the delivery of health care, the application of ethical analysis to address concerns about its use is warranted.

Advances in Healthcare Technology

All approaches to ethics seek to answer the questions "What should we then do?" and this is a particularly pertinent question when applied to healthcare technology that extends life without ensuring quality of life. Examples of past advances include hemodialysis and left ventricular assist devices (LVADs), both of which were conceived as interventions to maintain life until definitive treatment in the form of a kidney or heart transplant took place. The use of these technologies in patients as an ongoing treatment rather than a bridge to transplant means that patients experience an additional burden of treatment to derive the benefit of a longer lifespan. For many patients, this is tolerable, but if the patient's existence with such interventions does not meet their individual definition of quality of life, they have a right to refuse such therapy or to discontinue it after it has begun. Honoring the doctrine of informed consent, the healthcare team must ensure that the patient and family understand both the risks and benefits of technology-driven care and their impact on the disease and on the patient.

In critical care settings, patients with a complex mix of health problems often require an extensive array of healthcare technology. For instance, an older patient with coronary artery disease and chronic lung disease who develops sepsis may require invasive monitoring, mechanical ventilation, consults with specialists, and a long period of rehabilitation when the acute phase resolves. Restoration to the prior functional status may not be feasible if the patient's age and underlying health conditions have compromised his resiliency. Moral uncertainty may surface in the healthcare team around the justice of using resources in this way, particularly given the unequal distribution of healthcare resources in our society.

There is additional uncertainty around some forms of technology, such as continuous renal replacement therapy (CRRT) and extracorporeal membrane oxygenation

(ECMO) because the evidence to support their use remains mixed. The application of these interventions is appropriate if they meet the mutual goals of the patient, the family, and the healthcare team, but careful consideration and extensive discussion are warranted, particularly when the patient's prognosis is poor.

Electronic Health Record

In 2011, the Medicare and Medicaid Electronic Health Record Incentive Program, established by the Centers for Medicare & Medicaid Services, began offering incentives for hospitals and providers who demonstrated meaningful use of EHRs. These incentives lead to the rapid implementation of electronic documentation in most healthcare settings. The use of EHRs can improve quality of care for patients by providing some strategies to prevent errors and facilitate communication across healthcare settings. However, because incentives drove this implementation, many EHR systems were designed to meet federal requirements for meaningful use and not necessarily designed around healthcare workflow.

While EHR appropriately facilitates sharing patient information among the healthcare team, storing patient information electronically also creates risks. Individuals with access to the EHR who view information about patients they are not caring for are violating patient privacy. Whole groups of patients are affected when systems that house EHRs are hacked. An additional concern is the "copy forward" strategy for documentation that offers a short cut for entering patient information and introduces the risk that the note does not reflect the patient's current status but is information carried over from previous patient interactions. To address this problem, some institutions have eliminated the copy forward function completely. The EHR is thus an example of healthcare technology with the potential to improve the delivery of care and at the same time, introduce new ethical issues that require thoughtful and deliberate action.

Social Media

Another example of technology advancing before guidelines for its use are established is social media, which includes Internet-based social networks, blogs, wikis, and podcasts. These forms of communication can be beneficial in allowing healthcare professionals to share ideas or patients and families to garner support from those who are geographically distant. However, the use of social media also introduces ethical concerns for nurses and other members of the healthcare team. The ease of transmitting information to a large audience with a single post means that inappropriate communication about a patient or colleague has a much broader impact. Violations range from intentional bullying of colleagues to unintended disclosure of patient information when seeking emotional support after a challenging shift. The ability to

create photos or videos with a smart phone also introduces a risk for violating patient privacy.

Patient and family use of social media can generate problems for the healthcare team. Reliance on blogs or wikis for health information can be a barrier to effective patient education. Patients and families may also seek to contact members of the healthcare team through social networks. Online relationships of this kind can erode the boundaries between the nurse's personal and professional lives. Patients and families may use social media to learn private information about a nurse or they may expect the nurse to provide support that exceeds the parameters of the nurse's professional role.

Principles of Management

This discussion provides an overview of some of the ways in which technology impacts ethical issues in health care. Further innovations are likely to advance healthcare delivery but will also require careful consideration to determine the full range of impact on patients and the healthcare team. Some strategies for nurses that facilitate resolution of the ethical issues generated by evolving technology include:

- Use peer-reviewed journals and clinical practice guidelines to develop and maintain an accurate understanding of the indications for the technology you use
- Be honest with patients and families when they ask about the effectiveness of healthcare technology
- When uncertain about the use of a particular intervention or procedure, ask providers to clarify the rationale and expected outcome of the treatment
- Refer to hospital policies on the use of EHRs and avoid inappropriately accessing patient information
- Be deliberate in turning away from the computer to make eye contact with patients and families, observe their nonverbal communication, and demonstrate your interest in their needs
- Review the American Nurses' Association Social Networking Principles Toolkit which includes a poster of six key tips for guidance on the appropriate use of social media
- Avoid sharing information about specific patient situations in any electronic format other than the EHR

Patient Advocacy

Patient advocacy is an essential role of the nurse, as emphasized in provision 3 of the *Code of Ethics for Nurses*. Although there are many models for defining and interpreting the relationship between the nurse and the patient and no model can thoroughly describe its complexity and uniqueness, the patient advocacy role offers an essential description of the moral nature of this relationship.

The term advocacy refers to the use of one's own skills and knowledge to promote the interests of another. Nurses, through their education and experience, can interpret healthcare information and understand the impact of disease and medical interventions in a unique way. A nurse acts as a patient advocate by applying this unique understanding to ensure that the patient's beliefs and values guide the plan of care. The nurse does not impose personal values or preferences when acting as an advocate, but instead guides the patient or surrogate decision maker through values clarification, identification of the patient's best interests, and the process of communicating decisions. Thus, the patient or surrogate is empowered by the nurse to participate in the healthcare plan.

Assuming the role of patient advocate is not without risk. Nurses may find that obligations to oneself, the patient, the patient's family, other members of the healthcare team, or the institution are in conflict and have competing claims on nursing resources. The COVID-19 pandemic highlighted one such challenge in that nurses faced the obligation to protect themselves and their families from infection while also having an obligation to care for patients. These situations are intensely troubling to nurses and the support of colleagues is essential to resolving these dilemmas. In circumstances of conflict, nurses can clarify the nature and significance of the moral problem, engage in a systematic process of moral decision making, communicate concerns openly, and seek mutually acceptable resolutions. A framework within which to identify and compare options provides the necessary structure to begin the process of ethical resolution.

THE PROCESS OF ETHICAL ANALYSIS

When faced with ethical issues, nurses are more likely to achieve facilitation and mitigation of a dilemma when a consistent process is applied. A structured approach to ethical dilemmas reduces the risk of overlooking relevant contextual features and invites thoughtful reflection. While the individual nurse can hone and practice the skill of ethical analysis, a more robust process involves including others. Through a casual conversation with a colleague or a formal consult with an institution's ethics committee, nurses can engage others in discussing ethical issues and working toward a resolution. Whenever the situation falls outside of the comfort of the nurse, they should seek guidance from their institutional ethics resource. While there are a variety of ethical decision-making processes, there are three simple questions each nurse can ask to explore ethical elements in the situations they face:

1. What does the nurse think should be done and why?
2. What reasonable views can others hold about the situation that are different from the nurse's position?
3. Can the nurse find a third option that respects both/all sides?

For example, take the case of an actively dying patient on invasive treatments with a surrogate that wants "everything" to be done.

1. The nurse thinks the patient's dying process should be respected and all treatments prolonging the patient's death should be stopped. All interventions should focus on the patient's comfort.
2. The patient's surrogate wants "everything" to be done to allow a final visit from the patient's sibling who arrives in 24 hours. When the nurse learns this, by asking, "can you tell me more? What does *everything* mean to you?" The nurse finds this request to continue treatments for a short time reasonable.
3. After a care conference, while clinicians will continue current treatment, the patient's treatments will not be escalated and CPR will not be performed, pain medications will be given to ensure comfort until the patient's sibling arrives or the patient's body fails. After the sibling arrives, they plan to transition to focus solely on the patient's comfort and end treatments prolonging the dying process. This option respects both parties and was not an option available before.

The process of including recognition of reasonable disagreement can improve communication and ultimately facilitate the ethical issues to find a shared path forward. Nurses should also consider reaching out to their ethics committee or service for complex questions or ones they are unable to resolve.

ESSENTIAL CONTENT CASE

Applying the Process

The patient, an 82 year old with hypertension, atrial fibrillation, multi-infarct dementia, and chronic kidney disease presents with a large intracranial bleed, on warfarin. Her prognosis is very poor. The patient's son who is her primary caregiver is distraught and wants to stay at her bedside at all times. The unit has an open visitation policy and requires that all visitors wear a mask. The son initially complies with this policy but his mother's nurse, Maria, finds that he frequently removes the mask and must be reminded to replace it. After one such encounter, the son becomes angry, and verbally abusive. When Maria attempts to explain how the mask policy protects patients like his mother, he throws the hairbrush he had been using with the patient toward her and storms out, punching the wall as he goes.

Sharon, the nurse on the next shift witnesses this behavior and becomes fearful of the patient's son. She recognizes her obligation to provide the best care possible to her patient and that best practice usually includes supporting family involvement. At the same, she notes she has an obligation to herself, her team, and the other patients on the unit to maintain a safe and calm environment. She begins a deliberate analysis of the situation applying the nursing process:

Case Question 1: What information does Sharon need to gather?

Case Question 2: What kind of ethical problem is this?
(A) Moral distress
(B) Ethical dilemma
(C) Ethical Uncertainty
(D) Locus of authority

Case Question 3: What options for action should Sharon consider?

Case Question 4: How can Sharon examine this problem using ethics?

Case Question 5: What steps are involved in implementing a chosen action?

Case Question 6: After taking action, what criteria will Sharon use to evaluate the outcome?

Answers

1. All persons deserve to be safe. Safety includes physical, psychological, and emotional safety. Important sources of guidance for Sharon include her unit's policy on visitation, and the institution's policy on managing violent family members. Many organizations have de-escalation protocols or teams that can support nurses caring for potentially violent patients or families. Sharon can also seek input from her manager, particularly if there is no written policy that applies to this situation. Sharon can seek input from Maria about the son's behavior prior to this outburst and any assessment she has conducted regarding the son's understanding of the patient's prognosis. While the report she receives from Maria will also include clinical details, these may be less pertinent to the ethical analysis. Essentially, the patient has a very poor prognosis, which is a key relevant fact. Ideally, Sharon can also gather information by asking the son questions if he is calm and able to converse without presenting a threat.

2. Answer is option B. This problem, as Sharon frames it, is an ethical dilemma. She sees two opposing but equally justifiable options. The principle of beneficence and her obligation to provide the best possible care support allowing the son to visit the patient. However, she also has a duty to herself and to the other patients on the unit to prevent potential harm and this means asking the son not to visit to prevent violent outbursts. Sharon cannot both allow and not allow the son at the bedside.

3. Sharon recognizes that she must consider actions beyond the two that are in conflict. The following are some of the options she considers:

   - Tell the son that he cannot visit the patient under any circumstances.
   - Allow the son to visit, ignore his outbursts and his nonadherence to the mask policy.
   - Tell the charge nurse that she is uncomfortable with this assignment and cannot care for this patient.
   - Talk to the manager about having hospital security on the unit in case the son becomes violent. Restrict the son to visiting only during hours when security is available.
   - Allow the son to visit whenever he can but assess him at every point of contact for the risk of violent behavior.
   - Contact the social worker for help creating a Safety Agreement with the son that indicates explicit expectations for all people, the son, and the staff, including complying with the mask policy and a commitment to maintain safety by avoiding disrespectful and violent actions. The inability to maintain safety will result in the end of visitation and may limit future visits.
   - Call a member of the pastoral care team to talk to the son about his feelings and appropriate outlets.
   - Schedule a conference with members of the healthcare team and the son. Allow the son to verbalize his feelings.
   - Offer emotional support and also explain how his behavior with Maria is inappropriate and cannot be repeated.
   - Call a member of hospital administration to come to the unit and speak with the patient's son.

4. The next stage of the planning process is to examine the options through a selected framework. If Sharon adopts a principle-based approach and considers her primary duty to the patient, she may eliminate the options of telling the son that he cannot visit under any circumstances or refusing to take the assignment. These options fail to meet the best interests of the patient. At the same time, simply ignoring the son's outbursts places her own safety at risk which ultimately does not benefit the patient either. A principle-based approach may support the option of seeking a security presence on the unit or contracting with the son as these options uphold Sharon's duty to the patient and her duty to protect herself.

   A care-based perspective would examine these options based on their impact on the relationships in the situation. The relationship between the patient and the son is of course important, though the patient is currently unable to actively engage in that relationship because of her intracranial bleed. The relationship between the son and the healthcare team is newly formed and at high risk due to the fear engendered by the son's outburst. Sharon believes that bringing the team together with the son is probably the best action to take to establish a better relationship. In discussing the situation with members of the healthcare team, she suggests that a family conference include an assurance that the team wants what is best for his mother, and a clear description of expectations with regard to his behavior.

5. When applying a process for ethical analysis, taking the chosen action is an essential step. A key aspect of many of the options identified by Sharon is that they involve other members of the healthcare team. Resolution of ethical problems is rarely through independent action and often involves collaboration with colleagues, patient's families, or members of the hospital

administration. If Sharon is unable to take the chosen course of action due to resistance from her colleagues or other barriers, she is at risk for moral distress.

6. Once action is taken, Sharon will evaluate the effect on all involved parties. Her goal in conducting the analysis and taking action was to provide the son with appropriate access to the patient while also ensuring her own safety and the safety of her colleagues. If her evaluation shows that there are still gaps, for instance, if she or other members of the healthcare team continue to feel afraid of the son's violent behavior, additional action is needed.

SELECTED BIBLIOGRAPHY

Rushton CH; Schoonover-Shoffner K, Kennedy, MS. A Collaborative State of the Science Initiative: Transforming Moral Distress into Moral Resilience in Nursing. Am J Nurs 117(2):p S2-S6, February 2017. | DOI: 10.1097/01.NAJ.0000512203.08844.1d

American Medical Association, Decisions for Adult Patients Who Lack Capacity, Code of Medical Ethics Opinion 2.1.2. https://code-medical-ethics.ama-assn.org/ethics-opinions/decisions-adult-patients-who-lack-capacity

American Nurses Foundation. *Mental Health & Wellness Survey 3*. 2021. https://www.nursingworld.org/practice-policy/work-environment/health-safety/disaster-preparedness/coronavirus/what-you-need-to-know/pulse on the nations-nurses-covid-19-survey-series-mental-health-and-wellness-survey-3-september-2021/

American Nurses Foundation. *COVID-19 Impact Assessment Survey—The Second Year*. 2022. https://www.nursingworld.org/practice-policy/work-environment/health-safety/disaster-preparedness/coronavirus/what-you-need-to-know/covid-19-impact-assessment-survey---the-second-year/

Anderson WG, Puntillo K, Cimino J, et al. Palliative care professional development for critical care nurses: a multicenter program. *Am J Crit Care*. 2017;26:361-371.

Appelbaum PS. Assessment of patients' competence to consent to treatment. *N Engl J Med*. 2007;357:1834-1840.

Beauchamp TL, Childress JF. *Principles of Biomedical Ethics*. 8th ed. Oxford, England: Oxford University Press; 2019.

Bosslet GT, Pope TM, Rubenfeld GD, et al. An Official ATS/AACN/ACCP/ESICM/SCCM policy statement: responding to requests for potentially inappropriate treatments in intensive care units. *Am J Respir Crit Care Med*. 2015;191(11):1318-1330.

Brunnquall D, Michaelson CM. Moral hazard in pediatrics. *Am J Bioeth*. 2016;16(7):29-38.

Butler CR, Webster LB, Diekema DS, et al. Perspectives of triage team members participating in statewide triage simulations for scarce resource allocation during the COVID-19 pandemic in Washington State. *JAMA Netw Open*. 2022;5(4):e227639. doi: 10.1001/jamanetworkopen.2022.7639

Charland LC. *The Stanford Encyclopedia of Philosophy Decision Making Capacity 2008*; Fall 2014 Edition: http://plato.stanford.edu/archives/fall2014/entries/decision-capacity/. Accessed March 5, 2015.

Crutchfield P, Gibb TS, Redinger MJ, Ferman D, Livingstone J. The conditions for ethical application of restraints. *Chest*. 2019 Mar;155(3):617-625. doi: 10.1016/j.chest.2018.12.005. Epub 2018 Dec 19. PMID: 30578755.

Curtis JR, Burt RA. Point: the ethics of unilateral "do not resuscitate" orders: the role of "informed assent." *Chest*. 2007;132:748-751; discussion 755-746.

Curtis JR, Kross EK, Stapleton RD. The importance of addressing advance care planning and decisions about do-not-resuscitate orders during Novel Coronavirus 2019 (COVID-19). *JAMA*. Published online March 27, 2020. doi: 10.1001/jama.2020.4894

DHHS Privacy Rule. http://www.hhs.gov/ocr/privacy/. Accessed August 23, 2022.

DiGangi Condon KA, Berger JT, Shurpin KM. I've got the power: nurses' moral distress and perceptions of empowerment. *Am J Crit Care*. 2021;30(6):461-465. doi: 10.4037/ajcc2021112

Doherty RF, Purtilo RB. *Ethical Dimensions in the Health Professions*. 6th ed. St. Louis, MO: Elsevier Saunders; 2016.

Epstein EG, Delgado S. Understanding and addressing moral distress. *Online J Issues Nurs*. 2010;15(3), Manuscript 1. http://www.nursingworld.org/mainmenucategories/ethicsstandards/courage-and-distress/understanding-moral-distress.html

Epstein EG, Haizlip J, Liaschenko J, Zhao D, Bennett R, Marshall MF. Moral distress, mattering, and secondary traumatic stress in provider burnout: a call for moral community. *AACN Adv Crit Care*. 2020;31(2):146-157. doi: 10.4037/aacnacc2020285

Epstein B, Hamric A. Moral hazard and moral distress: a marriage made in purgatory. *Am J Bioeth*. 2016;16(7):46-48.

Gilligan C. Moral orientation and moral development. In: Kittay EF, Meyers DT, eds. *Women and Moral Theory*. New York: Rowman & Littlefield Publishers, Inc; 1987:19-33.

Hamric AB, Wocial LD, Epstein EG. *Transforming Moral Distress into Moral Agency. Panel Presentation*. Minneapolis, MN: ASBH Annual Conference; 2011.

Hiler C, Hickman R, Reimer A, Wilson K. Predictors of moral distress in a US sample of critical care nurses. *Am J Crit Care*. 2018;27(1):59-66.

Institute of Medicine. *Crisis Standards of Care: A Systems Framework for Catastrophic Disaster Response: Volume 1: Introduction and CSC Framework*. Washington, DC: The National Academies Press, 2012, 1-73 to 1-75. doi: 10.17226/13351

Jecker N. *Ending Midlife Bias: New Values for Old Ages*. New York: Oxford University Press; 2020.

Jones-Bonofiglio K, Nortjé N, Webster L, Garros D. A practical approach to hospital visitation during a pandemic: responding with compassion to unjustified restrictions. *Am J Crit Care*. 2021; 30(4):302-311. doi: 10.4037/ajcc2021611

Kon AA, Davidson JE, Morrison W, et al. Shared decision making in ICUs: an American College of Critical Care Medicine and American Thoracic Society Policy Statement. *Crit Care Med*. 2016;44:188-201.

Kon AA. Informed non-dissent: a better option than slow codes when families cannot bear to say "let her die." *Am J Bioeth*. 2011;11(11):22-23.

Kon AA, Shepard EK, Sederstrom NO, et al. Defining futile and potentially inappropriate interventions: a policy statement from the Society of Critical Care Medicine Ethics Committee. *Crit Care Med*. 2016;44(9):1769-1774. doi: 10.1097/CCM.0000000000001965

Lachman V. Social media: managing the ethical issues. *Medsurg Nurs*. 2013;22(5):326-329. http://www.nursingworld.org/MainMenuCategories/EthicsStandards/Resources/Social-Media-Ethical-Issues.pdf

Lohman D, Schleifer R, Amon JJ. Access to pain treatment as a human right. *BMC Med.* 2010;20:8.

Marshall MF, Epstein EG. Moral hazard and moral distress: a marriage made in purgatory. *Am J Bioeth.* 2016 Jul;16(7):46-48. doi: 10.1080/15265161.2016.1181895. PMID: 27292850.

McBride S, Tietze M, Robichaux C, Stokes L, Weber E. Identifying and addressing ethical issues with use of electronic health records. *Online J Issues Nurs.* 2018;23(1), Manuscript 5. doi: 10.3912/OJIN.Vol23No01Man05.

Morley G, Field R, Horsburgh CC, Burchill C. Interventions to mitigate moral distress: a systematic review of the literature. *Int J Nurs Stud.* 2021;121:103984. doi: 10.1016/j.ijnurstu.2021.103984

Robichaux C, ed. *Ethical Competence in Nursing Practice.* New York: Springer Publishing Company; 2016.

Rushton CH. Moral resilience: a capacity for navigating moral distress in critical care. *Adv Crit Care.* 2016;27(1):111-119.

Searight HR, Gafford J. Cultural diversity at the end of life: issues and guidelines for family physicians. *Am Fam Physician.* 2005 Feb 1;71(3):515-22. PMID: 15712625.

Shannon, S.E. (2016), The Nurse as the Patient's Advocate: *A Contrarian View.* Hastings Center Report, 46: S43-S47. doi: 10.1002/hast.632

Ulrich B, Lavandero R, Woods D, Early S. Critical care nurse work environments 2013: a status report. *Crit Care Nurse.* 2014;34(4):64-79.

Ulrich B, Barden C, Cassidy L, Varn-Davis N. Critical care nurse work environments 2018: findings and implications. *Crit Care Nurse.* 2019;39(2):67-84. doi: 10.4037/ccn2019605

Ulrich B, Cassidy L, Barden C, Varn-Davis N, Delgado SA. National nurse work environments—October 2021: a status report. *Crit Care Nurse.* 2022;42(5):58-70. doi:10.4037/ccn2022798

Ulrich C, Grady C, eds. *Moral Distress in the Health Professions.* New York: Springer International Publishing; 2017. https://link.springer.com/book/10.1007%2F978-3-319-64626-8.

United States. The Belmont report: Ethical principles and guidelines for the protection of human subjects of research. Bethesda, MD: The Commission; 1979.

Vaughn L. *Bioethics: Principles, Issues, and Cases.* New York, NY: Oxford University Press; 2010.

Wenar, Leif, "Rights," *The Stanford Encyclopedia of Philosophy* (Fall 2015 Edition), Edward N. Zalta (ed.). https://plato.stanford.edu/archives/fall2015/entries/rights. Accessed January 6, 2018.

Wocial LD, Hancock M, Bledsoe PD, Chamness AR, Helft PR. An evaluation of unit-based ethics conversations. *JONA's Healthc Law Ethics Regul.* 2010;12(2):48-54.

Professional Codes, Standards, and Position Statements

American Association of Critical-Care Nurses. *AACN Standards for Establishing and Sustaining Healthy Work Environments.* 2nd ed. 2016. https://www.aacn.org//media/aacn-website/nursing-excellence/standards/hwestandards.pdf

American Association of Critical-Care Nurses. *AACN Scope and Standards for Progressive and Critical Care Nursing Practice* (under Standard 5: Ethics). https://www.aacn.org/~/media/aacn-website/nursing-excellence/standards/aacn-scope-and-standards-for-progressive-and-critical-care-nursing-practice.pdf

American Association of Critical-Care Nurses. *Position Statement on Ethical Triage and End of Life Care.* https://www.aacn.org/policy-and-advocacy/~/link.aspx?_id=AA57E2D53B4B4CF3B0D351A02CD97AB5&_z=z

American Association of Critical-Care Nurses. *Position Statement on Moral Distress in Times of Crisis.* https://www.aacn.org/policy-and-advocacy/~/link.aspx?_id=0383CD301F394CBE80C3A3DC5D3BD0E1&_z=z

American Nurses Association. *Code of Ethics for Nurses.* 2015. http://www.nursingworld.org/MainMenuCategories/EthicsStandards/CodeofEthicsforNurses

Evidence-Based Guidelines

Bosslet GT, Pope TM, Rubenfeld GD, et al. An official ATS/AACN/ACCP/ESICM/SCCM policy statement: responding to requests for potentially inappropriate treatments in intensive care units. *Am J Respir Crit Care Med.* 2015;191(11):1318-1330. https://www.atsjournals.org/doi/abs/10.1164/rccm.201505-0924ST

Davidson J, Aslakson RA, Long AC, et al. Guidelines for family-centered care in the neonatal, pediatric and adult ICU. *Crit Care Med.* 2017;45(1):103-128. https://journals.lww.com/ccmjournal/Fulltext/2017/01000/Guidelines_for_Family_Centered_Care_in_the.12.aspx

National Consensus Project for Quality Palliative Care. *Clinical Practice Guidelines for Quality Palliative Care,* 4th ed. Richmond, VA: National Coalition for Hospice and Palliative Care; 2018. https://www.nationalcoalitionhpc.org/ncp

World Health Organization. *National Cancer Control Programmes: Policies and Management Guidelines.* 2nd ed. WHO, Geneva, Switzerland; 2002.

Online References of Interest: Related to Legal and Ethical Considerations

American Association of Critical Care Nurses. *Recognizing & Addressing Moral Distress;* 2020. https://www.aacn.org/~/media/aacn-website/clincial-resources/moral-distress/recognizing-addressing-moral-distress-quick-reference-guide.pdf

American Association of Critical Care Nurses Clinical Resources on Moral Distress: https://www.aacn.org/clinical-resources/moral-distress

American Nurses Association Ethics Resources. http://www.nursingworld.org/ethics/. Accessed August 23, 2022.

The Hastings Center. http://www.thehastingscenter.org/. Accessed August 23, 2022.

U.S. National Library of Medicine, Bioethics Information Resources. https://www.nlm.nih.gov/bsd/bioethics.html. Accessed August 23, 2022.

PATHOLOGIC CONDITIONS

II

CARDIOVASCULAR SYSTEM

9

Barbara Leeper

KNOWLEDGE COMPETENCIES

1. Identify indications for, complications of, and nursing management of patients undergoing coronary angiography and percutaneous coronary interventions.

2. Describe the etiology, pathophysiology, clinical presentation, patient needs, and principles of

management of patients with ischemic heart disease.

3. Discuss the etiology, pathophysiology, clinical presentation, patient needs, and principles of management of patients in shock, heart failure, and hypertensive crisis.

SPECIAL ASSESSMENT TECHNIQUES, DIAGNOSTIC TESTS, AND MONITORING SYSTEMS

Assessment of Chest Pain

Obtaining an accurate assessment of chest pain is an important aspect of differentiating cardiac chest pain from other sources of pain (eg, musculoskeletal, respiratory, anxiety). Ischemic chest pain, caused by lack of oxygen to the myocardium, must be quickly identified for therapeutic interventions to be effective. The most important descriptors of ischemic pain include precursors of pain onset, quality of the pain, pain radiation, severity of the pain, what relieves the pain, and timing of onset of the current episode of pain that brought the patient to the hospital. Each of these descriptors can be assessed using the "PQRST" nomogram (Table 9-1). This nomogram prompts the clinician to ask a series of questions to help identify the characteristics of the chest pain.

Coronary Angiography

Coronary angiography is a common and effective method for visualizing the anatomy and patency of the coronary arteries. This procedure, also known as cardiac catheterization, is used to diagnose atherosclerotic lesions or thrombus in the coronary vessels. Cardiac catheterization is also used for evaluation of valvular heart disease (including stenosis or insufficiency), atrial or ventricular septal defects, congenital anomalies, and myocardial wall motion abnormalities (Table 9-2).

Procedure

Prior to cardiac catheterization, the patient is kept NPO for at least 6 hours, to minimize the risk of aspiration in the event that emergency intubation is required during the procedure. NPO may indicate everything except medications, which are taken with small sips of water on the day of the procedure. Typically, if the patient is on insulin or taking oral hypoglycemics, the doses may need to be adjusted the day of the procedure. Benadryl may be administered prior to beginning the procedure as a precautionary measure against allergic reaction to the dye. Aspirin, clopidogrel, or other platelet inhibitor agents may be administered to prevent catheter-induced platelet aggregation during the procedure. Typically, patients remain awake during the procedure, allowing them to facilitate the catheterization process by controlling respiratory patterns (eg, breath holding during injection of radiopaque dye to improve the quality of the image). An anxiolytic agent, such as lorazepam or diazepam, is frequently administered during the procedure to decrease anxiety or restlessness.

TABLE 9-1. CHEST PAIN ASSESSMENT

	Ask the Question	Examples
P (Provoke)	What *provokes* the pain or what precipitates the pain?	Climbing the stairs, walking; or may be unpredictable—comes on at rest
Q (Quality)	What is the *quality* of the pain?	Pressure, tightness; may have associated symptoms such as nausea, vomiting, diaphoresis
R (Radiation)	Does the pain *radiate* to locations other than the chest?	Jaw, neck, scapular area, or left or right arm
S (Severity)	What is the *severity* of the pain (on a scale of 1-10)?	On a scale of 1-10, with 10 being the worst, how bad is your pain?
T (Timing)	What is the *time of onset* of this episode of pain that caused you to come to the hospital?	When did this episode of pain that brought you to the hospital start? Did this episode wax and wane or was it constant? For how many days, months, or years have you had similar pain?

An intracoronary catheter is inserted through a "sheath" or vascular introducer placed in a large artery, most commonly the femoral artery or the radial artery (Figure 9-1). If inserted via the femoral artery, the catheter is advanced into the ascending abdominal aorta, across the aortic arch, and into the coronary artery orifice located at the base of the aorta. If inserted through the radial artery, the catheter is then advanced into the brachial artery, through the subclavian artery, across the aorta, and into the coronary artery orifice located at the base of the aorta. There are pros and cons to transfemoral approach and the radial approach. The femoral approach has a higher risk of bleeding, longer hospital stay, chance of pseudoaneurysm, and clot formation. Also the femoral artery is the sole source of blood to the leg. With the radial approach,

TABLE 9-2. INDICATIONS FOR CARDIAC CATHETERIZATION

Right Heart
- Measurement of right-sided heart pressures:
  - Suspected cardiac tamponade
  - Suspected pulmonary hypertension
- Evaluation of valvular disease (tricuspid or pulmonic)
- Evaluation of atrial or ventricular septal defects
- Measurement of AVO_2 difference

Left Heart
- Diagnosis of obstructive coronary artery disease
- Identification of lesion location prior to CABG surgery
- Measurement of left-sided heart pressures: Suspected left heart failure or cardiomyopathy
- Evaluate for wall motion abnormalities
- Evaluation of valvular disease (mitral or aortic)
- Evaluation of atrial or ventricular septal defects

there are less trained providers, smaller arterial diameter, a longer procedure time, and risk of fistula, and severe vasospasm. With either approach, during the procedure, ionic dye, visible to the observer or operator under fluoroscopy (x-ray), is then injected into the coronary arterial tree via the catheter. If the cardiac valves, septa, or ventricular wall motion is being evaluated, the catheter is advanced directly into the left ventricle, followed by injection of dye. During a right heart catheterization, the catheter is inserted through the femoral vein, threaded up to the inferior vena cava, passed through the right ventricle, and advanced into the pulmonary artery.

Interpretation of Results

The coronary vascular tree consists of a left and a right system (Figure 9-2). The left system consists of two main branches, the left anterior descending (LAD) artery and the left circumflex (LCx) artery. The right system has one main branch, the right coronary artery (RCA). Both systems have a number of smaller vessels that branch off these three primary arterial vessels. An obstruction of 75% or more in a coronary artery or one of its major branches is considered clinically significant stenosis. If there is significant disease in only one of the major arteries, the patient is said to have single-vessel disease. If two major vessels are affected, the patient has two-vessel disease. If significant disease exists in all three major coronary arteries, the patient has three-vessel disease. Frequently, the microvasculature, or smaller vessels branching off the major coronary artery, may also have blockages. It is common to refer to these multiple lesions as diffuse disease.

A cineventriculogram is obtained by radiographic imaging during the injection of dye after advancing the

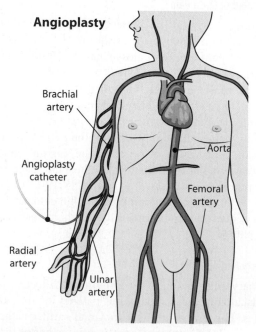

Figure 9-1. Cardiac catheterization insertion sites.

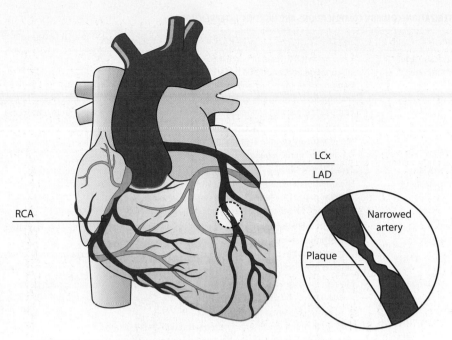

Figure 9-2. Coronary artery circulation with a coronary vessel narrowed by plaque formation.

catheter from the aorta, through the aortic valve, and into the left ventricle. A cineventriculogram provides information on ventricular wall motion, ejection fraction, and the presence and severity of mitral regurgitation and aortic regurgitation. Ejection fraction, the percentage of blood volume ejected from the left ventricle with each contraction, is the gold standard for determining left ventricular function and is helpful in selecting treatment strategies. A left ventricular ejection fraction (LVEF) normal value is 55% to 70%. The LVEF is one of the most important predictors of long-term outcome following acute myocardial infarction (AMI). Patients with ejection fractions less than 20% have nearly 50% 1-year mortality. Another important measurement is the pressure in the left ventricle at the end of diastole. This is called "left ventricular end-diastolic pressure (LVEDP)." It, too, is an important determinant of ventricular function and is considered to be a predictor of morbidity and mortality in patients with heart failure (HF) and those undergoing cardiac surgery. The normal LVEDP is 6 to 12 mm Hg.

Complications

During cardiac catheterization, a number of complications may occur, including dysrhythmia; coronary artery vasospasm; coronary artery dissection; allergic reaction to the dye; atrial or ventricular perforation from the catheter resulting in pericardial tamponade; bleeding at the insertion site, embolus to an extremity, a lung, or, rarely, the brain; acute closure of the left main coronary; myocardial infarction (MI); or cardiac arrest. Common management and prevention strategies for catheterization complications are summarized in Table 9-3. Cardiac catheterization may include treatment

with percutaneous coronary interventions (described later in this chapter).

PATHOLOGIC CONDITIONS

Acute Coronary Syndromes

Myocardial ischemia is the lack of adequate blood supply to the heart, resulting in an insufficient supply of oxygen to meet the demands of the heart muscle. This supply-demand mismatch, known as *ischemia,* is most often caused by thrombus formation at a site of atherosclerotic plaque rupture within a coronary artery. Decreased oxygen supply to myocardial tissue may cause a variety of symptoms such as chest discomfort (angina), shortness of breath, diaphoresis, and nausea. *Unstable angina,* defined as angina that is of new onset, increasing frequency, or occurring at rest, and AMI are referred to as acute coronary syndrome (ACS), which form the spectrum of acute ischemic heart disease.

Etiology and Pathophysiology

Intracoronary thrombus formation, and the resulting obstruction of coronary blood flow, is the pathophysiologic mechanism of acute ischemic heart disease. Preexisting atherosclerosis and spasm of the smooth muscle wall of the coronary arteries, termed *fixed obstructions,* may also contribute to reduced flow. In some situations, coronary artery spasm may play a major role, unrelated to underlying atherosclerosis, causing MI. These occurrences are sometimes associated with cocaine use in young patients.

Thrombus formation in the coronary arteries begins with the fissuring and rupture of atherosclerotic plaque in

TABLE 9-3. CARDIAC CATHETERIZATION: COMMON COMPLICATIONS AND NURSING INTERVENTIONS

Complication	Intervention
Local bleeding due to catheter site artery damage (hematoma, hemorrhage, pseudoaneurysm)	Keep patient flat; head of bed (HOB) < 30°. Discontinue unfractionated heparin infusion if present. Compress the artery just above the incision (pedal pulse should be faint). Monitor for hypotension, tachycardia, or arrhythmia. Embolectomy or vascular repair may be deemed necessary following groin ultrasound.
Coronary artery dissection	Stent will typically be placed during procedure. Monitor for arrhythmia or tamponade. Administer unfractionated heparin.
Tamponade due to perforation of the heart or bleeding due to antiplatelet medications	Typically this will be evident in the catheter laboratory at the time of perforation. Hypotension after procedure completed—often earliest sign. Monitor patient for equalization of cardiac pressures. Emergency surgery may be required for repair.
Peripheral thromboembolism	Extremity will exhibit pain, pallor, pulselessness, paresthesias, and paralysis; may also be cool to touch. Unfractionated heparin or other anticoagulant should be continued. Thrombolytic therapy may be administered directly to the clot using a tracking catheter. Surgical intervention may be necessary.
Thromboembolism: CVA due to embolus	Monitor for signs and symptoms of neurologic compromise including speech patterns, orientation, vision, equal grips and pedal pushes, and sensation.
Pulmonary embolism	Provide supplemental O_2. Monitor for adequate arterial oxygen saturation and respiratory rate. Continue administration of unfractionated heparin or other anticoagulant IV. Direct thrombolytic therapy may be administered using a tracking catheter; direct extraction of the clot may also be attempted. Ventilation-perfusion scan, computed tomography scan, or pulmonary arteriograms may be done to verify thrombus location.
Arrhythmia	Direct irritation of the ventricular wall by the catheter tip poses the greatest risk; post-procedure risk is extremely low. Monitor the patient in lead V_1.
Infection	Use aseptic technique for all dressing changes. Monitor catheter insertion sites for erythema, inflammation, heat, or exudate. Monitor patient temperature trends.
Pulmonary edema due to recumbent position, stress of angiographic contrast, or poor left ventricular function	Elevate HOB 30°. Administer diuretics as necessary. Consider use of flexible sheath or brachial access.
Acute tubular neurosis and renal failure	Hydrate patient well prior to and following procedure with continuous infusion of normal saline (typically 8 hours before and 8 hours after at 100 mL/h). Monitor for elevations in serum creatinine.
Vasovagal reaction	Administer pain medications prior to sheath removal. Monitor BP and heart rate before and after sheath removal, then every 15 minutes for four times after removal.

the vessel wall of the coronary artery (Figure 9-3). A continuous, dynamic process occurs whereby plaque may become unstable during periods of active accumulation of more lipid into the core of the plaque. The plaque then ruptures, dispelling its contents into the lumen of the coronary artery and causing activation of clotting factors at the site of plaque rupture. The rupture of plaque and resultant thrombus formation may eventually occlude the coronary artery.

Although most people have some degree of atherosclerotic plaque formation by age 30, the vast majority of these plaques are considered "stable." The smooth fibrous caps that cover these plaques allow adequate blood flow through the coronary arteries, and are not prone to development of unstable angina or MI. In young, growing plaques, the fibrous cap may become thin and rupture, resulting in unstable angina, ischemia, or MI.

A variety of factors predispose a plaque to fissure and rupture. Characteristics of plaque at increased risk for rupture include:

- *Location of the lesion in the vascular tree:* Areas of greater turbulence of flow and dynamic activity during the cardiac cycle are at higher risk.
- *Size of the lipid pool within the plaque:* A large amount of lipid inside the plaque core is more likely to be associated with plaque disruption.
- *Infiltration of the plaque with macrophages:* Macrophages are thought to weaken the integrity of the fibrous cap of the plaque, making it more susceptible to rupture.

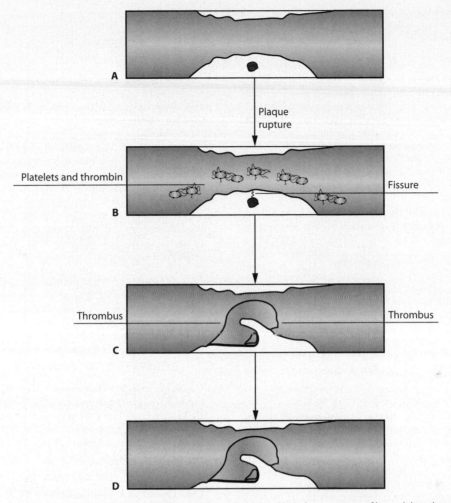

Figure 9-3. Atherosclerotic plaque formation. **(A)** Stable plaque. **(B)** Plaque with cap disruption. **(C)** Moderate amount of layered thrombus. **(D)** Occlusive thrombus.

Clinical assessment, stress testing, and even cardiac catheterization do not provide information about the contents of the plaque and therefore identification of the risk of rupture is challenging. Plaque rupture may be caused by a number of environmental or hormonal factors, known as *triggers* (Table 9-4). These triggers may precipitate an acute coronary event. Some of the triggers for atherosclerotic plaque rupture can be manipulated or controlled, such as blood pressure (BP), blood glucose level, and stress. In the clinical setting, management of these variables may decrease the risk for AMI, reinfarction, and reocclusion. They are closely monitored.

During the coronavirus 2019 pandemic, there were patients who were severely ill with the SARS-CoV-2 virus and were found to have acute cardiac injury identified by elevated high-sensitivity troponin levels. Many of these patients had underlying risk factors for cardiovascular disease. Mortality rates were higher in this group of patients. Studies have demonstrated that Coronavirus 2019 is associated with an extremely high inflammatory burden that produces vascular inflammation, macro and microvascular thrombosis,

myocarditis, and cardiac dysrhythmias. Recommendations are to treat the myocardial injury according to the evidence-based guidelines.

TABLE 9-4. HORMONAL AND ENVIRONMENTAL TRIGGERS OF PLAQUE RUPTURE

Acute	Chronic
Hemodynamic Reactivity	**Basal Hemodynamic Forces**
• Morning increase in BP	• Increased resting BP
• Morning increase in heart rate	• Increased resting heart rate
• Physical exertion	
• Emotional stress	**Basal Hemostatic Variables**
• Exposure to cold	• Location of the plaque
	• Size of the lipid pool within the
Hemostatic Reactivity	core plaque
• Increased coronary blood flow	• Degree of macrophage infiltration
velocity	of the plaque
• Increased viscosity of blood	
• Decreased tPA activity	**Chronic Risk Factors**
• Increased platelet aggregation	• Gender (male > female)
	• Increasing age
Vasoreactivity	• Diabetes mellitus
• Increased plasma epinephrine	• Hypercholesterolemia
• Increased plasma cortisol	• Cigarette smoking

ESSENTIAL CONTENT CASE

Unstable Angina

A 62-year-old man presents to the emergency department (ED) with complaints of pain in his chest and jaw. The pain, originally occurring only with exertion and resolving with rest, became increasingly persistent over the past 2 to 3 days. On the evening of his arrival, the patient experienced a 15-minute episode of severe pain while watching television. This episode he characterized as a "tight, burning feeling in my chest, and an aching in my jaw" that did not vary with respiratory effort and was accompanied by diaphoresis, nausea, and shortness of breath.

On arrival to the ED, his pain and nausea had resolved, pulse oximetry showed oxygen saturation of 98% on room air, and his vital signs were:

BP	148/86 mm Hg
HR	90 beats/min
RR	18 breaths/min
T	37.6°C orally

On physical examination, heart sounds were normal, without S3, S4, or murmurs. Initial diagnostic tests revealed:

- ECG: Normal sinus rhythm with nonspecific ST-T wave changes
- Chest x-ray: Normal cardiac silhouette, clear lungs

A more detailed assessment of his history revealed increasing dyspnea on exertion and fatigue for the previous 6 months. Despite these symptoms, he had continued his daily 2.5-mile walking routine, sometimes experiencing shortness of breath several times during the walk. The patient reported smoking cigarettes in the past, one pack per day for 20 years, but quit 25 years ago. No ankle swelling, nocturnal dyspnea, or orthopnea were reported, nor was he aware of any family history of cardiac problems, coronary artery disease, diabetes, or hypertension.

He was started on aspirin based on his history and the likelihood of underlying coronary artery disease. He was then admitted for observation and evaluation of cardiac enzymes (see section on cardiac enzymes).

	CK-M B	Troponin I
ED	5% (<5%)	0.4 ng/mL (<.06 ng/mL)
4 hours later	5% (<5%)	0.4 ng/mL (<.06 ng/mL)

Six hours after presenting to the ED, the patient had recurrent tightness in his chest. An ECG showed T-wave inversion in the anterior leads. Sublingual nitroglycerin 0.4 mg was administered every 5 minutes with complete relief of the pressure following the second tablet. An unfractionated heparin infusion was started. Subsequent cardiac enzymes showed:

	CK-MB	Troponin I
8 hours	4% (<5%)	0.4 ng/mL (<.06 ng/mL)
12 hours	4% (<5%)	0.4 ng/mL (<.06 ng/mL)

Other laboratory results were normal with the exception of elevated cholesterol and triglycerides on the lipid panel. Following receipt of these results, he was scheduled for an exercise tolerance test.

The ECG recorded a heart rate of 118 beats/min after 6 minutes of exercise. Onset of chest tightness during the last minute of exercise was described as similar to that which brought him to the hospital and correlated with 1.5-mm ST depression in leads V4 to V6. A cardiac catheterization was scheduled.

Coronary angiography showed a 75% obstruction of the LAD artery and 90% obstruction of the diagonal branch of the same artery. LVEF was 55%. A coronary angioplasty (PTCA) was performed on both lesions.

Case Question 1: What monitoring is the highest priority during the patient's ED stay?
(A) Obtain repeat ECGs every 4 hours
(B) Continuous ECG/ST-segment monitoring for signs of MI
(C) Monitor platelet levels every 6 hours
(D) Assess breath sounds every 2 hours

Case Question 2: What diagnosis is suggested by the finding of ST-segment depression and T-wave inversion on the ECG?
(A) Non–ST-segment elevation MI
(B) ST-segment elevation MI
(C) Coronary spasm
(D) Pericarditis

Case Question 3: Following the PTCA, what critical complication is the patient at risk for?
(A) Increased heart rate of 115 beats/min
(B) Hypotension
(C) 4 mm ST-segment elevation in leads V3-V4
(D) All of the above

Answers
1. B is the correct answer. Continuous ST-segment monitoring will reveal ischemic changes sooner when compared to intermittent ECGs.
2. A is the correct answer. Non–ST-segment MI is characterized by ST-segment depression and/or T-wave inversion in the setting of chest pain and increased cardiac biomarkers. Both coronary spasm and pericarditis can cause ST-segment changes on the ECG.
3. C is the correct answer. The new onset of 4 mm ST-segment elevation in leads V3-V4 is an indication of acute coronary closure following the interventional procedure. Hypotension and sinus tachycardia may also be present but are nonspecific signs.

When these triggers combine to cause plaque rupture, the lipid pool is exposed and a rough surface on the intima of the vessel wall occurs, stimulating the local effects of hormonal and immune factors and initiating thrombus formation. At the same time, the fibrinolytic system is stimulated, creating a dynamic process of simultaneous attempts to form and dissolve the clot. Because of the dynamic nature of the clotting process, the thrombus may be completely or only partially obstructive, or may fluctuate intermittently between the two stages. Regardless of the maturity of the clot, the process of thrombus formation may lead to obstruction of blood flow, diminishing oxygen delivery to distal myocardium and creating a mismatch between the supply of and demand for oxygen.

Because the underlying pathology of the ischemia-related diagnoses is the same (plaque rupture and thrombus formation), ischemic heart disease encompasses the entire spectrum of coronary events that are referred to as ACS. ACS represents a continuum of clinical events that may result from the supply-demand mismatch including unstable angina, non–ST-segment elevation myocardial infarction (NSTEMI), or ST-segment elevation myocardial infarction (STEMI) (Figure 9-4).

Following a decrease in oxygen supply to the myocardium, the cell membranes lose their integrity and fluid moves into the cell. The cell is no longer able to regulate its internal and external environment. The cell dies, releasing cytotoxic substances into the bloodstream. When they die, cardiac myocytes release significant amounts of myoglobin, troponin I and T, and cardiac-specific creatine kinase (CK-MB). Laboratory testing that shows elevated levels of these cardiac markers confirms the MI diagnosis.

Clinical Presentation

Clinical presentation across the spectrum of ACS is similar, with slight differences depending on the involved vessels (Table 9-5).

1. Pain or discomfort, usually in the chest (see Table 9-1)
   - Pressure or tightness in the chest
   - Jaw or neck pain
   - Left arm ache or pain
   - Epigastric discomfort
   - Scapular back pain
2. Nausea/vomiting
3. Hemodynamic instability
   - Hypotension (systolic BP < 90 mm Hg or 20 mm Hg below baseline)
   - Low cardiac index (CI) (<2.0 L/min/m2)
   - Elevated pulmonary artery diastolic (PAD) and/or pulmonary artery occlusion pressure (PAOP), if PA catheter present
   - Skin cool, clammy, diaphoretic
4. Dyspnea
5. Dysrhythmias/conduction defects
   - Left bundle branch block (LBBB)
   - Tachycardia/bradycardia
   - Frequent premature ventricular contractions
   - Ventricular fibrillation
6. Anxiety, sense of impending catastrophe
7. Denial
8. Recent use of cocaine can be a cause of AMI due to coronary artery vasoconstriction

Some patient populations are predictably different in their description of chest discomfort, such as women and those with diabetes. Women frequently present with symptoms that are more vague, such as feeling tired, short of breath, and a lack of energy. Women may deny their symptoms for longer periods of time than men, delaying their arrival to the ED and often rendering them ineligible for thrombolytic therapy. In addition, women are typically postmenopausal when signs and symptoms of atherosclerotic disease become apparent. This predominantly older patient population may face additional challenges such as fear of the inability to care for oneself following MI, and additional chronic health problems.

Patients with diabetes are another patient population with atypical symptoms when experiencing an MI. Patients with diabetes often develop atherosclerotic disease early and their experience of pain may be altered due to neuropathy. Coronary artery disease in this patient population is diffuse, and poor distal vascular anatomy is common. Lesion morphology in diabetic patients is also more difficult to revascularize, using either percutaneous or surgical methods.

Diagnostic Tests
Unstable Angina

1. *12-lead electrocardiogram (ECG):* Transient changes may occur and resolve; most commonly T-wave inversion or ST-segment depression.
2. *Cardiac enzymes* (Troponin [I or T], CK-MB): Normal, helpful in diagnosing unstable angina versus AMI.

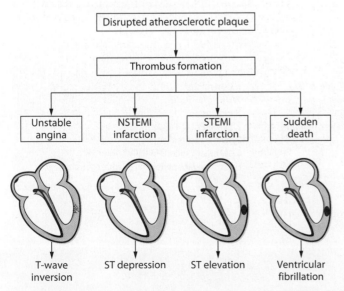

Figure 9-4. Pathophysiologic steps leading to acute coronary events.

TABLE 9-5. CLINICAL PRESENTATION OF MYOCARDIAL ISCHEMIA AND INFARCTION

Type MI	Arterial Involvement	Muscle Area Supplied	Assessment
Anteroseptal	LAD	Anterior LV wall, Anterior LV septum Apex LV Bundle of His Bundle branches	↓ LV function → ↓ CO, ↓ BP ↑ PAD, ↑ PAOP S₃ and S₄, with HF Rales with pulmonary edema
Posterior septal lateral	RCA circumflex branches (right and left)	Posterior surface of LV SA node 45% AV node 10% Left atrium Lateral wall of LV	Murmurs indicating VSD (septal) PA catheter to assess R to L shunt in VSD Signs/symptoms of LV aneurysm with lateral displaced PMI leading to signs and symptoms of mitral regurgitation
Inferior	RCA	RV, RA SA node 50% AV node 90% RA, RV Inferior LV Posterior VI septum Posterior LBBB Posterior LV	Symptomatic bradycardia: ↓ BP, LOC changes, diaphoresis. ↓ CO ↑ PAD ↑ PAOP Murmurs: associated with papillary muscle dysfunction, mid/holosystolic Rales, pulmonary edema, nausea
Right ventricular infarction	RCA	RA, RV, inferior LV SA node AV node Posterior IV septum	Kussmaul sign JVD Hypotension ↑ SVR, ↓ PAOP, ↑ CVP S₃ with noncompliant RV Clear breath sounds initially Hepatomegaly; peripheral edema; cool, clammy, pale skin

(continued)

TABLE 9-5. CLINICAL PRESENTATION OF MYOCARDIAL ISCHEMIA AND INFARCTION (CONTINUED)

ECG Changes	Likely Arrhythmias	Possible Complications
Anteroseptal Indicative ST elevation with or without abnormal Q waves in V_{1-4} Loss of R waves in precordial leads	RBBB, LBBB AV blocks Atrial fibrillation or flutter Ventricular tachycardia (VT) Tachycardia (septal)	Cardiogenic shock VSD Myocardial rupture Heart blocks may be permanent (LBBB) High mortality associated with this location of MI
Anteroseptal Reciprocal ST depression In II, III, aVF		
Lateral Indicative ST elevation I, aVL, V_{5-6} Loss of R wave and ↑ ST in I, aVL, V_{5-6}	Bradycardia Mobitz I (posterior)	RV involvement Aneurysm development Papillary muscle dysfunction Heart blocks frequently resolve
Posterior Indicative Tall, broad R waves (>0.04 second) in V_{1-3} ↑ ST V_4R (right-sided 12 lead, V_4 position)		
Posterior Reciprocal ST depression in $V_{1,2}$, upright T wave in V_{12} (Note: Posterior MI diagnosed by reciprocal changes)		
Inferior Indicative ↑ ST segments in II, III, aVF Q waves in II, III, aVF	AV blocks; often progress to CHB which may be transient or permanent; Wenckebach; bradyarrhythmias	Hiccups Nausea/vomiting Papillary muscle dysfunction MR
Inferior Reciprocal ST depression in I, aVL, V_{1-4}		Septal rupture (0.5%-1.0%) RV involvement associated with atrial infarcts especially with atrial arrhythmias
Right Ventricular Indicative 1- to 2-mm ST-segment elevation in V_4R ST- and T-wave elevation in II, III, aVF Q waves in II, III, aVF ST-elevation decreases in amplitude over V_{1-6}	First-degree AV block Second-degree AV block, type I Incomplete RBBB Transient CHB Atrial fibrillation VT/VF	Hypotension requiring large volumes initially to maintain systemic pressure. Once RV contractility improves fluids will mobilize, possibly requiring dieresis

- *High-sensitivity troponin*: Chronic, stable elevations may indicate increased risk of acute coronary events.
3. *Cardiac catheterization:* Not recommended in the acute setting, except in the case of continued pain/discomfort without relief from nitroglycerin. Catheterization results may be normal, or with visible atherosclerotic disease that is not completely occlusive.

Myocardial Infarction

1. *12-lead ECG:* Thirty-five percent of patients with AMI have ST-segment elevation on their initial ECG (see Chapter 18, Advanced ECG Concepts). The label "STEMI" is used in this situation. Approximately 65% of those with AMI have no ECG changes.
2. *Creatine kinase* (CK and CK-MB) (Figure 9-5).
   - Total CK > 150 to 180 mcg/L.
   - MB band > 10 ng/mL or > 5% of total.
   - Peaks at 12 hours after symptom onset.
   - CK-MB isoforms have better sensitivity and specificity for detecting MI within the first 6 hours.
3. *Troponin T:* Compare to laboratory reference range
   - Begins to increase 3 to 5 hours after symptom onset
   - Remains elevated for 14 to 21 days

4. *Troponin I:* Compare to laboratory reference range
   - Begins to increase 3 hours after onset of MI
   - Peaks at 14 to 18 hours
   - Remains elevated for 5 to 7 days
5. High sensitivity Troponin (hs-cTn)
   - A single hs-cTn below the level of quantitation can rule out AMI in patients who present more than 2 hours after symptom onset. The sensitivity declines 12 hours after symptom onset.
   - A single positive hs-cTn is sensitive for AMI but not specific; interpret with other clinical data.
   - Serial assessment of hs-cTn may be required, based on time of presentation and patient risk.
6. *Cardiac catheterization:* Ventricular wall motion abnormalities (also may be seen by echocardiography); total occlusion of one or more coronary arteries.

Principles of Management of Acute Coronary Syndromes

Because most complications of acute ischemic heart disease directly result from reduced coronary flow, a primary objective in patient management is to optimize blood flow to the myocardium. Additional goals are to prevent complications of ischemia and infarction, alleviate chest discomfort/pain, and reduce anxiety.

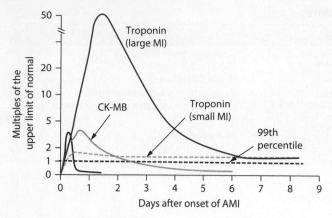

Figure 9-5. Timing and levels of biomarkers associated with heart injury. (*Data from Antman EM. Decision making with cardiac troponin tests.* N Engl J Med. *2002;346:2079; and Jaffe AS, Babiun L, Apple FS. Biomarkers in acute cardiac disease: the present and the future.* J Am Coll Cardiol. *2006;48:1.*)

Optimize Blood Flow to the Myocardium

Regardless of whether a patient presents with unstable angina or AMI, restoration and maintenance of coronary blood flow are important to improve patient outcomes. Interventions to optimize blood flow to the myocardium include pharmacologic measures, such as antiplatelet or antithrombin agents, and mechanical measures, such as percutaneous coronary revascularization (eg, angioplasty, stent, or other) or coronary artery bypass grafting (CABG). Refer to Table 9-6 for evidenced-based guidelines for AMI. The intervention selected and the optimal timing of the intervention depends on whether the occlusion of the artery is total or partial. This determination must be made as accurately and as quickly as possible, as a totally occluded artery will soon result in tissue necrosis or MI (see Figure 9-6 for algorithm on acute chest pain management). All unstable arteries benefit from the following interventions to stabilize the artery and optimize coronary perfusion. In addition, all patients with ACS should be treated with statin and anti-platelet therapy unless there is a contraindication.

Medical Management

1. Decrease activity of coagulation system with pharmacologic therapy (Figure 9-7):
   - Antiplatelet agents: aspirin, glycoprotein IIb/IIIa receptor blocking agents (eg, abciximab [Reopro®], eptifibatide [Integrilin®], and tirofiban [Aggrastat®]), thienopyridine agents (eg, clopidogrel [Plavix®] or tacagrelor [Brilinta®])
   - Antithrombin agents: indirect (eg, unfractionated heparin, low-molecular-weight heparin), direct (eg, bivalirudin [Angiomax®])
2. Increase ventricular filling time (decrease heart rate):
   - Beta-blockers (not indicated for cocaine-induced AMI)
   - Bed rest for 24 hours

TABLE 9-6. EVIDENCED-BASED PRACTICE: ACUTE CORONARY SYNDROME— ST-ELEVATION MI AND NON–ST-ELEVATION MI

Diagnosis
- Diagnosis of AMI is based on two of three findings:
  1. History of ischemic-like symptoms
  2. Changes on serial ECGs
  3. Elevation and fall in level of serum cardiac biomarkers
- Of AMI patients, 50% do not present with ST-segment elevation. Other indicators:
  1. ST-segment depression may indicate NSTEMI
  2. New LBBB
  3. ST-segment depression that resolves with relief of chest pain
  4. T-wave inversion in all chest leads may indicate NSTEMI with a critical stenosis in the proximal LAD

Acute Management
- Optimal time for initiation of therapy is within 1 hour of symptom onset. Rarely feasible due to delay in treatment-seeking behavior[a]
- Initial ECG should be obtained within 10 minutes of emergency department arrival
- Oxygen if $SaO_2 < 90\%$, nitroglycerin, and aspirin should be administered if not contraindicated

Reperfusion strategy: STEMI only:
  1. If non-PCI capable hospital, fibrinolytic agent should be initiated within 30 minutes of arrival if no contraindication
  2. If PCI capable hospital, primary PCI to be done, culprit vessel should be opened within 90 minutes of arrival

Reperfusion strategy for NSTEMI:[b]
  1. Fibrinolytics not recommended
  2. PCI to be done within 24 hours of arrival
- Weight-based heparin or low-molecular-weight heparin[a]
- Antiplatelet therapy
- IV beta-blocker should be given within 12 hours of arrival[a]
- Lipid-lowering agent (statin) should be initiated[a]

Data from [a]O'Gara, Kushner, Ascheim, et al (2013), [b]Amsterdam et al (2014).

3. Decrease preload:
   - Nitrates
   - Diuretics
   - Morphine sulfate
4. Decrease afterload:
   - Angiotensin-converting enzyme (ACE) inhibitors if EF ≤ 40%
   - Hydralazine
5. Decrease myocardial oxygen consumption (MVO_2):
   - Beta-blockers
   - Bed rest for 24 hours

In addition to the interventions listed above, totally occluded arteries require immediate reperfusion therapy, such as fibrinolysis, angioplasty, or CABG, to effectively restore blood flow to the coronary artery. In the event of left main coronary artery stenosis or three-vessel disease, urgent or emergent CABG is usually considered. In the acute setting, for STEMI, fibrinolytic therapy is often the fastest, most universally available method for reperfusion if a catheterization laboratory is not available or operational 24 hours a day. The indications, contraindications, and common complications of fibrinolytic therapy are listed in Tables 9-7 and 9-8. In those settings where the catheterization laboratory is operational 24 hours a day, primary PCI is indicated. Studies have indicated that primary PCI may be associated with better

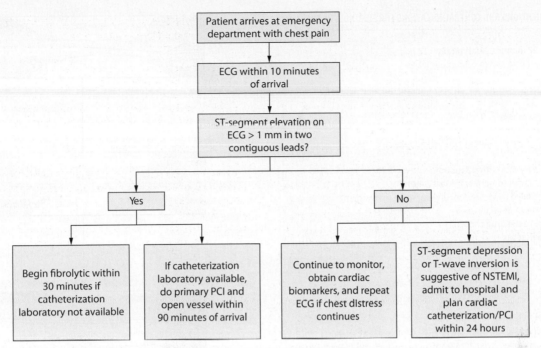

Figure 9-6. Algorithm for management of acute chest pain.

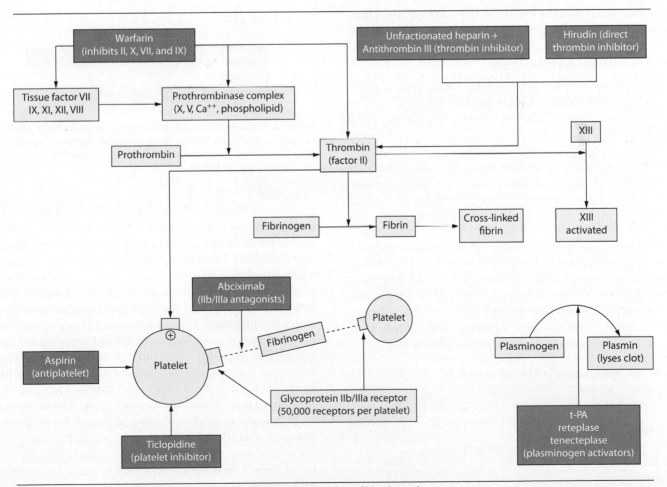

Figure 9-7. Coagulation sequence and site of antithrombotic/antiplatelet activity.

TABLE 9-7. INDICATIONS AND CONTRAINDICATIONS FOR FIBRINOLYTIC THERAPY

Indications
- Chest pain > 20 minutes, but typically <12 hours
- ST elevation ≥ 1 mm in two contiguous leads
- LBBB
- High-risk patients with chest pain > 12 hours in duration may still be candidates if pain persists

Absolute Contraindications
- Active internal bleeding
- History of intracranial bleeding, cerebral neoplasm, or other intracranial pathology
- Stroke or head trauma within 3 months
- Intracranial or spinal surgery in the last 2 months
- Severe uncontrolled hypertension, unresponsive to treatment
- Suspected aortic dissection
- Known allergy to the drug chosen

Relative Contraindications
- Dementia
- Ischemic stroke > 3 months ago
- Active peptic ulcer
- Prolonged traumatic CPR > 10 minutes
- Major surgery < 3 weeks ago
- Traumatic puncture of noncompressible vessel
- Pregnancy or 1 month postpartum
- History of uncontrolled hypertension
- Significant hypertension systolic > 180 or diastolic > 110

outcomes and fewer complications than with the use of fibrinolytic agents.

Percutaneous Coronary Interventions

Percutaneous coronary interventions (PCIs) include percutaneous transluminal coronary angioplasty (PTCA), insertion of one or more stents, and coronary atherectomy. PCI is one treatment option for patients with ACS and is performed in conjunction with cardiac catheterization. In PTCA, also termed *angioplasty* or *balloon angioplasty,* the catheter tip has is balloon apparatus that can be used to revascularize the myocardium (Figure 9-8). The catheter tip is advanced, generally over a guidewire, into the coronary artery until the balloon is positioned across the atherosclerotic lesion in the vessel. Once properly positioned, the balloon is inflated, resulting in fracture and compression of the atherosclerotic plaque, improving blood flow through the vessel. As a result, the degree of stenosis is reduced. This allows a higher rate and volume of blood flow through the vessel improving perfusion of the tissues, which translates clinically into fewer symptoms of angina and better exercise tolerance.

TABLE 9-8. COMPLICATIONS OF FIBRINOLYTIC THERAPY

Complication	Percentage Occurrence
Groin bleeding, local (compressible external)	25-45
Intracerebral bleeding	1.45
Retroperitoneal bleeding (noncompressible internal)	1
Gastrointestinal bleeding	4-10
Genitourinary bleeding	1-5
Other bleeding	1-5

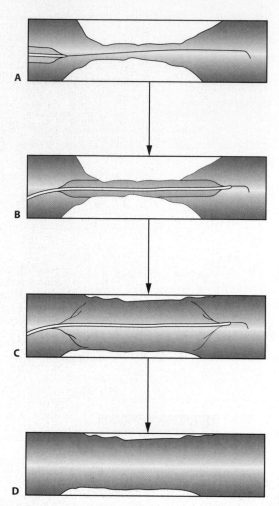

Figure 9-8. Percutaneous transluminal coronary angioplasty (PTCA). **(A)** PTCA catheter being advanced into the narrowed coronary artery over a guidewire. **(B)** Catheter position prior to balloon inflation. **(C)** Balloon inflation. **(D)** Coronary vessel following catheter removal.

Complications

Angioplasty is associated with the same complications found during cardiac catheterization (described earlier in this chapter). In addition, complications related to manipulation of the coronary artery itself may also occur. The most common serious complications include a 2% to 10% incidence of complete occlusion of the vessel ("abrupt closure"), AMI (1%-5% incidence), and the need for emergency coronary artery bypass surgery (1%-2% incidence). The most important predictor of complications of MI and abrupt vessel closure is reduced coronary flow through the lesion prior to the procedure. A universal scale, the thrombolysis in myocardial ischemia (TIMI) scale, is used to quantify this rate of coronary flow. The scale rates the coronary blood flow as follows: no perfusion, penetration without perfusion, partial perfusion, and complete perfusion.

Other Percutaneous Coronary Interventions

In addition to balloon angioplasty, a number of other devices are commonly used for percutaneous coronary

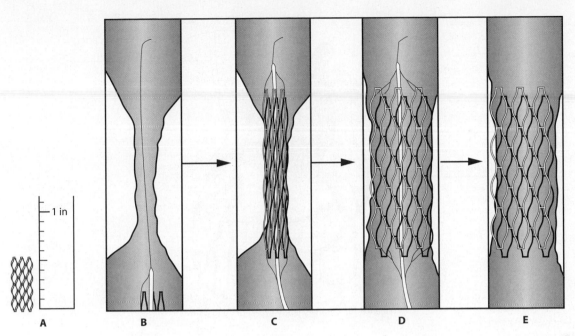

Figure 9-9. Intracoronary stent. **(A)** Size of stent device when fully deployed. **(B)** Insertion of stent into a narrowed area of a coronary artery on a balloon-inflatable catheter. **(C)** Inflation of the balloon catheter to expand the stent. **(D)** Inflation complete with stent fully expanded. **(E)** Stent following removal of balloon catheter.

revascularization. Intracoronary stents are small metallic mesh tubes placed across the stenotic area and expanded with an angioplasty balloon (Figure 9-9). Once expanded, the tube is permanently anchored in the vessel wall. Stents are effective in decreasing the rate of abrupt vessel closure seen with traditional PTCA. Some stents are coated with a drug that is bonded to a material on the stent causing the drug to be released directly on to the arterial wall over several months to years. These drug-coated stents have been shown to significantly reduce the restenosis rate associated with metal stents. Atherectomy catheters and lasers are used infrequently; however, patient outcomes are not significantly better than those achieved with traditional balloon catheters and stent deployment and may result in higher rates of complication, including AMI. Each of these devices may offer advantages over traditional balloon angioplasty catheters in situations involving specific vascular anatomy (eg, ostial lesions) or lesion morphology (eg, high degree of calcified plaque).

Surgical Management

CABG involves surgical revascularization in patients with ACS. CABG is performed both electively, as well as emergently, and may be performed either following an MI or to treat coronary artery disease before the patient experiences an MI. The CABG procedure in which a graft is placed in the coronary arterial tree to perfuse the area beyond the occlusion, requires *induction* with general anesthesia, and may require initiation of cardiopulmonary bypass (blood is diverted outside of the body to a pump that mechanically oxygenates the blood before returning it to the arterial circulation) (Figure 9-10).

The use of stabilizer devices permits CABG to be performed on some patients without cardiopulmonary bypass. The heart continues to beat while the surgeon places a device over the coronary artery site where the bypass graft is to be anastomosed, which stabilizes the small area allowing for suturing to occur. This is often referred to as *beating heart surgery* or "off pump" coronary artery bypass (OPCAB). In some situations, the surgeon may choose to use a minimally invasive approach with or without robotic support. This approach uses smaller incisions and avoids the traditional median sternotomy. The graft, generally the left internal mammary artery or the saphenous vein from the leg, or less often, the radial artery, is inserted past the distal end of the blockage in the coronary artery and, in the case of a leg vein graft and radial artery graft, anastomosed to the aorta. Multiple grafts may be inserted based on the number of blockages present and the availability of viable insertion sites in the patient's native coronary tree.

Indications

The indications for CABG are based on patient outcome following this procedure have been intensively reviewed. In general, patients with three-vessel disease, poor LVEF (<35%), or significant disease in the left main coronary artery have lower long-term morbidity and mortality with surgical revascularization (CABG) compared to medical therapy or percutaneous interventions such as angioplasty or stent. Patients with diabetes who have multivessel disease also fare better following CABG than following percutaneous interventions including drug-eluting stents. CABG may also be indicated as an emergent "rescue" procedure in

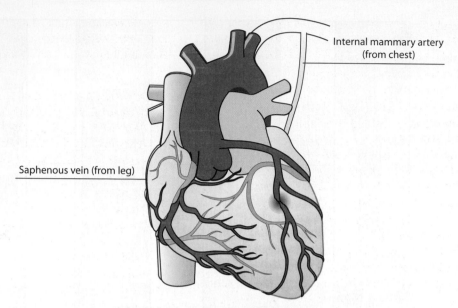

**Internal mammary artery
(from chest)**

Saphenous vein (from leg)

Figure 9-10. Coronary artery bypass grafting (CABG).

patients whose coronary artery severely dissects or fractures during an attempted percutaneous procedure. Mechanical complications of an AMI may also be an indication for surgical intervention.

Contraindications

Several populations of patients may be considered poor candidates for coronary bypass, including the very elderly, debilitated patients, patients with severely diseased distal coronary vasculature (eg, those with diabetes), and patients with extremely low LVEF (eg, <5%-15%). Patients with low ejection fractions often have difficulty being weaned from cardiopulmonary bypass following the procedure. Other contraindications are those related to general anesthesia risk, including pulmonary edema, severe chronic obstructive pulmonary disease, or pulmonary hypertension.

Postoperative Management

The following is a general overview of the early postoperative management of CABG patients.

1. *Maintain hemodynamic stability:* A variety of cardiac medications are administered to maintain hemodynamic stability in the first 24 hours postoperatively. Hemodynamic monitoring may be invasive using a pulmonary artery catheter, minimally invasive using a central line or arterial line, or completely noninvasive. Interpretation of postoperative hemodynamic status is best done with the patient's preoperative hemodynamic status in mind, as some of the values may be significantly elevated or abnormal at the patient's baseline. The following hemodynamic values may serve as guides for inotropic and vasopressor administration along with intravascular fluid

therapy. In general, values greater or lower than the following require intervention:

- Mean arterial pressure: 70 to 80 mm Hg
- CI: 2.0 to 3.5 L/min/m^2
- PAD/PAOP: 10 to 12 mm Hg (may be used to evaluate need for volume replacement; however, research has demonstrated that there is not a relationship between pressures and the intravascular volume status.)
- Central venous pressure (CVP): 5 to 10 mm Hg (may be used to evaluate need for volume replacement; however, research has demonstrated that there is not a relationship between pressures and the intravascular volume status.)
- HR: Intrinsic or paced rhythm in the range of 80 to 100 beats/min to keep CI ≥ 2.0.
- If radial artery graft used, monitor for arterial spasm. Use a prophylactic nitroglycerin drip and nitro paste if indicated.

2. *Maintain ventilation and oxygenation:* Ventilation and oxygenation are maximized in the early postoperative period with mechanical ventilation. Within 2 to 12 hours, most patients have recovered from the anesthesia effects and are sufficiently stable to allow weaning from mechanical ventilation and extubation. Frequently, younger, hemodynamically stable patients are extubated in the or soon after arriving in the ICU. Individuals with preexisting pulmonary problems may require longer periods of intubation until weaning can be successfully accomplished. Following weaning and extubation, supplemental O_2 therapy usually is required for 1 to 2 days to maintain Pao_2 or Sao_2 in normal ranges. Postoperative atelectasis and pleural effusions are common occurrences

after cardiopulmonary bypass, usually requiring frequent pulmonary interventions (eg, coughing and deep breathing, incentive spirometry, ambulation) to maintain ventilation and oxygenation.

3. Prevention of postoperative complications:

- *Bleeding from vascular graft anastomosis sites:* Frequent monitoring of mediastinal tube drainage, hematocrit, and coagulation status; avoidance of even brief periods of hypertension.
- *Cardiac tamponade:* Frequent assessment for signs and symptoms of tamponade, which include tachycardia, SOB, anxiety/decreased LOC, pulsus paradoxus, decreased mediastinal tube drainage, increased CVP, PAD, and PAOP (note: these are often within 2-3 mm Hg of each other). This is called equalization of pressures or diastolic plateau and is accompanied by muffled heart tones, decreased BP, and cardiac output. Also, monitor closely for cardiac tamponade after epicardial wire removal.
- *Infection:* Antibiotics may be used prophylactically for 24 to 48 hours; temperature spike within 24 hours postoperatively is not abnormal.
- *Cardiac dysrhythmias:* ECG and continuous ST-segment monitoring, treat unstable rhythms, maintain K^+ and Mg^+ within normal limits with IV replacement.
- *Relief of postoperative pain and anxiety:* Analgesic administration is typically required to ensure pain relief (opioids and NSAIDS), especially to facilitate ambulation, coughing, and deep breathing.
- If median sternotomy is performed, ensure sternal precautions are implemented, for example, avoid hyperextension of chest (arms and shoulders pulled posteriorly).
- Facilitate early mobility once the patient is extubated and determined to be hemodynamically stable, eg, dangle, out of bed to a chair, and ambulation.

Preventing Complications Associated With Coronary Obstruction

Complications associated with acute coronary syndromes include recurrent ischemia, infarction or reinfarction, onset of HF, and dysrhythmias.

1. *Prevent recurrent ischemia, infarction, or reinfarction:* Continue pharmacologic interventions such as antiplatelet and antithrombin agents and statins. Assess for recurrent angina with frequent chest pain assessment and serial 12-lead ECG and continuous ST-segment ischemia monitoring (see AACN Practice Alert: Ensuring accurate ST-segment Monitoring).

2. *Continuously monitor for dysrhythmia:* Monitor for 24 to 72 hours following an ischemic episode.

3. *Minimize potential for HF:* Minimize myocardial oxygen consumption with the administration of beta-blockers, limit physical activity (bed rest), and avoid increases in metabolic rate (eg, fever). Reduce left ventricular afterload with the administration of ACE inhibitors and hydralazine.

Alleviating Pain

Pain relief improves coronary flow by decreasing the level of circulating catecholamines, thereby decreasing BP (afterload) and heart rate (myocardial oxygen consumption). Nitrates typically relieve anginal pain by dilating coronary arteries and increasing blood flow, thereby improving myocardial oxygenation and directly treating the source of the pain. Another pharmacologic intervention commonly used to relieve pain in ischemia is morphine sulfate. Although morphine is a potent narcotic that has been criticized for masking cardiac pain, it is also a potent vasodilator and effectively vasodilates coronary as well as peripheral arteries, resulting in mild afterload reduction. Severe pain, unrelieved with nitrates or a combination of nitrates and morphine, is typically an indication for immediate PCI if available, or transfer to a referring institution for emergency PCI.

Reducing Anxiety

The reduction of anxiety in ischemic heart disease is important for a number of reasons. The most important physiologically is the reduction of catecholamine secretion and decrease in sympathetic tone following relaxation in the anxious patient. This effect has been shown to decrease the incidence of dysrhythmias and promote vasodilation and afterload reduction. Decreasing anxiety may also increase the patient's ability to process new information regarding his or her diagnosis, and to better understand instructions for tests or procedures that will be done.

Relief of pain typically is most effective in reducing patient anxiety. In the event that pain is not relieved with nitroglycerin, or fibrinolytics in the initial treatment of ischemia, pain relievers such as morphine sulfate or anxiolytics such as midazolam or lorazepam (short- or intermediate-acting benzodiazepines, respectively) are usually effective.

A number of interventions may be done at the bedside to promote relaxation, including specific relaxation and imagery techniques, meditation, music therapy, and the use of relaxation applications or audio files. Providing the patient and family with adequate information regarding unfamiliar surroundings, when the provider may be available to speak with them, possible "unknowns" such as tests or procedures, and important expectations such as visitation guidelines help provide a sense of security and facilitates relaxation by increasing the patient's level of comfort with the situation. Offering the patient opportunities for control in the acute setting also alleviates anxiety. Examples include the timing of simple activities such as visitor presence, bathing, and eating.

HEART FAILURE

Heart failure (HF) is a broad term referring to the inability of the heart to maintain an adequate cardiac output to meet the oxygen and metabolic requirements of the body. The

TABLE 9-9. CLINICAL SIGNS AND SYMPTOMS SPECIFIC TO RIGHT- AND LEFT-SIDED HEART FAILURE

Right Heart Failure	Left Heart Failure
Signs and Symptoms of Hepatic Congestion	**Signs and Symptoms of Pulmonary Congestion**
JVD	Pulmonary edema
Liver enlargement and tenderness	Rales
Positive hepatojugular reflex (pressure on liver increases JVD)	Atrial fibrillation or other atrial arrhythmias secondary to atrial distension
Dependent edema	Pulsus alternans (every other beat diminished)
Ascites	
Decreased appetite, nausea, vomiting	Dyspnea
Cardiac Pressures	Cough
Increased RV pressure	Hyperventilation
Increased RA pressure	Dizziness, syncope, fatigue
Heart Sounds	**Cardiac Pressures**
S_3 (early sign)	Increased LV and LA pressure
S_4 (may also present)	Increased pulmonary artery pressures
Wide split S_2	**Heart Sounds**
Pansystolic murmur at lower left sternal border secondary to stretching of tricuspid ring	S_3 and (occasionally) S_4
	Pansystolic murmur at apex secondary to mitral regurgitation

impairment may be due to either impaired left ventricular or right ventricular dysfunction. In some cases, both chambers are impaired, referred to as biventricular failure. A number of disorders may contribute to the development of HF, with coronary atherosclerosis, hypertension, valvular heart disease, and cardiomyopathy as the most common causes. While the underlying causes are diverse, the pathophysiologic process of heart failure is the same.

Left ventricular failure is more common than right ventricular failure. However, interest in right ventricular failure has increased because of the advances in the management of pulmonary hypertension, improved diagnostic technologies, and increased implantation of left ventricular assist devices (VADs) and other mechanical assist devices for cardiogenic shock. Refer to Table 9-9 for signs and symptoms comparing left and right ventricular failure. Management of right ventricular failure is directed toward the primary cause with a focus on right ventricular preload, afterload, and myocardial contractility. When medical management is not sufficient, right ventricular mechanical circulatory support may be implemented.

Etiology and Pathophysiology

Although HF refers to any cardiac insufficiency, left ventricular systolic dysfunction is the most common disorder. The pathophysiology of HF is a three-stage process, beginning with an initial insult to the myocardium, followed by a compensatory neurohormonal response, and resulting in the clinical syndrome known as HF, characterized by exhaustion of compensatory mechanisms. Regardless of the precipitating event, the physiologic progression of the syndrome, once initiated, is the same.

Two forms of heart failure involving the left ventricle have been described, systolic dysfunction and diastolic dysfunction. Systolic dysfunction is characterized by impaired myocardial contractility resulting in the inability of the ventricles to contract forcefully to eject blood out to the body, particularly when increases in cardiac output are needed to support the tissue oxygen demands. This is associated with a reduced ejection fraction (≤40%) and is frequently described as **H**eart **F**ailure with a **r**educed **E**jection **F**raction (HFrEF). The ventricles are often dilated contributing to mitral and tricuspid valvular insufficiency. The left ventricular end-diastolic pressure and left atrial pressure are not elevated. Patients with an ejection fraction in the range of 41% to 49% are described as **H**eart **F**ailure with **m**ildly **r**educed **E**jection **F**raction (**HFmrEF**). Patients with heart failure who have recovered myocardial contractility with an ejection fraction ≥50% are described as **H**eart **F**ailure with **imp**roved **E**jection **F**raction (**HFimpEF**).

Diastolic dysfunction is characterized by the inability of the left ventricle to "relax" or stretch slightly to accommodate arterial blood coming in from the lungs. The impaired muscle compliance results in higher left ventricular and left atrial pressures. The higher pressures are reflected back into the pulmonary vascular bed contributing to pulmonary vascular congestion. The ventricle is able to maintain its contractility resulting in a normal ejection fraction. This form of heart failure is often described as **H**eart **F**ailure with a **p**reserved **E**jection **F**raction (HFpEF). Echocardiogram findings for patients with HFpEF may include a thickened muscle wall. Patients with HFpEF are often older, more likely to be female and have a history of hypertension. Figure 9-11 is a comparison of the ejection fraction with the two types of heart failure.

Left ventricular systolic dysfunction is the most common form of heart failure. Once the initiating event occurs, a number of adaptive mechanisms occur in an effort to maintain an adequate cardiac output to meet the body's needs. In a normal heart, impaired ventricular contraction will cause a reduction of stroke volume and incomplete emptying of the left ventricle. The result is an increase in the volume of blood in the ventricle at the end of diastole (end-diastolic volume or EDV) which increases the stretch of the myocardial muscle fibers resulting in an increased contractile force and associated increase in stroke volume. This mechanism is impaired in systolic failure from myocardial injury. Instead of a greater contractility, the increase in left ventricular EDV increases LVEDP and stroke volume and cardiac output are reduced. The compensatory mechanisms for the reduction of stroke volume and cardiac output include sympathetic nervous system activation, ventricular remodeling, and neurohormonal activation.

Sympathetic Nervous System Activation

As cardiac output decreases and the sympathetic nervous system is activated, alpha-1 receptors are stimulated, resulting in arteriolar and venous vasoconstriction. This adaptive response

HF Diagnosis and EF

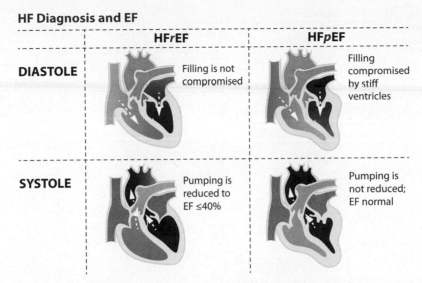

Figure 9-11. Comparison of Ejection Fractions for Systolic and Diastolic Heart Failure. (*Reproduced with permission from American Association of Critical Care Nurses.*)

initially increases venous return to the heart, increases left ventricular EDV, stretching the myocardial cells and increasing stroke volume and thus improving cardiac output. As demonstrated in the Frank-Starling curve, the improvement in stroke volume with increased left ventricular EDV levels off, as overstretching of the ventricle occurs. This results in left ventricular decompensation and myocardial hypertrophy. Of note, ventricular stretching leads to an increased release of brain natriuretic peptide (BNP) from granules in the ventricular cells resulting in an increased release of BNP in the serum. Increased BNP levels are a biomarker of severity of ventricular failure.

Ventricular Remodeling

In response to increased vascular volume and decreased myocardial function (loss of the Frank-Starling response, see Figure 9-12), the left ventricle dilates and hypertrophies.

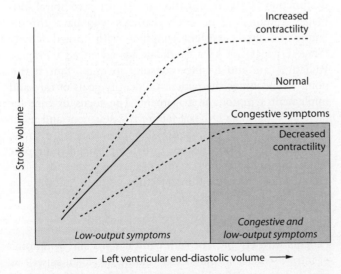

Figure 9-12. Frank-Starling curve.

This distortion of the normal left ventricular anatomy causes mitral regurgitation and further left ventricular dilatation. Activation of angiotensin II, a by-product of the renin-angiotensin-aldosterone system (RAAS), systemically and in the endothelial cells of blood vessels, directly induces myocyte hypertrophy as well. The result of these factors is decreased left ventricular reserve (stretch), increased preload (high residual volume in the ventricle following systole), and further mitral regurgitation.

Neurohormonal Response

In response to decreased stroke volume/cardiac output and decreased renal perfusion, several neurohormonal systems are activated. These include:

1. *Adrenergic nervous system:* Adrenergic nervous system activity is heightened in the setting of impaired ventricular function as a direct result of baroreceptor stimulation. These baroreceptors mediate the sympathetic nervous system, which in turn stimulates the beta-1 receptors. This results in an increase in heart rate and contractility.

2. *Renin-angiotensin-aldosterone system:* Decreased renal perfusion stimulates the release of renin, increasing the production of angiotensin I and II, and the release of aldosterone. The result is peripheral vasoconstriction, elevation of the blood pressure, and increased peripheral vascular resistance thereby increasing cardiac workload and reducing cardiac output. The kidneys retain sodium and water causing an increased intravascular volume contributing to further increases in cardiac workload (see Figure 9-13). The ventricle begins to dilate and hypertrophy. The sympathetic nervous system continues to be activated to increase cardiac output and maintain flow to the vital organs.

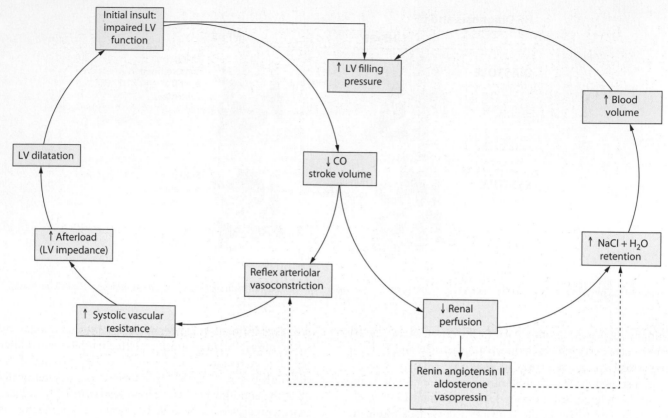

Figure 9-13. Compensatory mechanisms of HF.

3. *Arginine vasopressin (AVP) system:* AVP is a potent vasoconstrictor that is normally inhibited by stretch receptors in the atria during atrial distension. In HF, these receptors are less sensitive, causing a decrease in AVP inhibition. AVP activation leads to systemic vasoconstriction, and increased afterload, which is the pressure the ventricle must work against to eject blood out to the system. Increased AVP activity also inhibits free water excretion causing hypoosmolarity, and, impairs autoregulation of further AVP production.

4. *Atrial natriuretic peptide (ANP):* ANP is a counter-regulatory hormone that opposes all three of the above systems, resulting in vasodilation and sodium excretion. ANP is produced in response to atrial distension and results in decreased formation of renin, decreased effects of angiotensin II, decreased release of aldosterone and vasopressin, and enhanced renal excretion of sodium and water. Figure 9-13 demonstrates the effects of the compensatory mechanisms in heart failure.

The Progression of Heart Failure

The clinical expression and course of HF are determined by the extent of the initial myocyte damage, the severity of volume overload, and the patient's neurohormonal response to these changes. There will be progressive deterioration of

cardiovascular functioning due to the relationship between the compromised left ventricular function and cardiac afterload. Dilation of one or both ventricles occurs leading to mitral or tricuspid (or both) insufficiency, and the onset of intraventricular conduction disturbances. The most common cause of death in these patients is ventricular fibrillation.

The HF syndrome is characterized by periods of decline interrupted by periods of stability. It is a situation in which dysfunction begets dysfunction in a downward spiral ultimately culminating in death. Patients who have chronic failure and have persistent symptoms with limited activity (Stage D) may not be a candidate for advanced therapies. Palliative care and hospice consults are important at this point to encourage the patient to identify goals of care and implement symptom management. The focus of care for patients with Stage D heart failure is assessment and management of symptoms, addressing psychosocial distress, promoting quality of life, and providing caregiver support while aligning with the patient's preferences for end-of-life. Figure 9-14 describes the trajectory of heart failure as a chronic life-limiting disease.

Clinical Presentation

Patients with HF present with clinical signs and symptoms of intravascular and interstitial volume overload, as well as manifestations of inadequate tissue perfusion. Figure 9-15

Integrating Palliative Care Throughout The Heart Failure Trajectory

Chronic Care	Crisis Care	Terminal Care

Supporting patients, families/informal caregivers.
Information, communication, shared decision making.

Diagnosis

Death

Assess and optimize:
- Evidence-based treatment
- Sign & symptoms
- Spiritual, psychosocial & physical needs
- Comorbidities

Discuss:
- HF & self-care
- Role of patient, family & informal caregivers

Planning near future:
- Explore preferences & expectations
- Discuss trajectory & challenges to individualize prognosis

Advanced care planning:
- Prepare management during crisis

Assess and optimize:
- Possible reason deterioration/reversible precipitants
- Evidence-based treatment
- Signs & Symptoms
- Spiritual, psychosocial & physical needs
- Coordination of intensified care

Discuss:
- Preferences & possibility for treatment & care
- Role of patient, family and informal caregivers

Planning near future:
- Consider deprescribing and anticipatory prescribing
- Palliative needs assessment
- Consider referral to specialist palliative care team

Advanced care planning:
- Re-discuss HF trajectory
- Revisit advanced care plan
- Initiate end-of-life discussion

Assess and optimize:
- Signs & symptoms
- Spiritual, psychosocial and physical needs

Discuss:
- Preferences for treatment, care & place of care
- Discuss and decide regarding device deactivation (taking laws & culture into consideration)
- Deprescribing & anticipatory prescribing

Planning near future:
- Prepare & explain the dying process
- Increase practical & emotional support for patient, family and caregivers

Advanced care planning:
- Resuscitation status clarified
- Focus to ensure a good death
- Bereavement support

Figure 9-14. The trajectory of heart failure. (*Reproduced with permission from Hill L, Prager Geller T, Baruah R, et al: Integration of a palliative approach into heart failure care: a European Society of Cardiology Heart Failure Association position paper. Eur J Heart Fail. 2020;22(12):2327-2339.*)

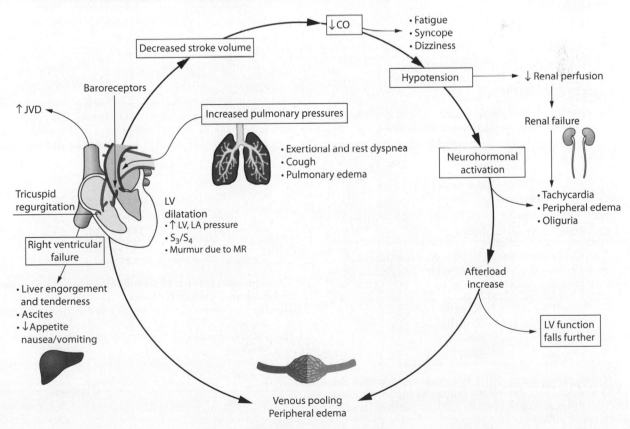

Figure 9-15. Clinical features of HF.

shows how the clinical features of heart failure coincide with altered cardiac function. Common findings in HF include:

- Dyspnea (especially with exertion, commonly severe in the acute setting)
- Paroxysmal nocturnal dyspnea
- Worsening exercise tolerance
- Pulmonary edema (pronounced crackles)
- Jugular venous distention (JVD)
- Chest discomfort or tightness
- Peripheral edema
- Cool, pale, cyanotic skin
- Oliguria
- Reported weight gain
- Fatigue

Signs and symptoms of heart failure may vary in individuals depending on which ventricle is primarily involved (see Table 9-9).

Because subjective assessment of symptoms and their severity may vary from clinician to clinician, classification systems are used to standardize symptom severity and evaluate the evolution and progression of HF. The American College of Cardiology and the American Heart Association developed a staging system that addresses the evolution and progression of HF. A second system, known as the New York Heart Association (NYHA) Functional Classification System, is used to provide systematic assessment of patient status and to benchmark improvement or deterioration from initial evaluation (Table 9-10).

TABLE 9-10. CLASSIFICATION OF CARDIOVASCULAR DISEASE

AHA/ACC Stages of Heart Failure	
Stage A:	Patients at high risk for HF due to the presence of conditions strongly associated with the development of HF. Asymptomatic.
Stage B:	Patients with structural disease, such as previous MI, but have never shown signs or symptoms of HF.
Stage C:	Patients with structural heart disease who have current or prior symptoms of HF.
Stage D:	Patients with advanced structural heart disease and marked symptoms at rest in spite of optimal medical therapy and who require specialized interventions.

New York Heart Association Functional Classification	
Class	
I	Patients with cardiac disease but without resulting limitations of physical activity. Ordinary physical activity does not cause undue fatigue, palpitations, dyspnea, or anginal pain.
II	Patients with cardiac disease resulting in slight limitation of physical activity. They are comfortable at rest. Ordinary physical activity results in fatigue, palpitations, dyspnea, or anginal pain.
III	Patients with cardiac disease resulting in marked limitation of physical activity. They are comfortable at rest. Less than ordinary physical activity causes fatigue, palpitations, dyspnea, or anginal pain.
IV	Patient with cardiac disease resulting in inability to carry on any physical activity without discomfort. Symptoms of cardiac insufficiency or of the anginal syndrome may be present even at rest. If any physical activity is undertaken, discomfort is increased.

ESSENTIAL CONTENT CASE

Heart Failure

A 75-year-old man presents to the ED with diaphoresis and severe dyspnea. Initial assessment revealed the following:

RR	32 breaths/min
BP	110/90 mm Hg
HR	110 beats/min, irregular
JVD	Bilateral 7-mm elevation
Lungs	Bibasilar crackles throughout the lower lobes
Cardiovascular	S1, S2 with an S3

A pulse oximeter revealed 93% oxygen saturation. Laboratory work, including an arterial blood gas sample, was done with the following results:

Pao_2	60 mm Hg
$Paco_2$	28 mm Hg
pH	7.51
Sao_2	93%

Oxygen was initiated at 4 L/min via nasal cannula. An ECG was done and showed left ventricular hypertrophy and LBBB. His chest x-ray showed an enlarged cardiac silhouette and bilateral infiltrates.

A dobutamine infusion was started at 2.5 mcg/kg/min, and furosemide 40 mg IV was given. Cardiac catheterization was performed the next morning with the following findings:

LAD	95% occlusion
RCA	50% occlusion
LCx	75%
EF	28%

Impaired Myocardial Contractility

Case Question 1: What effect will the dobutamine infusion and the dose of furosemide have?
(A) Increase myocardial contractility and reduce ventricular preload
(B) Increase myocardial contractility and reduce ventricular afterload
(C) Reduce myocardial contractility and increase ventricular preload
(D) Increase myocardial contractility and increase ventricular afterload

Case Question 2: Following the initiation of dobutamine and administration of furosemide, you would expect which of the following to occur?
(A) HR 120 beats/min; RR 36 breaths/min; Spo_2 83%
(B) HR 110 beats/min; RR 24 breaths/min; SpO_2 95%
(C) HR 95 beats/min; JVD Bilateral 7-mm elevation; RR 32 breaths/min
(D) BP 105/80 mm Hg, HR 130 beats/min; SpO_2 75%

Case Question 3: Based on the ECG and cardiac catheterization results, what additional intervention would benefit this patient?
(A) Implantation of a HeartMate 3™ LVAD as destination therapy
(B) Ventricular aneurysmectomy/reconstruction surgery
(C) Mitral valve repair
(D) Insertion of a dual-chamber biventricular pacemaker

Answers
1. A is the correct answer. Dobutamine is a positive inotrope and will increase myocardial contractility and cardiac output. It has some vasodilator effects and may cause the diastolic pressure to drop. Furosemide will reduce preload by promoting diuresis. All of this will reduce the amount of work the heart has to do.
2. B is the correct answer. He has diuresed, cleared some of the fluid in his lungs and his respiratory rate is slowing and pulse oximetry is improving.
3. D is the correct answer. LBBB causes ventricular dyssynchrony, indicating the ventricles do not contract simultaneously causing the cardiac output to decrease. Implanting a biventricular pacemaker will cause the ventricles to contract simultaneously and improve cardiac output. He is not a candidate for a left ventricular device at this time and a surgical procedure is not indicated.

A number of conditions, both cardiac and noncardiac, are similar to HF in their clinical presentation and are ruled out as possible diagnoses in the initial assessment. These conditions include MI, pulmonary disease, dysrhythmias, anemia, renal failure, nephrotic syndrome, and thyroid disease.

Diagnostic Tests

- *12-lead ECG:* Acute ST-T wave changes, low voltage, left ventricular hypertrophy, atrial fibrillation or other tachyarrhythmias, bradyarrhythmias, Q waves from previous MI, LBBB
- *Chest x-ray:* Cardiomegaly, cardiothoracic ratio more than 0.5
- *Complete blood count:* Low red cell count (anemia)
- *Urinalysis:* Proteinuria, red blood cells, or casts
- *Creatinine:* Elevated
- *Albumin:* Decreased
- *Serum sodium and potassium:* Decreased
- *BNP:* Elevated
- *Left/right cardiac catheterization:* Reduced LV wall motion, elevated LVEDP, elevated PAP, CI less than 2.0 L/min/m^2, AV valve incompetence.
- *Echocardiography:* Dilated left ventricle, right ventricle, or right atria; hypertrophied left ventricle; AV valve incompetence; diffuse or segmental hypocontractility; atrial thrombus; pericardial effusion; LVEF less than 40%, valve disease including mitral regurgitation, tricuspid regurgitation, aortic insufficiency or aortic stenosis.
- *Radionuclide ventriculography:* More precise measure of right ventricular dysfunction and LVEF.

Principles of Management for Heart Failure

Acute management of HF has changed dramatically over the past decade, from an emphasis on the micromanagement of hemodynamic parameters, primarily using positive inotropes, to an emphasis on functional capacity and long-term survival with the use of neurohormonal blocking agents. This shift is due to a better understanding of the neurohormonal response and the dependence of the body on these mechanisms for compensation in low output states. Goals of patient management in HF revolve around four general principles: (1) treatment of the underlying cause (eg, ischemia, valvular dysfunction), (2) management of fluid volume overload, (3) improvement of ventricular function, and (4) patient and family education.

Limiting the Initial Insult and Treating the Underlying Cause

The most effective, but often the most difficult, management strategy for HF is to limit the damage done by the initial insult. This limitation of myocardial damage and cell loss maximizes the amount of viable ventricular muscle, myocardial contractility, and overall ventricular function.

- Patient with AMI receives immediate treatment either with fibrinolytic therapy if eligible or transfer to the cardiac catheterization laboratory for primary PCI (see the previous section on acute coronary syndromes).
- Patients with persistent ischemia may benefit from revascularization as a preventive measure against eventual tissue necrosis.
- Valve replacement or repair or other surgical corrections (ventricular reconstruction surgery) is undertaken as soon as possible to prevent prolonged overstretching of the ventricular myocardium.

Management of Fluid Volume Overload

Decrease preload by administering diuretic therapy, limiting dietary sodium, and restricting free water.

- Diuretics are initiated according to the severity of the patient's signs and symptoms. More severe symptoms require intravenous therapy and loop diuretics, and less severe symptoms may be managed adequately on loop diuretics. Thiazide diuretics may be added later if the patient does not respond to the loop diuretics.

- Sodium and fluid intake are monitored carefully, with sodium not exceeding 2 g/day and free water not exceeding 1500 mL in a 24-hour period. Obtain nutrition consult to reinforce sodium and water restrictions. Educate the patient and family about restricting sodium and free water after discharge.
- Serum sodium and potassium are monitored on a regular basis to prevent inadvertent electrolyte imbalances (each day or two in the acute setting, depending on the aggressiveness of therapy).
- Use daily weights to evaluate for changes in fluid status.

Improvement of Left Ventricular Function

Improvement in left ventricular function is accomplished by decreasing the workload on the heart with preload and afterload reduction and by augmenting ventricular contractility. Ventricular function is often measured in the acute setting by monitoring CI or CO directly. As has been demonstrated by a number of large clinical trials, traditional micromanagement of hemodynamic variables, such as CI with inotropic agents, may be detrimental to long-term patient outcomes. Current recommendations do not advocate this as an initial management strategy, though short-term therapy in patients with decompensated HFrEF and low cardiac output resulting in end-organ hypoperfusion, and limited longer-term use may be appropriate.

- Decrease preload (manage fluid overload, above).
- Decrease afterload by administration of pharmacologic therapy, including ACE inhibitors and vasodilators. ACE inhibitors are recommended in all HF patients with a left ventricular EF less than 40% unless otherwise contraindicated. Contraindications to ACE inhibitor therapy include previous intolerance, potassium greater than 5.5 mEq/L, hypotension with systolic BP less than 90 mm Hg, and serum creatinine greater than 3.0 mg/dL. Cautious initiation of low-dose therapy in patients with contraindications may still be considered. Vasodilators may also be used in conjunction with diuretics and ACE inhibitors if further afterload reduction is necessary. Nitrates are often used concomitantly with ACE inhibitors and diuretics to augment afterload reduction, especially in the case of underlying atherosclerotic disease, the largest single contributor to HF. Angiotensin receptor blockers (ARBs) may be used if the patient does not tolerate the side effects of an ACE inhibitor (eg, cough).
- ACE inhibitors and beta-blockers are considered cornerstone therapy for HF in an effort to reverse the remodeling of the left ventricle. Aldosterone antagonists may be used as add-on therapy. Isosorbide

dinitrate and hydralazine may be effective, dinitrate and hydralazine may be an effective alternative. Digoxin has been shown to improve symptoms but is no longer considered to be first-line therapy unless paroxysmal atrial fibrillation or atrial flutter is present. Digoxin may be used to control the ventricular rate in this situation.

- The angiotensin receptor neprilysin inhibitors (ARNIs) are used in the management of heart failure with reduced ejection fraction. Sacubitril/valsartan (Entresto) is an example of this class of medications. It contains an ARB and a neprilysin inhibitor. The neprilysin inhibitor improves renal blood flow and promotes the loss of sodium. The ARB lowers blood pressure and reduces myocardial workload. Studies have demonstrated this medication reduces morbidity and mortality in heart failure as well as reduces hospital readmissions related to heart failure.
- Beta-blockers are also used to reduce the incidence of ventricular tachycardia (VT) and ventricular fibrillation, the most common cause of death in HF patients. Recommended beta-blockers for the management of HF include carvedilol, metoprolol, and bisoprolol. Caution is taken when initiating a beta-blocker in a patient with reactive airway disease.
- An emerging class of medications for the management of heart failure are the sodium-glucose co-transporter 2 inhibitor medications. Originally approved for patients with type II diabetes, dapagliflozin (Farxiga®) has been approved for patients with heart failure with and without diabetes because of its beneficial effect on cardiovascular outcomes. Primarily this class of medications reduce mortality and hospital readmissions in patients with heart failure. The exact mechanisms responsible for their effect are unclear and continue to be investigated. It is known that they promote diuresis/natriuresis, reduce afterload by lowering the blood pressure among several other potential effects.
- *Dual-chamber biventricular pacemaker/implantable cardioverter defibrillator (ICD):* Approximately 60% of patients with HFrEF develop LBBB. In the presence of LBBB, the right and left ventricles no longer contract simultaneously but in a series. This causes the intraventricular septum to shift inappropriately, interfering with the aortic and mitral valve functioning. There have been several studies demonstrating significantly improved outcomes (quality of life, survival rates, etc) with the use of a dual-chamber biventricular pacemaker, also called cardiac resynchronization therapy. This technology stimulates both ventricles simultaneously, causing both to contract at the same time resulting in a narrowing of the QRS complex and improved myocardial contractility and cardiac output. Often the pacing technology is combined with an ICD because sudden cardiac death related to VT/fibrillation is the most common cause of death in these patients.

- Cardiac assist devices (left ventricular, right ventricular, or both) can provide temporary maintenance or preservation of ventricular function, especially as a bridge to recovery, bridge to cardiac transplantation, or as destination therapy (discharge to home). These devices may be inserted percutaneously via the femoral artery or femoral vein, or surgically using the medial sternotomy or thoracotomy approach (see Chapter 19, Advanced Cardiovascular Concepts). Left ventricular apical cannulation allows ambulation and physical rehabilitation. Technological developments have contributed to the development of small axial flow pumps allowing many to be implanted with the drive line (power source) exiting the skin. Risks related to insertion of these devices include infection, peripheral embolization including stroke, and, for some, long-term weaning difficulties in the event that an organ donor is not available. At the time of this writing, the HeartMate 3™™ and HeartWare™ are approved for destination therapy (eg, a replacement for heart transplant).
- *Intra-aortic balloon pump (IABP):* Femoral or axillary artery cannulation with the IABP allows for ventricular support, but restricts the patient to bed rest (femoral primarily) and compromises arterial flow to the cannulated limb. (For more on IABP, see Chapter 19, Advanced Cardiovascular Concepts.)
- *Minimally invasive catheter-based micro-axial flow VADs:* These (Impella® or TandemHeart®) are frequently used to reduce either right or left ventricular afterload and myocardial work. They may be inserted through the femoral or axillary artery across the aortic valve into the left ventricle or are introduced via the femoral vein into the right atrium and through an atrial septostomy, and positioned in the left atrium for left ventricular support. For right ventricular support, the device is advanced from the femoral vein into the right atrium and out into the pulmonary artery. As with the IABP, if the access is via the femoral artery, the patient is restricted to bed rest.
- *Ventricular reconstruction:* Many patients with end-stage HF have a previous history of coronary artery disease and MI, resulting in the development of a ventricular aneurysm on the anterior wall of the left ventricle. A surgical procedure can be performed removing the aneurysm, reducing the size of the ventricle, resulting in increased contractility and cardiac output. Studies have shown that some patients experience improvement in physical functioning and NYHA functional class following this procedure.
- *Extracorporeal membrane oxygenation (ECMO):* ECMO is also a treatment for severely decompensated heart failure patients who are in cardiogenic shock. This is used as a bridge to recovery, a bridge to a VAD, or a bridge to transplant. The use of this technology is limited to ICU settings with access to resources that can provide it.

Patient Education

Patients who present with HF to the critical care unit have high acuity levels, require more intensive interventions, and have an increased need for emotional support surrounding the serious nature of the hospital admission. Previous admissions for HF make patients more aware of the serious nature of acute episodes. Patient education, which is appropriately addressed in the acute care setting, includes the following:

- Both patient and family may require crisis interventions. The nurse may help by encouraging the verbalization of fears related to role adaptations or changes in family responsibility, lifestyle alterations and limitations, and death and dying. The completion of advanced directives and discussion of goals of care are initiated if not previously addressed.
- Family involvement in the critical care phase is strongly encouraged, including assistance with activities of daily living such as bathing, and "patterning" of daily activities to allow for frequent periods of rest and spacing of exertional activity. In addition, family involvement in reading or other leisure activity with the patient is often restful and relaxing, and may be useful as a diversional activity. If possible, the family is also present for reinforcement of patient teaching regarding the medical regimen, the importance of fluid and sodium restriction, and the need for daily weights.

Shock

Shock is the inability of the circulatory system to deliver enough blood to meet the oxygen and metabolic requirements of body tissues. This clinical syndrome may result from ineffective pumping of the heart (cardiogenic shock), insufficient volume of circulating blood (hypovolemic shock), or massive vasodilation of the vascular bed causing maldistribution of blood (distributive shock). Although strategies for patient management vary according to the underlying pathophysiology, the basic definition of shock as ineffective or insufficient oxygen delivery to meet the needs of body tissues remains consistent.

Etiology, Risk Factors, and Pathophysiology

The ineffective delivery of oxygen to the tissues leads to cellular dysfunction, rapidly progressing to organ failure, and finally to total body system failure. The cause of the initial onset of the shock syndrome may be from any number of underlying problems, including heart problems, fluid loss, and trauma. Because the body responds in the same way, differences between cardiogenic, hypovolemic, and distributive shock are obvious to the clinician only after the initial assessment has provided key information about the patient's acute illness. Given the history and physical examination

TABLE 9-11. CAUSES OF CARDIOGENIC SHOCK

Coronary Causes
- MI with resultant cell death in a significant portion of the ventricle
- Rupture of ventricle or papillary muscle secondary to MI
- Dysfunctional ischemic—"shock ventricle"—which occurs as a result of myocardial ischemia, not involving cell death, and is therefore transient

Noncoronary Causes
- Myocardial contusion
- Pericardial tamponade
- Ventricular rupture
- Arrhythmia (PEA—pulseless electrical activity)
- Valvular dysfunction resulting in ventricular congestion
- Cardiomyopathies
- End-stage HF

TABLE 9-12. CAUSES OF HYPOVOLEMIC SHOCK

Sources of External Loss of Body Fluid
- Hemorrhage (loss of whole blood)
- Gastrointestinal tract (vomiting, diarrhea, ostomies, fistulas, nasogastric suctioning)
- Renal (diuretic administration, diabetes, insipidus, Addison disease, hyperglycemic osmotic diuresis)

Sources of Internal Loss of Body Fluid
- Internal hemorrhage
- Movement of body fluid into interstitial spaces ("third spacing," often the result of bacterial toxin, thermal injury, or allergic reaction)

data, the clinician can classify shock into one of three major pathologic groups and proceed to further determine the patient's needs with the help of diagnostic testing. Interventions to treat shock are directed at the cause, so identifying the underlying pathophysiology is an essential step.

Cardiogenic Shock

In cardiogenic shock, the heart is unable to pump enough blood to meet the oxygen and metabolic needs of the body. Pump failure is caused by a variety of factors, the most common being coronary artery disease involving a larger portion of the ventricles. A number of other factors may cause pump failure, however, and are typically categorized as coronary or noncoronary causes (Table 9-11).

In all cardiogenic shock cases, the heart ceases to function effectively as a pump, resulting in decreases in stroke volume and cardiac output. This leads to a decrease in blood

pressure and tissue perfusion. The inadequate emptying of the ventricle increases left atrial pressure, which then increases pulmonary venous pressure. As a result, pulmonary capillary pressure increases, resulting in pulmonary edema.

Hypovolemic Shock

Hypovolemic shock occurs when there is inadequate volume in the vascular space. This volume depletion may be caused by blood loss, either internal or external, or by the vascular fluid volume shifting out of the vascular space into other body fluid spaces (Table 9-12). The loss of vascular volume results in insufficient circulating blood to maintain tissue perfusion.

The pathophysiology of hypovolemic shock is related directly to decreased circulating blood volume. When an insufficient amount of blood is circulating, the venous blood returning to the heart is insufficient. As a result, right and left ventricular filling pressures are insufficient, decreasing stroke volume and cardiac output. As in cardiogenic shock, when cardiac output is decreased, BP is low and tissue perfusion is poor.

ESSENTIAL CONTENT CASE

Shock Following AMI

A 49-year-old man was found slumped in his living room chair, cool and clammy but still breathing. His wife called 911. The EMS transported him to the local emergency room. On arrival, his vital signs were as follows:

BP	68/44 mm Hg
HR	122 beats/min
RR	33 breaths/min
T	36.1°C, orally
Sao_2	91%

Oxygen at 60% by facemask had been initiated in flight, as well as intravenous normal saline running wide open, 450 mL having already been infused. Norepinephrine was started at a rate of 0.05 mcg/kg/min. A stat ECG showed "tombstone" ST elevation in the anterior leads (V2, V3, V4), with reciprocal changes in leads II, III, and a VF. The patient was taken for immediate PTCA. On arrival to the cardiac catheterization lab, a pulmonary artery catheter

was inserted followed by a cardiac catheterization. Findings from the catheterization were as follows:

LAD	99% proximal lesion
RCA	70% mid lesion
LCx	Normal
LVEF	13%
Wall motion	Left ventricular akinesis

An angioplasty with a drug-eluting stent was deployed to the proximal LAD and another to the mid-RCA. Following the procedure, the patient was admitted to the ICU.

On arrival to the ICU, the nurse obtained hemodynamic parameters as follows:

PA	45/25 mm Hg
RA	15 mm Hg
PAOP	22 mm Hg
CO	4.0 L/min
CI	1.5 L/min/m²

Case Question 1: What is the most likely cause of the patient's shock?
(A) Hypovolemic
(B) Distributive
(C) Cardiogenic
(D) Neurogenic

Case Question 2: What will be the primary goal caring for this patient after PCI?
(A) Reduce myocardial workload
(B) Dilate the pulmonary vascular bed
(C) Administer a diuretic
(D) Intubate the patient to improve oxygen delivery

Case Question 3: You anticipate the next intervention for this patient will be:

(A) Initiate a vasodilator to reduce afterload
(B) Give volume to improve preload
(C) Titrate the dopamine infusion up to 7.5 mcg/kg/min
(D) Insertion of an intra-aortic balloon

Answers
1. C is the correct answer. Based on his clinical presentation and the "tombstone" ECG changes, he has had an anterior wall infarction and is in cardiogenic shock.
2. A is the correct answer. The primary goal is to reduce myocardial workload allowing the heart to recover.
3. D is the correct answer. Based on the low cardiac output, insertion of an IABP will help reduce his cardiac workload and improve coronary perfusion. Giving volume at this point is not necessary and dopamine may cause his heart to work harder.

Distributive Shock

Distributive shock is characterized by an abnormal placement or distribution of vascular volume. There are three primary causes of distributive shock: (1) sepsis, (2) neurologic damage, and (3) anaphylaxis. In each of these situations, the pumping function of the heart and the total blood volume are normal, but the blood is not appropriately distributed throughout the vascular bed. Massive vasodilation occurs in each of these situations for various reasons, causing the vascular bed to be much larger than normal. In this enlarged vascular bed, the usual volume of circulating blood (approximately 5 L) is no longer sufficient to fill the vascular space, causing a decrease in BP and inadequate tissue perfusion. For this reason, distributive shock is also referred to as *relative hypovolemic shock*.

Of the distributive shock syndromes, septic shock is most commonly seen in the critical care setting. In the field or emergency department setting, anaphylaxis and neurogenic shock are also common and typically result from allergic reactions and trauma-related spinal cord injury.

Stages of Shock

Regardless of underlying etiology, all three types of shock (cardiogenic, hypovolemic, and distributive) activate the sympathetic nervous system, which in turn initiates neural, hormonal, and chemical compensatory mechanisms in an attempt to improve tissue perfusion (Figure 9-16). Cellular changes that occur as a result of these compensatory mechanisms are similar in all types of shock. Progression of these cellular changes follows a predictable, four-stage course.

Initial Stage

The initial stage of shock represents the first cellular changes resulting from the decrease in oxygen delivery to the tissue. These changes include decreased aerobic and increased anaerobic metabolism, leading to increases in serum lactic acid. No obvious clinical signs and symptoms are apparent during this stage of shock.

Compensatory Stage

The compensatory stage is composed of a number of physiologic events that represent an attempt to compensate for decreases in cardiac output and restore adequate oxygen and nutrient delivery to the tissues (Figure 9-17). These events can be organized into neural, hormonal, and chemical responses. The neural response involves the baroreceptors in the aortic arch and carotid arteries, detecting changes in the arterial BP, and responding by activating the vasomotor center of the medulla. Hypovolemia and resultant hypotension lead to activation of the sympathetic nervous system. The sympathetic nervous system initiates compensatory mechanisms causing peripheral vasoconstriction and elevation of the BP. Vasoconstriction of the peripheral circulation shunts blood to vital organs (autoregulation), reducing renal blood flow, which activates the hormonal response.

Hormonal responses include increased production of catecholamines and adrenocorticotropic hormone (ACTH) and activation of the RAAS. As a direct result of decreased renal blood flow, renin is released from the juxtaglomerular cells in the kidney, combining with angiotensinogen from the liver resulting in the production of angiotensin I. Angiotensin I, circulating in the blood, is converted to angiotensin II in the lungs. As was discussed in more detail in the HF section, this hormonal response results in direct peripheral vasoconstriction, in addition to release of aldosterone from the adrenal cortex and antidiuretic hormone (ADH) from the pituitary gland. Sodium and potassium retention, in conjunction with increased ADH, ACTH, and circulating catecholamines, effectively increases intravascular volume, heart rate, and BP, and decreases urine output.

Chemical responses during the compensatory stage are related to the respiratory ventilation-perfusion imbalance, which occurs as a result of sympathetic stimulation, redistribution of blood flow, and decreased pulmonary perfusion. A respiratory alkalosis ensues, adversely affecting the patient's level of consciousness and causing restlessness and agitation.

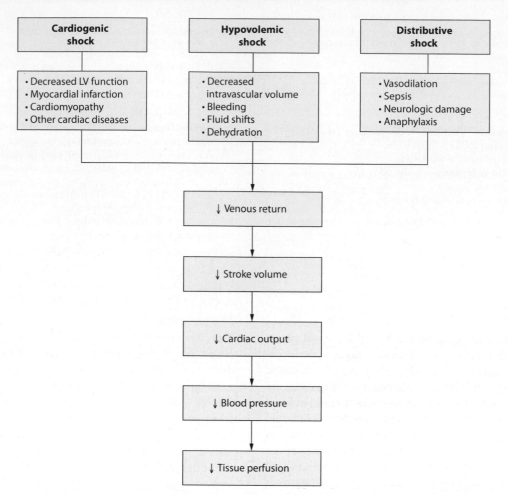

Figure 9-16. Pathophysiology of shock.

These compensatory mechanisms are effective for finite periods of time, which may vary depending on the individual and presence of comorbidities. Younger and healthier patients are more likely to survive a prolonged episode of shock. In the absence of vascular volume replacement, these intrinsic vasopressors eventually fail as a compensatory mechanism, and the patient enters the progressive, and finally refractory, stages of shock, usually resulting in death.

Progressive Stage

The progressive stage is characterized by end-organ failure due to cellular damage from prolonged compensatory changes. The compensatory changes, which supported BP and therefore tissue perfusion, are no longer effective and severe hypoperfusion ensues. Impaired oxygen delivery to the tissues results in multi-organ system failure, typically beginning with gastrointestinal and renal failure, followed by respiratory and/or cardiac failure and loss of liver and cerebral function (see Chapter 11, Multisystem Problems, for more on sepsis).

Refractory Stage

The refractory stage, as its name implies, is the irreversible stage of shock. At this stage, cell death has progressed to such a point as to be irreparable, and death is imminent.

Clinical Presentation

Clinical signs and symptoms vary, depending on the underlying cause of shock and the stage of shock in which the patient presents.

Initial stage: No visible signs and symptoms evident from ongoing cellular changes

Compensatory stage:

- Consciousness: Restless, agitated, confused
- Blood pressure: Normal or slightly low
- Heart rate: Increased (though neurogenic distributive shock leads to bradycardia)
- Respiratory rate: Increased (> 20 breaths/min)
- Skin: Cool, clammy, may be cyanotic—though massive vasodilation in distributive shock may make these signs absent
- Peripheral pulses: Weak and thready
- Urine output: Concentrated and scant (<30 mL/h)
- Bowel sounds: Hypoactive, possible abdominal distension
- Laboratory results:
  - Glucose: Increased
  - Sodium: Increased
  - Pao_2: Decreased
  - $Paco_2$: Decreased
  - pH: Increased

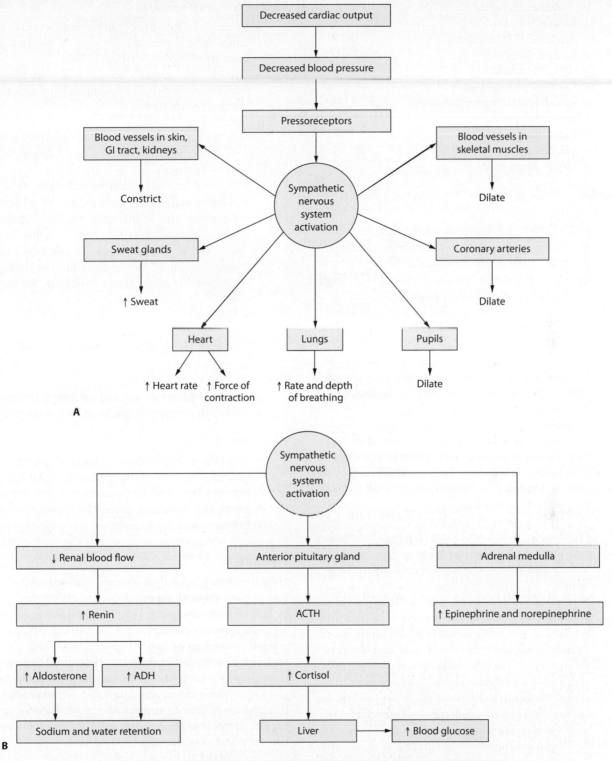

Figure 9-17. Compensatory response to shock. **(A)** Neural compensation. **(B)** Hormonal compensation.

Progressive stage:
- Consciousness: Unresponsive to verbal stimuli
  - Blood pressure: Inadequate (<90 mm Hg systolic)
  - Heart rate: Increased (>90 beats/min)
  - Respiratory rate: Increased, shallow
- Skin: Cold, cyanotic, mottled
- Peripheral pulses: Weak and thready, may be absent
- Urine output: Scant (<20 mL/h) and concentrated
- Bowel sounds: Absent
- Laboratory results:

- Amylase: Increased
- Lipase: Increased
- SGPT/SGOT: Increased
- Lactate: Increased
- CPK: Increased
- Creatinine: Increased
- Blood urea nitrogen: Increased
- Pao_2: Decreased
- $Paco_2$: Increased
- pH: Decreased
- HCO_3: Decreased

Diagnostic Tests

Cardiogenic

- ECG: Tachycardia, ventricular tachycardia, ventricular fibrillation, and underlying atrial fibrillation/flutter/heart block that contribute to shock
- Pulmonary arterial pressure: PAD/PAOP high (>12 mm Hg), RAP high (>8 mm Hg)
- Echocardiogram: Ventricular wall motion abnormalities, cardiac tamponade, ventricular rupture, valve disease
- Physical findings, in addition to the above: faint S1, S2, presence of S3-S4, a narrow pulse pressure, jugular venous distention, crackles in the lungs, and peripheral edema

Hypovolemia

- Presence of bleeding such as frank blood or black tarry stools, hematemesis, or saturated dressings.
- Risk factors for bleeding such as recent surgery or trauma, liver disease, NSAID use, or other risks for gastrointestinal bleeding
- Pulmonary arterial pressure: PAD/PAOP low (<8 mm Hg), RAP low (<5 mm Hg), right ventricular end-diastolic volume index low
- Ultrasound: Groin or retroperitoneal hemorrhage

Distributive

- Septic: WBC ≥ 12,000 or ≤ 4000, neutrophils > 10%, serum lactate > 4 mmol/L, positive blood cultures (in 50% of patients). Risk factors for septic shock include immunocompromised state and the presence or recent use of invasive devices (urinary catheter, endotracheal tube, central line)
- Anaphylactic: Arterial blood gas shows inadequate oxygenation history of allergen exposure, and ABG shows inadequate oxygenation
- Neurogenic: Computed tomography (CT) scan and magnetic resonance imaging (MRI) show spinal cord damage

Principles of Management for Shock

Differences in the underlying cause of shock lead to some variation in the principles of management. The basic goals of therapy for all forms of shock, however, include the need to correct the underlying cause of shock, improvement of oxygenation, and restoration of adequate tissue perfusion.

Correction of the Underlying Cause of Shock

- *Cardiogenic:* Remove coronary obstruction or correct tamponade, if present, and support ventricular contractility to increase cardiac output.
- *Hypovolemic:* Identify source and stop bleeding if possible; correct fluid shunting or third spacing with electrolyte management.
- *Distributive*
  - *Anaphylactic:* Intubate for oxygenation and treat the underlying allergic reaction using antidote or steroid therapy.
  - *Septic:* Administer fluid resuscitation, draw blood cultures and serum lactate; give broad-spectrum antibiotics and 30 mL/kg of fluid for hypotension; begin vasopressors if patient remains hypotensive; identify likely sources of infection including consideration of any invasive lines or devices (see Chapter 11, Multisystem Problems, for more on sepsis).
  - *Neurogenic:* Severing of the cord may be irreversible; however, intubation provides respiratory support while the underlying cause is identified.

Improve Oxygenation

- Assess for patent airway and intubate if necessary
- Administer oxygen to maintain Pao_2 > 60-70 mm Hg

Restore Adequate Tissue Perfusion

- Administer fluid volume expanders (normal saline, lactated Ringers solution, or plasmanate) in large rapid boluses. Type and cross-match for blood type and administer blood as necessary for hypovolemic shock.
- Initiate vasoactive therapy.

Hypertension

Hypertension is typically a chronic disease of BP elevation that is often masked, especially in the early years of onset, by lack of warning signs or symptoms. Hypertensive crisis is an acute episode or exacerbation, occurring infrequently in a small percentage of hypertensive patients and characterized by the pivotal effect the particular episode and its treatment may have on the patient's long-term outcome. In most cases, the numerical or absolute value of the arterial BP is less important than its impact on the individual's underlying risk of target organ damage, specifically cerebrovascular, coronary, and renal diseases.

Etiology, Risk Factors, and Pathophysiology

A number of clinical features are commonly associated with hypertension and many underlying etiologies may contribute to the progression of hypertensive disease. Modifiable risk factors include diabetes, smoking, dyslipidemia, obesity, and a sedentary lifestyle. While many patients have primary hypertension, sleep apnea and renal artery stenosis are two specific underlying conditions that can be treated to improve blood pressure management. The pathophysiology of hypertension is similar regardless of the underlying cause.

An acute hypertensive crisis begins with elevation of the systolic or diastolic BP causing a threat, direct or indirect, to an organ or body system. Acute, severe increases in pressure may cause serious, life-threatening cerebrovascular and cardiovascular compromise. Prolonged hypoperfusion of an organ system leads to ischemia, necrosis, and organ system failure.

Classification

Because of the increased risk of such events in all hypertensive patients, morbidity and mortality directly related to hypertension is high, and long-term, consistent therapy in all stages of hypertension is necessary. Hypertension can be described in stages or classified according to the value of the blood pressure (Table 9-13).

- *Elevated blood pressure:* Current guidelines define an elevated blood pressure as a SBP 120-129 and DBP < 80 mm Hg.
- *Stage 1 hypertension:* Hypertension characterized by an elevated SBP 130-139 mm Hg systolic or 80-89 mm Hg diastolic, in adults.
- *Stage 2 hypertension:* Hypertension is defined as a systolic BP ≥ 140 mm Hg or a diastolic BP ≥ 90 mm Hg.
- *Hypertensive crisis:* Hypertensive crisis is subdivided into "Urgencies" and "Emergencies." Hypertensive urgency is characterized by a systolic BP > 180 mm Hg and/or a diastolic BP > 120 mm Hg. Underlying pathophysiology, worsening primary hypertension, and nonadherence to antihypertensive therapy are all possible causes of hypertensive urgency. In addition, hypertensive crisis may occur in patients without a prior diagnosis of hypertension. Patients with hypertensive urgency do not have clinical evidence of new or worsening target organ damage. Hypertensive emergency is defined by a systolic BP > 180 mm Hg associated with target end-organ damage and/or a diastolic BP > 120 mm Hg associated with target end-organ damage. Both conditions require immediate intervention to lower blood pressure.
- *Special populations:* In pregnant women and in children, a less severe elevation in BP may result in significant end-organ damage and is therefore considered to be a "hypertensive crisis" at values much

lower than would be expected to be problematic in the average adult. The absolute value of the BP varies significantly depending on the situation and the individual involved; for example, preeclampsia, considered to be a hypertensive crisis in pregnancy, may occur at pressures as low as 130/100 to 160/100 mm Hg.

Clinical Presentation

Patients experiencing a hypertensive crisis may present with the following signs and symptoms.

- Headache
- Blurred vision
- Nosebleed
- Dizziness or vertigo
- Transient neurological changes such as change in speech or sensation, consistent with a transient ischemic attack (TIA)
- Chest or back pain indicating possible MI, or aortic dissection
- Shortness of breath, which may indicate pulmonary edema
- Fatigue, malaise, or generalized weakness
- Nausea and vomiting which may indicate elevated intracranial pressure
- Hematuria and dysuria

Physical examination of the patient with hypertensive crisis includes the following:

- Neurological exam: focal deficits may indicate a presence of stroke
- Cardiac exam: Diminished peripheral pulses or bruits, Carotid or abdominal bruit, Heart sounds with S3 and/or S4, systolic and/or diastolic murmurs
- Signs of gastrointestinal bleeding
- Respiratory exam; adventitious sounds consistent with pulmonary edema
- Funduscopic findings: Arteriovenous thickening, arteriolar narrowing, hemorrhage, papilledema, or exudates

Diagnostic Tests

- Computed tomography: of the brain to evaluate for stroke or head injury
- Computed tomography of the chest if aortic dissection is suspected
- Chest x-ray: Myocardial hypertrophy, pulmonary infiltrates
- Specific tests to target organ damage
  - Renal angiography
  - Coronary angiography
  - Carotid/cerebral angiography
- MRI: for further evaluation of cerebral vascular malperfusion
- Medication and substance use history may help determine the cause of hypertensive crisis

TABLE 9-13. CLASSIFICATION OF BLOOD PRESSURE FOR ADULTS

Blood Pressure Classification	SBP (mm Hg)	DBP (mm Hg)
Normal	< 120	And < 80
Elevated	120-129	< 80
Stage 1 hypertension	130-139	80-89
Stage 2 hypertension	≥ 140	≥ 90

Abbreviations: DBP, diastolic blood pressure; mm Hg, millimeters of mercury; SBP, systolic blood pressure.

Principles of Management for Hypertension

Management of the patient with acute exacerbation of hypertension, or hypertensive crisis, revolves around three primary objectives: (1) accurate arterial blood pressure measurement, (2) reduction of arterial pressure, and (3) preparation and planning for continuous and consistent outpatient follow-up.

Ascertain accurate arterial blood pressure measurement

Verify arterial BP, being sure to assess bilateral measurements with the correct cuff size if using sphygmomanometer, as well as orthostatic pressures if possible (lying and sitting up, if standing is not possible). Each measurement is 2 minutes apart and both right and left measurements are documented. If differences between the right and left measurements are greater than 10 mm Hg, the higher reading is used to gauge therapy. In most acute situations, priority is given to establishing a stable arterial access site for direct, invasive monitoring of BP (see Chapter 4, Hemodynamic Monitoring).

Initiate pharmacologic intervention

For acute high arterial pressure, intravenous pharmacologic intervention is the fastest, most effective means of reducing arterial BP. Several agents are used in the acute setting for management of hypertensive crisis (Table 9-14). Pharmacologic choices are based on the severity of BP elevation (immediate risk of stroke), the immediate risk of irreversible target organ damage (renal and hepatic function related to medication metabolism and clearance also is considered), and any confounding conditions or risk factors that are present (eg, the fetus in preeclampsia).

Immediate risks associated with hypertensive encephalopathy include dissecting aortic aneurysm, MI, or intracranial hemorrhage. Acute, severe hypertensive crises require urgent treatment at an appropriate pace to avoid rapid reduction that leads to ischemia. Guidelines recommend reducing the blood pressure by 25% in the first hour, and then to 160/100-110 over the subsequent 2 to 6 hours, before seeking a normal range in the following 1 to 2 days. These parameters and timeframes may be adjusted based on the patient's underlying pathology. For instance, patients with aortic dissection, severe preeclampsia, or pheochromocytoma may require more rapid blood pressure reduction, whereas treatment for hypertensive urgency in a patient with acute ischemic stroke may be more moderate, as a sudden drop

---

ESSENTIAL CONTENT CASE

Thinking Critically

A 52-year-old man, 4 days post anterior MI, is just transferred into the ICU from the general medical floor with severe shortness of breath. The initial assessment reveals the following:

HR	128 beats/min
BP	110/82 mm Hg
RR	36 breaths/min
T	37.6°C, orally
Pulse oximetry	88%
Lung sounds	Coarse, bilateral crackles in lower lobes, poor respiratory effort
Heart sounds	S1, S2, S3
Skin	Flushed, diaphoretic, 2+ pedal edema
ECG	Sinus tachycardia, with tall R-waves in V5-V6 indicating left ventricular hypertrophy

Case Question 1: What is the first priority in the care of this patient?
(A) Obtain an arterial blood gas measurement
(B) Initiate a furosemide infusion
(C) Prepare to administer high-flow oxygen
(D) Call a Code Blue

Case Question 2: What is the most likely underlying cause for this patient's respiratory compromise?
(A) Acute decompensated heart failure with pulmonary edema
(B) Abrupt onset of septic shock with adult respiratory distress syndrome
(C) Acute anxiety attack
(D) Hypovolemic shock

Case Question 3: Medical management of this situation would most likely include what interventions?
(1) Administration of a diuretic to reduce preload
(2) Initiation of a dobutamine infusion at 5 mcg/kg/min
(3) Consideration for mechanical support
(4) Consideration for intubation and ventilator support

(A) 1 and 3
(B) 1 and 2
(C) 3 and 4
(D) All of the above

Answers
1. C is the correct answer. Administration of high-flow oxygen provides higher oxygen delivery rates and may avoid the need for intubation. Higher oxygen delivery is necessary based on his high respiratory rate (36/min breaths) and pulse oximetry of 88%. Calling a Code Blue at this time is not necessary. Obtaining an arterial blood gas following intubation is recommended.
2. A is the correct answer. Given his recent anterior MI, decompensated heart failure and acute pulmonary edema is the most likely cause of his respiratory distress.
3. B is the correct answer. The diuretic will help reduce preload and pulmonary congestion. Dobutamine will improve myocardial contractility and improve cardiac output.

in atrial pressure can lead to cerebrovascular compromise. Other organ systems dependent on higher pressure for perfusion include the renal and coronary systems. A sudden, severe drop in systemic arterial pressure may result in ischemic episodes or acute renal failure.

For nonacute hypertension, dietary alteration and relaxation or biofeedback techniques may be used in addition to pharmacologic measures to reduce the morbidity and mortality of hypertension. Although these measures are most effective when employed long term as part of a cohesive outpatient follow-up program, initiating these strategies in the acute setting may help emphasize their importance.

Patient Education on Lifestyle Modification and Follow-up
Following control of hypertension in the acute phase, patient education is initiated regarding the serious and chronic nature of the disease. Target organs typically at risk include the brain, heart, kidneys, and eyes. Patients need to be aware to self-monitor for signs and symptoms of stroke or acute MI and to seek emergency care when symptoms occur. In addition, evaluation of kidney function in collaboration with a primary care provider is essential as it impacts the selection of antihypertensive agents. Patients can also self-monitor for visual changes that may indicate worsening hypertension.

Often, the clinician may have an opportunity in the acute stage to make an impact regarding the seriousness of uncontrolled hypertension and its potentially debilitating effects. Prior to beginning the educational process, assessment includes:

1. Family history of hypertension, cardiovascular disease, coronary artery disease, stroke, diabetes mellitus, and hyperlipidemia.
2. Lifestyle history including weight gain, exercise, and smoking habits.
3. Dietary patterns including high sodium, alcohol, and dietary fat intake or low-potassium intake.
4. Knowledge of hypertension and impact of previous medical therapy for hypertension (adherence, side effects, results, or efficacy).

TABLE 9-14. COMMON DRUGS USED TO MANAGE ACUTE HYPERTENSIVE EPISODES

Nitroprusside	• Dilates arterioles and veins • Administer IV at 0.5 to 10.0 mcg/kg/min (mix in normal saline only; 100 mg in 500 mL). Cover bottle with foil to avoid light exposure • Titrate up to desired BP, recognizing that the effect will be evident within 1 minute of change in dose
Nicardipine	• Calcium channel blocker • Administer 5 mg/h initially, titrate 2.5 mg/h at 5- to 15-minute intervals to a maximum dose of 15 mg/h
Nitroglycerin	• Dilates veins more than arterioles • Administer IV at a rate of 5 to 100 mcg/min. Maximum 100 mg in 100 mL NS or D_5 IV
Esmolol	• Beta-1 selective blocker and at higher doses inhibits B2 receptors in the blood vessels • Useful for treating hypertension • Administer 0.5 mg/kg over 1-minute loading dose followed by 50 mcg/kg/min infusion • Titrate to achieve desired lower BP • Onset of action within minutes • Peak effect in less than 5 minutes
Enalapril	• An ACE inhibitor • Administer IV at a rate of 5 mg/min
Labetalol	• Beta-receptor agonist (beta-blocker) • Particularly indicated in patients with suspected MI or angina • Administer 5 mg bolus over 5 minutes and repeat three times. IV drip may then be started
Clevidipine	• Calcium channel blocker/dihydropyridine • Dilates arterioles • Administer via infusion starting with 1-2 mg/h • Double dose every 90 seconds initially • Increase dose by less doubling when blood pressure goal is reached • Then increase time between adjustments to every 5-10 minutes • Maintenance infusion at 4-5 mg/h not to exceed 21 mg/h • Onset of action immediately

SELECTED BIBLIOGRAPHY

General Cardiovascular

Morton PG, Fontaine DK. *Critical Care Nursing: A Holistic Approach.* 11th ed. Philadelphia, PA: Wolters Kluwer; 2017.

Pickett JD, Bridges E, Kritek PA, Whitney JD. Passive leg-raising and prediction of fluid responsiveness: systematic review. *Crit Care Nurse.* 2017;37(2):32-47.

Sandau KE, Funk M, Auerbach A, et al. Update to practice standards for electrocardiographic monitoring in hospital settings: A scientific statement from the American Heart Association. *Circulation.* 2017;136:e273-e344. doi: 10.1161/CIR.0000000000000527

Zipes DP, Libby P, Bonow RO, Mann DL, eds. *Braunwald' Heart Disease: A Textbook of Cardiovascular Medicine.* 11th ed. Philadelphia, PA: Saunders Elsevier; 2018.

Coronary Revascularization

Anjum I, Khan MA, Aadil M, et al. Transradial vs transfemoral approach in cardiac catheterization: A literature review. *Cureus.* 2017;9(6):e1309. doi: 10.7759/cureus.1309

Hardin S, Kaplow R. *Cardiac Surgery Essentials for Critical Care Nursing.* 3rd ed. Sudbury, MA: Jones & Bartlett Publishing; 2020.

Lawton JS, Tamis-Holland JE, Sripal Bangalore et al. 2021 ACC/AHA/SCAI guideline for coronary artery revascularization: executive summary: a report of the American College of Cardiology/American Heart Association Joint Committee on Clinical Practice Guidelines. *J Am Coll Cardiol.* 2022;79(2):197-215. doi: 10.1016/j.jacc.2021.09.005

Levine GN, Bittl JA. Focused Update on Primary Percutaneous Coronary Intervention for Patients With ST-Elevation Myocardial Infarction. *JAMA Cardiol.* 2016;1(2):226–227. doi:10.1001/jamacardio.2016.0178

Acute Coronary Syndromes

Carey MG. Acute coronary syndrome and ST segment monitoring. *Crit Care Nurs Clin North Am.* 2016;(3):347-356.

Giustino G, Pinney SP, Anuradha L, et al. Coronovirus and cardiovascular disease, myocardial injury and ischemia. *JACC.* 2020;76(17):2011-2023.

Pelter MM, Kozik TM, Al-Zaiti SS, Carey MC. Differential diagnoses for suspected ACS. *Am J Crit Care.* 2016;25(4):377-378.

Sandoval Y, Fred S. Apple FS, Mahler, SA, et al. High-sensitivity cardiac troponin and the 2021 AHA/ACC/ASE/CHEST/SAEM/SCCT/SCMR guidelines for the evaluation and diagnosis of acute chest pain. *Circulation.* 2022;146:569-581

Thygesen K, Alpert JS, Jaffe AS, et al. Fourth universal definition of myocardial infarction (2018). *Circulation.* 2018;138:e618-e651.

Heart Failure

Albert NM. Right-sided heart failure. *American Nurse Journal.* 2021;16(5):6-11.

Beattie JM, Higginson IJ, McDonagh TA. Palliative care in acute heart failure. *Current Heart Failure Reports.* 2020;17:424-437.

Bloom MW, Greenberg B, Jaarsma T, Jaruzzi JL, et al. Heart failure with a reduced ejection fraction. *Nature Reviews: Disease Primer* 2017;3:17058.

Cross SH, Kamal AH, Taylor DH, Warraich HJ. Hospice use among patients with heart failure. *Cardiac Failure Review.* 20195(2):93-98.

Doty D. Ventricular assist device and destination therapy candidates from preoperative selection through end of hospitalization. *Crit Care Nurs Clin North Am.* 2015;27(4):551-564.

Fryer ML, Balsam LB. Mechanical circulatory support for cardiogenic shock in the critically ill. *Chest.* 2019;156(5):1001021.

Good VS, Kirkwood PL. *Advanced Critical Care Nursing,* 2nd ed. St Louis: Elsevier, 2018, pp 60-90.

Kitko L, McIlvennan CK, Bidwell JT, et al. Family Caregiving for individuals with heart failure: a scientific statement from the American Heart Association. *Circulation.* 2020;141(22):e864-e878. doi: 10.1161/CIR.0000000000000768

Lee CS, Auld J. Heart failure: a primer. *Crit Care Nurs Clin North Am.* 2015;27(4):413-425.

Leeper B. Right ventricular failure. *AACN Advanced Critical Care.* 2020;21(1):49-56.

Lopaschuk GD, Verma S. Mechanisms of cardiovascular benefits of sodium glucose co-transporter 2 (SGLT-2) inhibitors. *J Am Coll Cardiol.* 2020;5(6):632-644.

McCulloch B. Heart failure and atrial fibrillation. *Crit Care Nurs Clin North Am.* 2015;27(4):427-438.

Hypertension

Taylor DA. Hypertensive crisis: a review of pathophysiology and treatment. *Crit Care Nurs Clin North Am.* 2015;27(4):439-448.

Evidence-Based Practice Guidelines

Accurate dysrhythmia monitoring in adults. *Crit Care Nurse.* 2016;36(6):e26-e34. doi: 10.4037/ccn2016767

American Association of Critical-Care Nurses. *AACN Practice Alert: Ensuring Accurate ST-Segment Monitoring.* Aliso Viejo, CA: American Association of Critical-Care Nurses; 2016, December. Updated 5/17/2018, https://www.aacn.org/clinical-resources/practice-alerts/st-segment-monitoring

American Association of Critical-Care Nurses. AACN practice alert: obtaining accurate noninvasive blood pressure measurements in adults. *Crit Care Nurse.* 2016;36(3):e12-e16. Updated 5/1/2021 online at: https://www.aacn.org/clinical-resources/practice-alerts/obtaining-accurate-noninvasive-blood-pressure-measurements-in-adults

Amsterdam EA, Wenger NK, Brindis RG, et al. 2014 AHA/ACC guideline for the management of patients with non-ST-elevation acute coronary syndromes: executive summary: a report from the American College of Cardiology/American Heart Association Task Force on Practice Guidelines. *Circulation.* 2014;130(25):2354-2394.

Evans L, Rhodes A, Alhazzani W, et al. Surviving Sepsis Campaign: International Guidelines for Management of Sepsis and Septic Shock 2021. *Crit Care Med.* 2021;49(11):e1063-e1143. doi:10.1097/CCM.0000000000005337

Heidenreich PA, Bozkurt B, Aguilar D, et al. AHA/ACC/HFSA guideline for management of Heart Failure: A report of the American College of Cardiology/American Heart Association Joint Committee on Clinical Practice Guidelines. *Circulation.* 2022;145(18):e895-e1032.

Hillis LD, Smith PK, Anderson JL, et al. 2011 ACCF/AHA guidelines for coronary artery bypass surgery: executive summary: a report of the American College of Cardiology Foundation/American Heart Association Task Force on Practice Guidelines. *Circulation.* 2011;124(23):e652-e735.

James PA, Oparil S, Carter BL, et al. 2014 evidenced-based guideline for the management of high blood pressure in adults. Report from the panel members appointed to the Eighth Joint National Committee (JNC8). *JAMA.* 2014;311(5):507-520. doi:10.1001/jama.2013.284427, December 18, 2013.

Neumann FJ, Sousa-Uva M, Ahisson A, et al. 2018 ESC/EATS Guidelines of myocardial revascularization. *European Heart Journal.* 2019;40:87-165.

O'Gara PT, Kushner FG, Ascheim DD, et al. 2013 ACCF/AHA guidelines for the management of ST-elevation myocardial infarction: executive summary: a report of the American College of Cardiology Foundation/American Heart Association Task Force on Practice Guidelines. *Circulation.* 2013;127(4):529-555.

Peura JL, Colvin-Adams M, Francis GS, et al. Recommendations for the use of mechanical circulatory support: device strategies and patient selection: a scientific statement from the American Heart Association. *Circulation.* 2012;126:2648-2667.

ACC/AHA/AAPA/ABC/ACPM/AGS/APhA/ASH/ASPC/NMA/PCNA Guideline for prevention, detection, evaluation, and management of high blood pressure in adults. A report of the American College of Cardiology/American Heart Association Task Force on Clinical Practice Guidelines. *Hypertension.* 2017;70(6):1-112.

Yancy CW, Jessup M, Bozkurt B, 2013 ACCF/AHA guideline for the management of heart failure: executive summary. a report of the American College of Cardiology Foundation/American Heart Association Task Force on Practice Guidelines. *J Am Coll Cardiol.* 2013;62(16):1495-1539.

Yancy CW, Jessup M, Bozkurt B, et al. 2017 ACC/AHA/HFSA focused update on the 2013 ACCF/AHA/guideline for the management of heart failure: a report of the American College of Cardiology/American Heart Association Task Force on Clinical Practice Guidelines and the Heart Failure Society of America. *Circulation.* 2017;138(1):e137-e161.

RESPIRATORY SYSTEM 10

Kiersten N. Henry and Maureen A. Seckel

KNOWLEDGE COMPETENCIES

1. Identify various radiologic and pulmonary anatomic features relevant to interpretation of chest x-rays.
2. Describe different systems and principles of management for chest tubes.
3. Describe the etiology, pathophysiology, clinical presentation, patient needs, and principles of management of acute respiratory failure (ARF).
4. Compare and contrast the pathophysiology, clinical presentation, patient needs, and

management approaches for common diseases leading to ARF:
- Acute respiratory distress syndrome (ARDS)
- Acute respiratory failure
- Chronic obstructive pulmonary disease (COPD) exacerbation
- COVID-19 (SARS-CoV-2)
- Acute severe asthma
- Interstitial lung disease (ILD)
- Pulmonary hypertension (PH)
- Pneumonia
- Pulmonary embolism (PE)
- Venous thromboembolism (VTE)

SPECIAL ASSESSMENT TECHNIQUES, DIAGNOSTIC TESTS, AND MONITORING SYSTEMS

Chest X-Rays

Chest radiography is an important tool in respiratory assessment, providing visualization of the heart and lungs. Chest x-rays are a complement to bedside assessment. Critical care nurses need to know basic radiographic concepts and how to optimize portable chest x-ray technique, as well as how to systematically view a chest x-ray image.

Chest x-rays are obtained as part of routine screening procedures, when respiratory disease is suspected, to evaluate the status of respiratory abnormalities (eg, pneumothorax, pleural effusion, tumors), to confirm proper invasive tube placement (ie, endotracheal, tracheostomy, chest tubes, and pulmonary artery catheters), or following traumatic chest injury.

Basic Concepts

An x-ray is a form of electromagnetic radiation used by imaging machines to create radiographic images. Only a few rays are absorbed by air as beams pass through the atmosphere, whereas all rays are absorbed by metal as the beams attempt to pass through a sheet of metal. When nothing but air lies between the film cassette and the x-ray source, the radiographic image is blackness or radiolucency. If density increases, more beams are absorbed between the film cassette or detectors and the x-ray source, and the radiographic image is whiteness or radiopacity. As the x-ray beam passes through the patient, the denser tissues absorb more of the beam, and the less dense tissues absorb less of the beam. There are four distinct radiographic densities: white, light gray, darker gray, and black. Many institutions have replaced traditional x-ray film with detectors that convert the x-ray-energy to a digital radiograph. These images can then be stored and distributed in a digital format.

TABLE 10-1. BASIC X-RAY DENSITIES

Air/Gas (Black)
- Lungs, trachea, bronchi, alveoli
- Stomach, small intestines, bowel

Fat (Gray or Black)
- Breasts, marrow, hilar streaking

Soft Tissue/Fluid (Gray)
- Muscle, organs, soft tissues

Calcium/Bone/Metal (White)
- Ribs, scapulae, vertebrae
- Bullets, coins, teeth, ECG electrodes, barium

The lungs are primarily sacs of air or gas, so normal lung parenchyma looks black on chest films. Conversely, the skeletal thorax appears white, because bone is very dense and absorbs the most x-rays (Table 10-1). The heart and mediastinum appear gray because those structures are made up of mostly water and muscle or tissue. Breast tissue is made up of mostly fat and it appears whitish-gray. Structures of the thorax are made radiographically visible if they are surrounded by air. Conversely, they are obscured if adjacent to consolidation or fluid.

Basic Views of the Chest

The most common method of obtaining a chest x-ray is the posterior-anterior (PA) view. PA chest x-rays are typically done in the radiology department with the machine about 6 ft away from the x-ray film cassette and the patient standing with the anterior chest wall against the x-ray plate and the posterior chest wall toward the x-ray machine. The patient is told to take a deep breath and hold it as the x-ray beam is delivered through the posterior chest wall to the x-ray film cassette. The PA view results in a very accurate, sharp picture of the chest.

Critically ill patients are rarely able to tolerate the positioning requirements of a PA chest x-ray or the logistics of transport to the department. Most chest x-rays in critical care are obtained with an anterior-posterior (AP) view with the patient supine in bed, with or without back rest elevation. With portable AP chest films, the film cassette or digital sensor is placed behind the patient and the x-ray beam is delivered through the anterior chest to the film or sensor. The x-ray machine is only 3 ft away from the patient, which results in greater distortion of chest images, making the AP chest x-ray less accurate than the PA method. Of particular concern is that the heart size is enlarged on an AP film because of its anterior placement within the chest. When viewing chest x-rays, it is important to know whether a PA or AP view was used to avoid misinterpretation of heart size as cardiomegaly.

Placing the patient in a high Fowler position, or as erect as possible, with the thorax symmetrically placed on the film or sensor can help to minimize distortions. Explain the procedure to the patient and the need to avoid movement. All mobile objects lying on the anterior chest (such as ventilator tubing, safety pins, jewelry, ECG wires, nasogastric tubes, etc)

are removed or repositioned as possible. If the patient is unconscious, securing the forehead in a neutral position may be necessary, especially in the high Fowler position to avoid malpositioning of the head. If unable to leave the room, caregivers assisting with the chest x-ray need to protect themselves from radiation exposure by positioning themselves behind the x-ray machine or by using lead aprons covering the neck, chest, and abdomen. Nonessential staff and visitors should leave the room and remain at least 6 ft from the radiation source.

Other chest x-ray views include: (1) lateral views to identify normal and abnormal structures behind the heart, along the spine, and at the base of the lung; (2) oblique views to localize lesions without interference from the bony thorax or to get a better picture of the trachea, carina, heart, and great vessels; (3) lordotic views to better visualize the apical and middle regions of the lungs and to differentiate anterior from posterior lesions; and (4) lateral decubitus (cross-table) views, done with the patient supine or side-lying, to assess for air-fluid levels or free-flowing pleural fluid.

Systematic Approach to Chest X-Ray Interpretation

A systematic approach facilitates accurate interpretation of a chest x-ray film. It is important to first make sure that the images are properly labeled (correct name and medical record number) and to identify the right and left sides of the image. If previous images are available, place them next to the new images for comparison. View the chest x-ray from the lateral borders, moving to the medial aspects of the thorax and asking the series of questions found in Table 10-2.

Begin the chest x-ray analysis by comparing the right side to the left side using the following sequence (Figures 10-1 and 10-2): (1) soft tissues—neck, shoulders, breasts, and subcutaneous fat; (2) trachea—the column of radiolucency readily visible above the clavicles; (3) bony thorax—note size, shape, and symmetry; (4) intercostal spaces (ICS)—note width and angle; (5) diaphragm—dome-shaped

TABLE 10-2. STEPS FOR INTERPRETATION OF A CHEST X-RAY FILM

Step 1
Look at the different densities (black, gray, and white), and answer the question, *"What is air, fluid, tissue, and bone?"*

Step 2
Look at the shape or form of each density, and answer the question, *"What normal anatomic structure is this?"*

Step 3
Look at both right and left sides, and answer the question, *"Are the findings the same on both sides or are there differences (both physiologic and pathophysiologic)?"*

Step 4
Look at all the structures (bones, mediastinum, diaphragm, pleural space, and lung tissue), and answer the question, *"Are there any abnormalities present?"*

Step 5
Look for all tubes, wires, and lines, and answer the question, *"Are the tubes, wires, and lines in the proper place?"*

Adapted with permission from Urden L, Stacy KM, Lough M. Critical Care Nursing: Diagnosis and Management. 8th ed. St Louis, MO: Elsevier Mosby; 2017.

with distinct margins, right dome 1 to 3 cm higher than left dome; (6) pleural surfaces—visceral and parietal pleura appear like a thin hair-like line along the apices and lateral chest; (7) mediastinum—size varies with age, gender, and patient size; (8) hila—large pulmonary arteries and veins; (9) lung fields—largest area of the chest and most radiolucent; and (10) catheters, tubes, wires, and lines.

Normal Variants and Common Abnormalities

When the soft tissues are examined, the two sides of the lateral chest should be symmetric. A mastectomy makes one lung look more radiolucent than the other due to the absence of fatty tissue. The trachea should be midline, with the carina visible at the level of the aortic knob or second ICS. The most common cause of tracheal deviation is a pneumothorax, which causes a tracheal and mediastinal shift to the area away from the pneumothorax (Table 10-3; Figures 10-3 and 10-4).

Bony thorax inspection reveals general body build. Clavicles should be symmetric and may have an irregular notch or indentation in the inferior medial aspect of the clavicle called a rhomboid fossa, a normal variant. Deformities of the thorax can be detected, such as scoliosis, pectus excavatum (also called funnel chest), or pectus carinatum (also called pigeon chest). Decreases in the density (less white) of the spine, ribs, and other bones may indicate loss of calcium from the bones due to osteoporosis or long-term steroid dependency. Careful examination of the ICSs and rib angles may indicate pathology. Patients with chronic obstructive pulmonary disease (COPD) have widened ICS and the angle of the ribs to the spine increases to 90° instead of the normal 45° angle because of severe hyperinflation (see Figure 10-3). Conversely, narrowed ICS may be visible in patients with severe interstitial fibrosis. Old rib fractures, if present, are commonly visible along the lateral borders of the rib cage and appear as a "callus" or thickened area of the rib where scar has developed.

Elevation of the diaphragm can be a result of abdominal distention, phrenic nerve paralysis, or lung collapse. Depression or flattening of the diaphragm is demonstrated by the presence of 11 or 12 ribs on a chest x-ray. Flattening of the diaphragm indicates hyperinflation as in COPD or asthma. When the diaphragm is neither elevated nor depressed, 9 or 10 ribs are visible. Normal costophrenic angles can be seen where the tapered edges of the diaphragm and the chest wall meet. Because breast tissue can obscure the angles in women, these angles are more distinct in men. Obliteration or "blunting" of the costophrenic angle may occur with pleural effusion or atelectasis.

Identification of a pleural space on a chest x-ray is an abnormal finding (see Figure 10-4). The pleural space is not visible unless air (pneumothorax) or fluid (pleural effusion) enters it. These findings are commonly seen in the ICU population.

Two terms often heard regarding the appearance of the mediastinum on chest x-ray are *shifting* and *widening*.

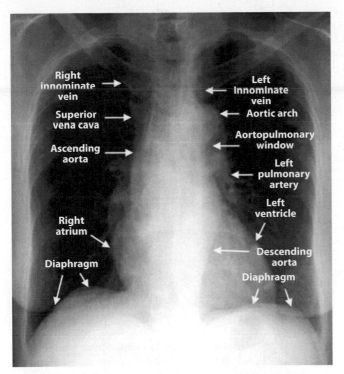

Figure 10-1. Normal chest x-ray with anatomical references. (*Reproduced with permission from Gay SB, Olazagasti J, Higginbotham JW, et al. Introduction to Chest Radiology. University of Virginia Health Sciences Center, Department of Radiology.*)

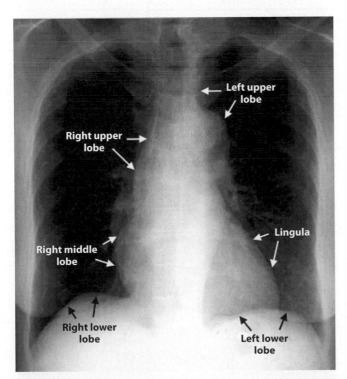

Figure 10-2. Normal chest x-ray with anatomical references. (*Reproduced with permission from Gay SB, Olazagasti J, Higginbotham JW, et al. Introduction to Chest Radiology. University of Virginia Health Sciences Center, Department of Radiology.*)

TABLE 10-3. CHEST X-RAY FINDINGS

Assessed Area	Usual Adult Findings	Remarks
Trachea	Midline, translucent, tubelike structure found in the anterior mediastinal cavity	Deviation from the midline suggests tension pneumothorax, atelectasis, pleural effusion, mass, or collapsed lung
Clavicles	Present in upper thorax and are equally distant from sternum	Malalignment or break indicates fracture
Ribs	Thoracic cavity encasement	Widening of intercostal spaces indicates emphysema; malalignment or break indicates fractured sternum or ribs
Mediastinum	Shadowy-appearing space between the lungs that widens at the hilum	Deviation to either side may indicate pleural effusion, fibrosis, or collapsed lung
Heart	Solid-appearing structure with clear edges visible in the left anterior mediastinal cavity; heart should be less than one-half the width of the chest wall on a PA film	Shift may indicate atelectasis or tension pneumothorax; if heart is greater than one-half the chest wall width, heart failure or pericardial fluid may be present
Carina	The lowest tracheal cartilage at which the bronchi bifurcate	If the end of the endotracheal tube is seen 3 cm above the carina, it is in the correct position
Main-stem bronchus	The translucent, tubelike structure visible to approximately 2.5 cm from hilum	Densities may indicate bronchogenic cyst
Hilum	Small, white, bilateral densities present where the bronchi join the lungs; left hilum should be 2-3 cm higher than the right hilum	A shift to either side indicates atelectasis; accentuated shadows may indicate emphysema or pulmonary abscess
Bronchi (other than main stem)	Not usually visible	If visible, may indicate bronchial pneumonia
Lung fields	Usually not completely visible except as fine white areas from hilum; fields should be clear as normal lung tissue is radiolucent; normal "lung markings" should be present to the periphery	If visible, may indicate atelectasis; patchy densities may be signs of resolving pneumonia, silicosis, or fibrosis; nasogastric tubes, pulmonary artery catheters, and chest tubes will appear as shadows and their positions should be noted
Diaphragm	Rounded structures visible at the bottom of the lung fields; right side is 1-2 cm higher than the left; the costophrenic angles should be clear and sharp	An elevated diaphragm may indicate pneumonia, pleurisy, acute bronchitis, or atelectasis; a flattened diaphragm suggests COPD; unilateral elevation indicates a pneumothorax or pulmonary infection; the presence of scarring or fluid causes blunting of costophrenic angles; 300-500 mL of pleural fluid must be present before blunting is seen

Reproduced with permission from Talbot I, Meyers-Marquardt M. Pocket Guide to Critical Assessment. St Louis, MO: CV Mosby; 1990.

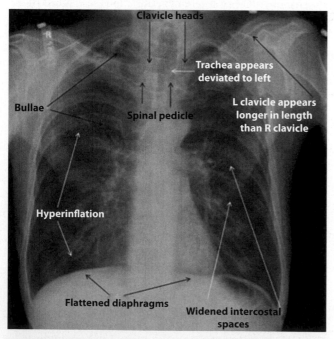

Figure 10-3. COPD, flattened diaphragms, hyperinflation, widened intercostal spaces, apical bullae, and chest rotation. (*Reproduced with permission from Siela D. Chest radiograph evaluation and interpretation. AACN Adv Crit Care. 2008;19(4):444-473.*)

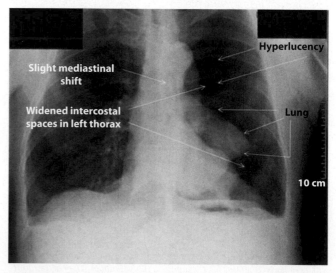

Figure 10-4. Left pneumothorax, hyperlucency, and widened intercostal spaces. (*Reproduced with permission from Siela D. Chest radiograph evaluation and interpretation. AACN Adv Crit Care. 2008;19(4):444-473.*)

Mediastinal structures, usually the trachea, bronchi, and heart, can shift with atelectasis, with the shift directed toward the alveolar collapse. Pneumothorax shifts the mediastinum away from the area of involvement. A widening of the mediastinum can indicate several pathologic conditions, such as cardiomegaly, aneurysms, or aortic disruption. Bleeding into the mediastinum, following chest trauma or cardiac surgery, also may cause widening of the mediastinum.

Heart size can be estimated on a PA film by comparing the ratio of the maximal horizontal cardiac diameter to the maximal horizontal thoracic diameter. A normal measurement is less than 50%. Greater percents are indicative of cardiac enlargement. This method for determining normal heart size is not accurate using an AP chest x-ray, the most common type taken in the critically ill.

The lung fields should be assessed for any areas of increased density (whiteness) or increased radiolucency (blackness), which can indicate an abnormality. Density increases when water, pus, or blood accumulates in the lungs, as in pneumonia (Figure 10-5). Increased radiolucency is caused by increased air in the lungs, as may occur with COPD. A fine line present on the right side of the lung at the sixth rib level (midlung) is a normal finding, representing the horizontal fissure separating the right upper and middle lobes.

Invasive Lines

Chest x-rays are frequently obtained in critical care to confirm proper placement of invasive equipment (endotracheal tubes, central venous and pulmonary artery catheters [PAC], intra-aortic balloons, nasogastric tubes, chest tubes). All invasive tubes have radiopaque lines running the length of the tube that are visible on the x-ray. When in the proper position, the endotracheal tube tip should be 4 to 6 cm above the carina with the patient's head in neutral

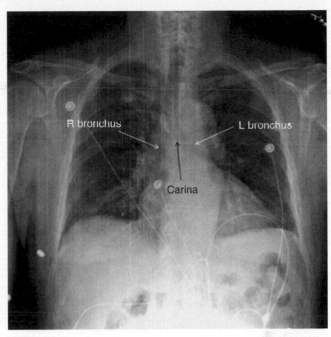

Figure 10-6. Carina and right bronchus. (*Reproduced with permission from Siela D. Chest radiograph evaluation and interpretation. AACN Adv Crit Care. 2008;19(4):444-473.*)

position (Figures 10-6 and 10-7). Flexion or extension of the patient's head causes a 2-cm change in the position of the tip of the endotracheal tube. Look for a thin white line in the trachea and follow it down to the level of the clavicles and measure the space between the end of the tube and the carina. The tip of the endotracheal tube is at least 3 cm distal to the vocal cords.

All lines should be identified and followed through their paths. The nasogastric tube runs the length of the esophagus with the tip of the tube beyond the gastroesophageal junction

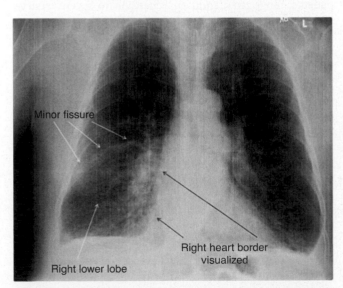

Figure 10-5. Right middle and lower lobe pneumonia with minor fissure visualized. (*Reproduced with permission from Siela D. Chest radiograph evaluation and interpretation. AACN Adv Crit Care. 2008;19(4):444-473.*)

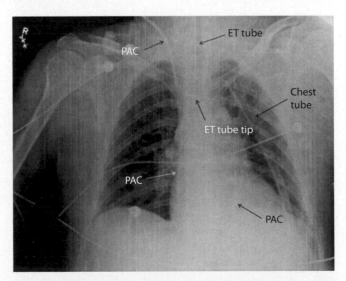

Figure 10-7. Pulmonary artery catheter (PAC), endotracheal tube (ET), and left chest tube. (*Reproduced with permission from Siela D. Chest radiograph evaluation and interpretation. AACN Adv Crit Care. 2008;19(4):444-473.*)

in the stomach. The stomach can be identified by the radiolucency just under the diaphragm on the left side, which is called the gastric air bubble. Small bore nasoenteric tubes may be positioned with the tip in the stomach or the small bowel depending on whether gastric or small bowel feedings are intended. Central line catheters are properly placed when the tip can be viewed in the superior vena cava. Pulmonary artery catheters run through the right atrium and right ventricle into the pulmonary artery. These can be difficult to identify at first, but be sure and look at both sides of the hila (right and left pulmonary arteries found on either side of the mediastinum). Chest tubes are visualized by viewing the radiopaque stripe and the location of the tip is dependent on whether the tube is inserted for air or fluid removal. The side holes should be positioned medial to the inner margin of the ribs.

Identify all items in the chest, such as temporary or permanent pacing wires, pacing generators, automatic implantable defibrillators, and surgical wires, drains, or clips (see Figure 10-7).

Helpful Hints

Chest x-rays should be taken after every attempt to insert central venous catheters to detect the presence of an iatrogenic pneumothorax. A common error is to mistake the area above the clavicles as a pneumothorax, especially on AP views.

Two common abnormal x-ray signs frequently discussed are the silhouette sign and the air bronchogram. For any structure to be visible, the density of its edge must contrast with the surrounding density. The loss of contrast is called the silhouette sign. It means that two structures of the same density have come in contact with each other and the borders are lost; for example, the heart is a muscle/water density, so if the alveoli near the left heart border fill with fluid, the two densities are the same and there is a loss of contrast and no left heart border. An air bronchogram is air showing through a greater density, such as water (Figure 10-8). The bronchi are not seen on a normal chest x-ray, except for the main-stem bronchi, because they have thin walls, contain air, and are surrounded by air in the alveoli (two structures of the same density). If water surrounds the bronchi, as in pneumonia and pulmonary edema, then the bronchi filled with air are in contrast to the water density and are visible.

Computed Tomography, Magnetic Resonance Imaging, and Bedside Ultrasonography

Computed tomography (CT) and magnetic resonance imaging (MRI) allow for the three-dimensional examination of the chest in situations where two-dimensional chest x-rays are insufficient. CT and MRI are particularly advantageous over chest x-rays to evaluate mediastinal and pleural abnormalities, particularly those with fluid collections. Pleural effusions or empyemas, malpositioned or occluded chest tubes, mediastinal hematomas, and mediastinitis are problems for which a three-dimensional view provided by CT and MRI are more sensitive than a chest x-ray.

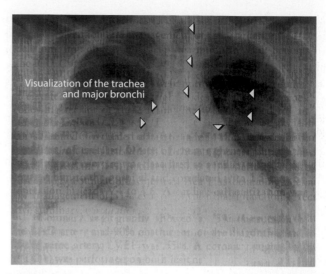

Visualization of the trachea and major bronchi

Figure 10-8. Air bronchogram. (*Reproduced with permission from Yale School of Medicine.*)

The need for transportation to the radiology department and positioning restrictions within the scanning devices pose certain risks to critically ill patients. Of particular concern is the automatic movement of patients during the procedure into and out of the scanning device. Accidental disconnection of invasive devices can easily occur if additional tubing lengths and potential obstructions are not considered. Decreased visualization of patients during the procedures requires vigilant monitoring of cardiovascular and respiratory parameters and devices, as well as establishing a method for conscious patients to alert nearby clinicians in case of difficulties. The strong magnetic field of MRI units may interfere with ventilator performance and a nonmagnetic ventilator is required.

MRI testing can be a frightening experience for the patient. Reactions, occurring in up to almost one-third of patients, range from mild apprehension to severe anxiety. These reactions can result in cancellation of the test or interference with its results. It is suggested that all patients receive basic information regarding the MRI procedure, including details of the small chamber they will be placed in, the noise and temperature they will experience, and the duration of the procedure. If possible, use of relaxation or music tapes, ear plugs or headsets, and the presence of a family member or friend should be considered. In addition, short-acting anxiolytics should be used for patients who need them.

Bedside ultrasonography is increasingly common in critical care as less expensive machines are available. Ultrasound can be performed quickly and easily and the information provided helps to confirm or rule out a suspected condition or a procedure-related complication. The transducer or probe produces sound waves along with echoes that are reflected back to produce two-dimensional images of tissue, fluid, and organs. Recent guidelines recommend ultrasound of the chest for the following situations: diagnosis of pleural effusion, identification of the location for drainage of a pleural effusion, rapid detection of pneumothorax, diagnosis of alveolar lung consolidation, and as an aide in central line insertion to prevent procedure-related complications. Advantages of ultrasound include its portability and rapid direct use at the bedside avoiding the need for patient transportation. Some disadvantages include the need for comprehensive training in obtaining and interpreting the images and the lack of availability in all critical care areas. The use of ultrasound during bedside procedures such as central venous catheter insertion is shown to decrease the number of procedural attempts and rate of complications due to increased accuracy of insertion.

CTPA and Ventilation-Perfusion Scans

Computed tomographic angiography (CTPA) is the gold standard imaging approach for diagnosis of pulmonary emboli. The CTPA is minimally invasive and requires a peripheral line through which to inject the contrast material. Images are acquired following contrast material injection, with an embolus appearing as a dark filling defect in the otherwise bright white contrast-dense pulmonary artery. CTPA has a high sensitivity and specificity for diagnosing PE and has replaced the more invasive pulmonary angiography.

While less common, ventilation-perfusion (V/Q) scans may also be used to diagnose PE if additional testing is needed or the CTPA is contraindicated. A V/Q scan is a nuclear medicine diagnostic tool that requires medical isotopes to be inhaled or injected in order to view the lungs and pulmonary arteries, respectively. Generally, the perfusion (or blood circulation) part of the test is done first. If there is no defect detected, the scan is read as "low probability." If the scan detects a defect, then the inhaled (ventilation) portion of the test is done. If no matching defect is seen in the lung, the test is interpreted as "high probability." But if a "matched defect" is noted (ie, there is a defect in the lung scan that corresponds with that of the perfusion scan), then the interpretation is "indeterminate" or "matched defect." This may be the result of an atelectasis, pneumonia, or other infiltrate where circulation to that inactive area of the lung is redistributed to other active areas, thus resulting in a "matched defect." In addition to the cumbersome nature of the V/Q scan, the critically ill patient may require both tests (perfusion and ventilation) rather than just one and the diagnostic yield is often poor.

Chest Tubes

Chest tubes are commonly used in critically ill patients to drain air, blood, or fluid from the pleural spaces (pleural chest tubes) or from the mediastinum (mediastinal tubes). Indications for chest tube insertion are varied (Table 10-4). The only absolute contraindication is in a lung that is adherent to the chest wall through the hemithorax. Relative contraindications may include patients with multiple adhesions, blebs, overlying skin infections, or coagulopathies. However, the emergent need for lung re-expansion may require careful evaluation of risk versus benefit on an individual patient basis including reversal of any coagulopathy if feasible. Pleural tube insertion sites vary based on the type of drainage

TABLE 10-4. INDICATIONS FOR CHEST TUBE INSERTION

Pneumothorax
- Open: Both chest wall and pleural spaces are penetrated.
- Closed: Pleural space is penetrated with an intact chest wall, allowing air to enter the pleural space from the lungs.
- Tension: Air leaks into the pleural space through a tear in the lungs, with no means to escape the space, leading to lung collapse.

Hemothorax (blood)
Hemopneumothorax (blood and air)
Post-thoracotomy
Pyothorax or empyema (pus)
Chylothorax (lymph)
Cholethorax (bile)
Hydrothorax (noninflammatory serous)
Pleural effusion (transudate or exudate)
Pleurodesis (installation of anesthetic or sclerosing agent)

Adapted with permission from Wiegand DI, ed. AACN Procedure Manual for Critical Care. *7th ed. Philadelphia, PA: Saunders; 2017.*

to be removed (air: second ICS, midclavicular line; fluid: fifth or sixth ICS, midaxillary line). Mediastinal tubes are placed during surgery, exiting from the mediastinum below the xiphoid process. Types of chest tubes include tube thoracostomy (traditional rigid tubes) or smaller percutaneously inserted catheters (pigtails).

Following insertion, chest tubes are connected to a closed drainage collection system that uses gravity or suction to restore negative pressure in the pleural space and facilitate drainage of fluid or air (Figure 10-9). Digital drainage systems may be utilized in patients with pneumothorax or following thoracic surgery. These systems allow objective monitoring of fluid drainage and air leak from the chest tube

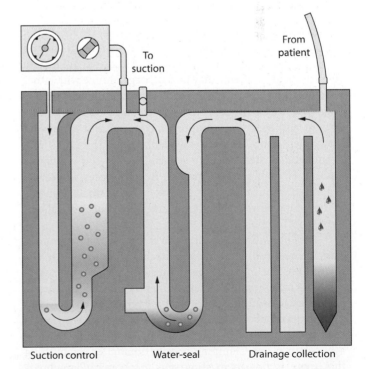

Figure 10-9. Disposable chest tube drainage system. (*Reproduced with permission from Luce JM, Tyler ML, Peirson DJ.* Intensive Respiratory Care. *Philadelphia, PA: WB Saunders; 1984.*)

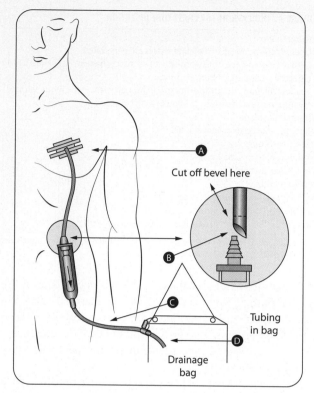

Figure 10-10. Heimlich chest drain valve with connection to drain bag. (*Courtesy ©Becton, Dickinson and Company.*)

Cut off bevel here

Tubing in bag

Drainage bag

while eliminating the need for connection to wall suction to maintain a predetermined pressure.

A Heimlich flutter valve is an alternative to the closed drainage system and consists of a one-way valve that allows air or drainage to collect in a vented drain bag (Figure 10-10). The indwelling pleural catheter (ie, PleurX catheter) also has a one-way valve and connects as needed to a drainage system (Figure 10-11). Patients may be discharged home with either a Heimlich flutter valve or an indwelling pleural catheter for long-term use. Connections to the drainage system must be airtight and secure for proper functioning and to prevent inadvertent entry of air into the pleural space (Figure 10-12). To maintain patency of the system, inspect the tubing for kinking or visible clot formation. In some cases, if a clot is visualized, gentle squeezing and releasing of small segments of the tubing between the thumb and index finger can alleviate the obstruction.

Patients with recurrent pneumothorax or effusion may undergo pleurodesis, in which a sclerosing agent is introduced into the pleural space through a chest tube. The resulting inflammation creates adherence of the lung to the chest wall, closing the space and reducing the risk of fluid and air accumulation. This procedure also involves clamping the chest tube for a defined interval while the sclerosing agent is in place. Clamping is only done after establishing that there is not an existing pneumothorax. Clamping a chest tube when a pneumothorax is present risks the development of tension pneumothorax, in which the air trapped

in the pleural space compromises the patient's ventilation and hemodynamic status.

Removal of the chest tube occurs when restoration of lung expansion and fluid or air removal has been accomplished and the underlying lung abnormality has resolved. An occlusive dressing at the chest tube removal site is typically used to prevent introduction of air into the pleural space until the skin has formed a protective seal. Analgesic administration is appropriate prior to removal; discomfort associated with removal is often as much or even greater than during insertion.

THORACIC SURGERY AND PROCEDURES

Thoracic surgery and procedures are terms inclusive of a number of procedures involving the thoracic cavity and the lungs. See Table 10-5 for definitions and indications. With the evolution of minimally invasive surgical techniques, thoracic surgery procedures such as pulmonary resection may be performed via laparoscopic or robotic techniques.

Principles of Management for Thoracic Surgery and Procedures

Management of the patient after lung surgery or post-procedure is similar to the patient with trauma to the chest. Refer to the section on thoracic trauma in Chapter 17, Trauma, with the following additions:

Pain Control

The thoracotomy incision is one of the most painful surgical incisions and pain control is an important factor in recovery and prevention of respiratory complications. The routine use of epidural catheters, intercostal blocks, intrapleural local anesthetic administration, or patient-controlled analgesia (PCA) narcotics has improved pain management significantly. These pain management strategies have evolved into enhanced recovery after surgery (ERAS) protocols which include interdisciplinary, perioperative strategies for reducing hospital stay and complication rates. Relaxation therapy, deep breathing exercises, and guided imagery may also be effective in helping to reduce pain and anxiety.

Positioning

- It was once thought that optimal ventilation and perfusion matching occurs when the "good lung" is positioned in the dependent position. While blood flow is improved to the dependent lung, patients actually recover best when they are frequently repositioned side-to-side to prevent atelectasis and other complications.
- Progressive mobility including sitting at the bedside or in a chair and assisted ambulation improves diaphragmatic excursion, enhancing ventilation and lung inflation.
- Deep breathing and use of incentive spirometry are encouraged regularly. These activities help promote lung re-expansion of collapsed lung tissue and prevent atelectasis.

Procedure Pack

Blue wrapping
around the following:

Gloves

Catheter valve cap

Blue emergency
slide clamp

Gauze pads

Foam catheter pad

**Vacuum Bottle with
Drainage Line**

White slide
clamp

500 ml
Plastic
vacuum
bottle

Green vacuum
indicator

Access tip
cover

Access tip

Drainage
line

Pinch
clamp

Self-adhesive
dressing

Alcohol pads

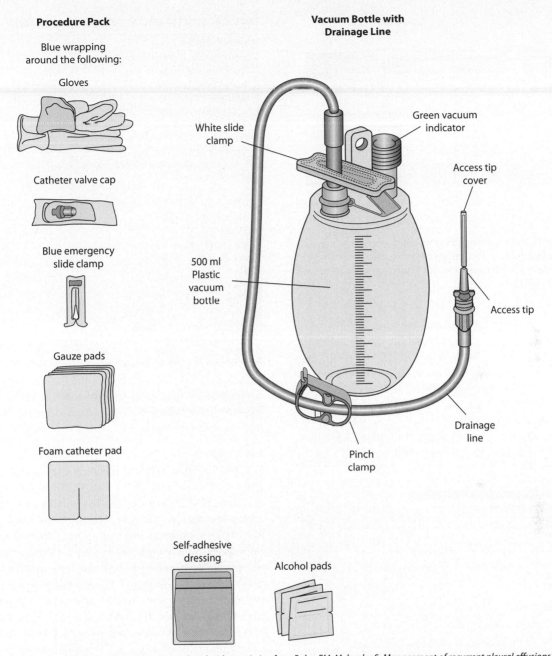

Figure 10-11. Components of a PleurX drainage kit. (*Reproduced with permission from Baker EM, Melander S. Management of recurrent pleural effusions with a tunneled catheter. Heart Lung. 2010;39(4):314-318.*)

Maintenance of Chest Tube System
See section "Chest Tubes" explained earlier.

PATHOLOGIC CONDITIONS

Acute Respiratory Failure

Each of the case studies below represents a common situation in a critical care unit—respiratory dysfunction. Rapid onset of respiratory impairment, which is severe enough to cause potential or actual morbidity or mortality if untreated, is termed *acute respiratory failure*. Although the origin of the respiratory failure may be a medical or surgical problem, the management approaches share similar features.

ARF is a change in respiratory gas exchange (CO_2 and O_2) such that normal cellular function is jeopardized. ARF may be primarily hypoxemia, with a Pao_2 less than 60 mm Hg, or primarily hypercapnia with $Paco_2$ greater than 50 mm Hg and a pH less than or equal to 7.30. Mixed ARF refers to situations in which both hypoxemia and hypercapnia occur. The Pao_2 and $Paco_2$ values that define ARF vary, depending on a variety of factors that influence the patient's normal (or baseline) arterial blood gas (ABG) values. Factors such as age, altitude, chronic cardiopulmonary disease, or metabolic

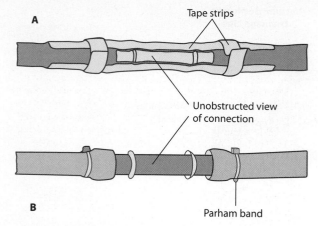

Figure 10-12. Methods for securing connections of chest tube and drainage system. **(A)** Tape. **(B)** Parham bands. *(Reproduced with permission from Kersten LD. Comprehensive Respiratory Nursing: A Decision-Making Approach. Philadelphia, PA: WB Saunders; 1989.)*

disturbances may alter the "normal" blood gas values for an individual, requiring an adjustment to the classic definition of ARF; for example, if $Paco_2$ levels in a 75-year-old man with COPD are normally 56 mm Hg, ARF would not be diagnosed until pH is less than or equal to 7.30.

Etiology, Risk Factors, and Pathophysiology

Many abnormalities can lead to ARF (Table 10-6). Regardless of the underlying cause, the pathophysiology of ARF can be

TABLE 10-5. THORACIC SURGERY AND PROCEDURES

	Definitions
Thoracic Surgery	
Pneumonectomy	Removal of entire lung
Lobectomy	Resection of one or more lobes of the lung
Wedge resection	Removal of small wedge-shaped section of lung tissue
Segmental resection	Removal of bronchovascular segment of the lung lobe
Bullectomy	Resection of emphysematous bullae
Lung volume reduction surgery (LVRS)	Resection of diseased and functionless lung tissue
Open lung biopsy	Resection of portion of lung for biopsy through a thoracotomy incision
Decortication	Surgical removal of pleural fibrous tissue and pus from pleural space
Video-assisted thoracic surgery (VATS)	Endoscopic procedure through small incision
Procedure	
Pulmonary stent	Device(s) placed by flexible or rigid bronchoscopes to keep airways open in the central tracheobronchial tree
Bronchoscopy (rigid or flexible)	Invasive procedure used to visualize the oropharynx, larynx, vocal cords, and tracheal bronchial tree for diagnosis and treatment
Thoracoscopy/ pleuroscopy	Visual examination of the structures of the chest, also utilized to obtain tissue and fluid samples

TABLE 10-6. CAUSES OF ACUTE RESPIRATORY FAILURE IN ADULT

Impaired Ventilation
- Spinal cord injury (C4 or higher)
- Phrenic nerve damage
- Neuromuscular blockade
- Guillain-Barré syndrome
- Central nervous system (CNS) depression
- Drug overdoses (narcotics, sedatives, illicit drugs)
- Increased intracranial pressure
- Anesthetic agents
- Respiratory muscle weakness or paralysis

Impaired Gas Exchange
- Pulmonary edema
- ARDS
- Aspiration pneumonia
- COVID-19

Airway Obstruction
- Aspiration of foreign body
- Thoracic tumors
- Asthma
- Bronchitis
- Pneumonia

Ventilation-Perfusion Abnormalities
- Pulmonary embolism
- Emphysema

organized into four main components: impaired ventilation, impaired gas exchange, airway obstruction, and ventilation-perfusion abnormalities.

Impaired Ventilation

Encephalopathy caused by metabolic alterations or medications such as narcotics and sedatives can suppress respiratory drive and lead to impaired ventilation. Conditions that disrupt the muscles of respiration or their neurologic control can impair ventilation and lead to ARF. Decreased or absent respiratory muscle movement may be due to fatigue from excessive use, atrophy from disuse, inflammation of nerves, nerve damage (eg, surgical damage to the vagus nerve during cardiac surgery), neurologic depression, progressive neuromuscular diseases such as Guillain-Barré or amyotrophic lateral sclerosis (ALS), or following administration of neuromuscular blocking agents. Impaired respiratory muscle movement decreases movement of gas into the lungs, resulting in alveolar hypoventilation. Inadequate alveolar ventilation causes retention of CO_2 and hypoxemia.

Impaired Gas Exchange

Conditions that damage the alveolar-capillary membrane impair gas exchange. Direct damage to the cells lining the alveoli may be caused by inhalation of toxic substances (gases or gastric contents), pneumonia, and/or other pulmonary conditions leading to two detrimental alveolar changes. The first is an increase in alveolar permeability, increasing the potential for interstitial fluid to leak into the alveoli and causing noncardiac pulmonary edema (Figure 10-13A). The second alveolar change is a decrease in surfactant production by alveolar type II cells, increasing alveolar surface tension, which leads to alveolar collapse (Figure 10-13B).

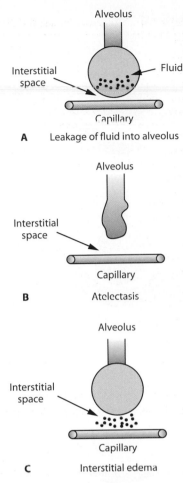

Figure 10-13. Pathophysiologic processes in ARF that impair gas exchange. **(A)** Increased alveolar membrane permeability. **(B)** Alveolar collapse from decreased surfactant production. **(C)** Increased capillary membrane permeability and interstitial edema.

Another cause of impaired gas exchange occurs when fluid leaks from the intravascular space into the pulmonary interstitial space (Figure 10-13C). The excess fluid increases the distance between the alveolus and the capillary, decreasing the efficiency of the gas exchange process. Interstitial edema also compresses the bronchial airways, which are surrounded by interstitial tissue, causing bronchoconstriction. Capillary leakage may occur when pressures within the cardiovascular system are excessively high (eg, in heart failure) or when pathologic conditions elsewhere in the body release biochemical substances (eg, serotonin, endotoxin) that increase capillary permeability.

Airway Obstruction
Conditions that obstruct airways increase resistance to airflow into the lungs, causing alveolar hypoventilation and decreased gas exchange (Figure 10-14). Airway obstructions can be due to conditions that: (1) block the inner airway lumen (eg, excessive secretions or fluid in the airways, inhaled foreign bodies) (Figure 10-14A), (2) increase airway wall thickness (eg, edema or fibrosis) or decrease airway

circumference (eg, bronchoconstriction) as occurs in asthma (Figure 10-14B), or (3) increase peribronchial compression of the airway (eg, enlarged lymph nodes, interstitial edema, tumors) (Figure 10-14C).

Ventilation-Perfusion Abnormalities
Conditions disrupting alveolar ventilation or capillary perfusion lead to an imbalance in ventilation and perfusion. This decreases the efficiency of the respiratory gas exchange

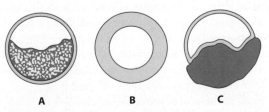

Figure 10-14. Mechanism of airway obstruction. **(A)** Fluid secretions present within airway. **(B)** Intraluminal edema narrowing airway diameter. **(C)** Peribronchial compression of airway.

ESSENTIAL CONTENT CASE

Postanesthesia

A woman is directly admitted to the surgical ICU following thoracic surgery for the removal of a malignant tumor of the right upper lobe. She is intubated and changed over from the transport ventilator to the ICU ventilator by respiratory therapy. A right pleural chest tube is draining minimal amounts of blood, with no evidence of air leaks or obstructions.

The patient is unresponsive to verbal and pain stimulation on admission. No spontaneous respirations are noted on the ventilator respiratory waveform screen or by physical assessment. Fifteen minutes after arrival to the unit (assist control ventilation [AC] of 10 breaths/min, tidal volume of 8 mL/kg, positive end-expiratory pressure [PEEP] of 5 cm H_2O, 0.40 fraction of inspired oxygen [FiO_2]), arterial blood gas (ABG) shows:

PaO_2	145 mm Hg
$PaCO_2$	41 mm Hg
pH	7.38
HCO_3	24 mEq/L

Case Question 1: What ventilator changes do you anticipate will be made?

Case Question 2: What missing assessment items in report from anesthesia do you need to continue to care for this patient?

Answers
1. Patient is oxygenating adequately with PaO_2 of 145 mm Hg and FiO_2 should be titrated down to maintain a PaO_2 goal of 60 to 70 mm Hg.
2. Since the patient is unresponsive without spontaneous respirations, additional history is obtained from anesthesia regarding anesthetic agents used, analgesia, and sedation use in the operating room, and any use of neuromuscular blocking agents. Assessment for an acute neurological event also needs to be considered.

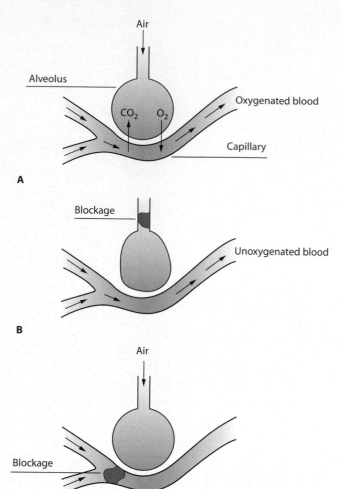

A

B

C

Figure 10-15. Pathophysiologic processes in ARF from ventilation-perfusion abnormalities. **(A)** Normal ventilation and perfusion relationship. **(B)** Decreased ventilation and normal perfusion. **(C)** Normal ventilation and decreased perfusion.

process (Figure 10-15A). In an effort to keep the ventilation and perfusion ratios balanced, two compensatory changes occur: (1) to avoid wasted alveolar ventilation when capillary perfusion is decreased (eg, with PE), alveolar collapse occurs to limit ventilation to alveoli with poor or absent capillary perfusion (Figure 10-15B); and (2) to avoid capillary perfusion of alveoli that are not adequately ventilated (eg, with atelectasis), pulmonary arteriole constriction (ie, hypoxic vasoconstriction) occurs and shunts blood away from hypoventilated alveoli to normally ventilated alveoli (Figure 10-15C). As the number of alveolar–capillary units affected by these compensatory changes increases, gas exchange eventually is negatively affected.

Each of these pathophysiologic changes results in inadequate CO_2 removal, O_2 absorption, or both. The severity of ARF can be further increased when anxiety or delirium develop, a common consequence of severe dyspnea and

hypoxemia. These symptoms increase oxygen demand and the work of breathing, further compromising O_2 availability for crucial organ function and depleting respiratory muscle strength.

Clinical Presentation

Signs and Symptoms

- Hypoxemia (PaO_2 < 60 mm Hg)
- SpO_2 < 90%
- Hypercarbia ($PaCO_2$ > 50 mm Hg
- Tachypnea
- Dyspnea
- Abnormal breath sounds (crackles, wheezes)
- Use of accessory muscles of respiration
- Restlessness
- Confusion
- Diaphoresis
- Anxiety
- Irritability

- Tachycardia progressing to arrythmias or bradycardia as respiratory failure progresses
- Hypertension progressing to hypotension as respiratory failure progresses
- Somnolence (late)
- Cyanosis (late)
- Loss of consciousness (late)
- Pallor or cyanosis of skin
- Manifestations of primary disease (see description of individual diseases discussed later)

Diagnostic Tests

- ABGs—PaO_2 less than 60 mm Hg and $PaCO_2$ more than 50 mm Hg, with pH less than or equal to 7.30 or PaO_2 and $PaCO_2$ in abnormal range for that individual
- Tests specific to underlying cause (see description of individual diseases discussed later).

Principles of Management for Acute Respiratory Failure

The management of the patient in ARF revolves around four primary areas: improving oxygenation and ventilation, treating the underlying disease state, reducing anxiety, and preventing and managing complications.

Improving Oxygenation and Ventilation

Most causes of ARF are treatable, with a return of normal respiratory function following resolution of the pathophysiologic condition. Aggressive support of respiratory function is required until there is resolution of the underlying condition.

1. Provide supplemental O_2 to maintain PaO_2 greater than 60 mm Hg. The use of noninvasive methods for O_2 administration (high-flow nasal cannula or face masks) is preferable if acceptable PaO_2 levels can be achieved. Continued hypoxemia despite noninvasive O_2 delivery methods necessitates intubation and mechanical ventilation.
2. Improve ventilation with the administration of bronchodilators, suctioning, positioning, and mobilization as indicated. Noninvasive ventilation such as continuous or bilevel positive airway pressure (CPAP or BiPAP) may improve respiratory muscle mechanics and decrease $PaCO_2$ retention.
3. Intubate and initiate mechanical ventilation if noninvasive methods fail to correct hypoxemia and hypercarbia or if cardiovascular instability develops. In patients with COPD exacerbation, a trial of noninvasive positive pressure mechanical ventilation may be appropriate prior to intubation. The mode of mechanical ventilation, rate, and tidal volume vary, depending on the underlying cause of respiratory failure and a variety of clinical factors. Modes of ventilation that decrease the work of breathing (control, assist/control, SIMV with high minute ventilation [MV] rates, and pressure support [PS]) are

typically used for the first 24 hours because respiratory muscle fatigue is common. PEEP levels more than 5 cm H_2O may be required if FiO_2 levels above 0.5 are needed to treat hypoxemia. Closely monitor the cardiovascular status during increases of PEEP, which may decrease venous return and cardiac output. Institute analgesia and sedation for patient comfort. (See Chapter 6, Pain, Sedation, and Neuromuscular Blockade Management and Chapter 20, Advanced Respiratory Concepts: Modes of Ventilation for additional strategies.) Neuromuscular blockade may be needed initially to prevent ventilator dyssynchrony and to maximize gas exchange.

4. During suctioning, closely observe for signs and symptoms of complications: drop in oxygenation (SpO_2, SvO_2), cardiac dysrhythmias, respiratory distress (bronchospasm, increased respiratory rate), increased blood pressure or intracranial pressure, anxiety, pain, agitation, or change in mental status. Hyperoxygenate with 100% FiO_2, preferably by using the manual 100% FiO_2 button on the ventilator. An alternative is the use of a manual resuscitation bag (MRB) that delivers 100% O_2 and can be used with a PEEP valve when the ventilator PEEP levels are more than 5 cm H_2O. Suctioning is only performed when clinically indicated, and never on a routine schedule. The use of in-line suction catheters is encouraged as the catheters do not affect oxygenation as dramatically as complete disconnection and they decrease the potential contamination of the clinician doing the suctioning.
5. Prior to intrahospital transport, verify adequacy of ventilatory support equipment to maintain cardiopulmonary stability. Verify that PEEP levels are maintained during transport. Some ventilators used for transport do not have the capability to provide more advanced ventilatory modes (eg, PS, reverse inspiratory:expiratory (I:E) ratio, pressure release, pressure-regulated volume control). Thus when transitioning from an advanced mode to a more traditional mode prior to transport, allow for a brief "stabilization" period prior to leaving the critical care unit.

Treating the Underlying Disease State

Correction of the underlying cause of the ARF is done as soon as possible. See specific management approaches later in the chapter for selected disease state.

Reducing Anxiety

Maintain a calm, supportive environment to avoid unnecessary escalation of anxiety. Give brief explanations of activities and approaches being done to relieve ARF. Vigilance and presence of healthcare providers during anxious periods are crucial to avoid panic by patients and visiting family members. Assess for physiologic causes of anxiety, such as worsening hypoxia or hypercapnia before proceeding to treatment with anxiolytics or other interventions.

Teach diaphragmatic breathing to slow the rate and increase the depth of respirations. Place one hand on the patient's abdomen. Instruct the patient to inhale deeply, causing the hand on the abdomen to rise. During exhalation, have the patient feel the hand on the belly sink down toward the spine. Explain that the chest moves minimally. After a minute or two, ask the patient to place his or her hands on the belly to continue the exercise. If necessary, administer mild doses of anxiolytics (ie, lorazepam or alprazolam) that do not depress respiration. Use a validated sedation assessment tool to measure the patient's anxiety and evaluate the medication's effect.

Preventing and Managing Complications

The risk of ARF is not only the imminent danger of respiratory compromise but also the many complications that can result from the interventions required to treat ARF over a prolonged interval. Mechanical ventilation, immobility, and the use of invasive tubes and lines create risks for lung damage, pressure injury, and infection. Nursing interventions to minimize these risks include continuous monitoring, frequent repositioning, and aseptic technique. See Chapter 5, Airway and Ventilatory Management, for additional strategies to prevent the complications of mechanical ventilation and Chapter 11, Multisystem Problems for strategies to prevent hospital-acquired conditions.

- *Pulmonary aspiration:* Ensure proper inflation of endotracheal tube cuff at all times. Refer to additional prevention strategies for ventilator-associated pneumonia (VAP) in Table 10-15.
- *Gastrointestinal (GI) bleeding:* Protect gastric mucosa and increase gastric pH in ventilator patients by using stress ulcer prophylaxis and/or tube feedings after assessing the patient's risk for GI bleeding (see Chapter 14, Gastrointestinal System).
- *Barotrauma:* Avoid unnecessary increases in airway pressures (eg, patient/ventilator dyssynchrony, excessive coughing) and assess for signs and symptoms of pneumothorax, pneumomediastinum, and other barotrauma complications.
- *Volutrauma:* Prevent alveolar damage from excessive tidal volumes.

Acute Respiratory Distress Syndrome

The case study of the patient in a motor vehicle accident is typical of a patient who develops ARDS. ARDS has a very high morbidity and mortality. It is characterized by noncardiac pulmonary edema caused by increased alveolar capillary membrane permeability and usually affects both lungs. Hypoxemia refractory to increase in inspired oxygen is a hallmark of the condition. ARDS is defined as "mild," "moderate," and "severe" ARDS according to the Berlin definition of ARDS. This definition considers the

timing of the condition, the results of chest imaging, the origin of lung edema, and oxygenation status. The severity stratification of mild, moderate, and severe is based on the PaO_2/FiO_2 score and PEEP level. The PaO_2/FiO_2 ratio (also called P/F ratio) is calculated by dividing the PaO_2 by the FiO_2 (with a decimal; 50% = 0.5). The ARDS PaO_2/FiO_2 ratio definition is as follows.

- *Mild ARDS:* PaO_2/FiO_2 ratio 201 to 300 mm Hg
- *Moderate ARDS:* PaO_2/FiO_2 ratio 101 to 200 mm Hg
- *Severe ARDS:* PaO_2/FiO_2 ratio less than or equal to 100 mm Hg.

See Chapter 20, Advanced Respiratory Concepts: Modes of Ventilation, for more information on ARDS stratification.

Etiology, Risk Factors, and Pathophysiology

Risk factors for the development of ARDS can be categorized into conditions that lead to direct damage to the alveolar-capillary membrane (primary causes) and those that are thought to be mediated by cellular or humoral injury to the capillary endothelial wall (secondary causes) (Table 10-7). Whether primary or secondary causes, the pathologic processes involved in ARDS are characterized by excessive alveolar-capillary membrane permeability, interstitial edema, and diffuse alveolar injury (see Figure 10-13). Direct damage to the alveolar membrane can easily occur when toxic substances are inhaled, such as during fires or chemical spills.

Alveolar and interstitial edema, microatelectasis, and ventilation-perfusion mismatching in ARDS lead to severe hypoxemia and poor lung compliance ("stiff lungs"). In the setting of trauma and sepsis, this abnormality in microvascular permeability occurs in capillary beds throughout the body. Typically, this multisystem organ dysfunction is not clinically apparent, with clinical manifestations isolated to the respiratory system. When multiorgan dysfunction syndrome does occur, it is seen in ARDS patients who develop bacterial infections and sepsis (see Chapter 11, Multisystem Problems).

TABLE 10-7. PRIMARY AND SECONDARY CAUSES OF ARDS

Primary Causes (Direct Damage to the Alveolar Membrane)
- Aspiration
- Pulmonary contusion
- Near drowning
- Inhalation of smoke or toxic substances
- Pneumonia (viral such as influenza, coronavirus, along with bacterial)

Secondary Causes (Mediated by Cellular or Humoral Injury to the Capillary Endothelium)
- Sepsis
- Hypovolemic shock associated with chest trauma or sepsis
- Acute pancreatitis
- Fat emboli
- Trauma
- Disseminated intravascular coagulation (DIC)
- Massive blood transfusions

The ARDS process disrupts normal macrophage function and increases the risk of infection. Mortality and long-term disability from ARDS are high.

Clinical Presentation

Signs and Symptoms

- Dyspnea
- Tachypnea (rates often > 40 breaths/min)
- Use of accessory muscles of respiration
- Abnormal breath sounds (crackles, wheezes)
- Tachycardia
- Chest pain
- Cough
- Diaphoresis
- Anxiety
- Confusion

Diagnostic Tests

- Chest x-ray shows new, diffuse, bilateral pulmonary infiltrates without increased cardiac size
- PaO_2/FiO_2 less than or equal to 300 mm Hg
- Static compliance (tidal volume/inspiratory plateau pressure – PEEP) less than 40 mL/cm H_2O

Principles of Management for ARDS

Most of the management of ARDS is supportive care and the prevention of complications. To date, interventions to limit the disease progression or reverse the underlying structural defects are not known.

Improving Oxygenation and Ventilation

Interventions specific to ARDS to improve oxygenation and ventilation include the following:

1. Administer high FiO_2 levels with high-flow system using face mask or nasal cannula if able to oxygenate noninvasively.
2. Initiate mechanical ventilation if cardiovascular instability is present, severe hypoxemia persists, or if respiratory fatigue develops.
   - Oxygen support at high FiO_2 levels with PEEP is usually required to achieve an acceptable PaO_2 (>50 mm Hg). Monitor for hemodynamic compromise when using PEEP greater than 5 cm H_2O and titrate oxygen if possible to less than .6 to prevent secondary lung injury. The goal is not to achieve a normal PaO_2 but to keep it above 50 mm Hg.
   - Decrease work of breathing initially by using ventilator modes and ventilator rates to decrease respiratory effort by the patient.
   - Prevent "volutrauma." Studies have demonstrated that large tidal volumes, which contribute to high plateau pressures, cause damage to the alveoli if used for prolonged periods (48 hours) in patients with ARDS. The use of small tidal volumes (4-8 mL/kg predicted body weight) is recommended to maintain plateau pressures of 30 cm H_2O or less.

3. Sedation and analgesia may be necessary after intubation to maximize gas exchange and minimize oxygen consumption. "Patient/ventilator dyssynchrony" is a common complication of ventilatory support in the severely dyspneic, hypoxemic patient.
4. Short-term use of neuromuscular blockade when used early in severe ARDS may improve long-term outcomes. This early and brief use of paralytics is thought to decrease lung and systemic inflammation along with alveolar collapse or over distention. Sedation is required prior to and for the duration of neuromuscular blockade. (Refer to Chapter 6, Pain, Sedation, and Neuromuscular Blockade Management for additional information.)
5. While transfusions may improve oxygen-carrying capacity, evidence has shown that transfusion itself is a cause of ARDS and increases the risk of mortality (TRALI—transfusion-related acute lung injury). Transfusions are reserved for hemoglobin below 7 g/dL unless underlying cardiac disease exists.
6. Enteral is the preferred route of nutrition as it may help decrease bacterial translocation across the gut and provide prophylaxis for GI bleeding. (Refer to Chapter 14, Gastrointestinal System).
7. Use of prone positioning for greater than 16 hours a day is recommended in patients with severe ARDS and refractory hypoxemia (PaO_2/FiO_2 ratio < 100 mm Hg). Ventilation in the prone position recruits atelectatic regions of the lungs without increasing airway pressure.
8. Extracorporeal membrane oxygenation (ECMO) has been used in patients with severe ARDS in ECMO centers familiar with its use. Additional evidence is needed to make recommendations for or against its use along with ongoing research measuring clinical outcomes.

Reducing Anxiety

Same as previously described for ARF management.

Achieving Effective Communications

Refer to Chapter 5, Airway and Ventilatory Management for detailed discussion of communication techniques for intubated patients.

Maintaining Hemodynamic Stability and Adequate Perfusion

1. Patients with ARDS who require high levels of PEEP for oxygenation are at risk for hemodynamic instability due to the increased positive pressure in the thoracic cavity and its impact on the heart and large vessels. Vigilant monitoring including continuous cardiac monitoring and noninvasive hemodynamic monitoring is essential. Assessment of fluid balance takes into account both the patient's hemodynamic status and the need to minimize volume overload which will worsen pulmonary edema.
2. Vasoactive drugs may be required to maintain adequate perfusion.

Preventing Complications

In addition to complications listed for ARF:

1. ARDS patients are at higher risk for development of hospital-acquired pneumonias. Follow prevention strategies described later in the chapter. Prophylactic antibiotics have not been shown to decrease hospital-acquired pneumonia rates in ARDS patients. Meticulous attention to head of bed elevation, hand washing, oral care, and removal of invasive devices as soon as possible are key prevention strategies.

2. The incidence of barotrauma is particularly high in patients with ARDS due to the stress of positive pressure ventilation on damaged alveolar membranes.

3. Delirium, deep venous thrombosis (DVT), GI bleeding, poor nutrition, pressure injury, and device-related infections are complications of ARDS as these patients often require prolonged mechanical ventilation. Assessment and preventative strategies are part of the daily plan of care.

Acute Respiratory Failure in the Patient with Chronic Obstructive Pulmonary Disease

Individuals with COPD are at risk for ARF or COPD exacerbation due to progressive airflow limitation with chronic inflammatory airway and lung response. Altered host defenses, increased secretion volume and viscosity, impaired secretion clearance and airway changes, and common pathophysiologic changes predispose the patient with COPD to acute exacerbations or episodes of ARF. The etiology, clinical presentation, and management of ARF in the COPD patient vary somewhat from ARF without chronic underlying pulmonary dysfunction. This section of the chapter highlights differences in ARF management in the patient with underlying COPD.

Etiology, Risk Factors, and Pathophysiology

Any systemic or pulmonary illness can precipitate ARF in patients with COPD. In addition to the etiologies of ARF listed in Table 10-6, diseases or situations that decrease ventilatory drive, muscle strength, chest wall elasticity, or gas exchange capacity, or increase airway resistance or metabolic oxygen requirements can easily lead to ARF in patients with COPD (Table 10-8). The most common precipitating events include:

- *Respiratory infection* (pneumonia, bronchitis): This is the most frequent trigger of COPD exacerbations. Respiratory infections can be caused by virus or bacteria. Common pathogens in patients with COPD include *Haemophilus influenza, Streptococcus pneumoniae, Moraxella catarrhalis,* and *Pseudomonas aeruginosa.*
- *Environmental factors:* Pollution, vaping, or smoking, including second hand smoke is an additional common cause of ARF.

TABLE 10-8. PRECIPITATING EVENTS OF ACUTE RESPIRATORY FAILURE IN COPD

Decreased Ventilatory Drive
- Oversedation
- Hypothyroidism
- Brain stem lesions

Decreased Muscle Strength
- Malnutrition
- Shock
- Myopathies
- Hypophosphatemia
- Hypomagnesemia
- Hypocalcemia

Decreased Chest Wall Elasticity
- Rib fractures
- Pleural effusions
- Ileus
- Ascites

Decreased Lung Capacity for Gas Exchange
- Atelectasis
- Pulmonary edema
- Pneumonia
- Pulmonary embolus
- Heart failure

Increased Airway Resistance
- Bronchospasm
- Increased secretions
- Upper airway obstructions
- Airway edema

Increased Metabolic Oxygen Requirements
- Systemic infection
- Hyperthyroidism
- Fever

- *Pulmonary embolus:* The high incidence of right ventricular failure in COPD increases the risk of pulmonary embolus from right ventricular mural thrombi. PE in patients with COPD exacerbations may contribute to respiratory compromise or it may be an incidental finding in these patients.
- *Pulmonary hypertension (PH):* The presence of secondary PH typically due to chronic hypoxemia, left heart failure, or sleep apnea may also be an additional risk factor for ARF.
- *Patient factors:* Other medical conditions such as heart disease or diabetes along with advanced age, previous hospitalizations, duration of COPD, productive cough, and history of antibiotic use are associated with increased risk.

The development of ARF in COPD patients places a tremendous burden on the pulmonary system. The chronic disease process leads to impaired ventilation, poor gas exchange, and airway obstruction. The additional burden of an acute disease process, even a relatively minor one, further impairs ventilation and gas exchange and increases airway obstruction. Compensatory mechanisms can easily be overwhelmed, with lethal consequences.

Clinical Presentation

Signs and symptoms are similar to ARF, but usually more pronounced.

Diagnostic Tests
- *Chest x-ray:* Evidence of COPD (flat diaphragms, hyperinflation of air fields), in addition to x-ray findings specific to the cause of the ARF (see Figure 10-3).
- *ABGs:* $Paco_2$ levels above the patient's baseline, which may be greater than 50 mm Hg during stable, chronic disease periods. Spo_2 levels below the patient's baseline, which may be maintained on room air or with home oxygen during stable periods.

Principles of Management for ARF in Patients With COPD

The presence of chronic respiratory dysfunction and an acute respiratory problem leads to some changes in the typical management of ARF. Treatment is directed at both the acute precipitating event and the chronic airflow obstruction problems associated with COPD.

Treating the Underlying Disease State

1. Increase airway diameter with bronchodilators and reduce airway edema with corticosteroids. Short-acting beta$_2$-agonists (SABA) with or without anticholinergic agents are recommended as the initial treatment (Table 10-9). Higher than usual doses may be necessary until the precipitating event is resolved.

TABLE 10-9. BRONCHODILATOR CATEGORIES FOR COPD

Category	Examples
Short-acting beta$_2$-agonists (SABA)	Albuterol Levalbuterol
Long-acting beta$_2$-agonists (LABA)	Arformoterol Formoterol Indacaterol Oladaterol Salmeterol Vilanterol
Short-acting anticholinergics or antimuscarinic (SAMA)	Ipratropium bromide Oxitropium bromide
Long-acting anticholinergics or antimuscarinic (LAMA)	Aclidinium bromide Glycopyrronium bromide Tiotropium Umeclidinium Glycopyrrolate Revefenacin
Combination SABA and SAMA	Fenoterol and ipratropium bromide Salbutamol and ipratropium bromide
Combination LABA and LAMA	Formoterol and aclidinium Formoterol and glycopyrronium Indacaterol and glycopyrronium Vilanterol and umeclidinium Olodaterol and tiotropium
Combination Corticosteroid, LABA, and LAMA	Fluticasone and vilanterol and umeclidinium Beclometasone and formoterol and glycopyrronium Budesonide and formoterol and glycopyrrolate
Methylxanthines	Aminophylline Theophylline

Systemic corticosteroids are used to decrease airway inflammation and thus bronchospasm. The steroids may also enhance secretion clearance.
2. Treat pulmonary infections with appropriate antibiotics.
3. Improve secretion removal. Strategies to improve secretion removal include adequate hydration, coughing, heated moist aerosolization, and mobilization. The routine use of chest physiotherapy is not supported by the literature and is not recommended. Secretions may be thick and tenacious. Monitor response to these therapies and discontinue them if no additional benefits are observed.

Improving Oxygenation and Ventilation

1. Correct hypoxemia (oxygen saturation < 90%) with small increases in Fio_2 levels, preferably with a controlled O_2 delivery device such as a Venturi mask. For patients with respiratory acidosis, noninvasive positive pressure ventilation via biphasic intermittent positive airway pressure (BiPAP), or continuous positive airway pressure (CPAP) is recommended. The goal is to maintain adequate arterial oxygenation (Pao_2 of 55-60 mm Hg or the patient's baseline values during nonacute situations) without significantly increasing $Paco_2$ levels.

   The administration of oxygen to COPD patients was once believed to eliminate the "hypoxic drive to breathe," creating a risk for hypercarbia, acidosis, and death. The hypoxic drive is responsible for approximately 10% of the total drive to breathe. Supplemental oxygen is usually necessary to prevent the deleterious effects of hypoxia and potential organ failure. Higher than necessary Fio_2 levels are avoided. The impact of Fio_2 on $Paco_2$ occurs by three physiologic mechanisms (see Table 10-10).

   Oxygen therapy in COPD patients is necessary to prevent hypoxia and organ failure and so is never withheld. Titration and considerations for noninvasive ventilation (NIV) or invasive mechanical ventilation in the COPD patient with CO_2 retention ($Paco_2$ > 50 mm Hg) are guided by the pH and $Paco_2$.
   - *Indications for NIV.* pH ≤ 7.35 and $Paco_2$ ≥ 45, severe dyspnea, or persistent hypoxemia. Improved ventilation is required to correct the acidosis in addition to oxygen therapy.
   - *Indications for invasive mechanical ventilation.* pH < 7.25, increasing $Paco_2$, and worsening hypoxia. Other indications include the following:
     - unable to tolerate NIV
     - post respiratory or cardiac arrest
     - decreased level of consciousness
     - aspiration or vomiting
     - hemodynamic instability
     - arrhythmias

TABLE 10-10. PHYSIOLOGIC EFFECTS OF OXYGEN IN COPD

Haldane effect	As hemoglobin becomes desaturated with oxygen, the affinity for carbon dioxide increases. The administration of oxygen then displaces carbon dioxide on hemoglobin and increases carbon dioxide levels in the plasma. Patients with COPD are unable to increase minute ventilation or "blow off" carbon dioxide. This leads to an increase in carbon dioxide, lowering the pH and resulting in a respiratory acidosis.
Hypoxic vasoconstriction	This physiologic adaptive mechanism is a response to a decrease in alveolar oxygen and moves capillary blood flow from a closed or atelectatic alveolus to an open alveolus. In patients with COPD, this adaptive mechanism no longer occurs. As a result, dead space ventilation or decreased perfusion (see Figure 10-15C) occurs with resulting increased carbon dioxide levels.
Decreased minute ventilation	As a result of increased dead space ventilation with resulting increased carbon dioxide, some COPD patients will decrease their minute ventilation. This decrease will further limit the patient's inspiratory reserve capacity.
Absorptive atelectasis	Increased oxygen levels cause a washout of alveolar nitrogen. This leads to collapse of smaller alveoli and decreased ventilation.

2. Position the patient to maximize ventilatory efforts and relaxation/rest during spontaneous breathing. A high Fowler position and leaning on an overbed table may be a position of comfort prior to intubation and mechanical ventilation.

3. Teach relaxation techniques and diaphragmatic, pursed lip breathing to decrease anxiety and improve ventilatory patterns. Anxiolytics and other sedatives are used cautiously to avoid decreasing MV.

4. Assist with implementing noninvasive ventilation if needed. The use of noninvasive ventilation in COPD patients with ARF is preferred as the initial mode of ventilation in most patients.

5. Monitor patients managed with supplemental oxygen or noninvasive ventilation for the need for intubation. Deterioration of mental status, hemodynamic instability, and inadequate response to initial therapy are all indications that intubation and mechanical ventilation are warranted. The patient's baseline pulmonary function and functional status, and the reversibility of the condition causing ARF are also factors in the decision to intubate. Weaning from mechanical ventilation is frequently more difficult, and in some cases not possible, in the presence of COPD. Informed discussions with the patient and family regarding intubation are essential. The presence of an advanced directive and designation of a power of attorney for healthcare decisions can help in guiding clinician's actions when patients are unable to make treatment decisions themselves (see Chapter 8, Ethical and Legal Considerations).

6. Close monitoring of COPD patients is also required following intubation and initiation of mechanical ventilation. Unlike other patients with ARF, patients with COPD must undergo slow correction of hypercarbia to avoid life-threatening alkalemia. This is because they generally have a higher than normal bicarbonate level secondary to the long-term metabolic compensation of the kidneys. CO_2 can be quickly decreased with mechanical ventilation resulting in alkalemia. The risk for auto-PEEP and barotrauma is higher in patients with COPD, necessitating smaller tidal volumes, lower respiratory rates, short inspiratory times, and long expiratory times.

Nutritional Support

1. Initiate enteral or oral feeding as soon as possible, once hemodynamic stability is achieved. Typically, patients with COPD have protein-calorie malnutrition, as well as low levels of phosphate, magnesium, and calcium. These chronic nutritional deficits lead to muscle weakness and may interfere with the weaning process, if mechanical ventilation becomes necessary. In addition, COPD patients who are malnourished have greater air trapping, lower diffusing capacity, and are less able to mobilize (see Chapter 14, Gastrointestinal System). Early enteral feeding (oral or by feeding tube) is essential to avoid further deterioration in their nutritional status during the acute illness.

2. In patients who are unable to eat, use enteral feeding rather than parenteral nutrition to decrease risk of infectious complications.

3. If used, noninvasive positive pressure ventilation makes oral feeding difficult and the insertion of a small bore nasoenteric tube may be necessary.

Preventing and Managing Complications

In addition to the complications associated with ARF, the following complications commonly are observed in COPD patients with ARF:

- *Arrhythmia:* High incidence of both atrial and ventricular arrhythmia in patients with COPD due to hypoxemia, acidosis, heart disease, medications, and electrolyte abnormalities. Cardiac monitoring and correction of the underlying cause is the goal, with pharmacologic treatment of arrhythmia only for life-threatening situations.

- *Pulmonary embolus:* Patients with COPD are at risk for venous thromboembolism. Observe for signs and symptoms and follow the treatment and prevention guidelines in patients presenting with COPD exacerbation.

- *GI distention and ileus:* Aerophagia is common in dyspneic patients, increasing the incidence of this complication.

- *Auto-PEEP and barotraumas* (if ventilated): High incidence, especially in the elderly and in individuals with high ventilation needs.

COVID-19 (SARS-CoV-2)

Coronaviruses are pathogens which cause a variety of mild to severe respiratory illnesses in children and adults. Some coronaviruses are referred to as "the common cold." SARS-CoV2 is a novel coronavirus discovered in 2019, and the disease it causes is COVID-19. A percentage of people infected with SARS-CoV2 develop a severe form of COVID-19 that leads to acute respiratory and multi-system failure. Because SARS-CoV2 was a new virus to humans and some infections led to few or no symptoms, the virus spread widely and rapidly. As the virus has spread, mutations with varying transmissibility and severity have developed leading to repeated surges in cases and subsequent hospital admissions with COVID-19.

Etiology, Risk Factors, and Pathophysiology

Transmission of COVID-19 occurs through close contact. Respiratory secretions are believed to be the vehicle of transmission, and individuals are at greater risk when they are within 6 feet of an infected person. The risk of secondary infection is highest in congregate living settings such as households, long-term care facilities, homeless shelters, and detention facilities, and in healthcare settings in which personal protective equipment was not utilized. COVID-19 has an estimated incubation period of up to 14 days from time of exposure, with a majority of individuals developing symptoms within 4 to 5 days of exposure, though these timeframes may vary with different variants. While COVID-19 is predominantly a pulmonary disease, the virus may affect multiple body systems, including cardiovascular (myocarditis, thromboembolism, heart failure), hematologic (hypercoagulability), renal (acute renal failure), and hepatic (acute liver failure).

Clinical Presentation

Patients presenting with COVID-19 infection vary from asymptomatic to severe symptoms or death (see Table 10-11). The severity of symptoms determines whether a patient may be managed in the home environment with isolation or requires hospitalization for respiratory interventions and inpatient therapy. Patients with underlying comorbidities or identified risk factors are at higher risk for progression to severe disease. These include age greater than or equal to 65, immunocompromising conditions, chronic lung disease, chronic kidney disease, cardiovascular disease, pregnancy, and diabetes.

Diagnostic Tests

- *Pulse Oximetry*: Patients presenting with severe COVID-19 infection often have pulse-oximetry readings that do not clinically correlate with their level of consciousness. Room air pulse oximetry readings may be lower than 70% to 80% in some otherwise healthy patients. Pulse oximetry may be utilized to determine oxygen requirement until an arterial blood gas can be obtained. The accuracy of pulse oximetry readings varies with skin pigmentation (See Chapter 5).

TABLE 10-11. CHARACTERISTICS OF DISEASE SEVERITY IN COVID-19 (SARS-CoV-2)

Asymptomatic Infection	An individual who has tested positive for COVID-19 via antigen or PCR testing without evidence of symptomatic disease.
Mild Disease	No pneumonia or dyspnea. Symptoms may include malaise, fever, sore throat, cough, myalgias, loss of taste and smell, nausea, vomiting, and/or diarrhea. These patients do not require hospitalization.
Moderate Disease	Evidence of respiratory disease on physical exam (abnormal lung sounds, tachypnea, cough) or chest x-ray. $Spo_2 \geq 94\%$ on room air.
Severe Disease	Evidence of pneumonia on chest x-ray. Dyspnea (respiratory rate ≥ 30 breaths/min), hypoxia ($Spo_2 \leq 93\%$), a partial pressure of oxygen: fraction of inspired oxygen (P:F) ratio of <300 mm Hg,, and/or a chest x-ray which shows >50% of the respiratory system with infiltrates in the first 24-48 hours.
Critical Disease	Respiratory failure, shock, and/or multiorgan dysfunction.

Data from COVID-19 Treatment Guidelines Panel. Coronavirus disease 2019 (COVID-19) treatment guidelines. National Institute of Health. Available at https://www.covid19treatmentguidelines.nih.gov/

- *Arterial blood gas:* In untreated severe disease, arterial blood gases will show hypoxemia (Pao_2 of less than 80), hypercarbia ($Paco_2$ greater than 45 mm Hg), with an overall respiratory acidosis (pH < 7.35).
- *SARS-CoV-2 test:* A variety of testing platforms exist for the diagnosis of COVID-19, including antigen and polymerase chain reaction (PCR) test. Testing is performed on a nasal, nasopharyngeal, or oropharyngeal swab sample.
- *Additional lab testing:* Additional lab tests which may be abnormal include leukocytes (decreased or elevated), elevation of markers of blood clotting (D-Dimer, ferritin, C-reactive protein), and elevation of markers of liver and renal function.
- *Chest x-ray:* In moderate to severe disease, the chest x-ray may show bilateral multifocal opacities consistent with COVID-19 pneumonia.

Principles of Management for COVID-19 Infection

Treatment is directed at improving oxygenation, decreasing inflammatory response, reducing organ dysfunction, and preventing thromboembolism. The science of COVID-19 management continues to evolve with research on the efficacy of new and existing therapies. These include steroids, antivirals, immunomodulators, and anticoagulants. Management of the patient with severe or critical COVID-19 infection may include noninvasive positive pressure ventilation such as high-flow nasal cannula or BIPAP. Patients who progress to respiratory failure may require mechanical ventilation, prone positioning, and vasoactive and sedative infusions in addition to COVID-19 therapeutics. Refer to the NIH COVID-19 Treatment Guidelines for the most updated recommendations. These recommendations are available online and are updated by a guideline committee that evaluates the evolving evidence on an ongoing basis. Vaccination against COVID-19 has proven to be effective in decreasing the risk of infection, hospitalization, and death.

Nonpharmacologic Interventions for the Spontaneously Breathing Patient Hospitalized with COVID-19

- *Self-proning*: Patients should be encouraged to reposition every 2 hours, moving from side to side, and to a prone or partially prone position. This recruits all areas of the lung to participate in oxygenation and ventilation and decreases the risk of atelectasis.
- *Incentive spirometry*: Incentive spirometry should be encouraged hourly while awake, to reduce the risk of atelectasis and pneumonia.
- *Oral care*: Patients may be on high levels of oxygen via high-flow nasal cannula or face mask. Frequent oral care will reduce dryness and decrease the risk of infection.
- *Psychosocial support*: Patients hospitalized with COVID-19 may experience anxiety related to their disease process and/or hypoxemia. They also experience isolation from family and friends due to their infection. Provide support, encouragement, and mechanisms such as tablets for video communication with family and friends.

Acute Respiratory Failure in the Patient with Asthma

Individuals with asthma are at risk for exacerbations that are characterized by a progressive increase in shortness of breath, cough, wheezing, or decrease in expiratory airflow. Acute severe asthma exacerbation, status asthmaticus, and asthma attack are also terms that have been used to describe this condition. Asthma differs from COPD in both pathophysiology and therapeutic response in that the airway restriction in asthma is reversible with aggressive and timely treatment (Figure 10-16) while COPD is a progressive disorder.

Etiology, Risk Factors, and Pathophysiology

Asthma exacerbations are first and foremost due to uncontrolled airway inflammation. Severe bronchospasm and increased mucus production both contribute to airway obstruction. Triggers vary and include infection, inhaled seasonal antigens, foods, exercise, or medications to name just a few. While triggers may stimulate an exacerbation of asthma, they are not causal.

Bronchoconstriction results from mediators released from mast cells including histamine, prostaglandins, and leukotrienes that contract the smooth muscle. Mucus plugging is thought to be due to eosinophils and shed bronchial epithelial cells as well as impaired mucus transport. Additionally, over time some patients may exhibit airway remodeling (thickening that contributes to airflow narrowing and airflow obstruction) especially if their airway inflammation

is not controlled. All of these contribute to the severe and often unrelenting nature of the asthma "attack." Some risk factors for the development of an acute severe asthma episode include frequent need for use of their "rescue" inhalers, recent illness, frequent past emergency room visits or hospitalizations, prior intubations and ICU admissions, noncompliance with medical therapy, and inadequate access to health care.

Clinical Presentation

Clinical findings are related to severe airflow obstruction and may include the inability to say a full sentence, shortness of breath, wheezing, pulsus paradoxus, use of accessory muscles of inspiration, diaphoresis, and need to maintain upright position. However, peak flow measurement is one of the best assessment tools for determining the severity of the exacerbation. A peak flow of less than or equal to 50% of expected or an absolute peak flow measurement of less than 100 L/min in an adult generally indicates severe bronchoconstriction, especially in combination with failure to respond to bronchodilator treatments. These patients are generally admitted to a critical care unit for monitoring and urgent therapy (see Figure 10-16).

Diagnostic Tests

- *Arterial blood gases*: Initial findings may show pH greater than 7.45, $PaCO_2$ less than 35 mm Hg indicating respiratory alkalosis, and mild to moderate hypoxia. In severe airflow obstruction, findings may progress to pH less than 7.35 and $PaCO_2$ greater than 50 mm Hg (respiratory acidosis).
- *Pulsus paradoxus*: A decrease of greater than 10 mm Hg in systolic blood pressure during inspiration.
- *Pulmonary function tests (PFTs)*: Forced expiratory volume in one second (FEV_1) of less than 20% or peak expiratory flow rate (PEFR) of less than 50% of predicted despite aggressive bronchodilator therapy.
- *SpO_2*: observe for hypoxia, monitoring trends in SpO_2 levels.

Principles of Management for Acute Severe Asthma and Asthma Exacerbations

Treatment is directed at decreasing airway inflammation, reversal of airflow obstruction, and correction of hypercapnia or hypoxemia if present.

Treat the Underlying Disease State

1. Reduce airway inflammation with edema with systemic corticosteroids and provide aggressive bronchodilation. Inhaled short-acting beta₂-agonist bronchodilators (eg, albuterol) are the drug of choice and may be provided continuously by nebulizer through a mouthpiece, mask, or if ventilated, through the ventilator circuit. Concomitant use of anticholinergic bronchodilators (eg. ipratropium)

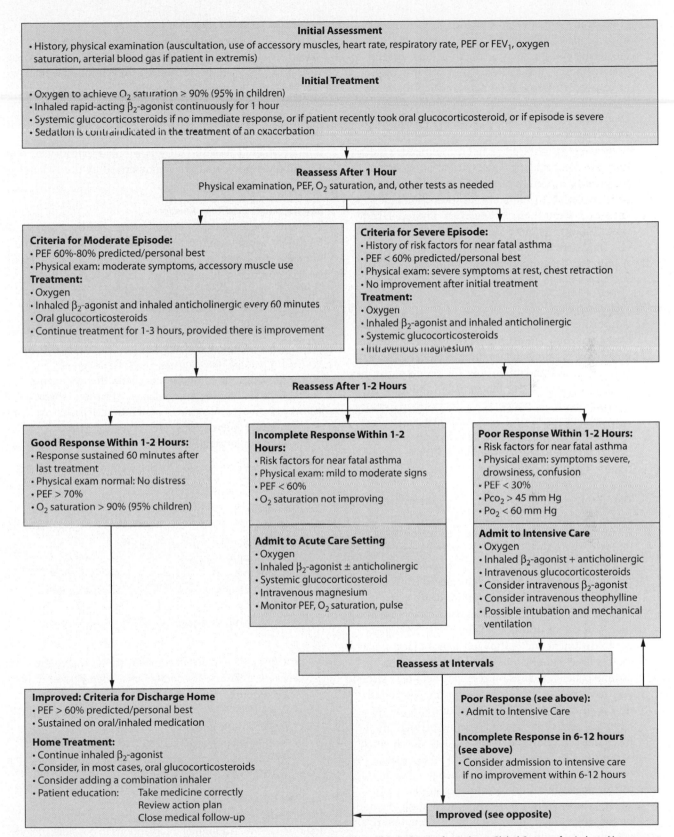

Figure 10-16. Management of asthma exacerbations in acute care facility. (*Data from Global Initiative for Asthma. Global Strategy for Asthma Management and Prevention.*)

is generally provided to enhance rapid reversal of bronchospasm. The use of magnesium sulfate is not recommended for routine use in asthma exacerbations, although it may be used in patients who fail to respond to initial treatment and have persistent hypoxemia. Intramuscular epinephrine should be considered in acute asthma with anaphylaxis and angioedema.

2. Routine use of antibiotics is not recommended unless there is strong evidence of respiratory infection.

3. Improve secretion removal: Generally, secretions will be easier to mobilize as bronchodilation is enhanced. Until then, strategies are limited. Hydration with intravenous fluids is often required to correct fluid deficits and loosen secretions.

4. Administer pneumococcal and influenza (seasonal) vaccines prior to discharge, if not already received.

Improving Oxygenation and Ventilation

1. Administer oxygen to correct hypoxemia: Severe hypoxemia may require high Fio_2 levels until an adequate oxygen saturation is obtained (90% or greater). Oxygen masks and high-flow O_2 systems may be used to deliver oxygen. Mechanical ventilation may be necessary if the patient does not respond to more conservative methods. Unlike COPD exacerbations, the use of noninvasive ventilation has not been effective in asthma exacerbation and can cause hyperinflation. Frequent monitoring of arterial blood gases is essential to monitor pH and $Paco_2$.

2. Position the patient to maximize ventilatory efforts and relaxation/rest during spontaneous breathing.

3. Relaxation techniques may be helpful to decrease anxiety and improve ventilatory patterns. Anxiolytics and other sedatives are not given unless the patient is intubated. Studies have demonstrated that doing so increases the potential for death.

4. If indicated, prepare the patient for intubation and mechanical ventilation. A patient who is not responding to treatment and is showing signs of fatigue may require urgent intubation. Ventilatory management of asthma patients focuses on restoring acid-base status and oxygenation while decreasing lung hyperinflation (known as dynamic hyperinflation in the spontaneously breathing patient and auto-PEEP in the mechanically ventilated patient). The development of auto-PEEP is due to the inability of the patient to exhale totally with each breath. When possible, monitor for auto-PEEP and for changes in plateau pressure measurements and use this information to guide pharmacologic and ventilator interventions. Low tidal volumes, low ventilator rates, short inspiratory times, and long expiratory times may help prevent hyperinflation. If this strategy is employed, the patient may require sedatives and sometimes paralytics to prevent dyssynchrony with the ventilator.

Preventing and Managing Complications

Patients with severe asthma exacerbations who require intubation are at risk for the same complications that all patients with ARF face. See the section on prevention and management of complications in the "Principles of Management for Acute Respiratory Failure," discussed earlier.

Interstitial Lung Disease

Interstitial lung disease (ILD) is a broad category of over 130 lung disorders that are characterized by fibrosis and/or inflammation of the lungs.

Etiology, Risk Factors, and Pathophysiology

The lung tissue or interstitium is damaged by a known or unknown causes leading to inflammation. The inflammation may include the alveolar space, small airways, blood vessels, and/or the pleura. Fibrosis and scarring then occur with resulting hypoxemia and "stiff lungs."

Some known causes include:

- Occupational and environmental exposure to irritants, asbestos, and silica
- Infections, tuberculosis, COVID-19
- Medications, amiodarone, chemotherapy agents
- Connective tissue or collagen disorders, rheumatoid arthritis, sarcoidosis, systemic sclerosis, systemic lupus erythematosus
- Genetic/familial

Unknown causes are classified as idiopathic pulmonary fibrosis (IPF).

Clinical Presentation
Signs and Symptoms
- Dyspnea
- Dry cough
- Clubbing
- Fine crackles or "velcro lungs" on auscultation
- Signs of right-sided heart failure
- Fatigue and weakness

Diagnostic Tests
- *Chest x-ray:* May be normal or show lung volume loss
- *High-resolution CT chest:* Classic description of honeycombing or "ground glass"
- *Lung biopsy:* May be indicated in some circumstances for definitive diagnosis
- *Serology:* For specific connective tissue diseases
- *PFTs:* Most of the disorders show a restrictive pattern with decreased lung volumes

Principles of Management
The management of ILD is similar to the management for ARF described above. Additional interventions to consider include:

- Smoking cessation (cigarettes and vaping) counseling and lifestyle changes to remove inhalation exposures
- Supplemental oxygen therapy in patients who demonstrate hypoxemia

- Discontinue and avoid using medications that can cause lung toxicity (eg, bleomycin, cyclophosphamide, nitrofurantoin, sulfasalazine, and amiodarone)
- Referral to pulmonary rehabilitation for monitored physical activity to prevent functional decline
- Medications specific to underlying cause:
  - Corticosteroids
  - Cytotoxic agents
  - Recent recommendations specific to IPF include two new oral medications that target specific pulmonary vascular growth factors: nintedanib or pirfenidone
- Referral to lung transplant center for evaluation
- Supportive care to improve symptom control and quality of life

Pulmonary Arterial Hypertension

Pulmonary arterial hypertension (PAH) is a progressive, life threatening disorder of the pulmonary circulation characterized by high pulmonary artery pressures (mean > 20 mm Hg) leading from the right side of the heart to the lungs. This persistent high pulmonary artery pressure ultimately leads to right ventricular failure. Patients with PAH in WHO Group 1 are often on a chronic regimen of therapy that should not be interrupted during hospitalization. Abrupt cessation of therapy can lead to rebound PH that can be fatal.

Etiology, Risk Factors, and Pathophysiology

PAH may result from a number of etiologies (Table 10-12). The pathophysiology is multifactorial with evidence that endothelial dysfunction leads to remodeling of the pulmonary artery vessel wall causing exaggerated vasoconstriction and impaired vasodilatation. The increase in pulmonary arterial pressure causes an increase in pulmonary vascular resistance, right ventricular dilation and hypertrophy, and decreased blood flow from the right side of the heart through the pulmonary vasculature. The result is a drop in the return of oxygenated blood to the left side of the heart. In PAH or WHO Class 1, the primary pathology is in the pulmonary vasculature. In WHO Class 2-5, the elevation in pulmonary artery pressure is secondary to other disorders such as left-sided heart disease, lung disease, chronic thromboembolic disease, or other causes. Distinction between PAH and PH is important because the treatment differs; most of the complex medications discussed later are indicated for PAH.

Clinical Presentation

Signs and Symptoms

Signs and symptoms include pallor, dyspnea, fatigue, chest pain, and syncope. Cor pulmonale or enlargement of the right ventricle can be a result of PAH and may lead to right ventricular failure (see Table 9-9). The diagnostic strategy is related to both establishing the diagnosis of PH versus PAH and if possible the underlying cause.

TABLE 10-12. WORLD HEALTH ORGANIZATION CLASSIFICATION OF PULMONARY HYPERTENSION[a]

Group	Main Classification	Diseases Included
1.	Pulmonary arterial hypertension (PAH)	PAH: Idiopathic, heritable, drug and toxin induced, associated with connective tissue disease, associated with HIV infection, associated with portal hypertension, associated with congenital heart disease, associated with schistosomiasis, long-term responders to calcium channel blockers, with overt features of venous/capillaries involvement, persistent PH of the newborn
2.	Pulmonary hypertension (PH) due to left heart disease	PH: Heart failure with preserved left ventricular ejection fraction (LVEF), heart failure with reduced LVEF, valvular heart disease, congenital/acquired cardiovascular conditions leading to post-capillary PH
3.	Pulmonary hypertension due to lung disease and/or hypoxia	PH: Obstructive lung disease, restrictive lung disease, other lung disease with mixed restrictive and obstructive pattern, hypoxia without lung disease, developmental lung disorders
4.	Pulmonary hypertension due to pulmonary artery obstruction	PH: Chronic thromboembolic disease, other pulmonary artery obstructions
5.	Pulmonary hypertension with unclear and/or multifactorial mechanisms	PH: Hematological disorders, systemic and metabolic disorders, others, complex congenital heart disease

Data from Simonneau G, Montani D, Celermajer DS, et al: Haemodynamic definitions and updated clinical classification of pulmonary hypertension. Eur Respir J. 2019;53(1):1801913.

Diagnostic Tests

- *Echocardiogram:* Valvular heart disease, left ventricular dysfunction, intracardiac shunts, right ventricular size, wall thickness and function, and tricuspid regurgitant jet velocity.
- *Chest x-ray:* Enlarged hilar and pulmonary arterial shadows and enlargement of the right ventricle.
- *12-lead ECG:* Right ventricular strain, right ventricular hypertrophy, and right axis deviation.
- *CTPA, ventilation-perfusion scan, or pulmonary angiogram:* These are done to rule out thromboembolism.
- *CT chest:* Assess for presence or absence of parenchymal lung disease.
- *6-minute walk test:* Measurement of distance used to monitor exercise tolerance, response to therapy, and progression of disease.
- *Right-heart cardiac catheterization:* Gold standard for diagnosis with vasodilator (adenosine, nitric oxide, epoprostenol) testing for benefit from long-term therapy with calcium channel blockers. Positive response is a decrease in mean PAP of 10 to 40 mm Hg with an increased or unchanged cardiac output (CO) from baseline values.

- *Serology testing:* Antinuclear antibodies.
- *Pulmonary function testing:* Used to rule out any other diseases contributing to shortness of breath.
- *Sleep study:* Done as a screen for sleep apnea, which may also contribute to the PH.

Principles of Management

Current treatment options aim to slow the progression of the disease and minimize symptoms.

- Provide anticoagulation therapy to prevent thrombosis and patient education about the long-term use of anticoagulants.
- Avoid beta-blockers, decongestants, or other medications that worsen PH or decrease right heart function.
- Encourage physical activity as tolerated, alternating periods of activity with periods of rest.
- Administer oxygen to treat hypoxemia and prevent increased pulmonary vasoconstriction due to low oxygen levels. Maintain SaO_2 greater than 90% if possible.
- Give diuretics to control edema and ascites if right-sided heart failure is present.
- Use calcium channel blockers in patients who show a positive response to vasodilator therapy during right heart catheterization.

Medical Treatment Options

Prior to 1995, there was no medical therapy for PAH other than continuous oxygen. Epoprostenol was the first medication for PAH and was approved in 1995. Patients must be preapproved through insurance for ongoing therapy and they must be able to self-administer. In general, these medications should not be stopped and require expertise in administration. There are five medication classifications. See Table 10-13 for examples.

- Phosphodiesterase inhibitors block phosphodiesterase type five, which is responsible for the degradation of cyclic guanosine monophosphate (cGMP).

TABLE 10-13. PULMONARY ARTERIAL HYPERTENSION MEDICATIONS

Category	Examples	Route
Phosphodiesterase inhibitor	Sildenafil	Oral, intravenous
	Tadalafil	Oral
Endothelin receptor antagonist	Bosentan	Oral
	Macitentan	Oral
	Ambrisentan	Oral
Prostacyclin receptor agonist	Selexipag	Oral
Soluble guanylate cyclase stimulator	Riociguat	Oral
Prostacyclin	Epoprostenol	Intravenous
	Treprostinil	Intravenous, subcutaneous Inhaled Oral
	Iloprost	Inhaled

Increased cGMP concentration results in pulmonary vasculature relaxation; vasodilation in the pulmonary bed and the systemic circulation (to a lesser degree) may occur.
- Endothelin receptor antagonists block the neurohormone endothelin from binding in the endothelium and vascular smooth muscle.
- Prostacyclin receptor agonists stimulate the endogenous production of prostacyclin to potentiate vasodilatation.
- Soluble guanylate cyclase stimulator acts synergistically with endogenous nitric oxide and also independently to produce vasodilatory effects, reduces pulmonary smooth muscle proliferation, and acts against platelet inhibition.
- Prostacyclin is a potent vasodilator of both systemic and pulmonary arterial vascular beds and is an inhibitor of platelet aggregation.

Surgical Treatment Options

- Atrial septostomy creates a right-to-left shunt to help decompress a failing right ventricle in select patients who are unresponsive to medical therapies. This also leads to significant hypoxemia in an already compromised patient.
- Pulmonary thromboendarterectomy for those with chronic thromboembolic pulmonary hypertension (CTEPH) to improve hemodynamics and functional status.
- Lung transplantation may be indicated when the PH has progressed despite optimal medical and surgical therapy.

Pneumonia

Respiratory infection is a common cause of ARF. Infections developed before hospitalization (community-acquired), during medical treatment (healthcare-acquired), and those acquired during hospitalization (hospital-acquired and ventilator-associated) can lead to significant morbidity and mortality, and require critical care management. A variety of respiratory infections occur in critically ill patients, including bronchitis and pneumonia. This section focuses on pneumonia, the most common respiratory infection and the most common cause of respiratory failure in critically ill patients.

Etiology, Risk Factors, and Pathophysiology

Infants, children, older adults, those with chronic cardiopulmonary disease, and immunocompromised individuals are at increased risk for pneumonia. In addition, immobility, decreased level of consciousness, and mechanical ventilation place hospitalized patients at high risk for development of pneumonias. These latter pneumonias are most commonly referred to as *ventilator-associated pneumonias* or *VAP*.

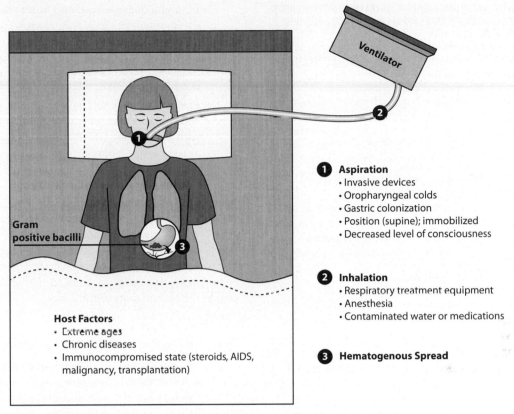

Figure 10-17. Pathogenesis of pneumonia.

Organisms that cause pneumonia enter the lungs by aspiration of nonsterile oropharyngeal or gastric contents, or inhalation of aerosols or particles containing the organisms, or hematogenic spread of the organism into the lungs from another site in the body (Figure 10-17). Most hospital-acquired pneumonias are due to aspiration of bacteria colonizing the oropharynx or upper GI tract. Pneumonia develops when the normal bronchomucociliary clearance mechanism or phagocytic cells are overwhelmed by the number or virulence of organisms aspirated or inhaled into the airways. The proliferation of organisms in the pulmonary parenchyma elicits an inflammatory response, with large influxes of phagocytic cells into the alveoli and airways and production of protein-rich exudates. This inflammatory response impairs the distribution of ventilation and decreases lung compliance, resulting in increased work of breathing and the sensation of dyspnea. Hypoxemia results from the shunting of blood through poorly ventilated areas of pulmonary consolidation. The inflammatory response leads to fever and leukocytosis.

Pneumonia also can develop through hematogenous spread, when organisms remote from the lungs gain access to the blood, become lodged in the pulmonary vasculature, and proliferate. Pneumonias with a hematogenous origin usually are distributed diffusely in both lung fields, rather than localized to a single lung or lobe.

Several factors present in critically ill patients increase the risk for the development of VAP. Aspiration of

oropharyngeal and gastric secretions is increased in the presence of tracheostomy tubes, endotracheal tubes, nasogastric tubes, poor GI motility, gastric distention, and immobility, all of which are common situations in critically ill patients. Treatments that neutralize the normally acidic gastric contents, such as antacids, H_2 blockers, proton-pump inhibitors, or tube feeding, increase the growth of gram-negative bacteria that can be directly aspirated into the lungs or spread to the lungs via the bloodstream.

The high frequency of gastric and pulmonary intubation further increases the risk for pneumonia. Within 24 hours of admission to a critical care unit, there is colonization of the pharynx with gram-negative bacteria. Approximately 25% of colonized patients develop a clinical infection (tracheobronchitis or pneumonia). Critically ill patients at high risk for hospital-acquired pneumonias are those immunocompromised from malignancy, AIDS, and chronic cardiac or respiratory disease; older adults; or those with depressed alveolar macrophage function (oxygen, corticosteroids).

Although a variety of similar organisms cause community-acquired and hospital-acquired pneumonias, their frequency distribution is different (Table 10-14). Of particular concern in hospital-acquired infections is the polymicrobial origin of the pneumonia and the potential for causative organisms to be resistant to antimicrobial therapy. Not surprisingly, during the COVID-19 pandemic in 2020, the standardized infection ratios (SIRs) for ventilator-associated events increased substantially.

TABLE 10-14. INFECTIOUS ETIOLOGIC AGENTS IN SEVERE COMMUNITY-ACQUIRED PNEUMONIA REQUIRING INTENSIVE CARE SUPPORT AND HOSPITAL-ACQUIRED PNEUMONIA IN CRITICALLY ILL PATIENTS

	Etiologic Agent (Decreasing Rank)
Community-acquired pneumonias	*Streptococcus pneumoniae*
	Staphylococcus aureus, Methicillin-resistant
	Staphylococcus aureus, Methicillin-susceptible
	Staphylococcus aureus
	Legionella species
	Mycoplasma pneumoniae
	Chlamydia pneumoniae
	Moraxella cararrhalis
	Haemophilus influenzae
	Gram-negative bacilli
	Viruses; Influenza, Parainfluenza, Adenovirus, Coronavirus
Ventilator-acquired pneumonias	*Staphylococcus aureus, Methicillin-resistant*
	Staphylococcus aureus, Methicillin-susceptible
	Staphylococcus aureus
	Pseudomonas aeruginosa
	Selected *Klebsiella* species
	Enterobacter species
	All *Streptococcus* species
	Haemophilus influenzae
	Escherichia coli
	Stenotrophomonas maltophilia
	Acinetobacter species
	Serratia species

Data from Metlay JP, Waterer GW, Long AC, et al. Diagnosis and Treatment of Adults with Community-acquired Pneumonia an Official Clinical Practice Guideline of the American Thoracic Society and Infectious Diseases Society of America. Am J Resp Crit Care Med. 2019;200(7):e45-e67. Weiner LM, Abner S, Edwards JR, et al. Antimicrobial-resistant pathogens associated with adult healthcare-associated infections: summary of data reported to the National Healthcare Safety Network, 2015-2017. Infect Control Hosp Epidemiol. 2020;41:1–18.

Development of a VAP is a serious complication in critically ill patients. Increased morbidity and mortality, in addition to increases in critical care and hospital lengths of stay and costs, make VAPs one of the most important sources of negative outcomes for critically ill patients.

Clinical Presentation

Signs and Symptoms

- Fever
- Cough, typically productive
- Purulent sputum or hemoptysis
- Dyspnea
- Pleuritic chest pain
- Tachypnea
- Abnormal breath sounds (crackles, bronchial breath sounds)

Diagnostic Tests

- Gram stain and culture of sputum for causative organisms. May require fiberoptic bronchoscopy with brush specimen or bronchoalveolar lavage specimen retrieval in situations where pneumonia responds poorly to empiric treatment. This may also be necessary early in admission in patients who are immunocompromised and susceptible to opportunistic organisms that require very specific antibiotic coverage.

- New or progressive infiltrates on chest x-ray. Infiltrates may be either localized or diffuse in nature (see Figure 10-5).

- Elevated WBC.

- Abnormal ABGs with initial finding of hypoxemia with hypocapnia which may progress to hypercapnia as respiratory failure progresses.

Principles of Management for Pneumonia

Treating the Underlying Disease

Appropriate empirical broad-spectrum antimicrobial therapy is based on an assessment of the most likely causative organisms until definitive culture results are obtained. Fluids are used to correct hypovolemia and hypotension, if present. Hypotension unresponsive to fluid therapy alerts the clinician to the potential for septic shock.

Improving Oxygenation and Ventilation

Similar to ARF management, with the following additions:

- Increased PEEP in the presence of focal pneumonia may exacerbate the ventilation-perfusion abnormalities by over-distending unaffected alveoli leading to increased capillary resistance and redistribution of blood flow to affected alveoli. These techniques are used with caution in pneumonia.

- Voluminous, tenacious respiratory secretions may require endotracheal intubation to assist with clearance. Chest physiotherapy may be helpful to increase secretion clearance, particularly when lobar atelectasis is present. Fiberoptic bronchoscopy may also be required to assist with secretion management.

Assessment and Surveillance

Although the signs and symptoms of VAP are known, clinical diagnosis is complicated by lack of specific and sensitive criteria. In 2013, the National Healthcare Safety Network lead by the Centers for Disease Control developed surveillance criteria for ventilator-associated events, which include ventilator-associated conditions (VACs), infection-related ventilator-associated conditions (IVACs), and possible or probable VAP (pVAP). These definitions were revised in 2021 and are shown in Figure 10-18. These definitions are less applicable to the clinical decisions about the care of patients with VAP and more useful for tracking rates of VAP and ventilator-associated event (VAE) so that the effectiveness of prevention strategies can be measured.

Preventing Ventilator-Associated Pneumonias

Because there are strategies that can prevent VAEs and VAP, rates of these conditions are indicative of the quality of care that patients receive. The cost of these complications is an additional consideration. It is estimated that a hospital-acquired pneumonia increases hospitalization 4 to 12 days,

Patient has a baseline period of stability or improvement on the ventilator, defined by ≥ 2 calendar days of stable or decreasing daily minimum* FiO_2 or PEEP values. The baseline period is defined as the 2 calendar days immediately preceding the first day of increased daily minimum PEEP or FiO_2.
*Daily minimum defined by lowest value of FiO_2 or PEEP during a calendar day that is maintained for > 1 hour.

After a period of stability or improvement on the ventilator, the patient has at least one of the following indicators of worsening oxygenation:
1) Increase in daily minimum* FiO_2 of ≥ 0.20 (20 points) over the daily minimum FiO_2 of the first day in the baseline period, sustained for ≥ 2 calendar days.
2) Increase in daily minimum* PEEP values of ≥ 3 cmH_2O over the daily minimum PEEP of the first day in the baseline period[†], sustained for ≥ 2 calendar days.
*Daily minimum defined by lowest value of FiO_2 or PEEP during a calendar day that is maintained for > 1 hour.
[†]Daily minimum PEEP values of 0-5 cmH_2O are considered equivalent for the purposes of VAE surveillance.

Ventilator-Associated Condition (VAC)

On or after calendar day 3 of mechanical ventilation and within 2 calendar days before or after the onset of worsening oxygenation, the patient meets <u>both</u> of the following criteria:

1) Temperature > 38°C or < 36°C, **OR** white blood cell count ≥ 12,000 cells/mm^3 or ≤ 4000 cells/mm^3.
AND
2) A new antimicrobial agent(s) (see Appendix for eligible antimicrobial agents) is started and is continued for ≥ 4 qualifying antimicrobial days (QAD).

Infection-related Ventilator-Associated Complication (IVAC)

On or after calendar day 3 of mechanical ventilation and within 2 calendar days before or after the onset of worsening oxygenation, ONE of the following criteria is met (**taking into account organism exclusions specified in the protocol**):
1) Criterion 1: Positive culture of one of the following specimens, meeting quantitative or semi-quantitative thresholds[†] as outlined in protocol, <u>without</u> requirement for purulent respiratory secretions:
   - Endotracheal aspirate, ≥ 10^5 CFU/mL or corresponding semi-quantitative result
   - Bronchoalveolar lavage, ≥ 10^4 CFU/mL or corresponding semi-quantitative result
   - Lung tissue, ≥ 10^4 CFU/g or corresponding semi-quantitative result
   - Protected specimen brush, ≥ 10^3 CFU/mL or corresponding semi-quantitative result
2) Criterion 2: Purulent respiratory secretions (defined as secretions from the lungs, bronchi, or trachea that contain ≥ 25 neutrophils and ≤10 squamous epithelial cells per low power field [lpf, ×100])[†] **PLUS** organism identified from one of the following specimens (to include qualitative culture, or quantitative/semi-quantitative culture without sufficient growth to meet Criterion #1):
   - Sputum
   - Endotracheal aspirate
   - Bronchoalveolar lavage
   - Lung tissue
   - Protected specimen brush
3) Criterion 3: One of the following positive tests:
   - Organism identified from pleural fluid (where specimen was obtained during thoracentesis or initial placement of chest tube and NOT from an indwelling chest tube)
   - Lung histopathology, defined as: 1) abscess formation or foci of consolidation with intense neutrophil accumulation in bronchioles and alveoli; 2) evidence of lung parenchyma invasion by fungi (hyphae, pseudohyphae, or yeast forms); 3) evidence of infection with the viral pathogens listed below based on results of immunohistochemical assays, cytology, or microscopy performed on lung tissue
   - Diagnostic test for *Legionella* species
   - Diagnostic test on respiratory secretions for influenza virus, respiratory syncytial virus, adenovirus, parainfluenza virus, rhinovirus, human metapneumovirus, coronavirus
[†]If the laboratory reports semi-quantitative results, those results must correspond to the quantitative thresholds. Refer to Table 2 and 3.

Possible Ventilator-Associated Pneumonia (pVAP)

Figure 10-18. Ventilator-associated events (VAEs) surveillance algorithm. (*Reproduced with permission from Centers for Disease Control and Prevention [CDC]. Device-associated module VAE. 2021. https://www.cdc.gov/nhsn/pdfs/pscmanual/10-vae_final.pdf.*)

and increases costs by $20,000 to $40,000 per episode. Prevention strategies (Table 10-15) include the following:

- Decrease the risk of cross-contamination or colonization via the hands of hospitalized personnel. Hand hygiene is the most effective strategy.

TABLE 10-15. EVIDENCE-BASED PRACTICE GUIDELINES FOR THE PREVENTION OF VENTILATOR-ASSOCIATED PNEUMONIA

Preventing Gastric Reflux
1. All mechanically ventilated patients, as well as those at high risk for aspiration (eg, decreased level of consciousness; enteral tube in place), should have the head of the bed elevated at an angle of 30°-45° unless medically contraindicated.[a,b,c]
2. Routinely verify appropriate placement of the feeding tube.[a]

Airway Management
1. Collaborate to identify patients where noninvasive positive pressure ventilation may be appropriate to prevent the need for intubation.[b]
2. If feasible, use an endotracheal tube with a dorsal lumen above the endotracheal cuff to allow drainage (by continuous or intermittent suctioning) of tracheal secretions that accumulate in the patient's subglottic area.[a,b,c]
3. Unless contraindicated by the patient's condition, perform orotracheal rather than nasotracheal intubation.[a]
4. ET cuff management: Before deflating the cuff of an endotracheal tube in preparation for tube removal, or before moving the tube, ensure that secretions are cleared from above the tube cuff.[a]
5. Use only sterile fluid to remove secretions from the suction catheter if the catheter is to be used for reentry into the patient's lower respiratory tract.[a]
6. Perform tracheostomy under aseptic conditions.[a]
7. Minimize sedation, perform daily spontaneous awakening trials daily assessment for readiness to wean, pair spontaneous breathing trials with spontaneous awakening trials.[c]

Oral and Skin Care
1. Develop and implement a comprehensive oral hygiene program.[a,c]
2. Chlorhexidine skin baths.[d]

Cross-Contamination
1. Hand washing: Decontaminate hands with soap and water or a waterless antiseptic agent after contact with mucous membranes, respiratory secretions, or objects contaminated with respiratory secretions, whether or not gloves are worn.[a]
2. Decontaminate hands with soap and water or a waterless antiseptic agent before and after contact with a patient who has an endotracheal or tracheostomy tube, and before and after contact with any respiratory device that is used on the patient, whether or not gloves are worn.[a]
3. Wear gloves for handling respiratory secretions or objects contaminated with respiratory secretions of any patient.[a]
4. When soiling with respiratory secretions is anticipated, wear a gown and change it after soiling and before providing care to another patient.[a]
5. Room-air humidifiers: Do not use large-volume room-air humidifiers that create aerosols (nebulizers) unless they can be sterilized or subjected to high-level disinfection at least daily and filled only with sterile water.[a]

Mobilization
1. Early exercise and mobility.[a,c]

Equipment Changes
1. Do not change routinely, on the basis of duration of use, the patient's ventilator circuit. Change the circuit when it is visibly soiled or mechanically malfunctioning. Periodically drain or discard any condensate that collects in the tubing. Do not allow condensate to drain toward the patient.[a,b,c]
2. Between use on different patients, sterilize or subject to high-level disinfection of all MRBs.[a]

[a]Data from Centers for Disease Control and Prevention (2004).
[b]AACN VAP Practice Alert (2017).
[c]SHEA/IDSA Practice Recommendations (2014).
[d]Robles MJ, Fonte J. Effect of chlorhexidine bath on the prevention of ventilator-associated pneumonia: a meta-analysis. Chest. 2019;155(4):123A.

- Decrease the risk of aspiration: Avoid supine positioning and keep the head of the bed elevated to 30° to 45° at all times, unless medically contraindicated. Use an endotracheal tube with a dorsal lumen above the endotracheal cuff to remove drainage with continuous suction. Suction above the endotracheal tube cuff before removing or repositioning the tube. Assess for, and correct, gastric reflux problems. See the AACN Practice Alert, Prevention of Aspiration in Adults.
- Use a progressive mobility protocol and in collaboration with other members of the healthcare team, promote exercise and mobility early in the course of a critical illness.
- Implement a comprehensive oral hygiene program that includes oral suctioning and teeth brushing.
- Implement a daily chlorhexidine bath protocol for ventilator patients.
- Maintain a closed system on ventilator/humidifier circuits, and avoid pooling of condensation or secretions in the tubing. Do not routinely change the ventilator circuit, except when visibly soiled or malfunctioning. Use sterile water or saline for use with any respiratory equipment.
- Use sterile technique for endotracheal suctioning and suction only when necessary to clear secretions from large airways.
- Provide nutritional support to improve host defenses and reduce the risk for pneumonia.
- Remove invasive devices and equipment as soon as possible. Assess weaning readiness daily with a spontaneous breathing protocol and limit the use of sedatives (see Chapter 5, Airway and Ventilatory Management and Chapter 6, Pain, Sedation, and Neuromuscular Blockade Management).

Pulmonary Embolism

Etiology, Risk Factors, and Pathophysiology

Pulmonary embolism is a complication of DVT, long bone fracture, or air entering the circulatory system. There are many risk factors for PE (Table 10-16). Critically ill patients are especially prone to pulmonary embolism due to the increase in risk factors associated with hospitalization.

Venous Thromboembolism

Virchow's triad describes a cluster of factors that predispose a patient to venous thromboembolism, including venous stasis (decreased mobility), hypercoagulability (cancer, heart failure, and blood clotting disorders), and vascular damage (trauma or surgery). Venous thrombi form at the site of vascular injuries or where venous stasis occurs, primarily in the leg or pelvic veins. Thrombi that dislodge travel through the venous circulation and can become wedged in a branch of the pulmonary circulation. Depending on the size of the thrombi, and the location of the occlusion, mild to severe obstruction of blood flow occurs beyond the thrombi.

TABLE 10-16. RISK FACTORS FOR THE DEVELOPMENT OF PULMONARY EMBOLISM

Thromboemboli
Obesity
Prior history of thromboembolism
Advanced age
Malignancy
Chemotherapy
Estrogen (estrogen replacement therapy or oral contraceptive use)
Immobility
Acute spinal cord injury with paralysis
Heart failure
Trauma
Pregnancy and postpartum
Surgery
Inherited thrombophilia
Central venous catheters
Inflammatory bowel disease
Nephrotic syndrome
Air Emboli
Surgery (neurosurgery, cardiothoracic, obstetrical/gynecologic, orthopedic, otolaryngological)
Pacemaker or defibrillator insertion
Radiologic procedures
IV contrast
Trauma
Positive pressure ventilation
Scuba diving
Hemodialysis
Central venous catheter insertion or removal
Fat Emboli
Long bone fracture and other fractures (pelvic, ribs, etc)
Intraosseous access
Chest compression
Lung transplantation
Liver disease
Pancreatitis
Lipid infusions
Sickle cell crisis
Cyclosporine administration

The primary sequela, and major contributor to mortality, of the PE is circulatory impairment. The physical obstruction of the pulmonary capillary bed increases right ventricular afterload, dilates the right ventricle, and impedes coronary perfusion. This predisposes the right ventricle to ischemia and right ventricular failure (cor pulmonale).

A secondary consequence of thromboemboli is a mismatching of ventilation to perfusion in gas exchange units beyond the obstruction (see Figure 10-15C), resulting in pulmonary arterial hypoxemia. This hypoxemia further compromises oxygen delivery to the ischemic right ventricle.

Air Emboli
Air or other nonabsorbable gases entering the venous system also travel to the right heart, pulmonary circulation, arterioles, and capillaries. A variety of surgical and nonsurgical situations predispose patients to the development of air embolization (see Table 10-16). Damage to the pulmonary endothelium occurs from the abnormal air-blood interface, leading to increased capillary permeability and alveolar flooding.

Bronchoconstriction also occurs with air embolization leading to impaired removal of carbon dioxide and hypercapnia.

Arterial embolization may occur if air passes to the left heart through a patent foramen ovale, present in approximately 30% of the population. Peripheral embolization to the brain, extremities, and coronary perfusion leads to ischemic manifestations in these organs.

Fat Emboli
Fat enters the pulmonary circulation most commonly when released from the bone marrow following long bone fractures (see Table 10-16). Nontraumatic origins of fat embolization also occur and are thought to be due to the agglutination of low-density lipoproteins or liposomes from nutritional fat emulsions. The presence of fat in the pulmonary circulation injures the endothelial lining of the capillary, increasing permeability and alveolar flooding.

Clinical Presentation
Because many of the signs and symptoms of PE are nonspecific, it is difficult to diagnosis. In critically ill patients, diagnosis is especially difficult due to alterations in communication and level of consciousness, and the nonspecific nature of other cardiopulmonary alterations.

Signs and Symptoms
- Dyspnea
- Pleuritic chest pain
- Cough
- Crackles
- Apprehension
- Diaphoresis
- Evidence of DVT
- Hemoptysis
- Tachypnea
- Fever
- Tachycardia
- Syncope
- Hypoxia
- Hypotension

Diagnostic Tests
- *Chest x-ray:* Evaluate for basilar atelectasis, elevation of the diaphragm, and pleural effusion, although most patients with PE have nonspecific findings on chest x-ray; diffuse alveolar filling may be seen in air embolism.
- *ABG analysis:* Hypoxemia with or without hypercarbia.
- *ECG:* Signs of right ventricular strain (right axis deviation, right bundle branch block) or precordial strain; sinus tachycardia.
- See earlier discussion of diagnostics for PE (CTPA and V/Q scans).

Principles of Management for Pulmonary Emboli
The key to reducing morbidity and mortality from PE is primarily prevention and secondarily early diagnosis and

treatment to prevent reembolization. Goals of care include the improvement of oxygenation and ventilation, improvement of cardiovascular function, prevention of reembolization, and prevention of additional pulmonary embolus. Some facilities have recently introduced a pulmonary embolism response team (PERT) to promote rapid interprofessional decision making in the early diagnosis and treatment of PE.

Improving Oxygenation and Ventilation

Oxygen therapy is usually effective in relieving hypoxemia associated with PE. When cardiopulmonary compromise is severe, mechanical ventilation may be required to achieve optimal oxygenation.

Improving Cardiovascular Function

Controversy exists as to the benefit of vasoactive drug administration (such as norepinephrine and/or inotropic agents) to improve myocardial perfusion of the right ventricle. In severe embolic events, where cardiac failure is profound, systemic thrombolytic agents are recommended. In patients with high bleeding risk or who have failed thrombolytic therapy, catheter-directed thrombolytic therapies or surgical embolectomy may also be warranted.

ESSENTIAL CONTENT CASE

Mechanical Ventilation

You are caring for a patient in ARF with the following interventions and findings:

- Mechanical ventilatory support (assist-control rate 10/min, tidal volume 440 mL, PEEP 15 cm H_2O, Fio_2 0.85)
- Pao_2 63 mm Hg
- MAP 68 mm Hg on vasoactive drug support (norepinephrine at 6 mcg/min)
- Neuromuscular blockade (cisatracurium)
- Sedation (midazolam)
- Pain Management (fentanyl)

Case Question 1: How might the level of PEEP this patient is receiving affect his response to suctioning?

Case Question 2: What precautions could you take to avoid or respond to potential complications?

Answers

1. When high levels of PEEP (>10 cm H_2O) are disrupted (such as during suctioning without an in-line catheter), functional residual capacity (the volume restored by PEEP) is lost and the alveoli lose their distending volume. A decrease in Pao_2 will ensue. High PEEP also increases risk for barotrauma with increased intrathoracic pressure which can lead to decreased venous return and decreased cardiac output (see Chapter 5 Airway and Ventilatory Management).
2. Hyperoxygenate the patient and use a PEEP valve on the MRB if not using an in-line suction catheter. Monitor hemodynamics for hypotension.

TABLE 10-17. ANTICOAGULANT AND THROMBOLYTIC MEDICATIONS

Category	Examples	Route
Unfractionated heparin	Heparin	Subcutaneous and intravenous
Low-molecular-weight heparin	Enoxaparin	Subcutaneous
	Dalteparin	Subcutaneous
Xa inhibitor	Fondaparinux	Subcutaneous
Vitamin K antagonist	Warfarin	Oral
Direct oral anticoagulants	Apixaban	Oral
Direct thrombin inhibitor	Dabigatran	Oral
Anti-Xa inhibitors	Apixaban	Oral
	Enoxaban	Oral
Thrombolytic	Alteplase	Intravenous

Preventing Reembolization

Several strategies are employed to prevent the likelihood of future embolization and cardiopulmonary compromise:

- Ambulation should not be limited in a patient with venous thromboembolism unless unrelated contraindications exist.
- Initial anticoagulation therapy is determined by patient comorbidities, provider assessment, and bleeding risk. Parenteral therapy may be initiated with unfractionated heparin or weight-based low-molecular-weight heparin. Intravenous therapy with unfractionated heparin is titrated to maintain a partial thromboplastin time (PTT) 1.5 to 2.5 times the control or anti-Xa level within a prescribed range. Patients on parenteral therapy will transition to a direct oral anticoagulant or vitamin K antagonist if there are no contraindications (Table 10-17).
- Insertion of vena cava filters to prevent emboli from legs, pelvis, and inferior vena cava from migrating to pulmonary circulation if anticoagulation therapy is contraindicated. Filters are placed percutaneously in the inferior vena cava if warranted.

Preventing Venous Thromboembolism

- An important recommendation for the prevention of VTE is awareness and access to a hospital prevention policy including risk assessment (Table 10-18). See AACN Practice Alert on Prevention of VTE.
- Assess the risk for VTE on admission to the unit and daily thereafter. Discussion also includes current VTE prevention intervention, risk for bleeding, and response to treatment.
- If ordered, apply graduated compression stocking or intermittent pneumatic compression (IPCs) (Figure 10-19; Table 10-19) and maintain in use at all times except when removed for correct fitting or skin assessment.
- Placement of prophylactic vena cava filters in high-risk patients who have a contraindication to anticoagulation.

TABLE 10-18. RISK FACTORS, ASSESSMENT, AND THROMBOPROPHYLAXIS FOR VTE

Risk Factors	Assessment of Risk and Thromboprophylaxis
• Active malignancy • Active rheumatic disease • Acute or chronic lung disease • Age • Central venous catheter • Congestive heart failure • Dehydration • Impaired mobility • Inflammatory bowel disease • Known thrombophilic state • Moderate to major surgery • Myeloproliferative disorders • Myocardial infarction • Nephrotic syndrome • Obesity • Oral contraceptives and hormone replacement therapy • Pregnancy or postpartum with immobility • Prior history of VTE • Sickle cell disease • Smoking • Trauma • Varicose veins or chronic stasis	**Low Risk** Ambulatory patients without additional risk factors or expected length of stay <2 days Minor surgery without additional risk factors (same-day surgery or <30 minutes) *Thromboprophylaxis* Early and aggressive ambulation **Moderate Risk** Most general, open gynecologic or urologic surgery Patients who are neither low risk nor high risk Acutely ill medical patients *Thromboprophylaxis* Pharmacologic prophylaxis with low-molecular-weight heparin, unfractionated heparin, or fondaparinux **Moderate Risk Plus Bleeding Risk** *Thromboprophylaxis* Mechanical thromboprophylaxis (pneumatic compression devices preferred), reassess bleeding risk daily, and initiate pharmacologic prophylaxis as soon as appropriate **High Risk** Post-surgical (hip/knee, abdominal/pelvic) Trauma (spinal cord/multiple major trauma) Hypercoagulable (active malignancy, hematologic disorders) Immobilized or limited mobility Critically ill and mechanically ventilated *Thromboprophylaxis* Pharmacologic prophylaxis with low-molecular-weight heparin, unfractionated heparin, oral vitamin K antagonist, or direct oral anticoagulant **High Risk Plus Bleeding Risk** *Thromboprophylaxis* Mechanical thromboprophylaxis (pneumatic compression devices preferred), reassess bleeding risk daily, and initiate pharmacologic prophylaxis (low-molecular-weight heparin or unfractionated heparin) as soon as appropriate

Data from Schünemann HJ, Cushman M, Burnett AE, et al: American Society of Hematology 2018 guidelines for management of venous thromboembolism: prophylaxis for hospitalized and nonhospitalized medical patients. Blood Adv. 2018;2(22):3198-3225 and AACN Venous Thromboembolism Prevention Practice Alert. Aliso Viejo, CA: AACN; 2016. https://www.aacn.org/clinical-resources/practice-alerts/venous-thromboembolism-prevention

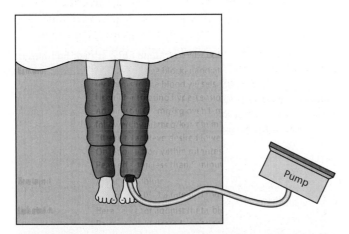

Figure 10-19. Intermittent pneumatic compression (IPC) device for prevention of DVT and PE.

TABLE 10-19. TIPS FOR SAFE AND EFFECTIVE USE OF INTERMITTENT PNEUMATIC COMPRESSION DEVICES

- Follow manufacturer recommendations for the correct fit including patient measurement.
- Include ongoing assessment for fit as changes in weight and fluid shifts occur.
- Monitor that the devices are on the patient whenever in bed and in correct placement with device turned on.
- Implement patient and family teaching regarding VTE and the role of mechanical prophylaxis.
- Ensure that devices do not impede ambulation.

- Early fixation of long bone fractures to prevent fat emboli.
- Early mobilization: As soon as hemodynamic stability is achieved, and there are no other contraindications to mobilization, activity level begins to increase by including sitting in a chair several times per day and short periods of ambulation.

SELECTED BIBLIOGRAPHY

Critical Care Management of Respiratory Problems

Abrams D, Brodie D. Extracorporeal membrane oxygenation for adult respiratory failure: 2017 update. *Chest.* 2017;152(3);639-649.

Bass S, Vance ML, Reddy A, et al. Bispectral index for titrating sedation in ARDS during neuromuscular blockade. *Am J Crit Care.* 2019;28(5):377-384.

Becker JC, Zakaluzny SA, Keller BA, et al. Clamping trials to thoracostomy tube removal and the need for subsequent invasive pleural drainage. *Am J Surg.* 2020;220:476-481.

Belli S, Prince I, Savio G, et al. Airway clearance techniques: the right choice for the right patient. *Front Med.* 2021;8:544826. doi:10.3389/fmed.2021.544826.

Binachon A, Grateau A. Allou N. Acute severe asthma requiring invasive mechanical ventilation in the era of modern resuscitation techniques: a 10-year bicentric retrospective study. *PLoS One.* 2020;15(10):e0240063. doi:10.1371/journal.pone.0240063.

Carlsson JA, Bayes HK. Acute severe asthma in adults. *J Med.* 2020;48(5):297-302.

Chastis V, Visintini S. Early mobilization for patients with venous thromboembolism: a review of clinical effectiveness and guidelines. Ottawa (ON): Canadian Agency for Drugs and Technologies in Health; 2018 Jan 17. Available from: https://www.ncbi.nlm.nih.gov/books/NBK531715/.

Chaudry P, Gadre SK, Schneider E. Impact of multidisciplinary pulmonary embolism response team availability on management and outcomes. *Am J Cardiol.* 2019;124:1465-1469. doi:10.1016/j.amjcard.2019.07.043.

Connor KA. Management of nosocomial pneumonia. *AACN Adv Crit Care.* 2018;28(1):5-10.

Cooper AS. Different durations of corticosteroid therapy for exacerbations of chronic obstructive pulmonary disease. *Crit Care Nurs.* 2019;39(6):78-80.

Dignani L, Toccaceli A, Lucertini C, Petrucci C, Lancia L. Sleep and quality of life in people with COPD: a descriptive-correlational study. *Clin Nurs Res.* 2016;25:432-447.

Dinic VD, Stojanovic MD, Markovic D, et al. Enhanced recovery in thoracic surgery: a review. *Front Med.* 2018;5(14):1-7. doi:10.3389/fmed.2018.00014.

Ebberts M. Competent management of patients receiving ECMO and CRRT. *Crit Care Nurs.* 2020;40(1):79-81.

Engkasan JK, Chan SC. Does non-invasive ventilation compared to invasive ventilation improve short term survival for acute respiratory failure in people with neuromuscular disease and chest wall disorders? A Cochrane Review summary with commentary. *Dev Med Child Neurol.* 2020;62(4):415-416.

Hanneman SK, Gusick GM, Hamlin SK, et al. Manual vs automated lateral rotation to reduce preventable pulmonary complications in ventilator patients. *Am J Crit Care.* 2015;24(1):24-32.

Khashkheli MS, Tabassum R, Awan AH. Effectiveness of magnesium sulphate in acute asthma: a retrospective study. *Anaesthes Pain Intensive Care.* 2017;21(4):458-462.

Kruse T, Wahl S, Guthrie PF, Sendelbach S. Place atrium to water seal (PAWS): assessing wall suction versus no suction for chest tubes after open heart surgery. *Crit Care Nurs.* 2017;37(4):17-28.

Loughran P. Ask the experts: stripping or milking of chest tubes. *Crit Care Nurs.* 2019;39(3):72-73.

Maselli DJ, Hardin M, Christenson SA, et al. Clinical approach to the therapy of asthma-COPD overlap. *Chest.* 2019;155(1):168-177.

McLenon M. Ask the experts: nursing assessment of tissue plasminogen activator for pulmonary embolism. *Crit Care Nurs.* 2018;36(4):73-74.

Mejza F, Gnatiuc L, Buist AS, et al. Prevalence and burden of chronic bronchitis symptoms: results from the BOLD study. *Eur Respir J.* 2017;50(5):1700621. doi:10.1183/13993003.00621-2017.

Montanaro J. Using a situ simulation to develop a prone positioning protocol for patients with ARDS. *Crit Care Nurs.* 2021; 41(1):12-24.

Porcel JM. Chest tube drainage of the pleural space: a concise review for pulmonologists. *Tuberc Respir Dis.* 2018;81:106-115. doi:10.4046/trd.2017.0107.

Powell B, Leeper B. Pulmonary hypertension: overview and case study. *AACN Adv Crit Care.* 2020;31(1):57-66.

Rigotti NA, Clair C, Munafo MR, Stead LF. Interventions for smoking cessation in hospitalized patients. *Cochrane Database Syst Rev.* 2015;5:CD001837. doi:10.1002/14651858.CDC001837.pub3.

Ritchie M, Brown C, and Bowling M. Chest tubes: indications, sizing, placement, and management. *Clin Pulm Med.* 2017;24:37-53. doi:10.1097/CPM.0000000000000188.

Robles MJ, Ponte J. Effect of chlorhexidine bath on the prevention of ventilator-associated pneumonia: a meta-analysis. *Chest.* 2019;155(4):123A.

Rochwerg B, Brochard L, Elliott MW, et al. Official ERS/ATS clinical practice guidelines: noninvasive ventilation for acute respiratory failure. *Eur Resp J.* 2017;50:1602426. doi:10.1183/13993003.02426-2016.

Seckel M, Remel B. Evidence-based practice: percussion and vibration therapy. *Crit Care Nurs.* 2017;37:82-83.

Smith RE, Shifrin MM. Critical care considerations in adult patients with influenza-induced ARDS. *Crit Care Nurs.* 2020;40(5):15-24.

Sole ML, Yooseph S, Talbert S, et al. Pulmonary microbiome of patients receiving mechanical ventilation: changes over time. *Am J Crit Care.* 2021;30(2):128-132.

Tan CW, Balla S, Ghanta RK, et al. Contemporary management of acute pulmonary embolism. *Semin Thorac Cardiovasc Surg.* 2020;32(3):396-403.

U.S. Department of Health and Human Services. Smoking Cessation: A Report of the Surgeon General, 2020. https://www.hhs.gov/sites/default/files/2020-cessation-sgr-full-report.pdf. Accessed September 20, 2021.

Yokoe DS, Anderson DJ, Berenholtz SM, et al. SHEA/IDSA practice recommendation: executive summary. A compendium of strategies to prevent healthcare-associated infections in acute care hospitals: 2014 updates. *Infect Control Hosp Epidemiol.* 2014;35:967.

Chest X-Ray Interpretation

Connolly MA. Black, white, and shades of gray: common abnormalities in chest radiographs. *AACN Clinical Issues.* 2001;12(2):259-269.

Corne J, Kumaran M. *Chest X-Ray Made Easy.* 4th ed. Edinburgh, SCT: Elsevier; 2016.

Godoy MC, Leitman BS, deGroot PM, Viahos J, Naidich DP. Chest radiography in the ICU: part 1; evaluation of airway, enteric, and pleural tubes. *Am J Roentgenol.* 2012;198:563-571.

Pezzotti W. Chest x-ray interpretation: not just black and white. *Nursing.* 2014;44(1):40-47.

Sanchez F. Fundamentals of chest x-ray interpretation. *Crit Care Nurse.* 1986;6:41-52.

Siela D. Advanced chest imaging interpretation of acute pulmonary disorders. *AACN Adv Crit Care.* 2014;25:365-374.

Coronavirus (COVID-19)

Alhazzani W, Evans L, Alshamsi F, et al. Surviving Sepsis Campaign guidelines on the management of adults with coronavirus disease 2019 (COVID-19) in the ICU: first update. *Crit Care Med.* 2021;49(3):e219-e234.

Allicock KA, Coyne D, Garton AN, Hare E, Seckel MA. Awake self-prone positioning: implementation during the COVID-19 pandemic. *Crit Care Nurs.* 2021:Apr 13:e1-e11. doi:10.4037/ccn2021153. Epub ahead of print.

Badulak J, Antonini MV, Stead CM, et al: Extracorporeal membrane oxygenation for COVID-19: updated 2021 guidelines from the extracorporeal life support organization. *ASAIO J.* 2021;67(5):485-495.

COVID-19 Treatment Guidelines Panel. Coronavirus disease 2019 (COVID-19) treatment guidelines. National Institute of Health. Available at https://www.covid19treatmentguidelines.nih.gov/. Accessed August 19, 2021.

McMichael TM, Clark S, Pgosjans S. COVID-19 in a long-term care facility—King County, Washington, February 27 March 9, 2020. *Morb Mortal Wkly Rep.* 2020;69(12):339.

Myall KJ, Mukherjee B, Castanheira AM, et al. Persistent post-COVID-19 interstitial lung disease. An observational study of corticosteroid treatment. *Ann Am Thorac Soc.* 2021;18(5):799-806.

Seckel MA. Awake self-prone positioning and the evidence. *Crit Care Nurs.* 2021;41(4):76-79.

Touchon F, Trigui Y, Prud'homme E, et al. Awake prone positioning for hypoxaemic respiratory failure: past, COVID-19 and perspectives. *Eur Resp Rev.* 2021;30:210022. doi:10.1183/16000617:0022-2021.

Weiner-Lastinger LM, Pattabiraman V, Konnor RY, et al. The impact of coronavirus disease 2019 (COVID-19) on healthcare-associated infections in 2020: a summary of data reported to the National Healthcare Safety Network. *Inf Control Hosp Epidemiol.* 2021. doi:10.1017/ice.2021.362.

Evidence-Based Practice Resources

American Association of Critical-Care Nurses Prevention of Aspiration in Adults. Aliso Viejo, CA: AACN; 2016. http://www.aacn.org. Accessed September 24, 2021.

American Association of Critical-Care Nurses Venous Thromboembolism Prevention Practice Alert. Aliso Viejo, CA: AACN; 2016. http://www.aacn.org. Accessed September 17, 2021.

Centers for Disease Control and Prevention. Guidelines for prevention of health-care-associated pneumonia, 2003: recommendations of CDC and the Healthcare Infection Control Practices Advisory Committee. *MMWR Recomm Rep.* 2004; 53(RR-3):1-35.

Criner GJ, Bourbeau J, Diekemper RL, et al. Prevention of acute exacerbation of COPD: American College of Chest Physicians and Canadian Thoracic Society Guideline. *Chest.* 2015;147:883-893.

Devlin JW, Skrobik Y, Gelinas C, et al. Clinical practice guidelines for the prevention and management of pain, agitation/sedation, delirium, immobility, and sleep disruption in adult patients in the ICU. *Crit Care Med.* 2018;46(9):e825-e873.

Ervin JN, Rentes VC, Dibble ER, et al. Evidence-based practices for acute respiratory failure and acute respiratory distress syndrome. A systematic review of reviews. *Chest.* 2020:158(6):2381-2393.

Erythropoulou-Kaltsidou A, Alkagiet S, Tziomalos K. New guidelines for the diagnosis and management of pulmonary embolism: key changes. *World J Cardiol.* 2020;12(5):161-166.

Fan E, Del Sorbo L, Goligher EC, et al. An Official American Thoracic Society/European Society of Intensive Care Medicine/Society of Critical Care Medicine Clinical Practice Guideline: mechanical ventilation in adult patients with acute respiratory distress syndrome. *Am J Respir Crit Care.* 2017;195:1253-1263.

Frankel HL, Kirkpatrick AW, Elbarbary M. Guidelines for the appropriate use of bedside general and cardiac ultrasonography in the evaluation of critically ill patients-part I: general ultrasonography. *Crit Care Med.* 2015;43:2479-2502.

Gattinoni L, Busana M, Giosa L, Macrì MM, Quintel M. Prone positioning in acute respiratory distress syndrome. *Semin Respir Crit Care Med.* 2019 Feb;40(1):94-100. doi:10.1055/s-0039-1685180 . Epub 2019 May 6. PMID: 31060091.

Global Initiative for Asthma. Global Strategy for Asthma Management and Prevention, 2021. www.ginathma.org. Accessed September 15, 2021.

Global Initiative for Chronic Obstructive Lung Disease. Global Strategy for the Diagnosis, Management, and Prevention of Chronic Obstructive Pulmonary Disease, 2021, https://goldcopd .org/2021-gold-reports/. Accessed September 15, 2021.

Good V, Kirkwood PL, eds. *Advanced Critical Care Nursing.* 2nd ed. St Louis, MO: Elsevier; 2018.

Holguin F, Cardet JC, Chung JF. Management of severe asthma: a ERS/ATS guideline. *Eur Respir J.* 2020;55:1900588. doi:10.1183/13993003.00588-2019.

Kalil AC, Metersky ML, Klompas M, et al. Management of adults with hospital-acquired and ventilator-associated pneumonia: 2016 Clinical Practice Guideline by the Infectious Diseases Society of America and the American Thoracic Society. *Clin Infect Dis.* 2016;63:e61-e111.

Klinger JR, Elliott G, Levine DJ, et al. Therapy for pulmonary arterial hypertension in adults. Update of the CHEST guideline and expert panel report. *Chest.* 2019;155(3):565-586.

Klompas M, Branson R, Eichenwalkd EC, et al. Strategies to prevent ventilator-associated pneumonia in acute care hospitals: 2014 update. *Inf Cont Hosp Epidemiol.* 2014;35(8):915-936.

Konstantinides SV, Meyer G, Becattini C, et al. 2019 ESC guidelines for the diagnosis and management of acute pulmonary embolism developed in collaboration with the European Respiratory Society (ERS). *Eur Heart J.* 2020;21(4):543-603.

Lyman GH, Carrier M, Ay C. American Society of Hematology 2021 guidelines for management of venous thromboembolism: prevention and treatment in patients with cancer. *Blood Adv.* 2021;5(4):927-974.

Metley JP, Waterer GW, Long AC, et al. Diagnosis and treatment of adults with community-acquired pneumonia. An official clinical practice guideline of the American Thoracic Society and Infectious Diseases Society of America. *Am Resp Crit Care Med.* 2019;200(7):e45-e67.

National Heart, Lung, and Blood Institute. 2020 focused updates to the asthma management guidelines, 2020. https://www .nhlbi.nih.gov/health-topics/all-publications-and-resources/ 2020-focused-updates-asthma-management-guidelines. Accessed September 20, 2021.

Ortel TL, Neumann I, Beyth R, et al. American Society of Hematology 2020 guidelines for management of venous thromboembolism: treatment of deep vein thrombosis and pulmonary embolism. *Blood Adv.* 2020;4(19):4693-4738.

Qaseem A, Exteandia-Ikobaltzeta I, Fitterman N, et al. Appropriate use of high-flow nasal oxygen in hospitalized patients for initial or postextubation management of acute respiratory failure: a clinical guideline from the American College of Physicians. *Ann Int Med.* 2021;174(4):977-984.

Raghu G, Remy-Jardin M, Myers JL, et al. Diagnosis of idiopathic pulmonary fibrosis. An official ATS/ERS/JRS/ALAT clinical practice guideline. *Am J Resp Crit Care Med.* 2018;198(5):e44-e68.

Raghu G, Rochwerg B, Zhang Y, et al. An official ATS/ERS/JRS/ ALAT clinical practice guideline: treatment of idiopathic pulmonary fibrosis. *Am J Respir Crit Care Med.* 2015;192. doi:10.1164/ rccm.201506-1063ST.

Schunemann HJ, Cushman M, Burnett AE. American Society of Hematology 2018 guidelines for management of venous thromboembolism: prophylaxis for hospitalized and nonhospitalized medical patients. *Blood Adv.* 2018;2(22):3198-3225.

Simonneau G, Montani D, Celermajer DS, et al. Haemodynamic definitions and updated clinical classification of pulmonary hypertension. *Eur Resp J.* 2019;53(1):1801913. doi:10.1183/13993003.01913-2018.

Stevens SM, Woller SC, Kreuziger LB, et al. Antithrombotic therapy for VTE disease: second update of the CHEST guideline and expert panel report. *Chest.* 2021. doi.org/10.1016/j.chest.2021.07.055.

Taylor BE, McClave SA, Martindale RG, et al. Guidelines for the provision and assessment of nutrition support therapy in the adult critically ill patient. *Crit Care Med.* 2016;44;390-438.

The ARDS Definition Task Force. Acute respiratory distress syndrome: the Berlin definition. *JAMA.* 2012;307:2526-2533.

US Preventive Services Taskforce (USPSTF). Screening for chronic obstructive pulmonary disease: US Preventative Services Task Force Recommendation Statement. *JAMA.* 2016;315:1372-1377.

Wedzicha JA, Miravittles M, Hurst JR, et al. Management of COPD exacerbations: a European Respiratory Society/American Thoracic Society Guideline. *Eur Respir J.* 2017;49:1600791. doi:10.1183/13993003.00791-2016.

Wiegand DL, ed. *AACN Procedure Manual for Critical Care.* 7th ed. St. Louis, MO: Elsevier Saunders; 2016.

MULTISYSTEM PROBLEMS

11

Sonya M. Grigsby

KNOWLEDGE COMPETENCIES

1. Identify the relationship between the cellular mediators and clinical manifestations of sepsis and septic shock.

2. Describe the etiology, pathogenesis, clinical manifestations, patient needs, and principles of management of sepsis and septic shock.

3. Compare and contrast the pathogenesis, clinical manifestations, patient needs, and management approaches for multisystem problems resulting from sepsis, septic shock, and overdoses.

4. Describe prone ventilation and nursing care for the prone patient.

5. Describe the symptoms and pharmacologic management of the patient experiencing alcohol withdrawal syndrome.

6. Describe treatment considerations for pressure injuries.

7. Identify factors related to the development of healthcare-associated infections (HAIs).

SEPSIS AND SEPTIC SHOCK

Sepsis is a serious global healthcare condition, affecting millions of patients annually. Older adults and those with underlying disease are disproportionally affected by sepsis. Despite advances in the treatment of infection, sepsis continues to be associated with high mortality rates, with 1 in 3 hospital deaths occurring in patients who experience sepsis (CDC, 2022). Early recognition and immediate treatment are key factors in reducing the impact of sepsis.

The basic elements of sepsis are infection, a dysregulated host response, and subsequent organ damage. A challenge in identifying patients with sepsis is that there is no single diagnostic test that indicates its presence. The diagnosis depends on analysis of an array of clinical data including abnormal vital signs, patient symptoms, physical examination findings, and lab values. Recognizing patients who are at risk for sepsis and closely monitoring their clinical status is essential to improving outcomes in the management of this disorder.

In 2016, the Third International Consensus Definitions for Sepsis and Septic Shock (Sepsis-3) defined sepsis as a dysregulated host response to an infection leading to life-threatening organ dysfunction. Septic shock, a subset of sepsis, occurs when patients with sepsis remain hypotensive after fluid resuscitation, require vasopressors, and have a serum lactate greater than 2 mmol/L. Hospital mortality from septic shock is over 40%.

Previous definitions of sepsis focused on the systemic inflammatory response syndrome (SIRS), which occurs in response to a clinical insult, such as an infection, inflammation, or injury. Most patients with sepsis have signs consistent with SIRS. However, SIRS is also present when a patient has an appropriate systemic inflammatory response to an infection or other insult and not a dysregulated response that can lead to organ dysfunction. A tool for identifying organ dysfunction is the Sequential Organ Failure Assessment (SOFA) (see Table 11-1). SOFA is not a screening tool for sepsis but may be used to assess the degree of organ dysfunction.

TABLE 11-1. SEQUENTIAL (SEPSIS RELATED) ORGAN FAILURE SCORE

System	Score				
	0	1	2	3	4
Respiration					
Pao$_2$/Fio$_2$, mm Hg (kPa)	≥ 400 (53.3)	< 400 (53.3)	< 300 (40)	< 200 (6.7) with respiratory support	< 100 (13.3) with respiratory support
Coagulation					
Platelets, × 10^3/μL	≥ 150	< 150	< 100	< 50	< 20
Liver					
Bilirubin, mg/dL (μmol/L)	< 1.2 (20)	1.2-1.9 (20-32)	2.0-5.9 (33-101)	6.0-11.9 (102-204)	> 12.0 (204)
Cardiovascular	MAP ≥ 70 mm Hg	MAP < 70 mm Hg	Dopamine < 5 or dobutamine (any dose)[b]	Dopamine 5.1-15 or epinephrine ≤ 0.1 or norepinephrine ≤ 0.1[b]	Dopamine > 15 or epinephrine > 0.1 or norepinephrine > 0.1[a]
Central nervous system					
Glasgow Coma Scale score[b]	15	13-14	10-12	6-9	< 6
Renal					
Creatinine, mg/dL (μmol/L)	< 1.2 (110)	1.2-1.9 (110-170)	2.0-3.4 (171-299)	3.5-4.9 (300-440)	> 5.0 (440)
Urine output, mL/day				< 500	< 200

Abbreviations: Fio$_2$, fraction of inspired oxygen; MAP, mean arterial pressure; Pao$_2$, partial pressure of oxygen.
[a]Catecholamine doses are given as mcg/kg/min for at least 1 hour.
[b]Glasgow Coma scale scores range from 3 to 15; higher score indicates better neurological function.
Reproduced with permission from Vincent JL, Moreno R, Takala J,et al: The SOFA (Sepsis-related Organ Failure Assessment) score to describe organ dysfunction/failure. On behalf of the Working Group on Sepsis-Related Problems of the European Society of Intensive Care Medicine. Intensive Care Med. 1996;22(7):707-710.

Etiology, Risk Factors, and Pathogenesis

The infection that causes sepsis may be bacterial, viral, fungal, or on rare occasions, rickettsial or protozoal. Immune and inflammatory responses to infection occur as natural processes that are protective. Figure 11-1 provides an overview of the events that comprise the dysregulated response in sepsis. As the figure demonstrates, a variety of immune mechanisms, when unchecked, lead to organ damage. These

include activation of polymorphonuclear cells (neutrophils), macrophages, platelets, and endothelial cells. These cells are either directly involved in the reaction, such as platelet aggregation which leads to microthrombi, or are stimulated to produce and release chemical mediators, such as cytokines or plasma enzymes that extend the dysregulated response.

The 2021 Sepsis guidelines recommend the use of screening tools to promote early identification of patients

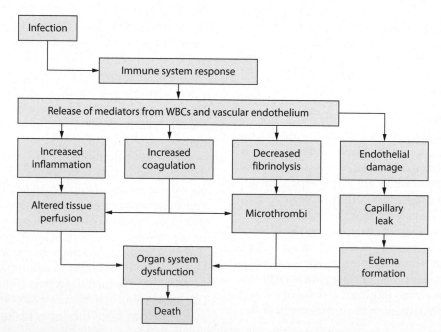

Figure 11-1. Interactive cascade of inflammation and coagulation leading to endothelium damage, diffuse thrombi, and organ system dysfunction. (*Reproduced with permission from Kleinpell R. New initiatives focus on prevention and early recognition of sepsis. Nurs Spectrum. 2004;17(12):24-26.*)

TABLE 11-2. SIRS CRITERIA

Two or more of the following
Temperature >38°C or <36°C
Heart rate > 90 beats/min
Respiratory rate ≥ 20 breaths/min or pCO_2 < 32
White blood cell count <4000 cells/mm^3 or >12,000 cells/mm^3 OR > 20% immature (band) forms

Data from Chakraborty RK, Burns B. Systemic Inflammatory Response Syndrome. 2022 May 30. In: StatPearls [Internet]. Treasure Island (FL): StatPearls Publishing; Jan 2022.

with sepsis and timely treatment. The recommendations advise using SIRS criteria (see Table 11-2) or applying the National Early Warning Score (NEWS), or the Modified Early Warning Score (MEWS) (see Table 11-3) to screen for sepsis. Institutions using these tools should establish specific parameters that prompt assessment and intervention. For instance, if two or more SIRS criteria are present or if the MEWS score is greater than 6, the patient has a risk for clinical deterioration and requires immediate attention. Incorporating sepsis screening tools into the electronic health record (EHR) may be one strategy that assists with early identification of sepsis.

Risk factors for the development of sepsis include malnutrition, immunosuppression, comorbidities, surgery, trauma, and prolonged antibiotic use. The presence of invasive devices including central lines, urinary catheters, and endotracheal tubes, also increases the risk for sepsis. Age is an important risk factor, as sepsis disproportionately affects the very young and the very old. Many infections leading to sepsis in critically ill patients are acquired during hospitalization and may be avoided with infection prevention tactics. Hand hygiene remains the single most effective method for preventing the spread of infection. Other measures such as meticulous mouth care to prevent ventilator-associated pneumonia, prompt removal of urinary catheters, and aseptic technique when handling central lines can help prevent sepsis in critically ill patients. Table 11-4 summarizes the nursing interventions to prevent, recognize, and ensure prompt treatment of sepsis.

Clinical Presentation

Early recognition of sepsis is crucial to ensure timely intervention such as broad-spectrum antibiotics and fluid resuscitation. When the nurse notes a change in patient status that indicates infection and the onset of sepsis, further assessment and collaboration with a provider are urgent priorities. Fever and leukocytosis are classic indications of infection, but other symptoms such as altered mental state, a change in wound drainage, or a new complaint of pain may also be an early indication of an infectious complication that warrants further assessment.

The clinical manifestations of sepsis result from altered perfusion to vital organ systems, due to the release of immune mediators. Skin changes such as pallor, cyanosis, mottling, or a hemorrhagic rash may indicate sepsis. Clinical signs of organ system dysfunction include alterations in the cardiovascular system (hypotension, tachycardia, dysrhythmias), the respiratory system (tachypnea, hypoxemia), renal function (oliguria, elevated creatinine), liver function (elevated ALT and AST, jaundice, coagulopathies), the hematologic system (thrombocytopenia), the gastrointestinal system, (ileus), and cognitive function (confusion, agitation).

The prognosis of sepsis depends on the number of organ systems affected and the severity of their dysfunction. Early identification and treatment are crucial to minimizing progressive organ dysfunction and improving patient outcomes. The Surviving Sepsis Campaign advises the use of sepsis bundles which provide a specific timeframe for implementing interventions in patients with suspected sepsis. The 2019 1-hour sepsis bundle from the Surviving Sepsis Campaign is listed in Figure 11-2. While interventions that comprise sepsis bundles may change as understanding of appropriate treatment evolves, the underlying principle of acting quickly to address hemodynamic instability is the crucial factor in improving patient survival.

Diagnostic Tests

There is no single biomarker that confirms a diagnosis of sepsis. The care of patients at risk for sepsis includes frequent

TABLE 11-3. MODIFIED EARLY WARNING SCORE (MEWS)

System	Score						
	3	2	1	0	1	2	3
Respiratory rate (bpm)	<8		9-11	12-20		21-29	>30
SpO_2 (%)	<91	92-93	94-95	>96			
Oxygen supplementation		Yes		No			
Systolic blood pressure (mmHg)	<90	91-100	101-110	111-200		200-219	>220
Heart rate (bmp)	<40		41-50	51-100	101-110	111-130	>131
Temperature (Celsius)		<35	35.1-36	36.1-38	38.1-39	>39.1	
Consciousness				A	V	P	U

Abbreviations: SpO_2, oxygen saturation; A, alert; V, responds to verbal stimuli; P, responds to painful stimuli; U, unresponsive.
Reproduced with permission from Balshi AN, Huwait BM, Noor ASN, et al: Modified Early Warning Score as a predictor of intensive care unit readmission within 48 hours: a retrospective observational study. Rev Bras Ter Intensiva. 2020;32(2):301-307.

TABLE 11-4. NURSING CARE OF PATIENTS WITH SEPSIS AND SEPTIC SHOCK

Recognize those at risk	Identify patients at risk for developing sepsis • Older adults • Immunocompromised patients • Patients undergoing surgical/invasive procedures • Patients with indwelling catheters • Mechanically ventilated patients
Monitor for sepsis	Signs of infection including • Fever or hypothermia, tachycardia, hypotension, tachypnea • Altered mental state • New complaint of pain • Adventitious breath sounds, increased oxygen requirement, new infiltrate on radiograph • Change in appearance of urine, pyuria, bacteria on urine culture • Change in wound appearance or drainage • Leukocytosis, thrombocytopenia on complete blood count (CBC) • Elevated blood glucose Signs of impaired organ perfusion • Hypotension, tachycardia, tachypnea • Elevated serum lactate • Skin mottling • prolonged capillary refill • Change in renal function: drop in urine output, elevated creatinine and blood urea nitrogen (BUN) • Change in liver function: elevated transaminases • Change in clotting: bruising, bleeding, elevated international normalized ratio (INR)
Collaborate with the healthcare team to initiate immediate resuscitation	• Circulatory support with fluids and vasopressors • Empiric antibiotics • Source control • Monitor and report patient response to treatment
Provide supportive care to patients with sepsis	• Frequent monitoring of hemodynamic status to determine patient response to treatment • Use supplemental oxygen or lung protective mechanical ventilation as indicated • Apply interventions in the ABCDEF bundle to prevent delirium • Provide enteral nutrition to prevent malnutrition and lower the risk of bacterial translocation • Give ulcer prophylaxis if risk factors for GI bleeding exist • Administer pharmacologic or mechanical interventions to prevent venous thromboembolism (VTE)
Patient/family-centered care	• Promote patient comfort, assess and treat pain, use a validated scale to guide the use of sedation • Assess patient/family understanding of diagnosis and prognosis • Participate in discussions of goals of care with the healthcare team and with the patient/family

Sepsis prevention	• Hand hygiene
	• Specific measures to prevent hospital-acquired infections include:
	  • Remove urinary catheters and central lines when no longer indicated
	  • Use aseptic technique when handling lines and catheters
	  • Facilitate weaning from mechanical ventilation through the use of spontaneous breathing trials, appropriate use of sedation, and early mobility as described in Chapter 5, Airway and Ventilatory Management
	  • Adhere to transmission-based precautions including the use of standard, contact, droplet, and airborne precautions as appropriate
	• Educate members of the healthcare team on prevention and recognition of sepsis

1. Measure lactate level.*
2. Obtain blood cultures before administering antibiotics.
3. Administer broad-spectrum antibiotics.
4. Begin rapid administration of 30 mL/kg crystalloid for hypotension or lactate ≥ 4 mmol/L.
5. Apply vasopressors if hypotensive during or after fluid resuscitation to maintain a mean arterial pressure ≥ 65 mm Hg.
* Remeasure lactate if initial lactate elevated (> 2 mmol/L).

Figure 11-2. The 2019 1-hour Sepsis Bundle lists the interventions to perform within the first hour of sepsis recognition. (*Reproduced with permission from Levy MM, Evans LE, Rhodes A. The Surviving Sepsis Campaign Bundle: 2018 Update. Crit Care Med. 2018;46(6):997-1000.*)

assessment with the aim of early recognition and prompt treatment. This assessment includes attention to common sources of infection with inspection of incisions and line insertion sites, and auscultation of the chest. Screening tools that identify signs of sepsis also support early recognition of this disorder (see Tables 11-2 and 11-3).

Diagnostic and laboratory assessment in sepsis include:

• *Serum lactate:* Tissues that are poorly perfused resort to anaerobic metabolism and produce lactate. Thus, a rise in serum lactate indicates poor perfusion and is associated with patient mortality. An elevated lactate level ranges from 1.6 to 2.5 mmol/L. Patients with a serum lactate equal to or greater than 4 mmol/L with evidence of infection should undergo urgent treatment for sepsis, though patients with lower lactate levels may also have the condition. A lactate greater than 2 mmol/L after fluid resuscitation indicates septic shock.

- *Complete blood cell count:* In response to infection, the white blood cell count may rise to greater than 12,000 cells/mm^3 or fall below 4000 cells/mm^3. A rise in the percent of bands, white blood cells released from the marrow before reaching maturity, to greater than 10%, indicates acute infection. The overactivation of platelets induced by the dysregulated response of sepsis can also lead to thrombocytopenia.

- *Serum creatinine and AST/ALT:* Elevations in creatinine indicate kidney hypoperfusion while elevated liver enzymes suggest liver hypoperfusion.
- *Chest x-ray:* May be normal or show signs of infiltrates/consolidation, particularly if pneumonia is the source of the sepsis.
- *Urinalysis:* May show pyuria and the presence of bacteria, particularly if infection in the urinary tract is the source of sepsis.
- *Culture and sensitivity:* Cultures of blood, urine, sputum, wound drainage, or other potential sources of infection may confirm the presence of bacteria or other pathogens.
- *CT scan, MRI, ultrasound:* May be indicated to identify the source of sepsis (such as an abscess, appendicitis, diverticulitis, bowel ischemia, cholecystitis).

ESSENTIAL CONTENT CASE

Sepsis

A 67-year-old man with a 6-year history of hypertension and a 30-pack-year smoking history was admitted to the ICU with a diagnosis of cirrhosis secondary to biliary obstruction. He underwent an exploratory laparotomy and cholecystectomy 3 days ago. He experienced an episode of hypotension 12 hours postoperatively, which resolved with IV crystalloid administration. He remains intubated on 40% FiO$_2$ and attempts at weaning have been complicated by hypoxemia.

He currently has an arterial line, central venous catheter (CVC), T-tube drain, and an indwelling urinary catheter. He is alert and following commands appropriately and moving in bed with little assistance. Physical examination reveals that his skin is pale, but warm, pulmonary auscultation is notable for bibasilar crackles, and cardiovascular exam is positive for 1+ pedal edema bilaterally. His abdomen is soft, nontender, and nondistended. His 5-inch midline abdominal wound requires dressing changes three times daily and is approximated with retention sutures. Current vital signs are:

T	38.6°C (101.0°F) core
HR	122 beats/min (sinus tachycardia)
RR	20 breaths/min
BP	82/54 mm Hg (MAP 63)
Spo$_2$	92%

Current laboratory results are:

ABG:	pH 7.30, Pao$_2$ 62, Paco$_2$ 46, HCO$_3$ 18, Sao$_2$ 94%
WBC:	22,000 (65% neutrophils, 50% segs, 12% bands)
Hemoglobin/hematocrit:	Hgb 13, Hct 39
Platelets:	40,000 (Baseline 300,000)
BMP:	Na$^+$ 140, K$^+$ 3.5, Cl 100, CO$_2$ 20, BUN 22, Creat 1.3 (Baseline Cr 0.9)
Liver function tests	AST 25, ALT 23
Total bili	2.7 mg/dL
Urine output	750 cc over last 24 hours

Case Question 1: What are this patient's risk factors for sepsis?

Case Question 2: What clinical manifestations may be suggestive of sepsis?

Case Question 3: What is his MEWS score?

Case Question 4: What actions should the nurse take based on this clinical information?

Answers
1. Postoperative status, intubated, invasive lines and catheters, and an abdominal wound requiring dressing changes are risk factors for sepsis in this patient.
2. Elevated temperature, leukocytosis with bandemia, sinus tachycardia, tachypnea, hypotension, thrombocytopenia, elevated creatinine, and a suspected source of infection are clinical findings consistent with sepsis.
3. Based on the clinical data given and the tool in Table 11-3, his MEWS is 9 which indicates a risk for clinical deterioration (scores > 6 indicate a risk).
4. In collaboration with the provider, the nurse will provide immediate interventions including drawing a lactate level to assess organ perfusion, collecting urine, blood, and sputum cultures to evaluate for sources of infection, initiating antimicrobial therapy and intravenous fluids, and performing frequent repeat assessments for further changes in his status. Based on the 2021 Sepsis Guidelines, checking the patient's capillary refill time should be included in these assessments. Further interventions will depend on the patient's response and may include ventilator changes, additional fluid, or vasopressor therapy to improve perfusion and reduce the risk of organ dysfunction.

Principles of Management of Sepsis and Septic Shock

Because sepsis is life threatening and prompt treatment impacts outcomes, the priority interventions are grouped and administered in a specific time interval. These groups of interventions are labeled "Sepsis Bundles" and can reduce the complexity and increase the rapidity of the healthcare team's response to sepsis. Figure 11-2 shows the 1-hour sepsis bundle which was revised in 2019 and lists the group of interventions that should be initiated within one hour of recognizing a patient has sepsis. The Surviving Sepsis Campaign (SSC) also offers the International Guidelines for the Management of Sepsis and Septic Shock, updated in 2021. The website, survivingsepsis.org, maintains a list of the most up-to-date information. The information below is based on evidence available at the time this text was written; however, research on sepsis management is ongoing and recommendations may change.

In general, the treatment of a patient with sepsis, or septic shock, consists of treating the underlying cause, providing fluid resuscitation, supporting dysfunctional organ systems, and applying evidence-based practices to prevent complications and meet goals of care.

Treating the Underlying Cause

The management plan begins with infection source control and administration of empiric, broad-spectrum antimicrobial therapy within the first 1 hour of symptom recognition. Identifying the source of infection is paramount, as therapy will not be successful without source control. Ideally, at least two sets of blood cultures are obtained prior to administering antibiotics but a delay in culture collection should not delay treatment. Institutional protocol dictates how cultures are collected and often include one set drawn percutaneously and one drawn through a vascular access device. Antibiotic administration must not be delayed. Even if the source of infection is not identified, antimicrobial agents are administered within the first hour of sepsis recognition. Once the source is identified and culture results are available, antimicrobial therapy is changed to provide more specific coverage. Source control interventions beyond antimicrobial therapy may include drainage of an abscess or the removal of an intravascular line, indwelling bladder catheter, vascular graft, or orthopedic device.

Fluid Resuscitation

The 2021 SSC guidelines recommend that patients with sepsis who have hypotension or lactate levels greater than or equal to 4mmol/L receive a fluid bolus of 30 mL/kg of balanced crystalloids within 3 hours of symptom recognition. As the Surviving Sepsis 1-hour bundle indicates, administration of fluids should begin within 1 hour of sepsis recognition. Administration of fluids increases intravascular volume thereby improving organ perfusion and reducing the risk of organ dysfunction and mortality. The goal of initial resuscitation is to reach a mean arterial pressure (MAP) of 65 mm Hg and to achieve a normal lactate level. Close monitoring is required to avoid excessive fluid administration.

While fluid resuscitation is recommended for all patients with potential sepsis, additional consideration is warranted in patients with acute respiratory distress syndrome (ARDS), heart failure, or chronic kidney disease, who may develop pulmonary edema. Patients with these comorbidities require close monitoring during fluid resuscitation. Patients who are already on high-flow oxygen may experience further respiratory compromise that requires intubation and mechanical ventilation. Following the initial bolus, most patients require ongoing fluid administration, but further decisions about volume administration are based on hemodynamic assessment of the patient.

The SSC guidelines emphasize that dynamic measures of a patient's hemodynamic status are preferred over static measurements. Dynamic measures include physical signs such as skin mottling, temperature of extremities, and delayed capillary refill time (CRT). Passive leg raise is an additional noninvasive assessment used to determine if a patient is likely to respond to further fluid resuscitation. Table 11-5 provides a list of static and dynamic hemodynamic measures that are used to determine if a patient with sepsis will benefit from additional infusion of fluids. See Chapter 4, Hemodynamic Monitoring, for a detailed discussion of hemodynamic monitoring.

Supporting Dysfunctional Organ Systems

While research is ongoing, there is currently no therapy available to prevent the dysregulated host response in sepsis and septic shock. Immediate administration of antimicrobials and removal of the source of infection may reduce the impact and duration of this response, but once set in motion, it may continue even after source control is achieved. For this reason, interventions aimed at supporting the affected organs are essential in the management of sepsis and septic shock.

Cardiovascular Dysfunction

The impact of the dysregulated immune response on the cardiovascular system includes myocardial dysfunction, systemic vasodilation, and increased capillary bed permeability. This combination of effects can lead to peripheral edema in the setting of low intravascular volume, and poor perfusion despite a normal or elevated cardiac output. Refractory hypotension during or after fluid resuscitation may indicate a need for intravenous vasopressors. Norepinephrine is the vasopressor of choice for sepsis and septic shock, according

TABLE 11-5. DYNAMIC AND STATIC HEMODYNAMIC MEASUREMENTS

Dynamic Measurements	Static Measurements
Pulse pressure variation	CVP
Systolic pulse variation	PAOP
Pleth variability index	Global end-diastolic volume
Stroke volume variation—via passive leg raise	Left ventricular end-diastolic volume
Inferior vena cava—visualized on ultrasound	

to the 2021 SSC guidelines. If the goal MAP of 65 mm Hg cannot be achieved with norepinephrine, vasopressin is added. Persistent hypotension in patients with cardiac dysfunction and sepsis warrants the addition of dobutamine, or switching to epinephrine.

Patients on vasopressors require close monitoring to ensure that the minimum dose to achieve the desired effect is used. Continuous monitoring for cardiac dysrhythmias, which may occur due to sepsis or due to the use of vasopressors, and frequent assessment of perfusion including blood pressure, end organ parameters, inspection for skin mottling, and capillary refill time are also essential elements of nursing care. Vasopressor support may be initiated peripherally to restore MAP until a central venous access is obtained. Insertion of an arterial catheter provides continuous arterial pressure measurement that facilitates therapeutic decisions based on real-time blood pressure information. Arterial and central venous access lines require meticulous nursing care to prevent infection. In addition, all invasive lines should be removed as soon as they are no longer needed to minimize the risk of complications.

The dysregulated immune response in sepsis may also lead to microthrombi, further impairing peripheral perfusion. In addition, patients with sepsis often have impaired mobility which increases the risk of thrombus formation. Because venous thromboembolism is a serious and sometimes fatal complication of sepsis, the 2021 Sepsis guidelines recommend the use of low-molecular-weight heparin to prevent clot formation, unless patients have a specific contraindication to this therapy.

Pulmonary Dysfunction

The systemic inflammation of sepsis leads to pulmonary vascular leak and microthrombi, which can lodge in the small vessels of the pulmonary system. As a result, patients with sepsis and septic shock can develop ARDS and require intubation and mechanical ventilation. The SSC guidelines support the use of low-tidal volume ventilation (6 mL/kg predicted body weight), the goal for plateau pressure less than or equal to 30 cm H_2O, and the use of positive end-expiratory pressure (PEEP) to minimize the risk of lung injury that can occur with high volumes and high Fio_2. Applying higher PEEP may facilitate gas exchange and increase Pao_2 by opening lung units. Prone positioning may also be appropriate in septic patients with ARDS. Further discussion of the management of ARDS can be found in Chapter 10 (Respiratory System) and Chapter 20 (Advanced Respiratory Concepts: Modes of Ventilation) of this book.

Because sepsis increases the demand for oxygen while ARDS reduces the supply, strategies to minimize oxygen consumption are key aspects of nursing care. These include:

- Controlling heart rate, respiratory rate, and temperature, in collaboration with provider
- Assessing and treating pain
- Preventing shivering

- Providing comfort measures, including verbal reassurance and explanations
- Consolidating activities to allow for periods of rest and promoting sleep at night
- Placing the patient on mechanical ventilation if clinically indicated, in collaboration with healthcare team
- Administering sedation guided by a standardized sedation assessment tool (see Chapter 6)

Renal Dysfunction

Renal dysfunction is a common sequela of sepsis and septic shock. It is monitored through evaluation of serum creatinine and electrolytes, and measuring urine output which normally is greater than 0.5 cc/kg/h. Patients with renal injury may need adjusted medication dosing, particularly with antibiotics. In some situations, renal dysfunction progresses and renal replacement therapy (RRT) is required; however, the SSC guidelines suggest careful consideration in implementing this intervention based on the associated poor patient outcomes. A full discussion of renal dysfunction and RRT can be found in Chapter 15 (Renal System) of this book.

Best Practices Based on Current Evidence

In addition to antibiotic administration, source control, fluid resuscitation, and managing organ dysfunction, the SSC guidelines also offer additional recommendations for the care of patients with sepsis. These include managing blood glucose, stress ulcer prophylaxis, VTE prophylaxis, judicious use of blood products, provision of enteral nutrition, and establishing goals of care with patients and families. Table 11-6 lists some of the recommendations of the 2021 SSC guidelines. The Society of Critical Care medicine offers an online tool for locating recommendations related to specific aspects of care. Healthcare professionals can click on items in the list to find relevant recommendations and guidance for specific aspects of patient care (https://www.sccm.org/Clinical-Resources/Guidelines/Guidelines/Surviving-Sepsis-Guidelines-2021#Recommendations).

Managing Blood Glucose

Control of glucose, maintaining a blood glucose less than 180 mg/dL and more than 90 mg/dL, can improve outcomes in some critically ill populations. The SSC 2021 guideline recommends initiating insulin if the patient has blood glucose levels above 180mg/dL. The use of intravenous insulin to maintain glycemic control requires frequent monitoring of blood glucose (eg, every 1-2 hours) and is a nurse-driven intervention.

Transfusions

While sufficient hemoglobin is necessary to ensure adequate oxygen-carrying capacity, the 2021 SSC guidelines suggest a restrictive strategy regarding transfusion. Frequent transfusions have been associated with increased morbidity and mortality in this patient population and therefore, the threshold for transfusion is often set at a Hgb of 7 g/dL. Exceptions

TABLE 11-6.   RECOMMENDATIONS FROM THE 2021 SURVIVING SEPSIS CAMPAIGN GUIDELINES FOR THE MANAGEMENT OF SEPSIS AND SEPTIC SHOCK

Resuscitation	Sepsis and septic shock are medical emergencies and resuscitation should begin immediately
	In adults with possible septic shock or a high likelihood for sepsis, give antimicrobials within one hour of recognition
	For adults suspected of having sepsis, check a serum lactate
	Administer 30 mL/kg of crystalloid within the first 3 hours
	Use dynamic measures to guide further fluid resuscitation
Goals of resuscitation	Achieve an MAP ≥ 65 mm Hg, and normalize lactate
Use of vasopressors	Use norepinephrine as a first-line vasopressor when appropriate fluid resuscitation does not achieve adequate MAP
	If the goal MAP ≥ 65 mm Hg is not achieved with norepinephrine, administer vasopressin and then epinephrine
	If the patient has cardiac dysfunction, use norepinephrine with dobutamine or epinephrine alone
	Reassess volume status frequently to guide further administration of fluids
Antibiotic therapy	Give empiric antibiotics within 1 hour of symptom recognition for adults with septic shock or a high likelihood for sepsis
	Conduct rapid assessment for infectious vs. noninfectious causes
	For patients without shock, where sepsis is possible, conduct rapid assessment for causes and give antimicrobials, if concern persists, within 3 hours
	Narrow antimicrobial therapy when the source of infection is identified and sensitivities are available
	Assess for de-escalation of antimicrobial daily
Steroids	Administer steroids to adults with septic shock who require ongoing treatment with vasopressor therapy
Blood products	Apply a restrictive transfusion strategy
Ventilation	Use high-flow nasal cannula over noninvasive ventilation in sepsis-induced hypoxemic respiratory failure
	For adults on invasive mechanical ventilation for sepsis-induced ARDS, use low tidal volumes and an upper limit goal for plateau pressures of 30 cm H_2O
	For adults with moderate to severe sepsis-induced ARDS, use higher PEEP rather than lower PEEP; use prone ventilation for more than 12 h/day, and use intermittent neuromuscular blockade rather than continuous infusion
	Use venovenous ECMO when conventional mechanical ventilation fails in an experienced center with infrastructure to support its use
Glucose control	Apply a protocol to address hyperglycemia in adults who have blood glucose values > 180 mg/dL
	Administer insulin with a goal of maintaining blood glucose < 180 mg/dL
Renal replacement	In adults with sepsis or septic shock and acute kidney injury, use either continuous or intermittent renal replacement therapy. Avoid the use of renal replacement therapy for sepsis-induced acute kidney injury in adults who do not have a definitive indication such as hyperkalemia, severe metabolic acidosis
Nutrition	Initiate early enteral feeding (within 72 hours) and advance as tolerated
Setting goals of care	Discuss goals of care, prognosis for achieving those goals, and level of certainty for the prognosis with patients and families, incorporating palliative care principles and as appropriate, end-of-life care planning as early as feasible, but no later than within 72 hours of ICU admission

For a complete list of 2021 Surviving Sepsis Campaign Guidelines, https://www.sccm.org/Clinical-Resources/Guidelines/Guidelines/Surviving-Sepsis-Guidelines-2021#Recommendations
Data from Evans L, Rhodes A, Alhazzani W, et al: Surviving Sepsis Campaign: International Guidelines for Management of Sepsis and Septic Shock 2021. Crit Care Med. 2021;49(11):e1063–e1143

may be needed for patients with significant comorbid conditions, such as an active or recent myocardial infarction.

Providing Nutritional Support

Enteral nutritional support is the gold standard and preferred route of specialized nutrition support delivery unless contraindicated. General guidelines for nutritional support include 25 to 35 kcal/kg/day for total caloric intake and 1.5 to 2.0 g protein/kg/day. Enteral nutrition is preferred to parenteral nutrition whenever possible and should be initiated within 72 hours. Early initiation of enteral nutrition maintains gut integrity, prevents intestinal permeability, and may reduce insulin resistance. It is helpful to have a nutrition specialist assist with nutritional planning.

Providing Psychosocial Support

Chapter 1, Assessment of Critically Ill Patients and Their Families, and Chapter 2, Planning Care for Critically Ill Patients and Their Families, discuss many aspects of psychosocial support. Especially important is the timely approach to goals of care discussions. The 2021 SSC guidelines recommend that a family conference to establish goals of care, and discuss prognosis be incorporated into the care of patients with sepsis and septic shock within 72 hours of ICU admission. The use of palliative care communication skills facilitates the effectiveness of these conversations.

Sepsis survivors may experience short- and/or long-term effects including cognitive or physical disabilities that persist for months to years. Because of the duration of their hospital admission, patients with sepsis have a risk of post-intensive care syndrome (PICS), discussed in Chapter 2. Diligent discharge planning and appropriate education are necessary to promote adherence. Timely, coordinated resources and early provider follow-up post hospital discharge may lead to reduced hospital readmissions. The 2021 sepsis guideline includes recommendations related to healthcare professionals' communication during transitions in care, acknowledging the importance of care continuity for sepsis survivors.

COVID-19

Coronavirus disease 2019 (COVID-19) led to surges in intensive care admissions and inpatient deaths. Severe COVID-19 overlaps symptoms exhibited by patients with septic shock and can include altered mental states, dyspnea, oliguria, tachycardia, coagulopathies, and multiorgan dysfunction. The SSC COVID-19 panel created guidelines which include best practice statements and strong recommendations in the care of critically ill ICU patients with COVID-19. In addition, the National Institutes of Health facilitates a COVID-19 Treatment Guidelines Panel to review evidence and provide up-to-date guidance online (https://www.covid19treatment guidelines.nih.gov/). Online publication means that the NIH guideline changes as our understanding of appropriate treatment for COVID-19 develops. Nurses and providers can promote best outcomes for their patients by frequently reviewing the guidelines for new information to guide their care. In addition to the priniciples of management described for sepsis, critical care for patients with COVID-19 includes infection prevention and control, fluid resuscitation, ventilation and prone positioning.

Infection Prevention and Control

Because the novel SARS-CoV2 virus that causes COVID-19 is spread through respiratory secretions, infection prevention and control is essential to protect healthcare workers, their families, and other patients. As our understanding of this virus is evolving, guidance for infection control has frequently changed, generating confusion and stress. Nurses must be aware of the policies and procedures that guide use of PPE in their clinical setting. Hospitals must be transparent about available supplies of PPE, the strategies in place for optimizing those supplies, and the plan to return to conventional use as soon as supplies permit. For a description of PPE use under conventional, contingency, and crisis standards, please see Chapter 23, Crisis Standards of Care.

The SSC COVID-19 guideline indicates that healthcare providers must be fitted for respirators (N95, PAPR, FFP2,) for aerosol-generating procedures, which are frequent events in critical care settings. Eye protection, gowns, and gloves in addition to respiratory protection are also key elements in the current advise for healthcare worker protection. In addition to PPE, engineering controls such as the use of negative pressure rooms and administrative controls such as cohorting infected patients are additional considerations. Because infection control guidance changes as understanding evolves, nurses should ask questions and seek information from reliable sources.

Fluid Resuscitation

Uncertainties about management strategies for COVID-19 remain, as immune responses and pathophysiologic pathways are not fully understood. Respiratory failure is the hallmark of severe COVID-19 and is marked by pulmonary edema due to increased capillary permeability resulting in susceptibility to resuscitation-induced lung congestion. Similar to the SSC guidelines for sepsis, the NIH COVID-19 guideline panel recommends basing decisions about fluid administration on dynamic measures of hemodynamic status, including skin temperature, capillary refile time, and lactate levels. In addition, the NIH guideline recommends the use of balanced crystalloids over unbalanced crystalloids and avoiding the use of albumin. Patients with persistent hypotension who cannot undergo further fluid resuscitation due to pulmonary edema should be started on vasopressors, and the recommended first-line agent is norepinephrine.

Ventilation

Severe illness in COVID-19 patients usually occurs 1 week after symptom onset and is characterized by dyspnea and hypoxia. Severe illness requires supplemental oxygen, including high flow and noninvasive ventilation, and close monitoring for respiratory decompensation. Signs and symptoms that indicate disease progression include changes in depth of ventilation, worsening tachypnea, adventitious lung sounds, and changes in mental status or ability to focus. COVID-19 patients can develop acute hypoxic respiratory failure, with low oxygen saturation levels despite supplemental oxygen, leading to the need for intubation and mechanical ventilation. Ideally, prior to the escalation to advanced respiratory support, the use of mechanical ventilation is discussed with the patient and their family to form a plan of care consistent with the patient's desired outcomes. If intubation is necessary and consistent with the patient's desires, an experienced provider performs the procedure in a controlled environment to reduce the risk of transmission of COVID-19. Nursing care to manage respiratory distress in COVID-19 infection is further discussed in Chapter 10.

Prone Ventilation

Prone positioning improves oxygenation in nonintubated and intubated patients with ARDS and COVID-19 when other modes of ventilation fail. Prone positioning allows for lung expansion, mobilization of secretions, and increased oxygenation. Improved ventilation and perfusion match results from redistribution of blood flow and recruitment of dorsal lung regions. In the supine position, ventral lung, heart, and abdominal organs increase pleural pressure resulting in dorsal lung compression; the prone position reverses this effect.

In some cases, patients are awake and able to reposition themselves, and so they can be encouraged to use prone positioning to improve ventilation and oxygenation. Prone ventilation in patients who are sedated or otherwise not able to move themselves requires coordinated, synchronized movements and is done slowly and methodically as a collaborative process with other team members. Careful attention to the process and communication among the team members is needed to prevent dislodgement of life-saving medical devices. Some institutions utilize proning teams to reposition patients and monitor their response. For patients with ARDS, the decision to initiate prone ventilation is based upon the severity of disease. Although prone ventilation is beneficial, it is not a rescue therapy and not all patients improve. Diligent nursing care is necessary to

TABLE 11-7. NURSING CARE OF THE PRONE PATIENT

Nursing Care of the Prone Patient
• Assess hemodynamic stability and oxygenation
• Administer sedation and neuromuscular blocking agents as ordered
• Provide eye care
• Provide oral care and suctioning as needed
• Use hydrocolloid dressings to bony prominences and face to prevent skin breakdown
• Secure the airway
• Empty drainage bags
• Place electrocardiogram electrodes on posterior chest
• Monitor response to prone positioning including hemodynamic and respiratory status
• Reposition every 2 hours to prevent pressure injuries
• Maintain inverse Trendelenburg position to prevent aspiration

prevent associated complications, such a pressure injuries (PIs), inadvertent removal of invasive lines, and aspiration. The patient is kept in the prone position for up to 18 hours and then placed supine for at least 6 hours. Table 11-7 lists nursing considerations in the care of critically ill patients undergoing prone positioning.

SUBSTANCE USE DISORDERS

The use of drugs and alcohol is pervasive and an important cause of multisystem disorders. Drug or alcohol overdoses maybe be deliberate or accidental and result in significant morbidity and mortality. Accidental overdose may involve one or multiple substances, and can be acute, such as inaccurate dosing of prescribed or over-the-counter medications or chronic, such as ongoing use of alcohol or opioids leading to tolerance and the need for higher doses to achieve the same effect. Data from the Centers for Disease Control and Prevention (CDC) shows that historically high rates of opioid prescribing peaked in 2012 and have declined since then, possibly due to increased provider awareness of the risk of overdose. Despite this change, deaths from opioid overdose increased 15% from 2020 to 2021, primarily due to a rise in synthetic opioids, such as fentanyl (CDC, 2022).

The priority of care when patients present with acute intoxication or overdose is maintenance of the patient's airway, breathing, and circulation. The level of intoxication or overdose varies with the element and amount ingested, the time until the patient is treated, the patient's age, tolerance to medications, and underlying comorbid conditions. Therefore, collecting data on the precepting event and close monitoring for clinical deterioration are also essential nursing actions.

Etiology, Risk Factors, and Pathophysiology

Alcohol Intoxication and Overdose

Alcohol overdose, often called alcohol poisoning is most often seen in persons with alcohol use disorder, in young persons who have not yet reached legal drinking age, or in combination with other drugs as a suicide attempt. There are four types of alcohol that can lead to overdose:

1. Ethanol (ethyl or grain alcohol)
2. Methanol (wood alcohol)
3. Ethylene glycol (antifreeze)
4. Isopropyl alcohol (rubbing alcohol, solvent, and de-icer)

The most common of these is ethanol overdose. Alcohol dissolves readily in the lipid components of the plasma membranes of the body, and thus crosses the blood-brain barriers quickly, affecting the central nervous system.

Most of the clinical effects of alcohol can be explained by the interaction with neurotransmitters and neuroreceptors in the brain. Alcohol binds directly to the gamma-aminobutyric acid (GABA) receptors in the central nervous system (CNS) and causes sedation. Ethanol levels over 300 to 400 mg/dL (blood alcohol levels of 0.3%-0.4%) are toxic and can lead to respiratory depression. Levels less than 50 mg/dL (a blood alcohol level of 0.05%) may cause a sense of relaxation but usually do not explain impaired judgment or altered behavior. A serum alcohol level of 80 mg/dL (a blood alcohol level of 0.08%) is the legal upper limit for driving a car in most of the United States. In the case of methanol intoxication, serum levels range from 50 mg/dL (mild intoxication) to 100 mg/dL (severe intoxication).

An important assessment for any one of the toxic alcohols is an increase in serum osmolality and serum osmolal gap that may or may not include a high-anion gap (eg, >12 mEq/L) metabolic acidosis. The serum osmolality is determined by the different solutes' concentration in the plasma. The osmolal gap is the difference between the measured plasma osmolality and the plasma calculated osmolality. Osmolal gaps are present when unmeasured osmotic solutes (eg, toxins, methanol, ethylene glycol) are in the plasma.

While all four types of alcohol intoxication can cause metabolic acidosis with an elevated osmolal gap, only methanol and ethylene cause high anion gap acidosis. Metabolic acidosis manifests as a decreased serum bicarbonate level and indicates that the generation of hydrogen ions exceeds the ability of the kidney to excrete them. The excess of systemic hydrogen ions leads to compensatory hyperventilation, as the body attempts to make the pH more alkaline. Refer to Chapter 5, Airway and Ventilatory Management, for further information on acid-base imbalance.

There are also differences in the way that the different types of alcohol affect patients. For instance, the metabolites generated by methanol intoxication are formaldehyde and formic acid, which cause optic nerve and central nervous system damage. Isopropyl alcohol intoxication is distinguished from other types of alcohol intoxication by the presence of ketoacids in both the urine and the serum. This usually leads to metabolic acidosis but sometimes due to rapid excretion of acetone, acidosis does not occur. Isopropyl alcohol is so rapidly absorbed that ingestion of as little as 150 mL can be fatal. The parent compound, rather than the metabolites, causes the toxicity.

Clinical Presentation

Excess ingestion of any type of alcohol causes central nervous system symptoms such as sluggish reflexes, emotional instability, or erratic behavior. Amnesia may result for events that occurred during the period of intoxication. Unconsciousness may occur before a person can ingest a fatal dose; however, in some cases, the rapid consumption of alcohol leads to death from respiratory depression or aspiration during vomiting. It is estimated that there are 1.3 million hospital admissions annually for problems related to alcohol. Patients who chronically use alcohol and are admitted for other reasons may experience severe withdrawal symptoms that require medical treatment and generally require longer hospital stays than patients without alcohol use disorder. On average, between 2015 and 2019, over 33,658 deaths were attributed to alcohol use (Centers for Disease Control and Prevention. Alcohol-Related Disease Impact (ARDI) application, 2022. Available at www.cdc.gov/ARDI.)

Signs and symptoms that are specific to each type of alcohol ingested include:

- *Acute ethanol intoxication:* Muscular incoordination, slurred speech, stupor, hypoglycemia, flushing, seizures, coma, depressed respirations, and hyporeflexia
- *Methanol intoxication:* Neurologic depression, metabolic acidosis, and visual disturbances
- *Ethylene glycol intoxication:* Neurologic depression, cardiopulmonary complications, pulmonary edema, and renal tubular degeneration
- *Isopropyl intoxication:* Neurologic depression, areflexia, respiratory depression, hypothermia, hypotension, and gastrointestinal distress

Diagnostic Tests

In patients with suspected alcohol overdose, the initial assessment includes checking blood glucose levels as hypo- or hyperglycemia may mimic intoxication. In addition, a history from either the patient, family member, friend, or the person who found the patient assists with determination of the type and volume ingested. Diagnostic studies may aid in determining the ingested agent and guiding the appropriate management. These include:

- *Ethanol and methanol serum levels:* These are elevated if these substances were ingested. Isopropyl serum levels are not performed as commonly as ethanol and methanol levels.
- *Urinalysis:* Oxalate crystals may be present in ethylene glycol intoxication and ketones may be evident in isopropyl alcohol ingestion.
- *Serum creatinine and blood urea nitrogen (BUN) levels:* These may be elevated due to renal dysfunction. These are not sensitive or specific for overdose.

- *Transaminases:* The hepatotoxic effects of certain types of alcohol lead to elevations in liver function tests. Serum ammonia level is also an important assessment, if patients exhibit a persistent altered mental state, have a history of liver impairment or high transaminase levels consistent with hepatotoxicity.
- *Serum glucose and electrolytes:* Patients with alcohol intoxication may develop hypoglycemia as alcohol interferes with glucose production. Electrolyte derangement and metabolic acidosis also occur with alcohol ingestion.
- *EKG and cardiac monitoring:* Patients with acute alcohol intoxication, particularly those with a history of chronic use, have a higher risk of cardiac arrhythmias.
- *Urine drug screen:* Patients who ingest alcohol may have also ingested other substances so concurrent intoxication may contribute to the clinical presentation.
- *Serum acetaminophen and salicylate levels:* If a patient uses alcohol and also ingests acetaminophen and salicylate, specific treatments are needed to mitigate the toxic effects of these agents, because of the risk of synergistic harm. Checking serum levels ensures prompt and appropriate management.
- *Thyroid function tests:* Thyroid deficiency may contribute to the symptoms of alcohol use and to underlying mood disorders that precipitate chronic use.

Treatment of Alcohol Overdose

The management of ethanol overdose is primarily supportive with the priority being assessment of the patient's ability to maintain their airway, breathing, and circulation. Intravenous fluids are often administrated as patients may be dehydrated from the diuretic effect of alcohol. Assessment for tolerance of fluid administration is a key consideration as patients who chronically use alcohol have a higher risk of heart failure. Thiamine is often administered to patients who present with alcohol intoxication or overdose, to treat potential thiamine deficiency, or Wernicke syndrome, a complication of alcohol use. Patients with alcohol levels above 100 mg/dL can exhibit impaired judgment and erratic behavior with higher levels associated with greater risk. Therefore, in caring for patients with acute alcohol intoxication, nurses and healthcare teams must also prioritize their own safety.

The use of ethanol, or preferably fomepizole, for alcohol dehydrogenase (ADH) inhibition is a mainstay in the management of toxicity due to ingestion of methanol and ethylene glycol. Ethanol can be administered orally or intravenously to maintain a blood concentration of 100 to 150 mg/dL to prevent metabolism of alcohols to toxic metabolites. Fomepizole is much preferred as it offers a predictable decline in the ethyl glycol levels without the sedating side effects associated with ethanol. Hemodialysis is sometimes necessary to remove alcohol and toxic metabolites and is continued until metabolic acidosis resolves. Folinic acid (leucovorin) is suggested in methanol poisoning to provide the cofactor for formic acid elimination.

Isopropyl alcohol does not have a reversal agent. Toxicity caused by isopropyl alcohol is treated with supportive measures. These patients may require mechanical ventilation, intravenous fluids, and in some cases, dialysis.

Alcohol Withdrawal Syndrome

Patients who chronically use alcohol may be admitted for management of alcohol withdrawal or they may be admitted for a different reason and develop withdrawal symptoms. Symptoms of alcohol withdrawal vary from mild anxiety to hallucinations and seizures which can be life threatening (Table 11-8). The time frame in which withdrawal symptoms emerge also varies and is influenced by the quantity and frequency of baseline alcohol consumption, comorbid conditions, older age, and concurrent liver disease. While many patients may experience withdrawal symptoms, only about 5% of patients suffer severe withdrawal, delirium tremens (DT). The symptoms of DT include disorientation, hallucinations, hypertension, tachycardia, agitation, and diaphoresis and they usually begin 48 to 96 hours after the last intake of alcohol. A complete history from the patient and/or family to determine the amount and frequency of alcohol ingestion assists in planning the care of a patient with alcohol use disorder. The time that alcohol was last ingested is also important to document, as this will assist in determining the most likely time frame of withdrawal symptoms. Measuring symptom severity with an alcohol withdrawal symptom assessment tool at regular intervals facilitates proactive treatment in those experiencing or at risk for withdrawal (Figure 11-3).

Most treatment regimens include the use of fluid, electrolyte, and nutrition replacement. Administration of thiamine can prevent or treat Wernicke encephalopathy, a type of encephalopathy caused by depletion of thiamine stores which is commonly seen in patients with alcoholism or those who are severely malnourished. Multivitamins, folate, and magnesium replacement are also common elements of the treatment regimen for those with alcohol withdrawal and are typically given intravenously initially due to the impaired gastric absorption by chronic alcohol use. Benzodiazepines are given in scheduled doses or as needed based on assessment of symptoms. Intermediate-acting benzodiazepines, such as lorazepam, are commonly preferred in acute and critical care settings. All benzodiazepines appear equally effective in the treatment of alcohol withdrawal syndrome. In moderate-to-severe withdrawal, long-acting agents may be preferred. Adjunctive medications may also be used in some cases to treat agitation or hallucinations, though caution is warranted in the use of haloperidol as it lowers seizure threshold and may prolong the QT interval. Dexmedetomidine or clonidine may be useful to decrease autonomic symptoms. See Chapter 7 for a further discussion of pharmacologic agents.

Discharge planning for patients who are admitted with alcohol withdrawal or exhibit withdrawal symptoms includes discussion of treatment options for substance use disorder. While alcohol use is prevalent across many cultures, the consequences of overdose and chronic use can be severe. Collaboration with case management and social work can facilitate transition to appropriate care.

TABLE 11-8. SYMPTOMS OF ALCOHOL WITHDRAWAL SYNDROME

Symptoms	Time of Appearance After Cessation Alcohol Use
Minor withdrawal symptoms: insomnia, tremulousness, mild anxiety, gastrointestinal upset, headache, diaphoresis, palpitations, anorexia	6-12 hours
Alcoholic hallucinosis: visual, auditory, or tactile hallucinations	12-24 hours[a]
Withdrawal seizures: generalized tonic-clonic seizures	24-48 hours[b]
Alcohol withdrawal delirium (delirium tremens): hallucinations (predominately visual), disorientation, tachycardia, hypertension, low-grade fever, agitation, diaphoresis	48-72 hours[c]

[a]Symptoms generally resolve within 48 hours.
[b]Symptoms reported as early as 2 hours after cessation.
[c]Symptoms peak at 5 days.
Data from Bayard M, McIntyre J, Hill KR, et al: Alcohol withdrawal syndrome. Am Fam Physician. 2004;69(6):1443-1450.

ESSENTIAL CONTENT CASE

Alcohol Overdose

A 19-year-old man is unresponsive after drinking at a party and his roommates bring him to the emergency department (ED). Initial assessment reveals a decreased level of consciousness, with decreased response to stimuli. His initial laboratory results reveal a serum alcohol level of 430 mg/dL. Current vital signs are:

T	36.5°C (97.8°F) rectal
HR	120 beats/min (sinus tachycardia)
RR	16 breaths/min
BP	92/70 mm Hg

Pulse oximetry 94% on room air

Case Question 1: What are the priority interventions for this patient?

Case Question 2: What information would help in guiding treatment?

Answers
1. Maintenance of airway, hemodynamic stabilization, obtain and maintain intravenous access, administer IV fluids, and provide detoxification.
2. Amount and type of alcohol ingested and time frame since ingestion.

Clinical Institute Withdrawal Assessment of Alcohol Scale, Revised (CIWA-Ar)

Patient: _____   Date: _____   Time: _____   (24 hour clock, midnight = 00:00)

Pulse or heart rate, taken for one minute: _____   Blood pressure: _____

NAUSEA AND VOMITNG – Ask "Do you feel sick to your stomach? Have you vomited?" Observation.
0 no nausea and no vomiting
1 mild nausea with no vomiting
2
3
4 intermittent nausea with dry heaves
5
6
7 constant nausea, frequent dry heaves and vomiting

TACTILE DISTURBANCES – Ask "Have you any itching, pins and needles sensations, any burning, any numbness, or do you feel bugs crawling on or under your skin?" Observation.
0 none
1 very mild itching, pins and needles, burning or numbness
2 mild itching, pins and needles, burning or numbness
3 moderate itching, pins and needles, burning or numbness
4 moderately severe hallucinations
5 severe hallucinations
6 extremely severe hallucinations
7 continuous hallucinations

TREMOR – Arms extended and fingers spread apart. Observation.
0 no tremor
1 not visible, but can be felt fingertip to fingertip
2
3
4 moderate, with patient's arms extended
5
6
7 severe, even with arms not extended

AUDITORY DISTURBANCES – Ask "Are you more aware of sounds around you? Are they harsh? Do they frighten you? Are you hearing anything that is disturbing to you? Are you hearing things you know are not there?" Observation.
0 not present
1 very mild harshness or ability to frighten
2 mild harshness or ability to frighten
3 moderate harshness or ability to frighten
4 moderately severe hallucinations
5 severe hallucinations
6 extremely severe hallucinations
7 continuous hallucinations

PAROXYSMAL SWEATS – Observation.
0 no sweat visible
1 barely perceptible sweating, palms moist
2
3
4 beads of sweat obvious on forehead
5
6
7 drenching sweats

VISUAL DISTURBANCES – Ask "Does the light appear to be too bright? Is its color different? Does it hurt your eyes? Are you seeing anything that is disturbing to you? Are you seeing things you know are not there?" Observation.
0 not present
1 very mild sensitivity
2 mild sensitivity
3 moderate sensitivity
4 moderately severe hallucinations
5 severe hallucinations
6 extremely severe hallucinations
7 continuous hallucinations

ANXIETY – Ask "Do you feel nervous?" Observation.
0 no anxiety, at ease
1 mild anxious
2
3
4 moderately anxious, or guarded, so anxiety is inferred
5
6
7 equivalent to acute panic states as seen in severe delirium or acute schizophrenic reactions

HEADACHE, FULLNESS IN HEAD – Ask "Does your head feel different? Does it feel like there is a band around your head?" Do not rate for dizziness or lightheadedness. Otherwise, rate severity.
0 not present
1 very mild
2 mild
3 moderate
4 moderately severe
5 severe
6 very severe
7 extremely severe

AGITATION – Observation.
0 normal activity
1 somewhat more than normal activity
2
3
4 moderately fidgety and restless
5
6
7 paces back and forth during most of the interview, or constantly thrashes about

ORIENTATION AND CLOUDING OF SENSORIUM – Ask "What day is this? Where are you? Who am I?"
0 oriented and can do serial additions
1 cannot do serial additions or is uncertain about date
2 disoriented for date by no more than 2 calendar days
3 disoriented for date by more than 2 calendar days
4 disoriented for place/or person

Total **CIWA-Ar** Score _____
Rater's Initials _____
Maximum Possible Score 67

The **CIWA-Ar** is not copyrighted and may be reproduced freely. This assessment for monitoring withdrawal symptoms requires approximately 5 minutes to administer. The maximum score is 67 (see instrument). Patients scoring less than 10 do not usually need additional medication for withdrawal.

Figure 11-3. Revised Clinical Institute Withdrawal Assessment for Alcohol (CIWA-Ar) scale. (*Adapted with permission from Sullivan JT, Sykora K, Schneiderman J, et al: Assessment of alcohol withdrawal: the revised Clinical Institute Withdrawal Assessment for Alcohol Scale (CIWA-AR)*, Br J Addict 1989;84(11):1353-1357.)

Drug Overdose

Drug overdose may involve any type of substance or medication, illicit, prescribed, or over the counter. Most overdoses involve analgesics (opioids, aspirin, and acetaminophen), antidepressants, sedatives, over-the-counter medications for cough and cold, and illegal drugs, such as cocaine, heroin, or methamphetamines. The CDC's National Center for Health Statistics noted that there were over 100,000 drug overdose deaths from April 2020 to April 2021 with 75,000 deaths related to opioids (CDC, 2022). Illegal diversion of prescribed opioids, illicit use of synthetic opioids, accidental overdose, and suicidal intent all contribute to the epidemic of opioid overdose deaths. In response to the dramatic rise in opioid deaths, the CDC issued opioid prescribing guidelines in 2016 and urged increased education for patients and providers about the risks of opioid use and the availability of alternative treatments for pain. In 2022, the CDC launched the *Facts on Fentanyl* campaign to raise awareness about the high potency of synthetic opioids (CDC, 2022).

Acetaminophen is also a significant cause of drug overdose. Easily available as a preparation to alleviate fever or pain, acetaminophen is also present in many combination medications, both over the counter and prescribed. Acetaminophen can cause hepatocellular damage that may be severe enough to require liver transplantation.

Illicit substances are often used intentionally to induce a relaxed state, elevate mood, or produce unusual states of consciousness. These effects are the result of chemical similarity to neurotransmitters such as serotonin, dopamine, or norepinephrine, which alters neurotransmitter-receptor interactions. With chronic use, adaptive changes in the neurotransmitter receptors occur, which means that higher doses of a drug are required to produce the same effect. Medullary inspiratory neurons are highly sensitive to depression by drugs, especially barbiturates and morphine, and death from an overdose of these agents is often secondary to respiratory arrest.

Clinical Presentation

The specific signs and symptoms of drug overdose depend on the substance ingested. However, there are several signs and symptoms that are commonly seen, including alterations in mental status, decreased or increased level of consciousness (LOC), behavioral changes, and respiratory depression. The signs and symptoms of overdose for specific agents are summarized in Table 11-9.

Diagnostic Tests

Diagnostic studies for patients following drug overdose may include the following:

- *Toxicology screening* typically consists of broad-spectrum tests and identifies the presence of substances such as amphetamines, barbiturates, benzodiazepines, and narcotics. Specific serum levels may be indicated if the substance is known. Serum acetaminophen and

TABLE 11-9. SIGNS AND SYMPTOMS OF OVERDOSE

Opioids	• Change in level of consciousness (LOC) • Respiratory depression, aspiration • Hypotension • Miosis • Decreased gastric motility
Barbiturates	• Decreased LOC • Hypothermia • Respiratory depression
Benzodiazepines	• Altered mental status • Respiratory depression • Weakness or tremors
Cocaine	• Hyperexcitability • Headache • Hypertension • Tachycardia • Nausea/vomiting, abdominal pain • Fever • Delirium, convulsions, coma
Phencyclidine (PCP)	• Violent behavior • Hallucinations • Seizures • Rhabdomyolysis • Hypertensive crisis
Tricyclics	• Seizures • Coma • Dysrhythmias, ECG changes • Heart failure • Shock
Salicylates	• Tinnitus • Vertigo • Vomiting • Hyperthermia • Altered mental status
Acetaminophen	• GI distress • Hepatotoxicity • Hepatic necrosis

salicylate levels are checked in all cases of suspected overdose as these require specific treatment.

- *Arterial blood gas* to evaluate oxygenation, ventilation, and the acid-base status, and measurement of the anion gap to determine the severity of metabolic derangement.
- *Serum glucose and electrolytes*, often abnormal because of overdose, are measured as they may contribute to the clinical presentation and require treatment.

Principles of Management for Overdose

The initial clinical evaluation of overdose is focused on resuscitating and stabilizing the patient. The principles of management include maintenance of a patent airway and adequate breathing, prevention of complications, elimination of ingested substances or toxic metabolites, and maintenance of hemodynamic stability. Specific treatment depends on the agent, route and amount of exposure, and the severity of overdose. Notification of the Poison Control Center is essential as they often have resources which provide specific guidance regarding appropriate treatment.

Airway and Breathing

1. Maintain adequate ventilation. Stimulate the patient to breathe, if needed. If the patient cannot breathe spontaneously to maintain oxygenation and prevent respiratory acidosis, intubation and mechanical ventilation may be required.
2. Monitor pulse oximetry and arterial blood gas values (see Chapter 10 for further explanation).
3. Position the patient with the head of the bed elevated at least 30°, unless contraindicated.
4. Suction the patient's airway as needed.

Circulation and Maintenance of Hemodynamic Stability

1. Ensure venous access (large-bore peripheral or central access).
2. Administer intravenous fluids to maintain intravascular fluid volume. Because opioid use can lead to vasodilation, patients may exhibit refractory hypotension. If volume expansion is not sufficient to maintain MAP more than or equal to 65, administration of vasopressors may be necessary.
3. Obtain a 12-lead ECG and maintain continuous cardiac monitoring. Dysrhythmias may be associated with drug overdose, such as supraventricular tachycardia and hypertension occurring with cocaine use. Collaborate with providers on medical management of dysrhythmias which may include beta-blockers, combined alpha and beta-blocker therapy, or calcium channel blockers.

Neurologic Depression

1. Measure glucose to exclude hypoglycemia and treat with 50% dextrose IV if necessary.
2. Evaluate for carbon monoxide poisoning by checking a carboxyhemoglobin level. If this is a concern, provide oxygen therapy if not already indicated.
3. Administer thiamine IV for Wernicke encephalopathy if there is a history that suggests concurrent alcohol use.
4. Administer antidotes for specific agents to reverse their effects. Naloxone IV or IM can be effective in opioid overdose and flumazenil can be used for benzodiazepine overdose. Caution is appropriate with flumazenil in those at risk for a seizure. If reducing the seizure threshold is too risky, intubation for airway protection may be preferable. In some cases, antidotes require repeat dosing if the patient experiences recurrent symptoms.

Catharsis, Clearing Drugs, and Antidotes

1. *Ipecac:* This agent is no longer recommended though it was once used to induce vomiting. There is little evidence that ipecac improves patient outcomes in poisoning cases. Patients are also at increased risk for aspiration, as they may become lethargic from drug overdose before the ipecac is effective. Furthermore, there is little evidence that ipecac prevents drug absorption or systemic toxicity.
2. *Gastric lavage:* Lavage refers to utilizing a nasogastric tube to remove stomach contents and decrease absorption of an orally ingested substance. Significant amounts of ingested agents can be recovered if lavage is used close to the time of ingestion. This method is less effective if performed more than 1 hour after ingestion due to the timing of gastric emptying. Gastric lavage is contraindicated in the management of ingested corrosive agents due to risk of esophageal injury and gastroesophageal perforation. It is also contraindicated with hydrocarbon ingestion because of the risk of aspiration-induced hydrocarbon pneumonitis.
3. *Activated charcoal:* Charcoal absorbs ingested toxins within the gut lumen, allowing the charcoal-toxin complex to be eliminated in the stool. Charcoal is not recommended for patients who have ingested caustic acids and alkalis, alcohols, lithium, or heavy metals. Charcoal is useful for most drug ingestions if it is used close to the time of ingestion (within 1 hour) as it only impacts the portion of drug that remains in the stomach.
4. *Hemodialysis and hemoperfusion:* Hemodialysis can be considered for severe poisoning due to methanol, ethylene glycol, salicylates, lithium, barbiturates, bromide, chloral hydrate, ethanol, isopropyl alcohol, procainamide, theophylline, salicylates, and heavy metals. Hemoperfusion, which involves the passage of blood through an absorptive-containing cartridge (usually charcoal), may be indicated for intoxication with carbamazepine, phenobarbital, phenytoin, and theophylline. Therapeutic plasma exchange has also been used to promote rapid lowering of the toxin level. Refer to Chapter 15, Renal System, for more information on renal replacement therapies.
5. Antidotes help counteract the effects of toxic agents by neutralizing them or by antagonizing their effects. Toxins and their specific antidotes include the following:
   - *Acetaminophen:* N-acetylcysteine
   - *Opiates:* Naloxone
   - *Benzodiazepines:* Flumazenil
   - *Digoxin:* Digibind
   - *Cyanide:* Kelocyanor
   - *Tricyclic antidepressants:* Sodium bicarbonate
   - *Beta-blockers or calcium channel blockers:* Glucagon and calcium
   - *Warfarin:* Vitamin K

Preventing Complications

1. Orient the patient to their surroundings.
2. Assess suicidality and implement 1:1 monitoring if appropriate.

3. Insert a nasogastric tube for gastric decompression and for delivery of charcoal or other antidotes, if indicated.
4. Keep the head of the bed elevated more than 30°, to prevent aspiration.
5. Provide support to the patient and family.
6. Monitor for signs and symptoms of end-organ damage, such as liver dysfunction from alcohol use, or cardiac dysfunction from cocaine.

PRESSURE INJURY

Pressure injuries are troubling complications of immobility for acute and critically ill patients. They increase length of hospitalization, recovery time, risk of infection, costs of care, and cause discomfort and disfigurement for patients. Of significance to the healthcare team is that PIs are thought to be preventable in most cases and are viewed as a reflection of the quality of care. As a result, starting in 2008, hospitals are not reimbursed for treatment of stage 3 and 4 pressure injuries that develop during an inpatient stay.

Hospital-acquired pressure injuries (HAPI) are a complication of hospital admission that increases length of stay and mortality. In the United States, between 1 and 3 million people are affected by PI each year, and 5% to 15% of hospitalized patients experience PI. Because of their association with quality of care and their financial impact, documentation of the presence of pressure injuries on admission and interventions to reduce the incidence are elements of nursing care.

A pressure injury (PI) is defined by the National Pressure Injury Advisory Panel (NPIAP) as an injury to the skin or tissue due to pressure or shear occurring in a localized area. When a person is immobile, the soft tissue is compressed between the skin and the bone. This can lead to ischemia and tissue death. Typically, a pressure injury occurs over a bony prominence such as the sacrum, hip or heel, but PI can occur anywhere soft tissue is compressed, including in areas where medical devices are applied. For instance, endotracheal tubes, nasogastric tubes, or blood pressure cuffs can lead to HAPI. The most common anatomical sites for pressure injuries to occur are the sacrum and heels.

There are several factors related to the risk of pressure injury development. In the critical care setting, immobility, poor perfusion, hypoxia, hypothermia, and use of vasoactive medications contribute to pressure injuries. Additionally, poor nutrition and dehydration contribute to pressure injury development because these conditions make tissue more vulnerable to damage. Older adults are at greater risk because of physiologic changes that occur to the skin and tissue with age, such as dermal thinning and the inability of tissue to distribute the mechanical load. Peripheral vasoconstriction during periods of hypotension or due to administration of vasopressors diverts blood away from the skin to more essential organs. Additionally, other comorbid conditions such as diabetes and peripheral vascular disease may increase risk for pressure injury development.

TABLE 11-10. PRESSURE INJURY CLASSIFICATION BRIEF GUIDE

Category/Stage 1 Pressure Injury	Intact skin with discoloration
Category/Stage 2 Pressure Injury	Partial-thickness tissue loss Wound bed is pink/red
Category/Stage 3 Pressure Injury	Full-thickness tissue loss extending into the subcutaneous tissue; slough/eschar may be present in the wound bed but does not obscure depth of the wound
Category/Stage 4 Pressure Injury	Full-thickness tissue loss; the muscle, bone, or tendon may be present in the wound bed; slough/eschar may be present in the wound bed but does not obscure depth of the wound
Unstageable– Unknown Depth	Full-thickness tissue loss; unable to visualize base of the wound due to slough or eschar
Deep Tissue Injury	Purple or maroon discoloration Intact skin Non-blanchable

Data from National Pressure Ulcer Advisory Panel. NPUAP Pressure Injury Stages.

According to the National Pressure Injury Advisory Panel, the six stages of pressure injuries (Table 11-10) are classified as follows:

Pressure Injury Stages

Stage 1

A stage 1 pressure injury is an area of intact skin with as nonblanchable erythema. The area may be painful, firm, soft, warmer, or cooler when compared to adjacent tissue, but the skin remains intact. Darkly pigmented skin may not have visible blanching so any change in color warrants further assessment for stage 1 pressure injury or for possible deep tissue injury. See Figure 11-4 for an illustration of stage 1 pressure injury.

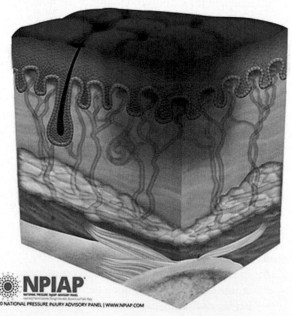

Figure 11-4. Stage 1 pressure injury. (*Reproduced with permission from National Pressure Ulcer Advisory Panel and European Pressure Ulcer Advisory Panel. Pressure Ulcer Prevention and Treatment: Clinical Practice Guideline. Washington, DC: National Pressure Ulcer Advisory Panel, 2009.*)

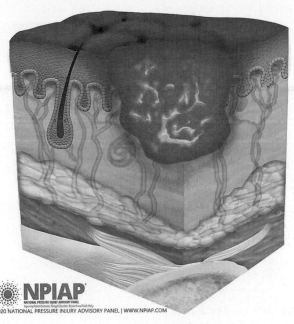

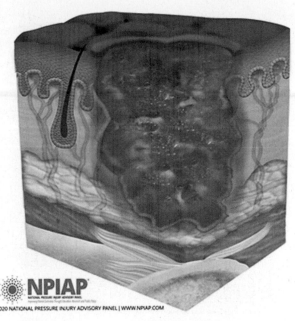

Figure 11-5. Stage 2 pressure injury. (*Reproduced with permission from National Pressure Ulcer Advisory Panel and European Pressure Ulcer Advisory Panel. Pressure Ulcer Prevention and Treatment: Clinical Practice Guideline. Washington, DC: National Pressure Ulcer Advisory Panel, 2009.*)

Figure 11-6. Stage 3 pressure injury. (*Reproduced with permission from National Pressure Ulcer Advisory Panel and European Pressure Ulcer Advisory Panel. Pressure Ulcer Prevention and Treatment: Clinical Practice Guideline. Washington, DC: National Pressure Ulcer Advisory Panel, 2009.*)

Stage 2

Stage 2 pressure injuries involve partial-thickness loss of dermis, or a shallow open area with a red-pink wound bed, without slough or bruising. An intact or open/ruptured serum-filled blister is also identified as stage 2 pressure injury. This stage should not be used to describe skin tears, tape burns, perineal dermatitis, maceration, or excoriation. See Figure 11-5 for an illustration of stage 2 pressure injury.

Stage 3

Stage 3 pressure injuries refer to full-thickness tissue loss. The wound bed may reveal subcutaneous fat, but bone, tendon, or muscle are not visible. Stage 3 pressure injury may exhibit slough but at least a portion of the wound is visible to demonstrate staging. See Figure 11-6 for an illustration of stage 3 pressure injury.

Stage 4

Stage 4 pressure injuries are full-thickness tissue loss in which bone, tendon, or muscle are visible. Like stage 3 PI, there may be slough or eschar on a portion of the wound. Stage 4 pressure injuries often demonstrate undermining and tunneling. The depth of stage 4 pressure injuries varies by anatomical location. Stage 4 pressure injuries can extend into muscle and/or supporting structures (ie, fascia, tendon, or joint capsules) making osteomyelitis a possible complication. Exposed bone/tendon is visible or directly palpable in stage 4 pressure injuries.

The depth of stage 3 and 4 pressure injuries varies by anatomical location. The bridge of the nose, ear, occiput, and malleolus do not have subcutaneous tissue so injury that reaches the tendon or bone occurs with shallow wounds

in these areas. In areas of greater adiposity, deeper wound may not expose tendon or bone and so would be classified as stage 3. Staging is not based on wound depth but rather on assessing the structures exposed by the wound. See Figure 11-7 for an illustration of stage 4 pressure injury.

Unstageable

A pressure injury that is unstageable is one in which full-thickness tissue loss is present but the wound base is covered by slough (yellow, tan, gray, green, or brown) and/or eschar

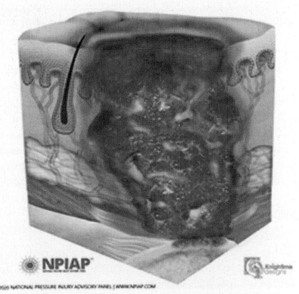

Figure 11-7. Stage 4 pressure injury. (*Reproduced with permission from National Pressure Ulcer Advisory Panel and European Pressure Ulcer Advisory Panel. Pressure Ulcer Prevention and Treatment: Clinical Practice Guideline. Washington, DC: National Pressure Ulcer Advisory Panel, 2009.*)

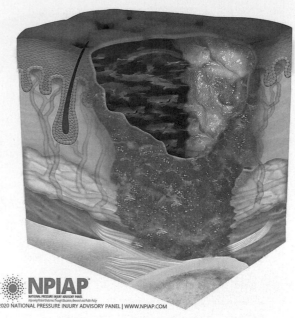

Figure 11-8. Unstageable pressure injury. (*Reproduced with permission from National Pressure Ulcer Advisory Panel and European Pressure Ulcer Advisory Panel. Pressure Ulcer Prevention and Treatment: Clinical Practice Guideline. Washington, DC: National Pressure Ulcer Advisory Panel, 2009.*)

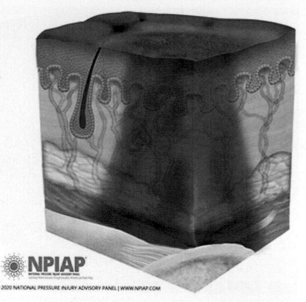

Figure 11-9. Deep tissue injury. (*Reproduced with permission from National Pressure Ulcer Advisory Panel and European Pressure Ulcer Advisory Panel. Pressure Ulcer Prevention and Treatment: Clinical Practice Guideline. Washington, DC: National Pressure Ulcer Advisory Panel, 2009.*)

(tan, brown, or black), impairing evaluation of underlying structures. Removal of slough or eschar is necessary if identifying the stage is required. In some cases, particularly with PI over the heels, the overlying eschar may provide a protective barrier that should be left intact. See Figure 11-8 for an image of unstageable pressure injury.

Deep Tissue Injury

Deep tissue injury is defined as a pressure-related injury to subcutaneous tissue that occurs under intact skin. The localized area may appear as a blister or discolored, purple, maroon, or deep red. The area may demonstrate temperature changes and/or tenderness. Deep tissue injury may be difficult to detect, particularly in individuals with dark skin tones. Evolution may include a thin blister over a dark wound bed. The wound may progress to stage 3 or 4 pressure injuries. Evolution may be rapid, exposing additional layers of tissue even with optimal treatment. These injuries may occur from medical devices such as oxygen saturation probes or may occur from prolonged positioning on hard surfaces, such as on the operating room table or interventional radiology table. See Figure 11-9 for an illustration of deep tissue injury.

COVID-19 Related Pressure Injuries

A subset of patients with COVID-19 or severe ARDS from another cause require prone positioning to improve respiratory mechanics and oxygenation. Patients remain in a prone position for up to 18 hours per day, alternating with an 86-hour supine position. Prone positioning increases the risk of HAPI and makes assessment for pressure injury challenging. Using appropriate support surfaces, protective dressings, and frequently repositioning the patient are key preventive strategies.

Principles of Management of Pressure Injury

Baseline assessment followed by frequent reassessment of patient's skin and their risk for pressure injury is an essential nursing practice in acute and critical care. Preventing HAPI requires consideration of the multisystem factors that generate the risk for injury. Nursing care to prevent PI includes attention to nutritional status, appropriate repositioning, and use of prophylactic dressings and pressure-reducing surfaces in accordance with institution policy.

The two most widely studied and validated risk assessment scales are the Braden© and Norton© scales. The Braden scale consists of six subcategories, sensory perception, moisture, activity, mobility, nutrition, and friction/shear. Each category is scored 1 (most at risk) to 4 (least at risk), with the exception of the friction and shear subcategory which is scored 1 to 3. The numbers are totaled, providing a score ranging from 4 to 23. A score less than 18 indicates risk for pressure injury development. The Norton score includes five parameters: physical condition, mental condition, activity, mobility, and continence. The rating for each category is 1 to 4 with a score potential of 5 to 20. For both the Braden and Norton scales, a low score indicates a greater risk for pressure injury development.

Due to the significant impact on morbidity and mortality of pressure injury, coupled with the economic impact, national strategies are in place for prevention. The Agency for Healthcare Research and Quality recommends that hospitals perform routine pressure injury prevalence surveys. By carefully tracking the incidence of pressure injuries, hospitals obtain real-time information to inform targeted implementation of prevention and treatment strategies.

Although the underlying relationship is uncertain, low body weight and malnutrition are risk factors for development of pressure injuries. Patients must have sufficient calories, fluid, and protein intake to reduce their risk. Evaluation and treatment for malnutrition, ideally by a registered dietician, may help prevent pressure injury development.

Repositioning should be scheduled for bed- and chair-bound patients at risk for pressure injury development. The patient's overall condition must be considered when repositioning. If the patient cannot be fully turned due to hemodynamic instability, then an advanced support surface can be used and slight adjustments in position provided. Support surfaces are used as adjunctive therapy and do not replace turning and repositioning. A pillow or a heel elevation device may be used to suspend heels off the surface of the bed.

The treatment of pressure injuries is complex and can vary based on the types of dressings available and the patients' underlying health. Prompt recognition and treatment are essential to limit the impact of pressure injury on a patient's overall prognosis. A wound care specialist should be consulted whenever possible to guide treatment and evaluate for possible debridement.

HEALTHCARE-ASSOCIATED INFECTIONS

The CDC reports that healthcare-associated infections (HAIs) occur in about 1 of every 31 inpatients. HAIs have been identified as one of the most serious patient safety issues in health care. Patients in critical care units are at an increased risk for catheter-associated urinary tract infections (CAUTIs), central line-associated bloodstream infection (CLABSI), hospital-acquired pneumonia (HAP), ventilator-associated events (VAE), and ventilator-associated complications (VAC). The etiology and treatment of HAP, VAE, and VAC are discussed in Chapter 10, Respiratory System.

CAUTI

CAUTIs result from the presence of an indwelling urinary catheter. Because infection can spread from the urinary tract into the bloodstream, the CDC reports that CAUTI is the leading cause of secondary hospital-associated bloodstream infections (BSIs). Patients that develop a bloodstream infection secondary to a CAUTI have an associated 10% mortality rate. Guidelines for the prevention of CAUTIs issued by the CDC outline several recommendations, including appropriate use and prompt discontinuation of indwelling catheters, sterile technique during catheter insertion, and maintaining a closed sterile drainage system. Table 11-11 further outlines evidence-based strategies to prevent CAUTI.

A variety of specialized catheters have been designed to reduce the risk of CAUTI. These include antiseptic-impregnated catheters and catheters coated with silver alloy or nitrofurazone. Several systematic reviews of the use of antimicrobial urinary catheters in the prevention of CAUTI have demonstrated a reduction in catheter-associated bacteriuria, but consensus on the economic benefit compared to standard catheter use has not been reached and further research is needed.

TABLE 11-11 EVIDENCE-BASED STRATEGIES FOR URINARY TRACT INFECTION PREVENTION

- Identify and assess indications for placement of indwelling urinary catheters, and consider alternative strategies
- Use aseptic technique for catheter insertion and seek assistance to ensure asepsis is maintained throughout the procedure
- Use the smallest catheter possible
- When caring for patients with indwelling catheters in place:
  - Use aseptic technique when handling the device
  - Secure the device
  - Ensure an unobstructed unidirectional flow of urine by avoiding kinks in the tubing and keeping the drainage bag below bladder level
  - Use a closed system and aseptic technique for taking urine samples
  - Empty the collection bag regularly
  - Use plain wipe bathing, and follow institutional protocol for cleaning the catheter regularly
- Discontinue indwelling catheters as soon as possible
  - Evaluate the need for indwelling catheter at least daily
  - Collaborate on the development of a surveillance program that tracks the number of urinary catheter days on the unit
  - Implement a nurse-driven protocol to regularly assess the indication for indwelling catheters and their ongoing use

Data from AACN Practice Alert: Prevention of Catheter Association Urinary Tract Infections in Adults. ©2017 American Association of Critical-Care Nurses.

Nursing care to reduce the risk of CAUTI includes assessment to determine if urinary catheter use is appropriate, consideration of alternative interventions such as external collection devises or periodic in and out catheterization, strict adherence to aseptic technique in managing the catheter, monitoring patients for signs of UTI, and teaching unlicensed personnel to handle the catheter and the collection bag appropriately. Removal of catheters when use is unnecessary is essential in preventing CAUTI. Nurse-driven protocols to reduce the duration of catheter use have effectively lowered CAUTI rates and shown a financial benefit.

CLABSI

Central venous catheters (CVCs) are frequently needed in critical care, but have associated risks, the most common being bloodstream infection. A central line-associated bloodstream infection (CLABSI) is defined as bacteremia in a patient with an intravascular catheter with at least one positive blood culture and clinical signs of infections (ie, fever, leukocytosis, and/or hypotension), with no apparent source for the BSI except the catheter. A BSI is associated with a central line if the line was in place during the 48-hour period before development of the BSI.

According to the CDC, there was a 50% decrease in the incidence of CLABSI from 2009 to 2014, most likely because of CLABSI prevention bundles. This trend reversed during the first year of the COVID-19 pandemic when CLABSI rates increased by 24%, with the greatest increase in intensive care settings (CDC, 2021). CLABSI thus continues to be a significant cause of morbidity and mortality in hospitalized patients. The most common mechanism of CLABSI is migration of the organism from the insertion site along the surface of the catheter and colonization of its distal port. CLABSIs can also occur from improper insertion techniques, lack of

TABLE 11-12. EVIDENCE-BASED STRATEGIES FOR CENTRAL LINE INFECTION PREVENTION

- Bathe critically ill patients with chlorhexidine preparation on a daily basis
- Use a checklist and if available an all-inclusive catheter kit for central line insertion
- Collaborate with providers to ensure infection prevention during central line insertion, including use of the subclavian vein, use of ultrasound guidance, and appropriate draping and skin preparation
- Perform hand hygiene prior to handling the device
- Use dressings over the insertion site that contain chlorhexidine
- Change loose, soiled, or damp dressings immediately. Change gauze dressings every two days and transparent dressings every 7 days.
- Disinfect catheter hubs, injection ports, or needleless connectors before accessing the catheter ("scrub the hub")
- Remove catheters when they are not needed
- Replace IV tubing every 7 days or according to hospital and unit protocol (unless tubing is used for blood, blood products, or lipid formulations)
- Additional approaches to consider, based on hospital and unit policy:
  - Use of antimicrobial-impregnated catheters
  - Use of antiseptic-containing hub/port protector
  - Use of vascular access teams
- Central lines should not routinely be replaced at scheduled intervals.

Data from Buetti N, Marschall J, Drees M, et al: Strategies to prevent central line-associated bloodstream infections in acute-care hospitals: 2022 Update. Infect Control Hosp Epidemiol. 2022;43(5):553-569.

an occlusive dressing, or contamination of the catheter hub or of the infusate administered through the device.

Several practices can reduce the incidence of CLABSI. These include using a standardized catheter insertion technique with skin prep such as chlorhexidine, careful maintenance of the catheter, and daily review of catheter necessity to ensure prompt removal. The use of antimicrobial-impregnated dressings may also reduce the incidence of CLABSI. Current CDC recommendations include use of CVCs coated with antibacterial or antiseptic agents when prolonged use (greater than 5 days) is expected, central line insertion bundles, daily chlorhexidine bathing of ICU patients with CVCs, chlorhexidine-impregnated dressings, proper hand hygiene, and careful disinfecting of catheter hubs. Table 11-12 outlines evidence-based strategies for CLABSI prevention.

Nursing interventions to prevent CLABSI include maximal barrier precautions during CVC insertion; ongoing care of the insertion site including sterile dressing changes; disinfection of CVC ports during blood sampling, infusion of intravenous fluids, and medication administration; intravenous tubing changes based on hospital and unit protocol; and monitoring of patients with CVCs for signs of infection. Nurses also assess the need for CVC placement and advocate for removal when no longer necessary.

Selected Infectious Diseases

Multi-drug-resistant organisms, or MDROs, are bacteria resistant to traditional antibiotic therapy. MDROs can cause serious local and systemic infections that can be severely debilitating and even life threatening. The most common MDROs include methicillin-resistant *Staphylococcus aureus* (MRSA), vancomycin-resistant *Enterococcus* (VRE), *Acinetobacter*, and

carbapenem-resistant *Enterobacteriaceae* (CRE). Hospitalization and prior use of antibiotics increases the risk for infection and colonization with MDROs. Patients with MDROs are placed on isolation precautions to prevent the spread of the organism to other patients. *Clostridium difficile (C. diff)* is often discussed with MDROs as infection with *C. diff* similarly occurs in the setting of antibiotic use, and requires special precautions to prevent transmission to other patients. According to the CDC, the prevalence of infections caused by MDROs and *C. diff* are on the rise largely due to overuse of antibiotics, making antibiotic stewardship a key intervention.

MRSA is a type of staphylococcal organism resistant to traditional antibiotic therapy, including methicillin, oxacillin, amoxicillin, penicillin, and cephalosporins. MRSA can be transmitted via personal contact with contaminated items such as dressings or other infected materials, and can be spread due to poor hand hygiene or use of contaminated equipment, such as stethoscopes.

VRE most commonly occurs in the hospital and long-term care settings. According to the CDC, risk factors for acquiring VRE include treatment with vancomycin, immunosuppression, recent surgery, presence of invasive devices, and/or prolonged courses of antibiotics, especially while hospitalized. VRE can be transmitted from person to person via contact due to poor hand hygiene or by touching contaminated surfaces.

CRE are a key concern in acute care settings because these bacteria do not respond to the most potent antibiotics available. While CRE can cause ventilator-associated pneumonia, BSI, and intra-abdominal abscesses, it is most often an infection of the urinary tract. The CDC estimates that up to half of patients who develop a CRE BSI will die as a result.

C. diff is also an important contributor to hospital-acquired infections and requires contact isolation. A spore-forming anaerobic bacillus, *C. diff* produces endotoxins that cause diarrhea and can lead to colitis, and, in vulnerable patients, sepsis. New strains of *C. diff* cause more severe disease and are less responsive to treatment. The single most important risk factor for *C. diff* is antibiotic use. Twenty percent of cases of *C. diff* resolve with antibiotic discontinuation; other cases require administration of metronidazole or vancomycin. Particular attention to hand hygiene is essential in limiting the spread of *C. diff*. Because the spores do not die with exposure to alcohol, healthcare professionals must perform meticulous hand washing with soap and water after exposure to patients with known or suspected *C. diff*.

HAI Prevention

The CDC has identified interventions necessary to control or eradicate MDROs and *C. diff*. These include administrative support, education, MDRO surveillance, infection control precautions, environmental precautions, and decolonization. Additionally, the CDC's Campaign to Prevent Antimicrobial Resistance recommends judicious use of antibiotics and avoiding excessive duration of antibiotic therapy.

Vigilance to prevent hospital-acquired infections among older adults is essential. Age-related changes in immune system function increase the risk of HAIs. In addition, older adults have comorbid conditions and often undergo transfers between different inpatient facilities creating a higher risk for infection with MDROs. Recognizing this risk, nurses monitor older adults for altered mental status, respiratory signs and symptoms, and changes in urination that may indicate infection even in the absence of a fever. Older adults who require long-term use of invasive devices such as central lines or urinary catheters require infection prevention education and may benefit from the support of home health nurses after discharge.

Nurses have an important role in preventing the spread of MDROs in the critical care setting. Hand hygiene is a significant intervention that applies to all patient care activities. Hand hygiene is performed before and after touching a patient, before aseptic procedures, after contact with body fluids, and after touching items in the patient's environment. In addition, nurses maintain transmission-based precautions for patients with confirmed MDRO or *C. diff* infection which includes donning gowns and gloves prior to entering patients' rooms and removing them before exiting. This procedure needs to be followed by all members of the healthcare team for each patient contact. It may be helpful to organize care to reduce the number of trips in and out of the patient room when transmission-based precautions are required. An additional consideration is the social isolation that patients on transmission-based precautions may face, and the use of electronic devices for video calls may be of benefit to allow interaction with loved ones while limiting their exposure.

Nurses collaborate with other members of the healthcare team to implement additional strategies that reduce the spread of MDROs. These include limiting the transport of patients with MDROs; using disposable equipment, disinfecting durable equipment; and ensuring cleaning and disinfecting of patients' rooms. Posted signs and education of staff, patients, and visitors are also essential in reducing the spread of MDROs and *C. diff*. Terminal room cleaning after discharge or transfer and including isolation precautions in hand-off communications are further nursing actions to reduce the spread of MDROs and C. *diff*.

SELECTED BIBLIOGRAPHY

Sepsis and Septic shock

AACN webinar: Update Your Practice With the 2021 Sepsis Guidelines. https://www.aacn.org/education/webinar-series/wb0064/update-your-practice-with-the-2021-sepsis-guidelines

American Association of Critical-Care Nurses. *Nurses on the Frontline of Sepsis*. https://www.aacn.org/clinical-resources/sepsis. Accessed November 28, 2022.

Alhazzani W, Evans L, Alshamsi F. et al. Surviving Sepsis Campaign Guidelines on the management of adults with Coronavirus Disease 2019 (COVID-19) in the ICU: first update. *Crit Care Med.* 2021;49(3):e219-e234. doi: 10.1097/CCM.00000000000004899

Balshi AN, Huwait BM, Nasr Noor AS, et al. Modified Early Warning Score as a predictor of intensive care unit readmission within 48 hours: a retrospective observational study. *Rev Bras Ter Intensiva.* 2020;32(2):301-307. doi: 10.5935/0103-507X.20200047

Center for Disease Control (2022). Sepsis. https://www.cdc.gov/sepsis/what-is-sepsis.html. Accessed October 4, 2022.

Chakraborty RK, Burns B. Systemic Inflammatory Response Syndrome. 2021 Jul 28. In: StatPearls [Internet]. Treasure Island (FL): StatPearls Publishing; 2022 Jan. PMID: 31613449.

Churpek MM, Snyder A, Han X, et al. Quick sepsis-related organ failure assessment, systemic inflammatory response syndrome, and early warning scores for detecting clinical deterioration in infected patients outside the intensive care unit. *Am J Respir Crit Care Med.* 2017;195(7):906-911. doi: 10.1164/rccm.201604-0854OC

Evans L, Rhodes A, Alhazzani W, et al. Surviving sepsis campaign: international guidelines for management of sepsis and septic shock 2021. *Crit Care Med.* 2021;49(11):e1063. doi: 10.1097/CCM.0000000000005337

Davidson J, Aslakson R, Long A, et al. Guidelines for family-centered care in the neonatal, pediatric, and adult ICU. *Crit Care Med.* 2017;45(1):103-128. doi: 10.1097/CCM.0000000000002169

Guerin C, Reigneier J, Richard JC, et al. Prone positioning in severe acute respiratory distress syndrome. *N Eng J Med.* 2013;368(23):2159-2168. doi: 10.1056/NEJMoa1214103.

Kazor A, Ronco C, McCullough, PlA. SARS-CoV-2 (COVID-19) and intravascular volume management strategies in the critically ill. *Proc (Bayl Univ Med Cent).* 2020;0(0):1-6. doi: 10.1080/08998280.2020.1754700

Kleinpell R, Schorr CA, Bulk RA. The new sepsis definitions: implications for critical care practitioners. *AMJ Crit Care.* 2016;25:457-464. http://ajcc.aacnjournals.org/content/25/5/457.full

McClave SA, Taylor BE, Martindale RG, et al. Guidelines for the provision and assessment of nutrition support therapy in the adult critically ill patient: Society of Critical Care Medicine (SCCM) and American Society for Parental and Enteral Nutrition (A.S.P.E.N.). *JPEN J Parenter Enteral Nutr.* 2016;40(2):159-211. http://journals.sagepub.com/doi/full/10.1177/0148607115621863.

Rubinsky M, Clark A. Early enteral nutrition in critically ill patients. *Dimens Crit Care Nurs.* 2012;31:267-274.

Shang Y, Pan C, Yang X, et al. Management of critically ill patients with COVID-19 in ICU: statement from front-line intensive care experts in China. *ANN Intensive Care.* 2020;10(73). doi: 10.1186/s13613-020-00689-1

Singer M, Deutschman CS, Seymour CW, et al. The Third International Consensus Definitions for Sepsis and Septic Shock (Sepsis-3). *JAMA.* 2016;315(8):801-810. doi:10.1001/jama.2016.0287.

Surviving Sepsis Campaign. *Hour-1 bundle: Initial Resuscitation for Sepsis and Septic Shock,* 2019. https://www.sccm.org/getattachment/SurvivingSepsisCampaign/Guidelines/Adult-Patients/Surviving-Sepsis-Campaign-Hour-1-Bundle.pdf?lang=en-US

Overdoses

Centers for Disease Control and Prevention. Alcohol Related Disease Impact (ARDI) application. 2022. www.cdc.gov/ARDI

Centers for Disease Control and Prevention. Prescribing Practices. 2019. https://www.cdc.gov/drugoverdose/deaths/prescription/practices.html

Centers for Disease Control and Prevention. U.S. overdose deaths in 2021 increased half as much as in 2020—but are still up

15%. 2022. https://www.cdc.gov/nchs/pressroom/nchs_press_releases/2022/202205.htm

Centers for Disease Control and Prevention. Now is the time to stop overdose deaths. Facts on fentanyl. 2022. https://www.cdc.gov/drugoverdose/featured-topics/overdose-prevention-campaigns.html

Cassidy EM, O'Sullivan I, Bradshaw P, Islam T, Onovo C. Symptom-triggered benzodiazepine therapy for alcohol withdrawal syndrome in the emergency department: a comparison with the standard fixed dose benzodiazepine regimen. *Emerg Med J.* 2011;29(10):802-804.

Centers for Disease Control National Center for Disease Statistics. Drug overdose deaths in the United States, 2001–2021, 2022. https://www.cdc.gov/nchs/data/databriefs/db457.pdf

Caputo F, Agabio R, Vignoli T, et al. Diagnosis and treatment of acute alcohol intoxication and alcohol withdrawal syndrome: position paper of the Italian Society of Alcohol. 2018. doi: 10.1007/s11739-018-1933-8.

Corfee FA. Alcohol withdrawal in the critical care unit. *Aust Crit Care.* 2011;24(2):110-116.

Cowan E, Su, MK. Ethanol intoxication in adults. 2021. Uptodate.com/contents/ethanol-intoxication-in-adults.

Dixon DW. Opioid abuse. *Medscape.* 2017. http://emedicine.medscape.com/article/287790-overview. Updated July 13, 2017. Accessed July 23, 2017.

Gallagher N, Edwards FJ. The diagnosis and management of toxic alcohol poisoning in the emergency department: a review article. *Adv J Emerg Med.* 2019;3(3):e28. doi: 10.22114/ajem.v0i0.153

Hoffman RS, Weinhouse GL. Management of moderate and severe alcohol withdrawal syndromes. UpToDate. 2021. Retrieved January 1, 2022 from uptodate.com/contents/management-of-moderate-and-severe-alcohol-withdrawal-syndromes.

Littlefield AJ, Heavner MS, Eng CC et al. Correlation between MMINDS and CIWA-AR scoring tools in patients with alcohol withdrawal syndrome. *Am J Crit Care.* 2018;27(4). doi: 10.4037/ajcc2018547

LaHood AJ, Kok SJ. Ethanol toxicity. https://www.ncbi.nlm.nih.gov/books/NBK557381/. Updated March 18, 2022. Accessed October 4, 2022.

Long B, Lentz S, Gottlieb M. Alcoholic ketoacidosis: etiologies, evaluation, and management. *J Emerg Med.* 2021;61(6):658-665. doi: 10.1016/j.jemermed.2021.09.007

Marraffa JM, Cohen V, Howland MA. Antidotes for toxicological emergencies: a practical review. *Am J Health Syst Pharm.* 2012;69(3):199-212.

NIH. Alcohol use in the United States. 2021. www.niaaa.nih.gov/publications/brochures-and-fact-sheets/alcohol-facts-and-statistics. Accessed May 23,2023.

O'Malley GF, O'Malley R. Alcohol toxicity and withdrawal. 2020. www.merckmanuals.com/professional/special-subjects/recreational-drugs-and-intoxicants/alcohol-toxicity-and-withdrawal

Rudd RA, Seth P, David F, Scholl L. Increases in drug and opioid-involved overdose deaths—United States, 2010–2015. *MMWR Morb Mortal Wkly Rep.* ePub: December 16, 2016. https://www.cdc.gov/mmwr/volumes/65/wr/mm655051e1.htm

Schutt RC, Ronco C, Rosner MH. The role of therapeutic plasma exchange in poisonings and intoxications. *Semin Dial.* 2012;25(2):201-206.

Stewart S, Swain S. Assessment and management of alcohol dependence and withdrawal in the acute hospital: concise guidance. *Clin Med.* 2012;12(3):266-271.

Taheri A, Dahri K, Chan P, et al. Evaluation of a symptom-triggered protocol approach to the management of alcohol withdrawal syndrome in older adults. *J Am Geriatr Soc.* 2014; 62(8):1551-1555.

Pressure Injuries

American Association of Critical-Care Nurses. 2022. https://www.aacn.org/education/webinar-series/wb0068/vasopressors-and-pressure-injury-risk-in-the-critically-ill

Agency for Healthcare Research and Quality. Preventing pressure ulcers in hospitals. https://www.ahrq.gov/professionals/systems/hospital/pressureulcertoolkit/putool3a.html. Accessed July 23, 2017.

Borojeny LA, Albatineh AN, Dehkordi AH, Gheshlagh RG. The incidence of pressure ulcers and its associations in different wards of the hospital: a systematic review and meta-analysis. *Int J Prev Med.* 2020;11:171. doi: 10.4103/ijpvm.IJPVM_182_19

Cox J. Predictors of pressure ulcers in adult critical care patients. *Am J Crit Care.* 2011;20:364-375.

Delmore BA, Ayello EA. Pressure injuries caused by medical devices and other objects: a clinical update. *Am J. Nurs.* 2017;117(12):36-25. https://nursing.ceconnection.com/ovidfiles/00000446-201712000-00026.pdf

National Pressure Injury Advisory Panel. NPIAP pressure injury stages. https://www.npuap.org/resources/educational-and-clinical-resources/npuap-pressure-injury-stages/

National Pressure Injury Advisory Panel Prevention and treatment of pressure ulcers/injuries: clinical practice guideline. 2019. https://guidelinesales.com/page/NPIAP

Mondragon N, Zito PM. Pressure Injury. [Updated 2021 Dec 9]. In: StatPearls [Internet]. Treasure Island (FL): StatPearls Publishing; 2022 Jan. https://www.ncbi.nlm.nih.gov/books/NBK557868/

Medicare. Hospital-acquired conditions. 2021. https://www.cms.gov/Medicare/Medicare-Fee-for-Service-Payment/HospitalAcqCond/Hospital-Acquired_Conditions

Team V, Team L, Jones A, Teede H, Weller CD. Pressure injury prevention in COVID-19 patients with acute respiratory distress syndrome. *Front Med.* 2020;7:558696. doi: 10.3389/fmed.2020.558696

Healthcare-Associated Infections

AACN Clinical Scene Investigator Academy. "Clean Cath Club." https://www.aacn.org/clinical-resources/csi-projects/clean-cath-club

AACN Practice Alert. Prevention of CAUTI in Adults. 2016. https://www.aacn.org/clinical-resources/practice-alerts/prevention-of-cauti-in-adults

Buetti N, Marschall J, Drees M, et al. Strategies to prevent central line-associated bloodstream infections in acute-care hospitals: 2022 update. *Infect Control Hosp Epidemiol.* 2022;43(5):553-569. doi: 10.1017/ice.2022.87

Centers for Disease Control and Prevention. Catheter-associated urinary tract infection. http://www.cdc.gov/HAI/ca_uti/uti.html

Centers for Disease Control and Prevention. Central line-associated bloodstream infection (CLABSI). https://www.cdc.gov/hai/bsi/bsi.html

Centers for Disease Control and Prevention. HAI data and statistics. https://www.cdc.gov/hai/data/index.html

Centers for Disease Control and Prevention. Healthcare infection control practices advisory committee. 2022. https://www.cdc.gov/hicpac/index.html

Cristina ML, Spagnolo AM, Giribone L, Demartini A, Sartini M. Epidemiology and prevention of healthcare-associated infections in geriatric patients: a narrative review. *Int J Environ Res Public Health.* 2021;18(10):5333. doi:10.3390/ijerph18105333

Infectious Diseases Society of America & Society for Healthcare Epidemiology of America. Healthcare-associated infections a compendium of prevention recommendations. 2022. https://www.guidelinecentral.com/guideline/12717/pocket-guide/13086/

Kleinpell RM, Munro CL, Giuliano KK. Targeting health care acquired infections: evidence-based strategies. *In: Patient Safety and Quality: An Evidence-Based Handbook for Nurses.* Agency for Healthcare Research and Quality. 2008. http://www.ncbi.nlm.nih.gov/books/NBK2632/

Richards B, Sebastian B, Sullivan H, et al. Decreasing catheter-associated urinary tract infections in the neurological intensive care unit: one unit's success. *Crit Care Nurse.* 2017;37(3):42-48. doi: 10.4037/ccn2017742.

Selected Infectious Diseases

Center for Disease Control and Prevention. Healthcare-associated infections: clinicians carbopenum resistant *Enterobacteriaceae* (CRE). 2019. https://www.cdc.gov/hai/organisms/cre/cre-clinicians.html

Centers for Disease Control and Prevention. 2020 National and State Healthcare-associated infections progress report. 2021. https://www.cdc.gov/hai/data/portal/progress-report.html updated 10/26/2021. Accessed October 4, 2022.

Centers for Disease Control and Prevention. *Clostridium difficile.* 2021. https://www.cdc.gov/cdiff/clinicians/index.html

Centers for Disease Control and Prevention. Intravascular catheter-related infection (BSI). 2015. https://www.cdc.gov/infectioncontrol/guidelines/BSI/index.html#rec2. Accessed October 4, 2022.

Centers for Disease Control and Prevention. *Methicillin-resistant Staphylococcus aureus.* 2020. https://www.cdc.gov/mrsa/healthcare/inpatient.html

Centers for Disease Control and Prevention. Multidrug-resistant organism management. 2015. https://www.cdc.gov/infection-control/guidelines/mdro/indcx.html

Centers for Disease Control and Prevention. VRE in healthcare settings. 2019. https://www.cdc.gov/hai/organisms/vre/vre.html

NEUROLOGIC SYSTEM

John C. Bazil and DaiWai Olson

SPECIAL ASSESSMENT TECHNIQUES, DIAGNOSTIC TESTS, AND MONITORING SYSTEMS

Although there is no single method of performing a neurological assessment, a systematic, orderly approach offers the best results. Knowledge of neurologic disease processes and neuroanatomy allows the critical care nurse to tailor the assessment to individual patients. Obtaining a comprehensive past medical history that includes any preexisting neurologic conditions in addition to a thorough history of the present illness or injury is essential. The time from injury to symptom onset, and identification of the mechanism of injury have important implications for diagnostic testing and treatment. The administration of any medications that may potentially alter the neurologic examination, especially sedatives and analgesics, should also be noted.

Serial assessments allow for detection of subtle changes in neurologic status. Detecting secondary brain injury (SBI) and early neurologic deterioration (END) permits rapid intervention and improves patient outcomes. The elements of a comprehensive neurologic assessment in the critical care unit can be broken down into the following components: level of consciousness (LOC), mental status, motor examination, sensory examination, and cranial nerve examination. A baseline examination should be established and subsequent assessments are compared against the baseline.

Level of Consciousness

A change in the LOC is often the first sign of END. There are multiple components to LOC including arousal, awareness, and responsiveness. *Arousal* refers to the state of wakefulness; *awareness* reflects the content and quality of interactions with the environment; and *responsiveness* refers to the ability to react to changes in the environment. Arousal reflects function of the reticular activating system (RAS) and brain stem; awareness indicates functioning of the cerebral cortex. LOC is assessed on all patients unless they are pharmacologically sedated and paralyzed. A change in LOC is the most important indicator of neurologic decline. Any change in the LOC requires further assessment or action from the healthcare team.

Observation of the patient's behavior, appearance, and ability to communicate is the first step in assessing LOC. If the patient responds meaningfully to the examiner without the need for stimulation, then the patient is described as *alert*. A patient may exhibit responsiveness

TABLE 12-1. COMPARISON OF GLASGOW COMA SCALE (GCS) AND FULL OUTLINE OF UNRESPONSIVENESS (FOUR) SCORES

Category	Score	GCS	FOUR Score
Eye response	4	Spontaneous eye opening	Eyelids open or opened, tracking, or blinking to command
	3	Eye opening to verbal stimuli	Eyelids open but not tracking
	2	Eye opening to painful stimuli	Eyelids closed but open to loud voice
	1	No eye opening	Eyelids closed but open to pain
	0		Eyelids remain closed with pain
Verbal	5	Oriented	
	4	Confused	
	3	Inappropriate words	
	2	Incomprehensible sounds	
	1	None	
Motor	6	Obeys commands	
	5	Localizes to pain	
	4	Withdraws to pain	Thumbs up, fist, or peace sign
	3	Flexion to pain	Localizing to pain
	2	Extension to pain	Flexion to pain
	1	No response	Extension to pain
	0		No response to pain or generalized myoclonus status
Brain stem reflexes	4		Pupil and corneal reflexes present
	3		One pupil wide and fixed
	2		Pupil or corneal reflexes absent
	1		Pupil and corneal reflexes absent
	0		Absent pupil, corneal, and cough reflexes
Respiration	4		Not intubated, regular breathing pattern
	3		Not intubated, Cheyne-Stokes breathing pattern
	2		Not intubated, irregular breathing
	1		Breaths above ventilator rate
	0		Breaths at ventilator rate or apnea

to auditory or physical stimuli. If stimulation is required, auditory stimuli are used first. If the patient does not rouse to auditory stimuli, tactile stimuli such as a gentle touch or shake are used, followed by painful stimuli if necessary to elicit a response. Accepted methods of central painful stimulus include squeezing the trapezius or another large muscle group. Care is taken to avoid tissue trauma. Supraorbital pressure is also an acceptable pain stimulus, but is not used if there is any suspicion of facial fracture. Using a sternal rub may result in a motor response that is difficult to interpret and often causes bruising. Nail bed pressure is a commonly used peripheral pain stimulus. Response to central stimulus is more indicative of cerebral function than peripheral stimulus. Certain responses to peripheral pain, such as the triple flexion response (stereotypical flexion of the ankle, knee, and hip), can result from a spinal reflex arc and thus may remain present even following death by neurologic criteria (brain death).

Glasgow Coma Scale (GCS) and the Full Outline of Unresponsiveness (FOUR) Score

Two scales used to stratify level neurologic function are the Glasgow Coma Scale and the Full Outline of Unresponsiveness Score. Table 12-1 lists the criteria and scoring for GCS and FOUR scales.

GCS

The GCS is often used to monitor neurologic status in critically ill patients because it provides a standardized approach to assessing and documenting LOC. Response is determined in three categories: eye opening, motor response, and verbal response. The best response in each category is scored, and the results are added to give a total GCS. Scores range from 3 to 15, with 15 indicating a patient that is alert, fully oriented, and following commands.

The eye-opening score reflects the amount of stimulation that must be applied for the patient to open his or her eyes. Spontaneous eye opening is the best response, followed by eye opening to verbal stimulation, then eye opening to painful stimulation. Scoring of the eye-opening section of the scale can be complicated by orbital trauma and swelling, and this is documented accordingly.

The verbal section of the GCS assesses a patient's ability to speak coherently and with appropriate content. Orientation to person, place, time, and situation is assessed. As mental status declines, orientation to time is lost first, followed by orientation to place. Orientation to person is seldom lost prior to loss of consciousness. Patients with an endotracheal tube or tracheostomy are sometimes assigned a verbal score of *T* and the total GCS is denoted as the sum of the eye opening and motor scores followed by *T*. Alternatively, the examiner assigns a verbal score based on estimation of the patient's abilities, often determined by noting the patient's response when presented with multiple choices.

The motor portion of the GCS is the most difficult to assess. Response in each extremity is tested, but only the best motor response is used in calculating a total score. The patient is first asked to follow a command such as "Hold up your thumb" or "Wiggle your toes." A patient who does not follow commands in his or her extremities may be locked in and should be asked to look up and down. In certain neurologic disorders (such as basilar artery stroke or high cervical spinal cord injury [SCI]), patients may be unable to follow commands with their extremities but still be awake and aware; assessing the ability to look up and down helps identify these individuals.

If the patient does not follow commands, the next step is to assess the response to pain stimuli in all four extremities. Upper extremity response to pain is described as localization, withdrawal, decorticate (flexor) posturing, or decerebrate (extensor) posturing. An attempt by the patient to push the stimulus away is clearly localization, but the response is not always easily apparent. Reaching across the midline of the body to a stimulus (eg, if the right arm comes up to the left shoulder when a left trapezius squeeze is applied) is scored as localization.

An easy way to remember decorticate and decerebrate posturing is that decorticate is "into the core," or flexion, and decerebrate is away from the body, or extension (Figure 12-1). Decorticate posturing signifies damage in the cerebral hemispheres or thalamus. Decerebrate posturing indicates damage to the midbrain or pons. The presence of posturing or a change from decorticate to decerebrate posturing requires immediate notification of the provider for further evaluation. Motor response to pain in the lower extremities is usually graded as withdrawal or triple flexion. In triple flexion, pain stimulus results in stereotypical flexion of the ankle, knee, and hip. This response can be differentiated from withdrawal by applying the pain stimulus to a different area of the lower extremity (eg, the medial aspect of the calf). If the response is withdrawal, the patient pulls away from the stimulus. If the response is triple flexion, the response is still stereotypical flexion at the ankle, knee, and hip.

Although the GCS is frequently used to monitor patients in the ICU, the information it provides is limited. In addition, the GCS has only been validated in patients with traumatic brain injury (TBI). Additional assessments are necessary to gain an accurate picture of neurologic functioning; these assessments are based on the type of disease process or injury and the part of the central nervous system (CNS) affected.

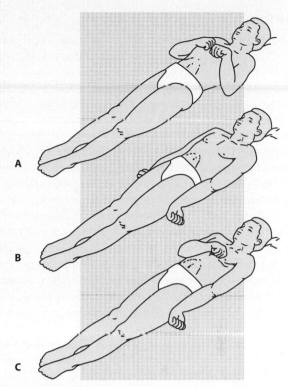

Figure 12-1. Abnormal motor responses. **(A)** Decorticate posturing. **(B)** Decerebrate posturing. **(C)** Decorticate posturing on right side and decerebrate posturing on left side of body. (*Reproduced with permission from Urden LD, Stacy KM, Lough ME*. Thelan's Critical Care Nursing: Diagnosis and Management. *St Louis, MO: Mosby; 2002.*)

FOUR Score

The FOUR score is another validated tool for the assessment of neurological patients. The FOUR score assigns a value of 0 through 4 in each of four categories: eye response, motor response, brain stem reflexes, and respiration. The scores in each category are added together to give a total score of 0 to 16. Lower scores are associated with more severe injury. Table 12-1 provides an overview of the FOUR score; critical care nurses who utilize this tool should seek additional information to assess verbal cognition. Because of the inclusion of brain stem reflexes and respiratory pattern, the FOUR score allows the clinician to identify changes in patients, such as those who are comatose with very limited responses.

The highest score given for eye response (4) indicates that the patient is able to track visual movements and either look up and down, open and close their eyes, or both. The patient who is unable to track visual movement is given a score of 3. Lower scores are based on eye opening to command (2), to pain (1), or no eye opening (0).

The highest score for motor response (4) is given to the patient who can either make a fist, make a peace sign, or give a "thumbs up" response to verbal command. Lower scores are given based on response to pain stimulus. A score of 3 is given if the patient touches the examiner's hand following pain stimulus. The patient who has flexion in response to pain is given a score of 2, versus extensor posturing (1), or no motor response to pain (0).

Mental Status

Although formal assessments of mental status exist, many critical care patients are unable to complete these assessments because of limited ability to communicate or decreased LOC. Orientation is the component of mental status most often evaluated in the critical care unit. Other components of mental status assessment such as attention/concentration, affect, memory, and reasoning are typically assessed informally by observing the patient throughout daily care. Short-term memory may be evaluated by giving the patient a list of three items and asking him or her to recall them later. However, deficits may also be noted in informal interactions as well.

Difficulty with speech production is *dysarthria* (weakness or lack of coordination of muscles of speech). A patient with dysarthria has slurred speech and is difficult to understand, but the content of the speech is appropriate. Dysarthria represents weakness or loss of coordination of the muscles of speech versus a problem with mental status. However, dysarthria often becomes apparent during assessment of mental status and thus is included here.

Difficulty with language is *aphasia*. The two major categories of aphasia are motor (Broca's aphasia and transcortical motor aphasia) and sensory (Wernicke's aphasia and transcortical sensory aphasia). Subtypes of aphasia include conduction (ie, understand but have poor speech repetition) and anomic (ie, cannot express the words they want to say). As shown in Table 12-2, testing for aphasia includes four elements: naming (can the patient name common items?); fluency (is the patient able to produce more than one or two words or sounds?); comprehension (can the patient understand the examiner?); and repetition (can the patient repeat what the examiner states?).

Delirium and Dementia

Delirium is an acute alteration in mental status. Delirium is usually rapid in onset, reversible, and is associated with poor clinical outcomes and increased hospitalization costs. Delirium is characterized by acute changes or fluctuations in mental status, inattention, and cognitive changes or perceptual disturbances. Delirium is described as hyperactive (restlessness, agitation) or hypoactive (flat affect, apathy, lethargy, and decreased responsiveness to the environment). Some patients present with a combination of hyperactive and hypoactive delirium. As described in Chapter 2, delirium is a complication of critical illness and is easier to prevent than treat.

Dementia is a progressive, irreversible loss of intellectual or cognitive abilities such as reasoning, math, or abstract thinking and develops more slowly than delirium. Delirium and dementia are not mutually exclusive; a patient with mild to moderate dementia may experience delirium in the unfamiliar environment of the intensive care unit. The Confusion Assessment Method for the intensive care unit is a valid tool to identify delirium in critically ill patients with or without mechanical ventilation but is limited when used in patients with neurologic injury. The Intensive Care Delirium Screening Checklist is also validated to assess for delirium but, similarly, can be complicated in patients with neurological diagnoses because the patient's responses may be due to the underlying diagnosis or sedation. Sedation may be stopped briefly to accurately evaluate the patient's mental state, or titrated to a lower sedation score, if safe to do so and ongoing mental status assessment is needed. Sedation scales are discussed in Chapter 6, Pain, Sedation, and Neuromuscular Blockade Management.

Contributing factors to the development of delirium include systemic illness (infection, fever, or metabolic dysfunction), inadequate pain control, electrolyte abnormalities, the administration of medications including benzodiazepines or opioids, sleep deprivation, immobility, and withdrawal from alcohol or other substances. Delirium is more common in older patients. The first step in treating delirium is to identify and remove reversible causes. The THINK mnemonic in which each letter stands for a potential cause of delirium can be helpful in this process (see Table 12-3).

Nursing strategies to prevent delirium and to decrease its effects include early mobility, reorientation, modulating environmental stimulation, providing appropriate cognitive activities, promoting normal sleep-wake cycles, ensuring that assistive devices such as hearing aids and glasses are available, treating pain, and facilitating family presence. Family members are educated about delirium and provided with guidance on how to interact with the patient (speak clearly and directly, provide frequent reorientation, and avoid multiple simultaneous conversations in the patient's room). Restraints are not used unless patient or staff safety is compromised, because they may add to the patient's confusion and risk for injury. In addition to environmental controls, medication changes, including avoiding

TABLE 12-2. APHASIA TESTING CATEGORIES

	Aphasia Type	Naming	Fluency	Comprehension	Repetition
Motor aphasia	Broca's	Unable	Unable	Intact	Unable
	transcortical motor	Unable	Unable	Intact	Intact
Sensory aphasia	Wernicke's	Unable	Intact	Unable	Unable
	transcortical sensory	Unable	Intact	Unable	Intact
Conduction aphasia		Unable	Intact	Intact	Unable
Anomic aphasia		Mixed	Intact	Intact	Intact

TABLE 12-3. THINK MNEMONIC FOR IDENTIFYING CAUSES OF DELIRIUM

Potential Causes of Delirium	
T stands for	Toxic situations (heart failure, kidney failure, liver failure, medications that cause delirium, shock, dehydration)
H stands for	Hypoxemia
I stands for	Infection and immobilization (altered mental state may be a sign of sepsis)
N stands for	Nonpharmacologic interventions (check with patient/family about hearing aids, glasses, consider sleep protocol, music, noise control)
K stands for	K^+ or other electrolyte abnormalities

Adapted with permission from Marta Render, MD – Deparmtent of Veteran Affairs Inpatient Evaluation Center (IPEC)

benzodiazepines and other agents linked to delirium are useful strategies. In patients with a primary neurological diagnosis, the use of sedative medications must be balanced with the need for ongoing neurological monitoring. See Chapter 6 for more information on the prevention and management of delirium, including application of the 2018 Clinical Practice Guidelines for the Prevention and Management of Pain, Agitation/Sedation, Delirium, Immobility, and Sleep Disruption.

Patients with organic brain disease, regardless of specific diagnosis, often exhibit challenging behaviors. Examples include agitation, emotional lability, and disinhibition. This can be very disconcerting to family members, especially when the patient has not exhibited these behaviors previously. Dealing with agitated, confused patients can also be frustrating and challenging for staff. Although medicating the patient can be necessary to keep the patient safe, many medications alter neurologic assessment, delay recovery, or even worsen symptoms. Environmental strategies such as decreasing noise and distractions may be very effective and are always used first. Encouraging family presence and supporting their role in responding to patient behaviors is also important. If medications are required, they are combined with environmental strategies and used at the lowest dose possible for the shortest time possible.

Motor Assessment

Motor assessment includes muscle size, tone, strength, and involuntary movements such as tics or tremors. Motor function is assessed in each extremity and evaluated for symmetry. In patients who are able to follow commands, the presence or absence of a pronator drift is an excellent indicator of upper extremity motor function. To assess for a pronator drift, instruct the patient to close their eyes and raise their arms with the palms facing the ceiling. A normal response is for the patient to maintain this position until told to stop. An abnormal response is when the arm drifts downward, or the palms rotate inward toward the body (pronation). Depending on the severity of weakness, the affected side may drift away from its initial position quickly or slowly, or the palm may simply begin to pronate (Figure 12-2).

Further assessment of upper extremity strength involves testing the deltoids, biceps, triceps, wrist flexion and extension, and intrinsic hand strength. Lower extremity testing includes the hamstrings, quadriceps, hip flexion and extension, knee flexion and extension, dorsiflexion, and plantar flexion. Strength is rated on a 5-point scale (Table 12-4). In patients who do not follow commands, motor assessment consists of first observing the patient for spontaneous movement. If necessary, a pain stimulus is applied and the patient's response is observed. The response is graded numerically as part of the GCS or FOUR score, but may also be described as purposeful, nonpurposeful, or no response.

In an awake and alert patient, complete motor assessment includes testing of coordination, which is an indicator of cerebellar function. Common testing mechanisms

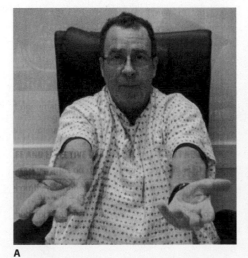 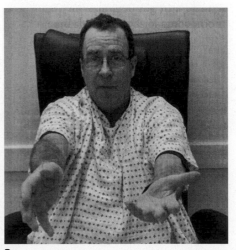

A   **B**

Figure 12-2. Assessment of pronator drift. Normal (panel **A**) and pronator drift (panel **B**). The patient is asked to hold his or her arms outstretched with the palms supinated and eyes closed. If weakness is present, the weak arm gradually pronates and drifts downward.

TABLE 12-4. EVALUATION OF MUSCLE STRENGTH

Grade	Definition
0	No movement
1	Muscle contraction only (palpated or visible)
2	Active movement within a single plane (gravity eliminated)
3	Active movement against gravity
4	Active movement against some resistance
5	Active movement against full resistance (normal strength)

applicable to the critical care environment include assessment of rapid alternating movements, finger-to-nose testing, and the heel slide test. To test rapid alternating movements, ask the patient to alternately supinate then pronate their hands as quickly as possible. In finger-to-nose testing, the patient is instructed to alternately touch their nose, then the examiner's finger. To assess the lower extremities, ask the patient to run the heel of their foot up and down the shin of the opposite leg. Patients with cerebellar dysfunction display decreased speed and accuracy on these tests.

Sensation

Sensory assessment is performed with the patient's eyes closed. Documentation of comprehensive sensory assessment is best accomplished using a dermatome chart (Figure 12-3). Areas of abnormal sensation can be marked and tracked over time. There are three basic sensory pathways: pain/temperature, position/vibration, and light touch. Light touch is the pathway most often assessed in the acute care setting, but it may be preserved even if lesions of the spinal cord exist because of overlapping innervation. Because most patients with intracranial lesions report altered sensation in an entire extremity or one side of the body, assessment of light touch is likely to identify these patients. Ask the patient to close their eyes, and lightly touch each extremity working distal to proximal. Trunk and facial sensation are also assessed.

When a more comprehensive assessment is indicated, testing for pain and position sense provides useful information. A cotton tip applicator with a wooden stem can be broken and used; the end with the cotton is dull and the broken end is sharp. Touch the patient's skin lightly in a random pattern and ask the patient to identify the sensation as sharp or dull.

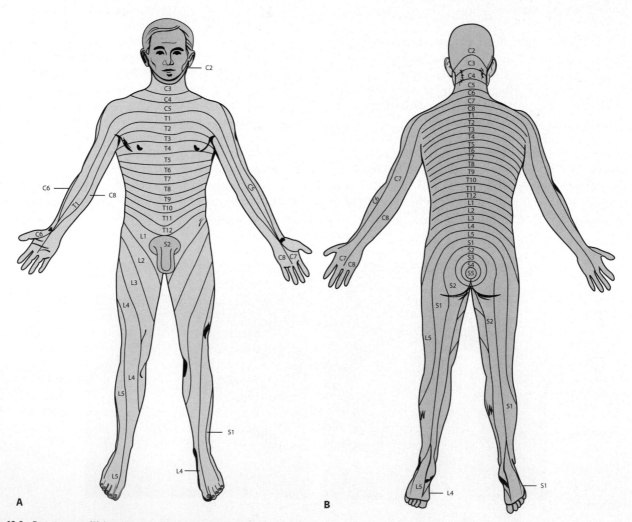

A   B

Figure 12-3. Dermatomes. **(A)** Anterior view. **(B)** Posterior view. (*Reproduced with permission from Urden LD, Stacy KM, Lough ME. Thelan's Critical Care Nursing: Diagnosis and Management. St Louis, MO: Mosby; 2002.*)

Two seconds should elapse between stimuli. To test position sense, or proprioception, move the patient's index finger or big toe up or down by grasping the digit laterally over the joints. Provide an example of both "up" and "down" positions prior to testing. Repeat these movements in a random order, with the patient's eyes closed, and ask the patient to identify whether the joint is up or down. Always return to the neutral position between movements and carefully grasp the digit to avoid giving the patient clues.

Cranial Nerve Assessment and Assessment of Brain Stem Function

Assessment of the cranial nerves provides an indication of the integrity of the nerves themselves and of brain-stem function. A screening examination based on pupillary response and protective reflexes (corneal, gag, cough) is conducted on all patients. Beyond that, the assessment is often customized to the individual based on pathology and the ability to participate in a more comprehensive examination. Patients with brain-stem, cerebellar, or pituitary lesions merit more extensive assessment because of the proximity of the cranial nerves to these structures. The assessments noted later are the most commonly performed tests of cranial nerve function in the critical care unit. Table 12-5 describes the primary function of the 12 cranial nerves.

Pupil Size and Light Reflex

Assessment of pupil size and reaction to light is performed in all patients and provides information about the function of cranial nerves II (optic) and III (oculomotor). Pupils are assessed for size (measured in millimeters), shape, and reaction to light.

TABLE 12-5. CRANIAL NERVE FUNCTION

Nerve	Function
I. Olfactory	Sense of smell
II. Optic	Visual fields, visual acuity
III. Oculomotor	Most extraocular eye movements, ability to elevate eyelid, muscular contraction of the iris in response to light
IV. Trochlear	Eye movement down and toward the nose
V. Trigeminal	Facial sensation, including cornea, nasal mucosa, and oral mucosa; muscles of chewing and mastication
VI. Abducens	Lateral eye movement
VII. Facial	Facial muscles, including eyelid closure; taste in anterior two-thirds of the tongue; secretion of saliva and tears
VIII. Vestibulocochlear	Hearing and equilibrium
IX. Glossopharyngeal	Gag reflex, muscles that control swallowing and phonation; taste in posterior third of tongue
X. Vagus	Salivary gland secretion; vagal control of heart, lungs, and gastrointestinal tract
XI. Accessory	Sternocleidomastoid and trapezius muscle strength
XII. Hypoglossal	Tongue movement

The pupillary light reflex (PLR) can be scored using a pupillometer or by observing the pupil change in reaction to light. Assessment of pupil size and reactivity may vary depending on the person performing the test. A pupillometer can help remove the subjectivity of the test. Pupillometers are noninvasive, handheld devices that provide an objective measurement of pupil size before and after a light stimulus, as well as the pupillary reactivity to light. The pupillometer is capable of providing automated measurement of one pupil at a time and therefore may not be an adequate substitute for evaluating the presence of anisocoria (unequal pupils). However, after completing paired measurements of both pupils within 30 seconds, the device can display a comparison of the pupillary size and reaction.

Both eyes are tested for direct and consensual response. To test direct pupillary response, shine a light into one eye and observe the response of the pupil in that eye. A normal response is brisk constriction followed by brisk dilation when the light is withdrawn. To test for consensual pupillary response, shine a light into one eye and observe the pupil of the other eye. It should constrict and dilate similarly. Assessing both direct and consensual response provides information about which cranial nerve (optic or oculomotor; and left or right) is affected.

Certain medications can affect pupil size and reactivity. For example, atropine can dilate the pupils and narcotics can cause them to become very constricted. Commonly used neuromuscular blockers do not affect pupillary reaction. Pupil changes are often seen late in the course of neurologic decline as increased intracranial pressure (ICP) leads to compression or stretching of cranial nerve III.

Corneal Reflex or Facial Movement/Sensation

The corneal reflex evaluates cranial nerves V (trigeminal) and VII (facial). This test is classically performed by assessing if the patient blinks when the examiner rapidly moves a finger toward the face ("blink to threat"). A drop of sterile saline applied to the eye can also be used as a stimulus; cotton wisps are avoided to reduce the risk of corneal abrasions. In alert patients, assessment of facial movement and sensation indicate deficits in cranial nerves V and VII. Movement is assessed by asking the patient to smile, puff out their cheeks with air, and raise their eyebrows. Assessment of facial sensation includes all three branches of cranial nerve V (the trigeminal nerve). Touching the forehead, then the cheek, and then the mandible can test the three distributions. Patients with cranial nerve VII dysfunction may be unable to close the eyelid on the affected side. Strategies to prevent corneal injury in such patients include the use of lubricating drops and ointments or taping the lid closed.

Gag and Cough Reflexes

The ability to swallow and the gag reflex are controlled by cranial nerves IX (glossopharyngeal) and X (vagus). To assess the gag reflex in a conscious patient, first explain the procedure and be sure the patient does not have a full stomach.

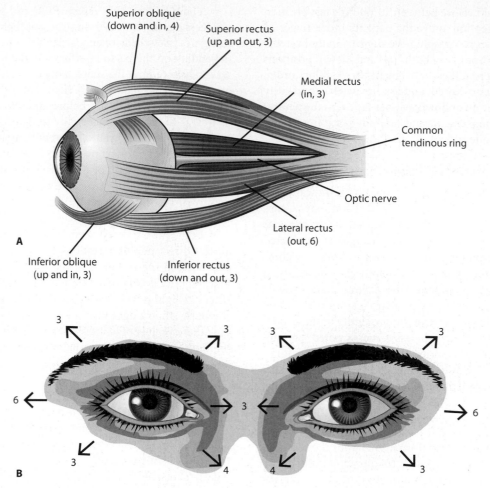

Figure 12-4. Extraocular eye movements. **(A)** Extraocular muscles. The eye movement controlled by the muscle is noted in parentheses, along with the associated cranial nerve supply. **(B)** The six cardinal directions of gaze and associated cranial nerves. (*Reproduced with permission from Urden LD, Stacy KM, Lough ME. Thelan's Critical Care Nursing: Diagnosis and Management. St Louis, MO: Mosby; 2002.*)

Ask the patient to open his or her mouth and protrude the tongue (this also provides partial assessment of cranial nerve XII, the hypoglossal nerve). Observe the palate for bilateral elevation when the patient says "ahhh." If the palate does not elevate symmetrically, lightly touch the back of the throat with a tongue blade and observe the response. Both the left and right sides should be tested. To assess the gag reflex in an unconscious patient, use a bite block to keep the patient's teeth separated, then stimulate the back of the throat with a suction catheter or tongue blade. Forward thrusting of the tongue and sometimes the head indicates an intact gag reflex. The cough reflex is also controlled by cranial nerves IX and X and can be assessed by noting spontaneous cough or cough in response to suctioning. Collectively, cranial nerves IX, X, XI, and XII make up the bulb of the brainstem (medulla oblongata), giving rise to the term "bulbar weakness" for patients with deficits associated with the lower cranial nerves.

Extraocular Eye Movements

Extraocular eye movements are controlled by muscles innervated by cranial nerves III, IV, and VI. To test extraocular movements, the patient is asked to follow an object (usually the examiner's finger) through six positions (Figure 12-4). A normal response consists of the eyes moving in the same direction, at the same speed, and in constant alignment (conjugate eye movement). Abnormal eye movements include nystagmus (a jerking, rhythmical movement of one or both of the eyes) or an extraocular palsy (eye movement in one or both eyes is inhibited in a certain direction). Mild nystagmus with extreme lateral gaze may be normal. Dysconjugate gaze, in which the eyes are not aligned, is an abnormal finding.

In unconscious patients, the oculocephalic and oculovestibular reflexes are used to test the portion of the brain stem that controls eye movement. Although these reflexes are not included in a typical critical care nursing assessment, it is useful to understand these reflexes and how they are assessed.

To test the oculocephalic reflex (doll's eyes), the patient's eyelids are held open by the examiner and the head is quickly rotated side to side. If the eyes deviate in the opposite direction from which the head is turned, then the pons is intact.

If the eyes do not move or movement is asymmetric, this is indicative of pontine dysfunction. The oculocephalic reflex is never evaluated in patients with suspected cervical spine injuries.

Evaluation of the oculovestibular reflex (cold calorics) is also commonly used to determine brain stem function in unconscious patients. After examination of the external canal for cerumen or perforation of the tympanic membrane, a bolus of cold water (iced water) is instilled into the ear. The amount of water used varies, but 30 to 50 mL is common. In a patient with intact brain stem function, conjugate deviation of the eyes toward the irrigated side occurs. Patients who have interrupted brain stem function either have no response or dysconjugate eye movement.

Vital Sign Alterations in Neurologic Dysfunction

Vital sign changes due to CNS dysfunction occur because of direct brain stem injury, decreased cerebral perfusion, or interruption of nerve pathways. Decreased perfusion causes ischemia and the body's response is to increase the blood pressure in an attempt to provide more oxygen and nutrients to the brain. Hypotension is rarely seen as an early response to primary brain injury. However, hypotension is observed in the terminal stages of brain stem dysfunction, and in patients with SCI due to loss of sympathetic tone. Abnormalities in heart rate and rhythm are common and can be a cause of neurologic decline because of clot formation or inadequate cardiac output, or may be a symptom of neurologic dysfunction (such as ST-segment abnormalities following subarachnoid hemorrhage [SAH]). Respiratory patterns vary widely. Some of the more common patterns are shown in Figure 12-5. Temperature is carefully monitored in patients with neurologic dysfunction, because hyperthermia (regardless of infectious or noninfectious etiology) causes increased cerebral metabolic demand. Hypothermia may result from injury to the brain stem, hypothalamus, or spinal cord.

Cushing response refers to a triad of vital sign changes seen late in the course of neurologic deterioration. The classic triad is marked by widened pulse pressure, bradycardia, and an irregular respiratory pattern. Cushing response is of minimal value in identifying early, significant changes in the patient's condition, but it is useful to be alert for components of Cushing response (eg, systolic hypertension or change in respiratory pattern).

Death by Neurologic Criteria

Death by neurologic criteria (brain death) indicates an irreversible loss of all functions of the entire brain, including the brain stem. The procedure that must be followed to declare a patient dead by neurologic criteria varies by state law and institutional policy. Conditions that must be ruled out as causes of coma prior to testing for death by neurologic criteria include the effects of CNS depressants, hypothermia, and severe metabolic or endocrine disturbance.

DIAGNOSTIC TESTING

Diagnostic testing includes imaging, laboratory testing, ultrasound, electroencephalography, direct measurement, and the physical examination. The three most common forms of imaging include computed tomography (CT), magnetic resonance imaging (MRI), and angiography.

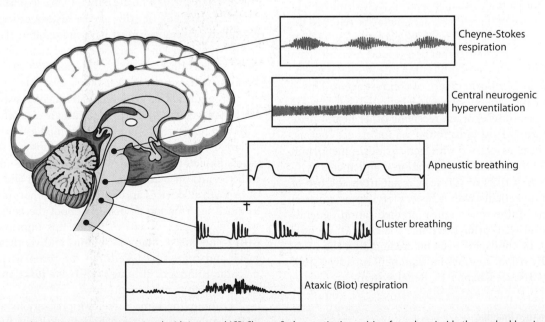

Figure 12-5. Abnormal respiratory patterns associated with increased ICP. Cheyne-Stokes respiration, arising from deep inside the cerebral hemispheres and basal ganglia; central neurogenic hyperventilation, from lower midbrain to middle pons; apneustic breathing, from middle to lower pons; cluster breathing, from upper medulla; and ataxic (Biot) respiration, from medulla. (*Reproduced with permission from Barker E.* Neuroscience Nursing: A Spectrum of Care. *St Louis, MO: Mosby; 2002.*)

Computed Tomography

Head (brain) and neck CT is a common diagnostic tool when neurologic dysfunction is suspected. CT scans are usually readily available and are noninvasive tests that identify most causes of acute neurologic deterioration, including bleeding, significant edema, and hydrocephalus. Acute bleeding and bony abnormalities such as fractures are better visualized with CT versus MRI. During a CT scan, an x-ray beam moves in a 360° arc around the patient as a detector measures penetration of the x-ray beam into tissue. Penetration of the x-ray beams vary based on tissue density. The computer translates the collected x-ray beams into a series of finely cut pictures showing bony structures, cerebrospinal fluid (CSF), and brain tissue in grayscale (quantified using Hounsfield units). Bone appears white because it is most dense. Lower-density components such as CSF (with a density similar to water) appear very dark gray; air appears entirely black. Brain tissue appears in varying shades of gray. The appearance of recent intracranial bleeding is white due to the relative density of blood; over time, the color darkens as the blood breaks down.

CT scanning can be performed with a contrast medium to allow for better visualization of lesions such as tumors, abscesses, or vascular abnormalities. Computed tomography angiography (CTA) uses scanning during intravenous (IV) contrast administration of a contrast medium to allow visualization of cerebral blood vessels. CTA is useful in the diagnosis of cerebral vascular anomalies, such as aneurysms, narrowed vessels, or an acute blockage causing an ischemic stroke. A three-dimensional reconstruction of the cerebrovasculature can be created from the images using a special computer program that subtracts other radiopaque structures (bone and tissue) from the images.

During CT, the patient is placed on a narrow table that is moved up into a donut-shaped gantry. Patient movement causes blurry images; therefore, sedation may be required for patients who are unable to lie still. In patients who receive contrast, assessment of renal function (blood urea nitrogen [BUN], creatinine, glomerular filtration rate [GFR]) is essential due to the nephrotoxic nature of contrast agent. This is especially true for patients who are dehydrated, have preexisting renal compromise, or are receiving other nephrotoxic agents. Because the administration of iodinated contrast medium has been associated with lactic acidosis, metformin should be held if contrast administration is anticipated.

The primary risks of CT scan result from the use of contrast agents. Patients with a history of allergic reaction to contrast or iodine may require premedication depending on the severity of prior reactions. If a contrast agent is administered, IV fluids are given before and after the study to decrease the risk of contrast-induced nephropathy (CIN). For more on CIN, see Chapter 15, Renal System.

Magnetic Resonance Imaging

MRI offers greater anatomic detail than CT scanning without using ionized radiation. The patient is placed in a strong magnetic field and controlled bursts of radio pulse waves are delivered, causing protons within atomic nuclei to resonate. The radiofrequency signals emitted by the resonating nuclei are then measured and used to construct digital images of the tissue. Cross-sectional images can be obtained in coronal, sagittal, and oblique planes. A contrast agent is sometimes administered, and to highlight areas where the blood-brain barrier (BBB) is disrupted. MRI scans are useful in diagnosing disorders of the brain stem, posterior fossa, and spinal cord, areas that are difficult to fully evaluate with CT. MRI also offers an advantage over CT in the identification of demyelinating disorders such as multiple sclerosis (MS) or other neurodegenerative diseases. Specific MRI sequences can be used to detect suspected lesions that cannot be seen on CT, such as early cerebral infarction and intramedullary tumors. Magnetic resonance angiography (MRA) uses a specialized computer program to highlight the cerebral vasculature. MRA is useful in the evaluation of suspected arteriovenous malformations (AVM), aneurysms, and cavernous angiomas. The time requirement for MRI scans is typically longer than that of CT scans, which is a disadvantage when seeking information to make urgent treatment decisions. In addition, access to the patient is significantly limited during an MRI.

All patients must be screened for the presence of implanted or embedded metal prior to MRI. Metallic objects inside the body may become dislodged or slip while the patient is in the large magnetic tube; this can cause patient injury. Most aneurysm clips are now made of nonferrous material and are safe for MRI; nevertheless, it is important to obtain additional information about any implanted devices prior to MRI, including when and where the device was placed. Orthopedic hardware may also be safe, depending on the part of the body being imaged and the length of time since the hardware was placed. Patients who are either unable to reliably complete the MRI screening or who have a history of impaled metal fragments or shrapnel must have radiographs taken prior to MRI. The MRI magnet can also damage internally magnetized units, such as cardiac pacemakers, causing them to malfunction. An MRI-safe pacemaker is now available.

Programmable VP shunts, frequently used for long-term management of hydrocephalus, are also affected by the MRI and may need to be reprogrammed following the procedure. Devices such as medication pumps and nerve/spinal cord stimulators may or may not be MRI safe and will need to be turned off before and reprogrammed after the procedure. With all devices and implants, it is important to obtain as much information as possible about the device type and when it was placed, and to report this information to the MRI technologist. Many IV pumps and ventilators contain metal and cannot be taken into the room where the MRI machine is located, although MRI-safe infusion pumps are now available at some institutions.

Of note, the same screening precautions apply to the staff member who accompanies the patient to MRI. Any card with a magnetic strip, such as a credit card or even an employee ID, will be damaged by the MRI magnet and should be removed prior to the staff entering the magnetic field radius. Patient education is important prior to scanning. Patients must be screened closely for any contraindications. In addition, all metal objects, such as jewelry, nonpermanent dentures, prostheses, hairpins, clothing with snaps or zippers, and electrocardiogram (ECG) electrodes with metal snaps must be removed. Transdermal medication patches may also need to be removed.

Additional preparation for an MRI includes advising the patient of the loud "booming" noise of the scanner. Inform the patient that the nurse or technician is able to view them while they are in the scanner and that they can talk over the intercom if they feel uncomfortable on the table or if any other concerns arise. Ensure the safety and comfort of the patients with safety belts and blankets for positioning. Patients who are claustrophobic may need anxiolytics or sedation. Open-sided MRI machines are available at some institutions and help decrease feelings of claustrophobia. Gadolinium-based contrast agents are sometimes administered in MRI and have been associated with nephrogenic systemic fibrosis (NSF) when given to patients with severe renal insufficiency; therefore, renal function must be assessed prior to administration. NSF causes fibrotic changes in the skin and other organs.

Cerebral (Catheter) Angiography

Although CTA and MRA are commonly used to assess the cerebrovasculature, catheter angiography remains the gold standard. Digital subtraction angiography is angiography of the cerebral vasculature and is similar to cardiac catheterization, wherein a computer program subtracts other radiopaque structures such as bone and brain tissue from the image in order to highlight only the vasculature. Angiography can be performed for both diagnostic purposes and therapeutic intervention. Blockages or abnormalities of the cerebral circulation can be visualized, aiding in the diagnosis of vascular malformations (such as aneurysms or AVMs) and arterial stenosis. Angioplasty (with or without stent placement) can be performed for narrowed cerebral vessels. Blood vessels can also be therapeutically embolized; this is sometimes done to decrease blood supply to a tumor prior to surgical resection or as treatment for an aneurysm.

During cerebral angiography, a catheter is placed in the femoral, brachial, or radial artery and threaded up into the carotid or vertebral arteries, and a radiopaque contrast material is injected. The flow of the contrast material is tracked using radiographic films and fluoroscopy. Patients are kept NPO for 6 hours prior to nonemergent angiography, and may need sedation during the procedure. The patient is under a sterile drape during the procedure so it is important to ensure that IV ports are easily accessible for medication administration. General anesthesia may be needed for uncooperative patients or during complex interventional procedures because the risk of vessel injury is increased if the patient moves their head during the procedure.

Potential complications include neurologic deficit due to injury to an intracranial vessel, allergic reaction to contrast, hematoma formation at the site of catheter insertion, vessel injury (dissection), retroperitoneal bleeding, and vessel spasm following injection of contrast. All patients undergoing cerebral angiography receive hydration because of the large amount of contrast agent used.

Following angiography, patients who undergo femoral artery catheterization are typically kept on bedrest with the head of bed flat to help prevent hematoma formation at the puncture site. In many cases, a special arterial closure device is used to promote clot formation and allow quicker mobility, typically after about 2 hours. Depending on the method of closure, the provider will place specific post-angiography orders that include how long the patient must remain flat. The arterial puncture site is monitored frequently for development of a hematoma, and the neurovascular status of the limb is also checked. Careful monitoring of vital signs and neurologic examination also aids in the detection of intra- or extracranial emboli or hemorrhage.

Transcranial Doppler Ultrasound

Transcranial Doppler (TCD) ultrasound studies allow the practitioner to measure the velocity of blood flow. TCD uses ultrasonic waves projected through the thinner parts of the skull bone and directed toward the major vessels. Structures within the skull are differentiated based on how much of the wave is reflected back to the probe. A Doppler effect is created when the probe detects moving structures, like red blood cells in a blood vessel. The velocity of blood flow can thus be calculated. TCDs are noninvasive and can be done at the patient's bedside. TCDs are used at many institutions to aid in the detection of vasospasm after aneurysmal subarachnoid hemorrhage (aSAH).

Lumbar Puncture

Lumbar puncture (LP) can be performed for diagnostic or therapeutic purposes. Diagnostic indications for LP include measurement of CSF pressure as an estimation of ICP and sampling of CSF for analysis when CNS infection, inflammation, or SAH is suspected. Therapeutic indications for LP include drainage of CSF and the placement of tubes for medication administration or ongoing CSF drainage. LP is used for diagnostic or therapeutic purposes in a number of disease processes, including meningitis, MS, Guillain-Barré syndrome (GBS), hydrocephalus, and SAH. Increased ICP is a theoretical contraindication to LP because of the risk for downward herniation of brain tissue due to the pressure gradient created when CSF is removed from the lumbar space. When increased ICP is suspected, a CT scan is performed prior to proceeding with the LP. Other contraindications include coagulopathy or infection in the area of skin through which the needle will be introduced. Although recommendations about duration vary based on the specific medication, anticoagulant and antiplatelet medications are frequently stopped when LP is planned.

When performing an LP, the clinician locates the L3 to L4 or L4 to L5 intervertebral space and injects a local anesthetic, followed by a hollow needle with a stylet into the spinal subarachnoid space. The risk of SCI is minimal because the actual cord ends at L1 and only nerve roots continue below. Proper patient positioning is critical; patients may require sedation if they are unable to remain still. The LP may be performed with the patient sitting up and leaning forward, but a lateral decubitus position is used for most critically ill patients. The patient lies on his or her side with the neck flexed forward and knees pulled up toward the chest. This position widens the intervertebral space, allowing the needle to pass through more easily. The needle is inserted and the stylet is removed. Outflow of CSF confirms that the needle is in the spinal subarachnoid space. A manometer is attached to the needle and used to measure an opening pressure. Pressures greater than 20 cm (200 mm) H_2O are considered abnormal. The amount of CSF drained varies based on the indication for the procedure, with smaller volumes needed for laboratory analysis than for treatment of hydrocephalus. If the purpose of the procedure is administration of medications or placement of a lumbar drain, the medications will be given or the drain will be placed once needle placement is confirmed by CSF outflow.

Normal CSF is clear and colorless. Infection and blood can change the appearance of CSF. In infection, CSF may be cloudy because of white blood cells and bacteria. Blood causes the CSF to be light yellow (xanthochromia), pink, red, or brown. Although some blood may be present if a small vessel was traumatized during needle insertion, this blood clears as more CSF is drained. Blood due to CNS hemorrhage does not clear. Common tests performed on CSF include analysis of cell counts with differential, glucose, protein, lactate, Gram stain, and culture with sensitivities. Special assays may be requested to look for specific inflammatory or demyelinating disease processes. Once the needle is removed, a small self-adhesive bandage is placed over the insertion site.

Post-procedure care varies with physician preference, hospital protocol, and whether or not the patient complains of headache, but it always includes monitoring the insertion site for bleeding, drainage, or hematoma development. Patients may complain of headache (due to loss of CSF), local pain at the insertion site, or pain radiating to the thigh (if a nerve root was hit during the procedure). Flat positioning and increased fluid intake are sometimes recommended after LP but have not been shown to reduce the incidence of post-LP headache. If headache does occur, these strategies are used in combination with analgesic administration. If the headache persists, an autologous blood patch may be used to stop continued CSF leakage.

Electroencephalography

The electroencephalogram (EEG) is a measurement of the brain's electrical activity. EEG is performed by attaching a number of electrodes to standard locations on the scalp. These electrodes are attached to a machine that amplifies and records the activity. EEG is useful in identifying seizure disorders, determining the anatomic origin of seizures, and evaluating causes of coma (structural vs. metabolic).

A routine EEG usually lasts 40 to 60 minutes with a portable machine for bedside use. The patient is instructed to lie still with their eyes closed. A mild sedative may be prescribed for restless or uncooperative patients, but the interpreter of the EEG must be aware of this because medications may cause changes in the recording. Documentation during the study is done by the technician and may include changes in blood pressure, changes in LOC, medications the patient is currently taking or has taken within 48 hours, patient movement or posturing, and any noxious stimuli introduced. It is best to plan nursing care around the time of the test so that no interventions are done during this examination. When the EEG is complete, the electrodes are removed and any medications that were held prior to the study are resumed.

In patients with symptoms that suggest seizure activity, such as intermittent twitching or fluctuating mental status, a prolonged EEG may be ordered in an attempt to correlate the symptoms with EEG findings. This type of EEG often lasts 24 hours or longer and requires the nurse to note any occurrences of the symptom or behavior thought to represent possible seizure activity. Most machines have a push-button system to allow the nurse to mark times that any seizure-like activity is noted; this allows for easier waveform-correlation by the interpreter.

In the setting of status epilepticus, continuous EEG monitoring may be used to guide treatment. Continuous monitoring is also used in the diagnosis and management of intractable or difficult-to-control seizures, usually in conjunction with video monitoring. Continuous EEG monitoring can also be helpful in identifying nonepileptic seizures. Rapid-EEG devices are becoming increasingly common and can be placed by nurses. Rapid-EEG is most commonly used when there is a high suspicion of new-onset seizure.

Electromyography/Nerve Conduction Studies

Electromyography (EMG) evaluates the electrical activity of skeletal muscle during activity and rest. Nerve conduction studies evaluate peripheral nerve function by measuring the transmission of electrical impulses after stimulation. Conditions in which these studies may aid diagnosis include critical care polyneuropathy or myopathy, myasthenia gravis (in which the neuromuscular junction is affected), and GBS. The patient may experience some pain related to insertion of the needle electrodes.

INTRACRANIAL PRESSURE: CONCEPTS AND MONITORING

The skull in adults is a partially closed, nondistensible compartment that contains three components: brain tissue/parenchyma (80%), blood (10%), and CSF (10%). The Monro-Kellie hypothesis suggests that to maintain a constant intracranial volume, an increase in any of the three components must be accompanied by a decrease in one or both of the other components. If this reciprocal decrease does not occur, ICP rises. Neuroscience researchers have questioned this hypothesis. The body is able to partially compensate for an increase in intracranial volume by displacement of intracranial venous blood, decreased production of CSF, arterial vasoconstriction, or displacement of CSF into the spinal subarachnoid space. ICP rises when these compensatory mechanisms fail.

Compliance refers to the change in volume needed to result in a given change in pressure and reflects the effectiveness of the compensatory mechanisms. With decreased compliance, a small increase in volume results in a large increase in ICP. Compliance is based on several factors, including the amount of volume increase and the time over which the increase occurs. Smaller increases in volume result in less increase in pressure. Increases in volume that occur over a long period of time are better tolerated than rapid increases because there is time for compensation to occur. Older adults typically have increased compliance because of cerebral atrophy. Increased ICP can result in cerebral hypoperfusion, ischemia, herniation, and eventually death.

Causes of Increased Intracranial Pressure

Increased ICP occurs as a result of cerebral edema, mass lesions, increased intracranial blood volume, or increased amounts of CSF. These factors often occur in combination. Pain, poor patient positioning (head and neck alignment), and nursing interventions such as suctioning have been associated with an increase in ICP.

Cerebral Blood Flow

The brain cannot store oxygen or glucose in significant quantities. Therefore, constant cerebral blood flow (CBF) is required to maintain cerebral metabolism. If CBF is insufficient, brain cells do not receive sufficient substrate to function and will eventually die. CBF is determined by blood pressure and cerebral vascular resistance.

Autoregulation refers to the ability of cerebral blood vessels to maintain consistent CBF by dilating or constricting in response to changes in blood pressure. Vasodilation occurs in response to decreased blood pressure; increased blood pressure results in vasoconstriction. In persons without neurologic disease, autoregulation allows consistent CBF when mean arterial pressure (MAP) is 60 to 160 mm Hg. In the injured brain, the autoregulatory response becomes less predictable. When autoregulation is impaired, CBF becomes dependent on systemic arterial pressure.

Cerebral vascular resistance can also be altered through chemoregulatory processes. An increase in the pressure of arterial carbon dioxide ($Paco_2$) produces a lower extracellular pH and causes dilation of cerebral vessels. Conversely, a decrease in $Paco_2$ raises pH and results in cerebral vasoconstriction. Vasodilation also results from Pao_2 levels less

than 50 or a buildup of metabolic by-products such as lactic acid. Other factors can decrease cerebral vascular resistance and thus alter CBF, including certain anesthetic agents (halothane, nitrous oxide), sodium nitroprusside, and some histamines.

Cerebral perfusion pressure (CPP) is a measurement of the pressure at which blood reaches the brain. CPP is an indirect reflection of CBF. It is calculated by subtracting ICP from MAP (CPP = MAP − ICP). Decreased CPP occurs as the result of an increase in ICP, a decrease in MAP, or both. A CPP of at least 50 to 70 mm Hg is necessary for adequate cerebral perfusion in adults. There is ongoing debate about where the arterial line transducer should be leveled when managing CPP. Some practitioners level the arterial line transducer at the foramen of Monro when calculating CPP to reflect the MAP in the cerebral vasculature versus systemic MAP, while others level the transducer at the phlebostatic axis. Follow institutional procedure to ensure consistency.

Cerebral Edema

Cerebral edema is an abnormal accumulation of water or fluid in the intra- or extracellular space, resulting in increased brain volume. Vasogenic edema results from increased capillary permeability of the vessel walls, which allows plasma and serum proteins such as albumin to leak through the BBB into the extracellular space (extravasation). Cytotoxic edema occurs when fluid collects inside the cells due to failure of cellular metabolism. This causes further breakdown of the cell membrane. Cytotoxic edema can lead to capillary damage, which then results in vasogenic edema. The time window for the formation of vasogenic edema differs than that of cytotoxic edema; vasogenic edema typically occurs days after the initial injury, whereas cytotoxic edema occurs much sooner within a period of hours.

Mass Lesion

Mass lesions (space-occupying lesions) in the brain parenchyma include brain tumors, hematomas, and abscesses. In addition to raising ICP, mass lesions can contribute to ischemia as they compress cerebral vessels.

Increased Blood Volume

Venous outflow obstruction can result from compression of the jugular veins (neck flexion, hyperextension, rotation) which then causes an increase in intracranial blood volume. Increased intrathoracic pressure or increased intra-abdominal pressure (Trendelenburg position, prone position, extreme hip flexion, Valsalva maneuver, coughing, high levels of positive end-expiratory pressure, endotracheal suctioning) also results in venous outflow obstruction. As discussed previously, cerebral vasodilation due to hypoxia, hypercapnia, increased metabolic demands, drug effects, or increased systemic blood pressure combined with autoregulatory failure cause an overall increase in intracranial blood volume.

Increased Cerebrospinal Fluid Volume

Approximately 500 mL of CSF is produced every day. CSF normally flows through the ventricular system into the subarachnoid space, where it is absorbed by the arachnoid granulations (Figure 12-6). Obstruction of CSF flow, decreased reabsorption of CSF, or increased production leads to increased intracranial CSF volume (hydrocephalus). Hydrocephalus is referred to as *communicating* or *noncommunicating* (also called obstructive). In meningitis or SAH, the arachnoid granulations may become clogged with cellular debris; this impairs CSF absorption and leads to communicating hydrocephalus. An example of noncommunicating hydrocephalus is obstruction of CSF flow due to a tumor or cyst in the third ventricle of the brain.

Clinical Presentation

Early signs of increased ICP include confusion, restlessness, lethargy, disorientation, headache, nausea and/or vomiting,

and visual abnormalities such as diplopia. Change in LOC is the most important indicator of elevated ICP. The patient may become unable to follow commands and develop motor deficits; abnormal posturing is an ominous sign. Changes in vital signs may occur. Increased systolic blood pressure is the body's attempt to maintain cerebral perfusion. As ICP worsens, alterations in heart rate or respiratory pattern may also emerge. Pupillary changes are usually late signs of increased ICP. Any of these signs and symptoms require immediate provider notification. Unless the cause of elevated ICP is known, a CT scan is ordered to evaluate for mass lesions (tumor, blood clot) or hydrocephalus.

Herniation

Prolonged elevation of ICP may result in cerebral herniation. Folds in the dura mater divide the intracranial cavity into several compartments. Herniation is the distortion

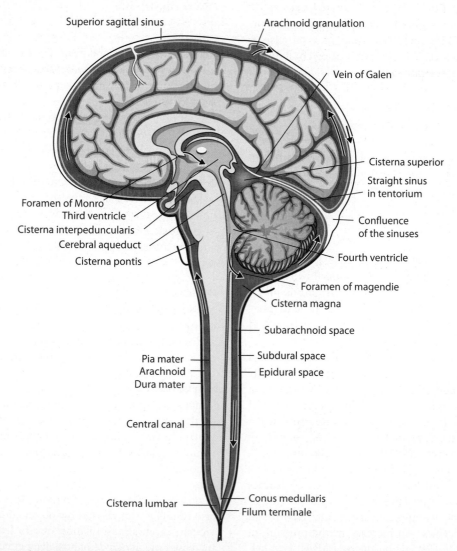

Figure 12-6. Flow of CSF/ventricular system. Drawing illustrates the ventricular system and other structures involved in CSF production, flow, and reabsorption. Arrows indicate the normal direction of flow of CSF. (*Reproduced with permission from Novack CR, Demarest RJ*. The Nervous System: Introduction and Review, *3rd ed. New York, NY: McGraw Hill; 1986.*)

and displacement of the brain from one compartment to another, which damages structures and decreases CBF through compression. Classic signs associated with herniation reflect pressure on the brain stem and surrounding structures. LOC deteriorates and the patient may demonstrate decorticate or decerebrate posturing. Compression or stretching of the oculomotor nerves (cranial nerve III) impairs pupil constriction and results in a large nonreactive pupil on one side. As compression continues, the other pupil also becomes large and nonreactive and vital sign changes (eg, Cushing response, altered respiratory pattern) occur. When any of these classic signs are noted, emergency action is needed to prevent brain death from occurring.

Invasive Monitoring of ICP

Intracranial pressure is most often measured via a catheter inserted into the ventricles, or a probe inserted into the brain parenchyma, but can also be measured in the subarachnoid space, epidural space, or subdural space (Figure 12-7). Use of an intraventricular catheter is considered the standard of care for ICP measurement. Several systems exist, but the basic setup includes a catheter, transducer (either external or integrated into the catheter), and collection device for CSF. The catheter is placed via a burr hole into the anterior horn of the lateral ventricle. The zero point of the drainage system is leveled at the external landmark of the foramen of Monro. If an external fluid-coupled transducer is in use, it will also be kept at the level of the foramen of Monro and zeroed to atmospheric pressure using manufacturer's specifications.

Different external landmarks for the foramen of Monro are reported in the literature (tragus, halfway between the outer canthus of the eye and the tragus, external auditory meatus); follow institutional protocols to maintain consistency among caregivers. The transducer senses the pressure exerted by the CSF in the ventricles and translates it into a waveform on the monitor. This system is referred to by several names, including *external ventricular drain (EVD), ventriculostomy,* and *intraventricular catheter.*

The advantage of using an intraventricular catheter for monitoring is that CSF can be drained, providing a treatment modality for increased ICP. The disadvantage is that ICP cannot accurately be measured when CSF drainage is occurring. Therefore, ICP measurements should never be recorded when the EVD is open to drain and the ICP waveform should be observed for at least 5 minutes with the EVD closed prior to recording an ICP value. CSF drainage is controlled by adjusting the height of the system relative to the foramen of Monro. The height of the fluid column in the drainage system creates hydrostatic pressure that opposes ICP. If the drainage system is raised, CSF drainage decreases; when the drainage system is lowered, CSF drainage increases. Rapid drainage of CSF can result in ventricular collapse, so CSF is drained in a controlled manner based on a predetermined ICP. This is accomplished by maintaining the drainage system at a specific height, such as 20 cm above the external landmark of the foramen of Monro, or by opening the system to allow CSF drainage only when the ICP exceeds a specified value. CSF drainage is monitored for amount and color. An occlusive dressing is maintained over the catheter insertion site.

Risks associated with intraventricular catheters include infection and hemorrhage caused by catheter placement. Sterile technique is essential when the catheter is placed and whenever the system is manipulated (eg, to sample CSF). Placement may be difficult in patients with decreased ventricular size due to shunting of CSF out of the cranium to compensate for increased ICP (eg, patients with diffuse cerebral edema due to TBI).

Intracranial pressure is also commonly monitored using a transducer inserted into the brain parenchyma. These monitors are easier to insert and have a lower rate of infection than intraventricular monitors. Leveling to the foramen of Monro is not required. Fiberoptic and strain-gauge transducers connect directly to an independent monitor, which provides an ICP reading. Other technology is available to monitor ICP, including some devices that allow re-zeroing after monitor insertion, but these are less commonly used in practice. Determining a target ICP depends on the individual and their injury. There is debate as to what constitutes a normal value, but a range of 0 to 15 mm Hg is often used as normal ICP in adults. In TBI patients, a target of <20-22 mm Hg is recommended.

ICP Waveforms

With continuous ICP monitoring, there are fluctuations in waveforms that correlate with specific physiologic events. Examination of these waveforms can be helpful in evaluating changes in the patient's condition.

The ICP pulse waveform is a continuous, real-time pressure display that corresponds to each heartbeat. The normal

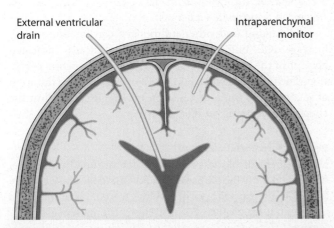

Figure 12-7. The two most common sites for ICP monitoring are via external ventricular drain (EVD) and intraparenchymal.

Arterial Pulse Waveform

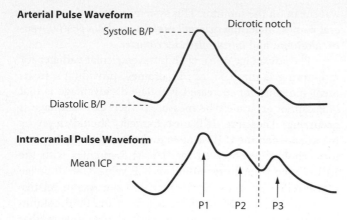

Figure 12-8. Arterial and intracranial ICP waveform (key components).

pulse wave has three or more defined peaks representing blood and CSF flow within the cranium:

- P1 (percussion wave) represents arterial blood flowing into the skull during systole
- P2 (tidal wave) reflects intracranial compliance
- P3 (dicrotic wave) represents the venous pulsation following systole

The pulse waveform at low and normal pressures is a descending saw-toothed pattern with a distinct P1 (Figure 12-8). As mean ICP rises, a progressive elevation of P2 occurs demonstrating decreased compliance. The result is the tidal (P2) wave appears more elevated than P1 (Figure 12-9).

Trend recordings compress continuous ICP recording data to reflect general trends in ICP over longer time periods (minutes to hours). Three distinct pressure waves have been identified (Figure 12-10). A waves (plateau waves) are sudden increases in pressure lasting 5 to 20 minutes. They begin from a baseline of an already elevated ICP (>20 mm Hg) and reflect cerebral ischemia. B waves are sharp, rhythmic oscillations of pressure (up to 50 mm Hg) occurring every 0.5 to 2 minutes. They are seen in relationship to fluctuations in the respiratory cycle, such as Cheyne-Stokes respirations. They are not clinically significant, but may progress to A waves. C waves are small rhythmic waves with pressures up to 20 mm Hg occurring 4 to 8 times per minute. They relate to normal changes in systemic arterial pressure, and their clinical significance is unknown.

Principles of Management of Increased ICP

Management focuses on early recognition of increased ICP. Interventions to reduce ICP are typically tiered. Mild or

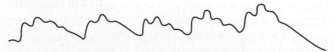

Figure 12-9. ICP waveform demonstrating decreased compliance.

nonacute ICP elevations may be treated less aggressively, whereas aggressive treatment is required if ICP rises suddenly or there is a significant change in the neurological assessment.

Monitoring Neurologic Status

Assess baseline neurologic signs, then reassess periodically and compare to previous findings. Include LOC, coma score, pupillary size and reaction to light, eye movement, and motor and sensory function. Assess vital signs and compare with previous findings to identify trends. In patients who are sedated for ICP management, the frequency of neurologic assessment may be decreased by provider in order to prevent ICP spikes related to stimulation. Assessment of pupillary size and reaction to light continue in sedated patients even if the patient is also receiving neuromuscular blocking (NMB) agents. Close monitoring of neurologic status facilitates the identification and treatment of complications, such as the development of an epidural or subdural hematoma. In these cases, surgical evacuation of the hematoma may be required. In cases of diffuse cerebral edema, a portion of the skull may be removed to increase compliance and allow the brain to swell outside the contained area of the skull. This procedure is referred to as a *craniectomy* or *decompressive hemicraniectomy*.

Adequate Oxygenation and Ventilation

Pao_2 and $Paco_2$ are maintained at normal levels, unless signs of herniation are present. For patients with impaired consciousness, intubation and mechanical ventilation may be required. Both hypercarbia and severe hypoxemia can result in cerebral vasodilation and increased ICP. Hyperventilation is not routinely used to decrease ICP because the resulting decrease in $Paco_2$ may lead to vasoconstriction, reduced cerebral perfusion, and ultimately cerebral ischemia. Controlled hyperventilation is sometimes still used in the setting of impending herniation to "buy time" for other measures to be implemented and take effect. Measures of cerebral oxygenation are useful in determining the impact of $Paco_2$ manipulation on cerebral metabolism (see Chapter 21, Advanced Neurologic Concepts).

Suctioning and other pulmonary care measures may increase ICP but are performed as clinically indicated because of the importance of oxygenation for cerebral perfusion. The patient is placed on 100% oxygen and the duration of suctioning is limited. Sedation may be used to blunt the effects of suctioning on ICP.

Blood Pressure and Fluid Management

Management of blood pressure is determined by the level of ICP and CPP. Blood pressure and CPP goals vary slightly based on disease process; in general, the goal is to maintain a CPP of at least 50 to 70 mm Hg. If the patient is hypotensive, infusions of non–glucose-containing fluids are preferred to ensure euvolemia. Vasopressors may be required to maintain CPP.

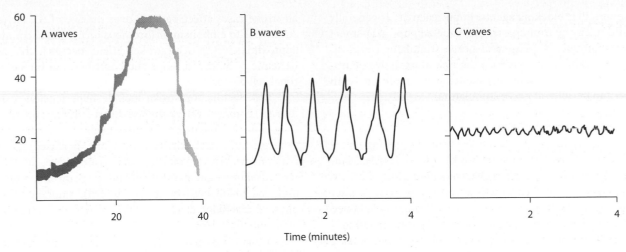

Figure 12-10. ICP trend recordings.

Positioning

Because the venous system of the brain is valveless, increased intrathoracic or intra-abdominal pressure reduces venous return and increases ICP. In general, elevating the head of the bed 30° optimizes ICP and CPP. Hip flexion is minimized. A bowel regimen is used to avoid constipation and abdominal bloating.

Neck positioning affects venous drainage and can raise ICP. The head and neck are maintained in a neutral position, avoiding flexion, hyperextension, or rotation. Cervical collars are applied carefully to avoid decreasing jugular venous return.

CSF Drainage

Although CSF drainage via an intraventricular catheter is often used as an intervention to lower ICP, there are no randomized controlled trials supporting this intervention. Drainage of small amounts of CSF may be used to decrease ICP in patients with an intraventricular catheter. The provider specifies the amount of drainage desired.

Minimizing Environmental Stimuli

Noise, temperature, and other noxious stimuli are carefully monitored and changed in response to the patient's needs. Limitation of visitors to decrease patient stimulation is not supported in the literature. Family members are encouraged to visit and speak quietly to patients and the ICP response is observed. If it is determined that stimulation is directly related to an increase in ICP, patient interactions can be modified if it is deemed necessary. Patient care activities (suctioning, bathing, turning) may be spaced out to avoid overstimulation and allow recovery time.

Preventing Increased Cerebral Metabolic Demand

Seizure activity increases cerebral metabolic demand and ICP. The prophylactic use of anticonvulsants during the first week of admission is common in neurologically impaired patients at risk for seizures. Additional information on the management of seizures is included later in this chapter.

Fever increases ICP by increasing metabolic demand. For each elevation of 1°C, cerebral metabolic demand increases by approximately 6%. Methods to normalize temperature include antipyretics, air- or water-filled cooling blankets, and intravascular cooling devices. Shivering also increases metabolic demand and is avoided.

Agitation also increases cerebral metabolic demand. Collaborate with other healthcare providers and the patient's family to maintain a calm, quiet environment. Agitation due to pain is managed through the use of analgesics. If analgesics or sedatives are used, short-acting agents are preferred because of the importance of ongoing neurological assessment. Careful monitoring of respiration in indicated since medications, such as opioids, can affect ventilation. Hypoxemia may cause increased ICP if neurons are deprived of oxygen.

Analgesia and Sedation

Analgesia and sedation are used to prevent elevation of ICP due to pain or agitation. Commonly used agents include fentanyl for analgesia and dexmedetomidine or midazolam for sedation. Propofol (a sedative hypnotic) is also commonly used because its short half-life allows for rapid awakening and evaluation of mental status. One of the side effects of analgesic and sedative medications is hypotension, careful use is required to avoid decreases in CPP. In addition, the use of propofol is limited by the associated risk of propofol infusion syndrome (PIS) if used for more than 48 hours. Limiting the duration of propofol infusion and using the lowest effective dose can reduce the risk of PIS. PIS includes bradycardia leading to asystole, metabolic acidosis, elevated triglycerides, and rhabdomyolysis.

Neuromuscular Blockade

Neuromuscular blocking agents may be used to prevent increases in intrathoracic and venous pressure that occur with coughing or patient-ventilator asynchrony. Sedation and analgesia are always used in conjunction with neuromuscular blocking agents. Pupil reactivity is generally not affected by neuromuscular blockade, so pupil assessment should continue. A peripheral nerve stimulator (train-of-four) should be used to reduce the risk of excessive neuromuscular blockade (refer to Chapter 6 for more on NMB agents and peripheral nerve stimulators).

Medications to Decrease Cerebral Edema

Osmotic diuretics reduce cerebral edema by pulling extracellular fluid from brain tissue into the blood vessels. Mannitol is commonly used and is given as a bolus dose of 0.25 to 1 g/kg body weight. Mannitol is administered using a filter because it crystallizes easily. Euvolemia is often maintained and electrolytes are closely monitored. Hypertonic saline is also used by many practitioners to increase serum osmolality and pull water into the vascular space.

Corticosteroids (eg, dexamethasone) are useful in decreasing cerebral edema associated with intracranial tumors. Steroids are generally not used in the management of cerebral edema related to TBI or stroke. Potential complications of steroid therapy include gastric irritation or hemorrhage and hyperglycemia.

Barbiturates

Barbiturate coma therapy is inconsistently used as a third-tier therapy for the management of refractory intracranial hypertension. Barbiturates decrease cerebral metabolism and CBF, which results in lower ICP. Complications associated with barbiturate coma include hypotension, myocardial depression, loss of thermoregulation, immunosuppression, and ileus.

Surgical Treatment

Close monitoring of neurologic status facilitates the identification and treatment of complications, such as the development of an epidural or subdural hematoma that leads to ICP. In these cases, surgical evacuation of the hematoma is likely to reduce ICP. In cases of diffuse cerebral edema, a portion of the skull may be removed to increase compliance and allow the brain to swell outside the contained area of the skull. This procedure is referred to as a craniectomy or decompressive hemicraniectomy.

Therapeutic Temperature Management

Avoiding hyperthermia can improve ICP control. Several large and ongoing clinical trials have been conducted to determine the optimal target temperature. Maintaining normothermia is the current standard of practice.

ACUTE ISCHEMIC STROKE

Etiology, Risk Factors, and Pathophysiology

Stroke is now the fifth leading cause of death in the United States and remains one of the top causes of disability worldwide. Prevalence increases with age; nearly 75% of all stroke cases affect patients over the age of 65. Ischemic stroke due to embolism or thrombus formation accounts for approximately 87% of all strokes. Edema occurs in the area of ischemic or infarcted tissue and contributes to further neuronal cell death.

Risk factors for stroke include hypertension, cardiac disease (coronary artery disease, heart failure, atrial fibrillation, endocarditis, patent foramen ovale, myocardial infarction, carotid artery disease), diabetes, increased age, race (African American), male gender, prior stroke, family history, dyslipidemia, hypercoagulability (cancer, pregnancy, high red blood cell counts, sickle cell), smoking, obesity, physical inactivity, alcohol or illicit drugs, and some forms of hormone therapy.

Transient ischemic attack (TIA) is an important warning sign for stroke. With a TIA, the patient develops stroke symptoms that resolve without tissue infarction. Although most TIAs resolve within minutes, an extensive workup to identify treatable causes is warranted to minimize the risk of subsequent stroke.

The pathophysiology of stroke varies based on the precipitating event. Thrombosis and embolism formation, described later, result in acute ischemic stroke.

Cerebral Ischemia

The human brain creates a high metabolic demand, consuming approximately 25% of a person's total metabolic consumption despite its relative size. The brain cannot store oxygen or glucose and therefore requires a constant blood flow to supply these nutrients. Homeostatic mechanisms work together to maintain this blood flow at a relatively stable rate (cerebrovascular autoregulation), but these mechanisms can be compromised, thereby altering the blood supply to the brain through several different processes.

Cerebral ischemia occurs when blood flow is altered long enough to cause tissue damage. Ischemic brain tissue can suffer necrosis as soon as 4 minutes after the disruption of glucose and oxygen supply. This damage can be global or focal and transient or permanent. Global cerebral ischemia is often caused by systemic hypotension (as seen in shock syndromes) and can also be transient in nature (as in vasovagal syncope or postural hypotensive episodes). Focal cerebral ischemia is commonly caused by obstruction of arterial blood flow to the brain as a result of a thrombus or embolus, vessel compression or torsion, vasospasm, infections (rare), or arterial stenosis.

If the ischemia is not reversed, neuronal cell death and infarction of brain tissue occurs, resulting in an ischemic stroke. Ischemic stroke symptoms are often focal, as the ischemia occurs in the region supplied by the artery affected. The *penumbra* is the area of tissue that surrounds the core ischemic area. The penumbra receives some blood flow from adjacent vessels (collateral circulation) but perfusion is marginal. If CBF is improved, the penumbra may still recover. Targeting the recovery of as much penumbra as possible is the overarching goal of stroke management.

ESSENTIAL CONTENT CASE

Acute Ischemic Stroke

A 59-year-old teacher is admitted to the ICU following fibrinolytic therapy for acute ischemic stroke. She has a history of atrial fibrillation and diet-controlled diabetes. For the last 3 weeks, she has complained to her husband about some minor heart palpitations, but has not been to the doctor. She developed left-arm hemiplegia, a left facial droop, and slurred speech while eating lunch at her desk. A student found the patient slumped against her desk when he returned to the classroom to retrieve a book. The student called 911. The paramedics established time of symptom onset by discovering that the student last saw her teacher normal about 20 minutes prior.

Upon arrival at the emergency department, she was quickly transported to head CT and the stroke team completed the necessary prefibrinolytic evaluation. No blood was present on CT, and recombinant tissue plasminogen activator was administered. On admission to the ICU, her left-arm weakness is beginning to resolve (strength 2/5) and her speech is almost normal. She is monitored in the ICU for 24 hours and diagnosed with atrial fibrillation. After 24 hours in the ICU, she is transferred to a telemetry bed in the stroke unit, where she is started on aspirin and later on an oral anticoagulant. She is discharged home after 4 days in the hospital, with outpatient occupational therapy.

Case Question 1: How would treatment priorities differ if the patient's CT had revealed an intracranial hemorrhage (ICH)?

Case Question 2: How often should vital signs and neurological assessment be performed for a patient who has received an IV thrombolytic for acute ischemic stroke?

Answers
1. If the CT scan showed bleeding, neither alteplase nor tenecteplase would be administered. Priorities of care would focus on controlling blood pressure, correcting coagulopathy, and supportive interventions.
2. Every 15 minutes for 2 hours after an IV thrombolytic agent is administered, then every 30 minutes for an additional 6 hours, then every hour until 24 hours have passed since the thrombolytic was given.

Thrombosis

Thrombosis is the most common cause of ischemic stroke and is usually due to atherosclerosis and the formation of plaque within an artery. A thrombus then forms at the site of the plaque and causes cerebral ischemia along the course of the affected vessel, which results in infarct if not quickly reversed.

Thrombosis due to atherosclerosis of large cerebral vessels results in large areas of infarct. Considerable edema often develops, further increasing ischemia by compressing areas surrounding the infarct. Significant functional deficits are common. If a thrombus forms in a smaller branching artery, a lacunar infarct develops. Lacunar infarcts result in smaller areas of neuronal cell death. Deficits are less apparent, unless the infarct is in a crucial area, such as the internal capsule. Patients with a history of atherosclerosis or arteritis are at highest risk for thrombotic strokes. Thrombotic strokes tend to develop during periods of sleep or inactivity, when blood flow is less brisk.

Embolism

Embolism refers to the occlusion of a cerebral vessel, most often by a blood clot but also by infectious particles, fat, air, or tumor fragments that came from a different part of the body. Heart disease leads to cerebral embolism when bacterial vegetations or blood clots that are easily detached from the wall or valves of the heart then travel to the brain and occlude a cerebral vessel. Chronic atrial fibrillation, valve disease, prosthetic valves, cardiomyopathy, and atherosclerotic lesions of the proximal aorta are common causes of embolism. Less common causes include atrial myxomas, patent foramen ovale, and bacterial endocarditis. The fragmented substance easily lodges at the bifurcation of the middle cerebral artery, sometimes breaking apart and traveling further into the cerebral vascular system. The onset of an embolic occlusion is rapid, with symptoms that develop without warning.

Clinical Presentation

Symptoms of stroke range from very mild to significant loss of functional abilities. Common signs and symptoms include focal weakness in an extremity or on one side of the body, sensory changes, difficulty speaking or understanding speech, facial droop, headache, and visual changes. Clinical presentation of stroke varies based on the area of ischemia or infarction. The National Institute of Health Stroke Scale (NIHSS) is often used to evaluate and monitor patients after stroke. NIHSS scores are predictive of stroke severity and outcomes. An overview of the NIHSS scoring system is presented in Table 12-6.

Stroke in a Cerebral Hemisphere

Signs and symptoms occur on the side of the body contralateral to the stroke. Weakness or paralysis occurs in one or both extremities, and sensory loss may also be noted. Visual field deficits are also contralateral to the lesion. The patient often displays an ipsilateral gaze preference, in effect "looking to the lesion." The left hemisphere is dominant in nearly 95% of right-handed individuals and over 80% of left-handed individuals. As the dominant hemisphere, it controls language functions and language-dependent memory. Dominant hemisphere strokes often produce receptive, expressive, or global aphasia. Nondominant hemisphere strokes often cause neglect syndromes, in which the patient becomes unaware of the environment and even their own body on the contralateral side.

Cerebellar or Brain Stem Stroke

Motor and sensory function may be impaired on one or both sides of the body. Loss of equilibrium, decreased fine

TABLE 12-6. NATIONAL INSTITUTES OF HEALTH STROKE SCALE (NIHSS)

Tested Item	Title	Response and Scores
1A	Level of consciousness	0—Alert 1—Drowsy 2—Obtunded 3—Coma/unresponsive
1B	Orientation questions (2)	0—Answers both correctly 1—Answers 1 correctly 2—Answers neither correctly
1C	Response to commands (2)	0—Performs both tasks correctly 1—Performs 1 task correctly 2—Performs neither
2	Gaze	0—Normal horizontal movements 1—Partial gaze palsy 2—Complete gaze palsy
3	Visual fields	0—No visual field defect 1—Partial hemianopia 2—Complete hemianopia 3—Bilateral hemianopia
4	Facial movement	0—Normal 1—Minor facial weakness 2—Partial facial weakness 3—Complete unilateral palsy
5	Motor function (arm) a. Left b. Right	0—No drift 1—Drift before 5 seconds 2—Falls before 10 seconds 3—No effort against gravity 4—No movement
6	Motor function (leg) a. Left b. Right	0—No drift 1—Drift before 5 seconds 2—Falls before 5 seconds 3—No effort against gravity 4—No movement
7	Limb ataxia	0—No ataxia 1—Ataxia in 1 limb 2—Ataxia in 2 limbs
8	Sensory	0—No sensory loss 1—Mild sensory loss 2—Severe sensory loss
9	Language	0—Normal 1—Mild aphasia 2—Severe aphasia 3—Mute or global aphasia
10	Articulation	0—Normal 1—Mild dysarthria 2—Severe dysarthria
11	Extinction or inattention	0—Absent 1—Mild (loss 1 sensory modality lost) 2—Severe (loss 2 modalities lost)

Additional information is available at http://www.ninds.nih.gov/disorders/stroke/strokescales.htm.
Data from Jauch EC, Saver JL, Adams HP, et al: Guidelines for the early management of patients with acute ischemic stroke: a guideline for healthcare professionals from the American Heart Association/American Stroke Association, Stroke 2013;44(3):870-947.

motor abilities, and nausea or vomiting are typical. Cranial nerve deficits are common and include dysarthria, nystagmus, dysphagia, and decreased cough reflex. Careful evaluation of airway protection and swallowing ability is essential to determine aspiration risk. Patients with severe deficits often require a feeding tube and potentially a tracheostomy. Because cortical injury is not present, patients maintain a normal mental status and level of alertness unless pressure in the posterior fossa leads to disruption of the RAS system.

In patients with cerebellar stroke, obstructive hydrocephalus may occur due to occlusion of the ventricular drainage system by edema. This is a medical emergency. Surgical decompression of the posterior fossa may be necessary, and an EVD may be placed.

Brain stem stroke because of basilar artery occlusion may result in quadriplegia and loss of facial movements (locked-in syndrome). Cognition is intact, and vertical gaze is maintained, therefore, these patients will be able to follow commands to look up or down. Early consultation with a speech-language pathologist is recommended for alternative communication strategies.

Diagnostic Tests

The goal of initial diagnostic testing in acute stroke is to rule out ICH, because treatments for hemorrhagic and ischemic stroke differ significantly. This is typically accomplished by performing a noncontrast head CT. CT scanning is available at most hospitals, can be performed quickly, and is an excellent tool for detecting intracranial bleeding. However, evidence of ischemia may not appear or may be very subtle on standard CT scanning until 12 to 24 hours after symptom onset. Specialized MRI scans (diffusion-weighted imaging, perfusion-weighted imaging) can detect areas of ischemia before they are apparent on CT. MRA detects areas of vascular abnormality as might be seen with clot owing to arterial dissection. Other tests that may be done acutely include cerebral angiography and carotid ultrasound. Transthoracic or transesophageal echocardiography is used to assess cardiac causes of stroke. Hypercoagulable states are detected through laboratory testing. All patients, who present with stroke receive a 12-lead ECG, are placed on cardiac monitoring for at least 24 hours, and undergo laboratory evaluation of cardiac biomarkers because of the strong correlation between cerebrovascular and cardiovascular disease. In addition, conditions that mimic stroke, such as hypoglycemia and seizure must be ruled out.

Principles of Management of Acute Ischemic Stroke

"Time is brain." Stroke is a medical emergency and is treated with the same urgency as acute myocardial infarction. The goals of treatment are to restore circulation to the brain when possible, stop the ongoing ischemic process, and prevent secondary complications. Management principles include the following:

Evaluation of Conditions That Mimic Acute Ischemic Stroke
Other conditions may mimic acute ischemic stroke and must be ruled out. The common causes of conditions that may present with stroke signs and symptoms ("stroke mimic")

include: seizure, systemic infection (urinary tract infection [UTI] in older adults), brain neoplasm, hyponatremia, hypo- or hyperglycemia, migraines, metabolic disorders, and conversion disorders. Hypoglycemia may cause stroke-like symptoms and is easily detected by using a glucometer to check blood glucose (point-of-care testing). Radiologic tests are performed on all patients with signs and symptoms of stroke to rule out intracranial bleeding.

Fibrinolytic Therapy

Fibrinolytic therapy is administered in an attempt to restore perfusion to the affected area. IV thrombolytic administration is considered in all patients who meet the inclusion/exclusion criteria (Table 12-7) and can be treated within 4.5 hours of the onset of symptoms. There are several additional exclusion criteria to IV thrombolytic therapy for patients who present >3 hours from symptom onset.

The recommended dose for alteplase is 0.9 mg/kg, with 10% of the total dose given as a bolus over 1 to 2 minutes followed by the remainder of the dose as an infusion over 1 hour. The maximum dose recommended is 90 mg. Tenecteplase is given as a single bolus dose of 0.25 mg/kg IV to a maximum dose of 25 mg. There is an increased risk of intracerebral hemorrhage following thrombolytic therapy administration and for this reason frequent serial neurologic assessments are essential. Vital signs and neurologic checks are done every 15 minutes for the first 2 hours, then every 30 minutes for 6 hours, and then hourly until 24 hours following initial treatment. If neurologic deterioration occurs, medication infusion is stopped, the physician is notified, and a stat head CT is performed to assess for bleeding. Following IV thrombolytic administration, antiplatelet or anticoagulant medicines are avoided for 24 hours. Placement of nasogastric tubes, bladder catheters, and invasive lines is delayed to decrease the risk of hemorrhage.

Endovascular Treatment

Endovascular treatment is an option for the treatment of acute ischemic stroke at some centers. However, the possibility of intra-arterial treatment should not delay the use of IV thrombolytics in patients who are eligible to receive it. Available endovascular therapies include intra-arterial fibrinolysis and mechanical clot extraction or disruption. These treatments, guided by cerebral angiography, must be performed by a physician specially trained in interventional neuroradiology and are not available at all centers. Although alteplase is not FDA approved for intra-arterial use, it is used for patients with middle cerebral artery occlusion who can be treated within 6 hours of the onset of symptoms and are not able to receive an IV thrombolytic medication. Mechanical thrombectomy using a special device may improve recanalization rates when used alone or in combination with fibrinolysis. Care of the patient following endovascular treatment for stroke includes standard post-angiogram monitoring, stroke-specific care, and other interventions as ordered by the physician.

TABLE 12-7. INCLUSION AND EXCLUSION CRITERIA FOR TREATMENT WITH THROMBOLYTICS AFTER ACUTE ISCHEMIC STROKE

Inclusion Criteria
- Diagnosis of ischemic stroke causing measurable neurological deficit
- Last known well or symptom onset <4.5 hours
- Aged ≥18 years

Exclusion Criteria
- Significant head trauma or prior stroke (<3 months)
- History of ischemic stroke (<6 weeks)
- Frank hypodensity on CT head scan (≥1/3 of the cerebral hemisphere)
- Clinical presentation suggestive of subarachnoid hemorrhage
- History of previous ICH within 3 months or current ICH
- Elevated BP (systolic ≥ 185 mm Hg or diastolic ≥ 110 mm Hg) despite aggressive treatment with IV antihypertensive agents (IV nicardipine, IV labetalol, IV hydralazine)
- Therapeutic LMWH dose within 48 hours of stroke symptoms and/or Anti-Xa > 0.3 (DVT prophylaxis dose is not a thrombolytic contraindication)
- Platelet count < 100,000/mm^3
- INR > 1.7, PT > 15, PTT > 40
- Presence of intra-axial intracranial neoplasm
- Use of direct thrombin inhibitors or direct factor Xa inhibitors within 48 hours of stroke symptoms
- Recent intracranial or intraspinal surgery (<30 days ago)
- Blood glucose concentration < 50 mg/dL without correction
- Infective endocarditis
- Active internal bleeding

Relative Exclusion Criteria/Special Consideration
- Only minor, non-disabling, and/or rapidly improving stroke symptoms (clearing spontaneously)
- History of stroke between 6 weeks and 3 months with limited parenchymal injury
- Hypodensity on CT head <1/3 of the cerebral hemisphere
- Pregnancy
- Renal and/or liver disease without abnormal coagulation factors
- Seizure at onset with postictal residual neurological impairments
- Major surgery or serious trauma within previous 14 days
- Recent gastrointestinal or urinary tract hemorrhage (within previous 21 days)
- Recent acute myocardial infarction (within previous 3 months)
- Arterial puncture at a non-compressible site in previous 7 days (example: axillary or subclavian arteries)
- Systemic malignancy with metastasis
- Acute or known bleeding diathesis
- Persistent neurological deficit after correction of hypoglycemia
- Aged <18 years
- Presence of extra-axial intracranial neoplasm (ie, meningioma)
- Presence of one or more AVMs without evidence of recent bleeding (past 4 weeks) or evidence of mass effect causing focal symptoms
- Cerebral aneurysms > 10 mm in size
- Acute pericarditis
- Other known, unruptured, or untreated intracranial vascular malformation
- Arterial puncture at noncompressible site within the last 7 days

Abbreviations: AVM, arteriovenous malformation; BP, blood pressure; CT, computed tomography; INR, international normalized ratio; IV, intravenous; LMWH, low-molecular-weight heparin; PT, prothrombin time; PTT, partial thromboplastin time.

Blood Pressure Management

Blood pressure management is essential after acute ischemic stroke because a marked or sudden decrease in blood pressure may significantly decrease cerebral perfusion. Acute ischemic stroke compromises cerebral autoregulation and makes CBF dependent on systemic blood pressure. The provider may elect to hold the patient's home antihypertensive

TABLE 12-8.   APPROACH TO BLOOD PRESSURE MANAGEMENT AFTER ACUTE ISCHEMIC STROKE IN PATIENTS WHO ARE CANDIDATES FOR REPERFUSION THERAPY

Patient Otherwise Eligible for Acute Reperfusion Therapy Except That BP is >185/110 mm Hg

- Labetalol 10-20 mg IV over 1-2 minutes, may repeat one time; or
- Nicardipine 5 mg/h IV, titrate up by 2.5 mg/h every 5-15 minutes, maximum 15 mg/h; when desired BP reached, adjust to maintain proper BP limits; or
- Other agents (hydralazine, enalaprilat, etc) may be considered when appropriate

If BP is not maintained at or below 185/110 mm Hg, do not administer rtPA.

Management of BP During and After rtPA or Other Acute Reperfusion Therapy to Maintain BP at or Below 180/105 mm Hg

Monitor BP every 15 minutes for 2 hours from the start of rtPA therapy, then every 30 minutes for 6 hours, and then every hour for 16 hours.

If systolic BP >180-230 mm Hg or diastolic BP >105-120 mm Hg:
- Labetalol 10 mg IV followed by continuous IV infusion 2-8 mg/min; or
- Nicardipine 5 mg/h IV, titrate up to desired effect by 2.5 mg/h every 5-15 minutes, maximum 15 mg/h

If BP not controlled or diastolic BP >140 mm Hg, consider IV sodium nitroprusside

Additional information is available at http://www.ninds.nih.gov/disorders/stroke/strokescales.htm

New guidelines for ischemic stroke were published in February 2017, but over 90 pages were subsequently retracted in April 2017. Thus, the recommendations published here do not reflect the 2017 guidelines. The reader is encouraged to update practice recommendations when definitive guidelines for the management of ischemic stroke are published.

Data from Jauch EC, Saver JL, Adams HP, et al: Guidelines for the early management of patients with acute ischemic stroke: a guideline for healthcare professionals from the American Heart Association/American Stroke Association, Stroke 2013;44(3):870-947.

medications to maximize CBF, especially in the first 24 hours after stroke. For patients who are not eligible for fibrinolytic therapy, blood pressure is not treated emergently unless the systolic blood pressure exceeds 220 mm Hg or the diastolic blood pressure exceeds 120 mm Hg. Because of the risk of hemorrhage, blood pressure management is more stringent in patients who are eligible for or who have received fibrinolytic therapy (Table 12-8).

Mobility

There is controversy related to the timing of mobility following a stroke. Current data suggests that very early (<24 hours) out-of-bed activity may be associated with worsened outcomes. However, early mobility (>24 hours following stroke) including in-bed active movement of extremities and gentle exercise is recommended.

Management of Increased ICP

Cerebral edema occurs in the area of infarct and may lead to increased ICP. For further discussion of treatment options, refer to the section on ICP. Osmotic diuresis using mannitol and hypertonic saline (up to 23.4% NaCl) may be used to reduce cerebral edema. Hemicraniectomy may be used to allow for expansion of cerebral edema and alleviate increased ICP in patients with large infarcts, particularly those in the area of the middle cerebral artery. Normothermia and mild hypothermia are treatment options depending on available resources. Aggressive treatment of fever is warranted to avoid increases in cerebral metabolic demand.

Glucose Management

Hyperglycemia is associated with worse outcomes after stroke and TBI. Although ongoing research seeks to define the optimal blood glucose target, current recommendations support lowering blood glucose to 140 to 180 mg/dL. Hypoglycemia is deleterious and must be avoided.

Preventing and Treating Secondary Complications

Patients are at significant risk for aspiration following stroke due to difficulty protecting their airway. Decreased LOC, facial weakness, and cranial nerve deficits contribute to this risk. Endotracheal intubation may be necessary during the acute phase. Some patients recover enough function to be extubated, but others may eventually need a tracheostomy. Dysphagia is very common after stroke, so careful assessment of swallowing ability is indicated before any oral intake. Most hospitals now have dysphagia screening protocols in place that support initial dysphagia screening by nursing staff. Consultation with the speech-language pathologist is indicated for patients who fail a nursing bedside dysphagia examination. Placement of a feeding tube may be necessary if the patient is unable to swallow safely.

Deep venous thrombosis (DVT) is a common complication in stroke patients and may lead to pulmonary embolism. Strategies to decrease risk include intermittent pneumatic compression devices, subcutaneous administration of low-dose anticoagulants, and early progression in physical activity.

In addition to pneumonia and DVT, patients with stroke are at risk for urinary tract infection (UTI). To reduce this risk, indwelling catheters are used only when medically necessary, the need is assessed daily, and they are removed as soon as possible. In patients without indwelling catheters, monitoring for urinary retention and assessment of postvoid residuals is important due to the risk of neurogenic bladder.

Preventing Recurrent Stroke

The use of antiplatelet and anticoagulant medications varies depending on the size of the infarct, presumed etiology, and whether or not the patient received fibrinolytic therapy. Patients are commonly placed on aspirin 24 to 48 hours after the initial event and the decision to use other antiplatelet or anticoagulant medications is made on an individual basis. Anticoagulation is typically not used in the acute phase of treatment because it increases the risk of hemorrhagic conversion (development of bleeding within the infarcted tissue), but it may be used in certain circumstances.

Carotid endarterectomy is the most common surgical procedure to prevent further ischemic strokes, but is not typically performed in the time period immediately following a stroke due to the risk of reperfusion injury and hemorrhage.

Stenosis may also be treated with angioplasty, with or without stent placement. Other strategies to prevent recurrent stroke include statins for dyslipidemia and behavior modification to address modifiable risk factors.

HEMORRHAGIC STROKE

Etiology, Risk Factors, and Pathophysiology

Approximately 15% of all strokes are hemorrhagic; either subarachnoid or intracranial. In SAH, bleeding into the subarachnoid space occurs, usually as the result of a ruptured aneurysm. Although SAH is a type of stroke, management issues vary significantly from ischemic stroke. Subarachnoid hemorrhage is discussed in Chapter 21, Advanced Neurologic Concepts. Here, *hemorrhagic stroke* refers to intraparenchymal bleeding (also called ICH).

Hypertension is the most common cause of ICH. Other causes include vascular malformations (arteriovenous or cavernous malformations), coagulopathy, amyloid angiopathy, tumor, vasculitis, venous infarction, and illicit drug abuse. Amyloid angiopathy is most common in patients older than the age of 70. It is a presumed diagnosis in older patients with repeated ICH, but can only be definitively diagnosed by deposits of beta-amyloid protein found in the vessel walls (usually on autopsy). AVM is a common cause of ICH in younger patients (ages 20-40). AVMs are congenital abnormalities in which a tangled mass of blood vessels is present in the brain. Within the AVM, the arterial and venous vasculatures connect without going through a capillary system. Following resolution of acute ICH, AVMs are treated with endovascular embolization, surgical resection, or stereotactic radiosurgery to prevent reoccurring bleeding.

In addition to direct tissue injury, the hematoma formed by ICH displaces nearby brain tissue and causes ischemia through compression. Edema occurs around the site of hemorrhage. If the ICH occurs deep within the cerebral hemispheres, it can rupture into the ventricle (intraventricular hemorrhage). The mortality rate is higher in hemorrhagic stroke than in ischemic stroke.

Clinical Presentation

ICH most often presents with a sudden onset of focal neurologic deficits often associated with a sudden severe headache, nausea/vomiting, decreased consciousness, and sometimes seizures. Neurologic deficits vary based on the area of the brain affected and are similar to the focal deficits experienced by patients with acute ischemic stroke.

Diagnostic Tests

ICH is most often diagnosed using CT scanning, although MRI is sometimes used. Tests that may be performed to determine the etiology of the hemorrhage include CTA, MRI/MRA, and cerebral angiography.

Principles of Management of Intracerebral Hemorrhage

Initial priorities of care for the patient with ICH include blood pressure control and correction of coagulopathy. This is considered a medical emergency, as bleeding can continue or recur for several hours after the initial event. IV medications are often required to treat elevated blood pressure and may be administered intermittently or continuously. Generally, the goal is to keep the systolic blood pressure between 140 and 160 mm Hg. Treatment of coagulopathy is based on the underlying cause of abnormal clotting. Fresh frozen plasma, platelets, vitamin K, or prothrombin complex concentrate may be ordered; regardless of the agent used, the goal is rapid correction of coagulopathy.

Operative management may or may not be indicated based on the size and location of hemorrhage. Cerebellar hemorrhage may require a suboccipital craniectomy to evacuate the clot and decrease pressure on vital structures. Intraventricular hemorrhage (IVH) may cause hydrocephalus, which is treated by placement of an EVD. Antiepileptic medications are recommended for patients who experience a seizure or who show electrographic evidence of seizure on EEG. These agents may also be administered to prevent seizures if the hemorrhage is in a part of the brain associated with seizure risk such as the temporal or frontal lobe.

Similar to patients with acute ischemic stroke, prevention of secondary complications is an essential element of nursing care for patients with ICH. Patients are at risk of aspiration and require careful monitoring of airway clearance, as well as assessment for dysphagia. Additional interventions include meticulous skin care, attention to bowel and bladder management, and strategies to prevent hospital-acquired infections.

SEIZURES

Etiology, Risk Factors, and Pathophysiology

Seizures are rapid, repeated bursts of abnormal electrical activity within the brain that result from an imbalance of excitatory and inhibitory impulses. Signs and symptoms depend on the location of the abnormal activity. A seizure may be a symptom or consequence of an underlying neurologic problem, such as a tumor, hemorrhage, trauma, or infection. Systemic disturbances such as hypoxia, hypoglycemia, drug overdose, and drug or alcohol withdrawal may also cause seizures. Many seizures are considered idiopathic, but treatable causes must be ruled out.

During a seizure, the metabolic demands of the brain for oxygen and glucose increase dramatically. The body tries to keep up with these increased requirements by increasing CBF. If CBF does not keep up with demand, neurons revert to anaerobic metabolism, which leads to secondary ischemia and brain injury.

Clinical Presentation

Clinical presentation varies based on the origin and extent of the brain's abnormal electrical activity. Seizures can be described as focal onset (starting in one area of the cerebral cortex and limited to one hemisphere), generalized (rapidly affecting both cerebral hemispheres), or of an unknown onset.

Focal Seizures

The term focal seizure is preferred over simple partial. If the patient remains aware (with or without the ability to speak), the seizure is termed *focal aware*. *Focal impaired* implies that the patient was unaware at some point during the seizure. Focal seizures may present with motor activity such as twitching or jerking in an extremity or one side of the face, sensory symptoms such as an unusual taste or smell, or autonomic sensations such as sweating or vomiting.

Patients with focal seizures may experience an aura (symptoms such as smelling burnt toast) that signal the onset of a seizure. Focal seizures may also present with automatisms (smacking the lips, chewing motions, or fidgeting), purposeless activity such as running or arm jerking, or a change in affect such as elation or fear. Focal seizures can progress to a bilateral generalized convulsive seizure.

Generalized Seizures

Generalized seizure replaces the terms *grand mal* and *petit mal*. Generalized seizures are characterized by abnormal electrical discharge that rapidly affects both hemispheres. Motor generalized seizure includes automatism, atonic, clonic, myoclonic, spasm, and hyperkinetic movements (below). Nonmotor seizure may include changes in cognitive, emotional, or sensory ability as well as autonomic behaviors.

- *Absence:* Sudden lapse of consciousness and activity that lasts 3 to 30 seconds. Commonly described as a staring spell.
- *Myoclonic:* Sudden, brief muscle jerking of one or more muscle groups. Commonly associated with metabolic, degenerative, and hypoxic causes.
- *Atonic* (also called drop attacks): Sudden loss of muscle tone.
- *Clonic:* Rhythmic muscle jerking.
- *Tonic:* Sustained muscle contraction.
- *Tonic-clonic:* Muscle activity varies between sustained contraction and jerking.

Unknown Onset Seizures

The type of seizure is determined by the first prominent sign or symptom. The term unknown onset seizure is used when the practitioner is unable to confidently identify the onset.

Patients are more likely to be injured during a generalized seizure than during a focal seizure and may complain of generalized muscle aches after the seizure stops if convulsions led to sustained muscle activity.

ESSENTIAL CONTENT CASE

Status Epilepticus

A 28-year-old man is admitted to the ICU for management of status epilepticus. He has a history of seizures following a TBI 4 years prior and takes levetiracetam. He has no obvious residual deficits of brain injury except mild to moderate short-term memory loss. Due to his memory loss, his wife manages his medications and reports that he consistently takes his levetiracetam. This morning his wife brought him to the emergency department (ED) after he experienced three seizures within 2 hours, and he had one more seizure in the ED. Soon after admission to the ICU for monitoring, he has a generalized tonic-clonic seizure.

Case Question 1: What are the initial priorities of care for this patient?
The seizure continues for several minutes, and the physician orders lorazepam. Despite receiving lorazepam, the patient continues to have seizure activity. He is intubated for airway management and a midazolam infusion is started. A loading dose of fosphenytoin is administered, and continuous EEG monitoring is initiated.

Case Question 2: What is the primary early adverse effect associated with fosphenytoin?
Seizure activity stops within 1 hour. The midazolam infusion is weaned over 24 hours with no return of seizure activity. He is successfully extubated and his mental status returns to baseline. He is continued on phenytoin and transferred to the acute care unit for continued adjustments of his antiepileptic medications.

Answers
1. Airway, breathing, and circulation are assessed first. In addition, patient safety is addressed by clearing objects out of the area and positioning the patient to allow drainage of oral secretions.
2. Fosphenytoin, similar to phenytoin, can cause treatment-resistant hypotension.

Status Epilepticus

Status epilepticus indicates prolonged or recurring seizures without a return to baseline mental status. The classic definition of status epilepticus is a seizure or series of seizures lasting longer than 30 minutes, but treatment is typically instituted much sooner and guidelines suggest a definition of seizure activity lasting longer than 5 minutes. Status epilepticus is a medical emergency with a significant mortality rate, higher in older adults or when the seizure is a symptom of an underlying acute process. There are two primary types of status epilepticus—convulsive status epilepticus and nonconvulsive status epilepticus. In convulsive status epilepticus, seizure activity is readily apparent using clinical observation. In nonconvulsive status epilepticus, no outward clinical seizures may be noted but consciousness is impaired and seizure activity is apparent on EEG. Status epilepticus is described as refractory if it continues despite initial treatment with a benzodiazepine and a second antiepileptic agent.

Diagnostic Testing

In the critical care environment, management of seizures in a patient without a history of epilepsy is aimed at stopping the seizure and then determining an underlying cause. Diagnostic testing for patients with seizures may include:

- *Laboratory testing* to identify electrolyte abnormalities or metabolic etiology.
- *CT* to assess for intracranial processes such as an ICH or tumor.
- *MRI* to look for structural lesions that may indicate a seizure focus.
- *LP* when an infectious process (eg, meningitis) is the suspected source of seizure activity.
- *EEG* to evaluate for seizure activity. Continuous EEG monitoring may be required, particularly in patients in status epilepticus. Epileptiform activity may be present on EEG even after the clinical seizure has stopped.
- *Continuous video monitoring* in conjunction with continuous EEG recordings correlate clinical phenomena with electrical activity in the brain.
- *Intracranial electrodes* in the evaluation of patients with intractable seizures to identify a focus or foci prior to surgical resection. Intracranial electrodes are inserted via burr holes or a craniotomy.

Principles of Management of Seizures

Management of the patient with seizures focuses on controlling the seizure as quickly as possible, preventing recurrence, maintaining patient safety, and identifying the underlying cause. Observation of seizure type, duration, and any precipitating factors is essential. Following a seizure, patients may experience a period of confusion and altered mental status that slowly resolves. They may complain of a headache or muscle aches. Todd's paralysis describes continued focal symptoms that can persist for up to 36 hours after a seizure. Because of the risk of missing underlying intracranial pathology, patients with focal neurologic deficits following a seizure are diagnosed with Todd's paralysis only after other causes have been ruled out.

Maintaining Patient Safety and Airway Management

The first priority is to protect the patient from injury. Ensure a safe environment during the seizure by clearing objects out of the area. Padded side rails are no longer considered routine care and are indicated only for patients at high risk. During a seizure, attempting to restrain patient movement may result in injury and is avoided.

Airway management assists with maintaining adequate cerebral oxygenation. Maintaining the airway may depend on stopping the seizure. Positioning the patient on his or her side decreases aspiration; supplemental oxygen is provided. Nothing should be placed in the patient's mouth during a seizure. ECG monitoring, continuous pulse oximetry, and blood pressure monitoring are required in patients with prolonged seizures. Hypoglycemia can induce seizure activity, so a glucose level is checked immediately and treated as appropriate.

Medication Administration for Prolonged Seizures and Status Epilepticus

The average seizure stops within 2 minutes without requiring medication. First-line treatment for patients with prolonged seizures or status epilepticus is the administration of a benzodiazepine such as lorazepam. The second medication given is typically levetiracetam, phenytoin, or fosphenytoin. Fosphenytoin is converted to phenytoin in the blood and is preferred because it causes less tissue injury should extravasation occur. Both agents can cause cardiovascular side effects, predominately treatment-resistant hypotension. Cardiac and respiratory status should be closely monitored. Valproate sodium and levetiracetam are also available in IV formulations and may be administered early in the course of management. Medications to treat seizures are discussed in more detail in Chapter 7, Pharmacology.

If seizure activity continues, a continuous infusion of midazolam is often ordered. Barbiturates may also be used but have significant cardiovascular side effects. Propofol can be effective in stopping seizures but prolonged use is limited because of the risk of PIP. In patients who receive neuromuscular blocking agents, either for intubation or as part of treatment for an underlying disease process, it is important to remember that neuromuscular blockers only stop the motor manifestations of seizure. The abnormal electrical activity in the brain and neuronal injury continues.

The prolonged muscle activity that occurs with convulsive status epilepticus may cause tissue breakdown and lead to rhabdomyolysis. Hydration is essential to avoid renal dysfunction.

Treatment Options for Patients With Seizures

Many patients benefit from ongoing medication for seizure control. Some common medications include levetiracetam, phenytoin, carbamazepine, oxcarbazepine, valproic acid, lamotrigine, and lacosamide. Approximately two-thirds of patients treated with medication are able to attain improved seizure control.

Some patients with seizures uncontrolled by medications may be helped by surgery to remove the seizure focus. These patients most often have seizures originating from the temporal lobe. Selection criteria include intractable seizures that significantly impact quality of life and are uncontrolled by medication, an identifiable unilateral focus of seizure activity, and seizure focus in an area where removal will cause no major neurologic deficit. A craniotomy is used to access and excise the seizure focus. The primary complications are hemorrhage and infection. Patients are kept on their previous seizure medications during the postoperative period. About 50% of patients become seizure free after surgery and an additional 30% experience a significant improvement in seizure control.

For patients with intractable seizures who do not have an identifiable focus, placement of a vagus nerve stimulator (VNS) may be considered. VNS reduces seizure duration, frequency, or intensity by providing intermittent electrical stimulation of the vagus nerve. The exact mechanism of action has not been determined. Roughly one-third of patients with VNS will experience a significant (>50%) reduction in the number of seizures. Adjunctive therapy with medication is generally indicated.

INFECTIONS OF THE CENTRAL NERVOUS SYSTEM

Meningitis

Meningitis is an acute inflammation of the meninges of the brain and spinal cord. Meningitis can be caused by bacteria, viruses, fungi, or parasites. Risk factors include immunocompromise, trauma, poor dentition, or surgery that disrupts the meninges or sinuses. Signs and symptoms include fever, headache, neck stiffness, irritability, vomiting, photophobia, changes in LOC, seizures, weakness, and cranial nerve deficits. Other signs of meningitis include Kernig sign (severe pain in the hamstring with knee extension when the hip is flexed 90°) and Brudzinski sign (involuntary flexion of the knees and hips when the neck is flexed). Many patients with meningococcal meningitis have a characteristic rash (petechial rash that progresses to purple blotches).

Diagnostic testing includes LP for opening pressure and CSF analysis, blood cultures, and other laboratory tests to look for infection. CT scanning is performed prior to LP in patients with papilledema or focal neurologic findings. Complications of meningitis include hydrocephalus, cerebral edema, and vasculitis. Nursing priorities include management of elevated ICP, implementation of seizure precautions, and prompt administration of antimicrobial therapy. Delays in antimicrobial therapy are associated with worse outcomes. Transmission-based isolation precautions may be required until the causative organism is identified and treated; notify the infection control practitioner and follow institutional guidelines.

Encephalitis

Encephalitis is inflammation of the brain parenchyma. There are many types of encephalitis, including arboviruses such as West Nile virus, but the most common type seen in most ICUs in the United States is encephalitis due to the herpes simplex virus (HSV). HSV encephalitis can result from a new infection, or a reactivation of a preexisting infection. Signs and symptoms include fever, focal or diffuse neurologic changes, headache, and seizures. HSV encephalitis predominately affects the inferior frontal and temporal lobes. Diagnostic testing includes MRI, EEG, and CSF analysis. The diagnosis is often presumed pending specialized testing of the CSF. Empiric therapy is started with an antiviral agent.

Intracranial Abscess

An *intracranial abscess* is a collection of pus in the brain and can be extradural, subdural, or intracerebral. The infective agent enters the brain through the bloodstream, via an opening in the dura (as may occur with a basilar or open skull fracture or following a neurosurgical procedure), or via direct migration from chronic otitis media, poor dentition, frontal sinusitis, or mastoiditis. Signs and symptoms typically develop over a few weeks and may include headache, seizures, fever, neck pain, focal neurologic signs such as hemiparesis, cranial nerve deficits, and change in LOC. Diagnostic testing includes CT with contrast administration, MRI, EEG, and potentially aspiration of the lesion for culture. Treatment includes prolonged antibiotic therapy (usually 6 weeks) and surgical drainage of the abscess.

NEUROMUSCULAR DISEASES

Although there are a number of neuromuscular diseases that may result in hospitalization, only a small number of these patients require admission to the critical care unit. Myasthenia gravis (MG), MS, Guillain-Barré syndrome, and amyotrophic lateral sclerosis often cause respiratory muscle weakness requiring mechanical ventilation and are briefly described.

Myasthenia Gravis

In myasthenia gravis, autoimmune-mediated destruction of acetylcholine receptors results in decreased neuromuscular transmission and muscle weakness. MG is a chronic disease with periodic exacerbations. Diagnostic testing includes laboratory testing for acetylcholine receptor antibodies, EMG, CT scanning of the chest to evaluate for abnormalities of the thymus, and serological antibody testing. Improvement in symptoms following edrophonium chloride injection is highly suggestive of MG. Adverse effects of edrophonium chloride include bradycardia, asystole, increased oral and bronchial secretions, and bronchoconstriction.

Patients with MG are admitted to the ICU when they require noninvasive mechanical ventilation or intubation during acute exacerbations. Respiratory muscle strength is assessed by measuring negative inspiratory force and vital capacity. Treatment includes IV immunoglobulin or plasma exchange in addition to supportive care. Long-term management may include the administration of anticholinesterase medications, thymectomy, or immunosuppression. Patients also need education about the triggers, including some classes of prescription medications, that can contribute to acute exacerbations. Priorities of nursing management during an acute exacerbation include close monitoring of respiratory status and prevention of secondary complications such as infections.

Multiple Sclerosis

Multiple sclerosis is a chronic disease characterized by immune-mediated damage to the myelin in the CNS. The etiology is unknown though there may be a genetic predisposition along with environmental triggers. Patients with MS may be admitted to the ICU with infections, pneumonia, or exacerbation of symptoms (especially neuromuscular respiratory weakness). The typical age of onset is 20 to 50 years of age and it affects women more than men. One-year mortality rates following ICU admission are nearly double those for MS patients not admitted to ICU (even after controlling for age and severity of MS).

Guillain-Barré Syndrome

Guillain-Barré syndrome causes progressive muscle weakness, sensory loss, and areflexia due to peripheral nerve demyelination. Symptoms generally start in the lower extremities and ascend. Diagnostic studies include LP and nerve conduction studies. Approximately 25% to 40% of patients require mechanical ventilation. Some patients experience autonomic instability characterized by variations in heart rate and blood pressure. Neuropathic pain related to inflammation and demyelination occurs and requires both pharmacologic and nonpharmacologic treatment. In addition to supportive therapy, patients may receive plasma exchange or IV immunoglobulin (IVIG). Most patients recover with minimal deficits, but may require weeks to months of hospitalization and rehabilitation. Nursing priorities include close monitoring of respiratory status and prevention of complications related to prolonged immobility.

Amyotrophic Lateral Sclerosis

ALS is a progressive disease that affects the motor neurons, causing muscle weakness without affecting sensation or cognition. Patients most commonly present with extremity weakness that is asymmetric and more pronounced distally. Bulbar symptoms such as dysarthria and dysphagia may be present initially, or may develop as the disease progresses. The rapidity of progression varies widely among patients. Eventually, ALS causes respiratory failure due to muscle weakness and decreased airway protection.

Patients with ALS may be admitted to the ICU when airway protection becomes problematic and complications such as pneumonia develop, or if they use assisted ventilation (bilevel positive airway pressure [BiPAP] or mechanical ventilation) at home and require admission for other complications or procedures. Because of the complexity involved in making treatment decisions in an irreversible disease process, consultation with palliative care for goals of care conversations is warranted. In addition, nursing care focuses on decreasing respiratory complications and other complications of immobility, controlling pain and other symptoms, and providing psychological support.

SELECTED BIBLIOGRAPHY

Acute Ischemic Stroke and Hemorrhagic Stroke

Boling B, Groves TR. Management of subarachnoid hemorrhage. *Crit Care Nurse.* 2019;39(5):58-67.

Boling, B, Keinath, K. Acute ischemic stroke. *AACN Adv Crit Care.* 2018;29:152-162.

Bösel J. Blood pressure control for acute severe ischemic and hemorrhagic stroke. *Curr Opin Crit Care.* 2017;23(2):81-86.

Muehlschlegel S. Subarachnoid hemorrhage. *Continuum (Minneap Minn).* 2018;24(6):1623-1657.

Nestor MA, Boling B. Reversing direct oral anticoagulants in acute intracranial hemorrhage. *Crit Care Nurse.* 2019;39(3):e1-e8.

Powers WJ, Rabinstein AA, Ackerson T, et al. Guidelines for the early management of patients with acute ischemic stroke: 2019 Update to the 2018 guidelines for the early management of acute ischemic stroke: a guideline for healthcare professionals from the American Heart Association/American Stroke Association. *Stroke.* 2019;50(12):e344-e418.

Tamburri LM, Hollender KD, Orzano D. Protecting patient safety and preventing modifiable complications after acute ischemic stroke. *Crit Care Nurse.* 2020;40(1):56-65.

Assessment and Diagnostic Testing

Derbyshire J, Hill B. Performing neurological observations. *Br J Nurs.* 2018;27(19):1110-1114.

Goeren D, John S, Meskill K, Iacono L, Wahl S, Scanlon K. Quiet time: a noise reduction initiative in a neurosurgical intensive care unit. *Crit Care Nurse.* 2018;38(4):38-44.

Lussier BL, Olson DM, Aiyagari V. Automated Pupillometry in Neurocritical Care: Research and Practice. *Curr Neurol Neuroscience Rep.* 2019;19(10):71.

Ungarian J, Rankin JA, Then KL. Delirium in the intensive care unit: is dexmedetomidine effective? *Crit Care Nurse.* 2019;39(4):e8-e21.

Evidence-Based Practice

Gunter EP, Viswanathan M, Stutzman SE, Olson DM, Aiyagari V. Development and testing of an electronic multidisciplinary rounding tool. *AACN Adv Crit Care.* 2019;30(3):222-229.

McNett M, Moran C, Johnson H. Evidence-based review of clinical trials in neurocritical care. *AACN Adv Crit Care.* 2018;29(2):195-203.

Tamburri L, Hollender K, Orzano D. Protecting patient safety and preventing modifiable complications after acute ischemic stroke. *AACN Crit Care Nurse.* 2020;40;56-65. https://www.aacn.org/education/publications/ccn/40/1/0056-patient-safety-protecting-patient-safety-and-preventing-modifiable-complications-after-acute-ischemic-stroke

Infections of the Central Nervous System

Chou SH, Beghi E, Helbok R, et al. Global incidence of neurological manifestations among patients hospitalized with COVID-19-A report for the GCS-NeuroCOVID Consortium and the ENERGY Consortium. *JAMA Netw Open.* 2021;4(5):e2112131.

Heming N, Mazeraud A, Verdonk F, Bozza FA, Chrétien F, Sharshar T. Neuroanatomy of sepsis-associated encephalopathy. *Crit Care.* 2017;21(1):65.

Toledano M, Davies NWS. Infectious encephalitis: mimics and chameleons. *Pract Neurol.* 2019;19(3):225-237.

Venkatesan A, Murphy OC. Viral encephalitis. *Neurol Clin.* 2018; 36(4):705-724.

Intracranial Pressure

Liu X, Griffith M, Jang HJ, et al. Intracranial pressure monitoring via external ventricular drain: are we waiting long enough before recording the real value? *J Neurosci Nurs.* 2020;52(1):37-42.

Olson DM, Parcon C, Santos A, Santos G, Delabar R, Stutzman SE. A novel approach to explore how nursing care affects intracranial pressure. *Am J Crit Care.* 2017;26(2):136-139.

Scarboro M, McQuillan KA. Traumatic brain injury update. *AACN Adv Crit Care.* 2021;32(1):29-50.

Tavakoli S, Peitz G, Ares W, Hafeez S, Grandhi R. Complications of invasive intracranial pressure monitoring devices in neurocritical care. *Neurosurg Focus.* 2017;43(5):E6.

Neuromuscular Diseases

Damian MS, Srinivasan R. Neuromuscular problems in the ICU. *Curr Opin Neurol.* 2017;30(5):538-544.

Mary P, Servais L, Vialle R. Neuromuscular diseases: diagnosis and management. *Orthop Traumatol Surg Res.* 2018;104(1S):S89-S95.

Morrison BM. Neuromuscular diseases. *Semin Neurol.* 2016;36(5): 409-418.

Williams L. Spinal muscular atrophy in the age of gene therapy. *AACN Adv Crit Care.* 2020;31(1):86-91.

Seizures

Picinich C, Kennedy J, Thind H, Foreman C, Martin RM, Zimmermann LL. Continuous electroencephalographic training for neuroscience intensive care unit nurses: a feasibility study. *J Neurosci Nurs.* 2020;52(5):245-250.

Wieruszewski ED, Brown CS, Leung JG, Wieruszewski PM. Pharmacologic management of status epilepticus. *AACN Adv Crit Care.* 2020;31(4):349-356.

Websites with More Information about Neurological Disorders

Epilepsy Foundation provides resources for health care professionals. https://www.epilepsy.com/living-epilepsy/epilepsy-and/professional-health-care-providers

Myasthenia Gravis Foundation of America provides resources for health care professionals. https://myasthenia.org/Professionals

National Multiple Sclerosis Society provides resources for healthcare professionals. https://www.nationalmssociety.org/For-Professionals/Clinical-Care

The American Heart Association's Get With The Guidelines ®—Stroke describes strategies to align in-hospital management of stroke with current evidence. https://www.heart.org/en/professional/quality-improvement/get-with-the-guidelines/get-with-the-guidelines-stroke

The National Institute of Neurological Disorders and Stroke provides fact sheets on a wide variety of neurological disorders. https://www.ninds.nih.gov/Disorders/Patient-Caregiver-Education/Fact-Sheets

13

HEMATOLOGIC AND IMMUNE SYSTEMS

Danya Garner

KNOWLEDGE COMPETENCIES

1. Analyze laboratory test results used to assess the status of the hematologic and immune systems:
   - Complete blood count (CBC)
   - White blood cell (WBC) differential
   - International normalized ratio (INR)
   - Activated partial thromboplastin time
   - D-dimer
2. Describe the etiology, pathophysiology, clinical presentation, patient needs, and interprofessional interventions for common hematologic problems in critically ill patients:
   - Anemia
   - Thrombocytopenia
   - Disseminated intravascular coagulation (DIC)
3. Contrast the clinical presentation, patient needs, and principles of management of the immuno-compromised patient with that of a patient with an intact immune response.

The hematologic and immune systems play a major role in the body's response to illness. Organs and tissues require a continuous supply of oxygen from the red blood cells (RBCs), while the white blood cells (WBCs) provide a first line of defense against infection and mount an immune response. The platelets and other coagulation components are essential for hemostasis. Assessment of these processes and treatment of hematologic and immune problems are an important part of patient management.

SPECIAL ASSESSMENT TECHNIQUES, DIAGNOSTIC TESTS, AND MONITORING SYSTEMS

A complete patient assessment guides the selection of screening tests for hematologic and immune problems. Historical data are particularly important and include family history, occupational exposures, lifestyle behaviors, travel, diet, allergies, past medical problems, surgeries, comorbid conditions, transfusion of blood or blood components, and recent and current medications. Abnormal physical assessment data from each body system collectively assist in the identification of risk factors or acute abnormalities pertinent to hematologic and immune function. In addition, a variety of laboratory tests including those listed in Table 13-1 assist the clinician to evaluate problems in these systems.

Complete Blood Count

The complete blood count (CBC) is a primary assessment tool for evaluation of the hematologic and immune status. The RBC count and RBC indices, along with the hemoglobin (Hgb) and hematocrit (Hct) levels, provide valuable information regarding the oxygen-carrying capacity of the blood. The total WBC count and the WBC differential reveal the body's ability to provide an immune response and to participate in the normal inflammatory process required for tissue restoration. Important information concerning hemostasis is obtained from the platelet count, with additional studies required to fully evaluate the coagulation process.

Red Blood Cell Count

The RBC count is determined by the number of erythrocytes per microliter of blood. Normal values for men are higher than for women. A decrease in the number of RBCs or in

TABLE 13-1. NORMAL VALUES FOR HEMATOLOGIC AND IMMUNE SCREENING TESTS[a]

Laboratory Test	Normal Value
RBC	Males: 4.2-5.4 million/μL
	Females: 3.6-5.0 million/μL
Hgb	Males: 14-17 g/dL
	Females: 12-16 g/dL
Hct	Males: 43%-52%
	Females: 36%-48%
RBC indices	
MCV	84-96 fL
MCH	28-34 pg/cell
MCHC	32-36 g/dL
RDW	11%-14.4%
Reticulocyte count	0.5%-1.5%
WBC	4500-10,500/μL
WBC differential (% of total)	
Neutrophils	50%-70%
Segmented	56%
Bands	0%-3%
Eosinophils	0%-3%
Basophils	0.5%-1.0%
Monocytes	3%-7%
Lymphocytes	25%-40%
T-cells	800-2500 cells/μL
T-helper (CD4) cells	600-1500 cells/μL
Cytotoxic T (CD8) cells	300-1000 cells/μL
Quantitative Immunoglobulins	
IgA	60-400 mg/dL
IgG	700-1500 mg/dL
IgM	60-300 mg/dL
IgE	3-423 IU/mL
Platelet count	150,000-400,000/μL
Bleeding time	3-10 minutes
INR	0.8-1.1
Therapeutic anticoagulation	2.0-3.0
aPTT	30-40 seconds
Therapeutic anticoagulation	1.5-2.5 times normal
ACT	70-120 seconds
Therapeutic anticoagulation	150-210 seconds
Fibrinogen	200-400 mg/dL
D-dimer	<1.37 nmol/L
Thromboelastogram (TEG)	
Reaction time (R time)	7.5-15 minutes
K time	3-6 minutes
a angle	45 degrees
Maximum amplitude (MA)	5 = 60 mm

Abbreviations: ACT, activated clotting time; aPTT, activated partial thromboplastin time; Hct, hematocrit; Hgb, hemoglobin; Ig, immunoglobulin; INR, international normalized ratio; MCH, mean corpuscular hemoglobin; MCHC, mean corpuscular hemoglobin concentration; MCV, mean corpuscular volume; RBC, red blood cell count; RDW, red blood cell distribution width; WBC, white blood cell count.
[a]*Normal values vary between laboratories. Refer to local laboratory standard values when interpreting test results.*

the amount of Hgb indicates anemia. Anemia can be due to many factors, including decreased production or increased destruction of RBCs, loss of RBCs by bleeding, vitamin B_{12} deficiency, and folate and/or iron deficiency. An increase in the total number of RBCs occurs as a compensatory mechanism in chronic hypoxia, as an adaptation to high altitude, iron overload, and in some malignant blood disorders. Further assessment of the ability of the bone marrow to produce RBCs is obtained by a reticulocyte count. Reticulocytes are immature RBCs that are released from the bone marrow. Normally they are present in the blood in small amounts. They mature in 1 to 2 days and prior to their maturation they are not as effective as mature red cells. When there is anemia or blood loss, the bone marrow produces more reticulocytes causing reticulocytosis (an increase in reticulocytes).

Hemoglobin

Hemoglobin is a complex iron-containing protein, which carries oxygen to body tissues and carbon dioxide back to the lungs. As the number of RBCs change, so does the Hgb content. A decline in Hgb to a level as low as 7 g/dL may be well tolerated in some patients, while in others, a decline can result in significant symptoms. The rate at which the decline in Hgb level occurs often influences the symptoms and tolerance of the patient. A decline that occurs gradually over time is often tolerated, whereas a rapid decline frequently results in more severe symptoms. Older adults and those with underlying cardiac or pulmonary disorders may become symptomatic with even small changes in the Hgb content of the blood.

Hematocrit

Hematocrit measures the RBC mass in relationship to a volume of blood and is expressed as the percentage of cells per 100 mL of blood. Multiplying the Hgb value by 3 gives an estimate of Hct. The Hct is particularly sensitive to changes in the volume status of the patient. It increases with fluid losses (hemoconcentration) and decreases with increased plasma volume (hemodilution). Interpretation of Hgb and Hct results must take into account the time the values were obtained in relationship to blood volume loss, fluid loss, and/or fluid administration; for example, values obtained immediately after an acute hemorrhage may appear normal, because compensatory mechanisms have not had time to restore plasma volume. Restoration of plasma volume by compensation or crystalloid resuscitation lowers the Hgb and Hct.

Red Blood Cell Indices

The RBC indices (mean corpuscular volume, mean corpuscular hemoglobin, mean corpuscular hemoglobin concentration, and RBC distribution width) are measurements of the size, weight, and Hgb concentration of the individual erythrocytes. These indices are useful in determining the etiology of anemia.

Total White Blood Cell Count

Leukocytes, or WBCs circulating in the blood, are measured as an indicator of the total number of WBCs in the body. Most WBCs are not sampled in a CBC because they are marginated along capillary walls, circulating in the lymphatic system, or residing in lymph nodes and other body tissues.

Increased WBCs, or *leukocytosis*, is usually caused by an elevation in one type of WBC. It is most often associated with a normal immune system response to an acute infection, but is also an expected result of other inflammatory processes. Increases in WBCs are known to have both positive and negative effects. Positive effects include phagocytosis of microorganisms in fighting an infection. Potentially destructive effects include the release of reactive oxygen species from neutrophils and excessive amounts of cytokines from macrophages causing damage of healthy tissue, and cell death. An abnormal production of leukocytes in the bone marrow occurs in leukemia.

Leukopenia refers to a decrease in the total WBC number. This occurs when bone marrow production is inhibited or when certain infections lead to rapid consumption of WBCs. The life span of a circulating WBC is only hours to days; therefore, a constant replacement process is necessary to prevent leukopenia and immune compromise, which can result in infection and harm to the patient.

White Blood Cell Differential

The differential is a measure of five different categories of leukocytes, with each type reported as a percentage of the total WBC count. The absolute count for each category of white cell (also referred to a cell line) is calculated by multiplying the percentage of each type of cell by the total WBC count. Increases or decreases in any one cell line help evaluate normal immune response and predict impaired immunity.

Neutrophils, or segmented neutrophils (also known as "segs"), are the primary responders to infection and inflammation in the body. They also are an accurate indicator of how the immune system is functioning. With active infections, the bone marrow also releases an immature form of neutrophil called a "band." Bands quickly mature into segmented neutrophils which have greater phagocytic properties to respond to infection. Leukocytosis is usually caused by an increased number of segmented neutrophils and is called neutrophilia. A "left shift" refers to leukocytosis with an increased percentage of bands. Neutropenia, or a decreased number of circulating neutrophils, places the body at increased risk for infection. An absolute neutrophil count (ANC = WBC × [% segmented neutrophils + % segmented bands] × 10) of less than 1000 cells/μL severely compromises immune system response, particularly to bacterial infections.

Monocytes are large phagocytic cells that circulate briefly in the blood before maturing into macrophages which then typically reside in body tissues. These leukocytes are important scavengers of microorganisms and other foreign materials. They also activate lymphocytes by presenting antigens to T cells.

Lymphocytes are the WBCs responsible for the body's adaptive (specific) immune responses. Subsets of T and B lymphocytes are assessed by specific cell counts. Lack of properly functioning lymphocytes or inadequate numbers of these cells places the body at risk for bacterial, viral, and fungal infections, and certain malignancies. The CD4 cell is a subset of lymphocytes. It is the target of human immunodeficiency virus (HIV) infection leading to the development of acquired immunodeficiency syndrome (AIDS).

Eosinophils increase in numbers and activity during parasitic infections and allergic responses. They attach to parasites and use enzymes to kill them. Increased percentages of these cells are also seen during an allergic response. Basophils are another WBC associated with allergy. They break down during allergic reactions, releasing their intracellular contents such as heparin and histamine, resulting in the allergic symptoms of itching, hives, erythema, swollen mucous membranes, etc.

Platelet Count

The platelet count is determined by the number of platelets per microliter of blood. Platelets are called *thrombocytes* because of their role in the initiation of blood coagulation at the site of damaged blood vessel walls. Two-thirds of the body's platelets are circulating in the blood, with the remaining one-third sequestered within the spleen. Thrombocytopenia (decreased number of platelets) is associated with increased risk of spontaneous bleeding and is caused by decreased production, increased consumption, or excessive destruction of platelets. Hypercoagulability of the blood can result from increased circulating platelets caused by proliferative disorders, malignancies, and inflammation. Qualitative assessment of platelet function is determined by the bleeding time.

Coagulation Studies

International Normalized Ratio

The INR evaluates the final coagulation pathway and the time it takes to form a blood clot. The INR is a calculation developed to standardize interpretation of a previously used test called the prothrombin time (PT). The PT and INR may be reported together, but the INR is the recommended parameter for establishing the therapeutic range for warfarin therapy. The INR is a general test of coagulation, and will be elevated in patients with liver disease, biliary tract disease, and those who are therapeutically anticoagulated with warfarin and sometimes in patients on direct oral anticoagulants as well. It is also elevated in patients with coagulopathies such as disseminated intravascular coagulation (DIC).

Activated Partial Thromboplastin Time

The activated partial thromboplastin time (aPTT) is reported in seconds and is used to evaluate fibrin clot formation stimulated by the pathways of coagulation. This test is used to screen for congenital coagulation disorders and for monitoring anticoagulation with unfractionated (IV) heparin therapy. Prolonged aPTT is also noted in persons with liver disease, vitamin K deficiency, and DIC.

Activated Coagulation Time

The activated coagulation time (ACT) is reported in seconds. The test is used most commonly to monitor effects of unfractionated heparin during and following cardiovascular procedures such as cardiopulmonary bypass and percutaneous coronary interventions. It is generally performed at the point of care.

Fibrinogen

The fibrinogen level is tested during evaluation for bleeding disorders. Fibrinogen is the plasma protein that becomes the fibrin clot. Plasma levels of fibrinogen may be increased during an inflammatory response, pregnancy, or acute infection. Decreased levels are present with liver disease and DIC.

D-Dimer

D-dimer is a very specific indicator of fibrinolysis, the natural process that breaks down fibrin clots. Levels of D-dimer are elevated in thrombotic disorders such as deep venous thrombosis (DVT) and pulmonary emboli (PE). Levels are also elevated during thrombolytic drug therapy and in DIC. It is important to recognize that in addition to pathological conditions, D-dimer is elevated postoperatively and any time a patient has clots that are being broken down by the fibrinolytic process.

Thromboelastogram

Thromboelastography (TEG) testing may be performed to assess clotting activity in patients with coagulopathies such as DIC. This test can be performed at the bedside to evaluate clot formation, clot strength, and breakdown (fibrinolysis).

Additional Tests and Procedures

After obtaining basic laboratory screening tests, additional diagnostic testing is necessary to identify specific disorders in hematologic and immune function. For patients with hematologic disorders, a bone marrow aspiration, or further studies of specific clotting factor assays may be performed. For those with suspected immune disorders, immunoglobulin quantification studies may be indicated.

Blood, sputum, urine, and wound specimens for Gram stain and culture help identify sources of infection. Molecular diagnostic techniques such as polymerase chain reaction (PCR) detect infectious agents not readily cultured, such as viruses. Noninvasive studies such as ultrasound may determine liver, spleen, or lymph node abnormalities. Radiologic procedures (radiographs, CT scans, arteriograms) may be needed to identify malignancy, infection, or hemorrhage.

Pathologic Conditions

Critically and acutely ill patients often have combined abnormalities involving the hematologic and immune systems. The patient with sepsis and subsequent DIC in the Essential Content Case in this chapter typifies this situation. Anemia, immune compromise, and coagulopathy are three distinct problems faced in the management of this patient. Each of these problems poses major threats to the patient's potential outcome and is evaluated separately.

Anemia

Etiology, Risk Factors, and Pathophysiology

Anemia is defined as a Hgb count less than 13.5 gm/dL in a man or less than 12.0 gm/dL in a woman and is the most common hematologic disorder. Its etiology may be classified into disorders of RBC production, increased destruction of RBCs, or acute blood loss.

A patient history gives important clues to the etiology of anemia. Decreased production may result from nutritional deficiencies in substrates necessary for RBC production such as iron, folic acid, or vitamin B_{12}. Those at high risk for iron deficiency anemia include children, adolescents, older adults, pregnant women, and patients with malabsorption syndromes. Folic acid deficiency is common in alcoholics. Dietary vitamin B_{12} deficiency may occur in strict vegetarians and also occurs due to a lack of intrinsic factors (postgastrectomy, gastric bypass, or with pernicious anemia) or Crohn disease. Another common cause of anemia is chronic blood loss from the gastrointestinal (GI) tract or from heavy menstruation. Daily blood testing in hospitalized patients may also contribute to anemia because the patient's bone marrow cannot keep up with the loss.

Anemia may be associated with chronic illnesses such as renal failure and cancer. Patients with renal failure experience anemia because of reduced production of the hormone erythropoietin. Without adequate erythropoietin, the bone marrow is not stimulated to produce RBCs. Cancer that specifically involves the bone marrow may replace normal bone marrow with malignant cells, disturb the development and maturation process of blood cells, and fill the marrow with immature cells that prevent RBC generation.

Anemia can also occur in cancer patients as a result of treatment-induced bone marrow suppression. Here the bone marrow fails to produce cells, sometimes causing a drop in all three types of blood cells (WBC, RBC, and platelets) known as *pancytopenia*. Medications such as chemotherapeutic agents and some antibiotics suppress the bone marrow and cause anemia. Other causes of anemia include radiation therapy to marrow-producing bones such as the sternum and other long bones in the body. In addition to renal failure and cancer, other chronic disease states may decrease the lifespan of RBCs leading to anemia when production of new cells by the bone marrow cannot keep up with the losses.

Hemolytic anemia results from excessive destruction of RBCs. This can occur episodically or chronically.

Abnormalities intrinsic to the RBCs are usually the result of hereditary causes of hemolytic anemia, such as sickle cell disease. Extrinsic sources of hemolysis include immune destruction from an adverse reaction to a medication or a blood transfusion, splenic disorders, damage by artificial heart valves, cardiopulmonary bypass, or use of an intra-aortic balloon pump.

Sickle cell anemia is an inherited Hgb disorder that results in chronic hemolytic anemia and occlusion of blood vessels. The problem is most prevalent in patients who identify as African American and can manifest itself as sickle cell trait, or the more serious sickle cell disease beginning in early childhood. During episodes of low oxygen tension or other stressors such as infection, the RBCs change their shape (to a sickle rather than rounded shape) and adhere to the endothelial lining of blood vessels where they activate coagulation. This results in hemolytic anemia, blood vessel occlusion, and ischemic pain in organs and tissues, a syndrome referred to as *sickle cell crisis*. Management of these crises often includes hospitalization for pain management, hydration, anticoagulation, and blood transfusion. Other complications of sickle cell disease include bone disorders, injury to the spleen, and stroke. Specialists in hematology are included in the management of patients with sickle cell anemia. General principles of management include infection prevention, nutrition, and pain management. Hydroxyurea is a cytotoxic drug that can reduce the number of painful crises and hospitalizations and increase survival. Hematopoietic cell transplantation is the only curative treatment option available.

Acute hemorrhage rapidly leads to anemia. Trauma, surgical blood loss, coagulopathy, GI bleeding, and bleeding related to anticoagulation are frequently encountered as causes of anemia in critically and acutely ill patient populations. With acute hemorrhage, both cellular components and plasma are lost simultaneously. The remaining cells are normal (normocytic, normochromic) and the main problem is an insufficient number of RBCs. Until volume replacement from fluid resuscitation or mobilization of fluids from extracellular sources occurs, a drop in Hct may not be appreciated. Following an episode of blood loss, the reticulocyte count will generally rise as newly produced immature RBCs are released into the circulation. Rapid loss of blood volume results in hypovolemic shock and cardiovascular instability, further reducing delivery of oxygen to body tissues.

Regardless of the etiology of an anemia, the critical effect of decreased RBCs and Hgb is a decrease in the oxygen-carrying capacity of the blood and a reduction in oxygen content. This may be tolerated if anemia develops slowly and the body can compensate, but may be life threatening if sudden blood loss occurs resulting in shock or cardiopulmonary collapse.

Clinical Signs and Symptoms

Clinical manifestations are related to the body's compensatory mechanisms that attempt to maintain perfusion of oxygen to vital tissues. Clinical manifestations may not be obvious until the Hgb level is less than 7 g/dL. As compensatory mechanisms are overwhelmed, serious signs and symptoms occur. Patients with pulmonary and cardiovascular system disease are less likely to tolerate the effects of anemia and will become symptomatic more quickly.

Cardiovascular

- Tachycardia, palpitations
- Angina
- Decreased capillary refill
- Orthostatic hypotension
- ECG abnormalities (arrhythmias, ischemic changes)
- Hypovolemic shock (hypotension, tachycardia, decreased cardiac output, increased systemic vascular resistance)

Respiratory

- Increased respiratory rate
- Dyspnea on exertion, progressing to dyspnea at rest

Skin/Musculoskeletal

- Pallor of skin and mucous membranes
- Dusky nail beds
- Decreased skin temperature

Neurologic

- Headache
- Light-headedness
- Ringing in the ears (tinnitus)
- Syncope
- Irritability/agitation
- Restlessness
- Severe fatigue

Abdominal

- Enlarged liver and/or spleen
- Anorexia, nausea, vomiting, pica (craving for inedible or non-nutritional items: ice, clay, soil, paper)

Principles of Management of Anemia

Management of the anemic patient must be guided by the severity of symptoms. Evaluating a change in Hgb and Hct includes assessment of the patient's clinical status and risk of active bleeding. Restoration of adequate blood volume to assure oxygen delivery to the tissues is a priority in critically and acutely ill patients. Identification of the etiology of anemia and resolution of the underlying cause is done simultaneously.

Improving Oxygen Delivery

Oxygen delivery is a product of the amount of Hgb in the blood, the saturation of the Hgb with oxygen, and the cardiac output. Management strategies focus on optimizing each of those components.

1. Administration of supplemental oxygen can increase oxygen saturation. Use of oxygen, particularly during activity, may minimize desaturation and dyspnea.

TABLE 13-2. SUMMARY OF CURRENT GUIDELINE RECOMMENDATIONS ON RED BLOOD CELL TRANSFUSION

1. Decisions regarding the need for transfusion of red blood cells should include assessment of the patient's clinical status, patient preference, and alternative therapy.
2. For hospitalized patients, including the critically ill, who are hemodynamically stable, a restrictive transfusion threshold of 7 g/dL should be used. A threshold of 8 g/dL is recommended for patients with preexisting cardiovascular disease and those undergoing cardiac or orthopedic surgery.
3. Regarding the storage time of blood, patients should receive units of blood selected at any time within the licensed dating period (standard issue).

Data from Carson JL, Guyatt G, Heddle NM, et al: Clinical Practice Guidelines From the AABB: Red Blood Cell Transfusion Thresholds and Storage. JAMA. 2016;316(19):2025-2035.

2. Adequate Hgb can be replaced in acute situations only by transfusion of RBCs. Transfusion of packed red blood cells (PRBCs) is considered when blood loss is severe, the patient is actively bleeding, or when the patient is very symptomatic. Table 13-2 lists the indications for transfusion.
3. Cardiac output can be optimized with volume replacement, including PRBCs, in situations of bleeding and hypovolemia. Other interventions to improve cardiac output may be guided by hemodynamic monitoring and are discussed in Chapter 4.
4. Monitoring vital signs, oxygen saturation, and subjective patient data before, during, and after a change in therapy or activity identifies the patient's ability to tolerate anemia.
5. Limiting strenuous activity and planning periods of rest are important nursing interventions for the anemic patient.

Identifying and Treating Underlying Disease State

Further diagnostic testing may be indicated to determine the etiology of anemia. Radiologic and endoscopic studies to locate sites of bleeding, particularly in the GI tract, may be necessary. Treatment of the underlying cause of anemia may include the following:

1. Administer recombinant human erythropoietin to restore bone marrow production of RBCs in chronic anemia. The response may take several weeks, so it may not be appropriate in situations in which acute correction of anemia is necessary. Chronic kidney disease patients may benefit from this treatment.
2. Supplemental oral or parenteral iron replacement may be indicated if iron deficiency anemia is present. Iron depletion is used therapeutically in treating porphyria and iron overload disorders.
3. Vitamin B_{12} and folic acid–related anemia may also require oral or parenteral supplementation.
4. Dietary consultation may be needed prior to discharge to help patients and families plan meals with foods high in iron, folate, or B_{12}.

Minimizing Iatrogenic Blood Loss and Reducing the Need for Transfusion

1. Use small volume collection tubes and microanalysis techniques.
2. Assess the need for routine and additional blood testing to decrease diagnostic blood loss.
3. Use blood salvage systems in surgical patients.
4. Assess the risk of GI bleeding and use prophylactic agents to reduce the risk of GI bleeding if indicated.
5. Screen all patients for anticoagulants and bleeding risk prior to procedures.
6. Accept normovolemic anemia in hemodynamically stable, asymptomatic patients.

Immunocompromise

Etiology, Risk Factors, and Pathophysiology

All patients in critical care and progressive care units have a high risk for infection because their defense mechanisms are limited by underlying disease, medical therapy, nutritional status, age, and/or physiological stress. The term *immunocompromised* is applied to patients whose immune mechanisms are defective or inadequate. The patient with immunocompromise is more likely to develop an opportunistic infection. Once infection develops, it may quickly progress to sepsis.

Immune system protection from infection is categorized into three levels: natural defenses, innate (general) immunity, and adaptive (specific) immunity. Natural defenses include having intact epithelial surfaces (skin and mucous membranes) with normal chemical barriers (pH, secretions) present and all protective reflexes (blink, swallow, cough, gag, and sneeze) intact. The invasive catheters and tubes used in critical and acute care units bypass these protective barriers and allow introduction of pathogens.

When natural defenses are bypassed or overwhelmed, the innate response to infection is activated. Phagocytic WBCs (neutrophils and monocytes) attack microorganisms marked by foreign proteins (antigens). The macrophages also play a key role in processing the invading antigen and presenting it to the lymphocytes involved in the adaptive immune response.

Lymphocytes (B cells and T cells) are responsible for the orchestration of an immune response specific to each microorganism based on its particular antigen. B lymphocytes create antigen-specific antibodies or immunoglobulins to aid in the recognition and destruction of the invading microorganism and to protect the body from future encounters with the antigen. This is called *humoral immunity*. T lymphocytes have different subsets of cells created to modulate the immune system response (including CD4 helper T cells) and cells that have cytotoxic properties, the CD8 T cells. The immune response of the T lymphocytes is called *cell-mediated immunity*. Both types of lymphocytes work closely together in a specific immune response. However, humoral immunity is the primary protection against bacterial invasion and cell-mediated immunity is effective against infection by viral and fungal organisms, and some malignancies.

Additionally, T cells are primarily involved in the rejection of foreign tissue and in delayed hypersensitivity reactions.

Deficiencies in immune system function can be categorized into primary, or congenital, immune system defects and secondary, or acquired, immune system dysfunction. Immune deficiencies may be pinpointed to a specific cell type, a specific antibody, or they may involve abnormalities in multiple components of the immune system. Secondary or acquired immunodeficiencies are the most likely type encountered in critical and acute care patients. Acquired immunodeficiency may be secondary to age, malnutrition, stress, chronic disease states, medications with immunosuppressive effects, cancer and its treatment, HIV infection, and other factors.

Today, an increased number of patients are undergoing organ transplantation and receiving immunosuppressive agents, in the transplant setting and treatment of autoimmune disorders and certain cancers. Patients who receive organ transplants require lifelong immunosuppressive drug therapy to prevent recognition and rejection of the transplanted tissue by the immune system. Patients typically receive a combination of drugs that affect various components of the immune response. Higher doses are required during the first weeks and months after the transplant. Depending on the type of transplant and the patient's history of rejection episodes, doses are decreased over time to minimize the risk of infection and other complications. Acute cellular rejection may be diagnosed by evidence of failure of the transplanted organ (such as elevated serum creatinine and decreased urine output in a kidney recipient) or by obtaining a biopsy diagnostic of rejection. Rejection is commonly treated by augmented immunosuppression, such as a series of doses of IV methylprednisolone. During and following treatment, these patients are at high risk for infection. Immunosuppressive agents are also used in the management of other disorders such as rheumatoid arthritis, lupus, and other autoimmune diseases.

As new regimens and new chemotherapy agents are used to treat cancer, many of these agents have the potential to produce significant bone marrow suppression and target the body's immune response. More aggressive chemotherapeutic treatment of cancer has led to higher numbers of patients with bone marrow suppression. These patients are at high risk for the development of complications, including pancytopenia, neutropenia, and sepsis.

Neutropenia refers to the state in which the ANC is less than 1500 or 1000 cells/μL, and severe neutropenia is usually defined as an ANC less than 500 cells/μL or an ANC that is expected to decrease to less than 500 cells/μL over the next 48 hours leading to increased susceptibility to infection and sometimes neutropenic fever and sepsis. Many factors contribute to the susceptibility of the neutropenic patient to develop an infection. This includes the cause and duration of neutropenia, functional capability of the existing neutrophils, the patient's defense mechanisms and natural barriers to infection, and endogenous and exogenous flora. The key to preventing severe infection and sepsis is patient education, early detection, and intervention.

Detection of infection in the immunocompromised patient may be difficult since the body's defense mechanisms are suppressed. Lack of neutrophils impairs the patient's ability to mount a vigorous inflammatory response, and classic signs and symptoms of infection may be diminished or absent. Redness, febrile response, or even the development of pus may not occur because purulent drainage is largely the result of dying neutrophils at the site of infection. The neutropenic patient can be severely infected and on the verge of becoming septic, and their only complaint may be malaise, somnolence, or pain.

Fever in this patient population is another key sign of infection and warrants aggressive investigation. Since development of fever may not be possible and some patients may even be hypothermic, the nurse must be keenly aware of other signs of sepsis including alterations in mental status, blood pressure, pulse, and respiratory rate that are the result of compensatory mechanisms. The rapid onset of sepsis in a neutropenic patient requires meticulous and frequent assessment to ensure early intervention, as these patients do not present or respond as those with a functional, normal immune system.

HIV is another disorder that leads to immunocompromise. It initially affects helper T cells, decreasing their number and function. This in turn has a profound effect on adaptive immunity. Following diagnosis, the CD4 cells are monitored, and a CD4 count of less than 200/μL is associated with a higher risk of complications. Viral load testing is also performed to measure the number of viral particles per microliter of blood. As patients receive antiretroviral therapy, the CD4 count may normalize and the viral load decrease. Patients with HIV may progress to having AIDS in which they are susceptible to opportunistic infections and certain malignancies. Antiretroviral therapy reduces the progression of HIV infection to AIDS and increases life expectancy. Patients with HIV may require hospital admission for the management of an opportunistic infection, an adverse reaction to antiretroviral therapy, or for a condition or surgery unrelated to their HIV infection.

Clinical Signs and Symptoms[1]

Local Evidence of Inflammation and Infection

- Redness
- Edema
- Warmth
- Pain
- Purulent drainage

---

[1]As noted earlier, immune-compromised patients may not show any of these clinical signs and symptoms of infection. The neutropenic patient may have very subtle signs of sepsis; thus heightened vigilance is necessary to expedite treatment.

General Evidence of Infection

- Fever or hypothermia
- Rigors or shaking chills
- Fatigue and malaise
- Changes in level of consciousness
- Lymphadenopathy
- Tachycardia
- Tachypnea

System-Specific Evidence

Neurologic

- Headache
- Nuchal rigidity
- Changes in mentation, agitation

Respiratory

- Cough
- Change in color, amount of sputum
- Dyspnea, orthopnea
- Pain in chest or pleura

Genitourinary

- Dysuria
- Urgency
- Frequency
- Flank pain
- Abdominal pain
- Cloudy and/or bloody urine

Gastrointestinal

- Nausea
- Vomiting
- Diarrhea
- Cramping abdominal pain
- Enlarged liver or spleen
- Oral or pharyngeal lesions

Principles of Management for Immunocompromised Patients

Patients at high risk for infection must be identified on admission. Measures to protect and strengthen immune system function are included in the plan of care. All healthcare team members must utilize measures to prevent the development of hospital-associated infections. Close monitoring for signs and symptoms of a local or systemic inflammatory response is especially important to ensure early detection of infection. Identification of the source and likely organisms causing infection allows for initiation of broad-spectrum, empiric antimicrobial coverage. Culture and sensitivity reports guide the choice of antimicrobials specific to the infecting organisms. Care is planned to reduce the risk of exposure to pathogens. Hand washing is the main intervention for the prevention of infection. Additionally, the number of lines, tubes, and drains is minimized when possible. Although central lines, indwelling catheters, and other devices are commonplace in critical care settings, the nurse must be vigilant to constantly evaluate the ongoing need for such devices.

Identification of Patients With High Risk of Infection

Risk factors for immunocompromise are as follows:

1. Neonates and older adults
2. Malnutrition
3. Use of medications with known immunosuppressive effects such as glucocorticoids, cancer chemotherapeutic agents, monoclonal antibodies, and transplant immunosuppressive agents
4. Recent radiation therapy to areas of the body that impact bone marrow production
5. Chronic systemic diseases such as renal or hepatic failure or diabetes
6. Diseases involving the immune system such as HIV infection
7. Loss of protective epithelial barriers through:
   - Oral or nasogastric intubation
   - Presence of pressure injuries
   - Burns
   - Surgical wounds
   - Skin and soft tissue trauma
   - Mucositis
   - Altered lymphatics (prior surgery removing lymph nodes)
8. Invasive catheters or prosthetic devices in place such as:
   - Intravascular catheters, including peripheral, central, and arterial lines
   - Indwelling urinary catheters
   - Endotracheal intubation and mechanical ventilation
   - Heart valve replacements
   - Orthopedic hardware such as artificial joints, pins, plates, or screws
   - Dialysis, apheresis catheters, shunts, fistulas, or grafts
   - Cardiovascular devices such as ventricular-assist devices, pacemakers, or implantable defibrillators
   - Ventricular shunts
9. Frequent hospitalizations

Implementing Measures to Protect and Strengthen Immune System Function

1. Take meticulous care of the skin and mucous membranes to prevent loss of barrier protection.
2. Use the enteral route for feeding to maintain caloric intake and normal gut function.
3. Avoid the use of indwelling urinary catheters or remove them as early as possible.
4. Minimize patient stress and the release of endogenous glucocorticoids by relieving pain or using alternative methods such as guided imagery or music for relaxation, and other comfort measures (positioning, massage).
5. Administer colony-stimulating factors (granulocyte colony-stimulating factor [G-CSF] or granulocyte/macrophage colony-stimulating factor [GM-CSF])

to stimulate bone marrow production of neutrophils and monocytes, when appropriate.

6. Administer medications for patients at risk for chemotherapy-induced bone marrow suppression as appropriate (such as trilaciclib for patients with small-cell lung cancer).

7. Administer granulocyte transfusion according to hospital protocol.

8. Administer prophylactic antimicrobials as appropriate (such as trimethoprim-sulfamethoxazole for prevention of pneumocystis pneumonia).

Implementing Measures to Prevent Infection

1. Educate patients, families, and colleagues about the importance of hand washing, the primary method of preventing hospital-associated infection. All personnel and visitors are to wash their hands before and after contact with the patient.

2. Use private rooms for patients at high risk. Use of protective attire such as masks may be employed according to specific hospital protocol.

3. Institute respiratory hygiene/cough etiquette for patients with signs of respiratory infection and appropriate isolation for known or suspected patient infection.

4. Adhere to strict aseptic technique in the care of intravascular catheters and during any invasive procedures.

5. Eliminate environmental sources of infection (eg, leftover fluids used for irrigations). Clean surfaces frequently with recommended disinfectant, including bedside table, equipment, and any surfaces where contamination is likely to occur.

6. Track the date and time fluids, tubings, and catheters are initiated and change them according to hospital protocol.

7. Provide healthy food choices and supplements if prescribed to enhance nutrition. Review hospital protocol regarding use of filtered water, appropriate cleaning of fresh fruits and vegetables, and other neutropenic precautions.

8. Encourage use of incentive spirometry, turning, deep breathing, and progressive mobility.

9. Promote recommended immunizations for preventable diseases such as influenza and pneumonia.

Early Detection of Local or System Inflammatory Response and Sepsis

1. Monitor the patient closely for signs and symptoms consistent with infection and sepsis and communicate abnormal findings to the interprofessional team.

2. Initiate the hospital's sepsis protocol, when indicated.

3. Collect specimens for culture and sensitivity from potential sources of infection (eg, urine, sputum, blood, stool, wound drainage).

4. Institute antibiotic therapy as directed. See Chapter 11, Multisystem Problems, for more information on the management of sepsis.

Coagulopathies

Etiology, Risk Factors, and Pathophysiology

Patients may develop coagulopathy due to disorders involving platelets, hemostasis, thrombosis, fibrinolysis, or a combination of abnormalities. Acquired disorders of coagulation, as opposed to inherited disorders, are more frequent in critical care and acute care units.

Thrombocytopenia

Platelets initiate the coagulation process at the site of blood vessel injury. Quantitative platelet disorders are associated with bleeding when the platelet count drops to less than 50,000/µL, especially if there is tissue trauma. Spontaneous bleeding is possible at counts of less than 20,000/µL, and counts of 5000 to 10,000/µL create a high risk for hemorrhage. Four general mechanisms are responsible for thrombocytopenia: (1) decreased production of platelets by the bone marrow, (2) shortened survival due to platelet utilization and destruction, (3) sequestration of platelets in the spleen, and (4) intravascular dilution of platelets during transfusion of multiple units of blood and components.

Thrombocytopenia may also be related to immune mechanisms. Drug-induced thrombocytopenia occurs when a drug causes an antigen-antibody reaction. This reaction leads to the formation of immune complexes that destroy platelets by complement-mediated lysis. There are several other types of immune-related thrombocytopenia that are seen in critical and acute care. Heparin-induced thrombocytopenia (HIT) is an immune-mediated reaction to heparin that results in the formation of antiplatelet antibodies that activate platelets and form clots. This then leads to platelet consumption and a precipitous drop in the platelet count. The patient may develop intravascular clotting resulting in clinical thrombosis. Venous thrombosis is most common and may result in limb ischemia and PE. When this syndrome is suspected, all heparin is stopped, and confirmatory testing for HIT antibodies is performed. Treatment options include administration of direct thrombin inhibitors such as argatroban. Patients diagnosed with HIT should not receive heparin again.

Immune thrombocytopenic purpura (ITP) is an acquired disorder that results in the production of IgG autoantibodies that attack glycoproteins on platelet membranes, destroying the platelets. This disorder was formerly called idiopathic thrombocytopenia, but was renamed when it was identified as an immune process. In adults, ITP may occur as a primary disorder or may be secondary to medications, viral infections, or autoimmune disorders such as systemic lupus erythematosus. For some, the cause may never be determined. Patients may develop petechiae, purpura, and epistaxis. Severe bleeding is possible, especially when the platelet count is less than 20,000/µL. Treatment options include glucocorticoids, intravenous immune globulin (IVIG), administration of rituximab, platelet stimulating agents, platelet transfusion, and in some cases, splenectomy.

Thrombotic thrombocytopenic purpura (TTP) is a syndrome characterized by thrombocytopenia, hemolytic anemia, renal failure, fever, and neurologic changes. The cause of this disorder is a deficiency of the enzyme ADAMTS13 leading to excessive platelet aggregation and binding to the endothelium of blood vessels. Patients with TTP develop widespread vascular occlusion in organs, as well as jaundice, purpura, petechiae, and bleeding. Acutely ill individuals may be treated with plasmapheresis.

Hemolytic-uremic syndrome is characterized by thrombocytopenia, hemolytic anemia, and renal failure. It is most often the result of infectious colitis and the toxin released from *Escherichia coli* 0157:H7. Children and older adults are most seriously affected by this syndrome, and will require hospitalization for supportive care including dialysis.

Patients may have adequate numbers of platelets but still have a bleeding tendency due to qualitative platelet disorders. Drug-induced suppression of platelet function is commonly associated with use of aspirin, clopidogrel, fish oil, vitamin E, and other agents. Renal failure, uremia,

ESSENTIAL CONTENT CASE

Sepsis and Disseminated Intravascular Coagulation

A 72-year-old Caucasian man is admitted to the medical intensive care unit (MICU) with hypotension, fever (102°F), vomiting, and altered mental status. He has a history of chronic lymphocytic leukemia (not currently on active treatment), prostatic hypertrophy, and peptic ulcer disease. He is disoriented to place and time. Initial assessment data include BP 80/62 mm Hg, HR 120 beats/min, RR 36 breaths/min and labored, and a small amount of cloudy urine per catheter. A dressing covering his intravascular venous port shows tan drainage and redness around the site. Nasogastric aspirate is coffee ground in appearance. His initial laboratory data include:

Hemoglobin	10.8 g/dL
Hematocrit	31%
WBC	13,000/μL, with 52% segmented neutrophils and 20% bands
Platelets	90,000/μL
Fibrinogen	175 mg/dL
INR	2.0
aPTT	60 seconds
D-dimer	2.05 nmol/L

Eight hours later, after administration of fluids and initiation of a norepinephrine infusion, the patient's BP is 102/84 mm Hg, heart rate is 104 beats/min, and respiratory rate is 24 breaths/min on continuous positive airway pressure (CPAP) via mask. The lab work is repeated.

Hemoglobin	8.2 mg/dL
Hematocrit	25%
WBC	11,500/μL
Platelets	92,000/μL
Fibrinogen	204 mg/dL
INR	1.8

Case Question 1: What are this patient's risk factors for hematologic and immune problems?

Case Question 2: What diagnostic testing should be done?

Case Question 3: Identify the therapeutic interventions that are the highest priority.

Case Question 4: Analyze the patient's initial lab work and outline how the values provide diagnostic information.

Case Question 5: Analyze the subsequent lab work and explain how results will be used to evaluate the response to interventions.

Case Question 6: Outline criteria and considerations for blood and transfusion therapy in this patient.

Case Question 7: What types of consultations should be ordered?

Case Question 8: What should the nursing assessment focus on?

Answers

1. The patient's leukemia and the treatment for it are risk factors for chronic immunosuppression and anemia. Prostate hypertrophy is a risk factor for urinary tract infection. Peptic ulcer disease is a risk factor for GI bleeding and subsequent anemia.
2. Diagnostic testing should include serial CBC to establish a trend in blood cell counts, Hgb and Hct, coagulation panel to evaluate clotting time, and cultures of urine, blood, and the intravascular access venous port.
3. Initial therapeutic interventions should include IV fluids, empiric antibiotics, oxygen, and use of the hospital's sepsis protocol.
4. The low Hgb and Hct indicate anemia. The elevated WBC with increased bands indicates acute infection in most patients, but may be chronically elevated in leukemia. A comparison with the patient's baseline WBC is needed. The low platelet count, low fibrinogen, high INR, and high aPTT suggest coagulopathy. The elevation in D-dimer indicates fibrinolysis, and is another indication of clotting abnormality.
5. The repeat Hgb and Hct indicate worsening anemia, and prompt further examination of the patient for active bleeding. The WBC count remains elevated, suggesting continuing infection. The platelets, fibrinogen, and INR have improved, indicating the patient is responding to interventions.
6. Blood transfusion is indicated for patients who are hemodynamically unstable and do not stabilize with administrations of IV fluids. Transfusions are also indicated when there is evidence of active bleeding and inadequate tissue oxygenation.
7. An infection disease consultation and notification of his medical oncologist team.
8. Assessment focuses on the evaluation of potential sources of infection and clinical manifestations of infection, anemia, and coagulopathy.

and adverse reactions to medications can also contribute to impaired platelet function in critically ill patients.

Disorders of Hemostasis

Disorders of hemostasis also occur due to inherited abnormalities of coagulation factors. Hemophilia types A and B are congenital deficiencies of factors VIII and IX. Von Willebrand disease represents a deficiency or dysfunction of the plasma protein of the same name. In acute bleeding, replacement of the deficient factor is essential to limit blood loss. Patients with these disorders may require critical or progressive care when undergoing routine surgical procedures or when hospitalized for other medical problems.

Acquired coagulation disorders can be associated with deficient coagulation factor production. This may be caused by a decreased intake of vitamin K, the vitamin essential for the formation of clotting factors II, VII, IX, and X. Intestinal malabsorption, liver disease, use of warfarin, or antibiotic therapy can all contribute to vitamin K deficiency, leading to prolonged INR. Because most coagulation factors are produced in the liver, patients with liver disease have deficiencies of fibrinogen and other factors in addition to deficiencies of the vitamin K–dependent factors.

Many of the medications used routinely in hospitalized patients have anticoagulant and antiplatelet effects. Therapeutic anticoagulation using heparin, warfarin, and other agents interferes directly with the clotting process. Heparin inhibits the final clotting pathway and its key procoagulant thrombin. Decreasing the dose or temporarily stopping a heparin infusion is usually adequate to control minimal bleeding. If bleeding is severe, the antidote to reverse heparin, protamine sulfate, may be administered intravenously. Low-molecular-weight heparin is associated with fewer bleeding and immunological complications. See Table 13-3 for a list of anticoagulants commonly used in acute care and

Figure 9-7 in Chapter 9 provides a summary of their mechanism of action.

Warfarin acts by inhibiting the production of vitamin K–dependent clotting factors. Effects from warfarin take several days to be observed after initiation of the drug, but may persist for many days following administration. The dose of warfarin is titrated to a goal INR, necessitating routine laboratory evaluation for the duration of treatment. Patients who take warfarin are advised to use caution in consuming foods high in vitamin K. If significant bleeding occurs while on warfarin, replacement of vitamin K–dependent factors with transfusion of fresh frozen plasma or prothrombin complex concentrate (PCC) may be necessary. PCC is a lyophilized powder containing pooled factors. It can be quickly reconstituted for emergency administration and does not require ABO blood typing. Administration of oral or IV vitamin K may also be helpful, but its effectiveness depends on the time needed by the liver to synthesize new clotting factors.

Direct oral anticoagulant (DOAC) agents such as rivaroxaban and dabigatran act by inhibiting factor Xa and thrombin. They do not require laboratory monitoring and do not have dietary restrictions and thus have a lower treatment burden than warfarin. Evidence to date demonstrates that DOACs are equally effective as warfarin in the prevention of thromboembolism but carry a similar risk for bleeding. At this time, only dabigatran has a Food and Drug Administration (FDA) approved reversal agent, idarucizumab.

Thrombolytic agents such as alteplase or reteplase are used to dissolve pathologic clots such as venous thrombi, PE, or acute ischemic stroke. They can also cause bleeding from sites where a protective clot previously formed. These agents are used in combination with other anticoagulants, and may precipitate obvious or occult bleeding. Patients who receive these potent thrombolytics and anticoagulants are monitored for any sign of bleeding complications.

DIC is a complex coagulopathy that affects patients who already have another critical illness. See Table 13-4 for a list

TABLE 13-3. ANTICOAGULANTS COMMONLY USED IN ACUTE AND CRITICAL CARE

Classification	Drug
Factor Xa and thrombin inhibitor	Heparin sodium
Direct thrombin inhibitor	Argatroban Bivalirudin (Angiomax) Dabigatran (Pradaxa)
Factor Xa inhibitor	Apixaban (Eliquis) Fondaparinux (Arixtra) Rivaroxaban (Xarelto)
Vitamin K antagonist	Warfarin (Coumadin)
Glycoprotein IIb/IIIa inhibitors	Abciximab (ReoPro) Eptifibatide (Integrilin) Tirofiban (Aggrastat)
Thrombolytic agents	Alteplase (Activase) Reteplase (Retavase)
Antiplatelet agents	Aspirin Clopidogrel (Plavix) Dipyridamole (Persantine) Prasugrel (Effient) Ticagrelor (Brilinta)

TABLE 13-4. ETIOLOGIES OF DIC

Infection and Sepsis
- Acute bacterial
- Acute viral, fungal, parasitic

Trauma
- Head injury
- Crushing injury
- Snake venom

Cardiovascular
- Shock
- Extracorporeal circulation

Obstetrical
- Eclampsia and pre-eclampsia
- Amniotic fluid embolism
- Abortion

Immunological
- Blood transfusion reaction

Neoplastic Disease
- Acute leukemia
- Metastatic cancer

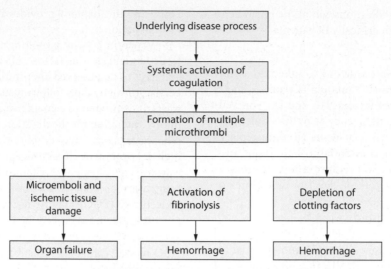

Figure 13-1. Clinical consequences of DIC.

of conditions that can precipitate DIC. The underlying condition triggers the release of proinflammatory cytokines, which activate the coagulation cascade and result in the formation of micro clots. The micro clots obstruct the capillaries of organs and tissues. This initiates a series of events that result in both bleeding and thrombosis. Figure 13-1 outlines the sequence of events that occur in DIC. Acute DIC and hemorrhage are seen in patients who are seriously ill with sepsis, traumatic injury, and extensive surgery. A chronic form of DIC and associated thrombosis may be seen in patients with cancer.

In DIC, stimulation of the clotting cascade rapidly depletes existing platelets and coagulation factors, consuming them faster than the body can replace them. Depletion of substrates of the coagulation process leaves the body at risk for spontaneous bleeding or hemorrhage from surgical sites, or even minimal trauma. Simultaneously, the multiple tiny clots formed in DIC flow to the small vessels where they are trapped. Microcirculatory thrombosis then leads to tissue ischemia, infarction, and organ dysfunction. Single or multisystem organ dysfunction may occur.

Activation of fibrinolysis in DIC releases the enzyme plasmin. Plasmin breaks down some of the fibrin in a physiologic attempt to open the microcirculation, and this produces fibrin degradation products, including D-dimer. Anticoagulant pathways are impaired, further interfering with the balance needed for appropriate hemostasis. Clots are unable to form at new sites of injury, and existing clots are dissolved, leading to bleeding from both old and new sites. Because of the complex pathophysiology, clinical manifestations of DIC are likely to include bleeding from multiple sites and evidence of organ ischemia due to microemboli. Ischemic injury to the skin may cause purpura and color changes in the hands and feet.

Diagnosis of DIC requires careful interpretation of coagulation panel results; there is no single definitive test. Table 13-5 lists the combination of results consistent with DIC. In many cases, absolute certainty regarding a diagnosis

of DIC may not be possible, especially in patients with other conditions, such as liver failure, that also cause coagulopathy. With or without a clear diagnosis of DIC, the primary goal of therapy is to treat the underlying condition. In addition, supportive care is provided with volume replacement and support of vital organ systems, including ventilatory assistance. Significant bleeding is managed with blood and component therapy.

Clinical Signs and Symptoms

Coagulopathy may be a subtle, occult process or a massive, obvious emergency. Assessment must encompass each body system, looking for evidence of abnormality in single or multiple components of the coagulation process.

Abnormal Platelet Numbers or Function

- Petechiae of skin or mucous membranes
- Spontaneous bleeding from gums or nose
- Thrombocytopenia
- Prolonged bleeding time

Abnormal Coagulation Factors

- Hemorrhage into subcutaneous tissue, muscle, or joints
- Ecchymosis, purpura
- Bleeding that is slow to improve with local pressure
- Prolonged INR, aPTT
- Decreased fibrinogen
- Decrease in level of specific coagulation factors

TABLE 13-5. LABORATORY RESULTS SUGGESTING DIC

Test	Abnormality
INR	Elevated
aPTT	Elevated
Platelet count	Decreased
Fibrinogen	Decreased
D-dimer	Increased

General Assessment for Bleeding or Decreased Organ Perfusion as a Result of Microthrombosis

Skin/Musculoskeletal

- Oozing of blood from multiple sites, including incisions, intravascular catheters
- Petechiae
- Purpura
- Ecchymosis
- Ischemic changes in toes, fingers, nose, lips, ears
- Pain, swelling, and limited joint mobility
- Increased size of body part, increased girth

Neurologic

- Changes in level of consciousness, pupils, movement, or sensation may indicate intracranial bleeding
- Impaired vision with retinal hemorrhage
- Headache

Gastrointestinal

- Blood in gastric aspirate
- Coffee ground emesis or gastric aspirate
- Melena or frank bloody stool
- Abdominal pain
- Enlarged liver or spleen

Genitourinary

- Hematuria
- Decreased urine output
- Vaginal bleeding

Cardiovascular

- Hypotension or labile blood pressure
- Hypovolemia and/or shock (with rapid loss of large volume of blood)

Principles of Management of Coagulopathies

The management of coagulopathy varies with the type and severity of the disorder. The overall goal of therapy is to restore normal hemostasis and prevent/treat hypovolemic shock. Supportive care focuses on the control and prevention of further bleeding and timely provision of therapeutic interventions.

Restoration of Normal Hemostasis

1. Administer blood and blood components to replace oxygen-carrying capacity, blood volume, and coagulation components. Transfusion is recommended for patients who are actively bleeding. Transfusion may also be indicated prior to invasive procedures or surgery, based on the preoperative evaluation.
2. Monitor patients for clinical response to transfusion. Positive outcomes include hemodynamic stability, increased oxygenation, and restoration of hemostasis.
3. Monitor for adverse reactions to transfusion. Table 13-6 describes the potential complications of administering blood and blood components. Patients receiving a large number of units of blood and components require additional monitoring for hypothermia, hypocalcemia from citrate in stored blood, and dilution of coagulation components.
4. Transfuse platelets as required to treat quantitative platelet disorders. Platelet dysfunction may improve if the offending agent, such as aspirin, is discontinued. Dialysis improves platelet function in patients with renal failure.
5. Acute replacement of coagulation factors can be accomplished with transfusion of fresh frozen plasma.

TABLE 13-6. COMPLICATIONS OF BLOOD AND BLOOD COMPONENTS TRANSFUSIONS

Type of Complication	Key Clinical Signs	Cause	Key Interventions
Acute febrile reaction	Temperature elevation ≥ 1°C or 2°F.	Preexisting antibodies against WBCs or action of cytokines.	Stop the transfusion. Administer antipyretics.
Acute allergic reaction	Urticaria, wheezing, possible anaphylaxis.	Preexisting antibodies.	Stop the transfusion. Administer antihistamines and steroids as indicated.
Transfusion-associated circulatory overload (TACO)	Dyspnea, tachypnea, crackles. Cardiogenic pulmonary edema.	Fluid volume overload.	Slow or stop transfusion. Administer diuretic.
Transfusion-related acute lung injury (TRALI)	Acute onset of hypoxemia and noncardiogenic pulmonary edema within 6 hours of transfusion.	Preexisting antibodies, cytokines, or microparticles within stored blood.	Aggressive respiratory support.
Acute hemolytic reaction	Fever, chills, dyspnea, tachypnea, hypotension, chest and back pain.	Immune destruction of transfused RBCs due to incompatibility of blood.	Stop transfusion. Notify provider and blood bank.
Immune modulation	Acute infections, eg, pneumonia.	Depression of immune cells.	Monitor for and recognize signs of infection.
Alloimmunization	Difficulty in cross-matching future blood transfusions or donor organs.	Antibodies to RBCs, WBCs, and platelets develop over time.	Monitor previously transfused patients for acute reactions.
Infection transmission	Clinical manifestations are usually delayed, and vary according to the infection.	Transmission of viral diseases such as HIV and CMV. Transmission of bacteria and other organisms.	Bacterial sepsis can lead to an acute reaction with fever, chills, and hypotension.

Cryoprecipitate replaces fibrinogen, factor VIII, and von Willebrand factor. PCC replaces vitamin K–dependent factors. Recombinant factor VIIa may be used for persistent hemorrhage.

6. Provide recombinant erythropoietin, iron, and B vitamins to patients with anemia to increase RBC production over time.

Controlling and Preventing Bleeding

1. Modify nursing care measures to minimize trauma and prevent skin and mucous membrane breakdown:
   - Provide gentle oral care.
   - Use electric razor or refrain from shaving.
   - Minimize use of automatic blood pressure cuffs to prevent skin trauma and subcutaneous bleeding; use manual cuffs.
   - Minimize peripheral blood sampling.
   - Avoid IM injections.
   - Use specialty mattress and pad side rails; avoid restraint use.
   - Handle patients gently when turning or moving.
   - Remove adhesive dressings with care.
   - Use low-suction setting to suction endotracheal tube and pharynx.
2. Modify nursing care procedures to control bleeding:
   - Minimize traumatic procedures; apply direct pressure afterward for at least 5 to 10 minutes or until bleeding has stopped.
   - Use ice packs on new hematomas or hemarthroses.
   - Do not dislodge or attempt to remove blood clots from areas of bleeding.
   - Control environment to prevent hypothermia which can worsen coagulopathy.

SELECTED BIBLIOGRAPHY

Anemia

American Association of Blood Banks. *Circular of Information for the Use of Human Blood and Blood Components.* Bethesda, MD: AABB; 2017.

American Society of Anesthesiologists Task Force on Perioperative Blood Management. Practice guidelines for perioperative blood management: an updated report by the American Society of Anesthesiologists Task Force on Perioperative Blood Management. *Anesthesiology.* 2015;122(2):241-275.

Carson JL, Guyatt G, Heddle MN, et al. Clinical practice guidelines from the AABB: red blood cell transfusion thresholds and storage. *JAMA.* 2016;316(19):2025–2035. http://jamanetwork.com. Accessed October 27, 2016.

Carlson JL, Stanworth SJ, Roubinian NR, et al. Transfusion thresholds and other strategies for guiding allogeneic red blood cell transfusion. *Cochrane Database Syst Rev.* 2016;10:CD002042.

Clifford L, Jia Q, Yadav H, et al. Characterizing the epidemiology of perioperative transfusion-associated circulatory overload. *Anesthesiology.* 2015;122(1):21-28.

Field JJ, Vichinsky EP, DeBaun MB. Overview of the management and prognosis of sickle cell disease. In: Schrier SL, ed. *Up-To-Date.* www.uptodate.com. Accessed May 10, 2017.

Fischbach F, Fischbach M, Stout K. *Fischbach's A Manual of Laboratory and Diagnostic Tests.* 11th ed. Philadelphia: Wolters Kluwer Health; 2021.

Gu Y, Estcourt LJ, Doree C, et al. Comparison of a restrictive versus liberal red cell transfusion policy for patients with myelodysplasia, aplastic anaemia, and other congenital bone marrow failure disorders. *Cochrane Database of Syst Rev.* 2015;10:1-4.

National Clinical Guideline Center. *Blood Transfusion.* London: National Institute for Health and Care Excellence (NICE); 2015. http://www.guidelines.gov. Accessed January 30, 2017.

Immunocompromised Patient

American Association of Critical Care Nurses. AANC Practice Alert: Prevention of aspiration in adults. 2016. http://www.aacn.org. Accessed May 10, 2017.

American Association of Critical Care Nurses. AACN Practice Alert: Prevention of catheter-associated urinary tract infections in adults. 2017. http://www/aacn.org. Accessed May 10, 2017.

Centers for Disease Control and Prevention. Core infection prevention and control practices for safe healthcare delivery in all settings—recommendations of the Healthcare Infection Control Practices Advisory Committee. 2017. http://www.cdc.gov/hicpac/recommendations/core-practices.html. Accessed March 27, 2017.

Crawford J, Becker PS, Alwan L., et al. NCCN clinical practice guidelines in oncology. Myeloid growth factors. *J Natil Compr Canc Netw.* 2018. https://www.nccn.org/guidelines/category_1. Accessed August 2, 2021.

Flowers CR, Seidenfeld J, Bow EJ, et al. Antimicrobial prophylaxis and outpatient management of fever and neutropenia in adults treated for malignancy. American Society of Clinical Oncology clinical practice guidelines. *J Clin Oncol.* 2013;31(6):794-819.

Foster M. Reevaluating the neutropenic diet: time to change. *Clin J Oncol Nurs.* 2014;18(2):239-241.

Masur H, Brooks JT, Benson CA, et al. Prevention and treatment of opportunistic infections in HIV-infected adults and adolescents: updated guidelines from the Centers for Disease Control and Prevention, National Institutes of Health, and HIV Medicine Association of the Infectious Diseases Society of America. *Clin Infec Dis.* 2014;58(9):1308-1311.

Rubin LG, Levin MJ, Ljungman P, et al. 2013 IDSA clinical practice guideline for vaccination of the immunocompromised host. *Clin Infect Dis.* 2014;58(3):e44-e100.

Spruce L, Connor R, Retzlaff KJ. Guideline for prevention of transmissible infections. In: *2015 Guidelines for Perioperative Practice.* Denver: Association of Perioperative Registered Nurses. http//:www.guidelines.gov Accessed May 7, 2017.

Taplitz, RA, Kennedy, EB, Bow, EJ, et al. Antimicrobial prophylaxis for adult patients with cancer-related immunosuppression: ASCO and IDSA clinical practice guideline update. *J Clin Oncol.* 2018;36(30):3043-3054.

Coagulopathy

Agency for Healthcare Research and Quality. Preventing hospital-associated venous thromboembolism: a guide for effective quality improvement. 2015. http://www.ahrq.gov/professionals/quality-patient-safety/patient-safety-resources/resources/vtguide/index.html.

American Association of Critical Care Nurses. AACN Practice Alert: Preventing venous thromboembolism in adults. 2016. http://www.aacn.org. Accessed May 10, 2017.

Coutre S, Crowther, M. Clinical presentation and diagnosis of heparin-induced thrombocytopenia. In: Leung LLK, ed. *UpToDate*. www.uptodate.com. Accessed May 7, 2021.

Coutre S, Crowther, M. Management of heparin-induced thrombocytopenia. In: Leung LLK, ed. *UpToDate*. www.uptodate.com. Accessed May 07, 2021.

Dirkes S, Wonnacott R. Continuous renal replacement therapy and anticoagulation: what are the options? *Crit Care Nurse*. 2016;36(2):34-40.

Dobesh PP, Fanikos J. New oral anticoagulants for the treatment of venous thromboembolism: understanding differences and similarities. *Drugs*. 2014;74:2015-2032.

Federici AB, Intini D, Lattuada A, et al. Supportive transfusion therapy in cancer patients with acquired defects of hemostasis. *Thromb Res*. 2014;133:S2, S56-S62.

Fontera JA, Lewin JJ, Rabinstein AA, et al. Guideline for reversal of antithrombotics in intracranial hemorrhage: a statement for healthcare professionals from the Neurocritical Care Society and Society of Critical Care Medicine. 2016. http://www.guidelines.gov. Accessed February 22, 2017.

George JN, Arnold DM. Immune thrombocytopenia (ITP) in adults: initial treatment and prognosis. https://www.uptodate.com/contents/immune-thrombocytopenia-itp-in-adults-clinical-manifestations-and-diagnosis. Accessed May 10, 2017.

Goforth CW, Tranberg JW, Boyer P, et al. Fresh whole blood transfusion: military and civilian implications. *Crit Care Nurse*. 2016;36(3):50-57.

Hunt BJ. Bleeding and coagulopathies in critical care. *N Engl J Med*. 2014;370:847-859.

Hurwitz A, Massone R, Lopez BL. Acquired bleeding disorders. *Emerg Med Clin N Am*. 2014;32:691-713.

Jones AR, Frazier SK. Consequences of transfusing blood components in patients with trauma: a conceptual model. *Crit Care Nurse*. 2017;37(2):18-30.

Kahn SR, Lim W, Sunn AS, et al. Prevention of VTE in nonsurgical patients: antithrombotic therapy and prevention of thrombosis, 9th ed. American College of Chest Physicians. *Chest*. 2012;141 (2 supp):e195S-e226S.

Katrancha ED, Gonzalez LS. Trauma-induced coagulopathy. *Crit Care Nurse*. 2014;34(4):54-63.

Kearon C, Akl EA, Ornelas J, et al. Antithrombotic therapy for VTE disease: CHEST guideline and expert panel report. *Chest*. 2016;149(2):315-352.

Leung LLK. Disseminated intravascular coagulation (DIC) in adults: Evaluation and management. In: Mannucci, ed. *Up-To-Date*. www.uptodate.com. Accessed June 12, 2021.

Levi M. Cancer-related coagulopathies. *Thromb Res*. 2014;133: S2,S70-S75.

Levi M. Diagnosis and treatment of disseminated intravascular coagulation. *Int J Lab Hematol*. 2014;36:228-236.

McEvoy MT, Shander A. Anemia, bleeding, and blood transfusion in the intensive care unit: causes, risks, costs, and new strategies. *Am J Crit Care*. 2013;22(6):eS1-eS13.

Menzin J, Sussman M, Nichols C, et al. Use of blood products in patients with anticoagulant-related major bleeding: an analysis of inhospital outcomes. *Am J Health-Syst Pharm*. 2014;71:1635-1645.

National Institute for Health Care Excellence (NICE). Detecting, managing and monitoring haemostasis: viscoelastometric point-of-care testing (ROTEM, TEG and Sonoclot systems). 2014. www.guidelines.gov.

Ozawa S, Nelson T. Clinical applications of prothrombin complex concentrate in blood management in patients. *Crit Care Nurse*. 2017;37(2):49-57.

Paterson TA, Stein DM. Hemorrhage and coagulopathy in the critically ill. *Emerg Med Clin N Am*. 2014;32:797-810.

Squizzato A, Hunt BJ, Kinasewitz GT, et al. Supportive management strategies for disseminated intravascular coagulation. An international consensus. *Thromb Haemost*. 2016;115:896.

GASTROINTESTINAL SYSTEM

14

Anna M. Alder

KNOWLEDGE COMPETENCIES

1. Describe the etiology, pathophysiology, clinical presentation, patient needs, and principles of management for:
   - Acute gastrointestinal bleeding
   - Liver failure
   - Acute pancreatitis
   - Bowel ischemia

   - Bowel obstruction
   - Bariatric Surgery and Weight Management
2. Identify nutritional requirements for enterally fed critically ill patients.
3. List important interventions to decrease the risk for aspiration pneumonia during enteral feeding.

PATHOLOGIC CONDITIONS

Acute Gastrointestinal Bleeding

Upper GI Bleeding

Bleeding from the upper gastrointestinal (GI) tract is a medical emergency associated with morbidity, mortality, and costly care. Prompt and decisive treatment is essential to improve outcomes. Upper GI bleeding is four times more common than lower GI bleeding. An acute upper GI bleed is suspected when patients present with syncope, hypotension, or abdominal tenderness, and report melanic stool, hematochezia, and blood or coffee-ground emesis. In addition to anemia, laboratory values typically show an elevation of the blood urea nitrogen (BUN) to creatinine ratio (>20:1). Although bleeding stops spontaneously in 80% to 90% of cases, patients presenting with sudden blood loss are at risk for hypotension, decreased tissue perfusion, and reduced oxygen-carrying capability. Many organ systems may be adversely affected.

Acute upper GI bleeding has a mortality of 6% to 15% and a high rate of reoccurrence. Many patients with bleeds are rebleeding from a previous upper GI tract lesion. A poor prognosis with upper GI bleeding is associated with age above 65, shock, overall poor health, active bleeding at the time of presentation, elevated creatinine or transaminases, onset of bleeding during hospitalization, and initial low hematocrit. Death is typically not a direct result of blood loss, but is related to age and comorbidities.

Etiology, Risk Factors, and Pathophysiology

A variety of abnormalities within the GI tract can be the source of upper GI bleeding (Table 14-1).

Peptic ulcer disease is the most common cause of upper GI bleeding. Fifty-five percent of patients with gastric ulcers and 39% of patients with duodenal ulcers are hospitalized for acute bleeds. The pathogenesis of peptic ulcer disease is related to hypersecretion of gastric acid, coupled with impaired GI tract mucus secretion. Normally, mucus protects the gastric wall from the erosive effects of acid. Peptic ulcers occur in the stomach and the duodenum and are characterized by a break in the mucosal layer that penetrates the muscularis mucosa (innermost muscular layer), resulting in bleeding. Peptic ulcers are more prevalent in those with a history of alcohol abuse, smoking, chronic renal failure, and nonsteroidal anti-inflammatory drug (NSAID) use. Infection of the mucosa by *Helicobacter pylori,* an organism naturally found in the GI tract, is strongly correlated with 90% to 100% of duodenal ulcers

TABLE 14-1. COMMON SOURCES OF UPPER GASTROINTESTINAL BLEEDING

Peptic Ulcer Disease
- Gastric ulcer
- Duodenal ulcer

Varices
- Esophageal
- Gastric

Pathologies of the Esophagus
- Tumors
- Mallory-Weiss syndrome
- Inflammation
- Ulcers

Pathologies of the Stomach
- Cancer
- Erosive gastritis
- *Helicobacter pylori* infection
- Tumors

Pathologies of the Small Intestine
- Peptic ulcers
- Angiodysplasia
- Aorto-enteric fistula

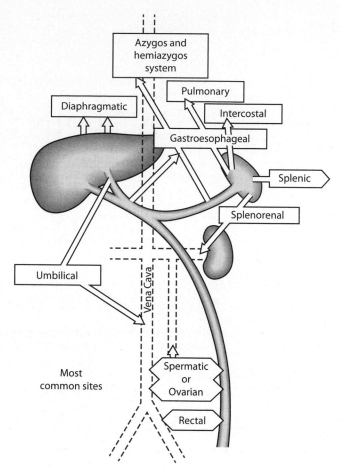

Figure 14-1. The liver with collateral circulation.

and 60% to 100% of gastric ulcers. However, the increased availability of over-the-counter NSAIDs also contribute to the high prevalence of the condition despite advances in medical management. Of note, many peptic ulcers are asymptomatic and patients can present with a bleeding ulcer without previous GI symptoms.

Gastroesophageal varices develop when there is increased pressure in the portal venous system of the liver. If blood cannot flow easily through the liver because of obstructive disease, it is diverted to collateral channels. These channels are normally the low-pressure vessels found in the distal esophagus (esophageal varices), the veins in the proximal stomach (gastric varices), and in the rectal vault (hemorrhoids) (Figure 14-1). Acute upper GI hemorrhage occurs when esophageal and/or gastric varices rupture from increased portal vein pressure (portal hypertension). Esophagogastric varices do not generally bleed until the portal pressure exceeds 12 mm Hg. Portal hypertension is most commonly caused by primary liver disease (see next section), liver trauma, or thrombosis of the splenic, mesenteric, or portal veins. Massive upper GI hemorrhage is associated with variceal bleeds.

Mallory-Weiss syndrome is a linear, nonperforating tear of the gastric mucosa near the gastroesophageal junction. The tear is the result of intra-abdominal pressure changes in the stomach that occur with forceful vomiting. Alcohol abuse and inflammatory conditions of the stomach and esophagus are associated with this disorder. Classically, these tears occur in alcoholic patients who experience intense retching and vomiting associated with binge drinking. However, they may also occur in any patient with a history of repeated emesis and other scenarios where the intra-abdominal pressure is suddenly increased.

Angiodysplasia refers to abnormal superficial blood vessels in the GI tract that are prone to bleeding. These abnormal vessels are associated with increased age. The potential

for the malformed vessels to bleed is exacerbated with aortic stenosis, chronic renal disease, liver disease, and Von Willebrand disease. This condition is commonly encountered in the outpatient setting and rarely requires admission to the intensive care unit (ICU).

Erosive gastritis describes gastric lesions that do not penetrate the muscularis mucosa. These are also referred to as stress ulcers. Stress-related ulcers occur frequently in hospitalized patients. Patients with respiratory failure and coagulopathies have an increased risk of bleeding from the ulcers. The onset of bleeding is sudden and is often the first symptom. However, the bleeding is often minimal and self-limited. The causes of gastritis are multifactorial (Table 14-2), but are most commonly associated with NSAID use, steroid intake, alcohol abuse, and physiologic conditions that cause severe stress (eg, trauma, surgery, burns, radiation therapy, severe medical problems). Alcohol and NSAIDs are known to directly disrupt the mucosal defense mechanisms of the stomach (Figure 14-2). Use of NSAIDs is particularly problematic in older adults and contributes to the increased incidence of symptomatic acute upper GI bleeding in this population. In the critical care population, particularly patients with neurological or burn injuries, Cushing and Curling stress ulcers may be

ESSENTIAL CONTENT CASE

Upper GI Bleeding

A 52-year-old man is admitted with reports of a 7-hour history of nausea and vomiting with recent emesis of large amounts of "bloody secretions" and frequent "maroon-colored" stools. His mental status is alert but confused. His friend reports that recently he has taken large amounts of NSAIDs due to an acute back injury. A gastric ulcer on the posterior wall of the stomach is diagnosed by upper endoscopy. Significant findings on his admission profile are:

Vital Signs

Blood pressure:	84/54 mm Hg lying, MAP 64
Heart rate:	132 beats/min; sinus tachycardia
Respiratory rate:	28 breaths/min
Temperature:	37.3°C (oral)

Respiratory
- Breath sounds clear in all lung fields but diminished

Cardiovascular
- S_1/S_2, no murmurs
- Extremities cool, diaphoretic; pulses present but weak

Abdomen
- Distended with hyperactive bowel sounds (BSs)
- Tender right upper quadrant, no rebound tenderness

Neurologic
- Slightly confused
- Anxious

Genitourinary
- 30 mL of amber cloudy urine following urinary catheter insertion
- Stools liquid maroon, guaiac positive

Arterial Blood Gases
- pH 7.33
- $PaCO_2$ 35 mm Hg
- HCO_3 16 mEq/L
- PaO_2 83 mm Hg on room air
- SaO_2 92%

Laboratory
- Hematocrit   22%
- Hemoglobin   6.0 g/dL
- White blood cell count   18,000/mm³
- Prothrombin time (PT)   11 seconds
- Activated partial   30 seconds thromboplastin time
- Platelet count   110,000/mm³
- Serum potassium   3.0 mEq/L
- Serum sodium   135 mEq/L
- Serum glucose   227 mg/dL
- Serum BUN   44
- Serum creatinine   1.9
- Liver function testing   Within normal limits

Case Question 1: Initial management of the patient with upper GI bleeding would include:
(A) Volume resuscitation
(B) Hemodynamic stabilization
(C) Identification of the site of bleeding
(D) Initiation of treatment to control bleeding within 24 hours of admission

Case Question 2: After the bleeding site is identified and bleeding is controlled, the drug of choice to treat a nonvariceal bleed is:
(A) Histamine receptor antagonists
(B) Proton pump inhibitors (PPIs)
(C) Antacids
(D) Octreotide/Somatostatin

Answers
1. The correct answer is (A). The fundamental goal for initial management of the patient is volume resuscitation. However, hemodynamic stabilization, identification of the bleeding site, and control of bleeding are all key points for managing the patient with upper GI bleeding. Vital signs are an important indicator of blood loss. If the patient is hemodynamically unstable, resuscitation begins with the administration of 2 to 3 L of crystalloid. Blood products are considered if the response is poor.
2. The correct answer is (B). PPIs are the drug of choice in this patient population as they lead to a more durable and sustained acid suppression. In randomized controlled clinical trials, PPIs are shown to decrease recurrent bleeding.

identified. However, they are rare and only occur in 1.5% of this population.

Regardless of the etiology, upper GI bleeding resulting in a significant and sudden loss of blood volume is associated with decreased venous return to the heart, and therefore a decrease in cardiac output (CO). The decrease in CO triggers the release of epinephrine and norepinephrine, causing intense vasoconstriction and tissue ischemia (Figure 14-3). In addition, aldosterone and antidiuretic hormones are released, resulting in sodium and water retention. The clinical signs and symptoms of upper GI hemorrhage are directly related to the effects of the decrease in CO and the vasoconstriction response typically seen in hypovolemic shock.

Clinical Presentation

History

Individuals may have a history of peptic ulcer disease, tobacco abuse, alcohol abuse, liver disease, severe physiologic stress,

TABLE 14-2. CAUSES OF GASTRITIS

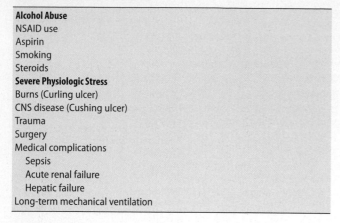

Alcohol Abuse
NSAID use
Aspirin
Smoking
Steroids
Severe Physiologic Stress
Burns (Curling ulcer)
CNS disease (Cushing ulcer)
Trauma
Surgery
Medical complications
Sepsis
Acute renal failure
Hepatic failure
Long-term mechanical ventilation

NSAID use, and anticoagulation or antiplatelet therapy. Older adults are at great risk for GI bleeding.

Signs and Symptoms

The response to blood loss depends on the rate and amount of blood loss, patient's age, overall health status, and the timing of the initial resuscitation. The patient may present with signs and symptoms that specifically demonstrate acute bleeding and hypovolemia and may also experience alternations in other systems.

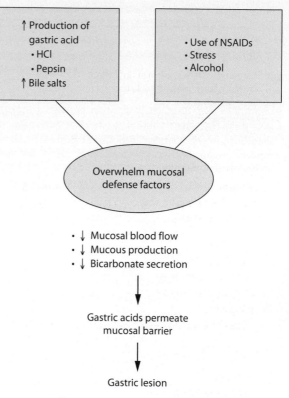

Figure 14-2. Pathogenesis of gastritis.

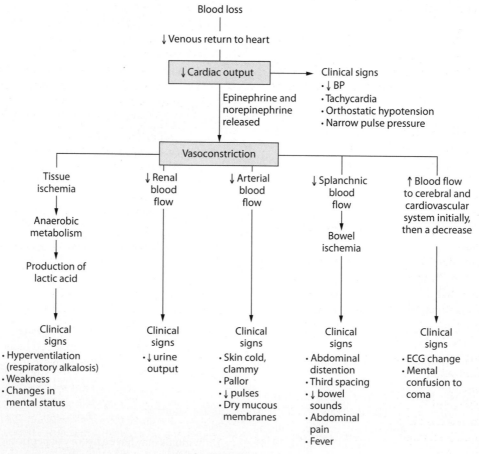

Figure 14-3. Hypovolemic shock.

Gastrointestinal signs and symptoms

- Hematemesis (bright red blood or coffee ground emesis)
- Hematochezia (red or maroon stools)
- Melena (black tarry stools)
- Nausea and/or early satiety
- Epigastric pain
- Abdominal distension or bloating
- Bowel Sounds increased or decreased

Signs and symptoms of hypovolemia

Hypotension (orthostasis suggests 30% blood volume loss) and altered hemodynamic values (see Chapter 4, Hemodynamic Monitoring).

- Tachycardia
- Decreased pulses
- Cold, clammy skin
- Dry mucous membranes
- Weakness
- Decreased urine output

Cognitive signs and symptoms

- Anxiety
- Mental status changes
- Restlessness

Respiratory and cardiovascular symptoms

- Rapid, deep respirations
- Electrocardiographic (ECG) changes consistent with ischemia (eg, ST-segment elevation, arrhythmias)
- Fever

Diagnostic Tests

- Hematocrit may be normal initially, then decreased with fluid resuscitation and blood loss. The hematocrit may not accurately reflect the actual volume of blood loss because of hemodilution and movement of extravascular fluid. The hematocrit decreases as extravascular fluid enters the vascular space in an attempt to restore volume. This process continues for 24 to 72 hours.
- Hemoglobin may also be normal initially, then decreased with fluid resuscitation and blood loss. It is considered slightly more reliable than hematocrit.
- White blood cell count is elevated due to inflammation.
- Platelet count may be decreased depending on the amount of blood loss.
- Serum sodium is usually elevated initially due to hemoconcentration.
- Serum potassium is usually decreased with vomiting.
- Serum BUN is mildly elevated.
- Serum creatinine is elevated.
- Serum lactate is elevated with severe bleeding.
- PT is usually decreased.

- Activated partial thromboplastin time (aPTT) is usually decreased.
- Arterial blood gases show respiratory alkalosis (early), then later metabolic acidosis with severe shock and hypoxemia.
- Gastric aspirate shows normal or acidotic pH and is guaiac positive.

Lower GI bleeding

Lower GI bleeding is defined as bleeding that originates distal to the ligament of Treitz (the thin band of tissue that connects the duodenum to the jejunum) and, unlike upper GI bleeding, has a lower morbidity and mortality. In fact, the bleeding resolves spontaneously in the vast majority of patients and the mortality rate is less than 5%. Distinguishing upper versus lower GI bleeding by origin is an important consideration because a rapid upper GI bleed may present as the presence of blood in the lower GI tract.

Lower GI bleeding is a common disorder in older adults and may be associated with a host of conditions including infection, hemorrhoids, cancer, diverticulitis, or vascular anomaly. Regardless of the source, lower GI bleeding typically presents as hematochezia. Bleeding sources within the left side of the colon often result in the presence of bright red blood whereas those from the right colon may be mixed with stool and present as a darker shade of red.

Principles of Management for GI Bleeding

The fundamental goal of initial treatment is volume resuscitation. The management of the patient with acute GI bleeding focuses on hemodynamic stabilization, identification of the bleeding site, and initiation of definitive medical or surgical therapies to control or stop the bleeding. Measures to decrease anxiety in this patient population are also indicated due to the severity and sudden onset of GI bleeding but sedatives are used sparingly if at all, particularly in patients with liver impairment. Patients should receive nothing by mouth (NPO) if endoscopy or other procedures are anticipated.

Hemodynamic Stabilization

The initial assessment of the patient with GI bleeding begins with a physical examination in which vital signs and mental status are the most reliable indicators of the amount of blood lost. In the presence of hemodynamic instability, resuscitation begins.

In addition to vital signs and physical assessment, risk stratification tools and laboratory findings help determine the severity of the bleed. The Glasgow Blatchford, Rockall, and AIMS65 scores can be used to anticipate patient outcomes. The Glasgow Blatchford score incorporates measures of BUN, Hgb, systolic BP, pulse, melena, syncope, liver disease, and/or heart failure while the Rockall includes age, shock, and morbidity. The Rockall score does have a secondary set of elements (age, shock, comorbidity, diagnosis, and stigmata of recent bleed) that can be reviewed post-endoscopy to further delineate risk. The AIMS65 score is used preprocedure and consists of five factors including albumin, INR, mental status, systolic BP, and age. The use of a risk assessment tool to stratify bleeding and associated mortality is recommended by several consensus groups. Additionally, meta-analyses demonstrate that factors such as active bleeding, hemoglobin less than 10 g/dL, systolic blood pressure less than 100 mm Hg, tachycardia, ulcer size more than 1 to 3 cm, and ulcer location (in the lesser gastric curvature or posterior duodenal bulb) are associated with poor patient outcomes.

1. Monitor and record cardiovascular status (blood pressure, heart rate including orthostatic changes), hemodynamic indices, and peripheral pulses.

2. Insert at least two large-bore intravenous (IV) catheters and begin fluid resuscitation with crystalloid solution (eg, normal saline or lactated ringer solution). Administer fluids to maintain mean arterial pressure (MAP) around 65 mm Hg or higher. Some patients may require temporary vasopressor support if the blood pressure fails to respond with IV fluid resuscitation. Intensive monitoring may be required for patients at risk for fluid overload.

3. Administer supplemental oxygen and monitor respiratory function. Airway protection with endotracheal intubation to prevent aspiration is indicated in patients with ongoing hematemesis or altered mental status.

4. Obtain blood for measurement of hematocrit, hemoglobin, and clotting studies, as well as for a type and cross-match for packed red blood cells (PRBCs). A Hgb less than 7 to 8 g/dL is considered a marker for transfusion. If the patient also has a history of unstable coronary artery disease or comorbid conditions, a higher threshold is typically used. In patients receiving multiple transfusions, monitoring ionized calcium levels is required as citrate, contained in the transfused blood, may lower calcium. Estimates for the amount of blood volume lost are most reliably guided by vital sign values and physical assessment (Table 14-3).

5. Administer prescribed IV colloids, crystalloids, or blood products until the patient is stabilized. After the administration of crystalloid fluids, blood products may be considered during the initial resuscitation if the hemodynamic response is poor. PRBCs are used to rapidly increase the hematocrit while providing less volume compared to infusions of whole blood. However, whole blood may be desired with severe hemorrhage as it provides more volume and also includes both plasma and platelets.

Each unit of PRBC increases the hematocrit by 2% to 3% and improves gas exchange. It may take up to 24 hours after blood is administered for changes to be reflected in the hematocrit values, especially if large amounts of crystalloid solutions were administered during the resuscitation period.

6. Monitor coagulation studies (eg, prothrombin time/partial thromboplastin time [PT/PTT], platelet count, and fibrinogen) to determine if transfusions of platelets or clotting factors will benefit the patient. Patients who receive multiple transfusions also require monitoring of ionized calcium levels as the citrate in blood products can lead to hypocalcemia.

7. Monitor fluid balance and renal function (intake and output, daily weight, BUN, creatinine, and hourly urine output). An elevated BUN:creatinine ratio may indicate poor renal perfusion but also occurs when blood is absorbed in the duodenum.

8. Placement of nasogastric tube (NGT) in patients with suspected acute upper GI bleeding is not recommended, as studies have failed to demonstrate a benefit to clinical outcomes. Use of gastric lavage is no longer used routinely to minimize bleeding. Some institutions use room temperature saline lavage to clear the stomach of blood, clots, or other particulate matter prior to endoscopy. Iced saline is no longer used as it lowers core temperature.

9. Position the patient with backrest elevation 30° to 45° to minimize aspiration associated with hematemesis.

10. Monitor temperature and maintain normothermia. Rapid fluid resuscitation, particularly with blood products, can lead to hypothermia which interferes with coagulation. Warming of fluids may be required to prevent hypothermia, if traditional measures are insufficient.

11. Administer medications such as IV octreotide and PPIs. Guidelines recommend that the initiation of PPIs should not be delayed before endoscopy and

TABLE 14-3. ESTIMATING BLOOD LOSS FROM ACUTE GI BLEEDING (ADVANCED TRAUMA LIFE SUPPORT CLASSIFICATION SYSTEM FOR HYPOVOLEMIC SHOCK)

	Class I	Class II	Class III	Class IV
Blood loss (mL)	Up to 750	750-1500	1500-2000	>2000
Blood loss (% Blood Volume)	Up to 15%	15%-30%	30%-40%	>40%
Pulse rate	<100	>100	>120	>140
Blood pressure	Normal	Normal	Decreased	Decreased
Pulse pressure (mm Hg)	Normal or increased	Decreased	Decreased	Decreased
Respiratory rate	14-20	20-30	30-40	>35
CNS/mental status	Slightly anxious	Mildly anxious	Anxious, confused	Confused, lethargy

high-dose PPI treatment should be continued for the first 72 hours post-endoscopy (when the patient is at the highest risk of rebleeding).

12. Prepare for urgent endoscopic therapy in patients with high-risk clinical features such as history of varices, bright red emesis, or Class III or IV hemorrhage. These patients may have improved outcomes when endoscopy is performed within 12 hours. Critically ill patients with active bleeding or altered mental status may be electively intubated to facilitate endoscopy and reduce aspiration risk. In patients at lower risk, endoscopy is usually performed within 24 hours of admission.

Identify the Bleeding Site

Although the history and physical examination are used to differentiate between upper and lower GI bleeding, endoscopic examination is required to determine the exact site of bleeding and to direct future therapy. Endoscopy allows early direct visualization of the upper GI tract during resuscitation measures.

1. Provide prokinetic agents, if required. The presence of blood in the upper GI tract can impede visualization of the site of bleeding. Prokinetic agents

facilitate gastric emptying of retained blood and may be administered prior to endoscopy. Meta-analyses demonstrate that when erythromycin is administered pre-endoscopy, visibility is improved and the need for a repeat procedure is reduced.

2. Administer sedation (eg, midazolam [Versed], propofol [Diprivan]) sparingly per institutional policy and initiate monitoring protocol.

3. Elevate the head of the bed to a 30° angle (if tolerated) and if intubated, maintain endotracheal tube (ET) cuff pressure to prevent aspiration.

4. Position the patient in a left lateral decubitus position, which facilitates scope placement, and helps to prevent aspiration of GI contents during endoscopy. Have oropharyngeal suction available at the bedside before the procedure begins.

5. Monitor for cardiac ischemia during the procedure (eg, draw troponin, assess for ST-segment changes [see Chapter 18, Advanced ECG Concepts], arrhythmias).

Institute Therapies to Control or Stop Bleeding

Definitive therapies to treat the bleeding depend on the cause. A general approach for treatment is summarized in Figure 14-4. Administration of PPIs is routine for patients

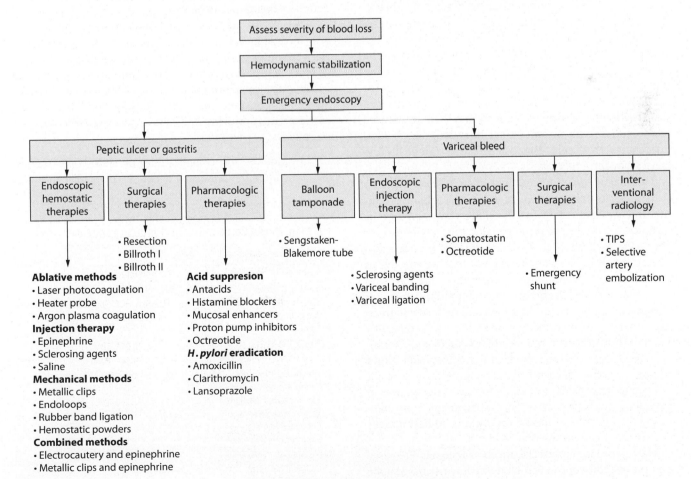

Figure 14-4. Upper GI bleeding treatment guide.

in whom an ulcer is suspected. The PPIs quickly neutralize acids and elevate gastric pH levels, which results in stabilization of the blood clot. An acidic environment will inhibit platelet aggregation and lyse an already formed clot.

In nonvariceal upper GI bleeding, endoscopic treatment is the modality of choice because it is the most effective method to control acute ulcer bleeding, prevent rebleeding, and it is relatively safe procedure. Although individual studies have been too small to show significant advantage for endoscopic therapy in reducing mortality, a meta-analysis indicates that endoscopic therapy prevents not only rebleeding but also death. While endoscopy carries a risk for complications including GI perforation, precipitation of bleeding, aspiration, adverse reactions to sedation medications including cardiac or respiratory compromise, and missed lesions, these rarely occur.

A variety of interventions are used via endoscopy and include ablative or coagulation therapy (laser, monopolar, bipolar, or multipolar electrocoagulation, and heater probe), pharmacologic therapy also known as sclerotherapy, and mechanical and combination therapies. Pharmacologic treatments are easy to use, inexpensive, and available in most settings. The goal is to control bleeding by tamponade, vasoconstriction, and/or an inflammatory reaction after the injection of the selected agent. A saline injection will compress the vessels. Sclerosants such as alcohol, ethanolamine, and polidocanol cause greater vascular thrombosis, but can result in tissue injury and necrosis and are used less frequently. Epinephrine (1:10,000-1:20,000) provides local tamponade, vasoconstriction, and improved platelet aggregation to promote hemostasis. It is the agent of choice in the United States to rapidly control the bleeding site. However, its effects will only last for 20 minutes and therefore is used in combination with an additional more durable thermal or mechanical treatment. Hemostatic sprays can be used to achieve short-term hemostasis.

Thermal coagulation methods such as electrocautery and argon plasma coagulation are examples of ablative treatments and are equally effective. Bleeding vessels can also be mechanically compressed using metallic clips, endoloops, or rubber band ligation. Metallic hemoclips are the mechanical treatment of choice and are shown to be as effective as other endoscopic techniques. Combination therapy with epinephrine injection has become the standard treatment for actively bleeding ulcers. Adding a second endoscopic treatment, either an ablative therapy or endoclips, significantly reduces the rate of recurrence, need for surgery, and mortality. It is no longer recommended to use epinephrine alone. If the patient rebleeds, a second attempt with endoscopic control may be considered before surgical intervention or angiography-guided intervention. Rebleeding is more common in patients with variceal bleeds and is highest initially after admission and for the first 24 hours.

The three-stage Forrest classification system is often used at the time of endoscopy to predict rebleeding risk based upon the visual characteristics of the GI lesion/ulcer. Patients with a high-risk for rebleed, as stratified by the Forrest classification system, are often hospitalized for 72 hours of treatment and evaluation. Depending on the risk severity, the patient may remain in the critical care setting during this time.

Treatment of a Mallory-Weiss tear is supportive therapy. Bleeding episodes are self-limited and the mucosa heals spontaneously within 72 hours in 90% of patients.

Significant bleeding from stress gastritis is rarely encountered. Critically ill patients with a history of gastritis, or those at risk for developing stress-related GI injury, benefit from prophylactic acid-suppressive therapy and from early enteral feeding to prevent bleeding. Invasive intervention is rarely required.

In patients with variceal bleeding, pharmacologic treatment to reduce portal hypertension may be considered as preparations are underway for emergent endoscopy. Somatostatin or its analogue octreotide are the vasoactive agents of choice. Continuous IV infusion of these agents can temporarily control bleeding so that resuscitation, diagnostic, and therapeutic measures can be completed. Pharmacologic treatments are summarized in Table 14-4. Both sclerotherapy and variceal banding or ligation are used during endoscopy to control variceal bleeding. Currently, balloon tamponade (Sengstaken-Blakemore [S-B] tube) is reserved for patients with massive hemorrhage. Once bleeding is controlled, more definitive therapies can be used.

Treatment of esophageal and gastric varices will also include antibiotic prophylaxis for spontaneous bacterial peritonitis (SBP) in patients with cirrhosis. A third-generation cephalosporin or fluoroquinolone is indicated, as bacteremia is often present in patients with variceal bleeding. Studies demonstrate that administering antibiotics to cirrhotic patients prior to endoscopy decreases infections and mortality.

1. Monitor for complications of endoscopic therapy and/or the sclerosing agents used to treat the ulcer or varix. Complications may include fever and pain

TABLE 14-4. PHARMACOLOGIC THERAPIES FOR ULCER DISEASE/GASTRITIS

Agent	Action
Antacids	Acid neutralizers

Histamine blockers
  Cimetidine
  Ranitidine
  Famotidine
  Nizatidine
	Block production of gastric acid (pepsin, HCl) by inhibiting the action of histamine

Cytoprotective agent sucralfate	Forms protective barrier over ulcer site

Proton pump inhibitors
  Omeprazole (Prilosec)
  Esomeprazole (Nexium)
  Lansoprazole (Prevacid)
  Rabeprazole (Aciphex)
  Pantoprazole (Protonix)-IV
	Suppress secretion of gastric acid

Mucosal barrier enhancers
  Colloidal bismuth
  Prostaglandins
	Protect mucosa from injurious substances

due to esophageal spasm, motility disturbances of the esophageal sphincter, and perforation. Systemic complications of endoscopic therapy and/or sclerosing agents also may occur and predominantly affect the cardiovascular and respiratory systems. Cardiovascular effects include heart failure, heart block, mediastinitis, and pericarditis. Respiratory effects include aspiration pneumonia, atelectasis, pneumothorax, embolism, and acute respiratory distress syndrome.

2. Institute pharmacologic therapies as prescribed to treat peptic ulcer disease or gastritis. The most common pharmacologic agents and their actions are reviewed in Table 14-4. PPIs are the drug of choice for the management of patients with nonvariceal bleeding. They provide a more durable and sustained acid suppression than histamine receptor antagonists. Treatment with PPIs is shown in randomized clinical trials to lead to a decrease in recurrent bleeding because of ulcer disease, need for transfusions, surgery, and the length of hospital stay. The traditional use of high-dose continuous IV PPIs for 3 days after successful endoscopic treatment for active bleeding continues (80 mg esomeprazole bolus, 8 mg/h continuous infusion). Yet, newer meta-analyses demonstrate the same benefits with IV BID dosing of 40 mg, until the patient is able to take oral medications. Oral PPIs are commonly recommended for months after an upper GI bleeding episode to allow for healing of the mucosa. Their use is especially beneficial in patients who use chronic NSAIDs or who have had *H. pylori* infection.

3. Administer pharmacologic therapies as prescribed to treat variceal bleeding (Table 14-5). Pharmacologic agents exert their effect by constricting splanchnic blood flow and thereby reducing portal pressure.

Shunt Procedure to Control Bleeding

When severe variceal bleeding cannot be controlled with endoscopic intervention, emergent portal decompression is achieved with the percutaneous transjugular intrahepatic portosystemic shunt (TIPS).

TABLE 14-5. PHARMACOLOGIC THERAPIES FOR VARICEAL UPPER GI BLEEDING

Drug	Action	Administration
Somatostatin	Inhibits splanchnic blood flow	250 mcg bolus then continuous IV infusion at 250 mcg/h
Octreotide	Reduces splanchnic blood flow thus resulting in decreased portal and variceal pressures	50 mcg bolus then IV infusion at 25-50 mcg/h (off-label use)
Nonselective beta-adrenergic blockers: propranolol, nadolol	Decreases cardiac output and reduces splanchnic flow (decreases portal hypertension)	Administered orally (or IV) to reduce resting pulse by 20% or to 55-60 beats/min

In the TIPS procedure, a stent is used to create a shunt between the hepatic vein and a branch of the portal vein. This decreases the pressure in the portal vein (decreases portal pressure) and subsequently on the varices to prevent rupture and bleeding.

The advantage of the TIPS procedure is that it is less invasive than surgery because the portal circulation is accessed via the right jugular vein. Contraindications to TIPS include severe-progressive liver failure, severe encephalopathy, polycystic liver disease, and severe right heart failure. Complications of the TIPS procedures include puncture of the biliary system, bleeding, infection, and clotting of the stent and stenosis. Postprocedural systemic failure (septic shock, renal failure) and hepatic encephalopathy (see next section) are also associated complications.

Nursing management of the patient undergoing TIPS includes:

1. Monitor blood pressure, ECG, and pulse oximetry throughout the procedure.
2. Administer preprocedure antibiotic coverage for gram-negative organisms as prophylaxis for sepsis.
3. Provide IV sedation according to institutional policy.
4. Provide pain medication (eg, fentanyl). Certain parts of the procedure, such as balloon dilation of the intrahepatic tract, can be painful.
5. Have lidocaine, atropine, and other emergency medications available to manage potential complications of the procedure. Due to the proximity of the hepatic vein to the right ventricle of the heart, ventricular ectopy can be induced during the procedure.
6. Have crystalloids, vasopressors, PRBCs, and fresh frozen plasma readily available to manage hypotension from sepsis, bleeding, or sedation.
7. Have continuous and intermittent suction ready to manage bleeding and airway patency.

An alternative to TIPS available at some institutions is the balloon-occluded retrograde transvenous obliteration (BRTO) procedure. The procedure involves the occlusion of blood flow to varices by inflating a balloon catheter and instilling a sclerosing agent. The procedure results in a blockage of blood to the varix and the shunting of blood through healthier veins. Further research is needed on the long-term results and effectiveness of BRTO.

Surgical Therapies to Stop Bleeding

Surgery is less common today and is reserved for patients with refractory disease or complications. Patients who experience life-threatening massive bleeding or who continue to bleed despite aggressive medical therapies are candidates for surgery. Surgical therapies include gastric resections such as antrectomy, partial gastrectomy, vagotomy, or combination procedures. An antrectomy or gastrectomy may be performed to decrease the acidity of the duodenum or stomach by removing gastric-acid secreting cells. A vagotomy decreases acid secretion in the stomach by dividing the

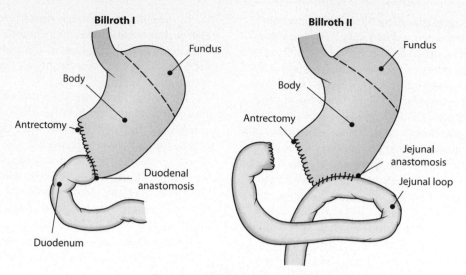

Figure 14-5. Billroth I and II procedures.

vagus nerve along the esophagus. Combination procedures are common and one example is the Billroth I, which is a vagotomy and antrectomy with anastomosis of the stomach to the duodenum. A Billroth II consists of a vagotomy, resection of the antrum, and anastomosis of the stomach to the jejunum (Figure 14-5). The latter is preferred over the Billroth I because it does not present the risk for dumping syndrome. Gastric perforations can be treated by simple closure.

Nursing considerations for patients undergoing surgery to treat GI bleed include:

1. Monitor for fluid and electrolyte imbalances postoperatively due to intraoperative fluid loss and the drains inserted to decompress the stomach or to drain the surgical site.
2. Provide for adequate nutrition to promote wound healing.
3. Monitor the appearance of the incision and surrounding tissue.
4. Document and report all wound drainage (color, amount, odor) and complaints of pain or tenderness.
5. Culture any suspicious drainage.
6. Monitor white blood cell count and temperature trends.

Reducing Anxiety

1. Encourage communication with a calm, interested, and patient-centered approach. If the patient is intubated, consider written communication or use of a communication board or electronic device.
2. Encourage the patient to identify and use coping skills used in past difficult situations. These may include family or caregiver presence, watching TV, listening to music, or relaxation techniques to alleviate anxiety. If visitation is restricted, consider alternative methods to facilitate connecting patients with their support network, including the use of electronic devices.

3. Offer appropriate reassurance, facts, and information as requested by the patient or family/caregiver. Explain the ICU routine and procedures and present information in terms that the patient or family/caregiver can understand. Repeat and rephrase the information as necessary. Allow time for questions.
4. As appropriate, help the patient establish a sense of control. Assist the patient to make distinctions among those things within their control (eg, bath time, visitor preferences) and those things that cannot be controlled (eg, need for vasopressors and monitoring equipment).
5. Guide the patient to use relaxation exercises and other diversion strategies to decrease anxiety.
6. Consider requesting consultation with other interprofessional members of the team (eg, case manager, spiritual care support, or other therapy as appropriate).

Liver Failure

Pathogenesis

The liver, the largest organ in the body, has a central role in regulating the body's metabolism. Metabolic functions include the synthesis of carbohydrates, fats, proteins, and vitamins for nutrition, energy, and key metabolic pathways. Additional processes performed by the liver include the formation of bile, bilirubin metabolism, synthesis of coagulation factors, and detoxification of drugs and toxins. Liver failure may be acute or chronic. Irrespective of the cause of liver injury, inflammation results in damage to hepatocytes, known as "hepatitis." Injured areas are surrounded by scar tissues leading to fibrosis, and after a period of time progressive fibrosis results in cirrhosis or replacement of the normal hepatic tissue with fibrotic tissue. Chronic liver failure is a slow deterioration that evolves over years leading to cirrhosis. Liver dysfunction potentially can be reversed early in the disease as the liver has a regenerative capability; however, fibrotic changes are irreversible resulting in chronic dysfunction and eventual end-stage liver disease.

Acute failure, also known as fulminant hepatic failure, results in a rapid deterioration of liver function in a person without prior liver disease. This cellular insult results in massive cell necrosis leading to a multiorgan dysfunction. Acute liver failure is rare and characterized by a coagulation abnormality (usually an INR ≥ 1.5) and encephalopathy occurring as the result of an insult without previous liver disease. The time between hepatic injury and presentation of either encephalopathy or coagulopathy is usually less than 2 to 6 weeks.

Etiology and Risk Factors

The leading cause of acute liver failure in the United States and Europe is acetaminophen overdose. Other causes include viral hepatitis (A, B, and E), thrombosis, and shock (Table 14-6). Survival in acute liver failure can be categorized into patients in whom intensive care enables recovery of hepatic function and patients who require liver transplantation. Common causes of chronic liver disease include nonalcoholic fatty liver disease (NAFLD), alcoholic liver disease, chronic hepatitis B and C, and hemochromatosis.

NAFLD and nonalcoholic steatohepatitis (NASH) are the most common causes of chronic liver disease in the Western world, and are becoming more prevalent in concert with increasing rates of obesity. The spectrum of liver disease associated with these syndromes can range from simple steatosis to hepatitis and advanced fibrosis and cirrhosis. They are associated with type 2 diabetes, hyperlipidemia, and metabolic syndrome. In contrast, alcoholic liver injury results from the toxic effects of ethanol on the hepatocytes. Similar to nonalcoholic fatty liver, alcoholic liver conditions may include a spectrum of associated conditions from steatosis to cirrhosis.

TABLE 14-6. COMMON CAUSES OF LIVER FAILURE

Viruses
Hepatitis A, B, C, D, and E
Herpes simplex
Epstein-Barr
Cytomegalovirus
Adenovirus
Parasites
Liver tumors
Toxic ingestion of drugs
   Acetaminophen
   Halothane
   Methyldopa
Toxic ingestion of chemicals and poisons
   Chlorinated hydrocarbons
   Phosphorus
Nonalcoholic fatty liver disease
Alcohol ingestion
Biliary disease
Cardiac disease
Hepatitis

TABLE 14-7. CLINICAL AND LABORATORY PATIENT SCORE FOR INCREASING ABNORMALITY AND SURVIVAL MEASUREMENT

Factor	1 point	2 points	3 points
Total bilirubin (molμ/L)	<34	34-50	>50
Serum albumin (g/L)	>35	28-35	<28
PT INR	<1.7	1.71-2.30	>2.30
Ascites	None	Mild	Moderate to severe
Hepatic encephalopathy	None	Grade I-II (or suppressed with medication)	Grade III-IV (or refractory)
	Class A	Class B	Class C
Total points	5-6	7-9	10-15
1-year survival	100%	80%	45%

The composite score of these factors is used to provide a severity grade. Grades are: Grade A 5-6, Grade B 7-8, Grade C 10-15.

Severity Scores

The Child-Pugh classification is a long-standing assessment tool to score hepatic function and estimate cirrhosis severity. This classification is based on two clinical variables and three biochemical tests (Table 14-7). Classes define well-compensated disease (Class A) to advanced decompensated disease (Class C).

The Model for End-Stage Liver Disease (MELD) score is another frequently used tool to measure disease severity. The MELD score is a calculation that incorporates age, international normalized ratio (INR), serum sodium, serum creatinine, and albumin. Additional points are included if the patient undergoes dialysis at least twice in a week. Scores range from 6 to 40 with a higher score associated with higher mortality risk. The MELD score is used by United Network of Organ Sharing (UNOS) to determine hierarchy of transplantation need.

Clinical Manifestations

Clinical manifestations are directly related to failure of the liver to perform important metabolic processes (Table 14-8). Complications of liver failure include jaundice, ascites, hepatic encephalopathy, hepatopulmonary syndrome, electrolyte imbalance, hepatorenal syndrome, and SBP.

Jaundice

Jaundice is secondary to excessive deposition of bilirubin in tissues including skin, mucous membranes, and sclera, resulting in the characteristic yellow discoloration. This deposition of bilirubin represents failure of the liver to adequately uptake, conjugate, and excrete bilirubin. Jaundice is typically evident when the bilirubin exceeds 2 to 3 mg/dL. The excessive bilirubin in the blood contributes to the urine darkness and pale or clay-colored stools. Pruritus from bile salt accumulation is a commonly associated and uncomfortable symptom.

Ascites

Cirrhosis is the most common cause of ascites, an abnormal collection of fluid in the peritoneal cavity. Increased pressure

TABLE 14-8. SEQUELAE OF LIVER FAILURE

Sequelae	Outcome	Clinical Manifestations
Impaired splanchnic hemodynamics	Portal hypertension	Varices, acute upper GI bleeding
	Hyperdynamic circulation	Increased CO, decreased SVR, decreased perfusion
Reduced liver metabolic processes	Altered fat, protein, and carbohydrate metabolism	Malnutrition, impaired healing
	Decreased phagocytic function of Kupffer cells	Infection
	Decreased synthesis of blood clotting components	Bleeding
	Decreased removal of activated clotting factors	Emboli
	Decreased metabolism of vitamins and iron	Impaired skin integrity
	Impaired detoxification	Increased ammonia, mental status changes, increased drug levels
Impaired bile formation and flow	Impaired bilirubin metabolism	Jaundice

in the portal system occurs secondary to fibrosis in the liver causing an obstruction to venous flow. This results in increased nitric oxide, vasodilation, and renal function compromise with sodium and water retention. Fluid shifts from the intravascular space into the peritoneal space. Decreased intravascular albumin levels and an increase in extravascular protein exacerbate the condition.

Hepatic Encephalopathy

Hepatic encephalopathy defines a spectrum of neuropsychiatric abnormalities that occur with liver failure. This condition most likely results from decreased hepatic clearance of cerebral toxins. Serum ammonia is most often implicated. Ammonia is produced by bacteria in the bowel and converted to urea in the liver for excretion through the kidneys. In liver failure, this function of the liver is impaired, allowing ammonia to directly enter the central nervous system. Because ammonia is neurotoxic, as serum ammonia levels rise, the patient often exhibits signs of impaired cerebral functioning or encephalopathy. These signs can range from minor sensory-perceptual changes such as muscle tremors, slurred speech, or slight mental status changes to marked confusion or profound coma. Asterixis is a common manifestation.

Classifications of deterioration in brain function have been used, from grade I (mild or episodic drowsiness, impaired concentration/intellect, but arousable and coherent); grade II (increased drowsiness, confusion, and disorientation, but able to arouse); grade III (very drowsy, agitated, disoriented, but able to respond to simple verbal commands); and grade IV (unresponsive coma with or without response to painful stimuli). Cerebral edema with elevated intracranial pressure can occur in up to 80% of patients with grade IV encephalopathy and carries a poor prognosis. The cause of cerebral edema is poorly understood. Patients with hepatic encephalopathy need to be carefully assessed for other causes of encephalopathy such as sepsis, uremia, acidosis, alcohol withdrawal, hypoxia, electrolyte abnormalities, and intracerebral bleed.

Hepatopulmonary Syndrome

A critical complication in liver failure, hepatopulmonary syndrome, occurs due to vascular dilation in the lungs leading to impaired gas exchange. Patients with hepatopulmonary syndrome may present with shortness of breath, cyanosis, arterial hypoxemia, and pulmonary edema. Mechanical ventilation may be necessary to provide oxygenation and ventilation. According to studies, hepatopulmonary syndrome has a wide range of prevalence (4%-47%) in cirrhotic patients. However, the critical nature of the condition is clear. Definitive medical treatment is not currently available. Liver transplantation may provide a cure.

Electrolyte Imbalance

A variety of electrolyte imbalances occur in liver failure. Hypoglycemia develops due to massive hepatic cell necrosis, leading to loss of glycogen stores and diminished glucose release. Hypokalemia may occur from inadequate oral intake, increased potassium losses from vomiting, or from medical interventions (eg, nasogastric suction or diuretic therapy). Hypomagnesemia commonly occurs in conjunction with hypokalemia as there is a close relationship between the movement of these electrolytes.

Hypocalcemia is a complication of multiple blood transfusions because the citrate used to anticoagulate stored blood may cause calcium depletion. Hypophosphatemia is also commonly associated with acute liver failure. The exact mechanisms remain unknown. Alkalosis and acidosis may both occur.

Hepatorenal Syndrome

Hepatorenal syndrome, a unique form of renal failure associated with severe liver disease, occurs in up to 40% of patients with advanced cirrhosis. This syndrome represents the most frequent fatal complication of liver failure. The pathogenesis of hepatorenal syndrome is multifactorial and includes portal hypertension resulting in splanchnic vasodilation and eventual sustained renal vasoconstriction and impaired renal perfusion. Precipitating events such as aggressive diuresis and SBP can cause an acute deterioration in renal function. Other than treating contributing conditions, the only definitive treatment for hepatorenal syndrome is liver transplantation. Renal function typically returns to normal after transplant. Without liver transplantation, hepatorenal syndrome is often fatal for the cirrhotic patient. Further research is needed regarding the use of vasoconstricting agents to reverse splanchnic vasodilation and improve outcomes.

Esophageal and Gastric Varices

Esophageal and gastric varices result from portal hypertension and develop in most patients with advanced cirrhosis. Mortality is significant and preventive measures including beta-blockers and endoscopic band ligation are of benefit (see previous section addressing upper GI bleeding). Similarly, prominent veins in the abdominal wall and around the umbilicus (caput medusa) may develop.

Spontaneous Bacterial Peritonitis

Spontaneous bacterial peritonitis (SBP) is an infected ascitic fluid collection, demonstrated by a polymorphonuclear (PMN) count more than 250 cells/mm^3 without an evident intra-abdominal source. SBP occurs in approximately one-quarter of patients admitted with chronic liver failure and ascites. While SBP is a common complication of liver failure, the overall incidence is decreasing due to prophylactic treatment in high-risk populations. A single microbial organism is usually responsible, such as *Escherichia coli*. It is theorized that intestinal translocation of organisms into the ascitic fluid results in infection.

Malnutrition

The liver performs many nutrition-related functions. They include metabolism of carbohydrates, fats, and proteins and storage of essential minerals such as iron, copper, and vitamins A, B$_{12}$, D, and K. In advanced hepatic failure, the impaired ability to synthesize and store glycogen results in rapid muscle loss even during brief periods of decreased nutrient intake. Patients with hepatic failure frequently require vitamin K supplementation to normalize PT and PTT. Patients with alcohol-related liver disease may require IV thiamine to prevent Wernicke encephalopathy.

Clinical Presentation of Liver Failure

History

- Exposure to contaminated food, water
- Exposure to blood, body fluids
- Alcohol abuse

Signs and Symptoms

Impaired Thought Processes

- Mental status changes (confusion, lethargy)
- Speech problems
- Behavioral changes
- Delirium
- Seizures
- Coma

Impaired Gas Exchange

- Hypoxemia
- Pulmonary edema

Fluid Volume Deficit or Excess

- Hypotension
- Skin cool, pale, and dry
- Urine output less than 30 mL/h (<0.5 mL/kg/h)
- Tachycardia
- Dry mucous membranes

Hyperdynamic Circulation

- Arrhythmias
- Fever
- Palmar erythema (flushed palms)
- Jugular vein distension
- Crackles
- Murmur
- Increased CO
- Decreased systemic vascular resistance

Altered Nutrition

- Decreased appetite
- Muscle wasting
- Nausea and vomiting

Impaired Liver Metabolism

- Jaundice/Icterus
- Dry skin
- Ascites

Diagnostic Tests

- Total bilirubin more than 1.5 mg/dL
- Aspartate aminotransferase (AST) more than 40 U/L
- Alanine aminotransferase (ALT) more than 60 U/L
- PT more than 13 seconds
- aPTT more than 45 seconds
- Fibrinogen less than 200 mg/dL
- Albumin less than 3.2 g/dL
- Ammonia more than 45 mg/dL
- Lactate dehydrogenase (LDH) more than 333 U/L
- Ultrasound, endoscopy, endoscopic retrograde cholangiopancreatography (ERCP), liver angiography/biopsy

Principles of Management for Liver Failure

The management of the patient with liver failure is centered on supporting cardiopulmonary status, supporting hematologic and nutritional functions of the liver, and preventing and treating complications.

Support Cardiopulmonary Status

1. Monitor fluid balance. The patient may have a fluid volume deficit related to portal hypertension, ascites, GI bleeding, or coagulation abnormalities. Fluid overload may be a problem related to sodium excess and hypoalbuminemia. Administer diuretics such as furosemide and spironolactone as prescribed. Weigh patient daily.

ESSENTIAL CONTENT CASE

Liver Failure

A 47-year-old man is admitted with a 3-day history of shortness of breath, increased confusion, nausea, and weakness. He has a history of upper GI bleeding from esophageal and gastric varices and was recently hospitalized for refractory ascites. He is diagnosed with liver failure due to alcohol abuse and is severely malnourished. Significant findings on his admission profile were:

History

Complaints of decreased appetite for the past 2 months; also complaints of nausea and weakness.

Vital Signs

Blood pressure:	89/52 mm Hg lying, MAP 64
Heart rate:	124, Sinus tachycardia with frequent PVCs
Respiratory rate:	32 breaths/min; shallow
Temperature:	37°C orally

Cardiopulmonary

- Dyspneic; using accessory muscles
- Crackles at the bases and coarse rhonchi throughout all lung fields
- S_3/S_4; no murmurs
- Extremities cool, weak pulses
- 4+ pitting edema lower extremities

Neurologic

- Alert, but disoriented to time and place
- Irritable

Abdomen

- Tense ascites, dull to percussion
- Hyperactive BSs in all four quadrants

Genitourinary

- Urine dark, amber, and cloudy (0.3 mL/kg/h via urinary catheter)
- Large hemorrhoid protruding from rectal vault
- Liquid stool; black; guaiac positive

Laboratory Data
Arterial blood gases on 2 L O_2 per nasal cannula

pH	7.49
$PaCO_2$	30 mm Hg
PaO_2	64 mm Hg
SaO_2	87%
HCO_3^-	32
Hematocrit	27%

Hemoglobin	8 g/dL
Aspartate transaminase (AST)	80 U/L
Alanine transaminase (ALT)	84 U/L
Bilirubin	2.5 mg/dL
PT	18 seconds
aPTT	45 seconds
INR	2.0
Fibrinogen	158 mg/dL
Albumin	2.8 g/dL
Potassium	3.0 mEq/L
Sodium	134 mEq/L
Creatinine	2.8 mg/dL
BUN	42 mg/dL
Glucose	80 mg/dL

Urine electrolytes

Sodium	5 mEq/L/day
Potassium	10 mEq/L/day

Case Question 1: Which complication of liver failure is this patient experiencing which contributes to a high risk of mortality?
(A) Hepatorenal syndrome
(B) GI bleeding
(C) Hepatic encephalopathy
(D) Ascites

Case Question 2: Which factor/s contribute/s to malnutrition in the patient with liver failure?
(A) Decreased oral intake
(B) Altered metabolism and storage of nutrients
(C) Altered mental status
(D) All of the above

Answers

1. The correct answer is (A). The most fatal complication of liver failure is hepatorenal syndrome. The risk for hepatorenal syndrome is evident with the low urine output, low BP, low Hgb/Hct, high BUN/creatinine, electrolyte abnormalities, and ascites.
2. The correct answer is (D). The liver metabolizes carbohydrates, fats, and proteins and also plays a key role in the storage of essential minerals, vitamins, and glycogen. When the liver is not able to synthesize and store glycogen, rapid muscle loss will occur. Altered mental status may lead to a decrease in oral intake which will further compromise nutritional status.

2. Monitor abdominal girth when ascites is present and assist with paracentesis if needed. Generally, paracentesis is done for patient comfort to reduce respiratory impingement by the ascites and painful tautness of the abdomen. Large-volume paracentesis is defined as removal of more than 5 L of fluid. This requires IV colloid replacement to prevent rapid re-accumulation of ascetic fluid and subsequent dehydration.

3. Monitor respiratory status and correlate with arterial blood gas results. Administer oxygen as ordered. Administer sedatives and analgesics cautiously. Assist the patient with maneuvers to improve oxygenation.

Support Hematologic, Nutritional, and Metabolic Functions of the Liver

1. Monitor for signs of bleeding (eg, gastric contents, stools, urine) and test for occult blood. Observe for petechiae and bruising. Monitor hematologic profile.
2. Administer blood and blood products as ordered.
3. Institute measures to prevent variceal bleeding as needed, including beta-blockers.
4. Institute measures to provide for safety and to minimize tissue trauma. Provide for frequent mouth care. Avoid use of rectal tubes.
5. Initiate oral nutrition supplementation or enteral nutrition (EN) as appropriate (see nutrition section of this chapter).
6. Monitor for signs and symptoms of infection. Maintain sterility of invasive lines and tubes. Maintain aseptic technique when performing procedures.

Preventing and Treating Complications

The most common complications of liver failure are hepatic encephalopathy, fluid and electrolyte imbalances, hepatorenal syndrome, and variceal hemorrhage.

1. Institute measures to prevent injury to the skin, particularly in conditions that result in third spacing such as ascites.
2. Limit the use of medications that are metabolized or detoxified by the liver, especially narcotics and sedatives.
3. Keep the head of bed elevated to prevent aspiration and improve breathing. However, to prevent compression of the lungs by ascites, elevate the patient's head by using the reverse Trendelenburg position when able.
4. Observe for changes in mentation. Institute safety measures if confusion is present. May require endotracheal intubation to protect airway.
5. Perform interventions to reduce ammonia levels. Lactulose is a first-line treatment to decrease gut ammonia production. It can be administered through a nasogastric tube, orally (if alert and without an endotracheal tube), or rectally via a rectal tube (if large friable hemorrhoids are not present). Use caution to avoid variceal rupture or tissue trauma is required with any tube insertion. Research demonstrates the efficacy of rifaximin in maintaining remission from hepatic encephalopathy. However, rifaximin is only available as tablets and is not appropriate for critically ill patients who cannot take medications orally. Perform frequent neurological assessments. Trending serum ammonia levels is not recommended as the levels rarely correlate with degree of encephalopathy.
6. Institute protocols for bleeding risk due to clotting abnormalities and acute upper GI hemorrhage due to variceal rupture (see previous section on acute gastrointestinal bleeding).

7. Definitive treatment for hepatorenal syndrome is liver transplantation. In critically ill patients, the use of albumin as an intravascular expander in combination with a vasoconstrictor is recommended and may result in improvement.

Artificial Liver Support Systems

Artificial liver support systems, currently available for investigational use only, may have a role in bridging patients with acute liver failure to transplant or providing support until regeneration of liver function occurs. The basic mechanism of artificial liver support systems is extracorporeal circulation of the patient's blood through filters that remove waste products normally filtered by the liver. These devices have not yet shown a decrease in mortality. Randomized trials are underway to optimize and assess the effectiveness of these devices.

Liver Transplantation

Liver transplantation has changed the survival of patients with liver failure. The decision to proceed with transplantation requires a detailed assessment and interprofessional review. The Model for End-Stage Liver Disease, or MELD scoring system, was adopted in 2002 as the index to determine transplant priority. In 2016, UNOS authorized the addition of serum sodium to the MELD calculation when considering transplantation status and established the current MELD score. A higher score is associated with higher mortality risk and subsequent greater priority for transplantation.

Acute Pancreatitis

Acute pancreatitis is inflammation of the pancreas resulting from premature activation of pancreatic exocrine enzymes, such as trypsin, phospholipase A, and elastase within the pancreas. The disease ranges in severity from a mild acute self-limiting form to severe and life threatening. Severe acute pancreatitis, occurring in approximately one-fifth of patients with pancreatitis, involves autodigestion and necrosis of the pancreas. This pancreatic injury triggers a systemic inflammatory response, which can lead to multisystem organ failure (see Chapter 11, Multisystem Problems). Pancreatitis is categorized into two forms: interstitial edematous pancreatitis, which has a 3% mortality rate, and necrotizing acute pancreatitis, which has a 17% mortality rate. For patients with severe acute pancreatitis with necrosis, the mortality rate is 30%.

The diagnosis of acute pancreatitis is based on at least two of the three following criteria: characteristic abdominal pain or epigastric pain that may radiate to the back; serum amylase or lipase values 2 to 4 times above the normal range; and characteristic findings on imaging, most often ultrasound imaging. In general, serum lipase is more sensitive than serum amylase as a marker of pancreatitis. However, neither is predictive of disease severity or indicative of disease progression. Amylase and lipase are only useful as diagnostic tools. Organ failure and pancreatic necrosis are the two most important markers of severity.

Scoring systems are recommended to accurately identify the severity of acute pancreatitis and determine the appropriate patient care setting. Some of these tools (such as Ranson, Modified Marshall, APACHE IV, and Glasgow-Imrie) have limited to no applicability upon admission and are best applied after full assessment at the 24- to 48-hour mark. Other scoring systems that offer an assessment of disease severity within the first 24 hours have demonstrated clinical usefulness. The Bedside Index of Severity of Acute Pancreatitis (BISAP) is one example. This tool is both accurate and easy to use. The score is calculated on five variables: (1) BUN greater than 25 mg/dL; (2) impaired mental status; (3) presence of two or more criteria of systemic inflammatory response syndrome; (4) age greater than 60; and (5) pleural effusion on imaging. Each variable provides one point and scores of 3, 4, and 5 are associated with higher hospital mortality with a score of 5 associated with ~22% rate of mortality.

Etiologies, Risk Factors, and Pathophysiology

The leading causes of acute pancreatitis are chronic alcohol use and gallstones/biliary tract disease (stones). Drug-induced pancreatitis occurs with less frequency but has been linked to metronidazole, tetracycline, azathioprine, and estrogens as well as others. Less common etiologies are hypertriglyceridemia, hypercalcemia, infectious, autoimmune, vascular, genetic mutations, pancreatic neoplasms, post-ERCP pancreatitis, and idiopathic causes. In fact, 15% to 20% of pancreatitis cases are designated as idiopathic after a complete workup proves inconclusive.

The pathogenesis of acute pancreatitis is not completely understood. The pancreas normally has a protective mechanism, an enzyme called trypsin inhibitor, to prevent activation of enzymes before they reach the duodenum, thereby preventing inflammation of pancreatic cells. Regardless of the etiology, the process of premature activation of pancreatic enzymes leading to local inflammation and possible necrosis is the defining characteristic of pancreatitis. The activated enzymes can also enter the systemic circulation via the portal vein and lymphatic system, which leads to stimulation of platelet-activating factor and humoral systems (kinin, complement, and fibrinolysis). These systems, which normally function to protect against infection, can generate a wide spread inflammatory response which results in damage to multiple organs (Table 14-9; see also Chapter 11, Multisystem Problems). Pancreatic abscess, pseudocyst, peripancreatic fluid collection, and necrosis are localized complications that may occur with fulminant forms of the disease. In severe acute pancreatitis, blood vessels in and around the pancreas may

TABLE 14-9. COMMON MULTISYSTEM COMPLICATIONS OF ACUTE PANCREATITIS

Pulmonary
Atelectasis
Acute respiratory distress syndrome
Pleural effusions
Cardiovascular
Cardiogenic shock
Neurologic
Pancreatic encephalopathy
Metabolic
Metabolic acidosis
Hypocalcemia
Altered glucose metabolism
Hematologic
Disseminated intravascular coagulation
GI bleeding
Renal
Prerenal failure

also become disrupted by microthrombi or enzymatic erosion of vasculature, resulting in hemorrhage.

Clinical Presentation

Signs and Symptoms

Pancreatic Inflammation

- *Acute pain:* Severe, relentless, knifelike; midepigastrium or periumbilical
- Abdominal guarding
- Rebound tenderness
- Nausea and vomiting
- Abdominal distention
- Hypoactive BSs

Fluid Volume Deficit

- Hypotension
- Tachycardia
- Mental status changes
- Cool, clammy skin
- Decreased urine output

Impaired Gas Exchange

- Decreasing Pao_2 (<60 mm Hg) and Sao_2 (<90%)

Diagnostic Tests

- Serum amylase more than 140 U/L
- Serum pancreatic isoamylase more than 50% (more sensitive than amylase)
- Serum lipase more than 160 U/dL
- Serum triglycerides more than 1000 mg/dL
- Urine amylase more than 14 U/h (indicative of increased serum amylase)
- Serum calcium less than 8.5 mg/dL
- Serum sodium less than 135 mEq/L
- Serum potassium less than 3.5 mEq/L
- Serum magnesium less than 1.5 mg/dL
- Increased ALT (>55 U/L), in gallstone pancreatitis
- C-reactive protein (>3 mg/L)
- Glucose more than 120 mg/dL

Imaging Studies

- Ultrasound abdomen, check for cholelithiasis or choledocholithiasis (but may be obscured by bowel gas)
- Computed tomography (CT), pancreatic protocol CT scan of abdomen
- Endoscopic ultrasound (EUS)
- ERCP
- MRI/magnetic resonance cholangiopancreatography (MRCP)

Principles of Management of Acute Pancreatitis

The management of the patient with acute pancreatitis centers on reducing the release of enzymes and treating complications that can occur with multisystem disease. Interventions within the first 24 hours are essential to improving outcomes including increased survival. These interventions include determining severity with a reliable scoring system, aggressive fluid resuscitation, and other supportive measures such as application of oxygen, intubation, and mechanical ventilation as needed. Patients who demonstrate signs of organ failure (severe acute pancreatitis) are cared for in a critical care unit. Patients who do not demonstrate improvement or in whom there is uncertainty about the diagnosis are considered candidates for CT or MRI/MRCP. At the time of this writing, there is no role for prophylactic antibiotics in patients with mild forms of acute pancreatitis. Additional principles of management include pain management, reducing pancreatic demands, and supporting other organ systems that may be failing due to the release of inflammatory mediators.

Fluid Resuscitation

Patients with acute pancreatitis experience significant hypovolemia as a result of third space losses, vomiting, and vascular permeability related to inflammatory mediators. Hypovolemia can compromise pancreatic circulation and increase the risk for pancreatic necrosis, so aggressive fluid and electrolyte replacement is essential in the initial management. However, after 48 hours, the amount and rate of fluid administration must take into account the risk of fluid overload and consequent compartment syndrome or pulmonary edema.

1. In adults, administer IV isotonic crystalloid fluids at rates of 5 to 10 mL/kg/h or greater if hypotensive with frequent reassessment of fluid needs, particularly within the first 12 to 24 hours. Caution is taken when treating patients with cardiovascular and renal conditions to diminish the risk of fluid overload. Monitor outcomes of fluid replacement therapy, including blood pressure, heart rate, intake and output, skin turgor, capillary refill, mucous membranes, and urine output (goal of greater than 0.5 to 1 mL/kg/h). See Chapter 4 for hemodynamic monitoring to assess fluid status.
2. Monitor for signs and symptoms of retroperitoneal hemorrhage (low hematocrit and hemoglobin levels).

Cullen sign is a bluish discoloration around the periumbilical area, and Grey Turner sign is a bluish discoloration around the flank, indicating blood in the peritoneum. Monitor for increasing abdominal girths.
3. Monitor electrolytes for imbalances related to prolonged vomiting or fluid sequestration. Calcium, sodium, magnesium, and potassium are most commonly affected. Monitor QT intervals on the electrocardiogram and implement seizure precautions with severe hypocalcemia. Hyperglycemia also may be present due to the stress response and impaired secretion of insulin by the islet cells in the inflamed pancreas. Glucose levels need frequent evaluation. If elevated, administer an insulin infusion with hourly glucose assessments and insulin adjustments, then subcutaneous insulin to obtain a normoglycemic state. Hyperglycemia decreases healing and increases infection risk.

Pain Management

Acute pain is a universal sign of acute pancreatitis. It is caused by peritoneal irritation from activated pancreatic exocrine enzymes, edema or distention of the pancreas, or interruption of the blood supply to the pancreas. Treatment of pain is a priority because it increases exocrine enzyme release by the pancreas, extending pancreatic inflammation and worsening hemodynamic instability.

1. Assess the degree of pain using a reliable pain-rating scale appropriate to the patient.
2. Administer analgesics. In the past, the use of opiate analgesics (eg, morphine, fentanyl) has been discouraged because of the potential for causing increased pressure on the sphincter of Oddi, which in turn may increase pain. Meperidine has been suggested as an alternative to other opioids. However, no outcome-based studies in patients with acute pancreatitis show that meperidine is superior. In addition, other opioids may provide better pain relief and do not have the seizure risk that occurs with meperidine. No studies or evidence exists to indicate morphine is contraindicated in acute pancreatitis. All analgesics are considered with an understanding of the risks and benefits to the individual patient. Regardless of what analgesic is prescribed, a pain rating scale is used to evaluate efficacy. In addition, scheduled doses, continuous infusions, and epidural analgesia are important to consider to maintain steady-state analgesia in patients with severe pain.
3. Assess patient anxiety and administer sedatives with analgesics.
4. Assist the patient in a position that promotes comfort. The knee-to-chest position, when possible, may decrease the intensity of the pain. (Refer to Chapter 6, Pain, Sedation, and Neuromuscular Blockade Management, for additional information on pain management.)

Preventing Pancreatic Stimulation

Preventing stimulation of pancreatic exocrine secretion is a priority to interrupt the cycle of pancreatic inflammation.

1. In mild pancreatitis, with decreasing pain, improving labs and no nausea/vomiting or ileus, it is recommended to initiate early oral feeding (generally within 24 hours) instead of keeping patients NPO. Success of early feeding has been demonstrated using a variety of diets (eg, low-fat, normal fat, and soft or solid consistency). Research has demonstrated no difference in mortality for early versus delayed feeding with patients experiencing acute pancreatitis.

2. In moderate to severe pancreatitis, EN with jejunal feedings is often preferred to prevent pancreatic stimulation and enzyme secretion and to meet nutritional and caloric needs. With improvement, oral intake may be initiated and advanced as tolerated. Research suggests that early enteral feeding improves outcomes and that oral, gastric, and jejunal feedings may all be feasible.

3. Parenteral nutrition (PN) is not necessary unless enteral feedings are not tolerated.

4. Administer pharmacologic agents as prescribed to block the secretion of pancreatic enzymes or facilitate nutrient absorption.

Treat Local Complications in the Pancreas

Local complications in the pancreas include peripancreatic fluid collections and pseudocysts, and necrotic collections (acute necrotic collection and walled-off necrosis). The Atlanta classification system is used to standardize recognition and definition of these complications. Percutaneous or stent therapies to drain the fluids in and around the pancreas and/or surgical resection or debridement may be required, especially if the pancreas becomes infected. Biliary ERCP and laparoscopic cholecystectomy are indicated for gallstone pancreatitis, once the pancreatic inflammation has abated.

Treat Multisystem Failure

Cardiopulmonary complications due to pancreatic enzyme–induced mediators are the most common multisystem problems. Pancreatic ischemia also promotes the release of myocardial depressant factor. This causes decreased myocardial contractility and CO. Surgical therapies such as a pancreatic resection may be performed to prevent systemic complications of acute necrotizing pancreatitis by removing necrotic or infected tissue. In some cases, a pancreatectomy may be performed.

1. Administer oxygen therapy to maintain arterial oxygen tension and oxygen saturation. Mechanical ventilation with adjunct therapies to promote maximal alveolar gas exchange is often used to manage acute respiratory distress syndrome (see Chapter 10, Respiratory System and Chapter 20, Advanced Respiratory Concepts: Modes of Mechanical Ventilation).

2. Administer fluids, inotropes, and other vasopressors to support myocardial contractility, CO, and blood pressure (see Chapter 11, Multisystem Problems, for more information on sepsis).

3. Institute measures to prevent infection. Monitor for signs and symptoms of sepsis and initiate appropriate treatment if indicated. Prophylactic antibiotics are not recommended (see Chapter 11, Multisystem Problems).

4. Manage coagulopathies (see Chapter 13, Hematologic and Immune Systems).

5. Treat acute kidney injury if a complicating factor (see Chapter 15, Renal System).

Intestinal Ischemia

Major disorders of the intestine include intestinal ischemia. Vascular occlusion or infarction of the mesenteric vessels is rare but catastrophic and will result in profound illness with a mortality rate of 50%. Intestinal ischemia may present as intestinal angina, ischemic colitis, or intestinal infarction. Ischemic colitis is the most common ischemic injury. Ischemia may be acute or chronic. Acute forms are due to sudden and complete arterial occlusion by emboli, thrombosis of atherosclerotic stenosis, small vessel occlusion, venous thrombosis, or significant vasoconstriction. Gradual occlusion is better tolerated as there is time for collateral circulation to form. Sudden or acute ischemia is poorly tolerated because the bowel is not protected by collateral circulation. There is an extensive mesenteric collateral circulation which protects against ischemic insults, allowing the intestine to tolerate up to a 75% reduction in blood flow for up to 12 hours. The colon is particularly susceptible to low-flow states, in particular, the splenic flexure, ileocecal junction, and rectosigmoid.

Etiology, Risk Factors, and Pathophysiology

Intestinal ischemia develops from a compromise in blood flow to the intestine, which is inadequate to meet metabolic demands. It is the result of hypoperfusion and reperfusion injury. Both the small intestine and the large bowel can be affected but ischemic colitis is the most common form of intestinal ischemia. Acute ischemic colitis affects segments of the colon with normal colon on either side of the affected area. The right colon is affected 25% of the time, transverse 10%, left 33%, distal colon 25%, and the entire colon 7%. Disease involving the right side of the colon is usually more severe with the patient at risk for having involvement of the small intestine. Three major arterial trunks—the celiac axis, superior mesenteric artery, and inferior mesenteric artery—comprise the splanchnic (intestinal) circulation. The superior mesenteric artery, the inferior mesenteric artery, and branches of the internal iliac arteries perfuse the colon.

An acute occlusion is usually the result of a cardiogenic embolus with the superior mesenteric artery most frequently affected. The tissue injury that occurs will result in the release of cellular contents and the by-products of anaerobic metabolism into the general circulation. The ischemic bowel loses protein, electrolytes, and fluid into the lumen and wall of the bowel. The third-space extracellular fluid loss decreases the circulating blood volume. Full-thickness necrosis leads to bowel perforation and peritonitis.

The underlying causes of intestinal ischemia are diverse and include decreased CO, hypovolemia, arrhythmias, hypercoagulable states, mechanical obstruction, vascular disease, and trauma. Predisposing medications include cocaine, cardiac glycosides, and alpha-stimulating sympathomimetic amines (epinephrine, norepinephrine). Older adult patients with systemic atherosclerosis are particularly at risk.

Clinical Presentation

Signs and symptoms will vary depending on the severity of the ischemia and area and length of intestine affected. The most common signs on admission to the hospital are hematochezia due to mucosal sloughing, abdominal pain, and diarrhea.

History

- Obstruction
- Diabetes mellitus
- Dyslipidemia
- Smoking
- Heart failure
- Aortic or coronary artery bypass surgery
- Shock
- Atrial fibrillation
- Atherosclerosis
- Medications: digitalis, diuretics, NSAIDs, catecholamines, and neuroleptics
- Recurrent nonspecific abdominal symptoms

Signs and Symptoms

- Peritoneal signs (abdominal guarding and rebound tenderness)
- Acute onset, colicky, severe left lower abdominal pain
- Pain out of proportion to abdominal examination findings
- Hematochezia (bloody stools)
- Nausea and vomiting
- Anorexia, early satiety
- Weight loss
- Urgent desire to defecate
- Diarrhea or constipation (or both)
- Abdominal distention
- Abdominal tenderness
- Cramping
- Post-prandial pain
- Decreased BSs
- Muscle rigidity
- Changes in vital signs including fever and tachycardia
- Changes in laboratory values including elevated lactate, leukocytosis, metabolic acidosis, elevated LDH

Diagnostic Tests

Diagnosis is based on clinical findings and supported by radiographic corroboration and colonoscopic evaluation. CT or CT arteriography (CTA) scan and magnetic resonance angiography (MRA) or ultrasound are useful in supporting clinical suspicion and for identifying potential complications. Catheter angiography can be used to confirm the diagnosis and to provide selective revascularization interventions.

Colonoscopy may also be considered with distinct efforts to avoid over-distending the fragile intestine. The colonoscopy can identify mucosal abnormalities; findings will depend on the stage and severity of the ischemia. The finding of hemorrhagic, dusky mucosa with patches of inflammation is typical. CT arteriography or MRA is indicated if acute mesenteric ischemia involving the small intestine is suspected. Interventional mesenteric arteriography may identify the site of occlusion and in addition can facilitate treatment with transcatheter thrombolysis, stent placement, or vasodilator infusion. A cardiac workup (ECG, Holter monitor, transthoracic echocardiogram, and cardiac catheterization if indicated) is done to exclude a cardiac source for an embolism. Laboratory serum markers have not proved to be valuable as a method of early detection of acute mesenteric ischemia.

Principles of Management for Intestinal Ischemia

Patient priorities revolve around treating the intravascular fluid volume deficit and avoiding the use of vasopressors. Generally, patients will respond to conservative supportive therapy. In elderly patients, and in those in whom treatment and surgical intervention is delayed, necrosis and death may ensue. Delayed treatment (>24 hours from the onset of symptoms) is associated with a mortality rate of more than or equal to 70%.

Medical treatment for intestinal ischemia will depend on the presentation and severity of the insult. Supportive care is provided with patients placed on bowel rest, antibiotics, and IV fluids. Systemic anticoagulation may also be considered for arterial and venous thrombosis and embolic disease. Hemodynamic status is optimized and vasoconstrictive drugs are avoided. The patient is monitored for signs of bowel necrosis such as persistent fever, leukocytosis, peritoneal irritation, or protracted pain or bleeding.

In the case of nonocclusive mesenteric insufficiency, a catheter infusion of a vasodilator, such as papaverine, into the superior mesenteric artery can be given intra-arterially at the time of arteriography. Spasm is considered the primary cause of this type of ischemia.

Exploratory laparotomy with thromboembolectomy or bypass of the occlusion (surgical revascularization) can be performed if the diagnosis is an acute mesenteric occlusion resulting from a clot or an atherosclerotic plaque. Surgery may also be indicated for peritonitis or clinical deterioration suggesting necrotic bowel (increasing abdominal tenderness, guarding, rebound tenderness, rising temperature, and/or paralytic ileus). Twenty percent of patients require surgical intervention for resection of the involved bowel. However, with current advances in endovascular treatments, surgical approaches are less frequent. The options for endovascular approaches, such as percutaneous transluminal angioplasty with stent placement, avoid the risks associated with an open surgical repair and are more common.

Bowel Obstruction

Bowel obstructions can lead to hospitalization for the management of fluid status, electrolyte abnormalities, and evaluation for surgical treatment. Intestinal transit can be affected by either a mechanical or functional obstruction. Mechanical obstructions can be due to lesions which block the internal lumen (luminal or intrinsic) or by lesions that compress the bowel lumen from the outside of the intestine (extrinsic). Mechanical obstructions can be further classified as either a small-bowel obstruction (SBO) or a large-bowel obstruction (LBO); and complete or partial. Complete obstruction always requires surgical management, whereas a partial obstruction can be managed conservatively with serial examinations and supportive treatment. Ileus and colonic pseudo-obstruction are categorized as functional obstructions.

Etiology, Risk Factors, and Pathophysiology
Small-Bowel Obstruction
Adhesions due to previous surgery are the most common cause of an SBO followed by malignant tumors (peritoneal implants), hernias, and inflammatory bowel disease. Adhesions account for approximately 70% of all SBO. Recent studies reveal that the incidence of SBO is lower in patients who have minimally invasive procedures versus open surgery. Evidence suggests patients with SBO have improved outcomes when they are admitted to the hospital under a surgical service who can intervene in a timely manner if needed.

Large-Bowel Obstruction
Colorectal cancer is the most common cause of an LBO in the United States with the descending colon and sigmoid colon being the most common sites of obstruction. Other causes of a mechanical (intraluminal) obstruction include fecal impaction and foreign bodies. Inflammation (diverticulitis or inflammatory bowel disease), ischemia, intussusception, and anastomotic stricture are also intrinsic etiologies. Extrinsic causes include hernias, abscess, volvulus, or tumors in adjacent organs. Adhesions are less likely to lead to obstruction of the large bowel; they are more common in the small bowel.

Early in the course of the obstruction, bowel motility and contractions will increase as the bowel attempts to push contents past the point of obstruction. This can account for diarrhea in the initial presentation. The intestine becomes fatigued, dilates, and contractions are less frequent and intense. Water and electrolytes accumulate in the bowel lumen and lead to dehydration and hypovolemia. Hypochloremia, hypokalemia, and metabolic alkalosis are not uncommon, especially if the patient is vomiting or has high large-volume nasogastric tube losses. Abdominal distention can compromise respiratory function. In general,

with either an SBO or LBO, a segment of the intestine may be excessively edematous or lumen malrotation may be present. These conditions can result in a blood supply that is compromised or strangulated. The blood supply can also be compromised by the increasing tension related to the abdominal distention. Ischemia may result and, if not treated, can lead to bowel necrosis. The cecum is the most common site of colonic ischemia or perforation, followed by the sigmoid colon.

Ileus
An ileus is intestinal distention and the slowing or absence of the passage of intestinal contents. It is a functional obstruction, so a mechanical cause cannot be identified. Common causes of an ileus are drug induced (anticholinergics, psychotropics, or opioids), metabolic derangements (hyperglycemia, hyperthyroidism), electrolyte abnormalities (such as hypokalemia), neurogenic, and infections. Ileus is most common after abdominal operations and often persists the longest after colon surgery.

Acute Colonic Pseudo-Obstruction
Pseudo-obstruction, also called Ogilvie syndrome, is a chronic condition of recurrent distention of the colon with signs and symptoms of obstruction, in the absence of a physical or mechanical cause. Acute colonic pseudo-obstruction (ACPO) is characterized by the absence of intestinal contractility. The exact cause remains unknown. It is commonly seen in hospitalized or institutionalized patients, older adults, and patients with chronic renal failure, respiratory, cerebral, or cardiovascular disease. It has an unknown prevalence and incidence, and as its name implies, it primarily affects the colon. It is diagnosed only after excluding mechanical LBO.

Clinical Presentation of Bowel Obstruction
Signs and symptoms will vary depending on the cause and location of the obstruction.

History
- Prior abdominal surgery
- Ischemia
- Hernia
- Abdominal cancer
- Abdominal radiation
- Inflammatory bowel disease

Signs and Symptoms
- Crampy or colicky abdominal pain; sometimes localized to periumbilical and epigastric regions, but usually diffuse
- Localized tenderness, rebound, guarding (suggesting peritonitis)
- Diarrhea
- Nausea and vomiting
- Failure to pass stool or flatus
- Abdominal distention

- Abdominal exam may show: visible peristalsis, hyperactive or absent BSs, tympany, and generalized tenderness
- Altered vital signs include: tachycardia, hypotension, fever

Diagnostic Tests

Plain films of the abdomen will demonstrate whether an obstruction is present. Dilated loops of bowel with air-fluid levels are characteristic in the proximal bowel; distal bowel is collapsed. A CT scan of the abdomen and pelvis with oral contrast will show the site of the obstruction, identify the transition zone, and often demonstrates the etiology. It is the diagnostic examination of choice. A small-bowel follow-through or enema study using water-soluble contrast solution may be necessary. Electrolyte disorders are common due to vomiting, diarrhea, lack of oral intake, and inflammatory mediators. The most common electrolyte abnormality is hypokalemia. The patient will exhibit either a metabolic or contraction alkalosis (renal sodium reabsorption in exchange for H^+) or metabolic acidosis (GI bicarbonate loss and hypovolemic tissue hypoperfusion).

Principles of Management for Bowel Obstruction

Treatment options will vary depending on the diagnosis. Initially, a nasogastric tube may be placed to decompress the bowel, the intravascular fluid volume deficit is treated with isotonic fluids, electrolyte abnormalities are corrected, bowel rest is initiated, and antiemetics and antibiotics are administered. Long intestinal tubes are no longer indicated and are associated with longer hospital stays and prolonged ileus. A rectal tube or colonic stent can be used to decompress the distal colon in patients with LBO. These interventions may serve as bridges to surgery or as palliative treatment. Studies demonstrate improved outcomes in bowel obstruction patients who receive prompt surgical consultation for symptoms of pain, nausea, and vomiting.

Treatment of an ileus consists entirely of supportive therapy. The most effective treatment is to address the underlying cause. Metabolic or electrolyte abnormalities are corrected and medications that may be contributing to the ileus are discontinued.

ACPO is treated with the administration of neostigmine, a parasympathomimetic agent. It is important that mechanical causes for the obstruction have been excluded before administering the drug. In the treatment of ACPO, 2.5 mg of neostigmine is given intravenously over 3 minutes. The pseudo-obstruction will resolve within less than 10 minutes with the patient passing stool and flatus. If no response occurs, the dose can be repeated 4 hours later. Bradycardia, bronchospasm, and hypotension are side effects of neostigmine and patients must be monitored with telemetry. Atropine is kept readily available. Patients with cardiac disease are not the candidates for this treatment. Patients who do not respond to neostigmine undergo a colonoscopy for decompression. Surgery is reserved for patients with signs of ischemia, perforation, or whose clinical status deteriorates.

The majority of SBOs will resolve spontaneously with supportive therapy, and therefore are managed nonoperatively. Surgical therapy is required to treat an LBO and may be necessary for up to 24% of patients with SBO whose symptoms don't resolve with supportive therapy. Strangulated obstructions are surgical emergencies and require immediate intervention. Surgical procedures for various types of obstructions may include lysis of adhesions, reduction of hernias, bypass of obstructions, and resection of affected intestine. Self-expandable metallic colon stents may be placed at the time of colonoscopy to decompress the colon and can be a bridge to elective surgery in patients with a malignancy. A permanent or temporary diverting ileostomy or colostomy may be performed. A flexible sigmoidoscopy can be used initially to decompress a sigmoid volvulus; definitive surgery follows.

Both LBO and SBO treatment may include the following components:

1. Administer colloids and crystalloids to treat the fluid volume deficit. Normal saline with potassium supplementation is the replacement fluid of choice. Monitor patient response to fluid resuscitation—hemodynamic parameters (MAP, heart rate), body weight, and intake and output. A urinary catheter may be placed to monitor urine output.

2. Administer antimicrobial therapy to treat intra-abdominal infection. Gram-negative aerobic and anaerobic coverage is appropriate.

3. Elevate the head of bed to promote lung expansion. Use of reverse Trendelenburg, if tolerated, is a preferred position as it minimizes abdominal compression due to flexion at the hips as seen in a sitting position. Assist with deep breathing exercises to promote lung expansion, mobilization of secretions, and relaxation.

4. Administer analgesics for pain as needed. However, avoid excess use of opiates to promote the return of peristalsis.

5. With severe nausea and vomiting, and/or the abdomen is distended, insert a nasogastric tube and apply and maintain suction to drain and decompress the upper GI tract.

6. Monitor and report signs and symptoms of ongoing infection, peritoneal signs, or deterioration in status. Multiple follow-up abdominal radiographs and serial clinical examinations are indicated. Classic symptoms associated with strangulated bowel are leukocytosis, fever, tachycardia, and severe abdominal pain.

7. Provide nutrition as prescribed. Early enteral therapy may be initiated at slow rates as this has been found to promote the return of peristalsis and may assist in maintaining the gut mucosal barrier function. EN is initiated with caution if bowel ischemia is suspected; total PN may be required.

Bariatric Surgery and Weight Management

Bariatric surgery is an option for weight reduction in obese individuals who have not been successful with conservative weight loss strategies such as lifestyle adjustments (diet, exercise, psychological or psychiatric intervention) or pharmacological therapy. At the time of this writing, there are a variety of endoscopic treatments emerging to help patients manage their weight. These procedures focus on reducing gastric volume (eg, intragastric balloon), slow gastric emptying (eg, gastroplication), or using bypass techniques (eg, implanting a temporary sleeve to mimic gastric bypass). Endoscopic bariatric and metabolic therapies (EBMT) represent innovative alternatives with fewer complications than surgical treatments and higher efficacy than pharmacotherapy (See Figure 14-6).

Bariatric surgery remains the most effective method of weight loss to date. Candidates for bariatric surgery include those patients with a body mass index (BMI) of 40, or a BMI between 35 and 40 in the presence of obesity-related comorbidities, such as diabetes, hypertension, obstructive sleep apnea, and cardiovascular disease.

Because all patients who have bariatric surgery are obese, and many have comorbid diseases, surgical recovery may be challenging. Diabetes mellitus, NAFLD, coronary artery disease, asthma, obstructive sleep apnea, and other conditions are more common among obese patients and require careful postoperative monitoring.

Surgical Procedure

There are three main types of weight loss surgery: restrictive, malabsorptive, and combined restrictive and malabsorptive. These procedures can be performed via either the laparoscopic or open approach. Laparoscopic is recommended because there is less pain, fewer wound complications, a shorter hospital stay, and quicker recovery. All procedures limit the volume of food eaten and alter gastric emptying. The risk for nutritional deficiencies will vary depending on the surgery performed. The restrictive procedures include the vertical banded gastroplasty (VBG), the laparoscopic adjustable gastric band (LAGB), and the laparoscopic sleeve gastrectomy (LSG). The malabsorptive procedures include the biliopancreatic diversion (BPD), biliopancreatic diversion with duodenal switch (BPD-DS), and duodenal switch (DS). The laparoscopic Roux-en-Y (LRYGB) is categorized as both restrictive and malabsorptive.

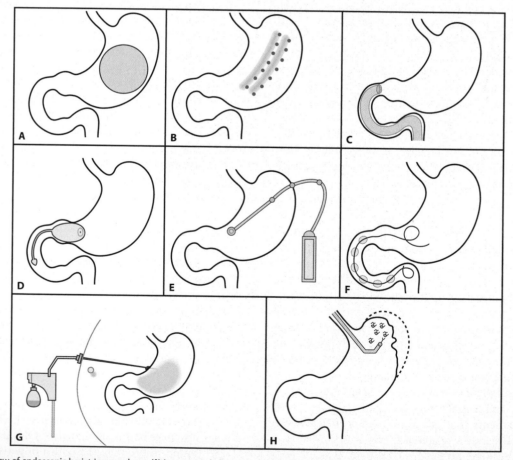

Figure 14-6. Overview of endoscopic bariatric procedures: (**A**) intragastric balloon placement, (**B**) endoscopic sleeve gastroplasty, (**C**) duodenojejunal bypass, (**D**) Transpyloric Shuttle, (**E**) electrical stimulation, (**F**) SatiSphere, (**G**) aspiration therapy, (**H**) Primary Obesity Surgery Endoluminal (POSE). (*Reproduced with permission from Král J, Machytka E, Horká V, et al: Endoscopic Treatment of Obesity and Nutritional Aspects of Bariatric Endoscopy. Nutrients. 2021;13(12):4268.*)

The VBG is done infrequently today, but was popular in the 1980s. The upper stomach near the esophagus is stapled vertically to create a small pouch. A band is placed to restrict the outlet from the pouch. With the LAGB, restriction is accomplished by placing an inflatable silicone band around the antrum of the stomach thereby creating a small pouch. The band is connected to an implanted reservoir under the skin, usually just below the rib cage. The pouch opening can be made smaller or larger by inflating or deflating the band via the reservoir.

The LSG, once considered a preliminary step toward LRYGB, has become an acceptable primary bariatric surgery. The procedure reduces the stomach to about 25% of its original size. The majority of the greater curvature of the stomach is removed. The open edges are stapled to form a sleeve or tube with a "banana" shape. The procedure permanently reduces the size of the stomach. Although it is described as a restrictive procedure, recent studies have identified similar metabolic effects as seen with the LRYGB. These effects could potentiate a sense of satiety for patients. Recent studies have shown weight loss after the LSG to be between that seen with the LAGB and LRYGB.

The BPD, BPD-DS, and DS are malabsorptive procedures. These surgeries carry the highest risk for nutritional deficiencies as they significantly alter digestion and absorption of protein, vitamins, and minerals. In general, there are three main components of these surgeries: a partial gastrectomy, the common or nutrient limb, and biliopancreatic limb. The common limb is a 50 to 100 cm portion of distal small bowel where limited digestion and absorption occur, while the biliopancreatic limb is created from the remainder of the proximal small bowel and functions to divert digestive juices to the nutrient or common limb.

The laparoscopic Roux-en-Y results in both restriction and malabsorption and is the gold standard surgery for treating obesity. The stomach is separated with a stapler and a 15-mL pouch is created. The small intestine is divided and the distal stomach, duodenum, and first part of the jejunum are bypassed. The distal end of the jejunum is anastomosed to the pouch (gastrojejunostomy) to allow for emptying while the proximal end is connected side to side to the jejunum (jejuno-jejunostomy) creating a 75- to 150-cm roux limb. The surgery also has a hormonal effect. Removing the gastric fundus, the primary site of ghrelin production, enhances weight loss by reducing appetite.

Principles of Management for Postoperative Bariatric Surgery

Standard nursing care following bariatric surgery includes assessment of vital signs and incisions, management of pain, pulmonary exercise, and venothromboembolism (VTE) prophylaxis. In addition to standard postoperative care, assessment for, and prevention of, complications inherent to the bariatric surgery procedure and the nuances of the bariatric patient are essential.

Respiratory Insufficiency

Airway obstruction and oxygenation problems are important postoperative concerns following bariatric surgery. Patients with obstructive sleep apnea preoperatively are at higher risk for postoperative respiratory problems. Patients with sleep apnea use their continuous positive airway pressure (CPAP) or bilevel positive airway pressure (BiPAP) machine while in the hospital to help minimize this risk. The increased risk of postoperative oxygenation problems from anesthesia and postoperative analgesics in this vulnerable group requires careful respiratory monitoring for 24 to 48 hours after surgery. Patients with asthma, a common comorbidity with obstructive sleep apnea, need to continue using inhaled medications during the postoperative period.

Assessment for Anastomotic Leaks

Leakage of gastric contents at the site of anastomosis is a potentially life-threatening complication and if not recognized early can lead to overwhelming sepsis. Signs and symptoms of an anastomotic leak include fever, left shoulder pain, tachypnea, and tachycardia. Thirst and hypotension are typically appreciated in progressive sepsis. Abdominal pain may occur, but the absence of it does not preclude the possibility of an anastomotic leak. The only sign of a leak may be unexplained tachycardia.

A leak is diagnosed with either a limited upper GI radiograph or a CT scan. A contained leak can be treated with percutaneous drainage. If the leak is not contained, the patient is returned to the operating room for definitive treatment. A leak could result in an intra-abdominal abscess. The key to treating a leak is to identify it early through watchful monitoring.

Once the upper GI radiograph or CT scan is clear, patients are typically able to begin a gastric bypass diet.

Nausea and Vomiting

Nausea and vomiting are not expected consequences of bariatric surgery. The cause may be mechanical or behavioral. Vomiting is generally very short lived as patients adjust to eating and drinking. Behavioral causes include eating too quickly, overeating, not chewing food well, drinking while eating, or a poor food choice. Dehydration may present as nausea. Anastomotic stricture or another mechanical cause of obstruction must be ruled out. Antiemetics are usually not helpful but may reduce retching that can put strain on the anastomosis and the incision line leading to complications. If the nausea is due to dehydration, the symptoms will resolve with the administration of IV fluids. Counseling the patient and addressing anxieties will assist with management of behavioral etiologies.

Prevention of Pulmonary Embolus

Patients having bariatric procedures are at high risk for pulmonary embolus (PE). Early ambulation postoperatively, which can be challenging in this patient population, reduces the risk of DVT and PE. In the immediate postoperative period, DVT and PE prevention requires a combination of subcutaneous weight-based pharmacologic prophylaxis, use of sequential compression devices, and a program of immediate and progressive mobilization. Optimal pain management is important not just for comfort, but to promote mobility. In patients with a prior history of DVT, PE, or a history of a clotting disorder, an inferior vena cava filter may be placed preoperatively.

Skin Care

The bariatric surgery patient is at high risk for skin breakdown and poor wound healing. Skin folds harbor moisture, bacteria, and yeast; in addition, the blood supply to adipose tissue is poor. The best skin care is prevention and includes daily inspection of the skin, frequent turning, early ambulation, and special attention to the positioning of catheters and drainage tubes so that they are not hidden within skin folds. Skin care needs to be thorough, paying special attention to the folds under the breasts, back, abdomen, and perineum, as well as the surgical sites or incisions.

Postoperative Medication Alterations

Another important consideration in the care of patients after bariatric surgery is the administration of medications. Because a portion of small bowel has been bypassed, absorption of medications will be impacted. Medications previously given as sustained-released formulations are given in regular-release form to compensate for the changes in absorption. Tolerance of the GI effects of some medications may be altered, and patients are carefully monitored for new or changing side effects.

Many bariatric patients also have hepatic insufficiency from NAFLD. Medication choices take this factor into account and patients are closely monitored for medication effects due to both limited hepatic function as well as decreased absorption.

Resumption of preoperative diabetic medications, both insulin and oral agents, is also carefully monitored. Requirements for glucose control change dramatically immediately after surgery and resuming preoperative doses may lead to hypoglycemia. Postoperatively, diabetic medications such as sulfonylureas and meglitinides are discontinued and insulin doses are adjusted to prevent hypoglycemia. Many patients are able to completely discontinue the use of diabetic medications, including insulin, after surgery.

Patient Education

Recovery from bariatric surgery is a lengthy and involved process, extending beyond surgical healing. Patient education is a critical part of acute nursing care. Patients are taught the signs and symptoms associated with an anastomotic leak before they go home since the leaks can occur weeks following surgery. Nutritional instruction and dietary progression is an important part of the process, and advancing diet properly may reduce nausea, vomiting, and other discomfort following surgery. Patients having malabsorptive procedures remain at long-term risk for vitamin and mineral deficiencies, and are best served by a sure understanding of long-term follow-up and dietary and vitamin/mineral supplementation. An interprofessional team should be utilized

for the treatment of obesity, including nutrition counseling, endocrinology, gastroenterology, psychiatry, psychology, physiotherapy, and fitness coaching.

NUTRITIONAL SUPPORT FOR CRITICALLY ILL PATIENTS

The negative consequences of malnutrition have been known for centuries, and there is substantial evidence that malnourished hospitalized patients have increased morbidity, compromised surgical outcomes, more ventilator days, and increased mortality rates.

There is accumulating evidence that the route of nutrition support can affect morbidity in the critically ill patient. Protocols and care bundles for the proper initiation and monitoring of patients on nutrition support may reduce complications.

It is recommended that patients undergo screening for malnutrition upon admission using validated tools. Traditional approaches that incorporate laboratory indicators or other markers (ie, albumin or pre-albumin) are not supported by scientific studies and are not recommended. EN is introduced within 24 to 48 hours of admission in critically ill patients who are unable to maintain sufficient oral intake. Gastric feedings are a reasonable approach if the jejunum is not readily accessible.

Nutritional Requirements

Current recommendations for feeding critically ill patients suggest approximately 25 cal/kg/day based on the patient's ideal body weight, or 27.5 total cal/kg/day in the presence of conditions that increase catabolism. A total of 1.2 to 1.5 g/kg/day of protein is also recommended. In severely malnourished patients, reduced calories (15-20 kcal/kg) are initiated to minimize electrolyte shifts from refeeding. When electrolytes are stable, progression to 30 or more cal/kg may be attempted to improve nutrition status. Close monitoring for tolerance is indicated. Controlled trials have demonstrated that overfeeding does not provide increased nutritional benefits, and actually has detrimental effects (Table 14-10).

TABLE 14-10. POTENTIAL CONSEQUENCES OF OVERFEEDING OF MACRONUTRIENTS[a]

Carbohydrate	Fat
Hyperglycemia	Impaired immune response
Synthesis and storage of fat	Fat overload syndrome with
Hepatic steatosis	neurologic, cardiac, pulmonary, hepatic, and renal dysfunction
Increased carbon dioxide production increasing minute ventilation	Thrombocyte adhesiveness
	Accumulation of lipid in the reticuloendothelial system (RES), leading to RES dysfunction

[a]Remember to look for additional sources of dextrose and fat, such as propofol, intravenous fluids (IVF), continuous venovenous hemodialysis (CVVHD), and peritoneal dialysis. Reproduced with permission from The University of Virginia Health System from Nutrition Support Traineeship Syllabus, University of Virginia Health System, Charlottesville, VA; Updated 2019.

Nutritional Case: Special Populations

Bariatric Surgery

Nutritional supplementation is standard therapy for all gastric-bypass operations. Ongoing monitoring and reinforcement of compliance is essential. Medication absorption is also altered in these patients. Ethyl alcohol (ETOH) absorption is enhanced, while sustained release and enteric-coated tablets may pass through undissolved or unutilized. The efficacy of drugs requiring a large volume of food or high-fat meal may be compromised (antifungals, antipsychotics).

Postgastrectomy Syndromes

Gastric resection can predispose patients to both nutritional intolerances and deficiencies. Intolerances include dumping syndrome, fat maldigestion, gastric stasis, and lactose intolerance. Nutrient deficiencies can develop months to years after gastric resections and can result in deleterious clinical consequences. Patients are at higher risk of developing osteoporosis and iron- and vitamin B_{12}–deficiency anemia. Decreased acid production and small bowel bacterial overgrowth most likely play a role in the latter two. Ongoing nutritional monitoring of these patients will prevent deficiencies and identify those in need of intervention.

Parenteral Nutrition

Parenteral nutrition may be indicated for malnourished patients and those at risk for becoming malnourished, only if the patient is unable to receive EN (Table 14-11). PN can be lifesaving in some cases, but is not without complications (including bloodstream infections) and is used only when EN is not feasible (Table 14-12). Prospective trials have demonstrated that the metabolic and infectious complications of PN outweigh the benefits in patients without significant malnutrition. Studies have demonstrated that even short-term PN, used to supplement EN in the ICU, does not enhance benefits and is associated with increased infectious complications and length of stay.

Enteral Nutrition

Current evidence suggests that EN is the preferred method of feeding the critically ill patient. It is associated with fewer infectious complications, is less expensive, confers some gut immune protection, and diminishes atrophy and attenuation of systemic response (Table 14-13). Patients that do not receive adequate amounts of EN have a greater need for rehabilitation services compared to patients receiving full feedings. To optimize EN, consider utilizing interprofessional team members, including registered dietitians, with knowledge and expertise in managing acutely ill patients.

Unfortunately, the delivery of EN is impeded by various situations that occur in critical care units; for example, EN may be stopped for diagnostic or therapeutic procedures, in patients who are hemodynamically unstable, or in those with clogged or dislodged enteral tubes (Table 14-14).

TABLE 14-11. INDICATIONS FOR PARENTERAL NUTRITION

Parenteral Nutrition Is Usually Indicated in the Following Situations:
- Documented inability to absorb adequate nutrients via the gastrointestinal tract. This may be due to:
    - Massive small-bowel resection/short-bowel syndrome (at least initially)
    - Radiation enteritis
    - Severe diarrhea
    - Steatorrhea
- Complete bowel obstruction or intestinal pseudo-obstruction
- Persistent ileus
- Severe catabolism with or without malnutrition when gastrointestinal tract is not usable within 5-7 days
- Inability to obtain enteral access
- Inability to provide sufficient nutrients or fluids enterally
- Pancreatitis accompanied by abdominal pain with jejunal delivery of nutrients
- Persistent GI hemorrhage
- Acute abdomen
- Lengthy GI workup requiring NPO status
- High-output enterocutaneous fistula (>500 mL) if enteral feeding ports cannot be distally placed
- Trauma requiring repeat surgical procedures

Parenteral Nutrition May Be Indicated in the Following Situations:
- Entero cutaneous fistula (<500 mL)
- Inflammatory bowel disease not responding to medical therapy
- Hyperemesis gravidarum when nausea and vomiting persist longer than 5-7 days and enteral nutrition is not possible
- Partial small bowel obstruction
- Intensive chemotherapy/severe mucositis
- Major surgery/stress when enteral nutrition not expected to resume within 7-10 days
- Intractable vomiting when jejunal feeding is not possible
- Chylous ascites or chylothorax

Reproduced with permission from The University of Virginia Health System from Nutrition Support Traineeship Syllabus, University of Virginia Health System, Charlottesville, VA.

Successful EN is also thwarted by experiential assumptions and practices, as well as beliefs about how the GI tract functions in critical illness. These unsupported practices are discussed below.

Gastric Residual Volume

Despite the publication of practice guidelines calling for clinicians to cease the checking of gastric residual volumes (GRVs), the practice continues. Reliance on isolated high residuals to determine GI tract malfunction may be counterproductive.

One of the physiologic functions of the stomach is to act as a reservoir and to control delivery of nutrients into the small bowel. This allows for maximal assimilation with

TABLE 14-12. CONTRAINDICATIONS FOR PARENTERAL NUTRITION

- Functioning gastrointestinal tract
- Treatment anticipated for <5 days in patients without severe malnutrition
- Inability to obtain venous access
- A prognosis that does not warrant aggressive nutrition support
- When the risks of PN are judged to exceed the potential benefits

Reproduced with permission from The University of Virginia Health System from Nutrition Support Traineeship Syllabus, University of Virginia Health System, Charlottesville, VA.

TABLE 14-13. BENEFITS OF ENTERAL FEEDING

- Stimulates immune barrier function
- Physiologic presentation of nutrients
- Maintains gut mucosa
- Attenuates hypermetabolic response
- Simplifies fluid/electrolyte management
- More "complete" nutrition than parenteral nutrition
- Less infectious complications (and costs associated with these complications)
- Stimulates return of bowel function
- Less expensive

Reproduced with permission from The University of Virginia Health System from Nutrition Support Traineeship Syllabus, University of Virginia Health System, Charlottesville, VA.

bile salts and pancreatic enzymes. A number of factors contribute to the GRV: endogenous secretions, normal gastric emptying, exogenous fluids, and the cascade effect.

Endogenous Secretions and Exogenous Additions

Two to four liters per day of saliva and gastric secretions are produced above the pylorus. Conservatively, this translates into 3 L of fluid that pass through the pylorus every 24 hours (an average of 125 mL/h). Once an enteral tube is positioned in the stomach, medications, water flushes, and EN add to this volume. Commonly in critical care, clinicians expect the stomach to be empty or only contain a very small amount of tube feeding or other liquid when checked. However, one

TABLE 14-14. COMMON BARRIERS TO OPTIMIZING ENTERAL NUTRITION DELIVERY

- Diagnostic procedures (feedings are stopped)
- Propofol (Diprivan) (calories from the lipid preparation must be calculated as part of the total kcal provided to prevent overfeeding—1.1 cal/mL infused)
- Enteral access issues (clogged/dislodged tubes or obtaining postpyloric access if needed)
- Feedings held due to drug-nutrient interactions
- Hypotensive episodes (patient is often flat in bed necessitating that feedings be turned off)
- Miscalculation of EN requirements
- "NPO" at midnight for tests, surgery, or procedures
- Conditioning regimes and/or therapies that require the feedings to be turned off
- Transportation off the unit
- Hemodialysis (EN is often stopped during hemodialysis if the patient is deemed unstable by the nurse, often after the patient experiences hypotension)
- Perceived or real "GI intolerance or dysfunction"
  Nausea/vomiting
  Complaints of fullness
  Abdominal distention
  Lack of bowel sounds (see Bowel Sounds)
  Diarrhea (see Diarrhea Table 14-18)
  Aspiration risk/no gag (see Aspiration)
  Gastric residual volume (see Gastric Residual Volume)

A note on checking GRV with jejunal tubes: There is no need to check a GRV with a jejunal tube; there is no "reservoir" to hold EN, hence the flow of EN distally begins immediately.

Reproduced with permission from The University of Virginia Health System from Nutrition Support Traineeship Syllabus, University of Virginia Health System, Charlottesville, VA.

study has demonstrated that 40% of healthy volunteers have an average GRV greater than 100 mL.

The Cascade Effect

The predominant position of critical care patients is supine, preferably with backrest elevation 30° or higher. In this position, the stomach partially splits over the spine and is mechanically divided into two parts, the fundus (proximal) and the antrum (distal). Because the fundus is the noncontractile portion of the stomach, contents fill the fundus until they "cascade over" the spine into the antrum and finally exit through the pylorus. Thus, if the patient's feeding port is in the proximal stomach or fundus when the GRV is checked, the aspirated GRV may be erroneous. The GRV in this case may be a function of the patient's supine positioning rather than decreased GI motility.

Checking Gastric Residual Volume

The routine practice of checking GRV has not been validated and is not supported by published clinical guidelines. Some of the factors that make the routine assessment of GRV questionable are listed below:

1. Type of tube (Salem sump vs Dobhoff-like feeding tube vs a gastrostomy)
2. Location of the gastrostomy on the patient's abdominal wall (fundus, antrum)
3. Position of the patient when GRV is checked (supine, right or left lateral decubitus, prone)
4. Method of aspiration (20-, 35-, 50-, 60-mL syringe vs gravity drainage vs low constant suction)
5. The volume of the aspirate obtained
6. Disposition of the aspirate (eg, reinfused or discarded)
7. The effects of GI stress prophylaxis medications (PPIs) on the production and volume of gastric secretions
8. Lack of data linking elevated GRV to pulmonary aspiration

The practice of measuring GRV is poorly standardized and should not be routinely incorporated into practice. GRV as a valid measure of EN tolerance or whether the amount of GRV is linked to the risk of aspiration pneumonia events has yet to be proven. Until more evidence is available, good clinical judgment is required when evaluating the need for obtaining and interpreting GRVs. While institutional protocols may vary regarding the use of GRVs, holding feedings for GRVs less than 500 mL is discouraged unless other signs of intolerance are clearly identified.

Aspiration as a Complication of Enteral Feeding

Aspiration is the passage of materials into the airway below the level of the vocal cords. The aspirated material may be saliva, nasopharyngeal secretions, bacteria, food, beverage, gastric contents, bile, or any other ingested substance.

The incidence of aspiration pneumonia from EN is unclear, because it is difficult to identify an aspiration event and definitions of aspiration vary. Commonly quoted aspiration pneumonia rates in EN patients are between 5% and 36%.

Detection

Several methods of evaluating patients for aspiration risk have been popularized through "conventional wisdom." These include the routine monitoring of GRVs (discussed above), evaluation of gag reflex, testing tracheal secretions for the presence of glucose, and the addition of blue food color to feeding formulas.

The gag reflex is the least reliable protective reflex in ensuring that aspiration does not occur. More important to airway protection are reliable cough and swallow reflexes.

The presence of glucose in tracheal secretions is not a specific or sensitive method of detecting aspiration of EN. Tracheal glucose can be positive in patients who are not receiving feeding. In addition, some EN formulas have low glucose concentrations and do not result in a positive test when aspirated.

Several studies have demonstrated that adding blue dye to feeding formulas is not a sensitive method for detecting aspiration and is not used to indicate aspiration of gastric contents. In addition, some food dyes are mitochondrial toxins leading the Food and Drug Administration to release a Public Health Advisory Report noting the toxicity associated with the use of FD&C Blue No. 1. As an alternative, some critical care units have incorporated validated tools to determine the risk of aspiration. Table 5-14 in Chapter 5 provides an example of a screening tool that can be used following extubation.

Reducing Aspiration Risk
Body Position

The position of the patient is one of the primary factors influencing aspiration risk (Table 14-15). Studies have confirmed that aspiration and pneumonia are significantly more likely when patients are supine with the head of the bed elevated at less than 30°. While the semirecumbent position with head of

TABLE 14-15. PREVENTION OF ASPIRATION

- Maintain backrest elevation of 30°-45° if no contraindication is present to that position.
- Use sedatives as sparingly as possible.
- For tube fed patients, verify appropriate placement of feeding tube every 4 hours.
- For patients receiving gastric feedings, assess for gastrointestinal intolerance every 4 hours.
- For tube fed patients, avoid bolus feedings if high risk for aspiration.
- Consult with provider about obtaining a swallow evaluation before oral feedings in recently extubated patients or those intubated for more than 2 days.
- Maintain endotracheal cuff pressures at appropriate level, and ensure that secretions are cleared from above the cuff before it is deflated.

Data from Prevention of Aspiration in Adults. Crit Care Nurse. 2016;36(1):e20-e24.

the bed elevations of greater than or equal to 30° cannot guarantee absolute protection against aspiration, it is a method that is inexpensive and relatively easy to accomplish and monitor. Strict use of semirecumbent position is the most consistent and potent means to reduce the likelihood of aspiration.

Tube Size and Placement Issues

The incidence of aspiration, and subsequently pneumonia, are not affected by the feeding tube size or whether the tube is placed through the nose, mouth, or a gastrostomy stoma. Regardless of the site, confirmation of accurate placement is essential.

Moreover, there is evidence that pulmonary injury during bedside placement of feeding tubes occurs more frequently than is generally appreciated. Using a method to provide feedback that the airway has been inadvertently intubated with the feeding tube can decrease the incidence of injury that may occur before the confirmatory radiograph is obtained. Several studies have reported that use of CO_2 detection, electromagnetic guidance, or a preliminary radiograph during placement decreases the incidence of inadvertent pulmonary intubation and injury. It is commonly believed that placing the tip of the feeding tube beyond the pylorus decreases the incidence of aspiration events. However, numerous studies and a meta-analysis on the topic note that it is unclear if a properly positioned jejunal tube can reduce aspiration risk.

The majority of critically ill patients in these studies received gastric tube feedings safely and effectively. In studies that used protocols for the prevention of aspiration, very low rates of aspiration pneumonia were demonstrated. From an evidence-based standpoint, the question of jejunal placement of feeding tubes and aspiration risk remains unanswered.

Considering the time and expense associated with jejunal placement of feeding tubes, it is reasonable to use the gastric route unless intolerance is evident. Exceptions to this approach include patients known to be at increased risk for aspiration due to altered anatomy (eg, esophagectomy) or dysmotility (eg, scleroderma, severe gastroparesis). These patients may benefit from a tube placed in the jejunum.

In congruence with the AACN Practice Alert, techniques to ensure proper placement of enteral tubes are recommended and include: (1) observe for signs of respiratory distress, (2) use capnography to detect inadvertent placement into the lungs, (3) measure pH of aspirates, and (4) observe for visual signs of gastric aspirate (refer to AACN practice alert for details). Tube placement is verified with radiologic assessment prior to any instillation of feedings, fluids, or medications. Placement is reassessed every 4 hours. The head of bed is raised to 30° to 40° and sedatives are used sparingly. These measures are associated with a reduction in untoward events.

Feeding Rate

The delivery rate of the feeding formula may influence aspiration and pneumonia. Bolus administration of 350 mL reduces lower esophageal sphincter pressure, which may precipitate reflux. Continuous EN (transpyloric feedings) has been associated with more rapidly attained feeding tolerance, but not a significant change in aspiration incidence. In one study, reduced aspiration events were associated with cyclic infusion feedings (16-hour cycle), compared to continuous feedings. The authors postulated that cyclic enteral feedings resulted in a reduction of gastric pH and subsequently prevented colonization of gastric contents. However, randomized trials have failed to demonstrate associations between gastric pH, gastric colonization, or pneumonia incidence between patients fed with cyclic versus continuous feedings.

Pharmacologic Interventions

Prokinetic medications have been evaluated to determine whether they improve EN tolerance. In critically ill patients, metoclopramide and erythromycin improve gastric emptying, but there are few data on the incidence of aspiration pneumonia associated with the use of these agents.

Bowel Sounds in Enterally Fed Patients

Auscultating the abdomen to determine the presence of BSs, and thus GI tract function, is a well-entrenched practice yet has never been validated as a marker of GI tract function. The absence of BS does not preclude the initiation of EN.

Careful initiation of EN in patients without BS may stimulate normal bowel function and the emergence of BS. Research suggests that enteral feeding initiated within the first 24 to 48 hours of ICU admission with or without the presence of BS is safe. Auscultation of BS in the clinical setting varies. Clinician assessment practices differ and include how the quadrants are auscultated, frequency of auscultation, time spent listening for sounds, and interpretation of the sounds. BSs are nonspecific markers and hence are best used in conjunction with the overall clinical assessment of the patient if used. Suggested approaches to assessment of GI function when BSs are absent can be found in Table 14-16.

Complications of EN: Nausea, Vomiting, and Diarrhea

Many factors contribute to nausea and vomiting in the critical care setting and include medications, the disease process, surgery, procedures, and bedside interventions (eg, placing a nasogastric tube and/or suctioning). After careful assessment and treatment of the underlying cause if possible (Table 14-17), antiemetic medications may allow the continuation of EN while making the patient more comfortable. If antiemetics and/or prokinetics are initiated, they are continued until symptoms abate. Scheduled versus as-needed antiemetics may increase efficacy and overall success.

Osmolality or Hypertonicity of Formula

Diarrhea in patients on EN is sometimes attributed to the use of hypertonic or hyperosmolar formulas, despite an absence

TABLE 14-16. SUGGESTED APPROACHES FOR GI ASSESSMENT OF GI FUNCTION WHEN BOWEL SOUNDS ARE ABSENT

- Assess need for, and volume of, gastric decompression (ie, compare volume aspirated to normal secretions above the pylorus expected over time frame between aspirations).
- Distinguish significance by differentiating those patients requiring:
  - Low constant suction
  - Gravity drainage
  - An occasional gastric residual check every 4-6 hours (small bowel aspirates should not be checked)
- Abdominal examination—firm, distended, tympanic.
- Presence of nausea, bloating, feeling full, vomiting.
- Evaluate whether patient is passing gas or stool.
- Compare clinical examination with the differential diagnosis, specifically high suspicion for abdominal process.
- Finally, after determining low risk from above, consider a trial of EN at low rate of 10-20 mL/h and clinically observe for any of the symptoms listed above.

Reproduced with permission from The University of Virginia Health System from Nutrition Support Traineeship Syllabus, University of Virginia Health System, Charlottesville, VA.

of data supporting this relationship. Diluting formula is thought to reduce this complication by lowering the tonicity and osmolality of the feeding. However, dilution of formula increases nursing time and the risk of contamination, and decreases the nutrient content of the feeding. Therefore, diluting gastric feeding formula is not recommended.

The practice of diluting jejunal feedings is also not scientifically supported. Some believe that full strength tube feeding will not reach isotonicity and therefore should not be delivered straight to the jejunum. However, the GI tract secretes gastric and pancreaticobilary juices (including bicarbonate) to ensure isotonicity. In patients who have received gastrectomies (all the food they eat is delivered directly from the esophagus into the jejunum), normal feedings (albeit smaller portions) are consumed without adverse consequences. Dilution of EN is avoided due to risks of bacterial contamination and confusion with water and feeding volumes.

TABLE 14-17. SUGGESTED APPROACHES TO REDUCE NAUSEA AND VOMITING IN ENTERALLY FED PATIENTS

1. Review medication profile; change suspected agents to an alternative.
2. Try a prokinetic agent or antiemetic—review orders for PRN vs scheduled doses as well as delivery method.
3. Switch to a more calorically dense product to decrease the total volume infused.
4. Seek transpyloric access of feeding tube.
5. Tighten glucose control to <200 mg/dL to avoid gastroparesis from hyperglycemia.
6. Consider analgesic alternatives to opiates.
7. If feeding into small bowel, vent gastric port (if available).
8. Consider a proton pump inhibitor in order to decrease sheer volume of endogenous gastric secretions (eg, omeprazole, lansoprazole, esomeprazole, pantoprazole, rabeprazole).
9. If bacterial overgrowth is a possibility, treat with enteral antibiotics.
10. Vent gastric port if available.

Reproduced with permission from The University of Virginia Health System from Nutrition Support Traineeship Syllabus, University of Virginia Health System, Charlottesville, VA.

Diarrhea

Diarrhea occurs in patients in the hospital setting regardless of how they are fed. EN is often implicated as a major cause of diarrhea. However, numerous studies suggest other compelling reasons for diarrhea, such as concurrent medications, especially liquid medications most of which contain sorbitol or have a very high osmolality and infectious agents (*Clostridioides difficile* in particular). A study on the effects of "fermentable, oligosaccharides, disaccharides, monosaccharides and polyols" (FODMAPs) in food suggests that they may adversely affect bowel activity. The study also found that the FODMAPs in many formulas are highly osmotic and fermentable by gut bacteria, which then may result in gas, bloating, cramping, and diarrhea. After potential causes for diarrhea have been ruled out (Table 14-18) and addressed, medications to slow GI motility may be warranted.

Flow Rates and Hours of Infusion

While typical infusion rates for the initiation of EN range from 10 to 50 mL/h with increases of 10 to 25 mL every 4 to 24 hours, nurses should follow institutional guidelines in their practice. Little science exists to confirm or refute the efficacy of such regimens. One study has demonstrated that continuous enteral feeding may be started at the final goal

TABLE 14-18. SYSTEMATIC APPROACH TO ASSESSMENT AND MANAGEMENT OF DIARRHEA IN ENTERALLY FED PATIENTS

- Quantify stool volume—determine if it is really diarrhea (>250 mL).
- Review medication list—look for elixirs or suspensions with sorbitol (not always listed on the ingredient list—may need to contact manufacturer).
- Try to correlate timing of diarrhea in relation to start of new medication(s) or change medications to enteral route once enteral access is obtained; common offenders include:
  –Acetaminophen and guaifenesin elixir
  –Neutra-Phos
  –Lactulose
  –Standing orders for stool softeners/laxatives
- Check for *Clostridium difficile* or other infectious etiologies.
- Try a fiber-containing formula or add a fiber powder (not in poorly perfused or dysmotile gut):
  –Few clinical studies
  –Supports the health of colonocytes
- Added Fructooligosaccharide (FOS) and Fermentable, Oligo-, Di-, Monosaccharides, and Polyols (FODMAPs) in some patients may precipitate or aggravate diarrhea.
- Once infectious causes are ruled out:
  –Consider an antidiarrheal agent such as Imodium (may need standing order vs PRN to be effective)
- Check for fecal impaction.
- Check total hang time of EN (should not exceed 8 hours—open systems only).
- Consider providing protein powders by bolus vs adding directly to formulas to decrease contamination risk.
- Check fecal fat as last resort; if negative it does not mean patient is not malabsorbing; if positive, however, there is need to evaluate further.
- Continue to feed.

Reproduced with permission from The University of Virginia Health System from Nutrition Support Traineeship Syllabus, University of Virginia Health System, Charlottesville, VA.

rate in critically ill patients without negative consequences. In the study, feedings started at goal-flow rate did appear to reduce the calorie deficit that frequently accrues in the hospitalized patient. Whether EN runs continuously, nocturnally, during the day, or is given as a bolus, is often institution specific. However, patient-specific factors may also dictate the feeding schedule. For instance, patients on insulin infusions may experience fewer hypoglycemic episodes on continuous infusions of EN.

It is difficult, in fact rare, to achieve goal volumes of EN in critically ill patients. Frequent interruptions in the delivery of EN are common (see Table 14-14). As a result, it is reasonable to consider "padding" flow rates by basing calculations on less than 24 hours to improve delivery of the desired dose. For example, instead of dividing the goal volume of 1800 mL by 24 hours, to arrive at a flow rate of 75 mL/h, divide by 22 hours to arrive at rate of 80 mL/h, assuming that there will be at least 2 hours during the day when formula infusion is interrupted.

Formula Selection

A vast array of EN formulas are available, including specialty formulas marketed for patients with diabetes, acute respiratory distress syndrome (ARDS), hepatic, and renal failure. Other formulas contain nutrients that may modulate immune function, or have nutrients in their most basic (elemental) form for patients with malabsorption syndromes. Medical nutrition products are not required to meet the same level of scientific scrutiny as medications before they are marketed. Adequate outcome data are not available to warrant the use of many of these expensive products. Prospective, randomized trials have demonstrated no advantages of specialized "pulmonary" or "glucose control" feeding formulas. In fact, in a large randomized multicenter trial of a specialized enteral formula with fish oil and antioxidants for patients with acute lung injury, mortality increased with the specialized feeding compared to standard products. Most critically ill patients may be fed with "standard" polymeric tube-feeding formulas. Most formulas provide between 1 and 2 cal/mL.

SELECTED BIBLIOGRAPHY

Acute Gastrointestinal Bleeding

Alhazzani W, Alenezi F, Jaeschke RZ, et al. Proton pump inhibitors versus histamine 2 receptor antagonists for stress ulcer prophylaxis in critically ill patients: a systematic review and meta-analysis. *Crit Care Med.* 2013;41(3):1-13.

Andreyev HJN, Davidson SE, Gillespie C, et al. Practice guidance on the management of acute and chronic gastrointestinal problems arising as a result of treatment for cancer. *Gut.* 2012;61:179-192.

Becq A, Rahmi G, Perrod G, Cellier C, Hemorrhagic angiodysplasia of the digestive tract: pathogenesis, diagnosis, and management. *Gastrointest Endosc.* 2017;86(5):792-806.

Biecker E. Portal hypertension and gastrointestinal bleeding: diagnosis, prevention and management. *World J Gastroenterol.* 2013;19(31):5035-5050.

Choi JY, Jo YW, Lee SS, et al. Outcomes of patients treated with Sengstaken-Blakemore tube for uncontrolled variceal hemorrhage. *Korean J Intern Med.* 2018;33(4):696-704. doi: 10.3904/kjim.2016.339

Dworzynski K, Pollit V, Kelsey A, et al. Management of acute upper gastrointestinal bleeding: summary of NICE guidance. *BMJ.* 2012;344:1-5.

El-Tawil AM. Management of non-variceal upper gastrointestinal tract hemorrhage: controversies and areas of uncertainty. *World J Gastroenterol.* 2012;18(11):1159-1165.

Hagel, AF, Heinz, A, Nägel, A, et al. The application of hemospray in gastrointestinal bleeding during emergency endoscopy. Gastroenterol Res Pract. 2017;3083481. doi:10.1155/2017/3083581

Hawks, MK, Svarverud, JE. Acute lower gastrointestinal bleeding: evaluation and management. *Am Fam Physician.* 2020;101(4):206-212.

Monteiro S, Cúrdia Gonçalves T, Magalhães J, Cotter J. Upper gastrointestinal bleeding risk scores: who, when and why? *World J Gastrointest Pathophysiol.* 2016;7(1):86-96.

Nishizawa, T, Suzuki, H. Propofol for gastrointestinal endoscopy. *United European Gastroenterol J.* 2018;6(6):801-805.

Sachar H, Vaidya, K, Laine L. Intermittent vs continuous proton pump inhibitor therapy for high-risk bleeding ulcers: a systematic review and meta-analysis. *JAMA Intern Med.* 2014;174(11):1755-1762.

Strate LL, Gralnek IM. American College of Gastroenterology clinical guideline: management of patients with acute lower gastrointestinal bleeding. *Am J Gastroenterol.* 2016;111(4):459-474.

Villanueva C, Colomo A, Bosch A, et al. Transfusion strategies for acute upper gastrointestinal bleeding. *N Engl J Med.* 2013;368:11-21.

Wang B, Zhang JY, Gong JP, et al. Balloon-occluded retrograde transvenous obliteration versus transjugular intrahepatic portosystemic shunt for treatment of gastric varices due to portal hypertension: a meta-analysis. *J Gastro Hepatol.* 2016;31(4):727-733.

Wilkins, T, Wheeler, B, Carpenter, M. Upper gastrointestinal bleeding in adults: evaluation and management. *Am Fam Physician.* 2020, 101(5):294-300.

Liver Failure

Baraldi O, Valentini C, Donati G, et al. Hepatorenal syndrome: update on diagnosis and treatment. *World J Nephrol.* 2015;4(5):511-520.

Charlton M, Levitsky J, Aqel B, et al. International Liver Transplantation Society consensus statement on immunosuppression in liver transplant recipients. *Transplantation.* 2018 May;102(5):727-743. doi: 10.1097/TP.0000000000002147. Erratum in: *Transplantation.* 2019 Jan;103(1):e37. PMID: 29485508.

Cosardereloglu C, Coscar A, Gurakar M, Dagher N, Gurakar A. Hepatopulmonary syndrome and liver transplantation: a recent review of the literature. *J Clin Transpl Hepatol.* 2016;4(1):47-53.

Dasher K, Trotter J. Intensive care unit management of liver-related coagulation disorders. *Crit Care Clin.* 2012;28(3):389-398.

Garcia-Tsao G, Abraldes J, Berzigotti A, Bosch J. Portal hypertensive bleeding in cirrhosis: risk stratification, diagnosis, and management: 2016 practice guidance by the American Association for the Study of Liver Diseases. *Hepatol.* 2017;65(1):310-335.

Kanjo A, Ocskay K, Gede N, et al. Efficacy and safety of liver support devices in acute and hyperacute liver failure: a systemic review and network meta-analysis. *Sci Rep.* 2021;11(4189). doi: 10.1038/s41598-021-83292-z

Karvellas C, Subramanian R. Current evidence for extracorporeal liver support systems in acute liver failure and acute-on-chronic liver failure. *Crit Care Clin.* 2016;32(3):439-451.

Leoni S, Tovoli F, Napoli L, Serio I, Ferri S, Bolondi L. Current guidelines for the management of non-alcoholic fatty liver disease: a systematic review with comparative analysis. *World J Gastroenterol.* 2018 Aug 14;24(30):3361-3373. doi: 10.3748/wjg.v24.i30.3361. PMID: 30122876; PMCID: PMC6092580.

Pericleous M, Sarnowski A, Moore A, Fijten R, Zaman M. The clinical management of abdominal ascites, spontaneous bacterial peritonitis and hepatorenal syndrome: a review of current guidelines and recommendations. *Eur J Gastroenterol Hepatol.* 2015;28(3):10-18.

Acute Pancreatitis

Crockett SD, Wani S, Gardner TB, et al. American Gastroenterological Association Institute Guideline on initial management of acute pancreatitis. *Gastroenterology.* 2018;154(4):1096-1101.

Jenkins A, Shapiro J. Clinical guideline highlights for the hospitalist: initial management of acute pancreatitis in the hospitalized adult. *J Hosp Med.* 2019 Dec 1;14(12):764-765. doi: 10.12788/jhm.3324. Epub Oct 23, 2019. PMID: 31634105.

Moggia E, Koti R, Belgaumkar AP, et al. Pharmacological interventions for acute pancreatitis. *Cochrane Database Sys Rev.* 2017;4. doi: 10.1002/14651858.CD011384.pub2

Intestinal Ischemia/Bowel Obstruction

Bower KL, Lollar DI, Williams SL, Adkins FC, Luyimbazi DT, Bower CE. Small bowel obstruction. *Surg Clin North Am.* 2018;98(5):945-971. doi: 10.1016/j.suc.2018.05.007

Brandt L, Feuerstadt P, Longstreth G. Blaszka M. ACG clinical guideline: epidemiology, risk factors, patterns of presentation, diagnosis, and management of colon ischemia (CI). *Am J Gastroenterol.* 2015;110:18-44.

Clair DG, Beach JM. Mesenteric Ischemia. *N Engl J Med.* 2016; 374:959-968.

Cudnik, MT, Darbha S, Jones J, Macedo J, Stockton SW, Hiestand BC. The diagnosis of acute mesenteric ischemia: a systematic review and meta-analysis. *Acad Emerg Med.* 2013;20(11):1087-1100. doi: 10.1111/acem.12254

Ten Broek RPG, Krielen P, Di Saverio S, et al. Bologna guidelines for diagnosis and management of adhesive small bowel obstruction (ASBO): 2017 update of the evidence-based guidelines from the world society of emergency surgery ASBO working group. *World J Emerg Surg.* 2018;13:24. Published 2018 Jun 19. doi: 10.1186/s13017-018-0185-2

Vogel J, Feingold D, Stewart D, et al. Clinical practice guidelines for colon volvulus and acute colonic pseudo-obstruction. *Dis Colon Rectum.* 2016;59:589-600.

Nutrition

Al-Dorzi HM, Arabi YM. Nutrition support for critically ill patients. *J Parenter Enteral Nutr.* 2021;45:S47-S59.

American Association of Critical-Care Nurses. AACN practice alert: initial and ongoing verification of feeding tube placement in adults. *Crit Care Nurse.* 2016;36(2):e8-e13.

American Association of Critical-Care Nurses. AACN practice alert: prevention of aspiration in adults. 2016. doi: 10.4037/ccn2016831

Karen L. Johnson, Lauri Speirs, Anne Mitchell, et al. Validation of a postextubation dysphagia screening tool for patients after prolonged endotracheal intubation. *Am J Crit Care.* 2018 Mar 1; 27(2):89-96. doi: 10.4037/ajcc2018483

McClave S, Taylor B, Martindale R, et al. Guidelines for the provision and assessment of nutrition support therapy in the adult critically ill patient: Society of Critical Care Medicine (SCCM) and American Society for Parenteral and Enteral Nutrition (A.S.P.E.N.). *JPEN J Parenter Enteral Nutr.* 2016;40(2):159-211.

Yasuda H, Kondo N, Yamamoto R, et al. Monitoring of gastric residual volume during enteral nutrition. *Cochrane Database Syst Rev.* 2021;9(9):CD013335. Published 2021 Sep 27. doi: 10.1002/14651858.CD013335.pub2

Online References of Interest

http://www.ginutrition.virginia.edu

Bariatric Surgery and Weight Management

C difficile—a rose by any other name... *Lancet Infect Dis.* 2019;19(5):449. doi: 10.1016/S1473-3099(19)30177-X

Král J, Machytka E, Horká V, et al. Endoscopic treatment of obesity and nutritional aspects of bariatric endoscopy. *Nutrients.* 2021;13(12):4268. Published 2021 Nov 26. doi: 10.3390/nu13124268

Ryan DH, Kahan S. Guideline recommendations for obesity management. *Med Clin North Am.* 2018 Jan;102(1):49-63. doi: 10.1016/j.mcna.2017.08.006. PMID: 29156187

Saltzman, JR, Feldman, M, Travis, AC. Approach to acute upper gastrointestinal bleeding in adults. *UpToDate.* October 4, 2021. Accessed March 12, 2022. https://www.uptodate.com/contents/approach-to-acute-upper-gastrointestinal-bleeding-in-adults

Tabesh MR, Maleklou F, Ejtehadi F, Alizadeh Z. Nutrition, physical activity, and prescription of supplements in pre- and post-bariatric surgery patients: a practical guideline. *Obes Surg.* 2019 Oct;29(10):3385-3400. doi: 10.1007/s11695-019-04112-y. Erratum in: *Obes Surg.* 2020 Feb;30(2):793. PMID: 31367987.

15

RENAL SYSTEM

Jie Chen

KNOWLEDGE COMPETENCIES

1. Describe the etiology, pathophysiology, clinical presentation, patient needs, and principles of management of acute kidney injury (AKI).

2. Differentiate between the three types of AKI:
   - Prerenal
   - Intrinsic renal
   - Postrenal

3. Compare and contrast the pathophysiology, clinical presentation, patient needs, and management approaches of life-threatening electrolyte imbalances:
   - Sodium (Na^+)
   - Potassium (K^+)
   - Calcium (Ca^{++})
   - Magnesium (Mg^{++})
   - Phosphorus (PO_4^-)

4. Differentiate between the indications for and the efficacy of the different types of renal replacement therapies.

5. Describe the nursing interventions for patients undergoing renal replacement therapy (RRT).

ACUTE KIDNEY INJURY

The most common renal problem seen in critically ill patients is the development of acute kidney injury (AKI), previously termed acute renal failure (ARF). AKI is the abrupt decrease in renal function with progressive retention of metabolic waste products (eg, creatinine and urea), and dysregulation of fluid, electrolytes, and acid-base homeostasis as results over the course of hours to days. AKI occurs in more than 50% of patients who are treated in the intensive care unit (ICU) setting and early data shows a higher incidence of AKI among patients with COVID-19. Mortality rates in patients with AKI range from 20% to 36%. Critically ill patients with AKI who are treated with renal replacement therapy (RRT) have a mortality rate of 50% to 60% and 5% to 20% of those who survive remain dialysis dependent at time of discharge. In addition, a history of chronic kidney disease (CKD) complicates the clinical course of any illness.

According to the Kidney Disease: Improving Global Outcomes (KDIGO) guidelines, the RIFLE criteria and Acute Kidney Injury Network (AKIN) criteria are appropriate classification systems for AKI. RIFLE is an acronym for: **R**isk of renal dysfunction, **I**njury to the kidney, **F**ailure of kidney function, **L**oss of kidney function, and **E**nd-stage kidney disease. KDIGO guidelines further define AKI as follows: increase in serum creatinine by ≥ 0.3 mg/dl within 48 hours, or increase in serum creatinine to ≥1.5 times baseline, which is known or presumed to have occurred within the prior 7 days, or urine output <0.5 mL/kg/h for 6 hours. Table 15-1 lists the RIFLE and AKIN criteria for comparison.

Etiology, Risk Factors, and Pathophysiology

For the purpose of determining an appropriate plan of care, AKI is often categorized into prerenal, intrinsic renal, or postrenal. These categories of AKI have different etiologies and laboratory findings. However, the common pathologic pathway is reduced glomerular filtration rate (GFR). In the acute and critical care setting, the most common factors that

TABLE 15-1. RIFLE AND AKIN CRITERIA FOR DIAGNOSIS AND CLASSIFICATION OF AKI

	RIFLE		Urine Output (common to both)	AKIN	
Class	SCr[a]			Stage	SCr[b]
Risk	Increased SCr to > 1.5 × baseline		Urine output < 0.5 mg/kg/h for > 6 h	1	Increase in SCr ≥0.3 mg/dL over 48 hours or increase in SCr to ≥150%-200% of baseline in a 7-day period
Injury	Increased SCr to > 2 × baseline		Urine output < 0.5 mg/kg/h for > 12 h	2	Increase in SCr to >200%-300% of baseline
Failure	Increased SCr to > 3 × baseline; or an increase of ≥ 0.5 mg/dL to a value of ≥ 4 mg/dL		Urine output < 0.3 mg/kg/h for > 12 h or anuria for > 12 h	3	Increase in SCr to >300% of baseline; or to ≥4 mg/dL with an acute increase of ≥0.5 mg/dL; or on RRT
Loss	Need for RRT for > 4 wk				
End Stage	Need for RRT for > 3 mo				

Abbreviations: AKI, acute kidney injury; AKIN, acute kidney injury network; RIFLE, risk, injury, failure, loss, end-stage disease; RRT, renal replacement therapy; SCr, serum creatinine.
[a]For RIFLE, the increase in SCr should be both abrupt (with 1-7 days) and sustained (>24 hours).
[b]For AKIN, the increase in SCr must occur in less than 48 hours.
Data from Palevsky PM, Liu KD, Brophy PD et al: KDOQI US Commentary on the 2012 KDIGO Clinical Practice Guideline for Acute Kidney Injury, Am J Kidney Dis 2013;61(5):649-672.

contribute to AKI include impaired renal perfusion, sepsis, and nephrotoxic agents, or a combination of those factors.

Prerenal Acute Kidney Injury
Physiologic conditions that lead to decreased perfusion of the kidneys, without intrinsic damage to the renal tubules, are identified as prerenal AKI (Figure 15-1). A decrease in renal arterial perfusion decreases the rate of blood filtration through the glomerulus. Pressure in the renal arteries is a key factor in perfusion and is determined by mean arterial pressure (MAP). When perfusion pressure falls to less than

80 mm Hg, protective autoregulation is lost, further decreasing glomerular filtration.

Renal tubular function, at this point, may remain normal. However, decreased GFR means that the kidneys are unable to adequately filter waste products from the blood. Consequently, more sodium and water are reabsorbed by the kidneys, resulting in oliguria. If the decreased perfusion state persists, damage to the renal tubules may occur, resulting in acute tubular necrosis (ATN), a form of intrinsic AKI. Prerenal AKI may be reversed by treating the underlying cause of decreased renal perfusion.

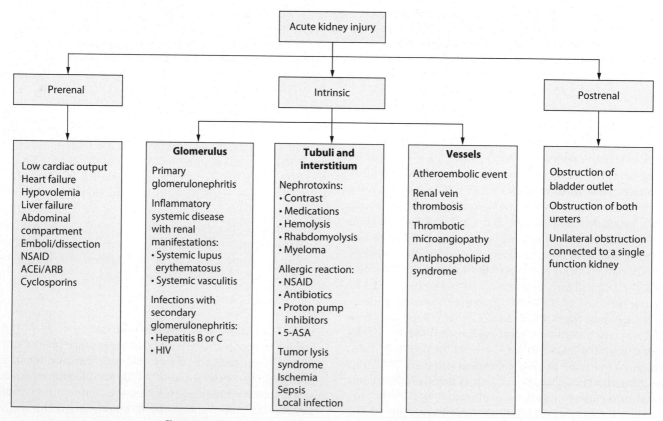

Figure 15-1. Causes of AKI, including prerenal, intrinsic, and postrenal conditions.

Intrinsic Renal Acute Kidney Injury

Physiologic conditions that cause damage to the renal tubule, glomerulus, or renal blood vessels are identified as intrinsic renal AKI (see Figure 15-1). Following prolonged decreases in renal perfusion, the kidneys gradually suffer damage that is not readily reversed with the restoration of renal perfusion. This results in ATN. ATN is the most common cause of AKI among hospitalized patients.

When the insult to the kidney is nephrotoxins (medications or other substances that cause direct damage to the kidney), the nephron damage occurs primarily at the tubular epithelial layer. Because this layer can regenerate, rapid healing is feasible once the nephrotoxic agent is removed. When the insult is ischemia, or inflammation, the damage occurs to the nephron's basement membrane which is not amenable to regeneration. Thus, these insults can lead to CKD. In healthy kidneys, the glomerulus acts as a filter, preventing the passage of large molecules into the glomerular filtrate. Damage to the glomerulus in intrinsic AKI allows protein and cellular debris to enter the renal tubules, leading to intraluminal obstruction, furthering kidney injury.

Contrast-Associated Acute Kidney Injury

Intrinsic AKI occurring within 48 hours of intravenous iodinated contrast material administration has been historically termed contrast-induced nephropathy (CIN). However, iodinated contrast material is not the only nephrotoxic factor causing AKI. In 2020, the American College of Radiology and the National Kidney Foundation endorsed the new terms contrast-associated AKI (CA-AKI) or post contrast AKI (PC-AKI) for any AKI occurring within 48 hours of intravenous contrast media administration. Retiring the term CIN was an acknowledgment of the challenge of isolating contrast as the single cause of AKI. The risk of CA-AKI is higher with procedures involving arterial contrast administration compared with the intravenous route. Recommendations applicable to intravenous contrast therefore may not apply to intra-arterial contrast media administration.

The primary risk factor for CA-AKI is impaired kidney function. Other risk factors include diabetes, age, hypotension, hypovolemia, albuminuria, congestive heart failure, and concomitant use of other nephrotoxic agents, such as nonsteroidal anti-inflammatory drugs and aminoglycosides. Contrast characteristics (osmolality, iconicity, and molecular structure) and high or repetitive doses of contrast also impact the risk.

CA-AKI is defined as a 25% increase in creatinine or an absolute increase of 0.5 mg/dL from baseline within 24 to 48 hours of intravenous contrast administration. The condition usually resolves in a few days. Patients may not experience oliguria as most cases of CA-AKI are mild. The pathophysiological changes are consistent with ATN, and the result of medullary hypoxia due to initial vasodilation followed by prolonged renal vasoconstriction, and direct epithelial cell injury from the contrast media.

ESSENTIAL CONTENT CASE

Contrast-Associated Acute Kidney Injury

A 74-year-old woman was admitted for substernal chest pain, shortness of breath, and weakness. She has a history of type II diabetes mellitus. She underwent diagnostic cardiac catheterization with successful angioplasty and placement of two stents. Postprocedure, an infusion of IV fluid was initiated. She is now 4 hours postprocedure and receiving normal saline at 200 mL/h. Vital signs are stable and she has had 50 mL urine output in total so far.

The next morning, serum creatinine has increased from a baseline of 1.2 mg/dL to 1.8 mg/dL. Urine output has remained marginal at 25 to 30 mL/h. Normal saline is continuing at 125 mL/h. The provider decides to keep her for one more day to monitor her renal status. On the second postprocedure day, serum creatinine remains at 1.8 mg/dL but urine output has increased to 35 to 40 mL/h. She is discharged to follow up in the office in 3 days and obtain lab work, including a BMP.

Case Question 1: What puts this patient at risk of CA-AKI?

Case Question 2: Why is the patient being discharged when the creatinine has not returned to baseline?

Answers
1. The risk factors for developing CA-AKI include a history of diabetes, advanced age, lack of hydration prior to using contrast medium, and the use of increased amounts of contrast media via arterial access (ie, related to the length of two procedures done at the same time).
2. The patient is discharged to be followed up as an outpatient because patient's creatinine has stabilized and research shows that creatinine returns to baseline within 5 to 7 days in most patients that develop CA-AKI. However, for patients with renal insufficiency, an episode of CA-AKI can lead to CKD. Therefore, emphasizing the close outpatient follow-up is a critical aspect of this patient's discharge instructions.

Postrenal Acute Kidney Injury

Physiologic conditions that partially or completely obstruct urine flow from the kidney to the urethral meatus can cause postrenal AKI (see Figure 15-1). Partial obstruction increases renal interstitial pressure, which in turn increases Bowman capsule pressure and opposes glomerular filtration. Complete obstruction leads to urine backup into the kidney, eventually compressing the kidney. With complete obstruction, there is no urine output from the affected kidney. Postrenal disease is not a common cause of AKI in critically ill patients but it is reversible and warrants consideration, particularly in patients with predisposing conditions such as urinary catheters, retroperitoneal tumors, or prostatic enlargement. The treatment for postrenal disease is focused on removing the obstruction.

Clinical Phases

There are three clinical phases of AKI, seen primarily as a result of intrinsic renal injury. The first, the oliguric phase, begins within 48 hours of the insult to the kidney. In intrinsic renal AKI, the oliguric phase is accompanied by a significant rise in blood urea nitrogen (BUN) and creatinine. The degree of elevation of these waste products is less pronounced in prerenal AKI. The most common complications seen in this phase are fluid overload and acute hyperkalemia. The oliguric phase may last from a few days to several weeks. The longer the oliguric phase continues, the poorer the patient's prognosis.

The diuretic phase follows the oliguric phase. During this phase, there is a gradual return of renal function. Although the BUN and creatinine continue to rise, there is an increase in urine output. The patient's state of hydration prior to the diuretic phase determines the amount of urine output. A patient who is fluid overloaded may excrete up to 5 L of urine a day and have marked sodium wasting. The average time in this phase is 7 to 10 days. Patients must be observed carefully for complications due to fluid and electrolyte deficits. If the patient receives dialysis during the oliguric phase, the diuretic phase may be decreased or absent.

The recovery phase marks the stabilization of laboratory values and can last for 3 to 12 months. Some degree of residual renal insufficiency is common following AKI. Some patients never recover renal function and progress to CKD or end-stage renal disease (ESRD, stage 5 CKD).

Clinical Presentation

The diverse causes of AKI determine the clinical presentation of the patient. Some patients may not experience any clinical symptoms and an increase in creatinine is detected on routine laboratory tests. In severe cases, AKI can cause multiple organ dysfunction and, therefore, manifests in a variety of ways. Uremia describes the clinical syndrome that accompanies the detrimental effects of renal dysfunction on the other organ systems. The clinical presentation of the patient with uremia reflects the degree of nephron loss and, correspondingly, the loss of renal function. Uremia can be corrected with dialysis and the decision for urgent dialysis is based on the patient's clinical presentation, not just lab values.

Signs and Symptoms

- Oliguria (<400 mL/day) or anuria (<100 mL/day)
- Tachycardia
- Heart murmur
- Pericardial friction rub
- Hypotension (prerenal)
- Hypertension (intrinsic renal)
- Jugular vein distension (intrinsic renal)
- Platelet dysfunction and bleeding
- Dry mucous membranes (prerenal)
- Edema
- Cool, clammy skin
- Pruritus
- Deep, rapid respirations
- Crackles or rales on lung auscultation
- Flank pain
- Hematuria
- Vomiting
- Nausea
- Lethargy
- Confusion
- Coma

Diagnostic Tests

Early detection of AKI is critical to prevent further decline in renal function. Laboratory tests are important in diagnosing AKI and evaluating the effectiveness of interventions to treat it. Serum creatinine is more specific to renal function while BUN is affected by many factors. In patients with AKI, there is a delay before a rise in serum creatinine and BUN, but these values are still commonly used to evaluate renal function by trending variations of daily levels. A plasma BUN/creatinine ratio greater than 20:1 suggests prerenal AKI as reduced kidney perfusion is associated with an increase in urea reabsorption. In intrinsic renal failure, the BUN and creatinine rise but the ratio often remains constant. Further testing such as the fractional excretion of sodium, described below is more reliable than the BUN: creatinine ratio in distinguishing between prerenal and intrinsic AKI.

Urinalysis is a useful and inexpensive test to evaluate renal function. Urine sodium values vary as the kidneys attempt to retain or excrete water. Urine specific gravity (SG) and osmolality identify the kidney's ability to excrete and concentrate fluid. Urinalysis findings are normal or near normal in prerenal AKI. An osmolality greater than 500 mOsmol/kg is suggestive of prerenal AKI. In contrast, early ATN presents with low urine osmolality as the kidneys lose their ability to concentrate urine. Muddy brown granular casts, epithelial cell casts, and free renal tubular epithelial cells are also seen on urinalysis in patients with ATN. Hematuria and dysmorphic red cells with or without red cell casts and proteinuria indicate glomerulonephritis, while pyuria with or without white cell casts is associated with interstitial nephritis. Low urine sodium levels (<20 mmol/L) are seen in prerenal AKI. In contrast, high urine sodium levels (>40 mmol/L) are seen in intrinsic renal AKI.

The fractional excretion of sodium (FeNa) is a valuable indicator of functional renal tubules. FeNa is less than 1% in prerenal injury and more than 1% in intrinsic renal injury with some exceptions, such as in patients with CA-AKI, rhabdomyolysis, liver failure, or cardiac failure. However, calculation of FeNa is not accurate in the setting of diuretic use. In that case, fractional excretion of urea (FeUrea) is used. FeUrea is less than 35% in prerenal injury and more than 35% in intrinsic renal injury.

There are several novel biomarkers of AKI. Urinary insulin-like growth factor-binding protein 7 (IGFBP7) and tissue inhibitor of metalloproteinase-2 (TIMP-2) can be detected at the bedside by using the commercially available and Food and Drug Administration (FDA)-approved NephroCheck Test (a urine test). The increase and decrease of IGFBP7 and TIMP-2 levels from baseline can be used to predict the development of AKI and renal recovery post-AKI events.

Radiologic tests also give important information about the kidneys. A kidney ultrasound may be used to evaluate existing renal disease and exclude postrenal AKI. Doppler ultrasound assesses the patency of the renal vasculature and presence of renal vascular diseases. Helical computed tomography (CT) without contrast can also be used to identify possible urolithiasis. Nuclear mercaptoacetyltriglycine-3 (MAG-3) scan can be used to evaluate renal perfusion and tubular function.

Renal biopsy is only considered when prerenal, ATN, and postrenal AKI have been excluded, and the etiology of the intrinsic renal AKI is still not clear. In these cases, the findings of renal biopsy are used to guide management. A biopsy may also be indicated when renal function does not improve for a prolonged period, and a long-term management plan needs to be made based on the results.

Post-biopsy care is determined by institutional policy and includes close observation for the risk of bleeding. Vital signs are checked frequently (initially every 15 minutes, and then every 30 minutes during the first 4-6 hour, and then every 4 hours overnight) and the patient is kept supine for 4 to 6 hours and then on bedrest for overnight observation. Nursing care also includes monitoring for blood clots in the patient's urine and asking about flank pain. Patients should be encouraged to drink plenty of fluids if there are no other contraindications.

Physical Assessment

Physical assessment related to the kidneys includes monitoring intake and output, daily weights, and noting a positive or negative fluid balance. Observation of the patient's urine for color, clarity, and odor adds to the assessment. Signs of volume overload may include pulmonary crackles, peripheral edema, jugular venous distention, or an S_3 heart sound. Volume deficit may be demonstrated by the presence of dry mucus membranes and weak peripheral pulses. Alterations in mental state may indicate uremia. The kidneys help control the internal environment of the body; therefore, when kidney function decreases, the critical care nurse may see changes in most, if not all, body systems.

Principles of Management of Acute Kidney Injury

The collaborative approach of the healthcare team to the treatment of patients with AKI begins with the recognition of AKI risk. The focus for those at risk is maintenance of adequate renal perfusion by maintaining an appropriate systemic blood pressure and avoiding renal injury such as from exposure to nephrotoxic agents. Careful monitoring of urine output, creatinine, and BUN are also essential nursing interventions.

Prevention of CA-AKI is also a key consideration, especially for those who have pre-existing AKI or an eGFR less than 30 mL/min/1.73 m^2 and are not undergoing maintenance dialysis. When the patient is able to tolerate it, prophylaxis with a normal saline infusion is preferred for isotonic volume expansion. The patient's volume status should be evaluated when deciding the amount to administer. The prophylaxis dose typically is given 1 hour before and continued 3 to 12 hours after intravenous contrast media administration. Patients who are considered to be at risk for CA-AKI may also receive oral acetylcysteine along with their hydration but its benefit is uncertain. In addition, nephrotoxic agents such as aminoglycoside antibiotics, nonsteroidal anti-inflammatory drugs, and chemotherapeutic agents should be held for patients at high risk for CA-AKI.

Once the patient develops AKI, the goal is to quickly reestablish homeostasis by treating the underlying cause. Management of AKI also includes correction of fluid imbalance, prevention, and correction of life-threatening electrolyte imbalances, treatment of metabolic acidosis, prevention of further renal damage, prevention and treatment of infection, and adequate nutrition. Educating patients and families as described in Chapter 2 is also a key element of the management of AKI.

Correction of Fluid Imbalance

Maintaining fluid balance in patients with AKI is a challenge. The simultaneous goals of providing enough fluid to ensure adequate renal perfusion and preventing excess fluid and volume overload require close attention. Assessment data that help to determine a patient's fluid status include trending of daily weight, measuring intake and output, especially urine output, and close monitoring of vital signs. Functional hemodynamics described in Chapter 4 (Hemodynamic Monitoring) may provide additional information about the patient's fluid balance. The following interventions are recommended in the management of fluid imbalance:

1. Calculate daily fluid needs. In prerenal disease, fluid replacement must be matched with fluid loss, both in amount and composition. Insensible fluid losses must be considered in this calculation (Table 15-2). Normal saline volume loading before a potential

TABLE 15-2. MINIMAL VOLUMES OF FLUID ASSOCIATED WITH INSENSIBLE FLUID LOSSES

Situation/Condition	Volume
Respiratory losses	500-850 mL/day (dependent on minute ventilation rate)
Fever (loss/°C elevation > 38.0)	200 mL
Diaphoresis	500 mL
Diarrhea	50-200 mL/stool

insult in patients at risk for renal dysfunction is a widely accepted practice. Additionally, volume expansion is beneficial in preventing a volume-depleted patient from progressing from prerenal AKI to intrinsic injury. In contrast, oliguric patients may not tolerate volume expansion. In some cases, during the oliguric phase, patients may require moderation of fluid intake, such as giving intravenous medications with the smallest possible volume of fluid. During the diuretic phase, the patient may require 1 to 4 L of fluid per day to prevent hypovolemia. The patient is frequently allowed to lose more fluid than is replaced in the diuretic phase, to facilitate fluid movement from the interstitial and intracellular spaces into the vascular space.

2. Obtain accurate intake and output measurements and include insensible losses in the measurements. Fluid therapy decisions are often based on the patient's clinical response.

3. Obtain daily weights. Body weight may decrease by 0.2 to 0.3 kg/day as a result of catabolism. If the patient's weight is stable or increasing, volume overload is suspected. If weight loss exceeds these recommendations, volume depletion or hyper-catabolism may be the cause.

4. Administer diuretics only when the patient is hypervolemic but non-anuric, and in consultation with nephrology. Increasing the dose of diuretics may be required to achieve optimal response. Potassium-sparing diuretics are typically avoided because potassium elimination is diminished with impaired GFR. Furosemide, a loop diuretic, is the most common diuretic used in AKI. It works by blocking sodium reabsorption in the renal tubules, thereby enhancing excretion of sodium and water. In patients who respond to diuretic use, furosemide is often given to treat fluid overload accompanied by hyperkalemia prior to initiating RRT. Furosemide is used cautiously in patients receiving aminoglycoside antibiotics because it potentiates the nephrotoxic effects of these medications and increases the risk of ototoxicity.

5. Institute RRT as needed. There are three types of RRT available. These include intermittent hemodialysis (IHD), peritoneal dialysis (PD), and several forms of continuous renal replacement therapy (CRRT). Each of these is described later in this chapter. Sustained low efficiency dialysis (SLED) also known as prolonged intermittent RRT (PIRRT) is considered one of the continuous therapies. CRRT is used in hemodynamically unstable patients who are not able to undergo the abrupt shifts in fluid status that occur with intermittent forms of dialysis.

Preventing and Treating Life-Threatening Electrolyte Imbalances

Electrolyte imbalances commonly occur in AKI, including hyperkalemia, hypocalcemia, hypermagnesemia, hyperphosphatemia, and bicarbonate deficiency. In AKI, the electrolyte status guides decisions about the type of fluid therapy and the initiation of RRT. The management of these electrolyte disorders is detailed later in this chapter.

Treating Acidosis

Patients with AKI often develop metabolic acidosis, with a compensatory mild respiratory alkalosis. A drop in serum bicarbonate is an indication of metabolic acidosis. On a basic metabolic panel, measures of carbon dioxide (CO_2) correlate to the serum bicarbonate level.

1. Administer sodium bicarbonate ($NaHCO_3$) as indicated. Treatment is usually not instituted until the serum bicarbonate level drops to less than 15 to 18 mEq/L. If patients have other indications for RRT, then treatment with $NaHCO_3$ may be deferred as acidosis may improve with that therapy. When using $NaHCO_3$, serum bicarbonate level and pH are reassessed frequently to evaluate the efficacy of treatment. Excessive administration of $NaHCO_3$ can cause metabolic alkalosis, hypocalcemia, and volume overload, especially for patients with lactic acidosis. Diuretics can be used for non-oliguric patients to prevent volume overload and enhance acid excretion.

2. If a patient is being dialyzed, using a dialysate containing bicarbonate will facilitate buffering of the patient's acidotic state. Dialysates containing bicarbonate are preferred to those with lactate.

Preventing Additional Kidney Damage

In AKI, medications metabolized or excreted by the kidney require adjustment to avoid excessive blood levels and potential nephrotoxicity. Particular attention must be given to medication scheduling related to RRT schedules. Medications may be eliminated at different rates in patients on RRT, altering the consistency of medication levels. As a result, selected medications, such as antibiotics, are often monitored with peak and trough levels (see Chapter 7, Pharmacology, for discussion of peak and trough levels). A clinical pharmacist is a helpful resource on appropriate medication selection, dosing, and monitoring during AKI.

1. Modify medication dosing. Because many medications are eliminated by the kidney, dosage and frequency are adjusted in patients with AKI. Medication dosing decisions depend on calculation of the patient's creatinine clearance, which, in turn, is based on the patient's gender, age, height, weight, and serum creatinine level. The phase of AKI and other concomitant treatments help determine the appropriate dose of medication.

2. Administer antihypertensive agents as needed. Patients with prerenal AKI are usually hypotensive, in which case medications previously taken for hypertension are held. Hypertension is a frequent

underlying health problem for many patients with AKI, often requiring concomitant use of several antihypertensive agents. Most antihypertensive agents are not removed by RRT. It is important to adjust the dosage schedule of antihypertensive agents to avoid hypotensive episodes during hemodialysis. Some antihypertensive agents, however, are eliminated by the kidney. Therefore, dialysis patients receiving these medications may require alterations in their dosages or frequency.

Preventing and Treating Infection

Patients with AKI are at high risk for infection and often require treatment with antimicrobial agents. Selection and dosing of antimicrobial agents are carefully considered to minimize the risk of additional kidney injury. Monitoring of both renal function and drug levels during antimicrobial therapy is necessary to avoid further renal damage. Also, different types of RRT affect drug removal differently and must be considered. Frequent assessment of surgical and line placement sites for signs of infection is imperative.

Maintaining Adequate Nutrition

In patients with AKI, the challenge in the management of nutritional status is to provide a balance between sufficient calories and protein to prevent catabolism, while avoiding problems, such as fluid and electrolyte imbalances that increase the requirement for RRT. The clinical nutritionist is an important resource for the healthcare team. The typical patient with AKI is hypermetabolic, with caloric needs potentially twice normal. Additional stresses, related to critical illness, can further elevate caloric requirements. Nausea and vomiting, common in uremia, may also decrease oral and enteral caloric intake. Adequate nutrition is essential to prevent infection by maintaining the integrity of the immune system and promoting wound healing and tissue repair. Hyperglycemia should be managed carefully to prevent exacerbating the risk for fluid and electrolyte imbalance and the long-term effects of high blood sugar on the renal system.

1. Restrict the patient's fluid, sodium, potassium, and phosphorus intake. Because patients with AKI cannot eliminate wastes, fluid, or electrolytes, their dietary intake of these substances is typically restricted. The degree of restriction depends on the cause and severity of the disease; for example, the level of sodium restriction is determined by the cause of AKI and the serum sodium level. Some causes of AKI lead to sodium wasting. This occurs when there is tubular damage or an appropriate response of the remaining, intact nephron to volume expansion. In other causes of AKI, sodium retention occurs. For instance, in prerenal AKI reabsorption of almost all of the filtered sodium is a compensatory response to decreased renal perfusion. RRT can correct abnormal sodium levels that occur in AKI. Phosphorus

may need to be restricted and calcium supplemented if the calcium level is low in conjunction with normal phosphorus levels.
2. Administer necessary vitamin supplements. Supplementation of folic acid, pyridoxine, and the water-soluble vitamins is often necessary.
3. Consult a dietitian for a diet plan. Dietary requirements change for patients depending on their renal status and the severity of their underlying condition. Although the precise role of nutrition in AKI is controversial, malnutrition is thought to increase morbidity and mortality. Recommendations in the 2016 Guidelines for the Provision and Assessment of Nutrition Support Therapy in the Adult Critically Ill Patient include early initiation of enteral feeding in critically ill patients who are unable to eat.

The usual approach to hypercatabolic states is to provide adequate proteins and carbohydrates for resynthesis of damaged or lost tissue. Protein requirements may range initially from 0.8 to 1 g/kg/day and increase with RRT to 1 to 1.5 g/kg/day to a maximum of 1.7 g/kg/day for patients on CRRT as amino acids are removed. Patients with AKI should not receive more than 30 kcal/kg/day nonprotein calories or 1.3 times the basal energy expenditure, calculated by the Harris-Benedict equation with 30% to 35% of energy coming from lipids. The enteral route is preferred unless contraindicated.

ELECTROLYTE IMBALANCES

The kidneys play a major role in the regulation of fluid and electrolyte balance in the body. Regulation of body fluids and electrolytes helps ensure a stable internal environment, resulting in maximal intracellular function. Any renal dysfunction results in abnormalities in both fluid and electrolyte balance.

Indications for treating electrolyte disorders vary from patient to patient. The signs and symptoms of any electrolyte imbalance are not necessarily determined by the degree of abnormality. Rather, the signs and symptoms are determined by the cause of the condition, as well as the magnitude and rapidity of onset. For many of the electrolyte imbalances, it is difficult to determine at precisely what level signs or symptoms may occur.

Sodium Imbalance: Hypernatremia and Hyperosmolar Disorders
Etiologies, Risk Factors, and Pathophysiology
Serum osmolality, a measure of the number of particles in a unit of blood volume, is an important indicator of fluid status. Because serum osmolality is determined primarily by the serum sodium level, evaluation of sodium levels provides valuable information about serum osmolality and potential excesses or deficits of total body water. A quick estimate of serum osmolality can be calculated by simply doubling the serum sodium value. Normal serum osmolality values are

285 to 295 mOsm/kg (calculated: 2[Na] mEq/L + serum glucose [mg/dL]/18 + BUN [mg/dL]/2.8). Abnormal serum sodium levels are classified as disorders of osmolality, with hyperosmolality referring to high sodium levels, which may be indicative of water deficit, or hypo-osmolality referring to low sodium levels, which may be indicative of water excess.

Critically ill patients often are at risk for disorders of osmolality, with children and older adults at highest risk. As a person ages, the hypothalamus becomes less sensitive to changes in osmolality and is, therefore, less able to alert the body to abnormalities through normal mechanisms. Additionally, the neurologic signs indicative of osmolality disorders are often missed or attributed to age rather than to a physiologic abnormality.

Hyperosmolar disorders are the result of a deficit of water. The causes of hyperosmolality include inadequate intake of water, excessive loss of water, and conditions that cause an inhibition of antidiuretic hormone (ADH). In the critically ill patients, hyperosmolar disorders develop because of inadequate intake, usually related to loss of consciousness or endotracheal intubation, and ADH inhibition, as manifested by diabetes insipidus in a patient with a head injury. The signs and symptoms seen are the results of the ensuing cerebral dehydration. Water is pulled from the intracellular space to enhance intravascular volume, leaving the cells dehydrated.

Clinical Presentation
Signs and Symptoms
- Lethargy
- Restlessness
- Disorientation
- Delusions
- Seizures
- Coma
- Oliguria
- Hypotension
- Tachycardia
- Thirst
- Dry mucous membranes

Diagnostic Tests
- Serum sodium more than 145 mEq/L
- Serum osmolality more than 295 mOsm/kg
- In patients who are hypovolemic from extrarenal losses: urine osmolarity more than 600 mOsm/kg with urine sodium less than 10 to 20 mEq/L
- In patients who are hypovolemic from renal loss: urine osmolarity 300 mOsm/kg or less with urine sodium more than 20 to 30 mEq/L

Sodium Imbalance: Hypo-osmolar Disorders
Etiologies, Risk Factors, and Pathophysiology
Hypo-osmolar disorders are the result of an excess of intravascular water and can occur when the patient is hypovolemic, euvolemic, or hypervolemic. The causes of hypo-osmolality

include excess intake or impaired excretion of water, excess ADH as in the syndrome of inappropriate ADH (SIADH), replacement of volume loss with pure water, and salt-wasting disorders. Hypo-osmolar disorders are extremely common in critically ill patients, often related to the use of 5% dextrose in water (D_5W) IV solutions which provide free water without sodium. Balanced fluid replacement is extremely important, particularly in patients who are hypovolemic. The neurologic signs and symptoms seen with hypo-osmolar or hyponatremic disorders are related to cerebral intracellular swelling, as water moves from the intravascular to the intracellular spaces to adjust for the change in concentration.

Clinical Presentation
Signs and Symptoms
- Confusion
- Delirium
- Headache
- Seizures
- Muscle twitching
- Coma
- Nausea
- Weight gain
- Anorexia
- Vomiting

Diagnostic Tests
- Serum sodium less than 135 mEq/L
- Serum osmolality less than 280 mOsm/kg

Potassium Imbalance: Hyperkalemia
Etiologies, Risk Factors, and Pathophysiology
Hyperkalemia occurs due to increased potassium intake, decreased potassium excretion, and redistribution of potassium from intracellular to extracellular fluid. Rarely is increased intake a sole cause of hyperkalemia, but in patients with decreased potassium excretion due to renal impairment, potassium intake is a contributing factor. The most common causes of hyperkalemia in the critically ill are AKI, cellular destruction (eg, from crush injuries), and excess supplementation. Serum potassium is a measure of the extracellular concentration of potassium, and the flow between the intracellular and extracellular spaces also affects this concentration.

Because cardiac tissue is sensitive to potassium levels, hyperkalemia often manifests first as changes in electrical conduction, demonstrated by changes on electrocardiogram (ECG) tracings. Elevated serum potassium levels alter the conduction of electrical impulses, particularly in cardiac and muscle tissue. These conduction abnormalities can lead to serious cardiac arrhythmias and death.

Clinical Presentation
Because potassium impacts normal neuromuscular and cardiac function, these systems are carefully evaluated when hyperkalemia is suspected. Tall or peaked T waves on ECG

represent cardiac membrane instability and the need for urgent treatment to correct hyperkalemia. It is important to note that a patient may be experiencing hyperkalemia and may have no symptoms or ECG changes.

Signs and Symptoms
- Vague muscle weakness
- Decreased deep tendon reflexes
- Flaccid paralysis
- Confusion
- Dyspnea
- Palpitations
- Chest pain
- Nausea or vomiting
- Diarrhea
- Cramping
- ECG changes correlate with changes in potassium levels as follows:
  - **5.5 to 6.5 mEq/L:**
    Tall, peaked T waves
    QT interval may shorten
    ST-segment depression
  - **6.5 to 8.0 mEq/L:**
    Peaked T waves
    Widened QRS
    Amplified R wave
    Prolonged PR interval
  - **>8.0 mEq/L:**
    Absence of P wave
    Progressive QRS widening
    Advanced AV block with ventricular escape rhythms, ventricular fibrillation, or asystole

Diagnostic Tests
- Serum potassium > 5.5 mEq/L.

Potassium Imbalance: Hypokalemia

Etiologies, Risk Factors, and Pathophysiology
Hypokalemia occurs with decreased potassium intake, increased potassium excretion or impaired conservation of potassium, excess or abnormal loss, and increased movement of potassium into the cells. In the critically ill patient, hypokalemia is often related to the use of diuretics and excessive losses through the gastrointestinal tract. Muscle weakness, including cardiac muscle, is the hallmark sign of hypokalemia. Asystole can result from severe hypokalemia. Depressed levels of serum potassium lead to increased irritability of cardiac muscle and neuromuscular cells. Serious cardiac arrhythmias and death may result from hypokalemia.

Clinical Presentation
Signs and Symptoms
- Weakness
- Respiratory muscle weakness, hypoventilation
- Paralytic ileus

- Abdominal distention
- Cramping
- Confusion, irritability
- Lethargy
- ECG Changes
  - Ventricular ectopy and flat, inverted T waves
  - QT interval prolongation
  - U-wave development
  - ST-segment shortening and depression

Diagnostic Tests
- Serum potassium less than 3.5 mEq/L

Calcium Imbalance: Hypercalcemia

Etiologies, Risk Factors, and Pathophysiology
The causes of hypercalcemia are either excess calcium entering the extracellular fluid or insufficient excretion of calcium through the kidneys. Approximately 90% of cases are caused by malignancy or hyperparathyroidism. Interpretation of calcium levels must consider that calcium exists in three forms, protein bound, ionized, and chelated. While most labs measure total serum calcium, ionized calcium is the physiologically active form and is often measured with arterial blood gas measurement.

Clinical Presentation
Signs and Symptoms
- Weakness
- Lethargy
- Confusion
- Coma
- Nausea or vomiting
- Anorexia
- Constipation
- Pancreatitis
- Dehydration
- Polyuria
- Nocturia
- Renal calculi
- Renal failure
- ECG Changes
  - Arrhythmias
  - Shortened QT interval

Diagnostic Tests
- Serum calcium more than 10.5 mg/dL

Calcium Imbalance: Hypocalcemia

Etiologies, Risk Factors, and Pathophysiology
True hypocalcemia is rare as it is defined as a decrease in ionized calcium level that is tightly regulated by parathyroid hormone and vitamin D. Total serum calcium concentration is affected by serum albumin level as 45% of calcium is bound to albumin, and by pH level which can either reduce the binding (acidosis) or enhance it (alkalosis). The causes of

hypocalcemia are classified into three categories: decreased absorption of calcium, increased loss of calcium, and decreased amounts of physiologically active calcium. Critically ill patients may develop hypocalcemia related to either hypoalbuminemia or hypoparathyroidism. The normal level of calcium is critical for normal cell function, neural transmission, membrane stability, bone structure, blood coagulation, and intracellular signaling. Symptomatic patients with classic clinical findings of acute hypocalcemia require immediate medical attention.

Clinical Presentation

Signs and Symptoms

- Positive Chvostek sign (twitching of the facial muscle in response to tapping the skin over the facial nerve)
- Positive Trousseau sign (carpopedal spasm in response to occlusion of circulation to the extremity for 3 minutes)
- Tetany
- Seizures
- Respiratory arrest
- Bronchospasm
- Stridor
- Wheezing
- Paralytic ileus
- Confusion
- Hallucination
- Increased irritability
- ECG Changes
  - Arrhythmias
  - Prolonged QT interval

Diagnostic Tests

- Serum calcium less than 8.5 mg/dL

Magnesium Imbalance: Hypermagnesemia

Etiologies, Risk Factors, and Pathophysiology

Renal failure is the most common etiology of hypermagnesemia in critically ill patients and results from an inability to excrete magnesium. Both neuromuscular and cardiac depressions are observed. Hypermagnesemia may also develop when magnesium intake is increased such as when antacids are overused, or in conditions that cause adrenal insufficiency, hypothyroidism, or hyperparathyroidism.

Clinical Presentation

Signs and Symptoms

- Respiratory depression
- Hypotension
- Diminished deep tendon reflexes
- Flaccid paralysis
- Drowsiness
- Lethargy
- ECG Changes

- Cardiac arrest
- Prolonged PR and QT intervals
- Widened QRS
- Increased T-wave amplitude
- Bradycardia

Diagnostic Tests

- Serum magnesium more than 2.1 mEq/L; however, patients remain asymptomatic until level more than 3 mEq/L

Magnesium Imbalance: Hypomagnesemia

Etiologies, Risk Factors, and Pathophysiology

Hypomagnesemia frequently occurs in critically ill patients and is often associated with hypocalcemia and refractory hypokalemia. Patients with alcoholism are also at risk for hypomagnesemia. Causes of hypomagnesemia include decreased intake, malabsorption, losses through the gastrointestinal tract such as diarrhea or acute pancreatities, or renal disorders that occur with nephrotoxic medications, in the diurectic phase of ATN and obstrutctive AKI. Proton pump inhibitor use is also associated with hypomagnesemia. Hypomagnesemia is common among postrenal transplant patients due to renal magnesium wasting.

Clinical Presentation

Signs and Symptoms

- Muscular weakness
- Positive Chvostek and Trousseau signs
- Nystagmus
- Seizures
- Tetany
- ECG Changes
  - Prolonged PR and QT intervals
  - Broad, flat T waves
  - Ventricular arrhythmias
  - Torsade de pointes

Diagnostic Tests

- Serum magnesium less than 1.6 mEq/L

Phosphate Imbalance: Hyperphosphatemia

Etiologies, Risk Factors, and Pathophysiology

Hyperphosphatemia can result from increased phosphate intake, decreased phosphate excretion, or a disorder that shifts intracellular phosphate to the extracellular space. The most common cause of hyperphosphatemia in all patients, including the critically ill, is renal injury; the regulation of phosphate in the body depends on the kidneys. Hyperphosphatemia is also seen in milk-alkali syndrome, vitamin D intoxication, hypoparathyroidism, rhabdomyolysis, and tumor lysis. Hyperphosphatemia is often associated with hypocalcemia.

Clinical Presentation
Signs and Symptoms

- Positive Trousseau or Chvostek sign
- Hyperreflexia
- Seizures

Diagnostic Tests

- Serum phosphate more than 4.5 mg/dL

Phosphate Imbalance: Hypophosphatemia

Etiologies, Risk Factors, and Pathophysiology

Hypophosphatemia occurs with hyperparathyroidism, correction of diabetic ketoacidosis, acute respiratory alkalosis, refeeding syndrome, and mesenchymal tumor-induced osteomalacia. Hypophosphatemia is frequently in conjunction with hypercalcemia and is common among renal transplant recipients.

Clinical Presentation
Signs and Symptoms

- Muscle weakness and wasting
- Fatigue
- Confusion
- Bone pain
- Tachycardia
- Anorexia
- Dyspnea
- Seizures

Diagnostic Tests

- Serum phosphate less than 2.5 mg/dL

Principles of Management for Electrolyte Imbalances

Hyperosmolar Disorders/Hypernatremia

1. Administer free water. Fluid replacement can be given orally, if feasible, or with intravenous administration of D_5W. The goal is to normalize the serum sodium level over a 48- to 72-hour period. A gradual return to normal avoids cerebral edema, which may lead to herniation, permanent neurologic deficit, or myelinolysis.
2. The amount of free water needed is to correct the water deficit and replace ongoing water loss.
3. During treatment, monitor sodium and serum osmolality levels frequently, and perform serial neurologic examinations in order to adjust the rate of correction safely.
4. For patients who are also hypovolemic, extracellular volume is restored with isotonic sodium chloride with concurrent use of free water.
5. In the setting of hypervolemia, a loop diuretic may be added to free water administration to increase renal sodium excretion. Those patients with AKI may require RRT for correction.

6. Administer desmopressin, an ADH analog in diabetes insipidus. A low sodium and low protein diet can help lower urine output in order to decrease water loss.

Hypo-osmolar Disorders/Hyponatremia

1. Restrict water intake. Mild, asymptomatic hyponatremia often is not treated or is treated only with a water restriction. This is the first-line therapy for patients with SIADH. Treatment should be focused on underlying causes in order to prevent further declines in serum sodium level.
2. Administer hypertonic saline (3%) only when severe or moderately severe symptoms present. It is important to avoid excessive correcting or sudden shifts in serum osmolality which can lead to osmotic demyelination syndrome. This syndrome consists of neurological symptoms and can be associated with irreversible brain damage.
3. Monitor sodium and urine electrolyte levels frequently. The target increase of serum sodium level is limited to 10 to 12 mEq/L over the first 24 hours, and to switch to isotonic saline when serum sodium reaches 125 mEq/L.

Hyperkalemia

Of all the potential electrolyte disorders, hyperkalemia is the most life threatening because of potassium's profound impact on the electrophysiology of the heart. Hyperkalemia is also a frequent indication for dialysis in AKI patients.

1. Initiate cardiac monitoring. Because hyperkalemia affects cardiac tissue, continuous ECG monitoring assists in recognizing cardiac manifestations of altered potassium levels.
2. Administer calcium salts, such as calcium gluconate in the setting of ECG changes. Calcium elevates the stimulation threshold, protecting the patient from the negative myocardial effects of hyperkalemia. The administration of calcium does not change serum potassium levels.
3. Administer hypertonic (50%) glucose and regular insulin intravenously. Insulin acts to drive potassium into the cells on a temporary basis, thereby protecting the heart from the effect of the elevated serum (extracellular) potassium level. Glucose is given to avoid hypoglycemia. All patients, especially patients with AKI, require glucose monitoring because the effects of insulin may be prolonged.
4. Administer medications such as loop or thiazide diuretics to increase renal excretion of extracellular potassium, or give cation-exchange resins, such as sodium polystyrene sulfonate (Kayexalate) to increase gastrointestinal excretion of potassium. Patients with impaired renal function have decreased response to diuretic therapy. Kayexalate

is administered orally or rectally. It is used in patients who have normal bowel function and are not at risk for constipation or impaction. Repeat dosing without a bowel movement can lead to intestinal necrosis.

5. Institute RRT. Hemodialysis may be necessary to rapidly remove potassium when the patient's potassium level cannot be controlled by other methods.

6. Restrict dietary intake of potassium by avoiding potassium-rich food. A dietary restriction is considered conservative management and is usually instituted in conjunction with other therapies.

7. Discontinue medications that inhibit renal potassium excretion, such as potassium-sparing diuretics, sulfamethoxazole-trimethoprim (Bactrim), and angiotensin-converting enzyme (ACE) inhibitors.

Hypokalemia

1. Administer potassium supplementation. Depending on the severity of the deficit and the patient's status, oral or IV replacements can be given. Ideally, IV supplementation of potassium is given through a central line due to the irritating nature of potassium to the tissues. Potassium replacement is given in at least 50 mL of fluid with no more than 20 mEq replaced per hour. It is common for patients to be unable to tolerate more than 10 mEq/h if the supplementation is given through a peripheral intravenous line.

2. Because potassium is primarily an intracellular cation, allow at least 1 hour after administration for the movement of the potassium into the cells before evaluating the serum potassium level. A level obtained too quickly after supplementation is completed may reflect an artificially high serum value. Hemolysis during blood draw may also result in an artificially high level.

3. Evaluate the patient's diuretic therapy. Patients with normal renal function who are on loop diuretics or thiazide diuretics may benefit from changing to potassium-sparing diuretics to prevent hypokalemia.

4. Replace magnesium if low. Correction of hypokalemia may not happen until hypomagnesemia is also corrected as magnesium deficiency exacerbates potassium wasting by increasing distal potassium secretion.

Hypercalcemia

1. Administer normal saline IV and diuretics. In the presence of normal renal function, normal saline infusion followed by loop diuretics reduces calcium reabsorption and enhances calcium excretion from the kidneys. Serum sodium, potassium, and magnesium levels are closely monitored, and replaced if needed.

2. Administer calcitonin. Calcitonin lowers serum calcium level by increasing renal calcium excretion and decreasing bone resorption. Calcitonin takes effect rapidly, but its effect is limited to first 48 hours. Therefore, it is beneficial for initial use in combination of hydration.

3. Administer bisphosphonates. Bisphosphonates are the preferred choice of treatment, especially in cancer-related hypercalcemia. They lower serum calcium by blocking bone resorption and calcitriol synthesis. They take 2 to 4 days to reach their maximum effect. Denosumab can be used in place of bisphosphonates for patients with impaired renal function.

4. Administer corticosteroids. Corticosteroids can be used to decrease absorption of calcium from the gastrointestinal tract in vitamin D toxicity or external synthesis of 1,25-dihydroxyvitamin D3. Dietary calcium and vitamin D intake are reduced as well.

5. Avoid calcium-rich food or calcium and vitamin D supplements.

6. Immobility worsens hypercalcemia so ambulation and weight-bearing exercise are encouraged.

7. RRT may be needed to effectively remove calcium.

Hypocalcemia

1. Administer calcium supplementation. IV calcium should be given to patients who demonstrate acute signs and symptoms of low serum calcium level. Calcium gluconate is preferred. Calcium chloride has higher concentration of elemental calcium, so it needs to be given through a central venous access with continuous monitoring. IV solution containing bicarbonate or phosphate should not be used with IV calcium in order to avoid calcium salt formation. Once serum calcium level is improved, oral calcium, such as calcium carbonate along with vitamin D should be initiated as a more effective and long-term regimen. Vitamin D is necessary for calcium to be absorbed from the gastrointestinal tract. Calcitriol is a form of vitamin D metabolite with rapid onset of action.

2. Oral calcium and vitamin D combination is usually a long-term regimen for patients with hypoparathyroidism.

3. Concurrent hypomagnesemia needs to be corrected before hypocalcemia can be effectively treated.

4. Institute seizure precautions. Patients with hypocalcemia are at risk for developing tetany and seizures.

Hypermagnesemia

1. Discontinue use of magnesium-containing antacids.

2. Administer normal saline and loop diuretics. If the patient has normal renal function, the administration of saline and diuretics promotes excretion of magnesium.

3. Administer calcium gluconate intravenously in order to antagonize neuromuscular and cardiovascular effects of magnesium.
4. Institution of RRT in patients with impaired renal function may be necessary.

Hypomagnesemia

1. Administer magnesium supplementation. Magnesium sulfate IV is given to patients with severe symptoms such as tetany, arrhythmias, or seizures. Those patients should be closely monitored. However, with IV infusion, the abrupt elevation of serum magnesium level partially inhibits magnesium reabsorption in the loop of Henle. Therefore, IV repletion is not sustaining.
2. Oral replacement is preferred for asymptomatic patients. However, the oral magnesium salts are not well tolerated as they cause diarrhea. Great caution should be taken with patients who have AKI or CKD.
3. Encourage a magnesium-rich diet, such as green vegetables, beans, nuts, and seeds.

Hyperphosphatemia

1. Limit oral phosphate intake.
2. Saline infusion increases phosphate excretion when kidney function is intact.
3. Administer phosphate binders as prescribed in patients with renal impairment, especially ESRD patients. They bind with phosphate in the intestine, limiting the absorption. The use of calcium-containing phosphate binders is restricted in the 2017 update to the KDIGO CKD Mineral and Bone Disorder guideline.
4. RRT is indicated with concurrent symptomatic hypocalcemia and impaired kidney function.

Hypophosphatemia

1. Administer phosphate supplementation. Supplementation can be administered by mouth or IV.
2. Discontinue use of phosphate binders.
3. Encourage a phosphate-rich diet, such as dairy products, meats, and beans.

RENAL REPLACEMENT THERAPY

For many years, IHD and PD were the only modalities of RRT available to manage renal failure with volume overload. Many critically ill patients cannot tolerate the rapid fluid and electrolyte shifts associated with conventional/intermittent hemodialysis (IHD) because of hemodynamic instability and cardiac arrhythmias. PD is associated with less abrupt shifts in fluid but cannot be used in patients with recent abdominal surgeries, respiratory distress, bowel diseases, or intra-abdominal infection.

Several alternative modalities to manage acute fluid volume overload and electrolyte disturbances have been introduced since 1977, beginning with continuous arteriovenous hemofiltration (CAVH). The further development of additional CRRTs offers more treatment options for the critically ill patient with renal injury and hemodynamic instability. These therapies include using a double-lumen venous access and a pump for continuous venovenous hemofiltration (CVVH) and the addition of dialysate for continuous venovenous hemodialysis (CVVHD). Continuous venovenous hemodiafiltration (CVVHDF) combines the principles of CVVH and CVVHD. Arteriovenous modalities are no longer used due to risks for embolization and bleeding associated with arterial access use. Compared to IHD, CRRT is a more efficient modality for hemodynamically unstable patients who need multiple intravenous medications with or without total parental nutrition as it has a higher net solute removal over 48 hours. Sustained low efficiency dialysis (SLED) involves using hemodialysis at lower flow rates usually over a 12-hour period at night. This therapy is suitable for the hemodynamically unstable patients who require multiple procedures that would interrupt CRRT.

The goals of any type of RRT are the removal of excess fluid and toxins and correction of electrolyte imbalances and metabolic acidosis. Each of the RRT modalities is able to accomplish that goal, with varying levels of efficiency. These homeostatic corrections are accomplished through the processes of diffusion (hemodialysis) and/or convection (hemofiltration). Diffusion, the process by which solutes move from an area of high concentration to one of a lesser concentration, provides for movement of fluids and electrolytes between blood and dialysate. Convection occurs as a result of the hydrostatic pressure gradient, which induces the filtration of plasma water across the membrane of the hemofilter. Substitution fluid is usually used to prevent excessive fluid removal. Bicarbonate can be added to the substitution fluid and dialysate as a buffer in patients with AKI.

Access

Before any type of RRT can be performed, access to the bloodstream, for IHD and CRRT or access to the peritoneum, for PD, is necessary. The type of access is determined by the reason for initiation and method of renal replacement. The access can be either temporary or permanent.

Permanent Vascular Access

Permanent access is achieved by placement of either an arteriovenous fistula or graft. A fistula is a surgically created anastomosis between an artery, usually the radial or brachial and an adjacent vein. This anastomosis allows arterial blood to flow through the vein, causing venous enlargement and engorgement. Arteriovenous grafts are placed in patients who do not have adequate vessels to create a fistula. A prosthetic graft is implanted subcutaneously and used to anastomose an artery to a vein.

Permanent access is necessary for patients requiring chronic dialysis. A period of maturation, usually 6 weeks, is necessary before the access can be used, and some fistulas do not achieve maturation. The maturation process involves dilation of the venous side and thickening of the vessel wall to permit repeated insertion of dialysis needles.

Temporary Vascular Access

Central venous catheters are used for patients presenting with AKI and for ESRD patients without permanent arteriovenous access or while waiting for the permanent access to mature. Temporary access to the bloodstream is obtained through cannulation of a large-diameter vein, with a large-bore, double-lumen catheter specifically designed for dialysis. These catheters are inserted and maintained like other arterial and central venous devices but are generally larger and reserved for dialysis treatments. Single-lumen catheters are not commonly used.

The catheters can be non-tunneled or tunneled. A non-tunneled catheter should be used when initiating RRT in patients with AKI that may be reversible. The tunneled catheter is associated with lower rates of infectious complications and can be used for extended periods of time (months to years) with meticulous attention to sterile technique.

Taking a patient-focused approach and based on expert opinion, the 2019 clinical practice guidelines from the National Kidney Foundation's Kidney Disease Outcomes Quality Initiative (KDOQI) considers a tunneled catheter to be a reasonable option for long-term use in some circumstances. These include patients with multiple failed AV access and no available options, limited life expectancy, or absence of AV access creation options due to a combination of inflow artery and outflow vein problems. The location for catheter placement is chosen to maximize blood flow and prevent kinking of the catheter with patient movement. The right internal jugular vein is the preferred site. The subclavian vein should be avoided because use of the subclavian site may lead to central vein stenosis and impede future permanent access. Femoral catheters are used when other accesses are not possible but are less desirable due to increased infection risk and impaired mobility. A temporary dialysis catheter is inserted with ultrasound guidance and a chest radiograph needs to be obtained promptly after placement and before first use, according to KDOQI recommendations.

Peritoneal Access

The International Society of Peritoneal Dialysis 2019 guidelines recommend silicone double-cuffed catheters with either a straight or coiled tip with either straight segment or preformed arc bend in the intercuff section. PD catheters are usually placed laparoscopically or under fluoroscopic guidance into the abdominal cavity and can be used immediately after placement. However, routinely PD is initiated 10 to 14 days post catheter placement to minimize the risk of leaking. If urgent start is needed, initially low volume should be used.

Dialyzer/Hemofilters/Dialysate

There are a variety of dialyzers and hemofilters available for use. The type of dialyzer or hemofilter chosen is determined by the patient's condition and the desired outcomes of the RRT. All dialyzers have a blood and dialysate compartment, separated by a semipermeable membrane. The dialyzer has two inlet ports and two outlet ports, one each for blood and dialysate. During hemodialysis, blood and dialysate are pumped through the dialyzer in opposite directions.

Hemofilters are made of highly permeable hollow fibers. These fibers are surrounded by an ultrafiltrate space and have arterial and venous blood ports. Plasma water and certain solutes are separated from the blood by the hemofilter and drained into a collection device.

Dialysate solution, used in any therapy that has dialysis as a component, is specifically designed to create concentration gradients that optimize the removal of wastes, restoration of acid-base and electrolyte balance, and maintenance of extracellular fluid balance. The specific solution is determined by the patient's condition and desired outcomes. Although standard solutions may initially be used, they can be tailored to meet the individual patient's needs and contain varying concentrations of sodium, potassium, magnesium, calcium, chloride, glucose, and buffers.

Procedures

Hemodialysis and Sustained Low Efficiency Dialysis

Initiation of hemodialysis or SLED through a temporary access is accomplished using a procedure called *coupling*. During coupling, the dialysis catheter and the dialysis circuitry are connected, using sterile technique. To initiate dialysis through a permanent access, two 14- or 16-gauge needles are inserted into the dilated vein of the fistula or the graft portion of the synthetic graft. One needle is considered arterial, used for blood outflow, and the other is considered venous, used for blood return.

The basic components of a hemodialysis system are shown in Figure 15-2. Blood, leaving the patient through the arterial needle, is pumped through the circuitry and returned to the patient through the venous needle. A blood pump moves the blood through the dialysis circuitry and dialyzer, allowing for different flow rates. Both arterial and venous pressures are monitored in the circuitry.

Peritoneal Dialysis

Peritoneal dialysis is accomplished through a series of cycles or exchanges. The dialysate, administered into the peritoneal cavity, remains in the cavity for a preset amount of time (dwell time) and then is drained. Each set of these activities is called a cycle or exchange. Dialysate flows into the peritoneal cavity by gravity, taking approximately 10 minutes for 2 L of fluid to infuse. During the dwell time, usually 4 to 6 hours, diffusion and convection occur across the peritoneal membrane. Dwell times are based on patient need. With an optimally functioning catheter, it takes 10 minutes for 2 L of

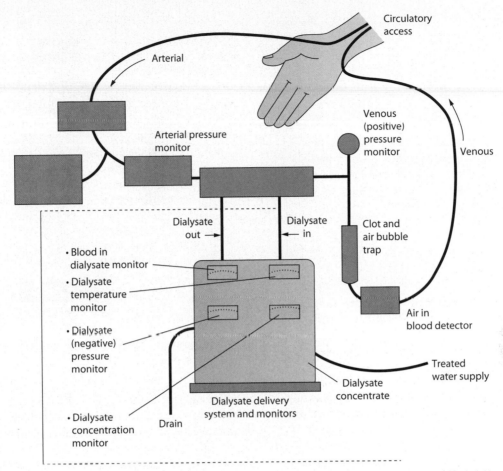

Figure 15-2. Components of a hemodialysis system. (*Reproduced with permission from Thompson JM, McFarland GK, Hirsch JE, et al: Mosby's Manual of Clinical Nursing. St Louis, MO: Mosby, 1989.*)

fluid to drain from the abdomen. Other forms of PD include continuous ambulatory peritoneal dialysis (CAPD) and continuous cyclic peritoneal dialysis (CCPD), although these forms are generally not used in AKI. However, if the patient uses this type of therapy at home for ESRD, it is possible that it will be continued during their hospital admission.

Continuous Renal Replacement Therapy

In CRRT, the blood lines are primed with a saline solution with or without an anticoagulant and then attached to the appropriate vascular access catheter arm (one for outflow and one for inflow). Blood is pumped from the outflow side and passes through the hemofilter. The use of anticoagulation (ie, unfractionated heparin or citrate) assists with blood flow and prolongs the filter life. The advantages and disadvantages of various anticoagulants used during CRRT are summarized in Table 15-3. The blood returns to the body via the inflow tubing after fluid and electrolytes are diffused into the ultra-filtrate. The ultrafiltrate is collected in a bag after removal.

In CVVHD, blood leaves the patient through the outflow catheter and is pumped through a dialyzer rather than a hemofilter. Wastes and fluid are removed and drained into an ultrafiltrate bag. The blood is then returned to

TABLE 15-3. ANTICOAGULANTS USED IN CRRT

Drug	Advantages	Disadvantages
Unfractionated heparin	Widely used, less expensive, shorter half-life, reversible, easy monitoring (aPTT or ACT)	Risk for bleeding, unpredictable action, heparin resistance, HIT
Low-molecular weight heparin	More reliable anticoagulation, reduced risk for HIT	Cumulative effect, expensive, anti-Xa monitoring needed
Citrate	Regional anticoagulation, low bleeding risk	Metabolic acidosis and hypocalcemia (especially in hepatic failure patients), hypernatremia, metabolic alkalosis
Alternative agents		
Argatroban		
Danaparoid	Safe and effective	Cost
Recombinant hirudin	Lack of experience in most centers	

Abbreviations: ACT, activated clotting time; aPTT, activated partial thromboplastin time; CRRT, continuous renal replacement therapy; HIT, heparin-induced thrombocytopenia.

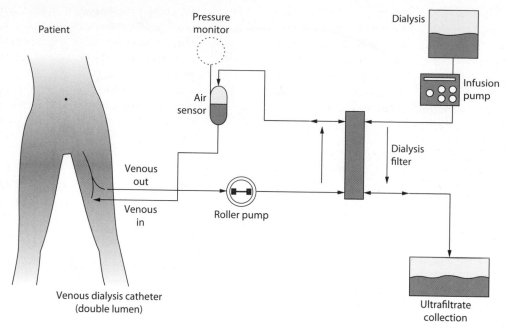

Figure 15-3. Components of a CVVHD system. (*Reproduced with permission from Strohschein BL, Caruso DM, Greene KA. Continuous venovenous hemodialysis. Am J Crit Care. 1994;3(2):92-99.*)

the body through the inflow catheter. The dialysate is pumped through the dialyzer countercurrent to blood flow. Figure 15-3 shows the basic setup of CVVHD. CVVH requires the use of a replacement fluid to replace part or all of the removed fluid. The replacement fluid can be infused pre- or postfilter. In CVVHDF, replacement fluids are given to maintain euvolemia.

Indications for and Efficacy of Renal Replacement Therapy Modes

Each type of RRT is indicated for different clinical situations to achieve identified goals. The goals of therapy are clearly delineated before selection of the type of therapy.

Intermittent Hemodialysis

Intermittent hemodialysis is implemented when urgent therapy is indicated for an acute situation, such as life-threatening hyperkalemia. IHD is contraindicated in patients with hemodynamic instability (although hypotension may be a relative contraindication), hypovolemia, coagulation disorders, or vascular access problems.

Considered the gold standard for the treatment of AKI and ESRD, IHD is the most effective of all of the RRTs. Fluid and uremic wastes can be eliminated from the body during a 4- to 6-hour treatment. Outpatient schedules for patients with ESRD usually involve three treatments per week. Approximately 200 mL of blood is utilized in the circuit in IHD, and this shift in blood volume can exacerbate hemodynamic instability.

Peritoneal Dialysis

Today, PD is rarely used for critically ill patients who need dialysis and are unable to tolerate the hemodynamic changes associated with hemodialysis. CRRT is used instead. PD may be performed in a patient who was on PD prior to admission and hospitalized with a critical illness. Utilizing the peritoneal membrane as the dialyzer, effective elimination of fluid and waste products can be achieved; however, PD is slower and less effective than hemodialysis.

PD is contraindicated in patients who have had recent or extensive abdominal surgery; who have abdominal adhesions, peritonitis, or respiratory distress; or who are pregnant.

Continuous Renal Replacement Therapy

CRRT is appropriate in patients with hemodynamic instability who require RRT. The specific type of CRRT is selected after considering the patient's fluid and electrolyte status, metabolic needs, and severity of uremia. The most commonly used forms of CRRT are CVVH, CVVHD, or CVVHDF as venous access has more predictable blood flow rate.

Continuous Venovenous Hemofiltration

The main objective of CVVH is fluid removal. Although large changes in blood chemistries are not expected, it is possible for a patient to achieve and maintain a stable volume and composition of electrolytes in the extracellular fluid. The higher the blood flow rate achieved in CVVH, the more solutes that can be removed. Because large volumes of fluid can be removed, the healthcare team has more flexibility in treating patients. Nutrition, a problem in many critically ill patients, can often be enhanced in these patients because nutrition can be provided without fear of fluid overload.

CVVH, in some institutions, has become the treatment of choice when patients have contraindications to IHD or PD.

Fluid shifts in CVVH are less rapid than in IHD, making CVVH an appropriate therapy when patients exhibit hemodynamic instability, especially hypotension. Other patients who may benefit from CVVH are patients with uncontrolled heart failure, pulmonary edema, severe burns, cerebral edema, or hepatorenal syndrome. Patients can be maintained on CVVH for several weeks until either long-term IHD can be initiated, or renal function improves. There are no absolute contraindications for CVVH. Unfortunately, the therapy has to be discontinued for transportation off the unit such as for selected diagnostic tests (eg, computed tomographic scans) and the continuous nature of the therapy limits mobility, particularly if a femoral access is used (eg, out of bed to chair).

Continuous Venovenous Hemodialysis

Continuous venovenous hemodialysis combines the principles of hemofiltration with a slow form of dialysis (see Figure 15-3). The indications for CVVHD are similar to those for IHD. Selection of CVVHD is generally made because a patient is unstable and not able to tolerate the rapid fluid and electrolyte shifts that occur with IHD. CVVHD provides an avenue for hemodynamically unstable patients to achieve a stable fluid and electrolyte balance without further compromise of their status. There are no absolute contraindications for CVVHD. Maintaining patency of the dialyzer is the key to successful CVVHD. Patients with coagulopathies require special monitoring if anticoagulation is used to prevent clotting in the circuit.

Slow Continuous Ultrafiltration

Slow continuous ultrafiltration (SCUF) is primarily for use in patients with a fluid volume excess and some degree of renal function. Because fluid removal is the primary goal, this procedure is performed without simultaneous fluid replacement. There is a minimal impact on the urea and creatinine levels.

General Renal Replacement Therapy Interventions

The frequency of RRT is on the rise. Although each therapy has unique characteristics, all require similar interventions.

1. Monitoring includes recording MAP, hourly intake and output and daily weights to assess fluid balance. Frequent analysis of acid-base balance and evaluation of serum chemistries for electrolyte levels are also required.
2. Monitoring with a pulmonary artery catheter or less invasive functional hemodynamic measurement guides fluid management. See Chapter 4, Hemodynamic Monitoring for more information.
3. With all forms of dialysis, prevention of infection is a key nursing consideration. Vascular access devices used for hemodialysis require meticulous sterile dressing changes and are not accessed for other purposes except in rare circumstances. Peritonitis is a common complication of PD, and sterile technique during exchanges and care of the insertion site is crucial. Frequent assessment for signs of infection promotes early treatment.
4. Clotting in the dialysis circuit is an additional complication that requires careful monitoring. Noting changes in the circuit pressure can identify clotting early and prevent blood loss due to changing out the circuit due to complete occlusion. Anticoagulation may be used to prevent clotting in the dialysis circuit and requires monitoring and dose adjustments.
5. The critical care nurse collaborates with the dialysis team in assuming responsibility for early recognition and initial interventions for patient and system problems. Interventions include adjusting the flow rate and the components of dialysate based on the patient's response.

Summary: Principles of Management

1. Early recognition of the signs and symptoms of AKI is essential in order to correct underlying causes and prevent further decline in renal function.
2. Close monitoring of patients' intake, output, and daily weight during different phases of AKI guides fluid administration, diuretic use, or initiation of RRT. CRRT is frequently utilized for patients who are hemodynamically unstable.
3. Electrolyte imbalance and metabolic acidosis can be life threatening and must be corrected in a timely manner. Frequent laboratory tests are warranted until homeostasis is reestablished.
4. Nephrotoxic agents need to be avoided in all patients with AKI if possible. Medications must be renally adjusted to prevent additional renal damage and drug toxicity. Removal of medications by CRRT in critically ill patients is determined by dialyzer type, CRRT mode, and prescription flow rates. Consultation with a pharmacist is needed.
5. Adequate protein and calories are important. Dietician consultation is helpful.

SELECTED BIBLIOGRAPHY

General Renal and Electrolyte

Cheungpasitporn W, Thongprayoon C, Kittanamongkolchai W, et al. Proton pump inhibitors linked to hypomagnesemia: a systematic review and meta-analysis of observational studies. *Renal Fail.* 2015;37(7):1237-1241.

Feehally J, Floege J, Tonelli M, Johnson R, eds. *Comprehensive Clinical Nephrology.* 6th ed. Philadelphia, PA: Elsevier Saunders; 2019.

Ketteler M, Block GA, Evenepoel P, et al. Executive summary of the 2017 KDIGO chronic kidney disease—mineral and bone disorder (CKD-MBD) guideline update: what's changed and why it matters. *Kidney Int.* 2017;92(1):26-36.

Molzhan A, Butera E, eds. *Contemporary Nephrology Nursing: Principles and Practice.* 2nd ed. Pitman, NJ: American Nephrology Nursing Association; 2007.

Muhsin SA, Mount DB. Diagnosis and treatment of hypernatremia. *Best Pract Res Clin Endocrinol Metab.* 2016;30(2):189-203.

Spasovski G, Vanholder R, Allolio B, et al. Clinical practice guideline on diagnosis and treatment of hyponatraemia. *Nephrol Dial Transplant.* 2014;Suppl 2:i1-i39.

Sterns R, Grieff M, Bernstein P. Treatment of hyperkalemia: something old, something new. *Kidney Int.* 2016;89(3):546-554.

Acute Kidney Injury

Balogun RA, Okusa MD. Fractional excretion of sodium, urea, and other molecules in acute kidney injury. *UpToDate.* Accessed January 30, 2022.

Davenport MS, Perazella MA, Yee J, Dillman JR, et al. Use of intravenous iodinated contrast media in patients with kidney disease: consensus statements from the American College of Radiology and the National Kidney Foundation. *Radiology.* 2020; 294(3):660.

Fiaccadori E, Maggiore U, Cabassi A, Morabito S, Castellano G, Regolisti G. Nutrition evaluation and management of AKI patients. *J Ren Nutr.* 2013;23(3):255-258.

Fisher M, Neugarten J, Bellin E, et al. AKI in hospitalized patients with and without COVID-19: a comparison study. *J Am Soc Nephrol.* 2020;31(9):2145-2157. doi:10.1681/ASN.2020040509

Hertzberg D, Ryden L, Pickering JW, Sartipy U, Holzmann M. Acute kidney injury-an overview of diagnostic methods and clinical management. *Clin Kidney J.* 2017;10(3):323-331.

Hoste EA, Bagshaw SM, Bellomo R, et al. Epidemiology of acute kidney injury in critically ill patients: the multinational AKI-EPI study. *Intensive Care Med.* 2015;41(8):1411-423.

Hoste EA, Schurgers M. Epidemiology of acute kidney injury: how big is the problem? *Crit Care Med.* 2008;36 (4Suppl): S146-S151.

Isaac S. Contrast-induced nephropathy: nursing implications. *Crit Care Nurse.* 2012;32(3):41-48.

Kidney Disease: Improving Global Outcomes (KDIGO) Acute Kidney Injury Work Group. KDIGO clinical practice guideline for acute kidney injury. *Kidney Int (Suppl).* 2012;2:1-138.

Palevsky PM, Liu KD, Brophy PD, et al. KDOQI US commentary on the 2012 KDIGO clinical practice guideline for acute kidney injury. *Am J Kidney Dis.* 2013;61(5):649-672.

Schonenberger E, Martus P, Bosserdt M, et al. Kidney injury after intravenous versus intra-arterial contrast agent in patients suspected of having coronary artery disease: a randomized trial. *Radiology.* 2019;292(3):664-672.

Srisawat N, Sileanu FE, Murugan R, et al. Variation in risk and mortality of acute kidney injury in critically ill patients: a multicenter study. *Am J Nephrol.* 2015;41:81-88.

Subramaniam RM, Suarez-Cuervo C, Wilson RF, et al. Effectiveness of prevention strategies for contrast-induced nephropathy: a systematic review and meta-analysis. *Ann Intern Med.* 2016;164(6):406-416.

Susantitaphong P, Cruz DN, Cerda J, et al. Acute Kidney Injury Advisory Group of the American Society of Nephrology. World incidence of AKI: a meta-analysis. *Clin J Am Soc Nephrol.* 2013;8(9):1482-1493.

Taylor BE, McClave, SA, Martindale RG, et al. Guidelines for the provision and assessment of nutrition support therapy in the adult critically ill patient: Society of Critical Care Medicine (SCCM) and American Society for Parenteral and Enteral Nutrition (A.S.P.E.N.). *Crit Care Med.* 2016;44(2):390-438.

Wood S. Contrast-induced nephropathy in critical care. *Crit Care Nurse.* 2012;32(6):15-23.

Renal Replacement Therapy

Crabtree JH, Shrestha BM, Chow K, et al. Creating and maintaining optimal peritoneal dialysis access in the adult patient: 2019 update. *Perit Dial Int.* 2019;39(5):414-436.

Golestaneh L, Richter B, Amato-Hayes M. Logistics of renal replacement therapy: relevant issues for critical care nurses. *Am J Crit Care.* 2012;21(2):126-130.

Lok C, Huber TS, Lee T, et al; KDOQI Vascular Access Guideline Work Group. KDOQI clinical practice guideline for vascular access: 2019 update. *Am J Kidney Dis.* 2020;75(4)(suppl 2): S1-S164.

Macedo E, Mehta R. Continuous dialysis therapies: core curriculum 2016. *Am J Kidney Dis.* 2016;68(4):645-657.

Nissenson AR, Fine RN. *Handbook of Dialysis Therapy.* 5th ed. Philadelphia, PA: Elsevier; 2017.

Tolwani A. Continuous renal-replacement therapy for acute kidney injury. *N Engl J Med.* 2012;367:2505-2514.

Wiegand, DL. Unit V: Renal System. In *AACN Procedural Manual for High Acuity, Progressive, and Critical Care,* 7th ed. Philadelphia, PA: Elsevier; 2016.

ENDOCRINE SYSTEM

16

Heather Roff

KNOWLEDGE COMPETENCIES

1. Outline the nursing management of patients receiving blood glucose monitoring.
2. Describe the etiology, pathophysiology, clinical presentation, patient needs, and principles of management for:
   - Hyperglycemic states
   - Diabetic ketoacidosis
   - Euglycemic diabetic ketoacidosis
   - Hyperosmolar hyperglycemic states
   - Acute hypoglycemia

- Syndrome of inappropriate antidiuretic hormone secretion
- Diabetes insipidus
- Hyperthyroidism and thyroid crisis
- Hypothyroidism and myxedema
- Adrenal cortex hypersecretion: Cushing syndrome, aldosteronism, adrenal insufficiency, and adrenal crisis
- Adrenal medulla and pheochromocytoma

PATHOLOGIC CONDITIONS

Pathologic endocrine conditions are managed in both the critical care and progressive care environments. By far, the most common are those associated with hyperglycemic and hypoglycemic states and to that end they are the major focus of this chapter. While not as frequently seen, the chapter also discusses selected pituitary and thyroid disorders.

HYPERGLYCEMIC STATES

Diabetes is a common comorbidity in hospitalized patients. This disease, along with the specter of hyperglycemia, is associated with significant increase in hospital morbidity and mortality. Additionally, many patients, without a history of diabetes, will develop hyperglycemia during their hospitalization.

Hyperglycemia occurs in hospitalized patients due to natural metabolic responses to acute injury and stress. During acute illness, the liver produces and releases glucose in response to glucocorticoids, catecholamines, growth hormone, and various cytokines (interleukin-6 [IL-6], interleukin-1a [IL-1a], and tumor necrosis factor-alpha). As a result, fat and protein are catabolized and blood glucose surges. Conditions such as myocardial infarction, stroke, surgery, trauma, pain, and sepsis may cause the release of these biological mediators and counterregulatory hormones. In essence, the greater the stress response, the higher the blood glucose will be. To help minimize the adverse outcomes associated with hyperglycemia, rigorous glucose monitoring and effective management of blood glucose are essential. This is usually accomplished in critically ill patients by frequent blood glucose testing paired with continuous infusions or intermittent corrective combined with nutritional doses of insulin. Infusion protocols, or standing order sets, are often used to standardize treatment and maintain glucose values in the targeted range.

Diabetic Ketoacidosis and Hyperglycemic Hyperosmolar

Diabetic ketoacidosis (DKA) and hyperglycemic hyperosmolar (HHS) are two extremes in the spectrum of decompensated diabetes. The diagnostic criteria utilized for DKA and HHS may vary slightly based on source. In general, DKA is defined as acute hyperglycemia (plasma glucose >250 mg/dL) with acidosis (arterial pH < 7.3), moderate ketonuria or ketonemia, and anion gap (>12 mEq/L), and HHS is classified as acute hyperglycemia (plasma glucose >600 mg/dL) without acidosis (nonketotic).

Diabetes is a metabolic disease that results in inadequate uptake of glucose by cells, resulting in hyperglycemia. The key disorder in type 1 diabetes mellitus (DM) is minimal or absent insulin secretion by the pancreas. This is often caused by an autoimmune activation where the immune system attacks and destroys the pancreatic beta islet cells that normally produce insulin. Type 2 DM usually occurs in older adults, but can occur in youth, and is associated with impaired insulin receptor sensitivity. Insulin production in type 2 DM may initially be normal, and then fall dramatically as the disease progresses. Although hyperglycemia is a shared feature, the etiology, risk factors, pathophysiology, and management priorities vary considerably for each classification of diabetes.

Etiology, Risk Factors, and Pathophysiology

Insulin is normally released from the pancreas by beta islet cells (Islets of Langerhans) in response to an increase in blood glucose. Insulin is necessary for cellular uptake of glucose by most cells in the body. Without insulin, the glucose fails to enter cells and accumulates in the blood, resulting in hyperglycemia and a vascular inflammatory state. Cells deprived of glucose begin to starve, triggering a mobilization of stored glucose via the breakdown of protein and fat (gluconeogenesis) and release of stored glucose from the liver (glycogenolysis). This triggers a complex series of physiologic processes that account for the major signs and symptoms associated with DKA and HHS.

Diabetic Ketoacidosis

The most common precipitating scenarios associated with DKA are underlying or concomitant infection (40%), missed insulin (25%), and newly diagnosed, previously unknown diabetes (15%). Other causes make up about 20% including myocardial infarction, stroke, trauma, and pancreatitis. Although DKA is primarily a complication of type 1 diabetes, it can occur (rarely) in some forms of type 2 diabetes under conditions of extreme stress and extreme hyperglycemia (Table 16-1). Primarily in the setting of increasing use of novel antidiabetic medications, although other causes may contribute, there is a growing incidence of euglycemic DKA (EDKA). EDKA, which can occur in both type 1 and 2 DM, is thought to account for approximately 10% of patients with DKA and poses diagnostic as well as therapeutic challenges given the characteristic hyperglycemia associated with DKA is not present.

In general, DKA is a biochemical triad of hyperglycemia, ketonemia, and metabolic acidosis with a large

TABLE 16-1. CAUSES OF DKA

Infections
Missed or Inadequate Doses of Insulin (Primarily Type 1 Diabetes)
Initial Presentation of Type 1 Diabetes
Clinical Stressors
• Trauma
• Surgery
• Pregnancy
• Kidney failure
• Liver failure
• Myocardial infarction/ischemia
Medication-Induced Impairment of Glucose Metabolism
• Thiazide diuretics
• Phenytoin
• Beta-blockers
• Calcium channel blockers
• Steroids
• Epinephrine
• Psychotropics
• Salicylate poisoning
• Sodium-glucose cotransporter 2 (SGLT2) inhibitors (may trigger euglycemic DKA)

anion gap, see Table 16-2. Mild DKA is typically characterized by hyperglycemia (>300 mg/dL), low bicarbonate level (15-18 mEq/L), and acidosis (pH < 7.30) with ketonemia and/or ketonuria. While definitions vary, moderate DKA can be categorized by worsening acidosis (pH < 7.20) and decreased serum bicarbonate (10-14 mEq/L), whereas severe DKA presents as a significant metabolic acidosis (pH < 7.1) and extreme loss of bicarbonate (<10 mEq/L). Patients presenting with mild DKA may be alert and responsive. In moderate DKA, increasing drowsiness occurs. Severe DKA is associated with a significantly decreased level of consciousness or coma.

DKA can develop in less than 24 hours. The initiating event in DKA is an insufficient or absent level of circulating insulin. This insulin deficiency results in increased fatty acid metabolism, increased liver gluconeogenesis (formation of glucose from amino acids and proteins), and increased secretion of counterregulatory hormones, including glucagon and the stress hormones (catecholamines, cortisol, and growth hormone). Counterregulatory hormones reduce the glucose-lowering effects of insulin, raise blood glucose, and are released in response to stress and other stimuli. The pathogenesis of DKA can be organized into three main components: fluid volume

TABLE 16-2. CALCULATION OF ANION GAP (NORMAL < 12 MEQ/L)[a]

$Na^+ - (Cl^- + HCO_3^-)$ = anion gap
Example from DKA case study:
$\qquad$ 130 − (94 + 11) = 25 mEq/L (anion gap acidosis)
Example from HHS case study:
$\qquad$ 152 − (121 + 20) = 11 mEq/L (no anion gap)

[a]Note: Potassium can be added to the sodium but because it is a small number, it is often excluded in the calculation.

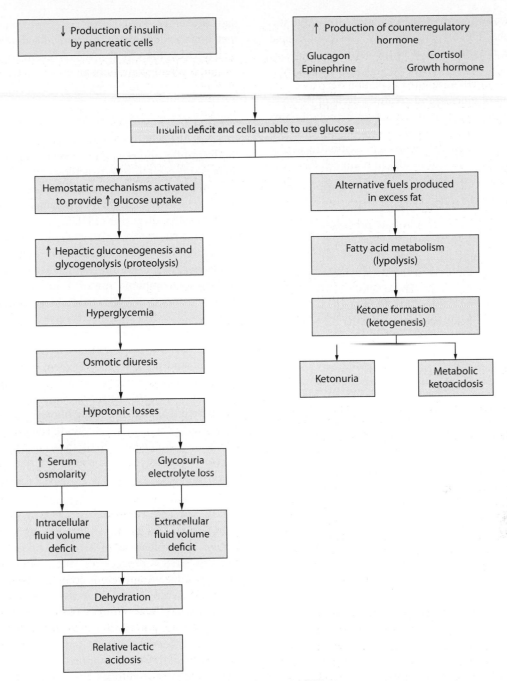

Figure 16-1. Pathogenesis of DKA.

deficit, electrolyte abnormalities, and acid-base imbalance (Figure 16-1).

Fluid Volume Deficit With Associated Electrolyte Imbalance in DKA

Because of the insulin deficiency, there is both hyperglycemia and increased amino acid release from cells. The stress response in the body leads to metabolic decompensation, and stress hormones further trigger a rise in plasma glucose and ketones. The hyperglycemia causes an osmotic diuresis and hypotonic losses leading to fluid volume deficits

(intracellular and extracellular) and electrolyte losses. As serum glucose exceeds the renal threshold, glycosuria results. In the absence of insulin, protein stores are also broken down by the liver into amino acids and then into glucose for energy. This further increases serum blood glucose, increases urine glucose, and worsens the osmotic diuresis and ketonemia. Urinary losses of water, sodium, magnesium, calcium, and phosphorus cause an increase in serum osmolality and decreased electrolyte levels. Potassium levels may be increased or decreased, depending on the amount of nausea and vomiting, acid-base balance, and fluid status of the patient. This hyperosmolality causes additional fluid shifts from the intracellular to the extracellular space, increasing dehydration. Hypovolemic shock can result from severe fluid losses in DKA. Volume depletion decreases glomerular filtration of glucose and creates a cycle of progressive hyperglycemia. The increase in serum osmolarity also is thought to further impair insulin secretion and promote insulin resistance. The altered neurologic status frequently seen in these patients is due primarily to brain cell dehydration and serum hyperosmolality.

Acid-Base Imbalance in DKA

Cells without glucose starve and initiate processes to access existing stores of fat and protein to provide energy for body processes (gluconeogenesis). Fats are broken down faster than they can be metabolized in the liver, which results in an accumulation of ketone acids. These ketone acids are usually cleared in peripheral tissues. If the ketogenic pathway is overwhelmed, ketone acids accumulate in the bloodstream where hydrogen ions (H^+) dissociate, causing a profound metabolic acidosis. Acetone is formed during this process and is responsible for the "fruity breath" found in these patients. Ketones can be quantitatively measured in both blood and urine.

Metabolic acidosis may be worsened with severe fluid volume deficits because hypovolemia is thought to result in tissue hypoperfusion creating production of lactic acids secondary to anaerobic metabolism although other physiologic mechanisms may also contribute to lactate production. Excess lactic acid contributes to an *increased anion gap* (increased body acids). Sodium, potassium, chloride, and bicarbonate are responsible for maintaining a normal anion gap in the body, which is normally less than 12 to 14 mEq/L (Table 16-2). The anion gap represents the difference between the cations (Na^+, K^+) and anions (Cl^-, HCO_3^-). Ketone accumulation, a by-product of gluconeogenesis, causes acidosis and further increases the anion gap, often more than 20 mEq/L (see DKA case study).

The normal physiologic response to metabolic acidosis is to produce bicarbonate to buffer the ketones and H^+ ions. The patient with DKA often has diminished bicarbonate levels because of the osmotic diuresis. The respiratory system attempts to compensate by blowing off carbon dioxide to restore normal blood pH. This explains the deep rapid breathing, called "Kussmaul respirations," often seen in these patients.

Metabolic acidosis also results in potentially life-threatening electrolyte imbalances. Serum potassium is elevated initially in DKA probably due to potassium shifts from the intracellular to the extracellular space because of the acidosis. Later, hypokalemia is common because of insulin-induced transfer of plasma potassium into cells and increased urinary excretion of potassium with the osmotic diuresis.

In the instance of EDKA, impaired gluconeogenesis, glycosuria, electrolyte abnormalities, severe dehydration, and worsening ketoacidosis all contribute to significant metabolic acidosis that can rapidly become life threatening. Unlike DKA, there is absence of serum hyperglycemia and despite severe dehydration, an excess lactic acid is not often present making initial recognition difficult.

Correction of Acid-Base Imbalance

In DKA, the administration of sufficient intravenous (IV) fluids, insulin, and potassium replacement per hospital protocol is sufficient to reverse acidosis in most cases. Use of IV sodium bicarbonate is not recommended for patients with a pH > 7.0 in DKA. Sodium bicarbonate is not administered to patients with a diagnosis of HHS.

Controversy has existed about use of sodium bicarbonate in DKA with severe acidosis, defined as a pH < 6.9. Guidelines from the American Diabetes Association (ADA) no longer recommend use of bicarbonate in severe acidosis. A systematic review of randomized controlled trials and case control studies evaluated the use of sodium bicarbonate, versus none, in patients with DKA with a pH between 6.9 and 7.2. There was no difference in normalization of hyperglycemia, and no difference in recovery time in the hospital. Thus, IV fluids, insulin, and potassium replacement per hospital protocol are the recommended strategies to correct acid-base imbalance in DKA. Although EDKA is increasing in incidence, there are no studies to suggest whether sodium bicarbonate should be utilized, thus, current practice is likely to remain consistent with the above recommendations as seen with DKA.

Hyperosmolar Hyperglycemic States

HHS is classified as hyperglycemia with profound dehydration in the absence of ketosis. The onset of hyperglycemia in HHS is progressive, often with a history of type 2 diabetes, meaning there is some circulating insulin. The extremely severe hyperglycemia in HHS results in profound extracellular fluid volume contraction, marked intracellular dehydration, and excessive loss of electrolytes. In addition, because there is some insulin secretion, lipolysis (fat breakdown) is suppressed. Therefore, there is no overproduction of ketones and no specific physical signs and symptoms of ketosis (no Kussmaul respirations, no excretion of ketones in the urine, abdominal pain, nausea, vomiting, or anorexia). Without obvious signs and symptoms, patients are unaware their blood glucose is rising and may be unaware of the need for treatment. Sustained osmotic diuresis results, leading to massive volume losses, electrolyte imbalance, and central nervous system (CNS) dysfunction. Mortality rates are higher with HHS, because of the severe volume loss and because it occurs more frequently in older adults. Death results from depression of vital body functions as cardiac and respiratory centers in the brain are depressed, cerebral edema occurs, with cardiovascular decompensation, acute kidney injury, and vascular embolism.

Clinical Presentation: Comparison of DKA/EDKA and HHS

DKA/EDKA	HHS
History	
DKA: Young adult or adolescent with history of type 1 DM or previously undiagnosed; preexisting infection is common, although can occur with type 2 DM EDKA: adults with history of type 2 DM with SGLT2 inhibitor therapy, may also be precipitated by pregnancy, pancreatitis, cirrhosis, surgery, infection, trauma	Older adult with history of type 2 DM, and preexisting chronic illness associated with decreased renal glucose excretion. Concurrent illness frequently precipitates viral infections or pneumonia
Signs and Symptoms	
Nonspecific: Polyuria, polydipsia, weakness, abdominal cramping, stupor, coma Specific: Nausea, vomiting, anorexia, Kussmaul respiration, fruity breath	Nonspecific: Polyuria, polydipsia, weakness confusion, coma Specific: None
Diagnostic Tests	
DKA: Serum glucose 250-800 mg/dL (usually <500) EDKA: serum glucose usually 100-180	Serum glucose At least 600 mg/dL often >1000 mg/dL
Serum osmolality <330 mOsm/kg/H_2O	Serum osmolality >350 mOsm/kg/H_2O
Ketoacidosis	Ketoacidosis

↓ pH
  Mild: pH 7.20-7.30
  Moderate: pH 7.10-7.19
  Severe: pH < 7.09
	Not a feature
	pH > 7.30

Serum HCO_3 < 15 mEq/L	Serum HCO_3^- > 15 mEq/L
Serum ketones > 2+	Serum ketones below 2+
Positive urine ketones	Minimal urine ketones
Positive anion gap > 12	Variable anion gap
Dehydration	Dehydration
Volume depletion (decrease intracellular and extracellular)	Severe volume depletion (intracellular and extracellular)
Kidney function	Kidney function
Increased BUN: creatinine ratio	Marked increase in BUN: creatinine ratio
Urine ketones +2	↓ GFR
Electrolyte depletion	Electrolyte depletion
Potassium, magnesium, phosphate, calcium	Potassium, magnesium, phosphate, sodium

Principles of Management for Hyperglycemic Emergencies

The monitoring and management of the patient in acute DKA including EDKA and HHS revolve around six primary areas:

- fluid replacement
- treatment of hyperglycemia
- electrolyte replacement
- treatment of any underlying disorders
- prevention and management of complications
- patient and family education

Refer to institutional guidelines, protocols, and order-sets for specific glucose monitoring, insulin therapy, and fluid and electrolyte repletion. An overview of these key aspects of care for patients with hyperglycemic conditions follows.

Blood Glucose Monitoring and Point-of-Care Testing

Effective glycemic control is vital for improved morbidity and mortality in critically and acutely ill patients. Frequent assessments of blood glucose levels are commonly performed at the bedside using small quantities of blood obtained from finger sticks, arterial lines, or central venous catheters. At the bedside, a drop of blood is placed onto a chemical reagent strip and inserted into a portable glucometer. This point-of-care (POC) glucometer bedside analysis allows for more rapid interventions to manage critical glycemic disorders than is possible from laboratory glucose analysis. Newer technologies have greatly enhanced both the usability and accuracy of bedside glucometers.

Despite the obvious benefits of POC glucometers and improved technology, inaccuracies of glucose measurements can occur. Studies of critically ill patients have reported significant discrepancies between glucometer POC values and laboratory glucose values. The acceptable discrepancy between glucometer values and laboratory values is ±15% for blood glucose values according to the United States Food and Drug Administration (FDA). Any large discrepancies between laboratory and the bedside glucometers must be investigated. This is particularly urgent in hypoglycemic states. There are many reasons for discrepancies in POC blood glucose values, but one important reason is that these glucometers were not originally developed or intended for use in critically ill and/or unstable patients. The FDA has released stricter industry guidelines for glucometer efficacy and identified acceptable ranges for POC and laboratory glucose value discrepancies.

Errors in blood glucose results may occur due to operator-introduced errors or patient condition. *Operator-introduced issues with POC testing*: A common source of error in glucose measurement is the incorrect operation of the glucometer device. Causes include the use of expired glucose reagent strips or insufficient blood application on the strip. Exogenous glucose contamination of blood samples can occur when venous sampling is obtained at a site above an IV infusion of a glucose-containing solution. All hospitals have written policies and procedures that describe POC standards of care. Generally, if there is an abnormal result with a POC glucometer, a blood sample is sent urgently to the clinical laboratory for verification. Tips for glucometer use are reviewed in Table 16-3.

Patient issues with POC testing: Several clinical conditions may influence POC glucose measurements. The accuracy of glucose measurement is affected by hypotension and vasopressor use that lead to inadequate tissue perfusion in fingers. Confounding factors in critical care that may result in erroneously low blood glucose values include

TABLE 16-3. TIPS FOR POINT-OF-CARE BLOOD GLUCOMETER USE

- Review the manufacturer's guidelines and hospital procedure before use. User error is the most common reason for inaccurate readings.
- Ensure that the glucometer is calibrated and clean before using.
- For patients with cold hands, warm hand in a warm blanket and let the hand hang down below the level of the heart so that blood can flow to the fingertips.
- Obtain a drop of blood and let it be drawn completely onto the reagent pad. Do not smear the blood.
- Use the side of the finger rather than the underpad as the side has fewer nerve endings (therefore less painful) and more capillaries providing a larger drop of blood.
- Correlate the glucometer device reading with the clinical assessment of the patient.
- Use universal precautions during the entire procedure.

low hemoglobin, high triglycerides, and hypoxemia. Clinical situations that may affect the accuracy of POC glucose monitoring are listed in Table 16-4.

In the future, continuous glucose monitoring (CGM) devices may offer a viable method of glucose monitoring for acute care settings. Subcutaneous CGM devices are used by millions of people with insulin-dependent DM in the outpatient setting. These devices use subcutaneous glucose sensors and have demonstrated that they optimize insulin therapy, metabolic control, and safety in the outpatient setting. Data from the CGM can be downloaded to a computer for a visual display of the patient's continuous glucose levels, as well as daily and weekly glucose trends. These devices also provide safety benefits as they come with hypo- and hyperglycemia alarms. Currently, only subcutaneous CGM monitoring is FDA-approved; in the future, IV glucose sensors are likely to be developed for use in critical care and acute care patients. Nurses should follow institutional policy in using patient's own devices for glucose monitoring.

Glucose Management With Insulin

A great deal of controversy has existed as to how tightly glucose should be controlled in the hospitalized patient. Earlier studies reported that tight glucose control using insulin infusions to maintain blood glucose target near 110 mg/dL improved morbidity and mortality in the postsurgical

TABLE 16-4. CLINICAL SITUATIONS THAT ALTER ACCURACY OF POINT-OF-CARE BLOOD GLUCOSE MEASUREMENTS

Blood glucose levels > 500 mg/dL or < 75 mg/dL
Inadequate tissue perfusion (hypovolemia and shock)
Vasoactive infusions
Low blood and skin temperature
Hct < 30% (false high reading) or > 55% *(false low reading)*
High blood triglycerides *(false low reading)*
High uric acid *(false low reading)*
High blood oxygen *(false low reading)*
Acetaminophen use *(false low reading)*

cardiovascular patient population. Unfortunately, "tight glucose control" was associated with an increased risk of severe hypoglycemia and higher mortality in a large randomized controlled trial named NICE-SUGAR. The current recommendations support moderate control, rather than tight glucose control. The ADA and American Association of Clinical Endocrinologists (AACE) jointly recommend a glucose target between 140 and 180 mg/dL in the critical care setting. The Society of Critical Care Medicine (SCCM) recommends a more conservative blood glucose target of 150 to 180 mg/dL for critically ill patients. In medical surgical units, the ADA/AACE recommends a blood glucose target between 100 and 180 mg/dL.

An insulin infusion is preferable in all hyperglycemic, critically and acutely ill patients, not just those experiencing DKA, including EDKA, and hyperosmolar hyperglycemic states (HHSs). Patients at greatest risk are those undergoing major cardiovascular surgery and organ transplants, those with decompensated diabetes (such as DKA and HHS), those in cardiogenic shock or kidney failure, and patients receiving high-steroid doses (Table 16-5). These patients often have increased hepatic glucose production, impaired insulin release and sensitivity, and widely fluctuating blood glucose and insulin needs.

Insulin infusion protocols: In critical illness, IV insulin infusions are preferred over subcutaneous insulin injections due to erratic tissue absorption in the presence of hypotension, generalized edema, and use of vasopressors. An effective insulin infusion protocol incorporates an algorithm that easily adapts to individual patient responses and attains the glucose target quickly with minimal hypoglycemic risk. Infusion rates are increased, decreased, or stopped temporarily based on blood glucose readings and the prescribed algorithm. Whatever protocol is used, it is important to consider the degree of insulin resistance. Patients who are highly insulin resistant may require a much higher hourly infusion rate.

Along with an insulin infusion, hyperglycemic patients will require a tandem infusion of 0.9% normal saline or 5% dextrose and 0.45% normal saline, at a rate commensurate with fluid requirements. A dextrose solution is preferred in patients with diabetes. Despite serum euglycemia, patients who experience EDKA are also treated with insulin infusions and simultaneous dextrose infusion to prevent hypoglycemia.

TABLE 16-5. COMMON INDICATIONS FOR IV INSULIN INFUSIONS

Hyperglycemia in critical illness
Diabetic ketoacidosis (DKA)
Euglycemic diabetic ketoacidosis (EDKA)
Hyperosmolar Hyperglycemic state (HHS)
Total parenteral nutrition
Post-cardiac surgery
Liver or pancreas transplant

TABLE 16-6. INSULIN ACTION CHART BY TYPE

Type	Onset	Peak	Duration
Rapid Acting (Bolus)			
Humalog (lispro)	<15 minutes	30-90 minutes	<5 hours
Novolog (aspart)	10-20 minutes	1-2 hours	3-5 hours
Apidra (glulisine)	10-15 minutes	0.5-1.5 hours	<3 hours
Humulin R (regular)	40-60 minutes	2-3 hours	4-6 hours
Novolin R (regular)	30 minutes	2-5 hours	8 hours
Intermediate (Basal)			
Humulin N (NPH)	2-4 hours	4-10 hours	14-18 hours
Novolin N (NPH)	90 minutes	4-12 hours	up to 24 hours
Long, "Peakless" (Basal)			
Lantus (glargine)	3-5 hours	minimal	22-26 hours
Levemir (detemir)	2-4 hours	minimal	13-20 + hours

Most patients also require simultaneous repletion of potassium as insulin is known to drive potassium into cells, especially into liver and muscle cells, which may increase the risk of hypokalemia.

Basal-bolus subcutaneous insulin: When the infusion is discontinued, subcutaneous insulin is often started using basal insulin to mimic normal pancreatic function. Basal insulin is also called long-acting insulin and controls blood glucose throughout the day. Bolus or correctional insulin is fast-acting insulin used to cover food intake and intermittent surges of blood glucose. It is essential that all patients with type 1 DM receive replacement insulin or DKA will ensue. Most hospitals have a protocol for the conversion from the IV insulin infusion to subcutaneous basal insulin with a bolus correction protocol for meals. The subcutaneous long-acting insulin is generally administered 1 to 2 hours before the IV infusion is stopped. This is to prevent hyperglycemia as the IV regular insulin disappears quickly from the bloodstream. Types of insulin are listed in Table 16-6. After discontinuation of the insulin infusion, POC blood glucose testing continues with meals and at bedtime in patients who are eating, or every 4 to 6 hours in patients who cannot take anything by mouth (NPO) or are receiving continuous enteral nutrition.

Hyperglycemia: Management Strategies

In DKA, including EDKA, and HHS, insulin replacement is always needed, although the requirements in DKA are typically lower than in HHS.

1. Regular insulin 0.15 U/kg as IV bolus.
2. Initiate low-dose IV insulin at a rate of 0.1 U/kg/h. If serum glucose does not fall by 50 to 70 mg/dL in the first hour, double insulin infusion on an hourly basis until glucose falls by 50 to 70 mg/dL.
3. Monitor serum glucose levels closely and titrate insulin infusion accordingly. Once the serum glucose falls

to 250 mg/dL, the insulin infusion is decreased to a rate of 2 to 4 U/h and the IV fluids changed to half normal saline with glucose (D5-1/2NS). This ensures that hypoglycemia does not occur during ongoing treatment of the acute condition. It is essential that insulin infusion continues in the patient with DKA until the serum pH is corrected to avoid intracellular hypokalemia. Additional glucose may be needed to achieve this outcome. A glucose-containing solution is also started in the patient with HHS when serum glucose reaches 250 to 300 mg/dL to protect against cerebral edema. Glucose-containing solutions should be started at the same time as the insulin infusion for patients experiencing EDKA and should continue until the anion gap closes after which basal insulin may be utilized to transition to correctional insulin therapies.

Fluid Replacement: Management Strategies

Replacement of intracellular and extracellular fluid volume deficits is a priority for DKA, including EDKA, and HHS to restore intravascular volume and prevent hemodynamic instability. Fluid replacement is often administered via two peripheral IVs, use of a central venous catheter is uncommon today except in the most critical situations. Initial volume replacement is based on assessment of vascular volume status.

1. Administer normal saline (0.9%). IV fluids are generally infused at rapid rates (1000-2000 mL in the first hour, 1000 mL in the second hour, and then at 500 mL/h) until fluid volume is restored or initially around 15 to 20 mL/kg/h. The blood glucose is expected to fall approximately 75 mg/dL per hour.
2. Some clinicians and clinical laboratories calculate a *corrected serum sodium* value from the measured serum sodium in hyperglycemic states. The corrected value adjusts for the dilution caused by fluid moving from the intracellular to the extracellular space and lowering the serum sodium. If the corrected sodium is normal or high, this suggests the patient is dehydrated and requires more fluid volume. The equation is shown in Table 16-7.
3. Titrate the rate of infusion based on blood glucose, urine output, and mean arterial blood pressure. Typically, the patient with HHS has more profound fluid volume deficits, but because the patient may be older and often has other underlying medical problems, the rate of fluid replacement needs to be carefully

TABLE 16-7. CORRECTION OF SERUM SODIUM LEVELS IN HYPERGLYCEMIA

$$\text{Corrected sodium} = (\text{serum sodium}) + 1.6 \times \left[\frac{\text{glucose (mg/dL)} - 100}{100} \right]$$

titrated. Serum glucose falls with initiation of fluids alone. It is critical that insulin therapy not be started without simultaneously correcting the fluid deficit. Otherwise, an acute loss of vascular volume, shock, and increased risk of mortality may occur.

4. When serum glucose reaches 250 mg/dL, change IV fluid to 5% dextrose with 0.45 NaCl at 150 to 200 mL/h. Maintain insulin therapy.

Electrolyte Replacement: Management Strategies

Electrolyte deficits are usually present in DKA, including EDKA, and HHS due to the osmotic diuresis. Hypokalemia may be masked by acidosis. Potassium levels rise approximately 0.6 mEq/L for every 0.1 drop in pH.

1. Administer potassium supplements based on serum levels and in accordance with hospital and unit protocols. Replacement of potassium is a priority during the correction of hyperglycemia to avoid hypokalemia during rehydration, when potassium moves into the cell along with glucose and insulin. To avoid cardiac arrhythmias associated with hypokalemia, the rate of insulin administration may be decreased or delayed until serum potassium levels are greater than 3.3 mEq/L. The rate of potassium chloride infusion is adjusted according to frequently monitored serum potassium levels and the urine output.

2. Monitor magnesium, calcium, potassium, and phosphate levels every 2 or 4 hours during rehydration. Hemodilution will further decrease serum electrolyte levels. Magnesium and calcium replacements are based on serum levels. Total body phosphorous levels are depleted due to osmotic diuresis. This may result in impaired cardiac and respiratory functions. Phosphate deficiencies are usually corrected with volume replacement. If needed, the administration of potassium phosphate 20 mEq/L is one method of phosphate replacement as it replaces both potassium and phosphate simultaneously. Electrolyte and fluid replacement are not administered in patients with severely impaired kidney function as this population often requires initiation of continuous or intermittent renal replacement therapy to ensure safety (see Chapter 15 on renal disorders for more on renal replacement therapy).

Preventing and Managing Complications

1. Monitor serum glucose, electrolytes (sodium and potassium), and arterial blood gases every 1 to 2 hours, if possible, until normal levels are attained.

2. Measure serum phosphate and magnesium initially and repeat as necessary.

3. Monitor temperature, blood pressure, heart rate, respiratory rate, pulse oximetry, urinary output, and central venous pressure (CVP; if central line inserted) at frequent intervals.

4. Evaluate neurologic status at frequent intervals. Institute seizure precautions if cerebral edema is suspected.

5. Institute measures to avoid aspiration in patients with altered mental status.

6. Titrate fluid replacement carefully to prevent fluid overload leading to worsening hypoxemia. Auscultate lung sounds and assess urine output.

7. Hyperosmolar patients are at risk for developing thrombosis and some patients may be on anticoagulants (see Chapter 10 for a discussion of VTE Prophylaxis).

Patient and Family Education

Teaching patients about self-management of diabetes is essential prior to discharge. Patients requiring ongoing glucose monitoring are evaluated for competency using the glucometer. It is important to first determine the patient's fasting glycemic goal. Underlying patient morbidities, cognitive skills, frailty, and age affect glycemic target goals. In a relatively healthy patient at home, a target fasting glucose between 85 and 140 mg/dL is usually acceptable. Target 2-hour postprandial, blood glucose levels are less than 180 mg/dL whenever possible. These goals are achieved through the use of oral hypoglycemic agents, insulin, and in outpatients, injectable incretins (ie, gastrointestinal hormones that increase the release of insulin from beta cells and enhance glucose metabolism). Accurate glucometer measurements are essential to safely achieve glycemic targets.

Before discharge to home, patients must teach-back how to self-monitor their blood glucose and to test blood levels before each meal and at bedtime, especially if on insulin therapy. Self-monitoring of blood glucose (SMBG) improves safety, especially if ongoing insulin dose adjustments are necessary. However, frequent glucose-monitoring schedules may not be feasible, and some patients may struggle with adherence to rigid self-monitoring schedules. Achieving an SMBG strategy that aligns with the patient's needs and goals is important.

The hemoglobin A1C is a blood test that is used to monitor blood glucose over time. The A1C measures the percentage of glucose absorbed by the red blood cells in a 3-month period, a process known as glycation. The ADA recommends the A1C be measured on all patients with diabetes or hyperglycemia admitted to the hospital, if it has not been measured in the prior 3 months. For ongoing control of blood glucose, the A1C target is approximately less than or equal to 6.5% for patients with diabetes. The intent is to achieve a balance between effective blood glucose control while avoiding hypoglycemic episodes.

Table 16-8 outlines required skills for diabetic management. Return demonstrations by the patient or designated caregiver are essential. Instruction regarding the need for routine medical follow-up and the availability of hospital and community resources are important components of the diabetes management plan. The patient is typically

TABLE 16-8. PATIENT EDUCATION: DIABETIC MANAGEMENT SKILLS

Blood glucose monitoring (which may include intermittent fingerstick or continuous ambulatory glucose monitoring)
Insulin administration
Meal planning and counting carbohydrates
Exercise therapy
Urine ketone testing
Sick day management
Recognition of signs and symptoms of hypoglycemia and hyperglycemia
Treatments for hypoglycemia and hyperglycemia
Management of a wearable insulin pump (if used)

Expected Outcomes

1. The patient or caregiver will be able to verbalize essential aspects of diet therapy, meal planning, exercise therapy, sick day management, signs and symptoms of hypoglycemia and hyperglycemia, and treatments for hypoglycemia and hyperglycemia.
2. The patient or caregiver will be able to demonstrate blood glucose monitoring, insulin administration, and urine ketone testing.

TABLE 16-9. CAUSES OF HYPOGLYCEMIA (PARTIAL LISTING)

Fasting Hypoglycemia
Excessive insulin dosage
Insulinomas (pancreas tumor)
Decreased need for insulin
  Decreased food intake
  Kidney failure/dialysis
  Liver failure
  Heart failure
Medications
  Oral hypoglycemic agents
  Salicylates
  Beta-adrenergic blockers
Postprandial Hypoglycemia
Excessive insulin effect
Gastric surgery
Other
Alcohol and alcohol binges

discharged on the inpatient insulin doses (via multiple-dose insulin or insulin pump). Sometimes a patient who was using preadmission insulin may resume the preadmission regimen unless an adjusted dose is required due to weight loss, decreased kidney function, or marked increase in exercise (typically less insulin is required with these conditions).

Particularly for patients with type 1 DM, education to prevent recurrent DKA is essential. Discuss precipitating factors such as infection and missed insulin doses. If available, contact a diabetes educator to help teach the skills needed to manage diabetes once the patient is stable and ready to receive information.

Patients with type 2 DM treated for HHS are usually discharged on oral medications to control blood glucose. Metformin is the principal medication prescribed for type 2 DM due to its insulin-sensitizing effects although sodium-glucose transport protein 2 (SGLT2) inhibitors have recently increased in utilization. Other medications may be added, and in some cases, a basal insulin is used. All hospitalized patients treated for hyperglycemia require follow-up with their primary care provider and/or an endocrinologist soon after discharge. This is especially true for patients with type 2 DM because of the known association with Metabolic Syndrome. The American Heart Association (AHA) describes Metabolic Syndrome as:

- *Abdominal obesity, defined as a waist circumference of greater than 40 inches in men, and greater than 35 inches in women.*
- *High triglycerides, defined as triglyceride blood level greater than 150 mg/dL.*
- *Low levels of high-density lipoprotein (HDL) cholesterol, defined as a blood level below 40 mg/dL in men or below 50 mg/dL in women.*
- *Hypertension, defined as a systolic blood pressure above 130 mm Hg, or diastolic blood pressure above 85 mm Hg.*
- *Fasting blood glucose above 100 mg/dL.*

Because many of the conditions in Metabolic Syndrome are treatable, it is important that patient teaching emphasizes management of the cardiovascular issues as well as diabetes-related health concerns.

Acute Hypoglycemia

Hypoglycemia is a low-blood glucose level and is considered an endocrine emergency. In hospitalized patients, an alert level of less than 70 mg/dL is often used. The ADA now defines clinically significant hypoglycemia as any value less than 54 mg/dL and severe hypoglycemia is defined as any low blood glucose value associated with cognitive impairment. Hypoglycemia results from the imbalance between glucose production and glucose utilization. Of the acute complications, hypoglycemia is most common in insulin-dependent (types 1 and 2) diabetics. Hypoglycemia also can occur with type 2 diabetics who are treated with oral hypoglycemic agents, especially the sulfonylureas: glipizide, glyburide, and glimepiride.

Etiology, Risk Factors, and Pathophysiology

Hypoglycemia can be divided into two categories: fasting hypoglycemia (>5 hours after a meal) and postprandial hypoglycemia (1-2 hours after a meal) (Table 16-9). *Fasting hypoglycemia* occurs when the normal physiologic response (gluconeogenesis and glycogenolysis) to a falling glucose level is altered and there is an imbalance in glucose production and utilization. Hypoglycemia in a hospitalized patient with diabetes is most commonly caused by excess insulin, or oral hypoglycemic agents, with insufficient caloric intake.

Glucose is the obligate fuel for the brain and CNS. The brain is unable to synthesize or store glucose and must rely on circulating plasma blood glucose levels for survival. As blood glucose declines rapidly, epinephrine, glucagon, glucocorticoids, and growth hormones are released. Patients exhibit

ESSENTIAL CONTENT CASE

Diabetic Ketoacidosis

An 18-year-old woman with known type 1 diabetes is in the emergency department (ED) with a diagnosis of DKA. She had run out of her basal insulin (glargine), and was only taking short-acting insulin to cover her meals. During the past 2 days, she had been experiencing flu-like symptoms, feeling unwell with abdominal cramping that she attributed to stress over her college examinations. She was brought to the ED by her roommates because she was drowsy and "acting drunk." Significant findings on her admission profile were:

Respiratory rate	38 breaths/min, deep ("fruity" breath)
Blood pressure	98/50 mm Hg
Heart rate	110 beats/min; sinus tachycardia
Temperature	38.7°C
Skin	Warm and flushed
Arterial blood gases	pH 7.09
Paco$_2$	24 mm Hg
Pao$_2$	88 mm Hg
HCO$_3$	11 mEq/L
Sao$_2$	94%
Serum glucose	440 mg/dL
Serum acetone	4+
Serum ketones	4+
Serum osmolality	310 mOsm/kg
Anion gap	25 mEq/L
Serum potassium	3.2 mEq/L
Serum BUN	28 mg/dL
Serum creatinine	1.5 mg/dL
Serum sodium	130 mEq/L
Serum magnesium	1.0 mg/dL
Serum phosphate	2.2 mg/dL
Serum chloride	94 mEq/L
White blood cell count	14,000/mm^3
Urine glucose	2+ (large)
Urine ketone	3+ (large)

Treatment: In the ED, a peripheral IV was started in her right arm and 1 L of 0.9% sodium chloride was infused over 1 hour. When this had infused, a new bag of 0.9% sodium chloride was hung at a rate of 250 mL/h. The low serum potassium level was replaced and potassium rechecked (now 4.0 mEq/L). She was then transferred from the ED to the critical care unit for intensive management of blood glucose, insulin, and assessment of ongoing neurological and metabolic status related to DKA. At this point, a second IV was started in her left arm. An IV insulin bolus was administered, and an insulin infusion started. Hourly blood glucose checks and serum potassium checks were started. Given her elevated white blood cell (WBC) count and elevated temperature urine and blood cultures as well as chest x-ray were obtained to evaluate for infectious sources.

After 24 hours, a total of 6 liters 0.9% sodium chloride was infused, blood glucose was now 298 mg/dL and was managed according to the hospital's DKA insulin protocol. Serum potassium, serum phosphorus, and serum magnesium were replaced per protocol. The anion gap had fallen to 17 indicating that the metabolic acidosis was resolving.

Six hours later, the blood glucose reached 250 mg/dL and the IV solution was changed to D5 .45% NS at 150 mL/h. Blood glucose checks continued.

The immediate plan of care was to continue the IV insulin infusion until the anion gap had closed. At that time, there was a transition to a basal-bolus insulin subcutaneous insulin regime with meals.

Case Question 1: Complete the following sentence: Intravenous isotonic 0.9% sodium chloride (normal saline) administered prior to insulin administration will
(A) not impact blood glucose levels
(B) dilute blood glucose levels
(C) dangerously raise serum sodium levels
(D) decrease serum potassium levels

Case Question 2: Sodium bicarbonate IV is indicated in DKA in which clinical situation?
(A) High anion gap
(B) pH more than 7.0
(C) pH less than 7.0
(D) Low anion gap

Case Question 3: In type 1 diabetes, a person can appear to be "acting drunk" because:
(A) Hyperventilation from Kussmaul ventilation reduces ketone bodies, lowers CO_2, and increases acetone in the bloodstream.
(B) Glucose interacts with glucagon to raise serum alcohol levels.
(C) In DKA, the gut microbiome has a fermentation effect that releases powerful peptides into the circulation that cross the blood-brain barrier making a person act inebriated.
(D) Glucose cannot enter the brain cells without insulin.

Answers
1. B
2. C
3. D

adrenergic symptoms—tachycardia, anxiety, sweating, trembling, and hunger. These symptoms can occur even if the blood glucose is normal but there is a sudden acute decline (ie, blood glucose level rapidly decreases to 80-90 mg/dL). In moderate to severe hypoglycemic reactions, the CNS is affected, signifying that the brain is being deprived of the glucose it needs.

Hypoglycemic unawareness is an autonomic neuropathy with potentially serious consequences. Hypoglycemic unawareness is defined as the loss of adrenergic symptoms of hypoglycemia that prompt a patient to act to prevent the progression of severe hypoglycemia and it results from alterations in counter-regulation physiology. Both type 1 and 2 diabetics may have deficiencies in counter-regulation systems.

Clinical Presentation

Signs and Symptoms

- Mild hypoglycemic symptoms (adrenergic response)
  - Diaphoresis (most common)
  - Tremors
  - Shakiness
  - Tachycardia
  - Paresthesia
  - Pallor
  - Excessive hunger
  - Anxiety
- Moderate to severe hypoglycemic symptoms (CNS or neuroglycopenic symptoms)
  - Headache
  - Inability to concentrate
  - Mood changes
  - Drowsiness
  - Irritability
  - Confusion
  - Impaired judgment
  - Slurred speech
  - Staggering gait
  - Double or blurred vision
  - Morning headaches
  - Nightmares
  - Psychosis (late)
  - Seizures
  - Coma

ESSENTIAL CONTENT CASE

Hyperosmolar Hyperglycemic State

A 72-year-old man was admitted to the MICU with a diagnosis of hyperglycemic crisis. He lives alone with his small dog with family living nearby. His daughter dialed 911 after finding her father confused and barely responsive at his home. She reported that he had experienced a cough for the past week. His history is significant for heart failure and type 2 DM. His daily medications include carvedilol 6.25 mg orally twice a day, Lipitor 40 mg orally once a day, lisinopril 20 mg orally once a day, furosemide (Lasix) 20 mg orally twice a day, KCl 20 mEq orally once a day, and glipizide 10 mg orally twice a day. On arrival in the ED with the paramedics, he is barely responsive and unable to answer any questions. He is maintaining an open airway with oxygen supplied via nasal cannula. Significant findings on his admission profile are:

Blood pressure	82/44 mm Hg; MAP 56 mm Hg
Heart rate	121 beats/min
Respiratory rate	14 breaths/min, shallow
Temperature	38.7°C
Skin	Dry, poor turgor; dry mucous membranes
ABG on 2 L/min O_2 per nasal cannula	pH 7.34
$Paco_2$	49 mm Hg
Pao_2	56 mm Hg
HCO_3^-	20 mEq/L
Sao_2	88%
Serum glucose	1467 mg/dL
Serum osmolality	362 mOsm/kg
Anion gap	11 mEq/L
Serum potassium	3.6 mEq/L
Serum BUN	41 mg/dL
Serum creatinine	2.2 mg/dL
Serum sodium	152 mEq/L
Serum phosphate	2.0 mg/dL
Serum chloride	121 mEq/L

Case Question 1. Blood glucose climbs higher in HHS than DKA because:

(A) The pancreas secretes small amounts of insulin in HHS but not in DKA, which raises blood glucose and delays the appearance of symptoms.
(B) Peripheral cellular resistance is protective in DKA but not in HHS which increases blood glucose and symptoms.
(C) Fast-acting insulin is contraindicated in DKA but not in HHS making blood glucose rise more quickly.
(D) The hyperosmolar component of HHS forces glucose into the cells delaying symptoms.

Case Question 2: The metabolic acidosis that can occur in HHS is caused by

(A) Ketone acidosis and accumulation of ketone bodies.
(B) Lactic acidosis caused by dehydration and decreased tissue perfusion.
(C) Respiratory acidosis due to decreased respiratory rate and low tidal volume.
(D) Metformin lactic acidosis.

Case Question 3: In hyperglycemic crisis, what is the blood glucose reduction target in the first hour using an insulin infusion?

(A) Decrease blood glucose by 150 to 200 mg/dL
(B) Normalize blood glucose as quickly as possible
(C) Decrease blood glucose by 50 to 70 mg/dL
(D) Maintain blood glucose by until 2 liters of crystalloid have infused

Answers
1. A
2. B
3. C

TABLE 16-10. PATIENT EDUCATION: FOODS WITH 10 TO 15 GRAMS OF CARBOHYDRATE EQUIVALENTS FOR TREATMENT OF MILD HYPOGLYCEMIC REACTIONS

4 oz orange juice
6 oz regular (non-diet) cola
3 glucose tablets
6-8 oz skim milk or milk with 2% fat
3 graham cracker squares
6-8 lifesavers
6 jelly beans
2 tbsp raisins
1 small (2-oz) tube of cake icing

Diagnostic Tests

- Serum blood glucose (blood test) less than 70 mg/Dl
- Fingerstick POC blood glucose less than 70 mg/dL
- Any low blood glucose value with cognitive impairment

Acute Hypoglycemic Management

The management of the patient with acute hypoglycemia depends on the severity of the reaction. Principles of management include normalization of blood glucose concentrations and patient teaching.

Normalization of Blood Glucose

Treatment of the hypoglycemia depends on its severity as described below.

Mild Hypoglycemia

1. Administer 10 to 15 g carbohydrate (Table 16-10). Follow in 10 minutes with another 10 to 15 g if the blood glucose does not improve.
2. Obtain a blood glucose measurement.
3. If the next meal is more than 2 hours away, provide a complex carbohydrate (ie, 4-oz milk).

Moderate and Severe Hypoglycemia

1. Administer IV glucose. The initial bolus is 50% dextrose (equivalent of 25 g glucose) followed by a continuous IV infusion until oral replacement is possible.
2. Monitor glucose levels frequently for several hours.

Prevention of Hypoglycemia

1. Teach the early signs and symptoms of hypoglycemia. Instruct the patient to always carry a source of fast-acting carbohydrate (see Table 16-10).
2. Advise the patient not to skip or delay meals and to limit alcohol to no more than 2-oz hard liquor, 8-oz wine, or 24-oz beer per day. It is advisable to never drink on an empty stomach.

Summary: Hyperglycemia and Hypoglycemia

Hypoglycemia and hyperglycemia are frequently encountered in critical and acute care. Hyperglycemia can result from multiple causes including: physiologic stress of critical illness, inadequate insulin in established diabetes, new

onset DM, DKA, or HHS. It is important to identify the cause of the hyperglycemia so that the correct treatment plan can be initiated. Most hospitals have protocols that outline treatment goals and procedures for hyperglycemia management. Hyperglycemia predisposes patients to increased infection and to worse cardiovascular outcomes. Achieving glycemic control is a priority intervention in critical care. In the setting of increasing utilization of newer oral antidiabetic agents, it is important to rapidly identify and treat EDKA to avoid worsening, life-threatening metabolic acidosis.

Hypoglycemia can be a life-threatening complication of critical illness. It may be precipitated by iatrogenic interventions such as too much insulin or inadequate nutrition. Vigilant monitoring of blood glucose levels is required to prevent neurologic complications or death from low blood glucose.

PITUITARY GLAND FUNCTION AND ASSOCIATED DISORDERS

The pituitary gland is a small gland, about the size of a pea, closely attached to the base of the brain by specialized nerve fibers. The pituitary gland has three lobes: anterior, intermediate, and posterior. The posterior gland is of particular interest in critical and progressive care because dysfunction can result in serious fluid and electrolyte disorders.

Antidiuretic hormone (ADH), also known as arginine vasopressin (AVP), is produced by the hypothalamus and is stored in the posterior pituitary gland. ADH exerts its primary effects in the distal collecting tubules of the kidneys where it acts upon vasopressin-2 (V2) aquaporin receptors to conserve water back to the bloodstream and decreasing serum osmolality. Osmoreceptors in the hypothalamus monitor changes in serum osmolality. An increase of osmolality by 2% leads to ADH release by the posterior pituitary. See Figure 16-2 for an illustration of normal function of the posterior pituitary, and release of ADH in response to dehydration (high serum osmolality) or overhydration (low serum osmolality). Clinical conditions involving the posterior pituitary and ADH include the syndrome of inappropriate antidiuretic hormone (SIADH) and diabetes insipidus (DI). Both of these conditions may require admission to a critical care because of serious fluid and electrolyte alterations.

Syndrome of Inappropriate Antidiuretic Hormone Secretion

Etiology, Risk Factors, and Pathophysiology

The syndrome of inappropriate antidiuretic hormone is characterized by excessive release of ADH unrelated to the serum osmolality. Normally, ADH release is controlled by this value (Figure 16-2). The serum osmolality blood test measures the concentration of electrolytes, glucose, and other osmotically active particles in the serum. SIADH is a syndrome of water intoxication and hyponatremia. There are numerous causes of SIADH (Table 16-11).

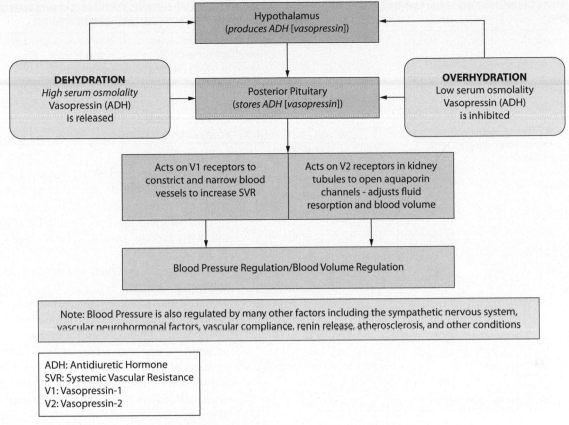

Figure 16-2. Hypothalamus-pituitary-vasopressin (ADH) actions.

Exogenous causes of SIADH: Vasopressin (ADH) can be produced by a variety of malignancies, most commonly small-cell carcinoma of the lung. Therefore, patients who develop "idiopathic" SIADH are screened for malignant tumors. SIADH is also commonly associated with pulmonary conditions, metabolic and traumatic neurologic disorders, and medications, particularly chlorpropamide, thiazide diuretics, opiates, and barbiturates.

Clinically, SIADH is distinguished by hyponatremia and water retention that progresses to water intoxication. The seriousness of the signs and symptoms depends on how fast the serum sodium falls. As water intoxication progresses and the serum becomes more hypotonic, brain cells swell, causing neurologic impairment. Without treatment, irreversible brain damage and death can occur.

Clinical Presentation

Early

- Urine volume decreased and concentrated
- Nausea
- Vomiting
- Headache
- Impaired taste
- Dulled sensorium
- Muscle weakness and cramps
- Anorexia

- Weight gain
- Crackles
- Dyspnea
- Increased CVP
- Weakness/fatigue

Late

- Confusion
- Delirium
- Aberrant respirations
- Hypothermia
- Coma
- Seizures

Diagnostic Tests

- Serum Na$^+$ less than 130 mEq/L
- Serum osmolality less than 280 mOsm/kg
- Increased urine osmolality more than 500 mOsm/kg
- Urine sodium more than 20 mEq/L
- Blood urea nitrogen (BUN) and creatinine decreased (hemodilution)
- Urine specific gravity (USG) more than 1.020

Management of SIADH

Principles of management depend on the severity and duration of the hyponatremia. Recognition of early clinical manifestations of SIADH is key to prevent life-threatening complications. Continued assessment of the neuromuscular,

TABLE 16-11. ETIOLOGIES OF SYNDROME OF INAPPROPRIATE ANTIDIURETIC HORMONE (SIADH)

Malignancies
Lung
Lymphoma
Gastrointestinal
Pulmonary Disorders
Positive pressure ventilation
Asthma
Pneumonia
Chronic obstructive pulmonary disease (COPD)
Acute respiratory failure
Tuberculosis
Neurological Disorders
Head trauma
Meningitis, encephalitis
Stroke
Brain tumors
Guillain-Barré syndrome
Medications
Vasopressin
Desmopressin
Thiazide diuretics
Opiates
Barbiturates
Nicotine
Antineoplastic drugs
Tricyclic antidepressants
Others
Acquired immunodeficiency syndrome (AIDS)

cardiac, gastrointestinal, and renal systems is important. Generally, treatment focuses on restricting fluids, replenishing sodium deficits, and in severe cases of hyponatremia using vasopressor-2 (V2) antagonist medications (also called vaptans), a class of diuretics that selectively eliminates water in the urine, and conserves sodium. Treatment of the underlying disorder is also a priority.

Fluid Restriction and Treating Hyponatremia in SIADH
Fluid restriction is the mainstay of treatment and, to be effective, a negative water balance must be achieved.

1. Treatment of mild hyponatremia (sodium level > 125 and < 135 mEq/L) includes fluid restriction of 800 to 1000 mL/day. This allows sodium level to correct over 3 to 10 days.
2. If severe neurologic symptoms of SIADH are present along with severe hyponatremia (<125 mEq/L), administer hypertonic 3% saline infusion slowly. To avoid osmotic demyelination syndrome (ODS) (formerly known as cerebral demyelination or central pontine myelinolysis), the goal is to only raise the serum sodium by 1 to 2 mEq/H, and no more than 10 to 12 mEq/L in 24 hours. *When the serum sodium has risen* above 125 mEq/L, isotonic saline (0.9%) is the usual IV fluid.
3. Frequent mouth care when fluid is restricted. An antiemetic may be necessary to manage nausea.
4. If fluid restriction alone is not effective at raising the serum sodium level, a V2 receptor agonist, also

TABLE 16-12. EXPECTED OUTCOMES FOR THE PATIENT WITH DIABETES INSIPIDUS OR SYNDROME OF INAPPROPRIATE ANTIDIURETIC HORMONE

Adequate fluid balance is maintained/restored as evidenced by
- Blood pressure within 10 mm Hg of patient baseline
- Heart rate 60-100 beats/min
- Normal skin turgor
- Peripheral pulses return to baseline
- Serum osmolality 275-295 mOsm/kg
- Serum sodium 135-145 mEq/L
- Urine osmolality appropriate for serum osmolality

known as vaptans, such as Tolvaptan, may be administered IV. Vaptans are medications that eliminate water while retaining salt and may be used with, or in place of, loop diuretics in dilutional hyponatremia. Oral vaptans are also available. See Chapter 7, Pharmacology.

5. When taking an oral diet, add salt to food and consult with a dietician.
6. Assess cardiovascular and respiratory functions closely to evaluate the effects of the excess volume on these systems. Right and left ventricular volumes may increase, causing heart failure and new-onset or exacerbation of atrial fibrillation. Tachypnea, reports of shortness of breath, and fine crackles are indicators of fluid overload and impending heart failure. Monitor neurologic status closely and protect the patient from self-harm. Institute seizure precautions as necessary.
7. Expected outcomes for the patient with SIADH are listed in Table 16-12.

Diabetes Insipidus

Etiology, Risk Factors, and Pathophysiology

Diabetes insipidus results from a group of disorders in which there is an absolute or relative deficiency of ADH (called *central DI*) or an insensitivity to its effects on the kidney tubules (called *nephrogenic DI*) (Figure 16-3). DI may complicate the course of critically and acutely ill patients and can result in acute fluid and electrolyte disturbances.

There are many causes of DI (Table 16-13). *Central DI* (also called neurogenic DI) results from damage to the hypothalamic/pituitary system. An absolute deficiency of ADH results in an impaired ability to concentrate urine and polyuria of several liters. The result is dehydration. Patients with head trauma or those who have had neurosurgery are at increased risk for up to 7 to 10 days after the injury. DI does not generally present for at least 48 to 72 hours after the initial hypothalamic or pituitary trauma.

Nephrogenic DI is characterized by kidney tubule insensitivity to ADH and develops because of structural or functional changes in the kidney. This results in impaired urine-concentrating ability and free water conservation. Nephrogenic DI is less dramatic than neurogenic DI in its onset and appearance and is usually managed in the outpatient setting.

In *central DI* the ability of the body to increase ADH secretion or respond to ADH is impaired. A high volume

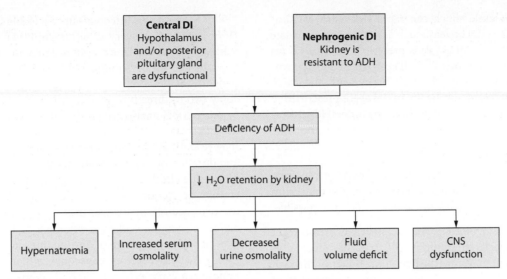

Figure 16-3. Pathogenesis of DI.

of dilute urine and increasing hemoconcentration is evident. Signs and symptoms of dehydration are often present when the thirst mechanism has been impaired or with inadequate fluid replacement. In addition, if a hyperosmolar state exists, intracellular brain volume depletion occurs as water moves from within the brain cells to the plasma. Typically, symptoms of central DI manifest when serum sodium levels exceed 155 mEq/L.

TABLE 16-13. EITOLOGIES OF DIABETES INSIPIDUS

ADH Insufficiency (Neurogenic Diabetes Insipidus [DI])
Familial (hereditary)
Trauma
Neoplasms
Infections
Tuberculosis
Cryptococcosis
Syphilis
Central nervous system infections
Vascular
Cerebral hemorrhage or thrombosis/embolism
Cerebrovascular aneurysm
Brain death
ADH Insensitivity (Nephrogenic DI)
Familial (hereditary)
Medication induced
Lithium
Demeclocycline
Glyburide
Colchicine
Amphotericin B
Gentamicin
Furosemide
Electrolyte disorders
Hypokalemia
Hypercalcemia
Kidney disease
Excessive water intake (secondary DI)
Excessive IV fluid administration
Psychogenic polydipsia (lesion in thirst center)

Clinical Presentation

ADH Deficiency

- Polydipsia (if alert)
- Polyuria (5-20 L in 24 hours)

Fluid Volume Deficit

- Persistent hypotension may initially present as orthostatic hypotension and progress to continuous vasopressor requirement
- Weight loss
- Tachycardia
- Decreased CVP
- Collapsed inferior vena cava (IVC) on ultrasound
- Poor skin turgor
- Dry mucous membranes

Intracellular Brain Volume Depletion

- Confusion
- Restlessness
- Lethargy
- Irritability
- Seizures
- Coma

Diagnostic Tests

- Water deprivation test (never in critical care)
- Serum sodium more than 155 mEq/L
- Serum osmolality more than 295 mOsm/kg/L
- Urine osmolality inappropriately low with high serum osmolality (<150 mOsm/kg/L)
- USG decreased
- BUN and creatinine increased (hemoconcentration)

Management of Diabetes Insipidus

The management of the patient in DI is directed at correcting the profound fluid volume deficit and electrolyte imbalances associated with this condition. If fluid losses are not replaced, hypovolemic shock can rapidly develop. Medications that simulate ADH release such as desmopressin acetate (commonly known as DDAVP) is prescribed to treat DI via IV, nasal spray, or oral routes. If DI has progressed to hypovolemic shock or in the setting of likely brain death, the use of continuous vasopressin may be the initial agent prescribed to address ADH repletion. As with other disorders, identification, diagnosis, and treatment of the cause of DI are priorities.

Fluid Volume Replacement

If the patient is alert and the thirst mechanism is not impaired, allow the patient to drink water to maintain normal serum osmolality. In many critically ill patients, this is not possible.

1. Administer hypotonic volume, such as dextrose 5% in water, quarter-strength or half-strength saline, IV as prescribed to restore the hypotonic fluid lost through diuresis. In severe DI, where large amounts of fluid replacement are required, the IV intake is usually titrated to urine output; for example, 400 mL of urine output for 1 hour is replaced with 400 mL IV fluid the next hour. Hypotonic saline solutions are preferred (quarter-strength or half-strength saline). Reduce the serum sodium by approximately 0.5 mEq/L every hour but no more than 12 mEq/L per day.
2. Monitor fluid status: Hourly urine outputs along with measurements of USG every 2 to 4 hours are done along with daily weight and strict intake and output. Monitor for signs of continuing fluid volume deficit. If the serum Na is more than 155 mEq/L, rehydration occurs over 48 hours. A serum sodium more than 170 mEq/L necessitates ICU care due to increased risk of seizures. Expected outcomes for the patient with DI are listed in Table 16-12.
3. Monitor neurologic status continuously. An altered level of consciousness indicates intracellular dehydration of the brain and hypovolemia.
4. Frequent electrolyte monitoring is recommended during the initial phase of treatment.

ADH Administration or Enhancement

In central DI, desmopressin (DDAVP), an ADH analogue, is the drug of choice and is available in subcutaneous, IV, intranasal, and oral preparations. Desmopressin acts on the distal tubules and collecting ducts of the kidney to increase water reabsorption and has very specific actions with little or no ADH-like activity elsewhere in the body. Vasopressin, the predecessor of desmopressin, may be utilized as a continuous infusion in the critically ill to aid in both treating ongoing shock and avoidance of iatrogenic hyponatremia associated with administration of ADH analogues. Vasopressin infusion should be considered when there is higher risk of iatrogenic hyponatremia given its relatively short half-life of 24 minutes instead of 158 minutes seen with DDAVP. Adjunctive therapies to enhance ADH release include nonhormonal agents such as chlorpropamide, carbamazepine, thiazides, and non-steroidal anti-inflammatory drugs (NSAIDs).

If the patient is unconscious, injectable DDAVP is given IV or IM 1 to 4 µg every 12 hours until therapeutic goals are achieved, such as a urine output of 2 to 3 mL/kg/h, USG 1.010 to 1.020, and serum sodium 140 to 145 mEq/L. In conscious patients, the nasal replacement route is given 10 to 20 µg by spray two to three times a day. It is important that DDAVP or other ADH analogues not be administered unless serum sodium is at least above 145 mmol/L, as serious hyponatremia may result. Oral formulations of ADH have a slower onset and duration of action and are not useful in acute situations. Major side effects to watch for include headache, abdominal cramps, or allergic reactions such as facial flushing. Monitor for overmedication, which may precipitate hypervolemia. Signs and symptoms of fluid volume excess include dyspnea, hypertension, weight gain, and angina. Iatrogenic hyponatremia is another serious consequence that when it develops rapidly can cause extreme cerebral edema and ODS. Therefore, close monitoring of serum sodium is necessary.

Summary: Pituitary Gland and DI/SIADH

The pituitary gland is a small pea-size gland that releases ADH to achieve water balance in the body. Alterations in fluid balance impact serum sodium levels. In central DI, the posterior pituitary produces little or no ADH resulting in excess urine output, hypernatremia, and life-threatening dehydration. In SIADH, the posterior pituitary produces excessive quantities of ADH unrelated to physiologic need, causing low urine output, water intoxication, and hyponatremia. Early recognition and prompt treatment are vital for survival.

THYROID GLAND FUNCTION AND ASSOCIATED DISORDERS

The thyroid gland has a shape that resembles a bow tie. The gland wraps around the trachea in the front of the neck. There are two lobes that are connected by a bridge of thyroid tissue called the isthmus. The thyroid gland secretes hormones associated with metabolism that are regulated by a feedback loop as shown in Figure 16-4.

In the normal thyroid feedback loop, the hypothalamus produces thyroid-releasing hormone (TRH), which stimulates the anterior pituitary to release thyroid-stimulating hormone (TSH), and based on the level of circulating hormones, the thyroid gland produces the thyroid hormones thyroxine (T_4) and triiodothyronine (T_3). T_4 is produced in greater quantity but T_3 is more biologically active. When needed, T_4 is converted to T_3 in the peripheral circulation, predominantly by the liver. In the circulation, T_4 and T_3 are protein-bound. Ultimately, these hormones are separated from their transport proteins so that metabolically active free-T_3 and free-T_4 can enter cells. Free-T_3 is the principal thyroid hormone inside cells. Disorders of the thyroid gland are caused by hypersecretion (hyperthyroidism and thyroid storm) and hyposecretion (hypothyroidism and myxedema).

Hyperthyroidism and Thyroid Storm

Hyperthyroidism, also known as thyrotoxicosis, is more common in women than men, occurring in about 2% of the

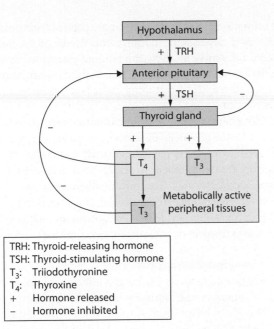

Figure 16-4. Hypothalamus-pituitary-thyroid hormone feedback loop.

female population (2 in 100), and in approximately 0.002% of the male population (2 in 1000). In this condition, the hyperactive thyroid produces too much thyroid hormone and is not regulated by the normal hypothalamus-pituitary-thyroid feedback loop as described in Figure 16-4.

Hyperthyroidism

The most common cause of hyperthyroidism is *Graves Disease*. This is an autoimmune condition where the immune system produces antibodies that bind to TSH receptors in the thyroid gland causing enlargement of thyroid follicular cells. This causes diffuse thyroid enlargement, with production of excess thyroid hormone, leading to suppression of TSH production from the pituitary gland. In response to the fall in TSH, the thyroid gland increases production of the thyroid hormones T_4 and T_3. On a laboratory blood test, the TSH level is low and circulating thyroid hormone levels are elevated. Hyperthyroidism can also develop after taking the antiarrhythmic medication amiodarone.

Iodine deficiency increases the risk of hyperthyroidism but is rare in wealthy countries, as salt has been supplemented with iodine since the 1920s. Thyroid hormones are involved in all cellular functions, and excess hormone increases metabolism usually leading to increased heart rate, increased temperature, and frequent bowel movements.

Thyroid Storm

Thyroid storm or thyrotoxic crisis is a life-threatening emergency with mortality up to 30%. It is a rare condition in developed countries, typically seen with undiagnosed or under-treated hyperthyroidism. Thyroid storm may be initiated by infection, surgery, or other acute illness. Because thyroid hormones are involved in all metabolic processes, an increase in thyroid hormone availability creates a hypermetabolic state with surges of sympathetic nervous system catecholamine release. This causes dangerously high heart rates,

treatment-refractory arrhythmias, increased blood pressure, high temperature, heat intolerance, diarrhea, anxiety, and mental status changes.

Thyroid Storm Management

Emergency management involves immediate administration of beta-blockers (propanol, esmolol) to blunt the sympathetic nervous system receptors, plus medications that block thyroid synthesis and block release of more thyroid hormone (methimazole, propylthiouracil). There are case-reports in the literature that a therapeutic plasma exchange (TPE) via apheresis may remove protein-bound T_3 and T_4. Dehydration occurs from fluids lost via the gastrointestinal tract and extreme diaphoresis. Volume resuscitation with monitoring of electrolytes is required. Fever is controlled with acetaminophen and comfort-cooling measures may increase comfort.

Hypothyroidism and Myxedema Coma

Hypothyroidism

As the name suggests, hypothyroidism signals an underactive thyroid with slowed metabolism. The most common cause of hypothyroidism is Hashimoto thyroiditis. This is an autoimmune condition where the immune system makes antibodies against healthy thyroid tissue. Amiodarone (antiarrhythmic medication) can also cause hypothyroidism. Amiodarone has a chemical structure that is similar to thyroxine and it also contains significant amounts of iodine. A high TSH blood level and symptoms of slowed metabolism (weight gain, fatigue, sensitivity to cold) are diagnostic symptoms. Hypothyroidism is more common in women than men. Ongoing critical illness is associated with a downregulation of the hypothalamic-pituitary-thyroid axis with lower levels of circulating thyroid hormones. The specific causes of this change are unknown.

Myxedema Coma

The terms myxedema coma or myxedema crisis are used to describe extreme hypothyroidism. Clinically this is observed as a decreased level of consciousness, respiratory failure, hypothermia, and often heart failure. The onset can be insidious and may only be discovered when a patient is admitted for another cause such as respiratory failure. Mortality can be 25% or higher. Hypothyroidism leads to an extreme hypometabolism that decreases basal metabolic rate, causes bradycardia, hypotension, and low cardiac output. Other clinical signs vary as some patients have periorbital edema, ascites, or pericardial effusion, and others may not.

Myxedema Coma Management

Pharmacologic replacement of thyroid hormone is essential. Levothyroxine (synthetic T_4) is administered to replenish hormone stores and increase the metabolic rate. Management involves supportive mechanical ventilation and meticulous nursing care to prevent complications such as hospital-acquired pressure injury (HAPI), ventilator-associated pneumonia (VAP), and sepsis.

Summary: Hyperthyroidism and Thyroid Storm, Hypothyroidism and Myxedema Coma

Severe thyroid dysfunction, whether hyperactive (thyroid storm) or hypoactive (myxedema coma), is rare as a primary diagnosis in critical care. However, it may be helpful to assess for the more common underlying thyroid conditions of hyperthyroidism or hypothyroidism by measuring the TSH level. The TSH value is low in hyperthyroidism, and high in hypothyroidism. This TSH test is useful when a patient who has been admitted for another reason has signs and symptoms not associated with the admitting diagnosis.

ADRENAL GLAND FUNCTION AND ASSOCIATED DISORDERS

The adrenal glands are located on top of the kidney. Although small, they are metabolically important for metabolic and hormonal health. The outer region, called the cortex, is responsible for secretion of glucocorticoids and aldosterone. The inner region, called the medulla, is responsible for secretion of the catecholamine epinephrine. Adrenal gland dysfunction can occur from either hypersecretion or hyposecretion of the hormones in either cortex or medulla (Figure 16-5).

Cushing Syndrome

Cushing syndrome can be primary or secondary. Primary Cushing syndrome is rare. It occurs when the adrenal cortex produces excessive amounts of the hormone cortisol. The origin may be a pituitary adenoma that produces excessive amounts of adrenocorticotropic hormone (ACTH) that stimulates the adrenal cortex to produce excessive cortisol. ACTH is a component of the hypothalamus-pituitary-adrenal feedback loop that normally regulates cortisol levels. A tumor of the adrenal gland that secretes excess cortisol can also lead to Cushing syndrome.

Secondary Cushing syndrome occurs when a patient is taking long-term glucocorticoids (steroids) for another medical condition. The medical conditions may include corticosteroids to prevent organ transplant rejection, various respiratory conditions, skin conditions, and chronic

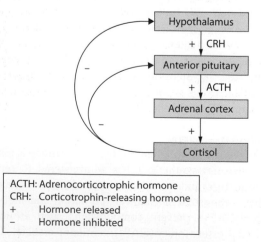

ACTH: Adrenocorticotrophic hormone
CRH: Corticotrophin-releasing hormone
+   Hormone released
−   Hormone inhibited

Figure 16-5. Hypothalamus-pituitary-adrenal cortex feedback loop.

inflammation. In this circumstance, patients are described as "steroid dependent" because the medications must be tapered off slowly to allow the adrenal glands to recover. If the corticosteroids are stopped abruptly, the patient may be plunged into a life-threatening crisis (see Addisonian crisis discussed later).

Whether Cushing syndrome is primary or secondary, the excess cortisol produces distinct features, including a round face, hirsutism (excess hair growth), fat accumulation on the upper back and abdomen, hyperglycemia, thin skin, bruises, fatigue, weakness, and a compromised immune system with increased vulnerability to infection. It is essential to know if a patient is steroid-dependent as abruptly stopping glucocorticoids leaves the patient without any stress-response protection.

Primary Cushing Syndrome Management

Primary or endogenous Cushing syndrome is rare. It results from a tumor of the pituitary gland that produces excess ATCH and can be removed surgically. Alternatively, an adrenal tumor may produce excess cortisol and surgical removal of the affected adrenal gland will resolve the problem.

Steroid-Dependent Patient Management

Secondary or exogenous Cushing syndrome occurs when a patient has been taking corticosteroids for prolonged periods, especially at high dosages. This creates unique challenges in treatment. When a steroid-dependent patient experiences an infection, trauma, surgery, or other medical condition, the adrenal gland cannot increase cortisol output. In this situation, their usual dose of corticosteroids may be inadequate. To compensate, a "stress steroid" regimen may be used to cover the physiologic stress of critical illness and associated procedures. Some hospitals have clinical guidelines/pathways to cover this situation. Addison crisis (discussed later) can be precipitated when glucocorticosteroids are abruptly stopped in a steroid-dependent patient. Corticosteroids are tapered off to avoid complications of cortisol deficiency.

Aldosteronism

The adrenal cortex also produces aldosterone, a mineralocorticoid hormone important in maintaining salt and water homeostasis. Aldosterone is a component of the renin-angiotensin-aldosterone system (RAAS). In primary aldosteronism, the adrenal cortex secretes excessive amounts of aldosterone unrelated to the RASS feedback loop. An adrenal cortex tumor (aldosteroma) is one of the causes of this rare condition. Patients can present with extreme hypertension, metabolic alkalosis, and life-threatening hypokalemia.

Aldosteronism Management

Emergency management is focused on reducing hypertension and replacing potassium and other electrolytes within normal limits. If the cause is an aldosteroma, resection of the adrenal tumor will be necessary. There are other causes of aldosteronism and an endocrinology consultation is recommended for a full diagnostic workup.

Addison Disease and Crisis

Adrenal insufficiency, also known as Addison disease, is caused by hyposecretion of glucocorticoids (cortisol) from the adrenal cortex. Simultaneously measuring the serum ACTH and the serum cortisol may confirm the diagnosis in this rare condition. An elevated ACTH with an extremely low cortisol level may be diagnostic. Addison disease can be a difficult diagnosis to make when there are other confounding comorbidities.

If the adrenal gland shuts down completely, this condition is known as an Addisonian crisis. Signature signs and symptoms include critical hypotension, hyperkalemia, hyponatremia, and hypoglycemia. Prompt recognition and intervention are vital to prevent demise.

Addisonian Crisis Management

As soon as the condition is recognized, emergency replacement with IV glucocorticosteroids is vital. Hydration with IV isotonic saline (0.9%) and electrolyte replacement are also priorities. Other supportive treatments will depend on the patient's level of consciousness, respiratory drive, and comorbidities. A thorough assessment by an endocrinologist is recommended once the initial crisis is managed.

Critical Illness-Related Corticosteroid Insufficiency

The physiologic stress associated with critical illness normally stimulates the adrenal gland to produce additional cortisol. However, in critical illness-related corticosteroid insufficiency (CIRCI), the adrenal gland does not respond, so that serum cortisol levels are inadequate to support a therapeutic stress response. Persistent elevation of inflammatory cytokines may be a precipitating and ongoing cause of CIRCI. Patients with CIRCI are vulnerable to infection with hypotensive shock, and to septic shock that is refectory to vasopressor catecholamines.

Diagnosis of CIRCI remains a challenge. Two tests may be helpful: (1) failure of the cortisol level to meaningfully increase ($\leq$9 mcg), at a 60-minute time-point following administration of an ACTH-cortisol stimulus (IV cosyntropin 250 mcg), suggests inadequate adrenal function; (2) a random plasma cortisol level below normal (<10 mcg/dL) suggests inadequate adrenal function.

Guidelines on the use of corticosteroids in critical illness were published by the major critical care medical societies in 2017. The Surviving Sepsis guidelines strongly recommend the use of fluids and antibiotics as first-line therapy to achieve hemodynamic stability (as described in Chapter 11, Multisystem Problems). If hemodynamic stability is not achievable with fluids, antibiotics, and vasopressors, IV hydrocortisone is considered. The 2017 CIRC guidelines also suggest IV hydrocortisone (<400 mg/day) for 3 days or longer at full dose for refractory septic shock. Corticosteroids are not recommended for sepsis without signs of shock.

The dilemma with pharmacologic glucocorticoids is to balance the known anti-inflammatory properties and potential for shock reversal, against depression of the immune system, and risk of secondary infection. Research on the role of steroids in managing sepsis and shock states is ongoing. For instance, a 2018 report on the ADRENAL trial showed that survivors of septic shock who received infusions of hydrocortisone recovered faster and were less likely to require a blood transfusion than those who received placebo. This same study did not demonstrate a reduced mortality with steroid versus placebo. Readers are referred to the full CIRCI treatment guidelines for more details about the conditions and circumstances under which corticosteroids may be helpful in critical care.

Pheochromocytoma and Catecholamine Crisis

The adrenal medulla normally produces two catecholamines: norepinephrine and epinephrine. In combination with the sympathetic nervous system, norepinephrine and epinephrine influence the heart and cardiovascular function. These catecholamines are used as infusions in critical care to mimic normal physiology.

Pheochromocytomas are tumors of the adrenal medulla that produce excessive amounts of norepinephrine and in some cases epinephrine. This can produce a catecholamine crisis manifested by extreme hypertension, tachycardia, hyperglycemia, and increased respiratory rate. Laboratory blood tests to measure the metanephrine level, or a 24-hour urine collection of daily metanephrine level, and imaging studies of the adrenal gland are performed as part of the diagnostic workup.

Pheochromocytoma Management

Definitive treatment requires removal of the tumor usually by minimally invasive laparoscopy. Before and throughout surgery, the blood pressure is aggressively managed with a combination of beta blockade and alpha blockade medications. Usually, hypertension is resolved by removal of the adrenal tumor.

Summary: Adrenal Gland Dysfunction

The adrenal glands are really two endocrine glands in one organ, the outer cortex and inner medulla. Most of the conditions associated with adrenal dysfunction are rare. Commonly seen conditions include Cushing syndrome, which results from excess glucocorticoids, whether endogenous (rare), or from exogenous medications (often seen). Adrenal insufficiency is believed to play a role in acute and chronic critical illness, especially in inflammatory shock states that are unresponsive to vasopressor infusions. Other conditions such as pheochromocytoma, or Addison disease are rarely encountered in critical care.

SELECTED BIBLIOGRAPHY

Blood Glucose Monitoring

American Diabetes Association. Clinical practice recommendations. *Diabetes Care.* 2017;40:S1-S135.

Schifman RB, Howanitz PJ, Souers RJ. Point-of-care glucose critical values: a Q-probes study involving 50 health care facilities and 2349 critical results. *Arch Pathol Lab Med.* 2016;140(2):119-124.

US Department of Health and Human Services. Blood Glucose Monitoring Test. Systems for Prescription. Point-of-Care Use. Guidance for Industry and. Food and Drug Administration Staff. Document issued on September 2020. https://www.fda.gov/regulatory-information/search-fda-guidance-documents/blood-glucose-monitoring-test-systems-prescription-point-care-use

Hyperglycemia, DKA, EDKA, and HHS

American Association of Clinical Endocrinology. *Diagnosis and Management of Hyperglycemic Crises: Diabetic Ketoacidosis and the Hyperglycemic Hyperosmolar State.* January 2019. AACE Inpatient Glycemic Control Resource Center; American Association of Clinical Endocrinology. https://pro.aace.com/sites/default/files/2019-01/Strategies-S3-Hyperglycemic-Emergencies.021017.pptx

American Diabetes Association. Standards of medical care in diabetes—2018. *Diabetes Care.* 2018;41:S1-S159.

Barski L, Eshkoli T, Brandstaetter E, Jotkowitz A. Euglycemic diabetic ketoacidosis. *Eur J Intern Med.* 2019;63:9-14. doi: 10.1016/j.ejim.2019.03.014

Benoit SR, Zhang Y, Geiss LS, Gregg EW, Albright A. Trends in diabetic ketoacidosis hospitalizations and in-hospital mortality—United States, 2000–2014. *MMWR Morb Mortal Wkly Rep.* 2018; 67(12):362-365. doi: 10.15585/mmwr.mm6712a3

Chua HR, Schneider A, Bellomo R. Bicarbonate in diabetic ketoacidosis—a systematic review. *Ann Intensive Care.* 2011; 1(1):23.

Plewa M, Bryant M, King-Thiele R. Euglycemic diabetic ketoacidosis. In *StatPearls*. StatPearls Publishing; 2021.

The NICE-SUGAR Study Investigators. Hypoglycemia and risk of death in critically ill patients. *N Engl J Med.* 2012;367: 1108-1118.

Umpierrez G, Korytkowski M. Diabetic emergencies—ketoacidosis, hyperglycaemic hyperosmolar state and hypoglycaemia. *Nat Rev Endocrinol.* 2016;12(4):222-232.

SIADH and Diabetes Insipidus

Ball S, Barth J, Levy M, Society for Endocrinology Clinical Committee. Society For Endocrinology endocrine emergency guidance: emergency management of severe symptomatic hyponatraemia in adult patients. *Endocr Connect.* 2016;5(5):G4-G6.

Cuesta M, Ortolá A, Garrahy A, Calle Pascual AL, Runkle I, Thompson CJ. Predictors of failure to respond to fluid restriction in SIAD in clinical practice; time to re-evaluate clinical guidelines? *QJM.* 2017;110(8):489-492.

Cuesta M, Thompson CJ. The syndrome of inappropriate antidiuresis (SIAD). *Best Pract Res Clin Endocrinol Metab.* 2016;30(2):175-187.

Hong GK, Payne SC, Jane JA Jr. Anatomy, physiology, and laboratory evaluation of the pituitary gland. *Otolaryngol Clin North Am.* 2016;49(1):21-32.

Levine JA, Karam SL, O'Connor C, et al. Central diabetes insipidus and chemotherapy: use of a continuous arginine vasopressin infusion for fluid and sodium balance. *AACE Clin Case Rep.* 2018;4(6):e487-e492. doi: 10.4158/ACCR-2018-0165

Robertson GL. Diabetes insipidus: differential diagnosis and management. *Best Pract Res Clin Endocrinol Metab.* 2016; 30(2):205-218.

Shepshelovich D, Schechter A, Calvarysky B, et al. Medication-induced SIADH—distribution and characterization according to medication class. *Br J Clin Pharmacol.* 2017;83(8):1801-1807.

Hyperthyroidism and Thyroid Storm

De Leo S, Lee SY, Braverman LE. Hyperthyroidism. *Lancet.* 2016; 388(10047):906-918.

McGonigle AM, Tobian AAR, Zink JL, King KE. Perfect storm: therapeutic plasma exchange for a patient with thyroid storm. *J Clin Apher.* 2018;33(1):113-116.

Hypothyroidism and Myxedema Coma

Fliers E, Bianco AC, Langouche L, Boelen A. Thyroid function in critically ill patients. *Lancet Diabetes Endocrinol.* 2015;3(10):816-825.

Gish DS, Loynd RT, Melnick S, Nezir S. Myxedema coma: a forgotten presentation of extreme hypothyroidism. *BMJ Case Rep.* 2016; 2016. doi:10.1136/bcr-2016-216225

Adrenal Gland, Cushing Disease, and Pheochromocytoma

Boonen E, Bornstein SR, Van den Berghe G. New insights into the controversy of adrenal function during critical illness. *Lancet Diabetes Endocrinol.* 2015;3(10):805-815.

Evans L, Rhodes A, Alhazzani W, et al. Surviving Sepsis Campaign: International Guidelines for management of sepsis and septic shock 2021. *Crit Care Med.* 2021;49(11):e1063-e1143. doi: 10.1097/CCM.0000000000005337

Gibbison B, López-López JA, Higgins JP, et al. Corticosteroids in septic shock: a systematic review and network meta-analysis. *Crit Care.* 2017;21(1):78.

Loriaux DL. Diagnosis and differential diagnosis of Cushing's syndrome. *N Engl J Med.* 2017;376(15):1451-1459.

Riester A, Weismann D, Quinkler M, et al. Life-threatening events in patients with pheochromocytoma. *Eur J Endocrinol.* 2015;173(6):757-764.

Critical Illness-Related Corticosteroid Insufficiency

Annane D, Pastores SM, Arlt W, et al. Critical illness-related corticosteroid insufficiency (CIRCI): a narrative review from a multispecialty task force of the Society of Critical Care Medicine (SCCM) and the European Society of Intensive Care Medicine (ESICM). *Crit Care Med.* 2017;45(12):2089-2098.

Annene D, Pastores SM, Rochwerg B, et al. Guidelines for the diagnosis and management of critical illness-related corticosteroid insufficiency (CIRCI) in critically ill patients (Part I): Society of Critical Care Medicine (SCCM) and European Society of Intensive Care Medicine (ESICM) 2017. *Crit Care Med.* 2017; 45(12):2078-2088.

Pastores S. Annane D, Rochwerg B; and the Corticosteroid Guideline Task Force of SCCM and ESICM. Guidelines for the diagnosis and management of critical illness-related corticosteroid insufficiency (CIRCI) in critically ill patients (Part II): Society of Critical Care Medicine (SCCM) and European Society of Intensive Care Medicine (ESICM) 2017. *Crit Care Med.* 2018; 46(1):146-148.

The ADRENAL Trial: Steroids in Septic Shock. 2018. http://rebelem.com/the-adrenal-trial-steroids-in-septic-shock/. Accessed February 16, 2018.

TRAUMA

17

Christopher Kolokythas and Janet Lee

KNOWLEDGE COMPETENCIES

1. Describe the mechanisms of traumatic injury and relate them to accurate assessment of overt and covert injuries.

2. Discuss the common physiologic and psychosocial effects on the patient and family caused by major traumatic injury.

3. Identify the specialized needs of the trauma patient in critical and progressive care units.

4. Integrate selected management principles to treat trauma patients with thoracic, abdominal, and musculoskeletal injuries.

Trauma is a leading cause of mortality worldwide and a significantly expanding public health problem in the United States. Injuries can occur by various insults and are classified as blunt or penetrating trauma. Common causes of trauma include motor vehicle accidents, falls, burns, poisonings, drownings, and violence. In 2019, the Centers for Disease Control and Prevention (CDC) identified unintentional injuries as the third leading cause of death and intentional self-harm (suicide) as the tenth leading cause of death for all age groups, gender, and ethnicities. Despite a high incidence of deaths, with over 210,000 reported per year, the rate of disability for trauma survivors is even higher. This chapter focuses on thoracoabdominal, musculoskeletal, and pelvic trauma. Traumatic brain injury (TBI) is the single largest cause of death from injury and is discussed in Chapter 21, Advanced Neurologic Concepts.

SPECIALIZED ASSESSMENT

The assessment of trauma victims requires a structured and systematic approach to determine injuries, especially life-threatening ones, and prevent further harm. Hospital admissions are sudden and unplanned for trauma victims, denying them the time for psychological preparation or stabilization of preexisting chronic conditions. Trauma patients are often young; however, there has been a rise in older patients admitted for trauma and whose comorbidities complicate their hospitalization. Traumatic injuries may be subtle, and complications are common. Without the appropriate assessment, minor injuries can evolve into devastating ones. The primary goals of the initial trauma assessment are identifying immediate life-threatening injuries and stabilizing the patient. Rehabilitation is frequently needed after injury, and a trauma victim's quality of life may never return to previous baseline status, especially for those who suffered traumatic brain or spinal cord injuries. Trauma takes a significant emotional and financial toll on all parties involved, including the patient, family, and society.

Management of traumatic injury in the initial phases of care occurs in tandem with assessment and typically begins before the patient's arrival to the hospital. Resuscitative efforts may include the insertion of an advanced airway, establishing intravenous (IV) access and administration of fluids, and pain control while simultaneously evaluating for obvious locations of injuries. Additional considerations in the assessment of traumatic injuries include identifying sources of bleeding. External hemorrhages are apparent and treated promptly, whereas due to the occult nature of internal bleeding, these may be missed on the primary survey.

A critical aspect of the trauma assessment is determining the injury based on the mechanism, whether blunt or penetrating trauma. Based on this information, an "index of suspicion" regarding potential injuries is formulated during the primary and secondary surveys. The overarching goal is to ensure that all injuries are accounted for, especially the obscured ones when developing the plan of care.

Primary, Secondary, and Tertiary Trauma Surveys

The initial management of trauma is often guided by identifying lethal physical findings that require immediate treatment. The primary and secondary surveys reveal immediate life-threatening injuries and direct the trauma team to develop an individualized resuscitation plan. The American College of Surgeons Advanced Trauma Life Support® course offers guidance on the initial care of the trauma patient.

Primary Survey

Upon the patient's arrival, the primary survey begins. All pertinent information from the prehospital survey is relayed, and a quick visual assessment is completed to determine obvious life-threatening injuries. These include, but are not limited to, uncontrolled external injuries, altered mental status, impaled objects, severe respiratory distress, and traumatic amputations. The primary survey serves to simultaneously assess and treat all life-threatening injuries using the ABCDE approach—Airway, Breathing, Circulation, Disability, and Exposure (Table 17-1).

Airway

Determining airway patency is the essential step in the primary survey. In conscious patients, having them talk provides key clues of both airway patency and mentation. Additionally, the airway assessment examines for possible obstruction, anatomy distortion, or other signs of respiratory distress. In unconscious patients or those with reduced levels of consciousness, the airway must be immediately secured through intubation or cricothyrotomy if unable to intubate.

Breathing

Following airway securement, the patient's breathing should be assessed by visual inspection of the chest, chest movement symmetry, rate and depth of respirations, respiratory effort, and physical assessment of the lungs and surrounding tissue.

Circulation

Next, circulation focuses on evaluating for hemorrhage and maintaining adequate perfusion through physical examination and diagnostic tools such as ultrasonography. The circulation assessment includes skin color and temperature, capillary refill time, and measuring pulse rate and blood pressure; concurrently, treatment may involve obtaining IV access, hemorrhage control, and resuscitation with fluid or blood products.

TABLE 17-1. PRIMARY SURVEY

Airway and C-spine	**Assessment** • Assess patency and airway obstruction **Management** • Basic airway maneuvers—jaw thrust or chin lift accompanied by assessment for foreign bodies in the airway • Insert nasopharyngeal airway or oral pharyngeal airway • Establish a definitive airway if necessary • Maintain C-spine in neutral position with an appropriate device while maintaining airway patency
Breathing	**Assessment** • Assess respiratory rate and depth after exposure of chest and neck area • Assure C-spine immobilization is maintained • Assess for injury to neck to include but not limited to deformity, tracheal deviation, subcutaneous emphysema, etc • Assess for chest wall motion and use of accessory muscle **Management** • Apply high-flow oxygen • Maintain airway by definite airway if necessary • Assure CO_2 and pulse oximetry monitoring with intubation • Alleviate tension pneumothorax or seal open pneumothorax

Circulation	**Assessment**
	• Identify source of hemorrhage—internal or external
	• Assess vital signs to include skin color, capillary refill, and pulses
	Management
	• Stop the bleeding
	  • external—direct pressure
	  • internal—locate source and need for operative intervention
	• Establish large bore IV access and obtain blood samples during this process
	• Initiate warmed isotonic (LR or NS) or colloid fluid resuscitation
	• Initiate warming measures to combat hypothermia

Disability	**Assessment** • Assess neurological status to include mental status, pupillary size, and response
Exposure	**Assessment** • Completely disrobe patient but avoid hypothermia

Disability

After the patient's critical injuries are stabilized, the patient's disability or neurologic function is addressed. Important considerations in this assessment are that patients with a Glasgow Coma Scale (GCS) score of 8 or less should have a definitive airway, and in all patients with unknown cervical spine injuries, immobilization should be maintained.

Exposure

The final step of the primary survey is exposure. All clothing is removed to identify any concealed injuries such as gunshot wounds (GSWs), lacerations, ecchymosis, or any other trauma. It is crucial to prevent hypothermia and keep the patient warm to avoid further complications.

Secondary Survey

The secondary survey begins after the patient's immediate life-threatening concerns are stabilized. It involves obtaining thorough history and physical examinations and a detailed workup of the patient to assess for any missed injuries (Table 17-2). Diagnostic tools such as radiographic imaging and laboratory tests are also part of the secondary survey. If the patient's status changes at any time during the secondary survey, the practitioner returns to the primary survey again

TABLE 17-2. SECONDARY SURVEY

Item to Assess	Establishes/Identifies	Assess	Finding	Confirm By
Level of consciousness	• Severity of head injury	• GCS score	• <8, severe head injury • 9-12, moderate head injury • 13-15, minor head injury	• CT scan • Repeat without paralyzing agents
Pupils	• Type of head injury • Presence of eye injury	• Size • Shape • Reactivity	• Mass effect • Diffuse brain injury • Ophthalmic injury	• CT scan
Head	• Scalp injury • Skull injury	• Inspect for lacerations and skull fractures • Palpable defects	• Scalp laceration • Depressed skull fracture • Basilar skull fracture	• CT scan
Maxillofacial	• Soft tissue injury • Bone injury • Nerve injury • Teeth/mouth injury	• Inspect for visible deformity, malocclusion • Palpation for crepitation	• Facial fracture • Soft tissue injury	• Facial bone x-ray • CT scan of facial bones
Neck	• Laryngeal injury • C-spine injury • Vascular injury • Esophageal injury • Neurologic deficit	• Visual inspection • Palpation • Auscultation	• Laryngeal deformity • Subcutaneous emphysema • Hematoma • Bruit • Platysmal penetration • Pain, tenderness of C-spine	• C-spine x-ray or CT • Angiography/duplex examination • Esophagoscopy • Laryngoscopy
Thorax	• Thoracic wall injury • Subcutaneous emphysema • Pneumo-hemothorax • Bronchial injury • Pulmonary contusion • Thoracic aortic disruption	• Visual inspection • Palpation • Auscultation	• Bruising, deformity, or paradoxical motion • Chest wall tenderness, crepitation • Diminished breath sounds • Muffled heart tones • Mediastinal crepitation • Severe back pain	• Chest x-ray • CT scan • Angiography • Bronchoscopy • Tube thoracostomy • Pericardiocentesis • TE ultrasound
Abdomen/flank	• Abdominal wall injury • Intraperitoneal injury • Retroperitoneal injury	• Visual inspection • Palpation • Auscultation • Determine path of penetration	• Abdominal wall pain/tenderness • Peritoneal irritation • Visceral injury • Retroperitoneal organ injury	• DPL/ultrasound • CT scan • Laparotomy • Contrast GI x-ray studies • Angiography
Pelvis	• Genitourinary (GU) tract injuries • Pelvic fracture(s)	• Palpate symphysis pubis for widening • Palpate bony pelvis for tenderness • Determine pelvic stability only once • Inspect perineum • Rectal/vaginal examination	• GU tract injury (hematuria) • Pelvic fracture • Rectal, vaginal, and/or perineal injury	• Pelvic x-ray • GU contrast studies • Urethrogram • Cystogram • IVP • Contrast-enhanced CT
Spinal cord	• Cranial injury • Cord injury • Peripheral nerve(s) injury	• Motor response • Pain response	• Unilateral cranial mass effect • Quadriplegia • Paraplegia • Nerve root injury	• Plain spine x-rays • CT scan • MRI
Vertebral column	• Column injury • Vertebral instability • Nerve injury	• Verbal response to pain, lateralizing signs • Palpate for tenderness • Deformity	• Fracture vs dislocation	• Plain x-rays • CT scan • MRI
Extremities	• Soft tissue injury • Bony deformities • Joint abnormalities • Neurovascular deficits	• Visual inspection • Palpation	• Swelling, bruising, pallor • Malalignment • Pain, tenderness, crepitation • Absence/diminished pulses • Tense muscular compartments • Neurologic deficits	• Specific x-rays • Doppler examination • Compartment pressures • Angiography

Reproduced with permission from Advanced Trauma Life Support Student Course Manual, 9th ed. American College of Surgeons; 2012.

to reassess the ABCDEs and look for additional or evolving decompensation.

Tertiary Survey

The tertiary survey provides a complete and comprehensive reexamination of the patient and reviews of all diagnostic tests. It usually occurs within 24 hours of the injury and serves as the final step of the trauma assessment to recap all obtained information and to determine the need for any further evaluation of the patient.

Diagnostic Studies

Ultrasound, Computed Axial Tomography, and Diagnostic Peritoneal Lavage

Hemorrhage from external and/or occult sources is a major concern and obtaining hemorrhage control with concurrent volume resuscitation is an initial priority in the primary survey. During the secondary survey, diagnostic studies such as ultrasound, computed tomography (CT), and diagnostic peritoneal lavage (DPL) assist in diagnosing occult thoracoabdominal hemorrhage.

Ultrasound is typically the first diagnostic tool when examining trauma patients. This noninvasive procedure is quick and readily available; however, its success in identifying injuries varies with the expertise of the user. Ultimately, it is not a replacement for more sensitive imaging studies such as CT scanning.

A CT scan, the gold standard for identifying specific injuries in patients with abdominal or thoracic symptoms, should be performed only when a patient is hemodynamically stable. Unstable patients with an inconclusive ultrasound that is unable to identify a source of bleeding may be candidates for DPL, angiography, or may require an immediate exploratory laparotomy. If a bleeding source is identified by ultrasound but the patient is hemodynamically unstable, this is considered an acute abdomen and an exploratory laparotomy is required.

Serial physical examinations coupled with ultrasounds are recommended to better evaluate some injuries. This is because the ultrasound examination is limited in identifying retroperitoneal, pancreatic, and pelvic injuries. For example, it is difficult for an ultrasound to conclusively differentiate between fluid (such as urine) and blood in the pelvic area. Refer to Table 17-3 for a comparison of ultrasound, CT, and DPL.

Cervical Spine Radiograph

A cervical spine (C-spine) radiograph is one of the first diagnostic tests obtained following the completion of the primary survey. Trauma patients are presumed to have a C-spine injury until the seven cervical vertebrae have been evaluated and determined to be intact. Patients with normal neurologic examinations and full range of motion of the cervical region can be cleared with clinical evaluation; however, patients with neurologic deficits or abnormal clinical evaluations require clearance with CT or magnetic resonance imaging (MRI) imaging. The CT scan is the gold standard for assessment of the C-spine. A hard cervical collar is applied to immobilize the neck and is used until the C-spine has been visualized radiographically and no injuries are found.

Radiographic Studies

Additional radiographic studies to determine the extent of injuries are performed after the primary survey is completed but should not delay resuscitation. Depending on the mechanism of injury, common x-rays may include chest and pelvis to rule out immediate life threats.

Whole-body CT imaging, or pan scanning, of the head, neck, chest, abdomen, and pelvis can be performed as an adjunct to the clinical exam to aid in determining underlying injuries. Early use of whole-body CT has shown to decrease morbidity and mortality in trauma patients but should be reserved for clinically stable patients.

Serial Examinations

Trauma patients require frequent reexaminations to ensure that all injuries are identified and to monitor for signs and symptoms of deterioration. Missed injuries may lead to pain, disability, and even death. Repeat assessments by the same provider are recommended for consistency, especially in traumatic brain and abdominal injuries, as internal bleeding may not be initially evident. Understanding the mechanism of injury and the specific injuries created by destructive blunt or penetrating forces provides the basis for accurate and focused assessments.

Mechanism of Injury

Determining the mechanism of injury provides the trauma team with a better understanding of possible occult injuries. The mechanism of injury describes how the injury occurred, the nature of the forces involved, and suspected tissue and

TABLE 17-3. INDICATIONS, ADVANTAGES, AND DISADVANTAGES OF COMMON DIAGNOSTIC TESTS FOR BLUNT ABDOMINAL TRAUMA

Procedure	Indications	Advantages	Disadvantages
DPL	Decreased BP with suspicion of internal hemorrhage	Easy, rapid, inexpensive	Invasive, unable to pinpoint location of injury, cannot evaluate retroperitoneum
Ultrasound (FAST)	Decreased BP with suspicion of internal hemorrhage	Easy, rapid, inexpensive, noninvasive, can be repeated	Sensitive to operator experience, unable to pinpoint location of injury, cannot evaluate retroperitoneum
CT scan	Normal BP with suspicion of internal hemorrhage	Can pinpoint which organ is damaged, including those in the retroperitoneum	Time consuming, costly, must lie flat

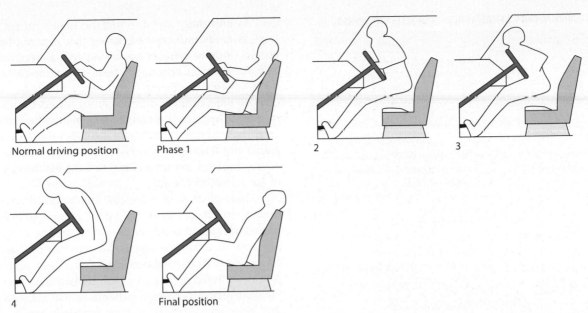

Normal driving position

Phase 1

2

3

4

Final position

Figure 17-1. Injury mechanism of an unrestrained driver. (*Adapted with permission from Holleran R, Wolfe A, Frakes M.* Patient Transport: Principles and Practice. *5th ed. St Louis, MO: Saunders/Elsevier; 2018.*)

organ damage. This knowledge is required when assessing a trauma patient at the scene of the accident, in the emergency department (ED), and in the critical or progressive care unit.

Injuries result when a body is exposed to an uncontrolled outside source of energy that disrupts the body's integrity and/or functional ability. Potential energy sources such as kinetic, penetrating, chemical, thermal, electrical, or radiating are all considered. The severity of the resultant injury is determined by several factors: the force or speed of impact, the duration of the impact or exposure, the total exposed surface area, and related risk factors such as age, gender, preexisting comorbidities, and alcohol/drug ingestion.

Mechanisms of injury are typically divided into two major categories: *blunt and penetrating. Blunt trauma* is defined as injuries that are not open to the atmosphere, and *penetrating* injuries are those in which the body has been pierced. Blunt trauma usually results from motor vehicle or motorcycle collisions, assaults, falls, contact sports injuries, pedestrian/vehicle collisions, or blast injuries. Assessment strategies useful in diagnosing blunt traumatic injuries include physical assessment, ultrasound, DPL, CT scanning, radiographic studies, angiography, blood count, and blood chemistry analysis. Penetrating trauma is commonly caused by GSWs or knives. It is important to recognize that the rate of mortality of penetrating trauma depends on the mechanism and location of the injury. For instance, mortality is higher in GSW injuries due to the velocity and energy displacement caused by the bullet.

Information related to the mechanism of injury helps determine patterns of injury. Common patterns assist clinicians in assessing trauma patients who cannot communicate pain or other symptoms. Patterns of injury are focused on during the primary and secondary surveys so that diagnostic tests are sequenced appropriately and accomplished efficiently and accurately. For example, in motor vehicle crashes, the common pattern of injury for the unrestrained driver includes the head, pelvis, chest, and extremities. Thoracic trauma is often due to impact with the steering wheel. Patterns of injuries to unrestrained passengers include craniofacial trauma resulting from hitting the head onto the windshield or posterior hip dislocations due to the knee hitting the dashboard at a high rate of speed (Figure 17-1). Fractures of the clavicle and humerus are more frequent among passengers, possibly because of the defensive reflex action of raising the arms before impact. Although the impact of seat belt use and airbags deployment lowers the risk of thoracic injury, they can still impart serious injuries based on the nature of the accident (Table 17-4).

Patterns of injury have also been identified for victims of falls and pedestrians struck by motor vehicles (Figure 17-2). Knowledge of these patterns of injuries helps prevent further damage or complications during resuscitation. For example, if a patient has sustained a head injury with a high suspicion of basilar skull fracture, an oral gastric tube is preferred over a nasogastric tube. This is because the nasogastric tube may be inadvertently passed through the fracture directly into the brain. A urinary catheter is not inserted if the mechanism of injury suggests bladder rupture or urethral trauma, and a more definitive examination such as the retrograde urethrogram or cystogram is warranted.

Physiologic Consequences of Trauma

Traumatic injuries unleash a cascade of vasoactive mediators, such as neurohormones, prostaglandins, and cytokines, which contribute to the body's stress response. However, in

TABLE 17-4. TRUNCAL AND CERVICAL INJURIES FROM RESTRAINT DEVICES

Restraint Device	Injury
Lap Seat Belt • Compression • Hyperflexion	• Tear or avulsion of mesentery (Bucket Handle) • Rupture of small bowel or colon • Thrombosis of iliac artery or abdominal aorta • Chance fracture of lumbar vertebrae • Pancreatic or duodenal injury
Shoulder Harness • Sliding under the seat belt ("submarining") • Compression	• Intimal tear or thrombosis in innominate, carotid, subclavian, or vertebral arteries • Fracture or dislocation of cervical spine • Rib fractures • Pulmonary contusion • Rupture of upper abdominal viscera
Air Bag • Contact • Contact/deceleration • Flexion (unrestrained) • Hyperextension (unrestrained)	• Corneal abrasions • Abrasions of face, neck, and chest • Cardiac rupture • Cervical spine • Thoracic spine fracture

Reproduced with permission from National Association of Emergency Medical Technicians (NAEMT).

severe multisystem trauma, these same mediators may exacerbate the stress response and contribute to complications and contribute to mortality. To lessen this response, the priorities of care should focus on supportive physiologic and psychosocial needs. Priorities include tissue oxygenation and the three main components of oxygen delivery: cardiac output, hemoglobin level, and oxygen saturation. The trauma patient undergoes continuous vital sign monitoring with an electrocardiogram (ECG), pulse oximetry, and capnography. Pain and anxiety are treated simultaneously.

As previously noted, traumatic injury results in fractures, wounds, and crushed tissues that may not be readily visible. Once the primary trauma survey has been completed and management begins, the head-to-toe, in-depth assessment (*secondary survey*) is initiated and used to create a detailed differential of injuries. From this, definitive care is planned. The nurse assists in stabilizing the patient with IV fluids and respiratory and circulatory support while also providing emotional support. The nurse has an integral role in addressing pain control and meeting the psychosocial needs of the patient and family.

Consequences of traumatic injury include blood loss, tissue destruction, intense pain due to damaged tissues, and altered oxygenation and ventilation. Therefore, airway management, fluid balance, aggressive pain control, and wound care are priorities. Stabilization of fractures and surgical repair of injured organs are accomplished in the early post-incident period. Although patients in the ED, critical care unit, or progressive care settings frequently have more than one injured system, a focus on one body system at a time assists in providing an organized management plan.

COMMON INJURIES IN THE TRAUMA PATIENT

Thoracic Trauma

Etiology and Pathophysiology

Thoracic trauma accounts for approximately 20% to 25% of all trauma-related deaths and includes injuries created by fractured ribs, blunt cardiac injury, vascular injury, and contused or punctured lung tissue. The most common mechanisms of injury to the chest are blunt trauma (from

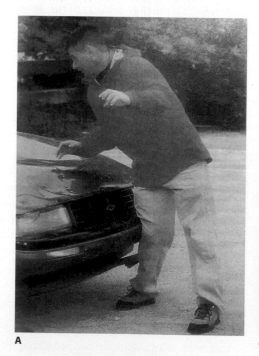

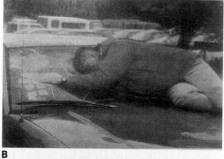

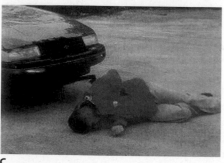

A   B   C

Figure 17-2. *Data from National Association of Emergency Medical Technicians [NAEMT].*

motor vehicle-related injuries and penetrating trauma from gunshots and stabbings. Common injuries associated with thoracic trauma are tension pneumothorax, open pneumothorax, hemothorax, pulmonary contusion, rib fractures, flail chest, cardiac tamponade, cardiac contusion, blunt cardiac injuries, and aortic disruption. Often a Focused Assessment with Sonography in Trauma (FAST) is performed early in the evaluative stage to scan for free fluid, which suggests bleeding in the peritoneal, pericardial, and/or pleural cavities. Ultrasound may also be used to evaluate the lungs for pneumothorax. The FAST examination and more specific diagnostic tools for thoracic and abdominal injuries are described below.

Tension pneumothorax: Accumulation of air within the pleural space due to injury or a laceration of the lung parenchyma may cause a tension pneumothorax. This occurs when the lung parenchyma is no longer intact, and air from the lung enters the pleural space but cannot exit. As air accumulates in the pleural space, the positive pressure collapses the lung and shifts the heart and great vessels to the opposite side of the chest. Signs and symptoms are severe respiratory distress, tachypnea, tachycardia, hypotension, hyperresonance and absence of breath sounds on the affected side, chest pain, and distended neck veins (may be flat in severely hypovolemic patients). A tension pneumothorax is a medical emergency. Management involves prompt detection and needle decompression to allow air to escape from the pleural space. A needle decompression consists of the insertion of a large bore angiocatheter, preferably a 14G to 16G and length of 4.5 cm in adults. The angiocatheter is inserted into the chest wall on the affected side, at the midclavicular line on the anterior portion of the chest between the second and third intercostal space. An alternate location is a lateral approach on the midaxillary line between the fourth and fifth intercostal space. However, according to recent data, the lateral approach may be less likely to be successful than the anterior approach. Regardless, the goal is to release the life-threatening tension. To that end, provider comfort and experience with the two approaches may guide the selection of the location. Once the needle decompression is performed as a lifesaving intervention, a chest tube is required as definitive treatment.

Open pneumothorax: An open pneumothorax, sometimes called a "sucking chest wound," is present when there is a passage of air in and out of the pleural space from the chest wall. This usually occurs when there is a penetrating injury to the chest wall caused by either a gunshot or stab wound. The definitive treatment for open pneumothorax is a chest tube; however, temporary management until a chest tube can be inserted includes using a three-sided dressing. This results in the closure of the dressing upon inhalation, so ambient air does not flow into the pleural space, and upon exhalation, air can escape from the pleural space. If the dressing is completely occlusive, a tension pneumothorax may occur. Should this happen, immediate removal of the dressing generally relieves the increased tension. However,

if the tension occurs with the three-sided dressing in place, a needle decompression may be done until a chest tube can be safely placed.

Hemothorax: A hemothorax is defined as blood in the pleural space. Rib fractures are typically the cause. Fracture of the clavicle (first rib) or the second rib is a very serious injury because the subclavian artery and vein are positioned directly under these ribs. A significant force is required to fracture these two ribs; thus, potential damage to the underlying vessels is considered dangerous and is carefully assessed. An initial chest x-ray demonstrating a widened mediastinum may be due to a tear in the aorta or one of its major branches. Hemothoraces can result in respiratory distress due to the compression of the lung parenchyma. If the hemothorax is large enough and the patient is experiencing respiratory difficulty, a chest tube is placed to drain the hemothorax. If the patient is hemodynamically unstable after chest tube placement, emergent interventions may include open thoracotomy immediately or exploratory surgery to gain control of the bleeding.

For other concerns of uncontrolled bleeding in thoracoabdominal trauma, another option is to attempt a resuscitative endovascular balloon occlusion of the aorta (REBOA). The REBOA procedure is a minimally invasive technique using an intra-aortic balloon occlusion catheter to temporarily occlude the large vessels contributing to bleeding. Once in the aorta, it is directed to the bleeding site to control bleeding and augment afterload in hemorrhagic shock states, a common cause of death after severe injuries. This is similar to an emergent open left thoracotomy to cross clamp the aorta. It can also be used with hemodynamic instability associated with severe pelvic injuries. In this case, the endovascular balloon occludes the lower descending portion of the aorta (called zone 3) versus a higher aortic level.

Pulmonary contusion: A pulmonary contusion is injury to the lung parenchyma, which commonly occurs after blunt injury to the chest. It consists of bleeding into the lung and alveolar space after the capillary membrane has been disrupted. Depending on the severity of the contusion, hypoxemia can occur, which may worsen several days after the injury with progression to respiratory failure and acute respiratory distress syndrome (ARDS). Pulmonary contusions are challenging to identify and diagnose during the initial trauma resuscitation because clinical findings may not become evident for several hours after the injury. Thus, knowing the mechanism of injury may help the healthcare team to anticipate such a complication. Frequent monitoring of oxygenation and ventilation with arterial blood gases (ABGs), pulse oximetry, and capnography is necessary to detect subtle changes in pulmonary status. Resuscitative management includes judicious use of IV fluids, support of oxygenation, pulmonary toilet, and mechanical ventilation, if necessary.

Fractured ribs: Fractured ribs are the most common injuries in blunt trauma. Fractured lower ribs can injure the liver or spleen, and upper rib fractures may puncture lung tissue. Pulmonary contusion, hemothoraces, and pneumothoraces are often associated with rib fractures. Management includes providing respiratory support and adequate pain control.

Flail chest: Flail chest may occur when several adjacent ribs are fractured in two places, creating a "floating segment" that may puncture the lung and compromise oxygenation and ventilation. Symptoms of flail chest include chest pain and shortness of breath. On observation, a flail chest is indicated by inward movement of the affected side of the chest during inspiration and outward movement during expiration, called "paradoxical breathing." This injury is best assessed when the patient is breathing spontaneously. Paradoxical breathing results in a notable increase in the work of breathing. In addition, the associated pain leads to splinted, shallow respirations, which results in atelectasis, pneumonia, and contributes to fatigue and respiratory failure. Mechanical ventilation may be necessary to stabilize the chest and support oxygenation and ventilation.

Cardiac injuries: Blunt trauma to the thorax may result in damage to the myocardium, coronary arteries, or structures of the heart (septum or valves). These injuries may be subtle and difficult to diagnose but are always suspected. The majority of patients are initially asymptomatic, but some have chest pain, which may be hard to differentiate from other thoracic injuries.

Chest x-ray, ECG, cardiac markers (especially troponin I), transthoracic echocardiography (TTE), and transesophageal echocardiography (TEE) assist in the identification of myocardial injuries both initially and also if the patient is unstable after resuscitative measures. Dysrhythmias also occur in patients with thoracic trauma. Sinus tachycardia, atrial fibrillation, and premature ventricular contractions are most common, while ventricular tachycardia and fibrillation are common with extensive myocardial damage.

Cardiac tamponade: A hemopericardium may result in cardiac tamponade and is a potentially life-threatening complication of both blunt and penetrating chest trauma. The pericardial membrane (sac) is ordinarily stiff and noncompliant. Bleeding into the pericardial sac (effusion) causes compression on the heart, compromising cardiac function and decreases cardiac output. The rate at which fluid accumulates around the heart in the pericardial sac determines whether the effusion will lead to compression of the heart or compensation (stretching of the sac and accommodation). A rapid accumulation of blood does not allow the pericardial sac to stretch, and the tamponade may lead to death unless it is rapidly identified and decompressed.

A chest x-ray may show an enlarged heart, but an echocardiogram is the gold standard for diagnosis. Signs such as tachycardia, jugular venous distension, hypotension, pulsus paradoxus, and finally, ventricular fibrillation and cardiac arrest may ensue. Rapid infusion of IV fluids followed by a pericardiocentesis or a cardiac window is the treatment.

Traumatic aortic disruption: An aortic disruption (partial or complete) is a surgical emergency and the most common cause of immediate death in the thoracic trauma patient population. A high index of suspicion and knowledge of the mechanism of injury, such as injuries associated with a high-speed motor vehicle collision, may result in an early diagnosis and improved outcomes. A widened mediastinum is typically seen on a chest x-ray. Historically, the standard for diagnosis was aortography (direct injection of contrast material into the aorta while x-rays are taken); however, current technological enhancements now allow for the confident use of TEE, CT scan, and MRI without the need for aortography. The patient's survival rate is directly related to how quickly this injury is diagnosed and operatively managed. These patients may require massive transfusions. If so, a Massive Transfusion Protocol (MTP) is initiated, which will be described later in this chapter.

Principles of Management for Thoracic Trauma

Management of the patient with chest trauma is individualized and includes several basic principles:

1. Support of oxygenation, ventilation, and cardiovascular status.
2. Monitoring and care of chest tube drainage and function.
3. Provision of optimal pain control, positioning, and physical care with attention to the promotion of wound healing.
4. Early mobility.
5. Prevention of complications such as infection.
6. Nutrition.

Ventilatory Support

The goals for ventilatory support of the trauma patient are the same as the ventilatory goals for any patient in the critical care or progressive care unit. Management focuses on improving oxygenation and ventilation, maintaining acid-base balance, decreasing the work of breathing, and preventing ventilator-associated conditions (VACs). Mechanical ventilation may be definitive or supportive, depending on the patient's injury and requirements. Supportive ventilatory care, which is provided if a patient can spontaneously ventilate, helps ease the work of breathing. Depending on the patient's injury and ventilatory needs, oxygen and positive pressure may be applied. This may be through a simple nasal cannula, high-flow nasal cannula, face mask, or a positive pressure mask. For patients who are unable to spontaneously ventilate, an advanced airway such as a laryngeal mask airway (LMA) or oral endotracheal tube (OETT) may be placed. In emergent situations where placement of the advanced airway is unobtainable, a cricothyrotomy may be performed. Definitive care, which would be required for long-term or permanent lung dysfunction, may require the patient to receive a tracheostomy.

The nurse's understanding of both traditional and newer modes and methods of mechanical ventilation is essential to accurately assess patient tolerance of the modes as well as the goals of therapy (see Chapter 5, Airway and Ventilatory Management and Chapter 20, Advanced Respiratory Concepts: Modes of Ventilation).

Monitoring Chest Tubes

Chest tubes are inserted in patients with chest wall injuries who develop complications from hemothorax, pneumothorax, pleural effusion, empyema, and those requiring a thoracotomy. Care of the patient with chest tubes includes observing for drainage characteristics, monitoring the quality and quantity of output, signs of a new or resolving air leak, and prevention of infection. Meticulous sterile technique, insertion site care, monitoring the placement security, and drainage system components and setup are key elements of chest tube management. Trauma patients may have draining wounds and suture lines adjacent to the chest tube site, which can make dressing changes more complicated. The vigilant surveillance for changes in drainage characteristics, infection monitoring and prevention, and ventilatory assessments are essential nursing functions for all trauma patients. (See Chapter 10, Respiratory System.)

Pain Control

Appropriate and effective pain control is essential for patient comfort and healing. Often thoracic injuries and pain result in chest wall splinting which can impede coughing and deep breathing. Both coughing and deep breathing are necessary to avoid atelectasis and pneumonia. Pain control may also allow for more effective spontaneous breathing and prevent the need for invasive mechanical ventilation in patients with milder degrees of thoracic trauma. Patient-controlled analgesia (PCA), epidural narcotic infusions, or local anesthetics may be used for aggressive pain control in the trauma patient to allow for deep inspiration, the use of incentive spirometers, and effective coughing and secretion clearance. These interventions are essential to avoid the progression of ventilatory failure and mechanical ventilation.

Patients report that chest tubes, suctioning, and turning are all extremely painful. Managing a patient's pain after trauma is humane and allows the patient to focus their mental and physical energy on healing. Pain may be controlled with various classes of medications. The most utilized drug class is opioids. They offer extreme flexibility in the administration route, onset, duration, and reversal. Opioids are powerful painkillers that carry the risk of impaired alertness, cognition, respiratory drive, and can cause hypotension, hypercapnia, and hypoxemia. Other types of useful medications include nonsteroidal anti-inflammatory drugs (NSAIDs), acetaminophen, muscle relaxers, and numbing medications like lidocaine.

A PCA provides the patient control of the timing and dosing of pain medication. Epidural PCA is commonly used in patients with single-location injuries, such as rib fractures, and may decrease the need for systemic pain medication, possibly preventing mechanical ventilation and is an important benefit in older trauma patients. Vigilant nursing care is essential because the epidural catheter may migrate from the pain site and not provide adequate pain relief. A patient's report of pain level and subsequent pain relief should be assessed hourly or more frequently as needed. Many critically or acutely ill trauma patients are unable to communicate their needs. Nonverbal pain scales are useful in monitoring patients' pain (refer to Chapter 6, Pain, Sedation, and Neuromuscular Blockade Management).

A variety of nonpharmacologic pain-reducing strategies are useful in patients with trauma, and the nurse may combine these with drug therapy for synergistic effect. Complementary, alternative, or integrative approaches can operate at the central level through cognitive distraction and relaxation, and peripherally by using positioning or application of heat and cold. Techniques such as guided imagery, talk therapy, meditation, sound and music therapy, acupressure, acupuncture, and energy healing are specialty adjuncts that can reduce pain medication requirements. See Chapter 6, Pain, Sedation, and Neuromuscular Blockade Management for more on pain and sedation.

Clear documentation of the strategies or combinations that work best for the individual is key for continuity of care. This approach requires an established communication system between the patient, family, nurse, and providers. Anxiety and sleeplessness contribute to the pain response and are addressed by asking the patients how they typically try to relax and by eliminating as much environmental noise as possible. Promoting rest and adequate sleep can reduce a patient's perception of pain and enhance their tolerance of pain (see Chapter 6, Pain, Sedation, and Neuromuscular Blockade Management and Chapter 7, Pharmacology.)

Positioning and Mobility

Early mobilization of the trauma patient promotes oxygenation, ventilation, and prevents other complications of immobility. This includes positioning the patient in and out of bed. Determining the best position to put a patient in depends on the injury and possible complications the nurse is treating and preventing. Positions to be considered include sitting, prone, and lateral decubitus. An example of how the concept of therapeutic positioning may be used by the nurse is to position the patient and evaluate for comfort as well as improvement in physical findings such as chest excursion, chest x-ray, respiratory rate, pulse oximetry values, ventilator tolerance, and if applicable, hemodynamic data. Continuous lateral rotation and/or prone positioning beds may be helpful for selected injuries or conditions, especially if the patient is experiencing difficulty in ventilation and oxygenation.

ESSENTIAL CONTENT CASE

Cardiac Tamponade

A 17-year-old woman with no past medical history is admitted to the ED after a stabbing × 2 to the upper posterior left side. She is lethargic and in no respiratory distress. Her pulse oximetry reading is 95%, HR 120 beats/min (sinus tachycardia), BP 105/85 mm Hg, and respiratory rate (RR) 24 breaths/min nonlabored. The team immediately provides supplemental oxygen with a 100% nonrebreather (NRB) and two large bore IV catheters with normal saline (NS) infusions. An emergent FAST examination does not reveal a cardiac tamponade or tension pneumothorax. After the infusion of 1.5 L of NS, the patient's pulse oximetry (Sao_2) reading is 97%, HR 98 beats/min (sinus rhythm), BP 118/80 mm Hg, and RR 20 breaths/min nonlabored.

The patient is transferred to the surgical intensive care unit (SICU) for 24-hour observation.

In the SICU, the patient continues to be lethargic but has a Glasgow Coma Scale (GCS) score of 15 and is arousable. She has no pain or distress but her skin is cool. Her tympanic temperature is 98.0°F. Her BP decreases to 75/65 mm Hg, with an HR of 110 beats/min. The NS infusion is increased to wide-open and the physician is called immediately. While the physician is on the way to the SICU, the nurses' reassessment finds clear breath sounds bilaterally and distant heart tones with jugular venous distention. The RR is 24 breaths/min with Sao_2 of 95% on 2 L nasal cannula. The nurse continues the IV boluses until the physician arrives. Upon arrival, the physician performs a FAST examination and orders a change in the oxygen to a 100% NRB.

The team suspects a tamponade but the repeat FAST examination results do not support their suspicion. The patient is unstable so a CT scan cannot be safely completed. Thus, the patient is prepared for emergency exploratory thoracotomy. In the OR, the patient was found to have a large posterior pericardial bloody effusion causing tamponade, which was subsequently decompressed. The patient then returns to the SICU postoperatively.

Case Question 1: Which of the following reasons best explains why NS was used versus a vasopressor when the patient's BP decreased?

(A) Dextrose solutions are hypotonic and do not expand the vascular bed as well as NS.
(B) The goal is to expand the intravascular volume to offset the pressure caused by the blood in the pericardial sac.
(C) Normal saline is an isotonic fluid.
(D) Vasopressors do not expand the intravascular space.
(E) All of the above.

Case Question 2: Why did two previous FAST examinations fail to show a cardiac tamponade?

(A) The FAST is not 100% predictive in all cases of tamponade.
(B) In cases of penetrating trauma to the chest an exploratory thoracotomy is the standard of care if symptoms of a tamponade persist despite negative FAST findings and if a CT scan cannot be done.
(C) The FAST is user dependent.
(D) All of the above.

Answers
1. Answer is option E: all the above.

Dextrose solutions may cause an increase in ICP as well as seizures in trauma patients, especially those who are altered mentally. The glucose in the IV fluids may eventually be absorbed and intravascular volume decreases resulting in a decrease in BP. Isotonic fluids (ie, NS, lactated ringers, or colloids) are necessary to expand intravascular volume thus assuring that the volume in the chambers of the heart always exceeds the volume that surrounds the heart. This prevents further heart compression (cardiac tamponade). Vasopressor use in trauma has been shown to increase mortality in the acute resuscitation phase. This is because vasopressors do not expand the intravascular volume.

2. Answer is D: all the above.

The FAST is just one tool used to diagnose tamponade and is limited in some cases. It is also user dependent. The CT scan is helpful but if the patient is unstable, it may not be safe to do. When these two tools do not definitively eliminate the possibility of a tamponade, yet other clinical findings such as vital signs suggest tamponade, an exploratory thoracotomy is necessary.

Abdominal Trauma

Etiology and Pathophysiology

Trauma to the abdomen may occur to organs in three distinct abdominal regions: peritoneal cavity, retroperitoneum, and pelvis. The anatomical location of the trauma will directly relate to the mechanism of injury. The two major mechanisms of injury will be from either blunt or penetrating traumatic mechanisms. When a patient falls off a ladder and their abdomen lands on a fence rail, this is an example of blunt trauma versus their abdomen landing onto a fence post, which punctures their abdomen, causing penetrating trauma. The organs most affected by blunt abdominal trauma are the spleen, liver, and kidneys. Most penetrating injuries occur anteriorly and the intestines are commonly injured. The types of injuries sustained include organ contusions, lacerations, fractures, vascular disruption and hemorrhage, and crush-type tissue damage. The presentation of abdominal trauma can be subtle on primary and secondary assessments, as other injuries may be more life threatening. It is the nurse's responsibility to continually reevaluate for the progression of symptoms, changes in the physical exam, and remain vigilant for evolving injuries.

Evaluation of Abdominal Trauma

Physical examination, the presence of pain, the FAST scan, and the abdominal CT scan are the main methods used to evaluate and diagnose abdominal injuries. These primary diagnostic tools are used to determine if the patient needs to go directly to the OR, angiography, or can be managed more conservatively with close monitoring. Vigilance in nursing assessment for covert changes and observance of trends are the key to identifying abdominal injuries. The major injuries nurses need to consider include: gastric perforation, bowel perforation, injuries to the greater vasculature of the abdomen, and solid organ or vascular injuries to the spleen, liver, pancreas, kidneys, bowels, or bladder.

Serial physical examinations are labor intensive, but essential to ensure detection of bleeding. The FAST examination is used to quickly and efficiently scan the abdomen at the bedside using ultrasound. Repeat FAST examinations may be done as often as necessary (especially during the resuscitation period) to determine a change in intraperitoneal bleeding. While diagnostic peritoneal lavage (DPL) and angiography may also be used for assessment, the FAST and the abdominal CT scan are the two diagnostic tools used most often in conventional trauma assessment. Abdominal CT scanning requires a hemodynamically stable patient, is more expensive, and incurs a higher radiation exposure than FAST examinations.

Historically, if the patient was unable to reliably confirm or deny the presence of abdominal pain, a DPL would be performed to evaluate for peritoneal injury. For patient safety during a DPL, a decompressed bladder and stomach are necessary to decrease the likelihood of nosocomial injury. To perform a DPL, a provider places a catheter just below the umbilicus and NS is infused. The bag is then lowered below the abdomen and the fluid is allowed to drain out. If the fluid comes out bloody or cloudy, there is a high probability of abdominal trauma. However, a DPL cannot evaluate for a retroperitoneal injury. A CT abdomen and pelvis would be required to investigate for a retroperitoneal injury. If a CT scan reveals an injury to an organ, the degree or "grade" of injury should be determined and a plan must be established with a trauma surgeon. A common grading scale widely used is that of the American Association for the Surgery of Trauma which includes scales for the spleen, liver, kidneys, and pancreas.

Damage to the spleen is one of the most frequently encountered blunt abdominal trauma injuries. Depending on the severity of splenic injury, interventions include nonoperative observation, splenic embolization, or splenectomy for a massively injured spleen. The liver is the second most injured organ in blunt trauma and runs the spectrum from minor injury to severe laceration, requiring operative repair and packing. The bowel, pancreas, and kidneys can be directly injured or sustain secondary injury as a result of poor perfusion and/or inflammation during the trauma, resuscitation, or the critical care phase of recovery.

Typically, presenting signs and symptoms in abdominal trauma include pain, hypotension, tachycardia, and hypovolemia. Complications from abdominal trauma are directly linked to the function of the gastrointestinal tract and include metabolic/nutritional alterations, infections such as peritonitis, and pancreatitis. Patients may require extensive

dressing changes if the wound is open or requires multiple surgeries for staged repair of the abdominal organs.

Principles of Abdominal Trauma Management

Selected principles of caring for the patient with abdominal trauma include monitoring for bleeding, infection prevention and management, and initiating early nutritional support (ie, within 24-48 hours) (see Chapter 14, Gastrointestinal System, for more on nutrition support).

Monitoring for Bleeding

Acute hemorrhage is commonly assessed and identified during the primary survey and frequently requires surgery. Occult bleeding may not be initially evident but later discovered during the secondary survey or during care provided by the nurse. Common abdominal injuries that may not initially exhibit early signs and symptoms of bleeding include liver laceration, splenic fractures, and slow retroperitoneal bleeds. In abdominal trauma, understanding the mechanism of injury and performing serial evaluations to detect changes from baseline are key components to assure rapid and effective treatment.

If the patient has concerns for continuous internal bleeding or has required a large volume of blood product resuscitation, it would be prudent to check laboratory tests frequently. Testing may include: complete blood count (CBC), basic metabolic panel (BMP), liver function tests (LFT), and coagulation panels (PT, PTT, INR, TEG, fibrinogen). Monitoring for medical reasons of hemorrhage or coagulopathy will help prevent exacerbating surgical or traumatic bleeding. The nurse is responsible for ensuring the patient does not have any apparent electrolyte disturbances, especially calcium after a large transfusion. Monitoring for worsening thrombocytopenia and hypofibrinogenemia can help the nurse assess for ongoing bleeding that may not be externally apparent. The nurse should also aim for normothermia, as hypothermia can worsen coagulopathy. Finally, the nurse should discuss with the provider an appropriate blood pressure goal and avoid extreme hypertension, as this may also worsen surgical bleeding. Additionally, monitoring the incision site and any surgical drains will help the nurse identify any continued bleeding.

The historical treatment of splenic injuries was splenectomy. However, conventional wisdom is to preserve the spleen if the patient is hemodynamically stable. Angiographic embolization of splenic vessels and close observation are more commonly employed. This allows the spleen to heal and preserves its valuable immunoprotective function. If a splenectomy is indicated due to massive injury, patients will require a polyvalent pneumococcal vaccine to prevent infection from pneumococci.

Hepatic, renal, and greater vessel bleeding also pose a major risk to the patient's survival. The principles of ongoing hemodynamic monitoring and support, continuous volume resuscitation, and frequent laboratory monitoring are the mainstay of nursing care when dealing with abdominal trauma. If a patient becomes hemodynamically unstable, the nurse is required to notify the provider and surgical team immediately. Additionally, they must prepare to support the hemodynamics of the patient, utilizing IV fluid boluses, blood transfusion, and vasopressors. When continuous bleeding is observed and the patient is requiring escalating amounts of vasoactive medications, the nurse should consult the surgical team for consideration for surgical exploration and management of the bleeding source.

Infection Prevention and Management

Abdominal trauma victims are at high risk for infection, even when surgery has not been performed. For all trauma patients, one of the major nursing care priorities after initial resuscitation is prevention, assessment, and management of infections. Traumatic wounds may be simple lacerations or abrasions from a motor vehicle crash or complex open abdominal surgical wounds that require packing and frequent trips to the OR. Care of the patient with a large abdominal wound is directed by the type of wound (open or closed), any indwelling devices such as catheters, stents, mesh, packing, and the degree of contamination due to the injury and surgery. Careful consideration is also given to the risks and benefits of empiric antimicrobial therapy in patients with contaminated wounds. Dressing changes are frequently performed by the nursing staff, which is when the nurse should assess for signs of infection and wound healing. The timing of dressing changes and the premedication for pain is another important role of the nurse. Trauma patients may have multiple sources of infection, some of which are hospital acquired. The presence of a central line, urinary catheter, endotracheal (ET) tube, nasogastric tube, chest tube, and IV lines all increase the risk of infection and potentially sepsis.

The general risk for infection for traumatic abdominal wounds revolves around a few concerns. The first concern is whether the wound was penetrating or not. If so, then the environment of the penetrating object should be assessed. A fence post covered in dirt will have a different microbial burden compared to a bullet or a spear used for deep-sea fishing. An infectious disease consultation will evaluate the potential burden of infection and decide on the appropriateness of empiric or prophylactic antibiotics.

The second concern to consider for infection risk is which surgical procedures, complications, or risk factors a patient has. If a patient had intra-abdominal spillage from a perforated bowel injury or biliary leak, the patient will have a risk for a gram-negative or anaerobic bacterial infection. If the patient had a surgical drain placed or a device placed internally, then it is possible to have a gram-positive bacterial infection.

The third concern to consider is if the patient is immunosuppressed. Multiple types of drugs and medical conditions could alter a patient's immune response to infection. Patients who have had a splenectomy are immunocompromised for the rest of their lives. Specific considerations for splenectomy patients involve postoperative prophylactic antibiotics, monitoring for continued bleeding, and determining the administration date of splenectomy vaccines.

Nutritional Support

Nutritional support in the trauma patient is an integral part of care. Management focuses on the route and timing of nutritional support. Other considerations include composition of nutrient formulation, nutrient indicators reflected by laboratory tests, tolerance of nutritional support, and the selection of enteral versus parenteral feedings. Trauma patients have increased metabolic needs due to a hypermetabolic stress response caused by severe injuries, wound healing, and/or sepsis.

Enteral nutrition is encouraged whenever possible at the earliest time after injury. Even a small amount of nutrition delivered via tube feeding to the gut may be beneficial. Enteral nutrition promotes gut health, immunologic function, and prevents bacterial translocation. A variety of metabolic derangements in the hypermetabolic trauma patient make nutritional support an early imperative. Insertion and maintenance of a feeding tube, percutaneous gastrostomy tube, or jejunostomy tube is often required after injury until the patient can be orally fed.

Total parenteral nutrition is recommended only if the gastrointestinal tract cannot be used within the first 7 days after injury. Accurate nutritional assessment conducted in collaboration with the nutritionist is critical as trauma patients are at risk of complications from overfeeding or underfeeding. Common clinical concerns of enteral feeding include as diarrhea, inappropriate withholding of tube feedings, and the risk of aspiration. See Chapter 14, Gastrointestinal System, for further discussion.

Musculoskeletal Trauma

Etiology and Pathophysiology

Approximately 70% to 85% of multisystem traumas involve the musculoskeletal system. Patients in critical or progressive care settings who have extremity or pelvic fractures often have other injuries due to the significant physical impact to the body. Motor vehicle trauma, falls, sports injuries, and industrial trauma are all frequent causes of musculoskeletal trauma. Victims of motorcycle crashes often have severe fractures with extensive soft tissue damage. Massive blood loss, edema of tissues, tissue destruction, and pain accompany musculoskeletal injuries. Major musculoskeletal injuries indicate that the body sustained significant forces. For example, a patient with long bone fractures above and below the diaphragm has an increased likelihood of associated internal torso injuries.

Compartment syndrome is a serious complication of extremity trauma as a result of contused tissue swelling in a specific muscle compartment (Figure 17-3). This may lead to lack of perfusion and nerve compression in the area. Muscle compartments are located in the forearm, leg, hand, foot,

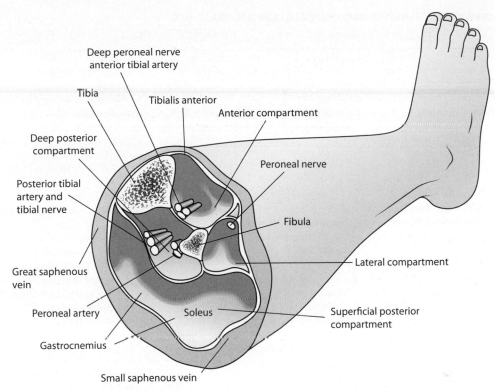

Figure 17-3. Compartments of the lower leg. (*Reproduced with permission from David Hayes, Fulton, MD, 2009.*)

thigh, abdomen, and chest. The nurse assesses for signs of compartment syndrome by performing repeated neurovascular checks. However, neurovascular assessment of the five Ps (pain, pallor, pulselessness, paresthesia, paralysis) may not provide accurate early assessment of rising compartment pressures.

Direct assessment of compartment pressures requires the use of a specialized needle that is inserted directly into the tissue compartment. The needle/catheter is attached to the transducer and the compartment pressures are evaluated and monitored. Even open fractures or open abdominal cavities may have significantly increased compartment pressures (normal pressure 0-8 mm Hg). Compartment syndrome is a medical emergency, and if the compartment pressures are high, a fasciotomy is required to relieve pressure. Acceptable pressure goals in an adult patient will depend on the anatomical location, the patient's clinical exam, and the surgeon. A standard pressure threshold for abdominal compartment syndrome is >20 mm Hg with accompanying signs of organ dysfunction. A standard pressure threshold for the hands is >10 to 15 mm Hg, and the extremities 30 to 40 mm Hg. If the patient's clinical exam exhibits signs of poor perfusion, lab abnormalities, or hemodynamic instability, a fasciotomy may be warranted with a lower threshold. A fasciotomy entails surgically opening the skin and fascia to relieve the pressure in a muscle compartment and is the treatment of choice for compartment syndrome. The primary goal of the fasciotomy is to improve perfusion and minimize ischemia and injury to distal tissues.

Additional nursing management consists of immobilization and keeping the extremity level with or below the heart. Elevation of the extremity can worsen the condition. In the event of a severe crush or vascular injury, there is a significant release of myoglobin from damaged and hypoperfused muscle tissue. Early detection of the condition rhabdomyolysis is essential. The nurse should monitor for dark urine, as this is myoglobin being released from the injured muscle and being cleared by the kidneys. This is treated with generous fluid resuscitation to prevent precipitation of myoglobin in the renal tubules, electrolyte imbalances, and possible acute kidney injury.

Principles of Musculoskeletal Trauma Management

Management of extremity trauma focuses on early stabilization of fractures to prevent further tissue damage, infection, bleeding, and disability. Complications from musculoskeletal trauma include immobility, which can lead to increased incidence of pulmonary emboli, fat emboli, venous thromboemboli (VTE), and pressure injury. Pain control to promote mobility and assessment of neurovascular status are key components to managing patients with musculoskeletal trauma (Table 17-5).

Fractures are repaired early after a traumatic injury to decrease further bleeding and to limit immobility and its complications (eg, VTE and pulmonary embolism). Guidelines for the management of VTE for trauma patients include pharmacologic prophylaxis (if able) and mechanical prophylactic devices, such as sequential compression devices, foot pumps, and vena cava filters (Table 17-6).

TABLE 17-5. PHYSICAL COMPLICATIONS RELATED TO IMMOBILITY COMMONLY SEEN IN TRAUMA PATIENTS

Body System	Complications	Pathophysiology	Prevention
Neurologic	Potentially affects all body systems from mentation to physical changes.	Caused by decreased level of consciousness; injury to cortex, motor, or sensory systems.	• Neurologic assessment. • Specific focus on the effects seen in other body systems. • Understand neurologic basis of complication.
Respiratory	Fatigue, decreased productivity, infection, pneumonia, respiratory acidosis.	Decreased respiratory movement, unable to mobilize secretions, alterations in blood gases.	• Assessment of respiratory status and changes in level of consciousness. • Mobilization of secretions by turning, coughing, and deep breathing; postural drainage, percussion, vibration, early ambulation, humidification, and hydration.
Cardiovascular	Orthostatic hypotension, fatigue, increased cardiac workload, thrombosis, embolus.	Increased heart rate, CVP, cardiac output, stroke volume in supine position; loss of supporting muscle tone resulting in venous stasis; orthostatic neurovascular receptors cannot adjust to position changes; hypercoagulability and external pressure to vessels.	• Cardiovascular assessment. • Encourage mobilization, exercise, range of motion, positioning. • Antiembolic devices. • Provide adequate hydration. • Avoid Valsalva maneuver.
Gastrointestinal	Anorexia, fatigue, malnutrition, constipation, impaction, bowel obstruction, diarrhea, dehydration.	Negative nitrogen balance and protein deficiency; stress; decreased appetite creates bowel intolerance; muscle weakness; diminished ability to apply abdominal pressure needed for evacuation; psychological factors and position for defecation may increase difficulty.	• Assessment of GI functioning, including baseline history of nutrition, exercise, and bowel habits. • Coordinate bowel plan with nutrition specialist. • Adequate hydration. • Positioning and privacy. • Gastrocolic reflex timing factors; use of digital stimulation. • Stool softeners and suppositories as bowel stimulants. • Adjust tube feedings to avoid constipation or diarrhea. • Small, frequent feedings to increase tolerance and decrease anorexia. • Encourage intake of protein, fluids, bulk forming foods.
Urinary	Urinary reflux, incontinence, urinary stasis, renal calculi, urinary tract infection.	Loss of effect of gravity, urinary stasis in renal pelvis; increased calculi formation from urine sediment in renal pelvis; diminished coordination of sphincters and muscles in supine position; bladder distention, overflow incontinence.	• Assess urinary tract function. • Promote movement and exercise. • Maintain fluid intake. • Decrease calcium intake, increase loss from bones. • Monitor distention and voiding patterns. • Prevent incontinence. • Use upright or sitting position for voiding if possible. • Intermittent catheters preferred to indwelling.
Musculoskeletal	Muscle atrophy, contractures.	Muscles shorten and atrophy; loss of ROM as supporting ligaments, tendons, and capsule lose mobility; loss of ROM becomes permanent; spasticity of antagonistic muscle with weakness of opposing muscle creates contracture.	• Ongoing assessment. • Passive, active, and active-assisted ROM exercises. • Appropriate positioning and body alignment in both bed and chair.
	Osteoporosis, stress fractures, heterotrophic ossification.	Normal bone-building activities depend on weight bearing and movement; increased destruction of bone, release of calcium; bone becomes porous and fragile; abnormal calcification over large joints may also occur.	• Calcium supplement to diet is not recommended. • Promote weight bearing.
Integumentary	Pressure injury; stages I-IV; risk of sepsis with infection due to pressure injury.	Prolonged pressure to skin diminishes capillary blood supply and stops flow of nutrients to cells; necrosis of cells results in skin injury and risk for infection.	• Assessment of skin integrity, nutritional status, and risk factors for breakdown. • Reposition; shift pressure and patient weight frequently. • Check for changes in blanching, sustained redness. • Keep off all red areas. • Massage at-risk areas to promote circulation. • Teach patient to inspect own skin and shift weight. • Increase protein in diet, monitor hydration status. • Take immediate, consistent action on any areas of potential injury.

TABLE 17-6. EVIDENCE-BASED PRACTICE: MANAGEMENT OF VENOUS THROMBOEMBOLISM IN TRAUMA PATIENTS

EVIDENCE-BASED PRACTICE: Venous Thromboembolism (VTE) Prevention	
Prevention (Expected Nursing Practice)	**Levels of Evidence**

1. Assess all patients upon admission to the critical care or progressive care unit for risk factors for VTE. Anticipate orders for (VTE) prophylaxis based on risk assessment (Level D)
2. Risk and treatment for VTE prophylaxis include:
   a. Acute medical patients: low-molecular-weight heparin (LMWH) or low-dose unfractionated heparin (LDUH) or fondaparinux (Level B)
   b. General surgery patients: LMWH, LDUH, or mechanical prophylaxis. Examples: antiembolism stockings/graduated compression stockings (GCSs), intermittent pneumatic compression devices (IPCDs), foot impulse devices (FIDs), also known as foot pumps (Level B)
   c. Critical ill patients: LMWH or LDUH (Level A)
   d. High risk for bleeding (trauma): mechanical prophylaxis (Level B)
   e. Use mechanical prophylaxis devices with anticoagulant-based treatment plans (Level D)
3. Discuss current VTE risk factors, the necessity for invasive lines (central venous catheter [CVC] or peripherally inserted central catheter [PICC]), and risk for bleeding (Level E)
4. Maximize mobility and reduce the time the patient is immobile (Level E)
5. Ambulatory patients are at risk for VTE (Level D)
6. Ensure mechanical prophylaxis devices are properly fitted and in use at all times except for skin assessment and cleaning (Level D)
	1. Level A: Meta-analysis of quantitative studies or meta-synthesis of qualitative studies with results that consistently support a specific action, intervention, or treatment (including systematic review of randomized controlled trials)
	2. Level B: Well-designed, controlled studies with results that consistently support a specific action, intervention, or treatment
	3. Level C: Qualitative studies, descriptive or correlational studies, integrative reviews, systematic reviews, or randomized controlled trials with inconsistent results
	4. Level D: Peer-reviewed professional and organizational standards with the support of clinical study recommendations
	5. Level E: Multiple case reports, theory-based evidence from expert opinions, or peer-reviewed professional organizational standards without clinical studies to support recommendations
	6. Level M: Manufacturer's recommendations only

Data from Hopkins AG. The trauma nurse's role with families in crisis. Crit Care Nurse. 1994;14(2):35-43.

Stabilizing Fractures

Improper handling or management of a patient with an injury to the musculoskeletal system may convert a simple problem into a much more serious problem. External fixation is used for pelvic fractures and lower limb fractures. Frequent sensation, movement, and vascular checks on affected extremities are essential. If the presence of pulses is in doubt, Doppler ultrasound is used at the bedside.

Pain Control

Pain control is best achieved with an individualized strategy of medications and nonpharmacologic therapies. Patients respond well when strict attention is paid to pain control and their own unique coping style is encouraged. Patients are expected to move in bed and get out of bed as soon as possible after an injury. Titrated pain medication is generally required to achieve this goal using PCA or a continuous infusion. Nurses are in a unique position to assess patient anxieties regarding the trauma and to promote adequate sleep and rest. Sleep deprivation from a noisy environment, stress, and unnecessary pain can exacerbate the patient's discomfort and delay rehabilitation.

COMPLICATIONS OF TRAUMATIC INJURY IN SEVERE MULTISYSTEM TRAUMA

General Concepts

The key to survival for patients with multisystem trauma is to limit the extent of complications and increase the delivery of oxygen to the tissues during the initial phase of resuscitation.

Historically, this has been called the "golden hour." The resuscitation goal is to prevent tissue oxygen deprivation due to hypoperfusion and identify and reverse the cause. Shock, by definition, is hypoperfusion which results in cellular hypoxia, organ dysfunction, and tissue death. Prompt reversal of hypoxemia and restoration of perfusion decreases the risk of developing complications related to shock. HR and BP are not considered adequate parameters to judge the effectiveness of resuscitation, as they indicate only the body's compensation for the stress of trauma and not the effectiveness of the resuscitation. Appropriate measures to evaluate during resuscitation should focus on assessing tissue oxygen delivery and tissue perfusion.

Monitoring signs of end organ function (e.g., mental status, urinary output, serum lactate) will assist the nurse in determining if adequate tissue perfusion is established. Serum labs, such as renal function (BUN, creatinine), lactate, and hepatic function labs (transaminases) may become elevated after the initial traumatic insult, related to the cellular damage caused by the shock from the injury. These lab values should be trended to ensure their return to baseline and return of normal cellular function.

To preserve adequate blood flow in the acutely injured trauma patient, permissive hypotension may be used. Permissive hypotension is based on the concept that resuscitation to attain normal BP may increase bleeding from a site that has already "clotted" through the normal clotting cascade process. If permissive hypotension is the goal, large volumes of fluid are not encouraged. Permissive hypotension may be effective in penetrating trauma but generally not with blunt trauma. If a TBI is suspected, permissive hypotension is contraindicated as perfusion to the brain is a priority (see Chapter 21, Advanced Neurologic Concepts).

Common complications of trauma include infection/sepsis, ARDS, and multiple organ dysfunction. They are discussed below (see also Chapter 10, Respiratory System and Chapter 11, Multisystem Problems).

Infection, Sepsis/Septic Shock, and Multiple Organ Dysfunction

Trauma patients are at high risk of developing an infection and consequently developing septic shock. Factors that contribute to this risk include the nature of the injury, the environment in which the injury occurred, the nonsterile conditions in which invasive devices are initially placed, and the multiple invasive procedures, including surgery, that are necessary for resuscitation, stabilization, and management. The emergent procedures performed during resuscitation are at best undertaken under clean conditions.

Infection

The classic signs and symptoms of infection are sometimes difficult to isolate in a recovering trauma patient. Fever, tachycardia, elevated white blood cell count, hyperglycemia, inflammation, pain, and a hyperdynamic state may be indicators of infection and sepsis. These assessment parameters are also common after injury, resuscitation, and during the healing process due to the stress response on the immune system. When clear identification of an infectious source is elusive, consideration is given to treating the most likely source of infection based on the clinical evidence, particularly if the patient exhibits hemodynamic instability. Sterile technique and hand hygiene are vital in this vulnerable patient population.

Sepsis and Septic shock

Understanding of the diagnosis and management of sepsis continues to evolve. Sepsis is defined as a dysregulated response to infection, which results in the release of many mediators, leading to end organ damage. While our understanding of sepsis continues to evolve, the guidelines updated in 2021 suggest the use of a validated tool such as SIRS, NEWS, or MEWS to screen for sepsis. When a patient is recognized as having sepsis, healthcare teams should collaborate to ensure the following actions are taken within 1 hour: obtaining blood cultures, administering broad-spectrum antibiotics, measuring the patient's lactate level, and starting fluid resuscitation and vasopressors if indicated. Early treatment is essential to offer the best possible outcome for the patient. The reader is referred to an in-depth discussion of sepsis in Chapter 11, Multisystem Problems.

Multiple Organ Dysfunction Syndrome

Multiple organ dysfunction syndrome (MODS) refers to progressive damage to two or more organs that may result in a permanent change in organ function. In the trauma patient, MODS may be due to infection and sepsis but also may occur as a result of excessive blood loss and hypoperfusion injury to the organs. Regardless of the etiology, unless hypoperfusion and shock are rapidly or adequately reversed, the organs sustain ischemia, inflammation, injury, and possibly infarction. The clinical presentation of organ dysfunction may have a rapid onset or take several days. Organ dysfunction is identified by signs and symptoms associated with organ failure such as ARDS, pancreatitis, acute kidney injury, and hepatic insufficiency. Delivering oxygen to the tissues by maintaining increased blood flow during resuscitation can decrease the duration of hypoperfusion, limit anaerobic metabolism, and avoid lethal complications.

Achieving adequate oxygen delivery to the tissues requires oxygen, hemoglobin, and sufficient cardiac output to meet cellular requirements. This is often accomplished with large volume fluid resuscitation or multiple blood transfusions in the trauma patient. MTPs are used to guide the use of large volumes of blood products (eg, the administration of more than 10 units of packed red blood cells within 24 hours). In such cases, multiple types of blood components (whole blood, packed red blood cells, fresh frozen plasma, cryoprecipitate, and platelets) are used. The different blood products address the restoration of the normal blood components.

It is recommended that when a trauma patient needs either a massive transfusion of blood products or fluids, the nurse administers these fluids via a fluid warmer to prevent hypothermia. Trauma patients suffering from hypothermia do not respond normally to the administration of blood and fluid resuscitation, and coagulopathy may develop or worsen. The concurrent presence of hypothermia, acidosis, and coagulopathy is known as the trauma triad or triangle of death. Mortality may be increased to over 90% if this combination of disorders is not reversed.

Trauma patients are at risk of experiencing significant complications after massive fluid/blood administration. Hypothermia, coagulopathy, acidosis, electrolyte imbalances, transfusion-related acute lung injury (TRALI), transfusion-associated circulatory overload (TACO), transfusion-associated immunomodulation (TRIM) (a down regulation of immune function or immunosuppression), and posttransfusion infections have all been attributed to massive fluid or blood replacement. Monitoring for and treating these complications are key components of trauma care.

Acute Respiratory Distress Syndrome

Patients with trauma have an increased incidence of ARDS (see Chapter 10, Respiratory System). Precipitating factors for ARDS in the trauma patient include direct or indirect injury to the lungs. Examples of direct injury include smoke inhalation, rib fractures causing lung laceration, aspiration, and large pulmonary contusions. Indirect injury may be due to sepsis, massive fluid and/or blood resuscitation, and prolonged hypoperfusion states (shock), which can lead to an inflammatory insult and alveolar infiltration.

Standard treatment for ARDS is supportive and includes mechanical ventilation, oxygen titrated to maintain PaO_2 more than or equal to 60 mm Hg, positive-end expiratory pressure (PEEP), and ventilatory modes and methods to recruit closed alveoli and decrease lung injury (see Chapter 20, Advanced Respiratory Concepts: Modes of Ventilation). In addition to mechanical ventilation, another method to improve oxygenation is positioning for optimal ventilation and perfusion. This is a unique challenge for the critically or acutely ill trauma patients because their traumatic injuries may preclude many positions; for example, the patient with an unstable pelvic fracture, a spinal cord injury, or lower extremity fractures may be difficult or impossible to turn. Finally, meticulous nursing care is necessary to prevent ventilatory-associated complications in all trauma patients receiving mechanical ventilation.

PSYCHOLOGICAL CONSEQUENCES OF TRAUMA

Any illness places stressors on patients and families, and this is often magnified in critically or acutely ill trauma patients. Trauma injury is by nature unexpected. It traditionally was more common in younger, healthy individuals, but is now seen widely throughout the lifecycle. Both the patient and the family can enter into a cycle of chaos and crisis. Common responses to trauma include anxiety, anger, fear, grief, loss, guilt, depression, denial, sleeplessness, and hopelessness.

Fear begins immediately as the awake trauma patient is transported from the scene. Fear is related to the unknown, the specifics of the injuries, the prognosis for the patient, and impacts on the patient's future, including body image, family, and career. Loss typifies the experience of trauma and can be characterized as loss of physical functioning, loss of quality of life, or even loss of significant others due to the traumatic event. Guilt may ensue as the patient may perceive responsibility for the event (directly or indirectly), and this may be overwhelming. Depression and denial are common coping mechanisms during personal crises and may be exhibited in a variety of ways by trauma victims. It is noted that although the injuries are sustained by the patient, the family members and friends are also frequently traumatized.

Monitoring the patient's psychological response to injury is as much the responsibility of the nurse as monitoring physiological parameters such as blood pressure. Just as there are long-term physiologic effects of a low BP (shock), there are long-term psychological effects of unmet or unidentified emotional needs. There are also psychoneuroimmunology responses that may impact physical recovery. Assessing the emotional response to injury is an important part of comprehensive care. Talk to the patient and listen to responses and perceptions. Help them identify and articulate concerns and fears.

Fear creates anxiety in the trauma patient, and unrelieved pain may worsen anxiety. With the intense monitoring and frequent care interruptions commonly present in the critical or progressive care environment, sleep may be minimal and fragmented. A vicious cycle is thus initiated whereby sleeplessness leads to an increased perception of pain, which in turn creates needless anxiety and inhibits sleep. Viewing these responses as cyclical emphasizes that the nurse may intervene anywhere in the cycle of responses and make a major impact on all three; for example, providing pain-relieving strategies that permit sleep automatically decreases anxiety. A focus on information sharing may ease the patient's mind so that sleep can occur, and pain perception decreases. The nurse has a significant role in intervening to stop this vicious cycle through a variety of holistic strategies.

All families of trauma patients experience a crisis. Families may have no idea of how to act or what the healthcare team expects of them. Clinicians have a key role in providing support and information to meet family needs and in identifying family coping mechanisms. Knowing the phases of family emotional response and suggested interventions is useful. Early assessment of family system structure, relationship process, and family functioning are keys to effective management of the psychosocial needs of the patient and family. Getting to know and working with family members in trauma care is essential and can be best facilitated with flexible visiting policies, and family presence during rounds, procedures, and codes when appropriate. Inviting family members to participate in decisions about the plan of care is also essential. Shared decision making is a key component of patient and family-centered health care. The healthcare team, the family, and the patient together can make decisions that are based on risk, clinical evidence, and outcomes as they relate to the patient's preferences and values.

SELECTED BIBLIOGRAPHY

General Trauma

American Association for the Surgery of Trauma. Injury Scoring Scale. 2009. https://www.aast.org/resources-detail/injury-scoring-scale. Accessed May 20, 2021.

American College of Surgeons. Advanced Trauma Life Support. 2021. https://www.facs.org/quality-programs/trauma/atls. Accessed June 22, 2021.

Beshay M, Mertzlufft F, Kottkamp HW, et al. Analysis of risk factors in thoracic trauma patients with a comparison of a modern trauma centre: a mono-centre study. *World J Emerg Surg.* 2020;15(1). doi: 10.1186/s13017-020-00324-1

Caputo ND, Stahmer C, Lim G, Shah K. Whole-body computed tomographic scanning leads to better survival as opposed to selective scanning in trauma patients. *J Trauma Acute Care Surg.* 2014;77(4):534-539. doi: 10.1097/ta.0000000000000414

Coles SJ, Erdogan M, Higgins SD, Green RS. Impact of an early mobilization protocol on outcomes in trauma patients admitted to the intensive care unit: a retrospective pre-post study. *J Trauma Acute Care Surg.* 2020;88(4):515-521.

Evans, L., Rhodes, A., Alhazzani, W. et al. Surviving sepsis campaign: international guidelines for management of sepsis and septic shock 2021. *Intensive Care Med.* 2021;47:1181-1247. doi: 10.1007/s00134-021-06506-y

Giancarelli A, Hobbs B, Sparks D, Motola D. Massive Transfusion for Coagulopathy and Hemorrhagic Shock. 2020. http://www.surgicalcriticalcare.net/Guidelines/Massive%20Transfusion%20Protocol%202020.pdf

Hamrick KL, Beyer CA, Lee JA, Cocanour CS, Duby JJ. Multimodal analgesia and opioid use in critically ill trauma patients. *J Am Coll Surg.* 2019;228(5):769-775.e1.

Holmstrom AL, Ott KC, Weiss HK, et al. Improving trauma tertiary survey performance and missed injury identification using an education-based quality improvement initiative. *J Trauma Acute Care Surg.* 2021;90(6):1048-1053. doi: 10.1097/ta.0000000000003152

Inaba K, Byerly S, Bush LD, et al. Cervical spinal clearance: a prospective Western Trauma Association Multi-institutional Trial. *J Trauma Acute Care Surg.* 2016;81(6):1122-1130.

Kochanek KD, Xu JQ, Arias E. *Mortality in the United States, 2019.* NCHS Data Brief, no 395. Hyattsville, MD: National Center for Health Statistics; 2020.

Lee RK, Gallagher JJ, Ejike JC, Hunt L. Intra-abdominal hypertension and the open abdomen: nursing guidelines from the Abdominal Compartment Society. *Crit Care Nurse.* 2020;40(1): 13-26.

Ley EJ, Brown CVR, Moore EE, et al. Updated guidelines to reduce venous thromboembolism in trauma patients: A Western Trauma Association critical decisions algorithm. *J Trauma Acute Care Surg.* 2020;89(5):971-981.

Long B, Koyfman A, Gottlieb M. Evaluation and management of acute compartment syndrome in the emergency department. *J Emerg Med.* 2019;56(4):386-397.

Martorella G. Characteristics of nonpharmacological interventions for pain management in the ICU: a scoping review. *AACN Adv Crit Care.* 2019;30(4):388-397.

Mowery NT, Gunter OL, Collier BR, et al. Practice management guidelines for management of hemothorax and occult pneumothorax. *J Trauma.* 2011;70(2):510-518.

Pelekhaty S, Gaasch S. Metabolic and nutritional management of the trauma patient. In: McQuillan KA, Flynn Makic, MB, eds. *Trauma Nursing: From Resuscitation Through Rehabilitation.* 5th ed. St. Louis, MO Elsevier; 2020: 251-276.

Rhodes A, Evans LE, Alhazzani W, et al. Surviving sepsis campaign: international guidelines for management of sepsis and septic shock: 2016. *Intensive Care Med.* 2017;43(3):304-377.

Taylor BE, McClave SA, Martindale RG, et al. Guidelines for the provision and assessment of nutrition support therapy in the adult critically ill patient: Society of critical care medicine (SCCM) and American Society for Parenteral and Enteral Nutrition (A.S.P.E.N.). *Crit Care Med.* 2016;44(2):390-438.

The Eastern Association for the Surgery of Trauma. Damage control resuscitation in patients with severe traumatic hemorrhage. East. org. https://www.east.org/education-career-development/practice-management-guidelines/details/damage-control-resuscitation-in-patients-with-severe-traumatic-hemorrhage. Accessed July 20, 2021.

The Eastern Association for the Surgery of Trauma. Monitoring modalities, assessment of volume status, and endpoints of resuscitation. East.org. https://www.east.org/education-career-development/practice-management-guidelines/details/monitoring-modalities-assessment-of-volume-status-and-endpoints-of-resuscitation. Accessed July 20, 2021.

ADVANCED CONCEPTS

III

ADVANCED ECG CONCEPTS

Carol Jacobson

18

KNOWLEDGE COMPETENCIES

1. Identify electrocardiogram (ECG) characteristics and treatment approaches for each of the following advanced dysrhythmias:
   - Supraventricular tachycardias (SVTs)
   - Wide QRS beats and rhythms
2. Using the 12-lead ECG, determine the following:
   - Bundle branch blocks
   - QRS axis
   - Patterns of myocardial ischemia, injury, and infarct

3. Identify effects of potassium and calcium imbalances on the ECG.
4. Identify ECG characteristics of single- and dual-chamber pacemakers during normal and abnormal functioning.
5. Identify ECG characteristics of Brugada syndrome (BrS) and long QT syndromes.

THE 12-LEAD ELECTROCARDIOGRAM

The 12-lead electrocardiogram (ECG) records electrical activity as it spreads through the heart from 12 different leads, which are in turn recorded by electrodes placed on the arms and legs, and in specific spots on the chest. Each lead represents a different "view" of the heart and consists of two electrodes. A bipolar lead has two poles—one positive and one negative. A unipolar lead has one positive pole and a reference pole that is a point in the center of the chest that is mathematically determined by the ECG machine. The standard 12-lead ECG consists of six frontal plane limb leads that record electrical activity traveling up/down and right/left in the heart, and six precordial leads that record electrical activity in the horizontal plane traveling anterior/posterior and right/left. Limb leads are recorded by electrodes placed on the arms and legs, and precordial leads are recorded by electrodes placed on the chest (Figure 18-1).

A camera analogy makes the 12-lead ECG easier to understand. Each lead of the ECG represents a picture of the electrical activity in the heart taken by the camera. In any lead, the positive electrode is the recording electrode or the

camera lens. The negative electrode tells the camera which way to "shoot" its picture and determines the direction in which the positive electrode records. When the positive electrode sees electrical activity traveling toward it, it records an upright deflection on the ECG. When the positive electrode sees electrical activity traveling away from it, it records a negative deflection (Figure 18-2). If the electrical activity travels perpendicular to a positive electrode, no activity is recorded. The standard 12-ECG records three bipolar frontal plane leads (leads I, II, and III) and three unipolar frontal plane leads (aVR, aVL, and aVF). In addition, there are six unipolar precordial leads: V_1, V_2, V_3, V_4, V_5, and V_6.

The three bipolar frontal plane leads are illustrated in Figure 18-3A. In each lead, the camera represents the positive pole of the lead. In lead I, the positive electrode is on the left arm and the negative electrode is on the right arm. Any electrical activity in the heart that travels toward the positive electrode (camera lens) on the left arm is recorded as an upright deflection and any activity traveling away from it is recorded as a negative deflection. In lead II, the positive electrode is on the left leg and the negative electrode is on the

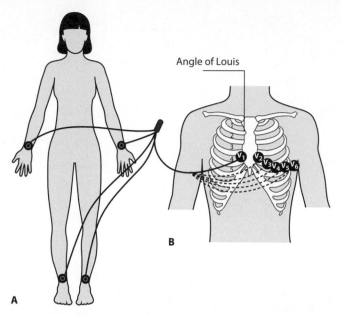

Angle of Louis

B

A

Figure 18-1. (A) Limb electrodes can be placed anywhere on arms and legs. Standard placement is shown here on wrists and ankles. **(B)** Chest electrode placement. V_1 = fourth intercostal space to right of sternum; V_2 = fourth intercostal space to left of sternum; V_3 = halfway between V_2 and V_4 in a straight line; V_4 = fifth intercostal space at midclavicular line; V_5 = same level as V_4 at anterior axillary line; V_6 = same level as V_4 at midaxillary line.

right arm. Any electrical activity traveling toward the left leg electrode (camera lens) is recorded as an upright deflection and any activity traveling away from it toward the right arm electrode is recorded as a negative deflection. In lead III, the positive electrode is on the left leg and the negative electrode is on the left arm. Any electrical activity coming toward the left leg electrode (camera lens) is recorded upright and any traveling away from it toward the left arm is recorded negative. The view of the heart by the bipolar leads can be compared to a wide-angle camera lens.

The three unipolar frontal plane leads, aVR, aVL, and aVF, are illustrated in Figure 18-3B. The camera represents the location of the positive electrode: on the right shoulder for aVR, on the left shoulder for aVL, and at the foot (left leg)

for aVF. The "negative end" of the unipolar lead is a reference spot in the center of the chest that is mathematically determined by the ECG machine. The same principles apply to unipolar leads: any electrical activity traveling toward the positive electrode is recorded as an upright deflection and any traveling away from it is recorded as a negative deflection. The six unipolar precordial leads are recorded from their locations on the chest as shown in Figure 18-3C. The view of the heart by unipolar leads can be compared to a telephoto lens on the camera, "zooming in" on the electrical activity in the heart.

The hexaxial reference system (or axis wheel) is formed when the six frontal plane leads are moved together in such a way that they bisect each other in the center (Figure 18-4A). Each lead is labeled at its positive end to make it easy to remember where the positive electrode is. In Figure 18-4B, the hexaxial reference system is superimposed over a drawing of the heart to illustrate how each lead views the heart.

The normal sequence of depolarization through the heart begins with an electrical impulse originating in the sinus node, high in the right atrium, and spreading leftward through the left atrium and downward toward the atrioventricular (AV) node, low in the right atrium (Figure 18-5A). Leads I and aVL, with their positive electrodes (camera lens) on the left side of the body, record this leftward electrical activity as an upright P wave, and leads II, III, and aVF, with their positive electrodes at the bottom of the heart, record the downward spread of activity as upright P waves. Lead aVR, with its positive electrode on the right shoulder, sees the electrical activity moving away from it and records a negative P wave.

As the impulse spreads through the AV node, no electrical activity is recorded because the AV node is too small to be recorded by surface leads. As the impulse exits the AV node, it moves through the bundle of His and enters the right and left bundle branches. The left bundle branch sprouts some Purkinje fibers high on the left side of the septum that carry the impulse into the septum and cause it to depolarize first in a left-to-right direction. The electrical impulse then enters the Purkinje system of both ventricular free walls

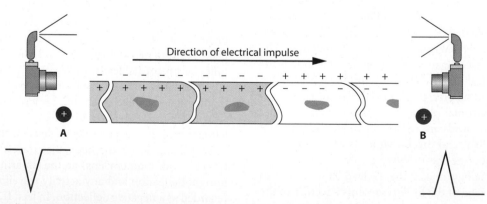

Direction of electrical impulse

A

B

Figure 18-2. A strip of cardiac muscle depolarizing in the direction of the arrow. A positive electrode at **(B)** sees depolarization coming toward it and records an upright deflection. A positive electrode at **(A)** sees depolarization going away from it and records a negative deflection.

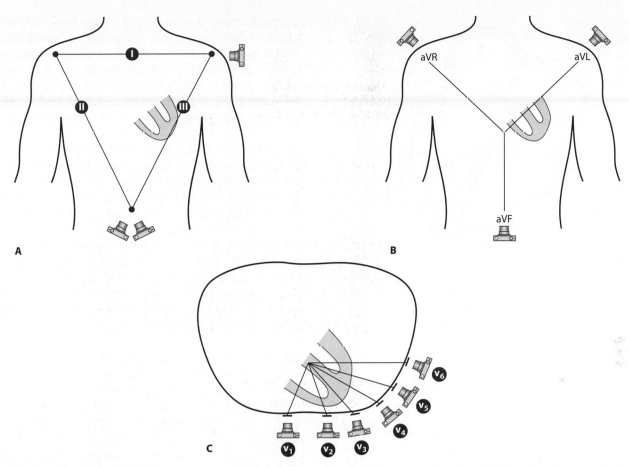

Figure 18-3. The 12 leads of the ECG. The camera represents the location of the positive, or recording, electrode in each lead. **(A)** Bipolar frontal plane leads I, II, and III. **(B)** Unipolar frontal plane leads aVR, aVL, and aVF. **(C)** Unipolar precordial leads V₁ to V₆.

simultaneously and depolarizes them from endocardium to epicardium, as shown by the small arrows through the ventricular wall in Figure 18-5A. The millions of electrical forces travel through the heart in three dimensions simultaneously,

but if averaged together they move downward, leftward, and posteriorly toward the large left ventricle, as indicated by the large arrow in the same figure. This large arrow represents the mean axis, which is the net direction of electrical

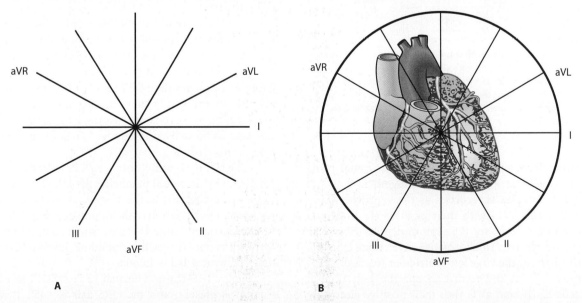

Figure 18-4. Hexaxial reference system (or axis wheel). **(A)** All six frontal plane leads bisecting each other. Each lead is labeled at its positive end. **(B)** The axis wheel superimposed on the heart to demonstrate each lead's view of the heart. Leads I and aVL face the left lateral wall; leads II, III, and aVF face the inferior wall.

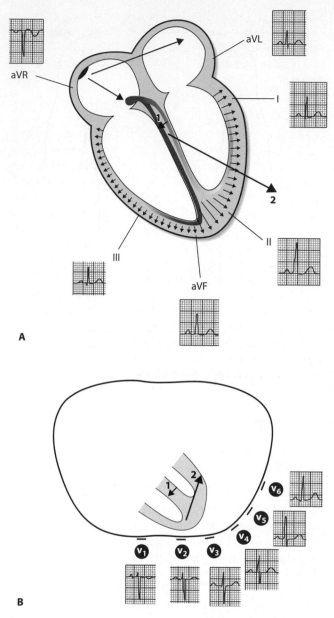

A

B

Figure 18-5. **(A)** Normal sequence of depolarization through the heart as recorded by each of the frontal plane leads. **(B)** Cross-section of the thorax illustrating how the six precordial leads record normal electrical activity in the ventricles. The small arrow (1) shows the initial direction of depolarization through the septum, followed by the direction of ventricular depolarization, indicated by the larger arrow (2).

electrical activity coming slightly toward them, they record a positive deflection. As the forces continue moving downward toward leads II, III, and aVF, an upright deflection (R wave) is recorded. Lead aVR, positive on the right shoulder, sees all activity moving away from it and records a negative deflection (QS complex). Figure 18-5A illustrates how the six frontal plane leads record normal electrical activity as it spreads through the atria and ventricles.

The six precordial leads record electrical activity traveling in the horizontal plane. Figure 18-5B illustrates the position of the precordial leads and how they record electrical activity as it spreads through the ventricles. Lead V_1 is located on the front of the chest and records a small R wave as the septum depolarizes toward it from left to right. It then records a deep S wave as depolarization spreads away from it through the thick left ventricle. As the positive electrode is moved across the precordium from the V_1 to the V_6 position, it records progressively more left ventricular forces and the R wave gets progressively larger. Lead V_6 is located on the left side of the chest and may record a small Q wave as the septum depolarizes from left to right away from the positive electrode, and it records a large R wave as electrical activity spreads toward the positive electrode through the thick left ventricle. Normal R wave progression means that the R wave becomes progressively larger from V_1 to V_6, or that the R wave in V_1 is a minimal part of the QRS complex and the R wave in V_6 is the dominant part of the QRS complex.

In addition to P waves and QRS complexes, the ECG records T waves as the ventricles repolarize. Normal T waves are slightly asymmetrical with an ascending limb that is more gradual than the descending limb. T waves are usually upright in leads I, II, and V_{3-6}, and negative in lead aVR. T waves can vary in other leads. A normal T wave is not taller than 5 mm in a limb lead or 10 mm in a chest lead. Tall T waves can indicate hyperkalemia or myocardial ischemia or infarction.

The ST segment begins at the end of the QRS complex (the J point) and ends at the beginning of the T wave. It is normally at the baseline (the isoelectric segment between the T wave and the next P wave) and should not stay on the baseline for longer than 0.12 seconds (Figure 18-6). The ST segment should gently curve upward into the T wave without forming a sharp angle. Normal ST-segment elevation and depression is discussed under "ST-Segment Monitoring" later in this chapter.

The U wave is sometimes seen following the T wave, and when present, it should be smaller than the T wave and point in the same direction as the T wave. U waves are thought to represent repolarization of the midmyocardial cells (M-cells) in the ventricles. Large U waves can be seen in hypokalemia and with certain drugs, like quinidine. Inverted U waves can indicate myocardial ischemia.

Figure 18-7 shows a normal 12-lead ECG. Normal sinus rhythm is present, and the QRS axis is +45°. P waves are normal (they are flat in V_2, but this is not necessarily abnormal), and T waves are normal. The QRS complex is normal

depolarization through the ventricles in the frontal plane when all the smaller arrows are averaged together.

The QRS complex is recorded as the ventricles depolarize. Leads I and aVL, with their positive electrodes on the left side of the body, see the septum depolarizing away from them and record a small negative deflection (Q wave). These leads then see the large left ventricular free wall depolarizing toward them and record an upright deflection (R wave). Leads II, III, and aVF, with their positive electrodes at the bottom of the heart, may not see septal activity at all and record no deflections. However, if these leads see septal

Lead II   Lead V₁

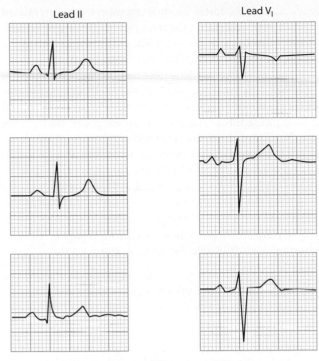

Figure 18-6. Normal ST segment and T waves.

(0.08-second wide), there are no abnormal Q waves, and R-wave progression is normal across the precordium. The ST segment is at baseline in all leads. This ECG is used for comparison as abnormalities are discussed throughout this chapter.

Axis Determination

The *hexaxial reference system* (axis wheel) forms a 360° circle surrounding the heart that by convention is divided into 180 positive degrees (+180°) and 180 negative degrees (−180°) (Figure 18-8). The normal QRS axis is defined as −30° to +90° because most of the electrical forces in a normal heart are directed downward and leftward toward the large left ventricle. Left axis deviation is defined as an axis of −31° to −90° and occurs when most of the forces move in a leftward and superior direction, as can happen in a variety of conditions, such as left ventricular hypertrophy, left anterior fascicular block, inferior myocardial infarction (MI), or left bundle branch block (LBBB) (Table 18-1). Right axis deviation is defined as +91° to +180° and occurs when most of the forces move rightward, as can happen in conditions such as right ventricular hypertrophy, left posterior fascicular block, and right bundle branch block (RBBB) (see Table 18-1).

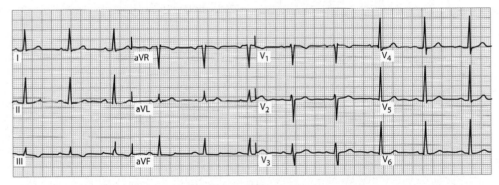

Figure 18-7. Normal 12-lead ECG.

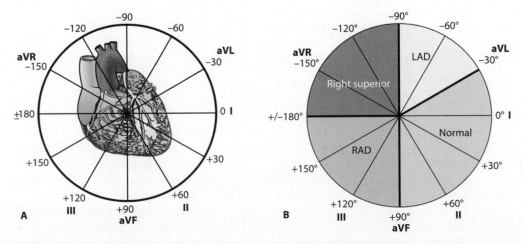

Figure 18-8. (A) Degrees of the axis wheel. **(B)** Normal axis = −30° to + 90°; left axis deviation = −31° to −90°; right axis deviation = +91° to +180°; right superior axis = −90° to −180°.

TABLE 18-1. SUMMARY OF CAUSES OF AXIS DEVIATIONS

Axis: −30° to +90°
- Normal

Left Axis Deviation: −31° to −90°
- Left ventricular hypertrophy
- Left anterior fascicular block
- Inferior myocardial infarction
- Left bundle branch block
- Congenital defects
- Ventricular tachycardia
- Wolff-Parkinson-White syndrome
- Obesity

Right Axis Deviation: +91° to +180°
- Right ventricular hypertrophy
- Left posterior fascicular block
- Right bundle branch block
- Dextrocardia
- Ventricular tachycardia
- Wolff-Parkinson-White syndrome

Right Superior Axis: −90° to −180°
- Ventricular tachycardia
- Ventricular pacing
- Bifascicular block

When most of the forces are directed superior and rightward between −90° and −180°, the term *right superior axis* is used. This axis can occur with ventricular tachycardia, ventricular pacing, and occasionally with bifascicular block.

The mean frontal plane QRS axis can be determined in a number of ways. The most accurate method is to average the forces moving right and left with those moving up and down because this represents the frontal plane, lead I is the "pure" right/left lead, and lead aVF is the "pure" up/down lead; it is easiest to use these two perpendicular leads to calculate the mean axis. Figure 18-9A shows the frontal plane leads of a 12-lead ECG. Leads I and aVF are shown enlarged along with the axis wheel with small dash marks along the axes of lead I and lead aVF (Figure 18-9B). These dash marks represent the small, 1-mV boxes on the ECG paper. To determine the mean QRS axis, follow these steps:

1. Look at the QRS complex in lead I and count the number of positive and negative boxes. Mark the net vector along the appropriate end of lead I on the axis wheel. In Figure 18-9B, the QRS complex in lead I is

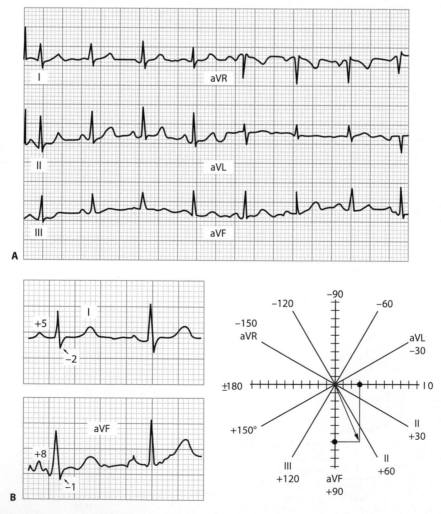

Figure 18-9. Calculating the mean QRS axis. **(A)** The six frontal plane leads of an ECG. **(B)** Leads I and aVF enlarged. See the text for instructions on calculating the axis using leads I and aVF on the axis wheel.

five boxes positive and two boxes negative, resulting in a net three boxes positive, or +3. Count three dash marks toward the positive end of lead I and put a mark on the axis wheel at that spot.

2. Look at the QRS complex in aVF and follow the same procedure as above. In this example, the QRS complex in aVF is eight boxes positive and has two very small negative deflections that equal approximately one box when combined, resulting in a net +7. Count seven dash marks along the positive end of aVF's axis and place a mark at that spot.

3. Draw a perpendicular line down from the mark on lead I's axis and a perpendicular line across from the mark on aVF's axis.

4. Draw a line from the center of the axis wheel to the spot where the two perpendicular lines meet. This line represents the mean QRS axis. In the example in Figure 18-9B, the axis is about +65°.

A quick but less precise method of axis determination is to place the axis in its proper quadrant of the axis wheel by looking at leads I and aVF, because these leads divide the wheel into four quadrants. As illustrated in Figure 18-10, if both of these leads are positive, the axis falls in the normal quadrant, 0° to +90°. If lead I is positive and aVF is negative, the axis falls in the left quadrant, 0° to −90°. If lead I is negative and aVF is positive, the axis falls in the right quadrant,

+90° to +180°. If both leads are negative, the axis falls in the right superior quadrant or "no-man's-land" −90° to −180°. Locating the correct quadrant is sometimes adequate, but because 30° of the left quadrant is considered normal, it is necessary to be more precise in describing the axis when it falls in the left quadrant. To "fine-tune" the axis when it is in the left quadrant, look at lead II. If lead II has a positive QRS, the axis is in the normal part of the left quadrant (0 to −30°); if it has a negative QRS, the axis is left deviated (−31° to −90°).

Using the ECG in Figure 18-11A, first place the axis in the appropriate quadrant by using leads I and aVF. Lead I is upright and aVF is negative, placing the axis in the left quadrant. However, because 30° of the left quadrant is considered normal, we need to fine-tune the axis to determine where within the left quadrant it actually falls. Since lead II is mostly negative, the axis is deviated to the left. The axis wheel shows how to count boxes in this example. The axis is −60°.

Using the ECG in Figure 18-11B, place the axis in the appropriate quadrant. Because lead I is negative and aVF is positive, the axis is in the right quadrant. The axis wheel shows how boxes are counted in this example. The axis is +130°.

Bundle Branch Block

When one of the bundle branches is blocked, the ventricles depolarize asynchronously. Bundle branch block is characterized by a delay of excitation to one ventricle and an abnormal spread of electrical activity through the ventricle whose bundle is blocked. This delayed conduction results in widening of the QRS complex to 0.12 second or more and a characteristic pattern best recognized in precordial leads V_1 and V_6 and limb leads I and aVL.

Normal ventricular depolarization as recorded by leads V_1 and V_6 is illustrated in Figure 18-12. The positive electrode for V_1 is located on the front of the chest at the fourth intercostal space to the right of the sternum, close to the right ventricle. The positive electrode for V_6 is located in the left midaxillary line at the fifth intercostal space, close to the left ventricle. Lead V_1 records a small R wave as the septum depolarizes from left to right toward the positive electrode. It then records a negative deflection (S wave) as the main forces travel away from the positive electrode toward the left ventricle, resulting in the normal rS complex in V_1. Lead V_6 may record a small Q wave as the septum depolarizes left to right away from the positive electrode. It then records a tall R wave as the main forces travel toward the left ventricle, resulting in the normal qR complex in V_6. When both ventricles depolarize together, the QRS width is less than 0.12 seconds.

Right Bundle Branch Block

The presence of a block in the right bundle branch causes a different spread of electrical forces in the ventricles and thus

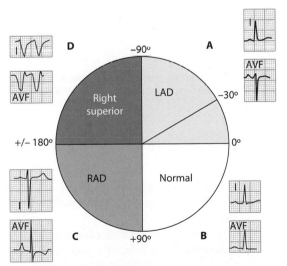

When the axis is in the left quadrant, look at lead II.
• If lead II has an upright QRS, the axis normal
• If lead II has a negative QRS, the axis is beyond −30° and there is left axis deviation

Figure 18-10. The four quadrants of the axis wheel. **(A)** Left axis deviation quadrant; lead I is positive and lead aVF is negative. When the axis falls in this quadrant, look at lead II: a positive QRS in lead II means the axis is in the normal portion of that quadrant (0° to −30°); a negative QRS in lead II means the axis in the left deviation portion (−31° to −90°). **(B)** Normal axis quadrant; leads I and aVF are both positive. **(C)** Right axis deviation quadrant; lead I is negative and lead aVF is positive. **(D)** Right superior quadrant; leads I and aVF are both negative.

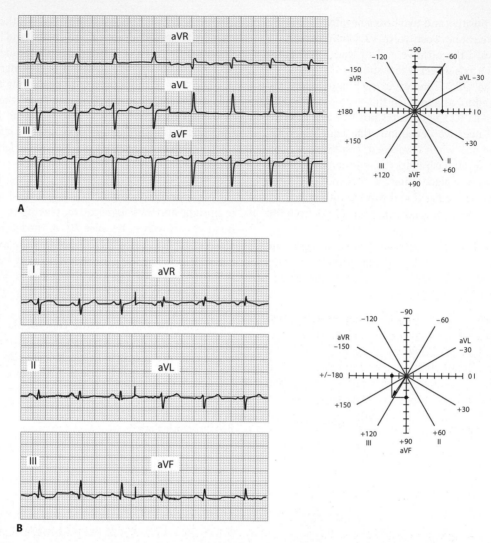

Figure 18-11. **(A)** Frontal plane leads demonstrating left axis deviation. Lead I is five boxes positive; aVF is two boxes positive and ten boxes negative for a net of −8. The axis is −60°. **(B)** Frontal plane leads demonstrating right axis deviation. Lead I is two boxes positive and four boxes negative for a net of −2; lead aVF is one box negative and four boxes positive for a net of +3. The axis is +120°.

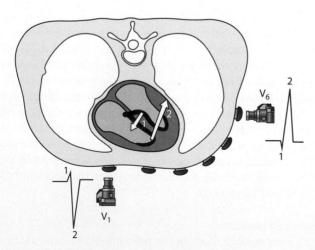

Figure 18-12. Normal ventricular depolarization as recorded by leads V_1 and V_6.

a different pattern to the QRS complex. Three separate forces occur, as seen in Figure 18-13A.

1. Septal activation occurs first from left to right (*arrow 1*), resulting in the normal small R wave in V_1 and small Q wave in V_6.
2. The left ventricle is activated next through the normally functioning left bundle branch. Depolarization spreads normally through the Purkinje fibers in the left ventricle (*arrow 2*), causing an S wave in V_1 as the impulse travels away from its positive electrode and an R wave in V_6 as the impulse travels toward the positive electrode in V_6.
3. The right ventricle depolarizes late and abnormally as the impulse spreads via cell-to-cell conduction through the right ventricle (*arrow 3*). This abnormal activation causes a wide second R wave (called R prime [R′]) in V_1 as it travels toward the positive electrode in V_1. It also results in a wide S wave in

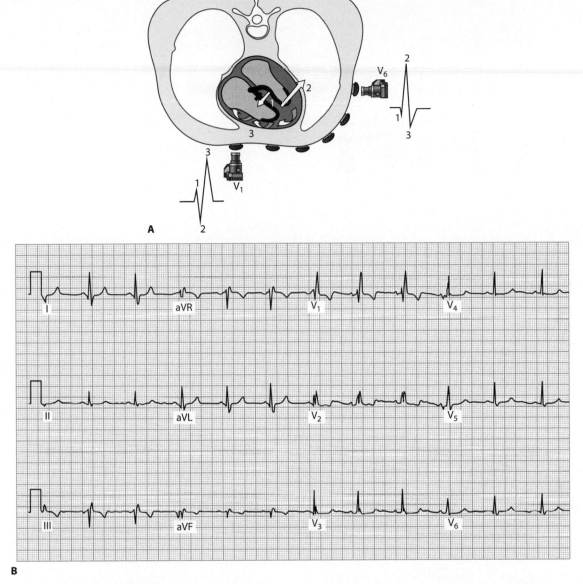

Figure 18-13. **(A)** Ventricular depolarization with RBBB as recorded by leads V_1 and V_6. **(B)** 12-lead ECG illustrating RBBB.

V_6 as it travels away from the positive electrode in V_6. Because muscle cell-to-cell conduction is much slower than conduction through the Purkinje system, the QRS complex widens to 0.12 seconds or greater.

RBBB can be recognized by a wide rSR′ pattern in V_1 and a wide qRs pattern in V_6, I, and aVL, because the positive electrode in these two limb leads is located on the left side of the body. The ECG in Figure 18-13B illustrates RBBB.

Left Bundle Branch Block

Figure 18-14 illustrates the spread of electrical forces through the ventricles when the left bundle branch is blocked. In LBBB, the septum does not depolarize in its normal left-to-right direction because the block occurs above the Purkinje fibers that normally activate the left side of the septum. This

results in the loss of the normal small R wave in V_1 and loss of the Q wave in V_6, I, and aVL. Two main forces occur in LBBB:

1. The right ventricle is activated first through the Purkinje fibers (*arrow 1*). Because the right ventricular free wall is so much thinner than that of the left ventricle, forces traveling through it are often not recorded in V_1. Sometimes a small, narrow R wave is recorded in V_1 during LBBB, and this wave is most likely the result of forces traveling through the right ventricular free wall.

2. The left ventricle depolarizes late and abnormally as the impulse spreads via cell-to-cell conduction through the thick left ventricle (*arrow 2*). This causes V_1 to record a wide negative QS complex as the impulse travels away from its positive electrode.

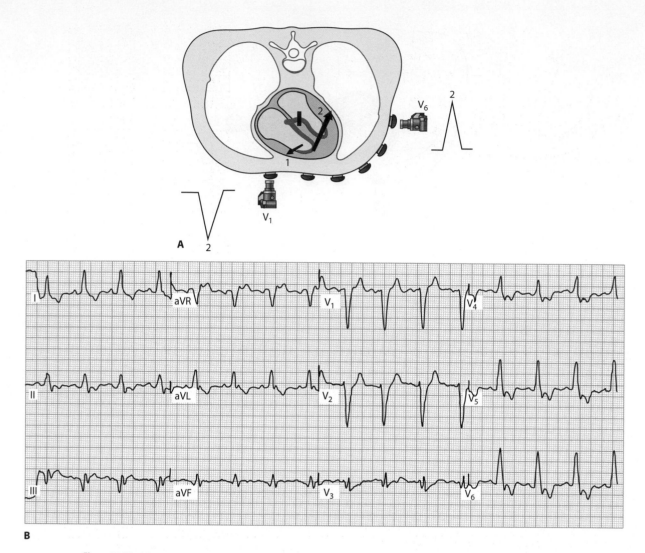

Figure 18-14. **(A)** Ventricular depolarization with LBBB as recorded by leads V_1 and V_6. **(B)** 12-lead ECG illustrating LBBB.

The lateral leads V_6, I, and aVL record a wide R wave as the impulse travels through the large left ventricle toward their positive electrodes. The QRS widens to 0.12 seconds or greater due to the slow cell-to-cell conduction in the left ventricle.

LBBB can be recognized by a wide QS complex in V_1 and wide R waves with no Q waves in V_6, I, and aVL. The ECG in Figure 18-14B illustrates LBBB.

Secondary ST Segment and T-Wave Changes in Bundle Branch Block

Whenever the ventricles depolarize abnormally as they do in bundle branch block, they also repolarize abnormally. This results in an ST segment and T wave that are directed opposite to the terminal portion (last half) of the QRS complex. For example, Figure 18-13 shows RBBB, in leads where the last part of the QRS is negative (eg, leads I, V_5, V_6) and the T wave is upright. In leads where the last part of the QRS is upright (eg, lead V_1), the T wave is negative. Figure 18-14 shows LBBB, and the leads in which the QRS is upright have

negative T waves (eg, leads I, V_4-V_6) while the leads with negative QRS complexes have upright T waves (eg, leads V_1, V_2). It is common for LBBB to present with ST elevation in leads V_1 and V_2 due to these secondary changes, which complicates the diagnosis of MI in the presence of LBBB. These same secondary T-wave changes are seen with ventricular beats, ventricular paced beats, and with ventricular preexcitation in Wolff-Parkinson-White (WPW) syndrome.

Acute Coronary Syndrome

The term *acute coronary syndrome* (ACS) refers to the pathophysiologic continuum that begins with plaque rupture in a coronary artery and ultimately results in cell necrosis (infarction), if the process is not arrested. ACS encompasses three distinct phases of this continuum: (1) unstable angina (UA), (2) non–ST-elevation MI (NSTEMI), and (3) ST-elevation MI (STEMI). The terms STEMI and NSTEMI refer to the presence or absence of ST elevation on the admission ECG in a patient who is having an MI as diagnosed by elevated

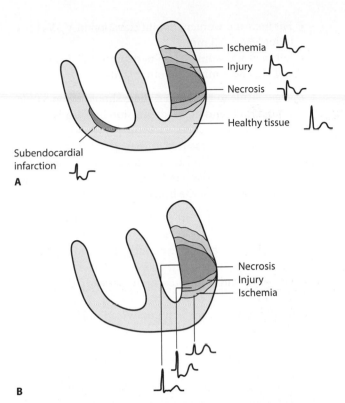

Figure 18-15. Zones of myocardial ischemia, injury, and infarction with associated ECG changes. **(A)** Indicative changes of ischemia, injury, and necrosis seen in leads facing the injured area. **(B)** Reciprocal changes often seen in leads not directly facing the involved area.

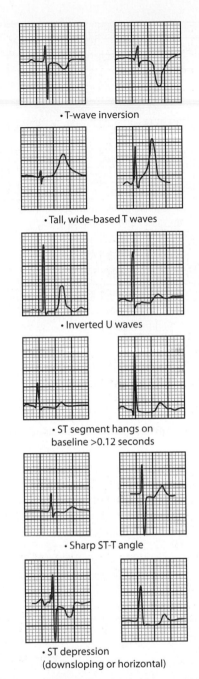

- T-wave inversion

- Tall, wide-based T waves

- Inverted U waves

- ST segment hangs on baseline >0.12 seconds

- Sharp ST-T angle

- ST depression (downsloping or horizontal)

Figure 18-16. ECG patterns associated with myocardial ischemia.

biochemical markers in the blood. Once an infarction has occurred, the terms Q-wave or non–Q-wave MI indicate the ultimate presence or absence of Q waves on the ECG.

MI can occur because of blockage of a coronary artery with thrombus or from severe and prolonged ischemia due to coronary artery spasm or unrelieved obstruction of a coronary artery. When infarction occurs, there are three "zones" of tissue damage, each producing characteristic changes on the ECG (Figure 18-15).

Myocardial ischemia can result in several changes on the ECG (Figure 18-16). The most familiar patterns of ischemia are horizontal or downsloping ST-segment depression of 0.5 mm or more, and T-wave inversion. Other indicators of ischemia include an ST segment that remains on the baseline longer than 0.12 seconds; an ST segment that forms a sharp angle with the upright T wave; tall, wide-based T waves; and inverted U waves. The ECG of patients who have *stable angina*, that is, angina that occurs with exertion or emotional stress and is relieved with rest or nitroglycerin, will sometimes show ST depression and/or T-wave inversion at rest, during pain episodes, or during exercise testing. However, the ECG may be normal in about 50% of patients who have stable angina.

Myocardial injury is most often indicated by ST-segment elevation in leads facing the infarcted area (Figure 18-17). The ST segment is measured at the J point (where the QRS complex joins the ST segment) or 60 msec after the J point

for continuous ST-segment monitoring. In clinical practice, the most common threshold values for ST-segment elevation in diagnosing MI is 2 mm in leads V_1-V_3, and 1 mm in all other leads. However, because the J point and ST segment position can vary depending on age, gender, and race, more specific recommendations for abnormal J point position have been recommended:

- For men 40 years of age and older: J point elevation 2 mm in leads V_2 and V_3, and 1 mm in all other leads.
- For men < 40 years of age: J point elevation 2.5 mm in leads V_2 and V_3.

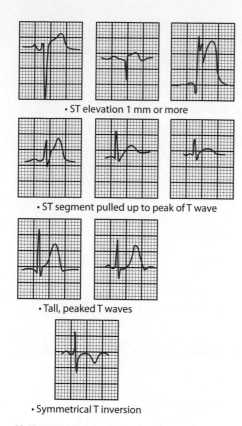

• ST elevation 1 mm or more

• ST segment pulled up to peak of T wave

• Tall, peaked T waves

• Symmetrical T inversion

Figure 18-17. ECG patterns associated with acute myocardial injury.

• For women: J point elevation 1.5 mm in leads V_2 and V_3, and 1 mm in all other leads.
• For men and women, J point elevation 0.5 mm in V_3R and V_4R (except for men <30 years of age where 1 mm of J point elevation in these leads is appropriate).

• For men and women, J point elevation in V_7-V_9 (posterior leads) 0.5 mm.
• For men and women, J point depression 0.5 mm in V_2 and V_3, and 1 mm in all other leads.

A general rule to remember: there should be no ST elevation in limb leads and no ST depression in V leads.

The diagnosis of acute ischemia/infarction is made when ST elevation is measured at the J point that equals or exceeds the above thresholds in two or more anatomically contiguous leads. Contiguous leads are neighboring leads that face the same area of the heart (Figure 18-5):

• Leads AVL and I are contiguous leads facing the lateral wall
• Leads II, AVF, and III are contiguous leads facing the inferior wall
• Leads V_1 and V_2 are contiguous leads that record septal forces
• Leads V_3 and V_4 are contiguous leads facing the anterior wall
• Leads V_5 and V_6 are contiguous leads facing the lateral wall

Other signs of acute injury include a straightening of the ST segment that slopes up to the peak of the T wave without spending any time on the baseline; tall, peaked T waves; and symmetric T-wave inversion.

Necrosis or death of myocardial tissue is indicated on the ECG by development of Q waves that are greater than 0.03 seconds wide or 25% of the ensuing R-wave amplitude (see Figures 18-5 to 18-7 for normal Q waves and Figures 18-18 and 18-19 for abnormal Q waves). Q waves can develop transiently with severe ischemia and with non–Q wave MI,

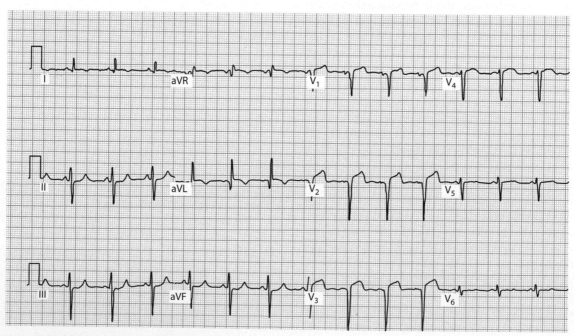

Figure 18-18. 12-lead ECG demonstrating acute anterior wall MI. Q waves are present in V_1 to V_3 and ST-segment elevation is present in V_1 to V_4. An abnormal Q wave is also present in aVL.

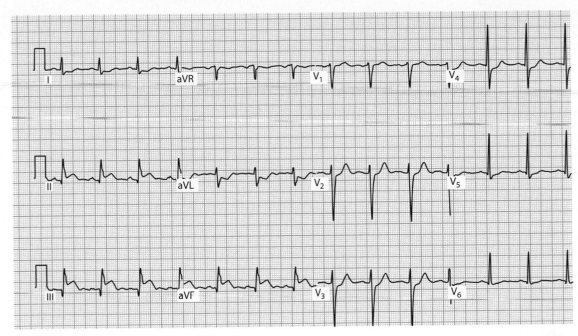

Figure 18-19. 12-lead ECG demonstrating acute inferior wall MI. ST elevation is present in II, III, and aVF; reciprocal ST depression is present in I, aVL, and V₂ to V₄. Q waves can be seen in III and aVF.

although Q waves are more commonly seen with necrosis that extends through the full thickness of the myocardial wall (transmural infarction). Necrosis that involves just the endocardial layer of the myocardium typically does not result in Q waves on the ECG and is referred to as a non–Q wave MI. In any case, the presence of abnormal Q waves is still considered to be ECG evidence of myocardial necrosis.

The ECG reflects the evolution of the infarction from the acute stage through the fully evolved stage. Very early MI often causes peaking and widening of the T waves followed within minutes by ST-segment elevation. ST-segment elevation can persist for hours to several days but resolves more quickly with successful reperfusion. Once the ST segment has returned to baseline, ECG evidence of the acute infarction stage is lost. Q waves appear within hours of pain onset and usually remain forever, although sometimes Q waves disappear with very early reperfusion. T-wave inversion occurs within hours after infarction and can last for months or remain inverted permanently. T waves often return to their previous upright position within a few months after acute MI. Thus, an *evolving infarct* is one in which serial ECGs show ST segments returning toward baseline, the development of Q waves, and T-wave inversion. The term *old infarction* or *infarct of undetermined age* is used when the first ECG recorded shows Q waves, ST segment at baseline, and T waves either inverted or upright, indicating that an MI occurred at some point in the past.

Following successful reperfusion of an acutely occluded coronary artery with percutaneous coronary intervention (PCI), the ST-segment elevation should resolve by 50% within 30 minutes. Patients whose ST segment resolves by <50% have higher rates of death, shock, and heart failure (HF). Similarly, T waves should invert along with ST segment returning toward baseline, and T waves should remain inverted for days to weeks. Early return of T waves to the upright position (pseudonormalization) or re-elevation of the ST segment may indicate reocclusion of the related artery and is not a good sign.

Locating the Infarction From the ECG

ST-segment elevation, Q waves, and T-wave inversion are recorded in leads facing the damaged myocardium and are called the *indicative changes of infarction*. Leads not facing the involved tissue often show changes related to the loss of electrical forces (depolarization and repolarization) in the damaged tissue. These leads record mirror-image changes that are called *reciprocal changes*. Figure 18-15 illustrates indicative and reciprocal changes associated with MI, and Table 18-2 lists leads in which indicative and reciprocal changes are found in each of the major types of MI.

TABLE 18-2. ECG CHANGES ASSOCIATED WITH MYOCARDIAL INFARCTION

Location of MI	Indicative Changes (ST Elevation)	Reciprocal Changes (ST Depression)
Anterior	V₁-V₄ (not necessarily all of these leads) aVR with proximal LAD occlusion	II, III, aVF, V5 with proximal LAD occlusion
Septal	V₁, V₂	V₅ with proximal LAD occlusion
Anterolateral	V₁-V₆, I, aVL	II, III, aVF
Inferior	II, III, aVF	I, aVL
Posterior	Posterior leads V₈, V₉	V₁-V₃
Lateral	I, aVL, V₅, V₆	II, III, aVF
Right ventricle	Right side leads V₃R-V₆R	

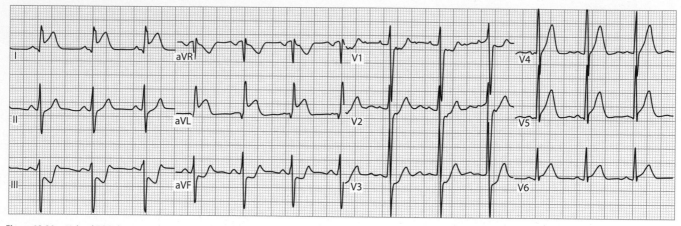

Figure 18-20. 12-lead ECG demonstrating acute lateral wall MI. ST elevation is present in leads I, aVL, V$_5$, and V$_6$ with reciprocal ST depression in leads II, III, aVF, V$_1$-V$_3$. The ST depression in V$_1$-V$_3$ is most likely due to coexisting acute posterior wall MI. Note the very large wide-based T waves in V$_4$-V$_6$, also a sign of acute injury.

Anterior wall MI is recognized by indicative changes in leads facing the anterior wall precordial leads V$_1$ to V$_4$ (see Figure 18-18). Reciprocal changes are often recorded in the inferior leads II, III, and aVF, and sometimes in V$_5$ with proximal left anterior descending (LAD) artery stenosis. Inferior wall MI is diagnosed by indicative changes in leads II, III, and aVF (see Figure 18-19), and reciprocal changes are often seen in leads I and aVL. Lateral wall MI presents with indicative changes in leads I, aVL, and/or V$_5$ and V$_6$, with reciprocal changes in leads II, III, and aVF (Figure 18-20). Posterior wall MI is less obvious because in the standard 12-lead ECG, there are no leads that face the posterior wall, and therefore there are no indicative changes recorded from the posterior wall. However, posterior wall infarction often accompanies inferior or lateral wall MI, so indicative changes from the inferior wall (Figure 18-21) or the lateral wall (Figure 18-20) are seen unless there is an isolated posterior wall infarction. The diagnosis is suspected when ST-segment depression is present in the anterior leads, especially V$_1$ and V$_2$ but often all the way to V$_4$. Reciprocal changes seen in these leads include a taller R wave than normal (mirror image of the Q wave that would be recorded over the posterior wall), ST-segment

depression (mirror image of the ST elevation from the posterior wall), and upright, tall T waves (mirror image of the T-wave inversion from the posterior wall). Posterior leads V$_7$, V$_8$, and V$_9$ should be recorded whenever posterior wall MI is suspected (Figure 18-22B).

Right ventricular MI occurs in up to 45% of inferior MIs; therefore, it usually is associated with indicative changes in the inferior leads II, III, and aVF (Figure 18-23). In addition, it is not uncommon to see ST elevation in V$_1$ as well, because V$_1$ is the chest lead that is closest to the right ventricle. ST elevation in V$_1$, together with ST elevation in the inferior leads, is suspicious for right ventricular MI. Another clue is discordance between the ST segment in V$_1$ and the ST segment in V$_2$. Normally, when the ST segment in V$_1$ is elevated, it is related to anterior or septal MI, in which case the ST in V$_2$ is also elevated. *Discordance* means that the ST segments do not point in the same direction—V$_1$ shows ST elevation while V$_2$ is either normal or shows ST depression. This finding is suspicious for right ventricular MI. The American Heart Association (AHA) and the American College of Cardiology (ACC) have recommended that right-sided chest leads V$_3$R and V$_4$R be recorded in all patients

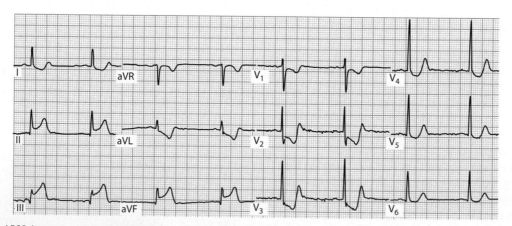

Figure 18-21. 12-lead ECG demonstrating acute inferior and posterior MI. ST elevation is present in leads II, III, and aVF (inferior leads), and ST depression is present in all of the V leads. ST depression in V$_1$ to V$_3$ is indicative of posterior MI. The ST depression in V$_4$ to V$_6$ is reciprocal to the inferior MI.

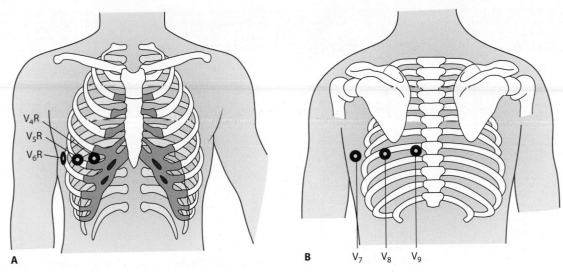

Figure 18-22. **(A)** Right side chest leads. V₄R at right fifth intercostal space, midclavicular line; V₅R at right fifth intercostal space, anterior axillary line; V₆R at right fifth intercostal space, midaxillary line. **(B)** Posterior leads: V₇ at posterior axillary line; V₈ at tip of scapula; V₉ next to spine.

presenting with ECG evidence of acute inferior wall infarction. Leads V_3R through V_6R develop ST elevation when acute right ventricular MI is present. Lead V_4R is the most sensitive and specific lead for recognition of right ventricular MI. Figure 18-22A shows location of right-sided chest leads and Figure 18-22B shows location of posterior leads.

Diagnosing MI in the Presence of Bundle Branch Block

Myocardial infarction alters the initial portion of the QRS complex and creates abnormal Q waves in leads facing the infarcted area. In addition, acute myocardial injury causes ST segment-elevation in leads facing the affected area. Bundle branch block causes similar changes in QRS morphology and secondary ST-T wave changes that can complicate the diagnosis of MI.

The diagnosis of MI in the presence of RBBB is the same as in patients with normal intraventricular conduction because the initial forces of depolarization are unchanged in RBBB. Therefore, the appearance of abnormal Q waves indicates acute MI just as it does in patients with normal conduction. In RBBB, secondary T-wave changes occur and T waves should be inverted in leads where the terminal portion of the

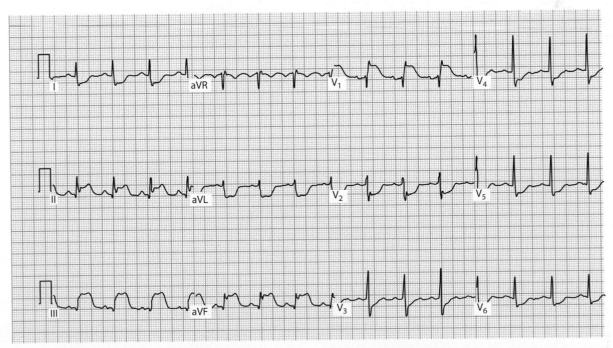

Figure 18-23. 12-lead ECG demonstrating acute right ventricular MI. ST elevation is present in II, III, aVF, and V₁; reciprocal ST depression is present in all other leads. Note the discordant ST elevation in V₁ and ST depression in V₂.

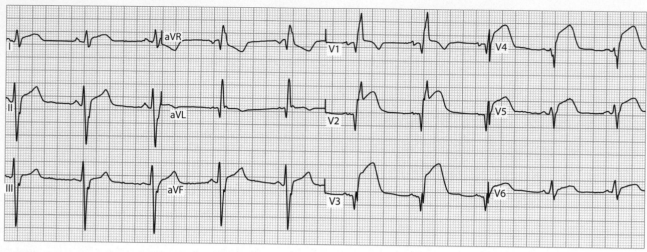

Figure 18-24. Acute anterior-lateral wall MI with RBBB. ST elevation is seen in leads I, V$_1$-V$_6$. Abnormal Q waves are present in V$_1$-V$_3$. The RBBB does not interfere with the ability to recognize this MI.

QRS is upright and upright in leads where the terminal portion of the QRS is negative. In the presence of RBBB, T waves that point the same direction as the terminal QRS complex indicate ischemia or injury. Figure 18-24 shows RBBB with an acute anterior-lateral wall MI.

The diagnosis of MI in the presence of LBBB is more complicated because LBBB alters both the initial and terminal portions of ventricular activation and produces secondary ST-T changes that can mimic MI. LBBB causes the septum to depolarize from right to left instead of from left to right, which causes a loss of the normal septal R waves in the anterior chest leads and creates a QS pattern in V$_1$ and V$_2$ that mimics septal infarction. The secondary ST and T-wave changes that occur in LBBB cause ST elevation in the anterior leads that mimics anterior wall MI. The following criteria help recognize ischemia or infarction in the presence of LBBB:

- ST elevation ≥ 1 mm in the same direction as the QRS complex (in uncomplicated LBBB, the ST segment is either isoelectric or directed opposite to the QRS)

- ST depression ≥ 1 mm in lead V$_1$, V$_2$, or V$_3$ (in uncomplicated LBBB, the ST is usually elevated slightly in these leads)
- ST elevation ≥ 5 mm in the opposite direction from the QRS complex (in uncomplicated LBBB, this secondary ST elevation is less than 5 mm)

While these criteria may help identify ischemia or infarction in the presence of LBBB, their sensitivity and specificity are low. It is helpful to have old ECGs available for comparison and look for changes in serial ECGs when a patient with chronic LBBB is suspected of having an acute MI. Figure 18-25 shows LBBB with signs of acute MI.

Unstable Angina and Non-ST Elevation Myocardial Infarction

Both UA and NSTEMI can present on the ECG with ST-segment depression and/or T-wave inversion. The differentiation between the two can only be made by assessing cardiac biomarkers, specifically troponin. In UA, initial troponin level is normal; in NSTEMI, the troponin is elevated. ST depression in multiple leads that occurs at rest

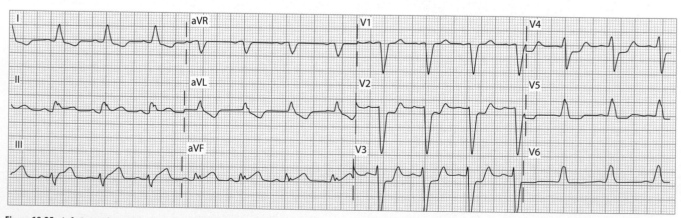

Figure 18-25. Inferior and possibly posterior MI with LBBB. The QRS and T waves are concordant in leads II and AVF where they should be discordant in uncomplicated LBBB; there is ST depression in leads V$_2$-V$_4$ where the ST segments should be slightly elevated leads with a predominantly negative QRS in uncomplicated LBBB.

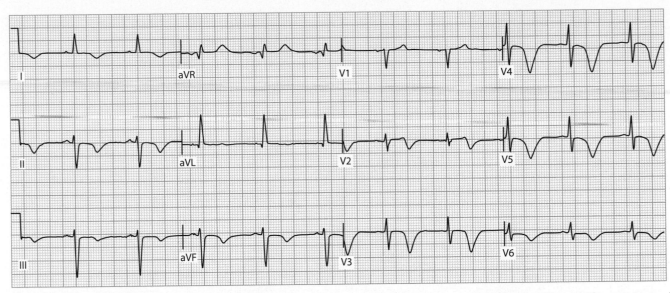

Figure 18-26. ECG of a patient with resting chest pain showing widespread and deep symmetrically inverted T waves indicating unstable angina (if troponin is normal) or NSTEMI (if troponin is elevated).

is associated with severe multivessel or left main coronary artery disease. Deep symmetrical T-wave inversion is not normal and can be seen with UA or NSTEMI. Terminal T-wave inversion refers to T waves that start out upright and then dip below the isoelectric line. This type of T-wave inversion seen in leads V_1-V_3 and sometimes to V_4 in a patient with chest pain at rest (UA), is called "Wellen's Warning" and is associated with significant proximal left anterior coronary artery stenosis. The presence of terminal T-wave inversion or deep symmetrical T-wave inversion in V_1-V_3 in a patient with chest pain should be considered indicative of LAD disease, and prompt catheterization is indicated. An ECG showing signs of ischemia (ST depression or T-wave inversion) in at least eight leads and ST elevation in leads AVR and/or V_1 can indicate significant left main coronary artery stenosis or significant triple vessel coronary disease. Figure 18-26 shows widespread T-wave

inversion in a patient with resting chest pain. Figure 18-27 shows ST depression or T-wave inversion in multiple leads, with ST elevation in AVR and V_1 in a patient with resting chest pain and a normal troponin.

Effects of Electrolyte Imbalances on the ECG

Electrolyte imbalances are diagnosed by measuring serum levels, but the ECG can be suggestive of electrolyte abnormalities. Recognizing potassium imbalances is particularly important because potassium is critical in regulating cardiac electrical activity. Magnesium abnormalities, especially hypomagnesemia, can contribute to QT prolongation and arrhythmias (torsade de pointes) and are most often associated with other electrolyte abnormalities. Sodium imbalances do not produce specific ECG changes. Potassium and calcium abnormalities can cause distinctive changes on the ECG and are reviewed here.

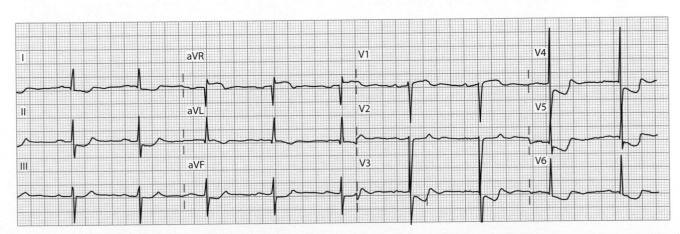

Figure 18-27. ECG of a patient with chest pain showing ischemic changes (ST depression or T-wave inversion) in leads I, II, AVL, AVF, V_2-V_6, and ST elevation in AVR and V_1. This is indicative of left main coronary artery disease or significant triple vessel disease.

ESSENTIAL CONTENT CASE

Acute MI

You are admitting a 56-year-old man complaining of 8/10 chest pain. His wife says he has been having intermittent chest pain associated with exertion for the last 6 months but has refused to see a physician. She says his pain usually goes away when he lies down, but today his pain occurred while sitting in a chair watching TV and is much more severe than usual. It has lasted for over an hour so she made him come to the ED.

This is his initial ECG on admission to ED:

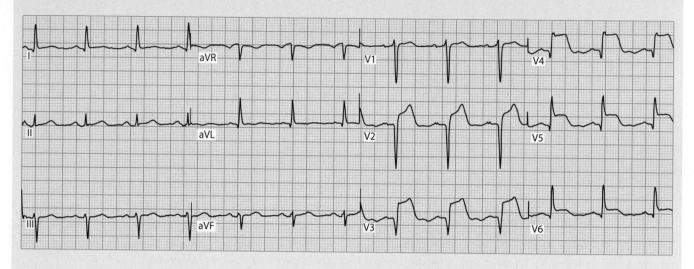

Question 1: What does his history of intermittent chest pain that is relieved by rest indicate?

Question 2: What is your interpretation of his admission ECG? Signs of ischemia/injury? Rhythm, QRS axis, bundle branch block?

He is transferred to the cardiac cath lab where he receives a stent to the LAD. This is his ECG recorded an hour after he returned to your unit following his PCI:

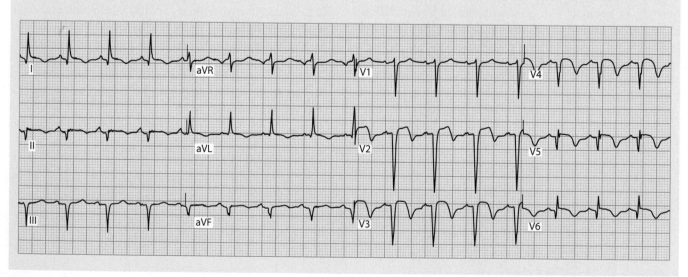

Question 3: What changes have occurred on his ECG after his procedure? Are you happy with this ECG?

The following day, this is his routine ECG:

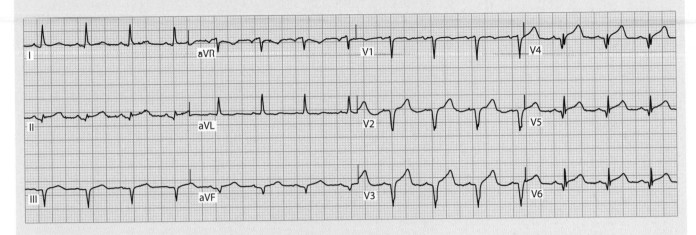

Question 4: What changes do you see? Are you happy with this ECG?

Answers

1. A history of intermittent chest pain that is brought on by exertion and relieved by rest is typical of stable angina.
2. His admission ECG shows an acute anterior-lateral wall MI with ST elevation and Q waves in leads V_2-V_6. The rhythm is sinus, the QRS axis is normal, and there is no bundle branch block.
3. The ECG following his PCI procedure shows that ST elevation has decreased by over 50% in leads V_3 and V_4, the leads that showed the highest ST elevation on admission. ST elevation has also decreased in V_2, V_5, and V_6 and T waves are inverted in V_2-V_6. The QRS axis has shifted slightly to the left. You should be happy with this ECG as it shows the expected ST resolution and T-wave inversion seen with successful reperfusion.
4. This ECG shows upright T waves in V_2-V_6 compared to inverted T waves in those leads following his PCI. This "pseudonormalization" of T waves could be an indicator of early reocclusion of his infarct-related artery and is NOT a good sign. Once T waves have inverted, they should remain inverted for weeks to months. He should be carefully assessed for pain and his physician should be notified. A return trip to the cardiac catheterization lab may be required.

Hyperkalemia

Normal potassium level is 3.5 to 5.0 mEq/L. Mild hyperkalemia is K^+ between 5.1 and 6.0 mEq/L, moderate hyperkalemia is K^+ between 6.1 and 7.0 mEq/L, and severe hyperkalemia is K^+ >7 mEq/L. As the potassium level progressively rises, serial ECG changes are usually seen, although it is not possible to determine the exact potassium level based on ECG changes (Figure 18-28). Some patients can have significant hyperkalemia without any ECG changes. The first change typically seen is tall peaked T waves and shortening of the QT interval. At a potassium of about 6.5 mEq/L, P waves begin to widen and flatten, the PR interval prolongs, and eventually P waves disappear. As the potassium rises >7mEq/L, there is progressive QRS widening with bizarre morphology and eventually the QRS merges with the T wave and appears as a sine wave pattern. Bradycardia, bundle branch blocks, and AV blocks can occur. Moderate to severe hyperkalemia can cause ST-segment elevation that can mimic MI. At very high levels, asystole, pulseless electrical activity, and death occur. Figure 18-29 is an example of hyperkalemia.

Hypokalemia

Hypokalemia, potassium levels less than 3.5 mEq/L causes flattening of T waves, ST depression, and enlarged U waves. The T wave often merges with the large U wave to create a T-U combination that prolongs the QT interval. Hypokalemia can cause ventricular ectopy and torsades de pointes (TdP) and potentiates digitalis toxicity. Figure 18-30 is an example of hypokalemia.

Hypercalcemia

Normal calcium levels vary with age, sex, and physiological status. In adults, a normal total Ca^{++} level is 8.9 to 10 mg/dL and a normal ionized (not attached to proteins) Ca^{++} level is 4.8 to 5.7 mg/dL. The primary ECG change that occurs with hypercalcemia is shortening of the ST segment which also shortens the QT interval. With severe hypercalcemia, Osbourn waves (also called J waves) may be seen as a notch at the end of the QRS complex. Figure 18-31 is an example of hypercalcemia.

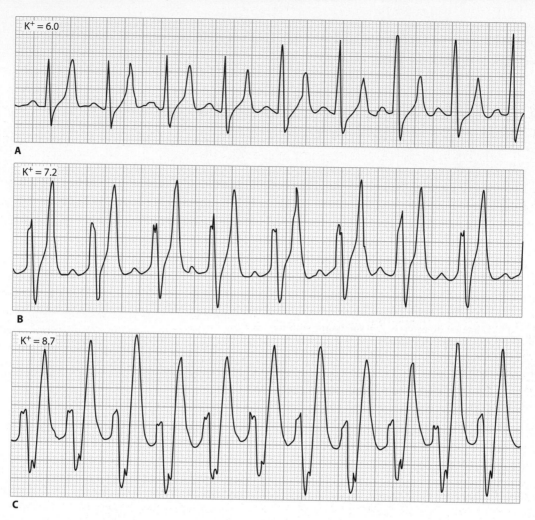

Figure 18-28. Rhythm strips showing the progressive changes of hyperkalemia. **(A)** Tall pointed T waves—usually the first sign. **(B)** QRS widens, T waves become even larger. **(C)** QRS even wider, P waves have disappeared.

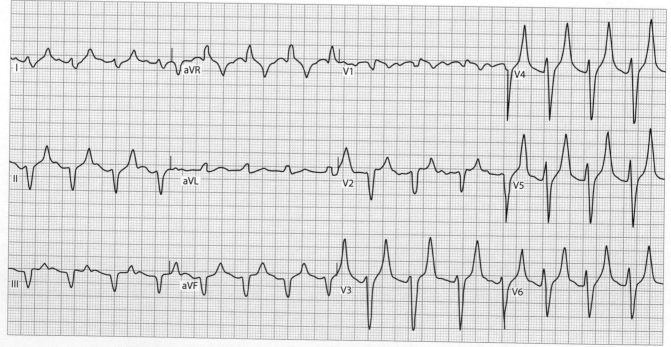

Figure 18-29. ECG of a patient showing large T waves of hyperkalemia. Potassium level was 7.8 mEq/L.

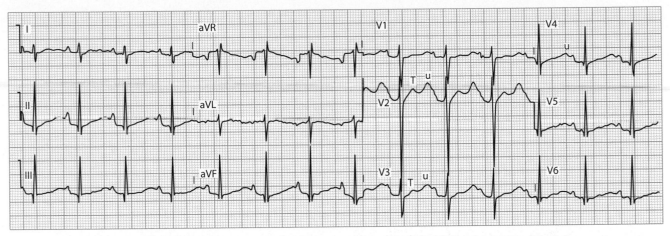

Figure 18-30. ECG showing large U waves and prolonged QT interval of hypokalemia. Potassium level was 2.6 mEq/L.

Hypocalcemia

Hypocalcemia prolongs the ST segment and thus also prolongs the QT interval. T waves usually remain normal. The long ST segment can also be seen in Type 3 Long QT syndrome, but T waves are often abnormal in that case. Figure 18-32 is an example of hypocalcemia.

Preexcitation Syndromes

Preexcitation means early activation of the ventricle by supraventricular impulses that reach the ventricle through an accessory conduction pathway faster than they travel through the AV node. Many people have tracts of tissue, often referred to as "bypass tracts" or "accessory pathways," that can carry electrical impulses directly from atria to ventricles, bypassing the delay in the AV node and causing early and abnormal depolarization of the ventricles. These accessory pathways can be found anywhere around the tricuspid or mitral valve rings. The most common type of preexcitation syndrome is the WPW syndrome, in which the impulse travels down the accessory pathway from the atria directly into the ventricles, completely bypassing AV node delay. Other anatomic connections exist that can bypass the normal AV

node delay or create connections between different parts of the conduction system and the ventricles and cause variations of the preexcitation pattern. Fibers originating in the atria and inserting into the bundle of His have been demonstrated anatomically and can result in a short PR interval and normal QRS complex (formerly called Lown-Ganong-Levine syndrome).

Wolff-Parkinson-White Syndrome

In WPW syndrome, the ventricle is stimulated prematurely by an electrical impulse traveling through the accessory pathway while the impulse simultaneously descends normally through the AV node (Figure 18-33A). Impulses travel faster through the accessory pathway because they bypass the normal AV node delay. Part of the ventricle receives the impulse early via the accessory pathway and begins to depolarize before the rest of the ventricle is activated through the His-Purkinje system. Early stimulation of the ventricle results in a short PR interval and a widened QRS complex as the impulse begins to depolarize the ventricle via muscle cell-to-cell conduction. Premature stimulation of the ventricle causes a characteristic slurring of the initial part of the QRS complex, called a delta wave. The remainder of

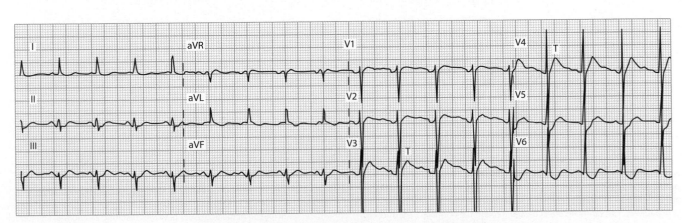

Figure 18-31. ECG showing hypercalcemia. Note very short QT interval.

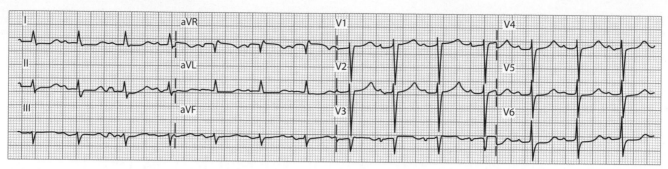

Figure 18-32. ECG showing hypocalcemia. Note long ST segment that prolongs the QT interval.

the QRS complex is normal because the rest of the ventricle is depolarized normally through the Purkinje system. This preexcitation results in ventricular fusion beats as the ventricles are depolarized simultaneously by the impulse coming through the accessory pathway and through the normal AV node. The degree of preexcitation varies, depending on the relative rates of conduction down the accessory pathway and through the AV node, and it determines the length of the PR interval and size of the delta wave (Figure 18-33).

WPW syndrome is recognized on the ECG by the presence of a short PR interval (<0.12 second) and delta waves in many leads. Figure 18-34 shows two examples of this type of pattern. Preexcitation syndromes are clinically significant because the presence of two pathways into the ventricle is a setup for reentrant tachycardias, which occur frequently in people with accessory pathways and are a part of the "syndrome" of WPW. See the section Supraventricular

Tachycardias later in this chapter for more information on dysrhythmias associated with accessory pathways.

Treatment

WPW syndrome does not require treatment unless it is associated with symptomatic tachycardias. Specific therapy depends on the mechanism of the tachyarrhythmia, the effect of drugs on conduction through the AV node and the accessory pathway, and on the patient's tolerance of the dysrhythmia. The section on supraventricular tachycardias later in this chapter discusses drug treatment of tachycardias associated with accessory pathways.

Radiofrequency (RF) catheter ablation of the bypass tract provides a cure for the tachyarrhythmias associated with accessory pathways in many patients. RF ablation is an invasive procedure that requires the introduction of several catheters into the heart through the venous and sometimes

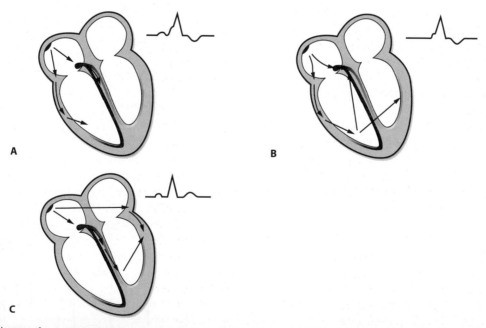

Figure 18-33. Varying degrees of preexcitation **(A)** Ventricles are activated by the impulse traveling through both the normal AV conduction system and the accessory pathway. Preexcitation of the ventricle via the accessory pathway results in a short PR interval and a delta wave on the ECG. **(B)** Maximal preexcitation as the ventricles are activated totally by the accessory pathway. The entire QRS is wide and the PR interval is so short that the P wave is on the upstroke of the QRS. **(C)** Concealed accessory pathway. The ventricles are activated through the normal AV conduction system with no participation of the accessory pathway, resulting in a normal PR interval and normal QRS complex.

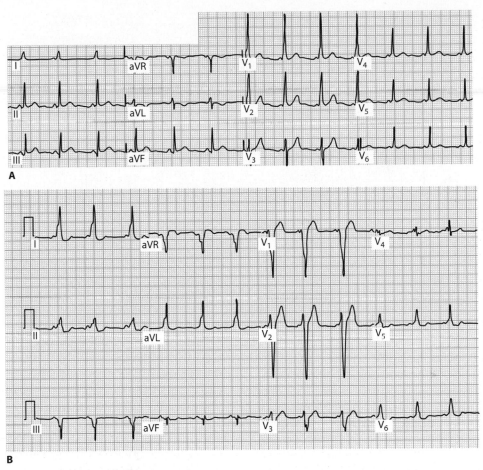

Figure 18-34. **(A)** 12-lead ECG demonstrating Wolff-Parkinson-White syndrome with short PR interval and delta waves. Lead V_1 is positive, indicating a posterior accessory pathway. **(B)** Wolff-Parkinson-White syndrome with short PR and delta waves with a negative V_1, indicating an anterior or right-sided accessory pathway.

arterial systems. An electrophysiology study is done first to record intracardiac signals and determine the mechanism of tachycardia. The electrophysiology study confirms the presence and location of the accessory pathway, participation of the pathway in maintaining the tachycardia, and conduction characteristics of the accessory pathway. A special ablation catheter is then positioned next to the bypass tract and RF energy is delivered through the catheter to the tract, destroying the tissue and preventing it from being able to conduct. Permanent tissue damage in the accessory pathway is the goal of RF ablation, and when successful, it prevents further episodes of tachycardia.

Brugada Syndrome

Brugada syndrome (BrS) is an inherited channelopathy involving mutations of the genes that regulate the function of sodium, calcium, or potassium channels in the cardiac cell membrane. Abnormalities of the SCN5A gene affecting sodium channels are the most common gene mutation associated with BrS. It is associated with a high incidence of VT/VF and sudden cardiac death (SCD) in people with structurally normal hearts. BrS is estimated to be responsible for at least 4% of all sudden deaths and at least 20% of sudden

deaths in patients with structurally normal hearts. SCD is the first symptom in about 4.6% of patients with BrS, but many people with the typical ECG pattern of BrS are totally asymptomatic. It is seen worldwide but is most prevalent in Southeast Asia, occurs most often in men (8:1 male-to-female ratio), and typically manifests in the third or fourth decade of life. Life-threatening arrhythmias usually occur at rest or during sleep.

BrS is characterized by ST-segment elevation and an RBBB-type QRS pattern in leads V_1 and/or V_2, typically without the dominant S waves in the lateral leads that is seen with true RBBB. Three patterns of ST elevation were initially described, but current consensus is that there are two patterns typical of BrS (Figure 18-35): (1) type 1 ECG pattern with a coved ST-segment elevation more than or equal to 2 mm, descending with an upward convexity into a negative T wave; (2) type 2 ECG pattern with a saddle-back shaped ST elevation of more than or equal to 0.5 mm followed by an upright or biphasic T wave. Only the type 1 pattern is considered diagnostic (Figure 18-36). BrS is diagnosed by the presence of a type 1 or coved-type ST-segment elevation in V_1 or V_2 recorded in the second, third, or fourth intercostal space either spontaneously or after drug testing with IV sodium

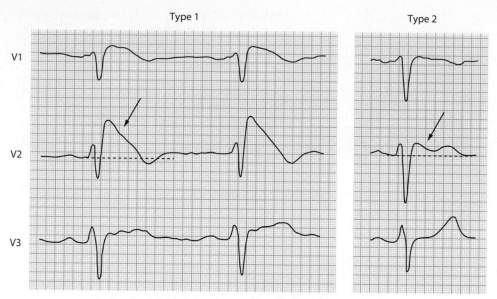

Figure 18-35. Two ECG patterns of Brugada syndrome. Type I shows the coved ST-segment elevation and T-wave inversion and is considered the diagnostic pattern. Type 2 shows the saddle-back type ST elevation with an inverted T wave in V_1 and upright T wave in V_2.

channel blockers. Previous diagnostic criteria required the presence of at least one of the following conditions: documented VF or polymorphic VT, a family history of SCD at a young age (<45 years), a type 1 ECG in family members, otherwise unexplained syncope, nocturnal agonal respiration, or inducibility of VT/VF with programmed electrical stimulation. The currently accepted definition of BrS no longer requires the presence of these additional criteria as long as the type I ECG pattern is present in V_1 or V_2. The diagnosis is also established when a type 2 ECG pattern present at baseline converts to the diagnostic type 1 pattern after sodium channel blocker administration. These characteristic ECG changes are transient or variable in some patients, thus the ECG can be nondiagnostic even when BrS is present.

The mainstay of therapy for BrS is an implantable cardioverter defibrillator (ICD). ICD implantation is a class I recommendation for survivors of cardiac arrest due to VF or hemodynamically unstable sustained VT not because of a reversible cause, and a class IIa recommendation for patients with BrS who have had syncope or documented VT. Quinidine is the only drug that has been shown to be effective in preventing ventricular dysrhythmias in patients with BrS. The best way to manage asymptomatic BrS patients is still debated.

The QT Interval and Long-QT Syndromes

The QT interval is measured from the beginning of the QRS complex to the end of the T wave and is used clinically as a reflection of ventricular repolarization time. The QT interval is heart rate dependent; it shortens at faster heart rates and lengthens at slower heart rates, therefore, the measured QT interval must be corrected for heart rate (QTc = QT corrected for heart rate). A normal QTc is less than 0.46 seconds (460 msec) in women and less than 0.45 seconds (450 msec) in men. A prolonged QTc indicates abnormally prolonged ventricular repolarization and is associated with TdP and SCD. The most commonly used method of correcting the measured QT interval for heart rate is the Bazett's formula:

QTc = measured QT interval divided by the square root of the preceding R-R interval (all measurements in seconds).

Figure 18-37 illustrates how to use the Bazett's formula. A QTc more than 500 msec increases the risk of developing TdP.

Long-QT syndrome (LQTS) can be acquired or congenital. The acquired type is usually due to medications that

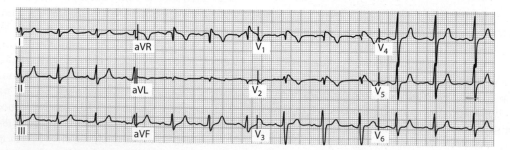

Figure 18-36. 12-lead ECG showing type I Brugada pattern in a young man with syncope.

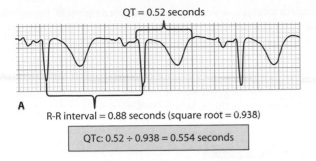

QT = 0.52 seconds

R-R interval = 0.88 seconds (square root = 0.938)

QTc: 0.52 ÷ 0.938 = 0.554 seconds

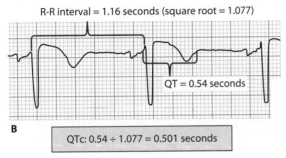

R-R interval = 1.16 seconds (square root = 1.077)

QT = 0.54 seconds

QTc: 0.54 ÷ 1.077 = 0.501 seconds

Figure 18-37. Two examples showing Bazett correction for measured QT intervals.

prolong ventricular repolarization or to electrolyte abnormalities, especially hypokalemia or hypomagnesemia. The congenital type is owing to gene mutations that affect ion channels on the cardiac cell membrane and is hereditary. Both types of QT-interval prolongation increase the risk of TdP and can be a cause of SCD.

Table 18-3 lists indications for QTc monitoring from the AHA practice standards for ECG monitoring in hospitalized patients.

Each facility should develop a protocol that defines a single consistent method of QT-interval monitoring that is used by all clinicians responsible for cardiac monitoring. The protocol should define the equipment used (manual or electronic), the method for determining the end of the T wave, the formula for heart-rate correction, criteria for lead selection, and require that whichever lead is chosen should be used for serial measurements in the same patient.

The American Association of Critical-Care Nurses (AACN) practice alert on dysrhythmia monitoring in adults lists the following guidelines for QT interval monitoring:

1. Measure QT interval and calculate QTc (rate-adjusted QT interval) by using the same lead where there is a T-wave amplitude of at least 2 mm and a clearly identified T-wave end.

2. Do not include a distinctly separate U wave in the measurement of the QT interval.

3. Assess and document QTc at least once per shift in patients who meet criteria for QT interval monitoring as identified in the American Heart Association Scientific Statement: Practice Standards for Electrocardiographic Monitoring in Hospital Settings. Also

TABLE 18-3. INDICATIONS FOR QTc MONITORING OF HOSPITALIZED PATIENTS BY PATIENT POPULATION

Drug Initiation
1. Patients with or without risk factors for TdP who are started on antiarrhythmic drugs with known risk for TdP (dofetilide, ibutilide, sotalol, disopyramide, procainamide, quinidine) (Class I) a. Factors determining duration of QTc monitoring: 1. QTc return to baseline 2. Drug half-life 3. Time to drug elimination dependent on hepatic or renal function 4. Presence of QT-related arrhythmias b. Continue monitoring for 48-72 hours for patients initiating or increasing dose of disopyramide, procainamide, quinidine, and sotalol.
2. Patients with or without risk factors for TdP who are started on antiarrhythmic drugs with possible risk for TdP (amiodarone, dronedarone, flecainide)—QT monitoring may be reasonable (Class IIb)
3. Patients with history of prolonged QTc or with general risk factors for TdP who are started on nonantiarrhythmic drugs with risk for TdP. a. QTc monitoring recommended with drugs with known risk (Class I) b. QT monitoring is reasonable with drugs with possible or conditional risk (Class IIa)
4. Patients without history of prolonged QTc or without general risk factors for TdP who are started on nonantiarrhythmic drugs with risk for TdP— QTc monitoring not indicated (Class III)

Targeted Temperature Management
1. QTc monitoring recommended until (Class I): a. Temperature normalized b. QTc interval in normal range c. No evidence of QT-related arrhythmias

Congenital LQTS
1. Patients with inherited LQTS who present with unstable ventricular arrhythmias—monitor until stabilization of ventricular arrhythmias (Class I)
2. Patients with inherited LQTS who have medically or metabolically induced prolongation of QTc—monitor until exacerbating medical or metabolic condition is reversed (Class I)

consider QTc monitoring as a routine practice in patients with one or more risk factors for TdP.

4. Assess QTc more frequently in patients with baseline QTc prolongation, the initiation or dosage increase of a drug that prolongs QTc, or in patients with other warning signs for TdP observed on the monitor.

5. Assess QTc before and after administration of a medication that prolongs the QTc by using the same lead, the same device, and the same formula for heart-rate correction.

6. Use QTc to differentiate TdP from polymorphic ventricular tachycardia (PVT) with normal QT interval.

7. Report a QTc greater than 0.50 seconds (500 msec) or any increase in the QTc of more than 0.06 second (60 msec) after administration of a QTc-prolonging medication. Report any new finding of a QTc greater than 0.50 seconds (500 msec).

8. Review the patient's medication list for actual or potential QT-prolonging medications whenever QT prolongation is a concern. Consider collaboration with a clinical pharmacist when reviewing the medication profile.

Acquired Long-QT Syndrome

The most common cause of acquired LQTS is pharmacologic therapy. Many medications prolong the QT interval by inhibiting potassium channels that are responsible for repolarization of cardiac cells. The most common classes of drugs that prolong the QT interval and cause TdP include antiarrhythmics, antibiotics, antipsychotic and antidepressant drugs, antihistamines, and gastric motility agents. A list of drugs commonly associated with TdP is available at www.crediblemeds.com but also may be found in selected drug references and/or hospital pharmacies. Episodes of TdP in the acquired form of LQTS are most commonly precipitated by short-long RR intervals, such as those caused by a ventricular premature beat (short cycle) followed by a compensatory pause (long cycle). Episodes of TdP are also associated with bradycardia or frequent pauses in the rhythm, thus, the acquired type is commonly referred to as pause-dependent LQTS.

The risk of developing TdP from medications increases in the presence of hypokalemia or hypomagnesemia, high doses or rapid intravenous (IV) infusion of QT-prolonging agents, or combined use of multiple medications that also prolong the QT interval or slow medication metabolism. Other risk factors for TdP include HF or myocardial ischemia, liquid protein weight-loss diets or starvation, bradycardia or sudden pauses in rhythm, acute neurological events (eg, subarachnoid hemorrhage), older age, female sex, and genetic predisposition to QT prolongation. Significant changes in QTc after initiation of a medication associated with TdP include an increase in QTc of more than 60 msec from the baseline QTc, or a QTc more than 500 msec. Other warning signs of TdP during medication administration include widening or distortion of the T wave, development of enlarged U waves or T-U waves, exaggerated T-U wave distortion on beats terminating pauses, T-wave alternans (alternating T-wave amplitude from beat to beat), and premature ventricular contraction (PVC) couplets or short runs of polymorphic VT occurring on the T wave of the beat terminating a pause.

Treatment of TdP includes identifying and managing the cause, discontinuing any causative agents, and correcting electrolyte imbalances. IV magnesium can be administered to control episodes of TdP until the cause is corrected.

Overdrive atrial or ventricular pacing at a rate of 80 beats/min or faster can prevent the pauses that may precipitate episodes of TdP and cause the QT interval to shorten as the heart rate is increased. Pacing and magnesium are temporary management strategies until the cause is eliminated. If TdP becomes sustained or degenerates into VF, defibrillation with an unsynchronized shock is required to terminate the episode.

Congenital Long-QT Syndromes

Congenital LQTS involves mutations in several genes that control potassium or sodium channels on cardiac cells. Fourteen different types of congenital LQTS have been identified and are named LQT1 through LQT14. The three most common are LQT1, LQT2, and LQT3, which are responsible for up to 90% of genotyped cases of LQTS. LQT1 and LQT2 are due to mutations of genes that affect potassium channel function (KCNQ1 and KCNH2), and LQT3 is because of mutations of the SCN5A gene that affects sodium channel function. The three main types of mutations all present with long QT intervals but differ from each other in several ways. The ECG in LQT1 often has wide, broad-based T waves that cause the prolonged QT interval, and dysrhythmia events often occur during physical activity, especially swimming or diving. In LQT2, the ECG often shows notched T waves in multiple leads, and dysrhythmia events are typically triggered by emotional upset or loud noises, such as alarm clocks or telephones. LQT3 usually shows long-ST segments, which are responsible for the long-QT interval, and dysrhythmia events commonly occur at rest or during sleep. T-wave abnormalities are often present in all three types. There is overlap between these types in terms of ECG and clinical presentation. Figure 18-38 illustrates the three main types of congenital LQTS.

Patients with congenital LQTS often present in childhood or in their teens. They may be asymptomatic and their LQTS is incidentally discovered when they are screened after a syncopal episode or when a family member is diagnosed with LQTS. Symptoms can range from palpitations and dizziness to seizures to cardiac arrest. The diagnosis is made by family history and a careful review of symptoms, triggering events if they can be identified, and the ECG. Genetic testing can identify the genotype and help direct therapy.

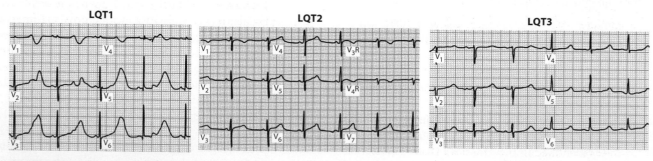

Figure 18-38. Representative V leads from the three major types of LQTS. The LQT1 patient is a 2-year-old girl who is in second-degree AV block with 2:1 conduction. The LQT2 patient is a 13-year-old girl who had a cardiac arrest at a slumber party. The LQT3 patient is a 17-year-old boy who had a "seizure."

Treatment depends on severity of symptoms and risk stratification. Lifestyle modifications include avoiding competitive sports and extreme exertion, especially swimming in LQT1 patients. Patients with LQT2 should avoid startling loud noises such as alarm clocks or telephones. Hypokalemia and hypomagnesemia must be avoided, and electrolyte loss due to vomiting, sweating, etc, should be replaced. All LQTS patients should avoid medications known to prolong the QT interval. Beta-blockers are the mainstay of medical therapy for all patients with LQTS and are especially effective in decreasing the incidence of exercise-induced events and SCD in LQT1 and LQT2 patients. They are less effective in LQT3. ICD implantation is a class I recommendation for any patient who has had a cardiac arrest owing to VT or VF in which no reversible cause is identified. ICD is a class IIa recommendation for patients with LQTS who have syncope and/or VT while receiving beta-blockers.

ADVANCED DYSRHYTHMIA INTERPRETATION

The study of cardiac rhythms provides a never-ending challenge to those interested in learning about dysrhythmias. In most basic ECG classes, the content presented is limited to basic rhythms originating in the sinus node, atria, AV junction, and ventricles, and to basic AV conduction abnormalities, all of which are described in Chapter 3 of this text. Rarely does time permit the inclusion of more advanced concepts. This section discusses some of these more advanced concepts of dysrhythmia interpretation and provides clues to aid in recognition of selected dysrhythmias not usually covered in a basic course.

Supraventricular Tachycardias

Supraventricular tachycardia (SVT) describes a rapid rhythm that arises above the level of the ventricles (atria or AV junction) or utilizes the atria or AV node as part of the circuit that maintains the tachycardia but whose exact origin is not known. Usually, SVT is used to describe a narrow QRS tachycardia where atrial activity (P waves) cannot be identified, and therefore the origin of the tachycardia cannot be determined from the surface ECG. The presence of the narrow QRS indicates the supraventricular origin of the rhythm and conduction through the normal His-Purkinje system into the ventricles.

Sometimes SVT conducts with bundle branch block, which results in a wide QRS but does not change the fact that the rhythm is supraventricular in origin. Thus, *SVT* can be used for narrow QRS tachycardias whose mechanism is uncertain or for wide QRS tachycardias that are known to be coming from above the ventricles.

SVTs can be classified into those that are AV nodal passive and those that are AV nodal active. *AV nodal passive SVTs* are those in which the AV node is not required for the maintenance of the tachycardia but serves only to passively conduct supraventricular impulses into the ventricles.

Examples of AV nodal passive dysrhythmias include atrial tachycardia, atrial flutter, and atrial fibrillation, all of which originate within the atria and do not need the AV node to sustain the atrial dysrhythmia. In these rhythms, the AV node passively conducts the atrial impulses into the ventricles but does not participate in the maintenance of the dysrhythmia itself. *AV nodal active tachycardias* require participation of the AV node in the maintenance of the tachycardia. The two most common causes of a regular, narrow QRS tachycardia are AV nodal reentry tachycardia (AVNRT) and circus movement tachycardia (CMT) using an accessory pathway, both of which require the active participation of the AV node in maintaining the tachycardia.

Atrial fibrillation is a supraventricular rhythm that is usually easily recognized because of its irregularity, but atrial tachycardia, atrial flutter, junctional tachycardia, AVNRT, and CMT can all present as regular, narrow QRS tachycardias whose mechanism often cannot be determined from the ECG. Because AVNRT and CMT are the most common causes of a regular, narrow QRS tachycardia, they are discussed in detail here.

Atrioventricular Nodal Reentry Tachycardia

In people with AVNRT, the AV node has two pathways that are capable of conducting the impulse into the ventricles. One pathway conducts more rapidly and has a longer refractory period than the other pathway (Figure 18-39A). In AVNRT, a reentry circuit is set, usually using a slowly conducting pathway just outside the body of the AV node as the antegrade limb into the ventricle and the faster conducting pathway in the AV node as the retrograde limb back into the atria (Figure 18-39C).

The sinus impulse normally conducts down the fast pathway into the ventricles, resulting in a normal PR interval of 0.12 to 0.20 seconds. If a PAC occurs and enters the AV node before the fast pathway with its longer refractory period has recovered its ability to conduct, the impulse conducts down the slow pathway into the ventricle because of its shorter refractory period (Figure 18-39B). This slow conduction causes the PR interval of the PAC to be longer than the PR interval of sinus beats. The long conduction time through the slow pathway allows the fast pathway time to recover, making it possible for the impulse to conduct backward through the fast pathway into the atria. This returning impulse may then reenter the slow pathway, which is again ready to conduct antegrade because of its short refractory period, thus setting up a reentry circuit within the AV node and resulting in AVNRT. Figure 18-39C illustrates the mechanism of the most common type of AVNRT in which antegrade conduction occurs over the slow pathway and retrograde conduction over the fast pathway. The resulting rhythm is usually a narrow QRS tachycardia because the ventricles are activated through the normal His-Purkinje system. P waves are either not seen at all or are barely visible peeking out at the tail end of the QRS complex because the atria and ventricles depolarize almost simultaneously (Figure 18-40A and B).

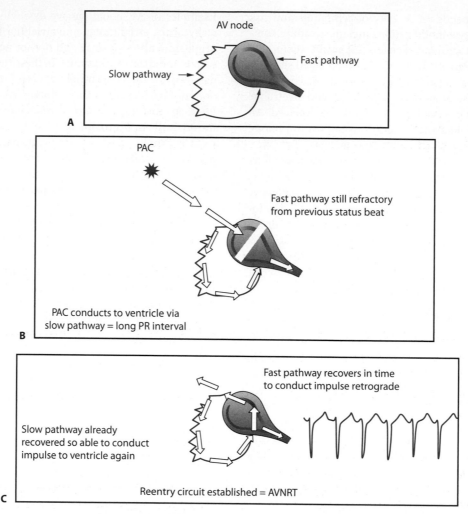

Figure 18-39. Mechanism of AVNRT. **(A)** Illustrates the dual AV nodal pathways responsible for AVNRT. The normal AV node is the fast-conducting pathway with a long refractory period; the slow-conducting pathway lies outside the AV node and has a shorter refractory period. **(B)** A PAC finds the fast pathway still refractory but is able to conduct through the slow pathway. **(C)** When the impulse arrives at the end of the slow pathway, it finds the AV node recovered and ready to conduct retrograde to the atria. The slow pathway has already recovered due to its short refractory period and is able to conduct the same impulse back into the ventricle. This sets up the reentry circuit and causes AVNRT.

In the presence of preexisting bundle branch block or rate-dependent bundle branch block, the QRS in AVNRT is wide.

In about 4% of cases of AVNRT, the impulse conducts antegrade into the ventricle through the fast pathway and retrograde into the atria through the slow pathway, reversing the circuit within the AV node. This reversal of the circuit in the AV node results in P waves that appear immediately in front of the QRS because atrial activation is delayed because of slow conduction backward through the slow pathway. These P waves are inverted in inferior leads because the atria depolarize in a retrograde direction.

Treatment
AVNRT is an AV nodal active SVT because the AV node is required for the maintenance of the tachycardia. Therefore, anything that causes block in the AV node, such as vagal stimulation or drugs like adenosine, beta-blockers, or calcium channel blockers, can terminate the rhythm. AVNRT is usually well tolerated unless the rate is extremely rapid.

Episodes can become frequent and, if not controlled with drugs, can interfere with lifestyle. Many people learn to stop the rhythm by coughing or breath holding, which stimulates the vagus nerve. Acute medical treatment involves administering any drug that blocks AV node conduction, but adenosine is usually used first because of its rapid effect, short duration of action, and lack of significant side effects. RF ablation can destroy the slow pathway and prevent recurrence of the dysrhythmia. Refer to Table 3-4 in Chapter 3 for recommendations on management of AVNRT.

Circus Movement Tachycardia
Circus movement tachycardia (CMT) is an SVT that occurs in people who have accessory pathways (see the section Preexcitation Syndromes earlier). *AV reentrant tachycardia (AVRT)* is also used to describe this dysrhythmia, but to avoid confusion between AVRT and AVNRT, *circus movement tachycardia* is used here.

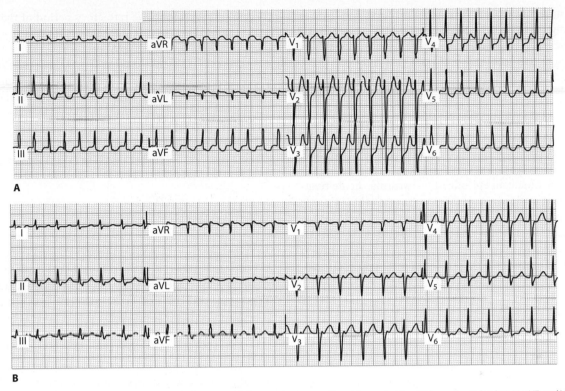

Figure 18-40. **(A)** AVNRT, rate 214. No P waves are visible. **(B)** AVNRT, rate 150. P waves distort the end of the QRS complex in leads II, III, aVF, and V_1 to V_3.

In CMT, an impulse travels a reentry circuit that involves the atria, AV node, ventricles, and accessory pathway. *Orthodromic* is used to describe the most common type of CMT, in which the impulse travels antegrade through the AV node into the ventricles and retrograde back into the atria through the accessory pathway (Figure 18-41A). The result is a regular, narrow QRS tachycardia because the ventricles are activated through the normal His-Purkinje system. In the presence of bundle branch block, a wide QRS pattern is present. Because the atria and ventricles depolarize separately, P waves, if visible at all, are seen following the QRS complex in the ST segment or between two QRS complexes, usually closest to the first QRS.

Antidromic describes the rare form of CMT in which the accessory pathway conducts the impulse from atria to

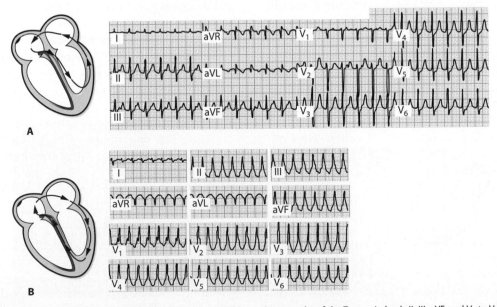

Figure 18-41. **(A)** Orthodromic circus movement tachycardia. P waves are visible on the upstroke of the T wave in leads II, III, aVF, and V_1 to V_3. **(B)** Antidromic circus movement tachycardia.

ventricles and the AV node conducts it retrograde back to the atria (Figure 18-41B). Antidromic CMT is a regular wide QRS tachycardia because the ventricles depolarize abnormally through the accessory pathway. This form of SVT is often indistinguishable from ventricular tachycardia on the ECG.

Treatment

CMT is an AV nodal active tachycardia because the AV node is necessary for maintenance of the dysrhythmia. Vagal maneuvers and drugs that block AV conduction can be used to terminate an episode of tachycardia. Acute treatment is aimed at slowing conduction through the AV node with a vagal maneuver or medications such as adenosine, beta-blockers, or calcium channel blockers, or at slowing accessory pathway conduction with antiarrhythmics such as procainamide or ibutilide. See Table 3-4 in Chapter 3 for recommendations for management of CMT.

Atrial Fibrillation in Wolff-Parkinson-White Syndrome

Atrial fibrillation occurs more frequently in people with accessory pathways than in the general population and can be life threatening. Atrial flutter and fibrillation are especially dangerous in the presence of an accessory pathway because the pathway can conduct impulses rapidly and without delay into the ventricles, resulting in dangerously fast ventricular rates (Figure 18-42). These rapid ventricular rates can degenerate into ventricular fibrillation and result in sudden death. When atrial fibrillation is the mechanism of the tachycardia in WPW syndrome, the QRS complex is wide and bizarre due to conduction of the impulses into the ventricle through the bypass tract. The ventricular response to the atrial fibrillation is irregular and very rapid, often approaching rates of 300 beats/min or more because of lack of delay in conduction through the accessory pathway. Atrial fibrillation with accessory pathway conduction must be recognized and differentiated from atrial fibrillation conducting through the AV node because treatment is different for the two situations. When accessory pathway conduction is known or suspected, flecainide, ibutilide, or procainamide are recommended

because they prolong the refractory period of the accessory pathway and slow ventricular rate, and they may convert the atrial fibrillation to sinus rhythm.

Verapamil often is used to slow AV conduction in atrial fibrillation conducting into the ventricles through the AV node, but it can be very dangerous and even lethal when used in the presence of an accessory pathway. Digitalis, verapamil, diltiazem, and IV amiodarone are contraindicated in preexcited atrial fibrillation because they can result in ventricular fibrillation. See Table 3-4 in Chapter 3 for management of preexcited atrial fibrillation.

Polymorphic Ventricular Tachycardias

Polymorphic ventricular tachycardia (PVT) refers to VT with unstable, continuously varying QRS morphology often occurring at rates of approximately 200 beats/min. It can occur in short repetitive runs, longer sustained runs, or can degenerate into VF and cause SCD. PVT can be classified based on whether it is associated with a normal or prolonged QT interval.

Polymorphic VT with a normal QT interval can occur in the presence of ventricular ischemia during ACS or following MI, although it is not a common dysrhythmia. Figure 18-43 shows PVT in a patient during acute anterior-wall MI. Therapy of PVT associated with ischemia should be directed toward relieving the ischemia by either surgery or PCI. Beta-blockers are recommended for PVT if ischemia is suspected. For recurrent PVT in the absence of a long-QT interval, IV amiodarone is useful and lidocaine may be helpful. If PVT becomes sustained or degenerates to VF, defibrillation with an unsynchronized shock is necessary. Table 3-6 in Chapter 3 summarizes recommendations for managing PVT.

Torsades de pointes (TdP) means "twisting of the points" and describes polymorphic VT that occurs with abnormal ventricular repolarization. This abnormal repolarization presents on the ECG as an abnormally prolonged QT or QTU interval. See the section on LQTSs in this chapter for more information on LQTSs.

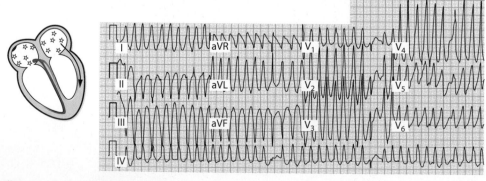

Figure 18-42. Atrial fibrillation conducting into the ventricle through an accessory pathway. Note the extremely short RR intervals in the V leads. QRS is fast, wide, and irregular.

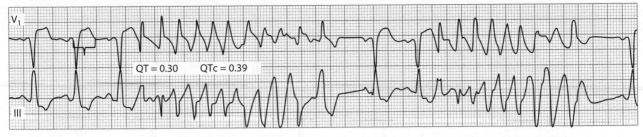

Figure 18-43. Polymorphic VT with a normal QT interval. This patient was having an acute MI (note ST elevation in lead V₁).

Characteristic ECG findings of TdP include: (1) markedly prolonged QT intervals with wide TU waves; (2) initiation of the dysrhythmia by an R-on-T PVC with a long coupling interval; and (3) wide, bizarre, multiform QRS complexes that change direction frequently, appearing to twist around the isoelectric line (Figure 18-44). Ventricular rate during TdP is commonly 200 to 250 beats/min. TdP is usually self-terminating and occurs in repeated episodes, but it can deteriorate into ventricular fibrillation. IV magnesium can be used to manage episodes of TdP until the cause can be corrected.

Differentiating Wide QRS Beats and Rhythms

Determining the origin of a wide QRS beat or a wide QRS tachycardia is one of the most common problems encountered when caring for monitored patients. A supraventricular beat with abnormal, or aberrant, conduction through the ventricles, can look almost identical to a beat that originates in the ventricle. The problem with aberration is that it can mimic ventricular dysrhythmias, which require different therapy and carry a different prognosis than aberrancy. Aberrancy is always secondary to some other primary disturbance and does not itself require treatment. Nurses must be able to identify accurately which mechanism is responsible for the wide QRS rhythm being observed whenever possible, initiate appropriate treatment when needed, and avoid inappropriate treatment.

Mechanisms of Aberration

Aberrancy is the temporary abnormal intraventricular conduction of supraventricular impulses. Aberration occurs whenever the His-Purkinje system or ventricle is still partly refractory when a supraventricular impulse attempts to travel through it. The refractory period of the conduction system is directly proportional to preceding cycle length. Long cycles are followed by long refractory periods,

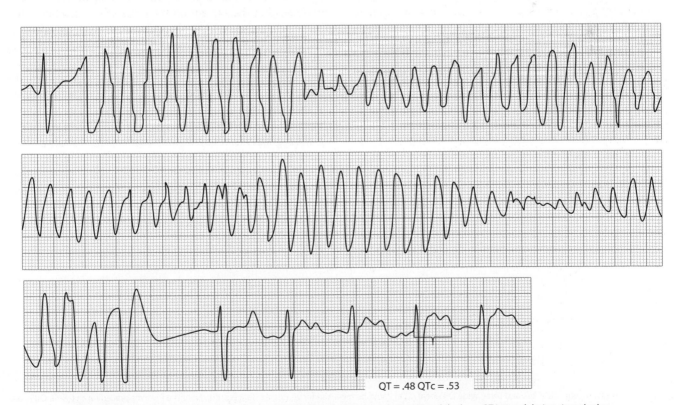

Figure 18-44. Torsades de pointes. Note characteristic "twisting" appearance during VT and the long-QT interval during sinus rhythm.

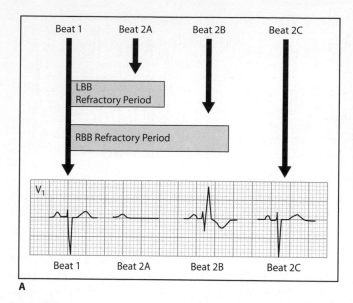

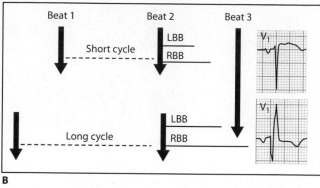

Figure 18-45. Mechanisms of aberration. **(A)** The right bundle has a longer refractory period than the left. Beat 2A occurs so early that it cannot conduct through either bundle branch. Beat 2B encounters a refractory right bundle and conducts with RBBB. Beat 2C falls outside the refractory period of both bundles and is able to conduct normally. **(B)** The refractory period of the bundle branches is proportional to preceding cycle length. Top: a short cycle results in shorter bundle branch refractory periods. Bottom: a long cycle causes longer refractory periods in the bundle branches. When beat 3 comes early following a short cycle (*top*), it can conduct normally, but when it comes early following a long cycle (*bottom*), the right bundle branch is still refractory and beat 3 conducts with RBBB.

and short cycles are followed by short refractory periods (Figure 18-45B). An early supraventricular beat, such as a PAC, may enter the conduction system during a portion of its refractory period, forcing conduction through the ventricles to occur in an abnormal manner. Beats that follow a sudden lengthening of the cycle may conduct aberrantly because of the increased length of the refractory period that occurs when the cycle lengthens. The right bundle branch has a longer refractory period than the left (Figure 18-45); therefore, aberrant beats tend to conduct most often with an RBBB pattern, although LBBB aberration is common in people with cardiac disease.

Electrocardiographic Clues to the Origin of Wide QRS Beats and Rhythms
P Waves

If P waves can be seen during a wide QRS tachycardia, they are very helpful in making the differential diagnosis of aberration versus ventricular ectopy. Atrial activity, represented by the P wave on the ECG and preceding a wide QRS beat

or run of tachycardia, strongly favors a supraventricular origin of the dysrhythmia. Figure 18-46 shows three wide QRS beats that could easily be mistaken for PVCs if not for the obvious presence of the early P wave initiating the run.

An exception to the preceding P-wave rule occurs with end-diastolic PVCs. *End-diastolic PVCs* occur at the end of diastole, after the sinus P wave has been recorded but before it has a chance to conduct through the AV node into the ventricle. Figure 18-47 shows sinus rhythm with an end-diastolic PVC occurring immediately after the sinus P wave. Here, the P wave preceding the wide QRS is merely a coincidence and does not indicate aberrant conduction. The PR interval is much too short to have conducted that QRS complex. In addition, the P wave preceding the wide QRS is not early; it is the regularly scheduled sinus beat coming on time. Thus, early P waves that precede early wide QRS complexes are usually "married to" those QRSs and indicate aberrant conduction, while "on-time" P waves in front of end-diastolic PVCs are not early and do not cause the wide QRS.

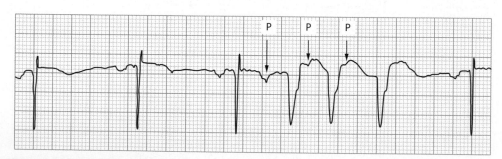

Figure 18-46. Sinus rhythm with PACs and three wide QRS beats that could be mistaken for ventricular tachycardia. Note the P waves preceding the wide QRS complexes, indicating aberrant conduction.

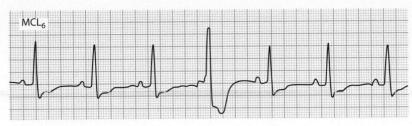

Figure 18-47. Sinus rhythm with an end-diastolic PVC. The P wave preceding the PVC is the sinus P wave that coincidentally occurs just before the PVC.

P waves seen during a wide QRS tachycardia also can be very helpful in making the differential diagnosis between SVTs with aberration and ventricular tachycardia. If P waves are seen associated with every QRS, the rhythm is supraventricular in origin (Figure 18-48A). P waves that occur independently of the QRS and have no consistent relationship to QRS complexes indicate the presence of AV dissociation, which means that the atria and the ventricles are under the control of separate pacemakers and strongly favor ventricular tachycardia (Figure 18-48B).

QRS Morphology

The shape of the QRS complex is very helpful in determining the origin of a wide QRS rhythm. When using QRS morphology clues, it is extremely important to examine the correct leads and apply the criteria only to leads that have been proven helpful. Many clinicians prefer to monitor with lead II because usually it shows an upright QRS complex and clear P wave. Lead II, however, has no value in determining the origin of a wide QRS rhythm. The single best dysrhythmia monitoring lead is V_1, followed by V_6 and V_2 in certain situations.

When applying QRS morphology criteria for wide QRS rhythms, it is helpful to first decide whether the QRS complexes have an RBBB morphology or an LBBB morphology. RBBB morphology rhythms have an upright QRS in lead V_1, while LBBB morphology rhythms have a negative QRS complex in V_1.

When dealing with a wide QRS rhythm of RBBB morphology (upright in V_1), follow these steps to evaluate QRS morphology (Figures 18-49 and 18-50A):

1. Look at V_1 and determine if the upright QRS complex is monophasic (R wave), diphasic (qR), or triphasic (rsR'). Monophasic and diphasic complexes favor a ventricular origin, if the left peak ("rabbit ear") is taller. A taller right rabbit ear does not favor either diagnosis. A triphasic rsR' is typical of RBBB aberration in V_1.

2. Look at V_6 and determine whether the QRS is monophasic (all negative QS), diphasic (rS), or triphasic (qRs). A monophasic or diphasic complex in V_6 favors a ventricular origin, and the triphasic qRs complex is typical of RBBB aberration in V_6.

If the QRS has an LBBB morphology (negative in V_1), follow these steps to evaluate morphology (Figures 18-49 and 18-50B):

1. Look at V_1 or V_2 (both are helpful in this case) and determine if the R wave (if present) is wide or narrow. A wide R wave of more than 0.03 seconds favors a ventricular rhythm, and a narrow R wave favors a supraventricular origin with LBBB aberration.

2. Next look at the downstroke of the S wave in V_1 or V_2. Slurring or notching on the downstroke favors

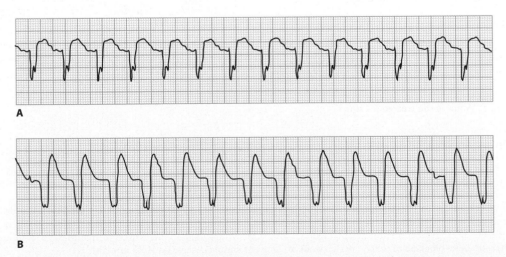

Figure 18-48. Two very similar, wide QRS tachycardias. **(A)** Sinus tachycardia, rate 115. P waves can be seen on the downslope of the T wave preceding each QRS, indicating a supraventricular origin of the tachycardia. **(B)** P waves are independent of QRS complexes, indicating AV dissociation, which favors ventricular tachycardia.

ESSENTIAL CONTENT CASE

Patient With Syncope

A 20-year-old patient was admitted with a head laceration after an episode of syncope with seizure. He had one previous episode of "fainting" about a month ago but did not seek medical care. His BP is 126/72 mm Hg, heart rate 50 beats/min, and complains of pain at the laceration site but is awake, oriented, and cooperative. This is the 12-lead ECG obtained as part of his workup for syncope:

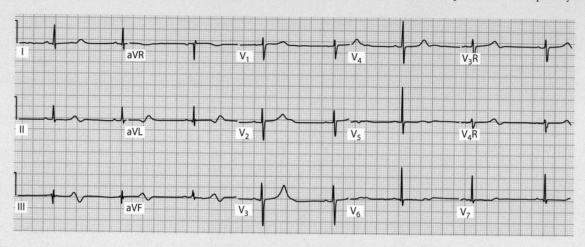

Case Question 1: What is your interpretation of this ECG, rhythm, QRS axis, and bundle branch block?

Case Question 2: Is there anything on the ECG that might indicate a cause of his "seizure?"
You put him on the bedside monitor and set the alarms. He remains stable for the next few hours, then you hear his monitor alarm. When you enter the room, he complains of extreme dizziness and says he feels like he might pass out. This is his rhythm on the monitor:

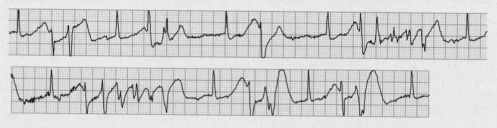

Case Question 3: What is this rhythm?

Case Question 4: What treatment is indicated for this rhythm acutely and long term?
In the next minute, the following rhythm appears:

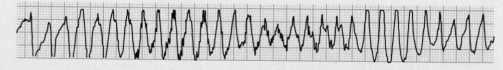

Case Question 5: What is the treatment now?

Answers
1. The rhythm is sinus bradycardia. The QRS axis is normal. There is no bundle branch block.
2. The QT interval is long, about 0.58 seconds (580 ms) in lead II and 0.60 seconds (600 ms) in lead V_2. The T waves are biphasic or notched. This is a form of congenital long-QT syndrome, which increases the risk of TdP and SCD. Patients often present with syncope, or seizures that are due to episodes of TdP that last long enough to result in loss of consciousness.
3. The basic rhythm appears to be sinus (narrow QRS beats) with PVC couplets and short runs of TdP.
4. Treatment of short runs of TdP includes IV magnesium or overdrive pacing to shorten the QT interval. Any drugs that might contribute to QT interval prolongation should be discontinued, and any electrolyte imbalances need to be corrected. Beta-blockers are the mainstay of long-term treatment of congenital long-QT syndrome. Patients who continue to have significant ventricular dysrhythmias on beta-blockers or who experience an SCD event should receive an ICD implant.
5. This strip represents a sustained run of TdP. Long runs that do not terminate spontaneously cause loss of consciousness and usually degenerate into VF. Defibrillation is the treatment for sustained TdP.

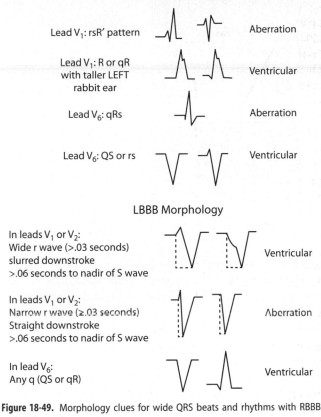

RBBB Morphology

Lead V₁: rsR′ pattern — Aberration

Lead V₁: R or qR with taller LEFT rabbit ear — Ventricular

Lead V₆: qRs — Aberration

Lead V₆: QS or rs — Ventricular

LBBB Morphology

In leads V₁ or V₂:
Wide r wave (>.03 seconds) slurred downstroke >.06 seconds to nadir of S wave — Ventricular

In leads V₁ or V₂:
Narrow r wave (≥.03 seconds) Straight downstroke >.06 seconds to nadir of S wave — Aberration

In lead V₆:
Any q (QS or qR) — Ventricular

Figure 18-49. Morphology clues for wide QRS beats and rhythms with RBBB and LBBB patterns.

a ventricular origin. LBBB aberration typically slurs on the upstroke if it slurs at all.

3. Measure from the onset of the QRS complex to the deepest part of the S wave in V_1 or V_2. A measurement of more than 0.06 seconds favors a ventricular rhythm and a narrower measurement favors LBBB aberration. Note that this measurement can be prolonged due to either a wide R wave or slurring on the downstroke of the S wave, either one of which favors the ventricular origin of the rhythm.

4. Look at V_6 and determine whether a Q wave is present. Any Q wave (either a QS or qR complex) favors a ventricular origin.

Concordance

Concordance means that all the QRS complexes across the precordium from V_1 through V_6 point in the same direction; positive concordance means they are all upright, and negative concordance means they are all negative (Figure 18-51A). Negative concordance favors a diagnosis of ventricular tachycardia when it occurs in a wide QRS tachycardia, and positive concordance favors ventricular tachycardia as long as WPW syndrome can be ruled out.

Fusion and Capture Beats

Ventricular fusion beats occur when the ventricles are depolarized by two different wavefronts of electrical activity at the same time. Fusion often results when a supraventricular

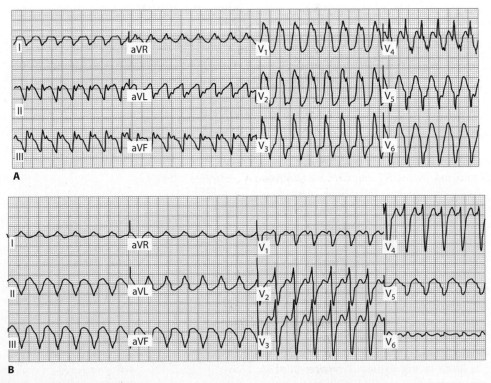

Figure 18-50. 12-lead ECG of ventricular tachycardia. **(A)** With RBBB morphology. Note monophasic R wave with taller left rabbit ear in V₁ and QS complex in V₆. **(B)** With LBBB morphology. Note wide R wave in V₁ and V₂, and qR pattern in V₆.

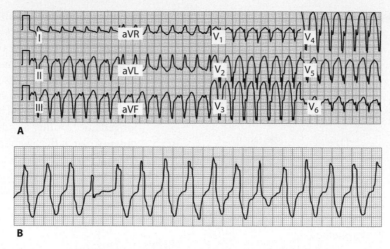

Figure 18-51. **(A)** 12-lead ECG of ventricular tachycardia with negative concordance. **(B)** Rhythm strip of ventricular tachycardia with fusion beats.

impulse travels through the AV node and begins to depolarize the ventricles at the same time that an impulse from a ventricular focus depolarizes the ventricles. When two different impulses contribute to ventricular depolarization, the resulting QRS shape and width are determined by the relative contributions of both the supraventricular and the ventricular impulses. In the presence of a wide QRS tachycardia, the presence of fusion beats indicates AV dissociation, which means that the atria and ventricles are under the control of separate pacemakers. Capture beats occur when the supraventricular impulse manages to conduct all the way into and through the ventricle, depolarizing ("capturing") the ventricle and resulting in a normal QRS in the midst of the wide QRS tachycardia. The presence of fusion and capture beats in a wide QRS tachycardia is strong evidence supporting the diagnosis of ventricular tachycardia, but they occur rarely and cannot be counted on to make the diagnosis. Figure 18-51B shows fusion beats in a wide QRS tachycardia. Helpful ECG clues for differentiating aberrancy from ventricular ectopy are summarized in Table 18-4.

ST-SEGMENT MONITORING

Many bedside monitors have software programs that allow for continuous monitoring of the ST segment in addition to routine dysrhythmia monitoring. In patients who have undergone thrombolytic therapy or a PCI procedure to treat acute MI, continuous ST-segment monitoring can detect ischemia related to reocclusion of the involved artery. ST-segment monitoring is also useful in detecting silent ischemia (ischemic episodes that occur in the absence of chest pain or other symptoms) that would otherwise go unnoticed with symptom and dysrhythmia monitoring alone. Early detection of ischemic changes is critical in identifying patients who need interventions to reestablish blood flow to myocardium before permanent damage occurs.

ST elevation in leads facing damaged myocardium is the ECG sign of myocardial injury. ST depression is often recorded as a reciprocal change in leads that do not directly

face the involved myocardium (see Table 18-2). In addition, ST depression can be recorded in leads facing ischemic tissue. Therefore, either ST elevation or ST depression indicates myocardium at risk for infarction. The sooner the artery is opened and blood flow reestablished to ischemic or injured tissue, the more myocardium is salvaged and the fewer complications and deaths occur.

Measuring the ST Segment

Clinically significant ST-segment deviation is defined as ST elevation or depression 1 mm or more from the baseline,

TABLE 18-4.   ECG CLUES FOR DIFFERENTIATING ABERRATION FROM VENTRICULAR ECTOPY

	Aberrancy	Ventricular Ectopy
P waves	Precede QRS complexes	Dissociated from QRS or occur at rate slower than QRS; if 1:1 V-A conduction is present, retrograde P waves follow every QRS
Precordial QRS concordance	Positive concordance may occur with WPW	Negative concordance favors VT; positive concordance favors VT if WPW ruled out
Fusion or capture beats		Strong evidence in favor of VT
QRS axis	Often normal; may be deviated to right or left	Right superior axis favors VT; often deviated to left or right
RBBB QRS morphology	Triphasic rsR' in V$_1$; triphasic qRs in V$_6$	Monophasic R wave or diphasic qR complex in V$_1$; left "rabbit ear" taller in V$_1$; monophasic QS or diphasic rS in V$_6$
LBBB QRS morphology	Narrow R wave (<0.04 seconds) in V$_1$; straight downstroke of S wave in V$_1$ (often slurs or notches on upstroke); usually no Q wave in V$_6$	Wide R wave (>0.03 seconds) in V$_1$ or V$_2$; slurring or notching on downstroke of S wave in V$_1$; delay of greater than 0.06 seconds to nadir of S wave in V$_1$ or V$_2$; any Q wave in V$_6$

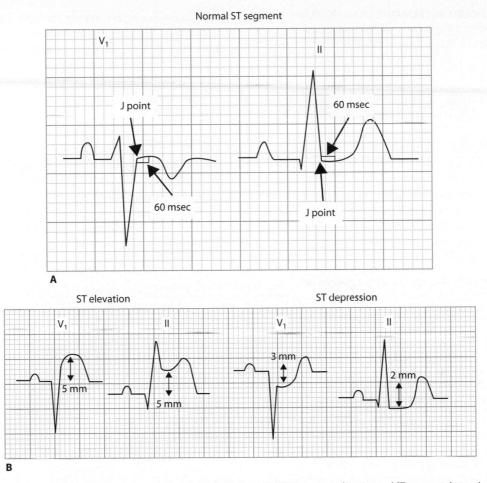

Figure 18-52. **(A)** Normal ST segment on the baseline in leads V$_1$ and II. **(B)** ST-segment elevation and ST-segment depression.

or isoelectric line, measured at the J point or 60 msec (0.06 seconds) after the J point. The J point is the point at which the QRS ends and the ST segment begins. Figure 18-52A illustrates a normal ST segment, and Figure 18-52B illustrates ST-segment elevation and depression.

ST-segment monitoring software in newer bedside monitors defines the baseline and the ST-segment measuring point. It also sets default alarm parameters so the equipment can audibly notify the nurse when the patient's ST segment falls outside the defined parameters. Most monitors allow the user to redefine the baseline, reset the J point, choose where the ST segment is measured, and change the alarm parameters to account for individual patient variations. The monitor then displays the ST-segment measurement in millimeters on the screen, and most monitors also allow for trending of the ST segment over specified time intervals.

Choosing the Best Leads for ST-Segment Monitoring

Some monitoring systems offer continuous 12-lead ECG monitoring, which eliminates the need to select the "best" leads to monitor for a given clinical situation. Most younger generation bedside monitors offer at least two leads for simultaneous ECG monitoring and some offer three leads. The best single lead for dysrhythmia monitoring is V$_1$, with V$_6$ being next best. Using two or three leads for ST-segment monitoring is optimal because a single lead may miss significant ST-segment deviations. Since most current bedside monitors allow for the use of only one V lead at a time, using V$_1$ as the dysrhythmia monitoring lead (or V$_6$ if V$_1$ is not available because of dressings, etc) means that limb leads must be used for ST-segment monitoring. The best limb leads are discussed below.

The best way to choose leads for ST-segment monitoring is to know the patient's "ischemic fingerprint." To determine the patient's ischemic fingerprint, obtain a 12-lead ECG during a pain episode or with inflation of the balloon during PCI and note which leads show the most ST-segment displacement (either elevation or depression) during the acute ischemic event. Choose the lead or leads with the most ST-segment displacement as the bedside ST-segment monitoring leads.

If no ischemic fingerprint is available, use a lead or leads that have been determined through research to be best for the artery involved (Table 18-5). The limb leads that have been shown to best detect ischemia related to all three major coronary arteries (right coronary, left anterior descending,

TABLE 18-5. RECOMMENDED LEADS FOR CONTINUOUS ECG MONITORING

Purpose	Best Leads
Dysrhythmia detection	V_1 (V_6 next best)
RCA ischemia, inferior MI	III, aVF
LAD ischemia, anterior MI	V_3 (or V_2; III, or aVF if V lead not available)
Circumflex ischemia, lateral MI	V_6, (I or aVL if V lead not available; III, aVF good reciprocal leads)
RV infarction	V_4R
Axis shifts	I and aVF together

and circumflex) are leads III and aVF. In the case of the right coronary artery (RCA), leads III and aVF directly face the inferior wall supplied by this artery and record ST elevation with inferior wall injury. The left anterior descending

and circumflex artery supply the anterior and lateral walls, respectively. Because these walls are not directly faced by leads III and aVF, ST-segment depression is recorded as a reciprocal change when anterior or lateral wall injury occurs. Table 18-6 summarizes critical elements of ST-segment monitoring.

CARDIAC PACEMAKERS

Chapter 3, Interpretation and Management of Basic Cardiac Rhythms, describes the components of a temporary pacing system and basic pacemaker operation. This section discusses single-chamber and dual-chamber pacemaker function and evaluation of pacemaker rhythm strips for appropriate capture and sensing.

TABLE 18-6. EVIDENCE-BASED PRACTICE: ST-SEGMENT MONITORING

Patient Selection

ST segment monitoring should be used judiciously and only in the highest-risk patients in order to avoid alarm fatigue.

Class I: There are no class I recommendations.

Class IIa: ST-segment monitoring is reasonable for the following types of patients:

- Early-phase ACS (<24 hours) for intermediate to high-risk NSTEMI or STEMI, while receiving definitive diagnosis. Initiate immediately and continue uninterrupted for 24-48 hours or until ruled out.[a]
- After MI without revascularization or with residual ischemic lesions. Initiate immediately and continue for 24-48 hours until no evidence of ongoing modifiable ischemia or hemodynamic or electrical instability.[a]
- Newly diagnosed left main coronary artery lesion (until revascularized).
- Vasospastic angina (can be useful to document transient ST-segment changes until diagnosed and stabilized).[a]
- After nonurgent PCI with complications or suboptimal results. Continue for ≥24 hours or until complication resolved.[a]
- Open heart surgery (intraoperatively).[a]

Class IIb: ST-segment monitoring may be considered for:

- After MI with revascularization of all ischemic lesions. Initiate immediately and continue for 12-24 hours after revascularization.[a]
- Apical ballooning (stress cardiomyopathy): until symptoms resolved.[a]
- During targeted temperature management (therapeutic hypothermia) procedure based on presumed cause of arrest.[a]
- Open heart surgery: immediately postoperatively in intubated and sedated patients until able to recognize and report new or ongoing ischemia.[a]
- Acute decompensated heart failure: only if possible ischemic origin (until precipitating event is successfully treated).[a]
- Stroke: only in patients with acute stroke at increased risk for cardiac events (24-48 hours).[a]

Electrode Application

- Make sure skin is clean and dry before applying monitoring electrodes.[a,b]
- Place electrodes according to manufacturer recommendations when using a derived 12-lead ECG system.[a,b]
- When using a 3- or 5-wire-monitoring system, place electrodes as follows:
  – Place arm electrodes in infraclavicular fossa close to shoulder[a,b] or on top or back of shoulder as close to where arm joins torso as possible.
  – Place leg electrodes at lowest point on rib cage or on hips.[a,b]
  – Place V_1 electrode at the fourth intercostal space at right sternal border.[a,b]
  – Place V_6 electrode in a straight line from V_4 at left midaxillary line.
- Mark electrode placement with indelible ink.[a,b]
- Change electrodes daily.[b]

Lead Selection

- Monitor all 12 leads continuously if ST segment mapping is available.[b]
- Use V_1 (or V_6 if V_1 is not possible due to dressings) for arrhythmia monitoring in all multilead combinations.
- Choose the ST-segment monitoring lead according to the patient's "ischemic fingerprint" obtained during an ischemic event whenever possible.[a,b] Use the lead with the largest ST-segment deviation (elevation or depression).[b]
- If no ischemic fingerprint is available, use either lead III[a,b] or aVF (whichever has tallest QRS complex) for ST-segment monitoring.
- Lead V_3 is the best lead for detecting anterior wall ST-segment deviation,[b] but it can only be used if the chest lead is not being used for arrhythmia monitoring in lead V_1.

Alarm Management

- Establish baseline ST level with patient in the supine position.[a,b]
- Set the ST alarm parameter in the highest risk patients 1 mm or less above and below the patient's baseline ST segment in all leads except for leads V_2 and V_3, where the upper alarm limit can be 1.5 mm from baseline in women and 2.0 mm from baseline in men.[b]
- Alarm limits should be adjusted based on patient risk, institution policy, and collaboration with care providers.

Data compiled from:

[a]*Sandau KE, Funk M, Auerbach A, et al. Update to practice standards for electrocardiographic monitoring in hospital settings. Circulation. 2017:136;e273-e344.*

[b]*AACN Practice Alert. Ensuring accurate ST segment monitoring. Crit Care Nurse. 2016;36:e18-e25.*

TABLE 18-7. PACEMAKER CODES

First Letter: Chamber Paced	Second Letter: Chamber Sensed	Third Letter: Response to Sensing	Fourth Letter: Rate Modulation	Fifth Letter: Multisite Pacing[a]
0 = None	0 = None	0 = None	0 = None	0 = None
A = Atrium	A = Atrium	I = Inhibited	R = Rate modulation	A = Atrial
V = Ventricle	V = Ventricle	T = Triggered		V = Ventricular
D = Dual (A&V)	D = Dual (A&V)	D = Dual (I&T)		D = Dual

[a]Multisite indicates either pacing in both atria or both ventricles or pacing multiple sites within a chamber.

Cardiac pacemakers are classified by a standardized five-letter pacemaker code that describes the location of the pacing wire(s) and the expected function of the pacemaker. Table 18-7 illustrates the five-letter code. The first letter in the pacemaker code describes the chamber that is paced (A = atrium, V = ventricle, D = dual [atrium and ventricle], 0 = none). The letter in the second position describes the chamber where intrinsic electrical activity is sensed (A = atrium, V = ventricle, D = dual, 0 = none). The letter in the third position describes the pacemaker's response to sensing of intrinsic electrical activity (I = inhibited, T = triggered, D = dual [inhibited or triggered], 0 = none). The fourth letter indicates the presence or absence of rate modulation, and the fifth letter describes multisite pacing functions. To know how a pacemaker should function, it is necessary to know at a minimum the first three letters of the code, which describe where the pacemaker is supposed to pace, where it is supposed to sense, and what it should do when it senses. The last two letters representing advanced pacemaker function are not covered in this text; see the recommended references at the end of the chapter.

Three types of temporary pacing are commonly used in critical care or telemetry settings. The first is transvenous pacing through a wire introduced into the apex of the right ventricle via a peripheral or central vein and set in the demand mode (sensitive to intrinsic ventricular activity). Ventricular pacing is always done in the demand mode to avoid the delivery of pacing stimuli into the vulnerable period of the cardiac cycle, which could induce ventricular tachycardia or fibrillation (see Chapter 3, Interpretation and Management of Basic Cardiac Rhythms). This type of pacing is described by the pacemaker code as a VVI pacemaker—it paces the ventricle, senses intrinsic ventricular electrical activity, and inhibits its output when sensing occurs.

The second type of pacing done in critical care or telemetry is temporary epicardial pacing (either atrial, ventricular, or dual chamber) via pacing wires attached to the atria and/or ventricles during cardiac surgery. If atrial pacing is done with no sensing of atrial electrical activity, also called asynchronous mode, the pacemaker operates as an A00 pacemaker—it paces the atria, does not sense, and therefore does not respond to intrinsic atrial activity. If atrial pacing is done with sensing of atrial electrical activity, also called the demand mode, the pacemaker operates as an AAI pacemaker—it paces the atria, senses atrial activity, and inhibits its output when it senses. Dual-chamber pacing can be done in several modes involving pacing and sensing functions in one or both chambers and described by the pacemaker code according to the mode chosen. The two most common dual-chamber modes used with temporary epicardial pacing (and occasionally with temporary transvenous pacing) are DVI (paces atria and ventricles, senses only in the ventricle, and inhibits pacing output when sensing occurs) and DDD (paces both chambers, senses both chambers, and either triggers or inhibits pacing output in response to sensing). The common dual-chamber pacing modes are listed in Table 18-8.

The third type of temporary pacing is external (transcutaneous) pacing. External pacing is done in emergency situations requiring immediate pacing when placement of a temporary transvenous pacing wire is not feasible. External pacing is not as reliable as transvenous or epicardial pacing and is used as a temporary measure until transvenous pacing can be instituted. External pacing is briefly described in Chapter 3, Interpretation and Management of Basic Cardiac Rhythms.

Evaluating Pacemaker Function

Evaluating pacemaker function requires knowledge of the mode of pacing expected (ie, VVI, AAI); the minimum rate of the pacemaker, or pacing interval; and any other programmed parameters in the pacemaker. The basic functions

TABLE 18-8. DUAL-CHAMBER PACING MODES

Mode	Chamber(s) Paced	Chamber(s) Sensed	Response to Sensing
DVI	Atrium and ventricle	Ventricle	Inhibited
VDD	Ventricle	Atrium and ventricle	Atrial sensing triggers ventricular pacing Ventricular sensing inhibits ventricular pacing
DDI	Atrium and ventricle	Atrium and ventricle	Inhibited
DDD	Atrium and ventricle	Atrium and ventricle	Atrial sensing inhibits atrial pacing, triggers ventricular pacing Ventricular sensing inhibits atrial and ventricular pacing

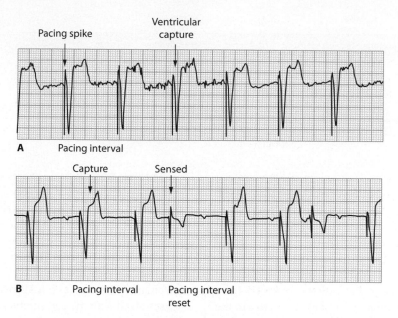

Figure 18-53. Normal VVI pacemaker function. **(A)** Pacing electrical activity ("pacer spike") followed by a wide QRS complex indicating ventricular capture. Pacemaker sensing cannot be evaluated because no intrinsic QRS complexes are present. **(B)** Pacemaker capture and sensing are both normal. Intrinsic QRS complexes are sensed, inhibiting ventricular pacing output, and resetting the pacing interval. Absence of intrinsic ventricular electrical activity causes pacing to occur with capture.

of a pacemaker include stimulus release, capture, and sensing. *Stimulus release* refers to pacemaker output, or the ability of the pacemaker to generate and release a pacing impulse. *Capture* is the ability of the pacing stimulus to result in depolarization of the chamber being paced. *Sensing* is the ability of the pacemaker to recognize and respond to intrinsic electrical activity in the heart. Pacemaker operation is evaluated according to these three functions. Single-chamber pacemaker evaluation is much less complicated than dual-chamber evaluation. Because single-chamber ventricular pacing is a very common type of temporary pacing in critical care and telemetry units, VVI pacemaker evaluation is discussed here.

VVI Pacemaker Evaluation

Stimulus release, capture, and sensing must all be assessed when evaluating VVI pacemakers. A VVI pacemaker is expected to pace the ventricle at the set rate unless spontaneous ventricular activity occurs to inhibit pacing. The set rate of the pacemaker, or *pacing interval,* is measured from one pacing stimulus to the next consecutive stimulus. Pacemakers have a *refractory period,* which is a period following either pacing or sensing in the chamber, during which the pacemaker is unable to respond to intrinsic activity. During

the refractory period, the pacemaker in effect has its eyes closed and is not able to see spontaneous activity. In a normally functioning VVI pacemaker, pacing spikes occur at the set pacing interval and each spike results in a ventricular depolarization (capture). If spontaneous ventricular activity occurs (either a normally conducted QRS or a PVC), that activity is sensed and the next pacing stimulus is inhibited. Figure 18-53A and B shows normal VVI pacemaker function.

Stimulus Release

Stimulus release depends on a pacemaker with enough battery power to generate the electrical impulse, and on an intact pacemaker lead system to deliver the electrical stimulus to the heart. The presence of a pacer spike on the rhythm strip or monitor indicates that the stimulus was released from the generator and entered the body. The presence of the spike does not indicate where the stimulus was delivered (eg, atria or ventricles), only that it entered the body somewhere. Total absence of pacing stimuli, when they should be present, can indicate a faulty pulse generator or battery, or a break or disconnection in the lead system. Pacing stimuli also can be absent when pacing is inhibited by the sensing of intrinsic electrical activity. Figure 18-54 illustrates total loss

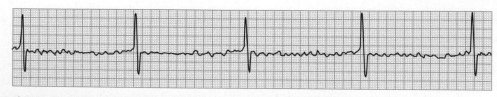

Figure 18-54. Absence of stimulus release in a patient with a permanent pacemaker. Underlying rhythm is atrial fibrillation with complete AV block and a very slow ventricular rate. The battery in the pacemaker generator was depleted.

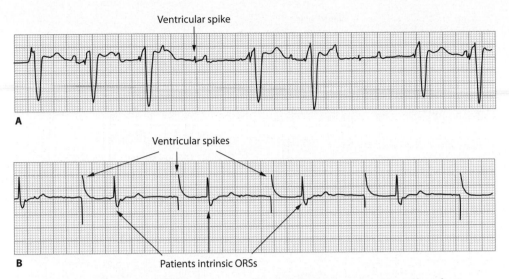

Figure 18-55. **(A)** VVI pacemaker with intermittent loss of capture. **(B)** VVI pacemaker with total loss of capture.

of stimulus release in a patient whose pacemaker battery was depleted.

Capture

Capture is indicated by a wide QRS complex immediately following the pacemaker spike and represents the ability of the pacing stimulus to depolarize the ventricle. Loss of capture is recognized by the presence of pacer spikes that are not followed by paced ventricular complexes (Figure 18-55). Causes of loss of capture include:

- Inadequate stimulus strength, which can be corrected by increasing the electrical output of the pacemaker (turning up the milliampere level).
- Pacing wire out of position and not in contact with myocardium, which can be corrected by repositioning the wire and sometimes the patient.
- Pacing lead positioned in infarcted tissue, which can be corrected by repositioning the wire to a place where the myocardium is not injured and is capable of responding to the stimulus.
- Electrolyte imbalances or medications that alter the heart's response to the pacing stimulus.
- Delivery of a pacing stimulus during the ventricle's refractory period when the heart is physiologically unable to respond to the stimulus. This problem occurs with loss of sensing (undersensing) and can be corrected by correcting the sensing problem (Figure 18-56A).

Sensing

Sensing of intrinsic ventricular electrical activity inhibits the next pacing stimulus and resets the pacing interval. Sensing cannot occur unless the pacemaker is given the opportunity to sense. It must be in the demand mode and there must be intrinsic ventricular activity that occurs for the pacemaker to have an opportunity to sense. In Figure 18-53A, sensing cannot be evaluated because there is no intrinsic ventricular

activity that occurs, and therefore the pacemaker is not given an opportunity to sense. In Figure 18-53B, the occurrence of two spontaneous QRS complexes provides the pacemaker with an opportunity to sense. In this example, sensing occurred normally, as indicated by the absence of the next expected pacing stimulus and resetting of the pacing interval by the intrinsic QRS complex.

Two sensing problems can occur: undersensing (Figures 18-56A and 18-57A) and oversensing (Figure 18-57B). Undersensing, also called "failure to sense" or "loss of sensing," can be caused by:

- Asynchronous (fixed rate) mode in which the sensing circuit is off. This problem can be corrected by turning the sensitivity control to the demand mode.
- Pacing catheter out of position or lying in infarcted tissue, which can be corrected by repositioning the wire. Pacing wire repositioning must be done by a physician; however, turning the patient onto his or her side sometimes temporarily works when the pacing wire loses contact with the ventricle.
- Intrinsic QRS voltage too low to be sensed by the pacemaker. Turning the sensitivity control clockwise or decreasing the sensitivity number increases the sensitivity of the pacemaker and makes it able to "see" smaller intrinsic electrical signals. Repositioning the wire sometimes helps.
- Break in connections, battery failure, or faulty pulse generator. Check and tighten all connections along the pacing system, and replace the battery if it is low. A chest x-ray may detect wire fracture. Change the pulse generator if problems cannot be corrected any other way.
- Intrinsic ventricular activity falling in the pacemaker's refractory period. If a spontaneous QRS complex occurs during the time the pacemaker has its eyes closed, the pacemaker cannot see it. This event occurs when the pacemaker fails to capture, which can allow

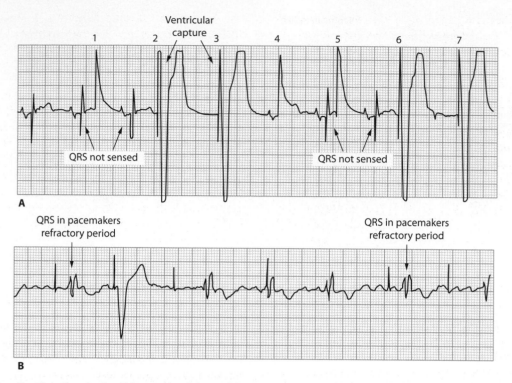

Figure 18-56. (A) Intermittent loss of sensing in a VVI pacemaker. Delivery of the pacing stimulus during the heart's refractory period makes it appear that capture is lost as well. Because the heart is physiologically unable to respond to the pacing stimulus when it falls in the refractory period, this is not a capture problem. Pacer spikes 1, 2, 5, and 6 should not have occurred; their presence is due to loss of sensing. Pacer spike 4 occurred coincident with the normal QRS complex, resulting in a "pseudofusion" beat, and does not represent loss of sensing. (B) Loss of capture in a VVI pacemaker. Only one pacer spike captures the ventricle. Two QRS complexes occur during the pacemaker's refractory period and thus are not sensed. This does not represent loss of sensing because the pacemaker has its "eyes closed" during the time intrinsic ventricular activity occurred.

an intrinsic QRS to occur during the pacemaker's refractory period. This problem is due to loss of capture and does not reflect a sensing malfunction (see Figure 18-56B).

Oversensing means that the pacemaker is so sensitive that it inappropriately senses internal or outside signals as QRS complexes and inhibits its output. Common sources of outside signals that can interfere with pacemaker function

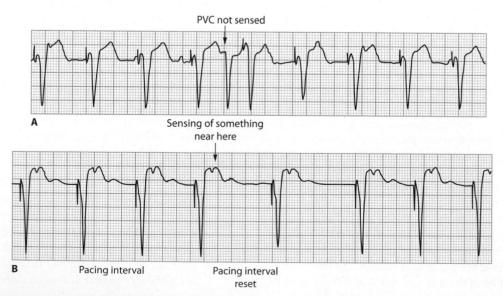

Figure 18-57. (A) Undersensing in a VVI pacemaker. The PVC is not sensed and pacing occurs at the programmed pacing interval, resulting in a pacemaker spike on the T wave of the PVC. (B) Oversensing in a VVI pacemaker. The pacing rate slows for two intervals, presumably due to sensing of something near the T wave, which resets the pacing interval from the point where sensing occurred.

include electromagnetic or RF signals, or electronic equipment in use near the pacemaker. Internal sources of interference can include large P waves, large T-wave voltage, local myopotentials in the heart, or skeletal muscle potentials (see Figure 18-57B). Because a VVI pacemaker is programmed to inhibit its output when it senses, oversensing can be a dangerous situation in a pacemaker-dependent patient, resulting in ventricular asystole. Oversensing is usually due to the sensitivity control being set too high, which can be corrected by turning the sensitivity dial counterclockwise (increasing the sensitivity number) and reducing the pacemaker's sensitivity. It is recommended that the sensitivity control be set between the 1 and 3 o'clock positions on the dial (about 2 mV) rather than all the way to the right, unless a higher sensitivity is required to make the pacemaker sense QRS complexes.

Stimulation Threshold Testing

The stimulation threshold is the minimum output of the pacemaker necessary to capture the heart consistently. The stimulation threshold changes over time. When the pacing lead is first placed, the stimulation threshold is usually very low. Over time, the threshold increases and it takes more output to result in capture. When caring for a patient with a temporary pacemaker, stimulation threshold testing should be done every shift until a stable threshold is reached. Once the threshold has been determined, set the output two to three times higher than threshold to ensure an adequate safety margin for capture. To determine the stimulation threshold, follow these steps:

- Verify that the patient is in a paced rhythm. The pacing rate may need to be temporarily increased to override an intrinsic rhythm.
- Watch the monitor continuously while slowly decreasing output by turning the output control counterclockwise.
- Note when the pacing stimulus no longer captures the heart (a pacing spike not followed by a paced beat).
- Slowly increase the output until 1:1 capture resumes. This is the stimulation threshold.
- Set the output two to three times higher than threshold (ie, if threshold is 2 mA, set output between 4 and 6 mA).

DDD Pacemaker Evaluation

Dual-chamber pacemakers have become very complicated, with multiple programmable parameters and varying functions depending on the manufacturer. It is impossible to present dual-chamber pacemaker function in detail in a single chapter. To understand dual-chamber pacemaker function, it is necessary to understand the timing cycles involved in dual-chamber pacing. More detailed information on dual-chamber pacemaker function is available in the references at the end of this chapter. In this section, the major timing cycles are defined and basic DDD pacemaker evaluation is covered in a very generic manner, because each pacemaker is different depending on the manufacturer. Dual-chamber pacemakers can function in a variety of modes (see Table 18-8). Because the DDD mode is most commonly used, basic DDD function is described here.

According to the pacemaker code, DDD means both chambers (atria and ventricles) are paced, both chambers are sensed, and the mode of response to sensed events is either inhibited or triggered, depending on which chamber is sensed. When atrial activity is sensed, pacing is triggered in the ventricle after the programmed AV delay unless intrinsic conduction to the ventricle occurs. When ventricular activity is sensed, all pacemaker output is inhibited.

The following timing cycles determine dual-chamber pacemaker function:

- *Pacing interval* (or lower rate limit): The base rate of the pacemaker is measured between two consecutive atrial pacing stimuli. The pacing interval is a programmed parameter.
- *AV delay* (or AV interval): The amount of time between atrial and ventricular pacing, or the "electronic PR interval." This is measured from the atrial pacing spike to the ventricular pacing spike and is a programmed parameter.
- *Atrial escape interval* (or VA interval): The interval from a sensed or paced ventricular event to the next atrial pacing output. The VA interval represents the amount of time the pacemaker waits after it paces in the ventricle or senses ventricular activity before pacing the atrium. The atrial escape interval is not a programmed parameter but is derived by subtracting the AV delay from the pacing interval. Its length can be estimated by measuring from a ventricular spike to the next atrial pacing spike.
- *Total atrial refractory period* (TARP): The period of time following a sensed P wave or a paced atrial event during which the atrial channel will not respond to sensed events (ie, "has its eyes closed"). The TARP consists of the AV delay and the PVARP (see later).
- *Post ventricular atrial refractory period* (PVARP): The period of time following an intrinsic QRS or a paced ventricular beat during which the atrial channel is refractory and will not respond to sensed atrial activity. PVARP is a programmable parameter but is not evident on a rhythm strip.
- *Blanking period*: The very short ventricular refractory period (VRP) that occurs with every atrial pacemaker output. The ventricular channel "blinks its eyes" so it does not sense the atrial output and inappropriately inhibits ventricular pacing. The blanking period is a programmable parameter but is not evident on a rhythm strip.
- *Ventricular refractory period*: The period of time following a paced ventricular beat or a sensed QRS during which the ventricular channel ignores intrinsic

ventricular activity (ie, "has its eyes closed"). VRP is a programmable parameter but is not evident on a rhythm strip.

- *Maximum tracking interval* (or upper rate limit): The maximum rate at which the ventricular channel will track atrial activity. The upper rate limit prevents rapid ventricular pacing in response to very rapid atrial activity, such as atrial tachycardia or atrial flutter. The maximum tracking interval is a programmable parameter and usually is set according to how active a patient is expected to be and how fast a ventricular rate is likely to be tolerated.

Because a dual-chamber pacemaker has both atrial and ventricular pacing and sensing functions, evaluation includes assessing atrial capture, atrial sensing, ventricular capture, and ventricular sensing. To evaluate dual-chamber pacemaker function accurately, it is necessary to know the following information: mode of function (ie, DDD, DVI), minimum rate, upper rate limit, AV delay, PVARP, and VRPs. In the real world of bedside nursing, this information is not always available, so we do the best we can with what we have. The following sections briefly discuss the issues of assessing atrial and ventricular capture and sensing in a dual-chamber pacing system.

Atrial Capture

Atrial capture, unlike ventricular capture, is not always easy to see. Often, the atrial response to pacing is so small that it cannot be seen in many monitoring leads, so we cannot rely on the presence of a P wave following every atrial pacer spike as evidence of atrial capture. If a clear P wave is present after every atrial pacemaker spike, atrial capture can be assumed. In the absence of a clear P wave, atrial capture can only be assumed when a normally conducted QRS complex follows an atrial pacer spike within the programmed AV delay. If the atrial spike captures the atrium and there is intact AV conduction, the presence of the normal QRS indicates that the atrium must have been captured for conduction to occur into the ventricles before the ventricular pacing stimulus was delivered. Because a DDD pacemaker paces the ventricle at a preset AV interval following atrial pacing, the presence of a ventricular paced beat following an atrial paced beat does not verify capture, because the ventricle paces at the end of the AV delay whether atrial capture occurs or not. Therefore, atrial capture can only be assumed when there is an obvious P wave after every atrial pacing spike or when an atrial pacing spike is followed by a normal QRS within the programmed AV delay.

Atrial Sensing

Atrial sensing is verified by the presence of a spontaneous P wave that is followed by a paced ventricular beat at the end of the programmed AV delay. If a P wave is sensed, it starts the AV delay and ventricular pacing is triggered at the end of the AV delay unless AV conduction is intact and results in a normal QRS. The presence of a normal P wave followed by a normal QRS only proves that AV conduction is intact, not that the pacemaker is sensing electrical activity in the atria. Therefore, atrial sensing is verified by a spontaneous P wave followed by a paced QRS.

Ventricular Capture

Ventricular capture is recognized by a wide QRS immediately following a ventricular pacing spike. Ventricular capture is much easier to recognize than atrial capture and is no different than with single-chamber ventricular pacing.

Ventricular Sensing

Ventricular sensing can only be verified if there is spontaneous ventricular activity present for the pacemaker to sense. Ventricular sensing is verified when an atrial pacer spike followed by a normal QRS inhibits the ventricular pacing spike, which is the same event that proves atrial capture. If a QRS is sensed before the next atrial pacing spike is due, both the atrial and ventricular pacing stimuli are inhibited and the VA interval (atrial escape interval) is reset.

Dual-chamber pacemakers are capable of operating in four states of pacing: atrial and ventricular pacing (AV sequential pacing state), atrial pacing with ventricular sensing, atrial sensing with ventricular pacing (atrial tracking state), and atrial and ventricular sensing. All four states of pacing can occur within a short period of time, and the timing cycles determine which state of pacing is done. Figure 18-58 shows the four states of dual-chamber pacing, and Figure 18-59 illustrates the basic principles of dual-chamber pacemaker evaluation.

Cardiac Resynchronization Therapy With Biventricular Pacing

Patients with chronic HF often have intraventricular conduction delays (especially LBBB) that result in ventricular dyssynchrony and impair cardiac function. This intraventricular conduction delay causes electrical and mechanical abnormalities in ventricular function that interfere with ventricular filling, impair cardiac output, worsen mitral regurgitation, and contribute to mortality in patients with HF. LBBB causes both electrical and mechanical abnormalities that result in ventricular dyssynchrony. Interventricular dyssynchrony refers to the time delay between right and left ventricular contraction, where the right ventricle (RV) depolarizes and contracts before the left ventricle (LV). Intraventricular dyssynchrony refers to the abnormal segmental contraction within the LV as it depolarizes late and abnormally in LBBB.

When the RV contracts before the LV, the septum depolarizes and contracts with the RV instead of with the LV. Since the septum normally contributes to LV ejection by contracting with the LV, normal septal function is lost in LBBB. Since the septum contracts with the RV, it is relaxed by the time the LV begins contracting, and increasing pressure in the LV causes paradoxical septal motion by pushing the septum into the RV. In LBBB, the papillary muscles that are responsible

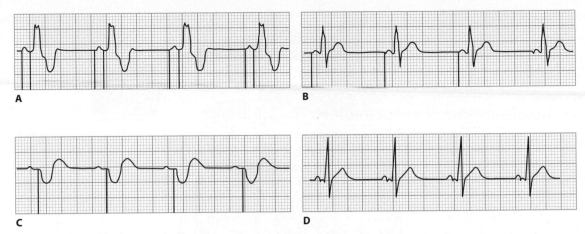

Figure 18-58. Four states of DDD pacing. **(A)** Atrial and ventricular pacing (AV sequential pacing state). **(B)** Atrial pacing, ventricular sensing. **(C)** Atrial sensing, ventricular pacing (atrial tracking state). **(D)** Atrial and ventricular sensing (inhibited pacing state).

for holding the mitral valve leaflets tight depolarize late and fail to keep valve leaflets from everting into the atria during LV systole, resulting in mitral regurgitation. The combination of paradoxical septal wall motion and mitral regurgitation contribute to the already reduced LV stroke volume that occurs in HF. Portions of the LV that are activated first contract before those portions that are activated late, creating mechanical dyssynchrony that reduces systolic function by about 20%, reduces stroke volume, increases wall stress, and delays relaxation.

Cardiac resynchronization therapy (CRT) is biventricular pacing aimed at improving electromechanical activity in the failing heart. The goals of CRT are to improve hemodynamics by restoring ventricular synchrony, and improve quality of life via symptom relief. CRT devices can be standalone pacemakers or combination ICD and biventricular pacemakers (CRT-D). Class I recommendations for CRT include patients with the following characteristics: HF with New York Heart Association (NYHA) class II, III, or ambulatory IV symptoms; left ventricular ejection fraction less than 35%; presence of significant intraventricular conduction delay (QRS duration > 150 msec); sinus rhythm; and symptoms in spite of optimal guideline directed medical therapy for HF. Class IIa indications include patients with LVEF less than 35% and NYHA class II, III, or ambulatory IV symptoms with QRS duration between 120 and 149 msec; those with non-LBBB pattern wide QRS of more than 150 msec;

those with atrial fibrillation who are likely to be near 100% ventricular paced; and those undergoing new or replacement device implantation with anticipated requirement for more than 40% ventricular pacing.

CRT is accomplished by placing standard pacing leads in the right atrium and into the right ventricular apex as is done for normal dual-chamber pacing. A third lead is advanced through the coronary sinus and into a lateral or posterior left ventricular vein for pacing of the LV (Figure 18-60).

The goal in biventricular pacing is to cause both ventricles to depolarize and contract simultaneously, thus eliminating the interventricular and intraventricular dyssynchrony that occurs during LBBB. The AV interval is often programmed shorter than intrinsic AV conduction in order to force the ventricles to pace rather than allowing intrinsic conduction to occur. Biventricular pacing causes both ventricles to contract simultaneously and allows the septum to contract with the LV. Controlling the AV delay restores the normal timing between left atrial and left ventricular contraction, allowing the LV papillary muscles to contract earlier and put tension on the mitral valve leaflets to reduce or prevent mitral regurgitation. Biventricular pacing allows the LV to complete contraction and begin relaxation earlier, which increases filling time and improves "atrial kick."

Electrocardiographic evaluation of biventricular pacemaker function is more complicated than single ventricle pacing from the right ventricular apex. Pacing from the

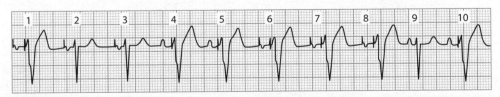

Figure 18-59. DDD pacemaker operating in all four states of pacing. Beats 1, 6, 7, and 8 illustrate AV sequential pacing (A pace and V pace); beats 2 and 3 illustrate atrial pacing and ventricular sensing; beats 4, 5, and 10 illustrate atrial sensing and ventricular pacing; beat 9 is an intrinsic beat with normal P wave and normal conduction to the ventricle. Atrial capture is proven evident in beats 1, 2, 3, 6, 7, and 8; atrial sensing is verified by beats 4, 5, and 10; ventricular capture is evident in beats 1, 4, 5, 6, 7, 8, and 10; ventricular sensing is verified by beats 2, 3, and 9.

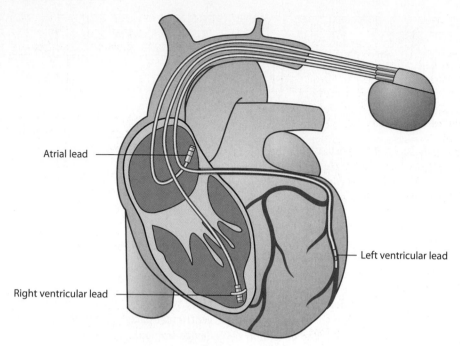

Atrial lead

Left ventricular lead

Right ventricular lead

Figure 18-60. Lead placement for biventricular pacing.

RV apex creates an LBBB pattern with a wide negative QRS complex in lead V_1. Left ventricular pacing is more complicated due to the fact that the LV lead can be placed in either a lateral or posterior LV vein and can be located in an apical or a basal site within the vein. The resulting QRS varies in morphology, depending on the location of the LV lead, but, in general, LV pacing produces an RBBB pattern with a wide upright QRS complex in lead V_1. It makes logical sense that pacing both ventricles simultaneously would result in a narrow QRS complex preceded by a pacemaker spike, but this narrowing is not always obvious with biventricular pacing. Loss of capture in one or the other ventricle should cause a change in the morphology of the paced QRS that would indicate single-chamber pacing from the ventricle that is still being captured. A shift in the frontal plane axis may also occur with loss of capture in one ventricle.

Some experts recommend recording four 12-lead ECGs at the time of implant: during intrinsic conduction, in the course of RV pacing with capture, in LV pacing with capture, and during biventricular pacing with capture in both ventricles. These ECGs should be examined to determine which lead best demonstrates an obvious difference between the four pacing states recorded, then the best lead should be used as the monitoring lead for pacemaker evaluation. Figure 18-61 shows leads V_1 and II recorded during intrinsic conduction, RV pacing, LV pacing, and bi-ventricular pacing. Note the similarity between the intrinsic QRS with LBBB and the RV paced QRS, which produces an "iatrogenic" LBBB pattern. The ventricular pacing spike is not visible in lead V_1 in LV pacing, and the QRS is negative during LV pacing in this patient as opposed to the more common upright QRS during LV pacing. The QRS during biventricular pacing is narrower than the intrinsic beats and the single-chamber paced beats. Lead V_1 would be a good monitoring lead for this patient due to the differences in QRS morphology among these four examples.

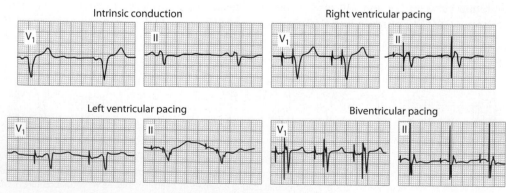

Intrinsic conduction

Right ventricular pacing

Left ventricular pacing

Biventricular pacing

Figure 18-61. ECG in biventricular pacing.

SELECTED BIBLIOGRAPHY

Electrocardiography

Bayes de Luna A, Goldwasser D, Fiol M, Bayes-Genis A. Surface electrocardiography. In: Fuster V, Harrington R, Narula J, Eapen Z, eds. *Hurst's The Heart*. 14th ed. New York: McGraw Hill; 2017.

Hanna EB, Gancy DL. ST segment depression and T wave inversion: classification, differential diagnosis, and caveats. *Cleve Clin J Med*. 2011:78:404-414.

Jacobson C, Marzlin K, Webner C. *Cardiovascular Nursing Practice 3rd ed: Cardiac Arrhythmias & 12 Lead ECG Interpretation*. Burien, WA: Cardiovascular Nursing Education Associates; 2021.

Mirvis DM, Goldberger AL. Electrocardiography. In: Zipes DP, Libby R, Bonow D, Mann G, Tomaselli G, eds. *Braunwald's Heart Disease: A Textbook of Cardiovascular Medicine*. 11th ed. Philadelphia, PA: Elsevier; 2019.

Sgarbossa EB, Pinski SL, Barbagelata A, et al. Electrocardiographic diagnosis of evolving acute myocardial infarction in the presence of left bundle-branch block. *N Engl J Med*. 1996;334:481-487.

Wiegand, DL, eds. Unit II: Cardiovascular. Section 6: Cardiac pacemakers and Section 8: Electrocardiographic leads and cardiac monitoring. In: *AACN Procedure Manual for High Acuity, Progressive and Critical Care*. 7th ed. St Louis, MO: Elsevier; 2017.

Acute Coronary Syndrome

Buller CE, Yuling F, Mahaffey KW, et al. ST-segment recovery and outcome after primary percutaneous coronary intervention for ST-elevation myocardial infarction. *Circulation*. 2008;118:1335-1346.

Moliterno DJ, Januzzi JL. Evaluation and management of non-ST-segment elevation myocardial infarction. In: Fuster V, Harrington RA, Narula J, Eapen ZJ, eds. *Hurst's the Heart*. 14th ed. New York, NY: McGraw Hill; 2017.

O'Gara P, Kushner FG, Ascheim DD, et al. 2013 ACCF/AHA guideline for the management of ST-elevation myocardial infarction. *Circulation*. 2013;127:e362-e425.

Patel MR, Singh M, Gersh BJ, O'Neill W. ST-segment elevation myocardial infarction. In: Fuster V, Harrington RA, Narula J, Eapen ZJ, eds. *Hurst's the Heart*. 14th ed. New York, NY: McGraw Hill; 2017.

Long QT Syndrome and Brugada Syndrome

Brugada J, Campuzano O, Arbelo E, et al. Present status of Brugada syndrome. *JACC*. 2018;72:1046-1059.

Kusumoto F, Bailey K, Chaouki A, et al. Systematic Review for the 2017 AHA/ACC/HRS Guideline for Management of Patients With Ventricular Arrhythmias and the Prevention of Sudden Cardiac Death. *J Am Coll Cardiol*. 2018 Oct, 72 (14) 1653–1676.

Priori SG, Wilde AM, Horie M, et al. HRS/EHRA/APHRS expert consensus statement on the diagnosis and management of patients with inherited primary arrhythmia syndromes. *Heart Rhythm*. 2013;10(12):1932-1963.

Dysrhythmias

Bradfield JS, Boyle NG, Shivkumar K. Ventricular arrhythmias. In: Fuster V, Harrington RA, Narula J, Eapen ZJ, eds. *Hurst's the Heart*. 14th ed. New York, NY: McGraw Hill; 2017.

Calkins H. Supraventricular tachycardia: atrial tachycardia, atrioventricular nodal reentry, and Wolff-Parkinson-White syndrome. In: Fuster V, Harrington RA, Narula J, Eapen ZJ, eds. *Hurst's the Heart*. 14th ed. New York, NY: McGraw Hill; 2017.

Jacobson C, Marzlin K, Webner C. *Cardiovascular Nursing Practice 3rd ed: Cardiac Arrhythmias & 12 Lead ECG Interpretation*. Burien, WA: Cardiovascular Nursing Education Associates; 2021.

Pacemakers

Barold SS, Herweg B, Giudici M. Electrocardiographic follow-up of biventricular pacemakers. *Ann Noninvasive Electrocardiol*. 2005;10(2):231-255.

Jacobson C, Marzlin K, Webner C. *Cardiovascular Nursing Practice 3rd ed: Cardiac Arrhythmias & 12 Lead ECG Interpretation*. Burien, WA: Cardiovascular Nursing Education Associates; 2021.

Kenny T. *The Nuts and Bolts of Cardiac Pacing*. Malden, MA: Blackwell Futura; 2005.

Swerdlow CD, Wang PJ, Zipes DP. Pacemakers and implantable cardioverter-defibrillators. In: Zipes DP, Libby P, Bonow RO, Mann DL, Tomaselli GF, eds. *Braunwald's Heart Disease: A Textbook of Cardiovascular Medicine*. 11th ed. Philadelphia, PA: Elsevier; 2019:780-806.

Upadhyay GA, Singh JP. Pacemakers and defibrillators. In: Fuster V, Harrington RA, Narula J, Eapen ZJ, eds. *Hurst's the Heart*. 14th ed. New York, NY: McGraw Hill; 2017.

Evidence-Based Practice

AACN Practice Alert. Accurate dysrhythmia monitoring in adults. *Crit Care Nurse*. 2016;36(6):e26-e34.

AACN Practice Alert. Ensuring accurate ST-segment monitoring. *Critical Care Nurse*. 2016;36(6):e18-e25.

Drew BJ, Ackerman MJ, Funk M. Prevention of Torsade de Pointes in hospital settings. *J Am Coll Cardiol*. 2010;55:934-947.

Epstein AE, DiMarco JP, Ellenbogen KA. ACC/AHA/HRS 2008 guidelines for device-based therapy of cardiac rhythm abnormalities: a report of the American College of Cardiology/American Heart Association Task Force on Practice Guidelines. *Circulation*. 2008;117:e350-e408.

Hancock EW, Deal BJ, Mirvis DM. AHA/ACCF/HRS recommendations for the standardization and interpretation of the electrocardiogram part V: electrocardiogram changes associated with cardiac chamber hypertrophy. A scientific statement from the American Heart Association Electrocardiography and Arrhythmias Committee, Council on Clinical Cardiology; the American College of Cardiology Foundation; and the Heart Rhythm Society. *Circulation*. 2009;119:e251-e261.

O'Gara P, Kushner FG, Ascheim DD, et al. 2013 ACCF/AHA guideline for the management of ST-elevation myocardial infarction. *Circulation*. 2013;127:e362-e425.

Page RL, Joglar JA, Caldwell MA, et al. ACC/AHA/HRS Guideline for the management of adult patients with supraventricular tachycardia: a report of the American College of Cardiology/American Heart Association Task Force on Practice Guidelines and the Heart Rhythm Society. *Circulation*. 2016;133:e506-e574.

Priori SG, Blomstrom-Lundqvist C, Mazzanti A, et al. 2015 ESC guidelines for the management of patients with ventricular arrhythmias and the prevention of sudden cardiac death. *Eur Heart J*. 2015;36:2793-2867.

Priori SG, Wilde AA, Horie M, et al. HRS/EHRA/APHRS expert consensus statement on the diagnosis and management of patients with inherited primary arrhythmia syndromes. *Heart Rhythm*. 2013;10:1932-1963.

Rautaharju PM, Surawicz B, Gettes LS. AHA/ACCF/HRS recommendations for the standardization and interpretation of the electrocardiogram part IV: the ST segment, T and U waves, and the QT interval. A scientific statement from the American Heart Association Electrocardiography and Arrhythmias Committee, Council on Clinical Cardiology; the American College of Cardiology Foundation; and the Heart Rhythm Society. *Circulation*. 2009;119:e241-e250.

Sandau KE, Funk M, Auerbach A, et al. Update to practice standards for electrocardiographic monitoring in hospital settings. *Circulation*. 2017:136;e273-e344.

Surawicz B, Childers R, Deal BJ, Gettes LS. AHA/ACCF/HRS recommendations for the standardization and interpretation of the electrocardiogram part III: intraventricular conduction disturbances: a scientific statement from the American Heart Association Electrocardiography and Arrhythmias Committee, Council on Clinical Cardiology; the American College of Cardiology Foundation; and the Heart Rhythm Society. *Circulation*. 2009;119:e235-e240.

Thygesen K, Alpert J, Jaffe A, et al. Fourth universal definition of myocardial infarction. *JACC*. 2018;72:2018-2231.

Tracy CM, Epstein AE, Darbar D. 2012 ACCF/AHA/HRS focused update of the 2008 guidelines for device-based therapy of cardiac rhythm abnormalities: a report of the American College of Cardiology Foundation/American Heart Association Task Force on Practice Guidelines. *Circulation*. 2012;126:1784-1800.

Wagner GS, Macfarlane P, Wellens H, et al. AHA/ACCF/HRS recommendations for the standardization and interpretation of the electrocardiogram: part VI: acute ischemia/infarction: a scientific statement from the American Heart Association Electrocardiography and Arrhythmias Committee, Council on Clinical Cardiology; the American College of Cardiology Foundation; and the Heart Rhythm Society. *Circulation*. 2009;119: e262-e270.

ADVANCED CARDIOVASCULAR CONCEPTS

19

Barbara Leeper

KNOWLEDGE COMPETENCIES

1. Describe the etiology, pathophysiology, clinical presentation, and patient needs in:
   - Cardiomyopathy
   - Valvular disease
   - Pericarditis
   - Aortic aneurysm
   - Cardiac transplantation

2. Compare and contrast the principles of management of:

   - Cardiomyopathy
   - Valvular disease
   - Pericarditis
   - Aortic aneurysm
   - Cardiac transplantation

3. Identify indications for, complications of, and nursing management of patients receiving intra-aortic balloon pump (IABP) and ventricular assist device (VAD) therapy.

PATHOLOGIC CONDITIONS

Cardiomyopathy

Cardiomyopathy is made up of a group of diseases involving destruction of the cardiac muscle fibers, causing either mechanical or electrical dysfunction resulting in a decreased cardiac output (CO). The body responds to this with initiation of several neuroendocrine responses including activation of the sympathetic nervous system and renin-angiotensin-aldosterone chain. The prevailing result is marked vasoconstriction, retention of sodium and water, and further myocyte injury. This process contributes to remodeling of ventricular myocytes and the downward spiral of cardiomyopathy. The cause of cardiomyopathy is often unknown. Cardiomyopathies are commonly classified into three types: dilated, hypertrophic, and restrictive (Figure 19-1).

Dilated cardiomyopathy, the most common type of cardiomyopathy, is commonly caused by coronary artery disease and is associated with impaired myocardial contractility and increased left ventricular end-diastolic pressures (LVEDPs). Coronary artery disease contributes to ventricular remodeling, thereby reducing ejection fraction. The two case studies

presented later in this chapter involve patients with dilated cardiomyopathy.

Hypertrophic cardiomyopathy may occur in both the young and the older adults. Hypertrophic cardiomyopathy is often categorized as obstructive or nonobstructive. Ventricular hypertrophy occurs in both types. The diagnosis of obstructive hypertrophic cardiomyopathy is made if hypertrophy of the intraventricular septum is also present. This is the congenital form and is often referred to as hypertrophic obstructive cardiomyopathy (HOCM). In the past, other terms used to describe this type of cardiomyopathy were idiopathic hypertrophic subaortic stenosis (IHSS) and asymmetric septal hypertrophy (ASH). The hypertrophied septum obstructs the left ventricular outflow tract just below the aortic valve, thereby limiting ejection. Blood volume is "trapped" within the left ventricular chamber.

Restrictive cardiomyopathy is the least common of the three types. A classic finding for this type of cardiomyopathy is ventricular fibrosis, often caused by infiltration of the cardiac myocytes with abnormal tissue such as sarcoid or amyloid disease. The fibrotic muscle tissue becomes very rigid with decreased compliance thus limiting distention during diastole.

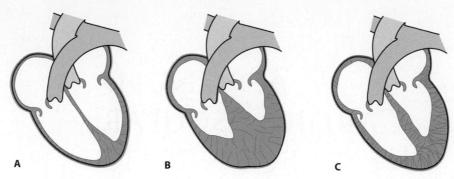

Figure 19-1. Types of cardiomyopathies. **(A)** Dilated (cardiac dilation and impaired contractility). **(B)** Hypertrophic (decreased size of ventricular chambers and increased ventricular muscle mass). **(C)** Restrictive (decreased ventricular compliance).

Etiology and Pathophysiology

A variety of conditions may cause or contribute to the development of cardiomyopathy (Table 19-1). As noted previously, coronary artery disease is the most common cause of dilated cardiomyopathy in the United States. Early studies show that myocardial cells are a target for COVID-19. There have been several reports worldwide of myocarditis occurring several weeks after the viral infection. The actual prevalence is unclear as researchers continue to investigate the impact of this virus.

Pathophysiology of Dilated Cardiomyopathy

Dilated cardiomyopathy begins with gradual destruction of the myocardial fibers, impairing myocardial contraction. As the disease progresses, left ventricular dilation occurs, with increased blood volume in the left ventricle at the end of diastole. Additionally, ventricular compliance is reduced which contributes to an increase in LVEDP and a decrease in SV and CO. Left atrial volume and pressure eventually increase as the atrium struggles to overcome the higher LVEDP and eject blood into the left ventricle. The increased left atrial pressure often leads to an increased pulmonary capillary pressure as the higher filling pressures are reflected back into the pulmonary vascular bed leading to the development of pulmonary hypertension. Right ventricular failure will eventually occur as the right ventricle has a limited capacity to increase its force of contraction against the higher pressures in the pulmonary vascular bed. Eventually, the right ventricle dilates along with the left ventricle. In addition, the atrioventricular valves (mitral and tricuspid) may develop insufficiency due to the dilated chambers stretching the papillary muscle and interfering with the closure of the valves.

Pathophysiology of Hypertrophic Cardiomyopathy

Patients with hypertrophic cardiomyopathy have a greatly thickened ventricular wall (see Figure 19-1). It is not uncommon for the ventricular chamber size to be dramatically reduced because of the hypertrophy. In obstructive cardiomyopathy, the intraventricular septum is also involved in the hypertrophic process, whereas in nonobstructive cardiomyopathy, the septum is relatively normal. Common causes of the nonobstructive form include aortic stenosis and hypertension. The hypertrophied ventricle becomes rigid, reducing ventricular compliance and distention. Myocardial contractility becomes impaired resulting in decreased stroke volume and CO. If HOCM is present, left ventricular systolic ejection will be compromised by obstruction of the outflow tract as the anterior leaflet of the mitral valve presses against an enlarged intraventricular septum. Stress is placed on the left atrium as it attempts to propel blood forward into the stiff left ventricle. It is not uncommon for left atrial enlargement to develop as the left atrium is forced to contract against high left ventricular resistance.

Pathophysiology of Restrictive Cardiomyopathy

The ventricles of patients with restrictive cardiomyopathy become rigid as fibrotic tissue infiltrates the myocardium. The stiffness of the ventricles decreases the compliance, or distensibility of the ventricles, thus limiting ventricular filling and increasing end-diastolic pressures. Myocardial contractility is

TABLE 19-1. ETIOLOGY OF CARDIOMYOPATHY

Dilated Cardiomyopathy
- Idiopathic
- Coronary artery disease
- Toxins, such as lead, alcohol, cocaine
- Chemotherapeutic agents
- Viral, bacterial, or fungal infections
- Chagas disease (parasitic)
- Peripartum or postpartum status
- Hemochromatosis
- Scleroderma
- Hypertension
- Microvascular spasm

Hypertrophic Cardiomyopathy
- Idiopathic
- Congenital
- Aortic stenosis
- Amyloidosis

Restrictive Cardiomyopathy
- Idiopathic
- Myocardial fibrosis
- Hypertrophy
- Amyloidosis
- Hemochromatosis
- Scleroderma

impaired, leading to decreases in CO. As with the other types of cardiomyopathy, atrial workload is increased as the atria attempt to propel blood forward into stiff ventricles. Often, the atrioventricular valves become insufficient and the pressures in the pulmonary vascular bed and peripheral venous bed increase, leading to peripheral edema.

ESSENTIAL CONTENT CASE

Cardiomyopathy—Case 1

A 56-year-old man was admitted to the emergency room with shortness of breath. His chest x-ray revealed an enlarged heart and pulmonary congestion. His 12-lead electrocardiogram (ECG) was consistent with left ventricular hypertrophy and his rhythm was atrial fibrillation (AF) with a ventricular rate of 102. Clinical findings included bilateral crackles auscultated one-third up from the bases, bilateral lower extremity, 4+ pitting edema to the midcalf, jugular venous distention (JVD), an S_3, and a systolic murmur heard best at the apex. An emergency echocardiogram showed impaired contractility of the dilated left ventricle.

Case Question 1: After the patient is admitted and his diagnosis is confirmed, the initial priority for his medical management is:
(A) Initiate inotropic support
(B) Obtain electrophysiology consult for a biventricular pacemaker workup
(C) Administer a diuretic to reduce fluid overload
(D) Administer carvedilol to control the ventricular rate

Case Question 2: The most likely cause of a systolic murmur in this patient is:
(A) Aortic stenosis
(B) Mitral insufficiency
(C) Tricuspid stenosis
(D) Pulmonic insufficiency

Answers
1. C is the correct answer. A diuretic is indicated to reduce his signs and symptoms of significant fluid overload.
2. B is the correct answer. The mitral insufficiency produces a systolic murmur (valve is leaking when it should be closed) that is heard best at the apex. Murmurs of the aortic and pulmonary valves are heard best at the second intercostal space on the right sternal border (aortic) and left sternal border (pulmonic). Murmurs from the tricuspid valve are heard at the fourth intercostal space at the left sternal border.

Clinical Presentation

Patients may be asymptomatic for lengthy periods of time (months to years) prior to being diagnosed with a cardiomyopathy. By the time patients develop symptoms, myocardial contractility may be significantly impaired. The heart rate (HR) increases initially as the heart attempts to maintain an adequate CO. As the disease progresses and/or during physical exertion, the impaired myocardium is no longer able to maintain an adequate CO to meet the metabolic demands of the tissues in spite of the increased heart rate.

ESSENTIAL CONTENT CASE

Cardiomyopathy—Case 2

A 32-year-old woman was admitted to the high-risk perinatal unit at 31 weeks' gestation with dyspnea and fatigue. She had bilateral, basilar crackles, and her oxygen saturation via pulse oximetry was 88%. An echocardiogram showed a markedly dilated left ventricle with diffuse hypokinesis and an ejection fraction of 20% to 25%.

A pulmonary artery catheter was placed and the following parameters were obtained:

Right atrial (RA)	12 mm Hg
PA	48/26 mm Hg
Elevated pulmonary artery occlusion pressures (PAOP)	24 mm Hg
CO	3.7 L/min
Cardiac index (CI)	1.8 L/min/m^2

A dobutamine infusion was initiated at 5 mcg/kg/min and oxygen was applied at 6 L/min via nasal cannula.

Case Question 1: The most likely medical diagnosis for this patient is:
(A) Hypertrophic obstructive cardiomyopathy
(B) Restrictive cardiomyopathy
(C) Peripartum cardiomyopathy
(D) Idiopathic cardiomyopathy

Case Question 2: Her hemodynamic profile indicates a low CI with possible volume overload as evidenced by:
(A) PA pressure 48/26 mm Hg
(B) RAP (12 mm Hg) and PAOP (24 mm Hg)
(C) EF 20% to 25%
(D) Spo_2 88%

Case Question 3: Your plan of care for this patient includes which of the following:
(A) Improve oxygen delivery to the tissues
(B) Increase myocardial contractility
(C) Careful management of preload as blood volume is normally 1.5 times higher during pregnancy
(D) Education about self-management of heart failure and coping strategies
(E) All of the above

Answers
1. C is the correct answer. Her symptoms presented at 31 weeks gestation.
2. B is the correct answer given her clinical presentation of dyspnea and the presence of bibasilar crackles confirming the cause of the elevated RAP and PAOP.
3. E is the correct answer. All of these strategies are important for the management of this patient.

Dilated Cardiomyopathy

1. Inability to maintain adequate CO
   - Fatigue
   - Weakness
   - Sinus tachycardia
   - Pulses alternans

- Narrowed pulse pressure
- Decreased CO

2. Increased left ventricular filling pressures (LVEDP)
   - Dyspnea
   - Orthopnea
   - Paroxysmal nocturnal dyspnea
   - Crackles
   - S3/S4
   - Dysrhythmias (atrial fibrillation (AF), ventricular tachycardia, or fibrillation)
   - Systolic murmur associated with mitral valve insufficiency
   - Abnormal hemodynamic profile:
     – Increased pulmonary artery systolic (PAS) and diastolic (PAD) pressures
     – Elevated pulmonary artery occlusion pressures (PAOPs)
     – Increased systemic vascular resistance (SVR)
     – Elevated V wave on PAOP waveform with mitral valve insufficiency

3. Increased right ventricular filling pressures
   - Peripheral edema
   - JVD
   - Hepatomegaly
   - Elevated V wave on the RA waveform and systolic murmur with tricuspid valve insufficiency

4. Increased atrial pressures
   - Palpitations
   - S_4 may develop as the atria attempt to eject blood into stiff ventricles
   - Atrial dysrhythmias may occur, such as premature atrial complexes (PACs) or AF, due to the increase in atrial pressure
   - Elevated A wave on PAOP waveform
   - Elevated RA pressures
   - Elevated A wave on the RA waveform

Hypertrophic Cardiomyopathy

1. Inability to maintain adequate CO
   - Angina
   - Syncope
   - Fatigue
   - Sinus tachycardia
   - Ventricular dysrhythmias including ventricular fibrillation
   - CO is initially normal, then decreases

2. Increased ventricular filling pressures
   - Dyspnea
   - Orthopnea
   - Dysrhythmias, such as premature ventricular contractions or ventricular tachycardia
   - Abnormal hemodynamic profile:
     – Elevated PAS and PAD pressures
     – Elevated PAOP pressure
     – Increased SVR

3. Increased atrial pressure
   - S_4 may develop as the atria attempt to eject blood into rigid ventricles
   - Atrial dysrhythmias may occur (eg, PACs, AF) due to the increase in atrial pressure
   - Palpitations
   - Elevated A wave on PAOP waveform
   - Elevated RA pressure

4. Left ventricular outflow tract obstruction
   - Systolic murmur as blood flows through a narrowed outflow tract owing to septal hypertrophy; heard at apex

Restrictive Cardiomyopathy

Signs and symptoms of restrictive cardiomyopathy and pericarditis are similar. Diagnosis can usually be made after an echocardiogram.

1. Inability to maintain adequate CO
   - Activity intolerance
   - Weakness
   - Sinus tachycardia
   - Dysrhythmias
   - Decreased CO/CI

2. Increased left ventricular filling pressures
   - Dyspnea
   - JVD
   - S_3
   - Narrowed pulse pressure
   - Systolic murmur with mitral valve insufficiency
   - Abnormal hemodynamic profile:
     – Elevated PAS, PAD, and PAOP pressures
     – Elevated SVR
     – Elevated V wave on PAOP waveform with mitral valve insufficiency

3. Increased right ventricular pressures
   - Peripheral edema
   - Hepatomegaly
   - Jaundice
   - JVD
   - Systolic murmur with tricuspid valve insufficiency
   - Kussmaul sign (increased neck vein distention with inspiration)
   - Elevated V wave on the RA waveform if tricuspid valve insufficient

4. Increased atrial pressures
   - Palpitations
   - S_4 may develop as the atria attempt to eject blood into rigid ventricles
   - Atrial dysrhythmias may occur (eg, PACs, AF) due to the increase in atrial pressure
   - Elevated A wave on PAOP waveform
   - Elevated RA pressure
   - Elevated A wave on the RA waveform

Diagnostic Tests
Dilated Cardiomyopathy

- *Chest x-ray:* Left ventricular dilation with potential enlargement and dilation of all four cardiac chambers
- *12-lead ECG:* ST-segment and T-wave changes; left axis deviation; left ventricular hypertrophy and bundle branch block (LBBB most common)
- *Echocardiography:* Dilated left ventricle with an increase in chamber size (other chambers may be enlarged also); diminished ventricular contractility; decreased septal wall movement; elevated ventricular volumes and decreased ejection fraction

Hypertrophic Cardiomyopathy

- *Chest x-ray:* Normal or left atrial and ventricular hypertrophy
- *12-lead ECG:* ST-segment and T-wave changes; septal Q waves due to septal hypertrophy; left ventricular hypertrophy
- *Echocardiography:* Thickened ventricular walls with a decrease in chamber size; left ventricular outflow obstruction created by thickened ventricular septum and motion of mitral valve leaflet

Restrictive Cardiomyopathy

- *Chest x-ray:* Normal or slight enlargement of left atria and ventricle
- *12-lead ECG:* ST-segment and T-wave changes; low QRS amplitude
- *Echocardiography:* Thickened ventricular walls; enlarged atria; diminished ventricular contractility; decreased ventricular volumes; elevated ventricular end-diastolic pressures

Principles of Management for Cardiomyopathy

The primary objectives in the management of cardiomyopathy are to treat the underlying cause (if known); maximize cardiac function; assist the patient and family members to cope with a debilitating, chronic disease; and prevent complications associated with cardiomyopathy.

Improvement of Cardiac Function

Dilated Cardiomyopathy

1. *Improve myocardial oxygenation:* As ventricular dilation occurs, ventricular wall tension increases, increasing the myocardial workload and oxygen consumption. Oxygen therapy is initiated as necessary to increase oxygen delivery. Pulse oximetry, mixed venous oxygenation saturation (SVO_2) or central venous oxygen saturation ($ScvO_2$), and arterial blood gases are helpful in guiding supplemental oxygen therapy.
2. *Increase myocardial contractility:* Inotropic agents including β1 receptor stimulating agents (eg, dobutamine) and phosphodiesterase inhibitors (eg, milrinone) produce a positive inotropic effect (eg,

strengthen myocardial contractility) and cause mild vasodilation, thereby reducing the workload of the failing ventricle.

3. *Decrease preload and afterload:* Diuretics decrease excess fluid and lower ventricular end-diastolic volumes. Fluid and sodium restrictions also may be necessary. Vasodilators (eg, isosorbide dinitrate, hydralazine) dilate arterial and venous vessels, decreasing venous return and resistance to ventricular systolic ejection (afterload).
4. *Administer beta-blockers* (eg, metoprolol, carvedilol, bisoprolol) to reduce the risk of sudden cardiac death (VF, VT), as well as prevent further deterioration of the myocytes.
5. *Administer angiotensin-converting enzyme (ACE) inhibitors, angiotensin II receptor blockers (ARBs), or angiotensin receptor neprilysin inhibitors (ARNIs)* to block the negative effects of angiotensin II on the cardiac cells, as well as reduce ventricular afterload. ARNIs are never given in conjunction with ARB or ACE inhibitor and are started only after a minimum of 36 hours has passed since the last ACE inhibitor or ARB dose.
6. *Mechanical cardiac assist devices* (eg, intra-aortic balloon therapy, VAD therapy), and in some critical situations, extracorporeal membrane oxygenation (ECMO), may be instituted to assist with improving CO/CI and oxygen delivery to the tissues.
7. *Dual-chamber biventricular pacemaker/implantable cardioverter defibrillator:* Refer to Chapter 9, section Improvement of Left Ventricular Function.
8. *Ventricular reconstruction procedure:* This is a surgical procedure focusing on removal of a ventricular aneurysm and scar tissue on the left ventricle, usually a result of a myocardial infarction (MI). The left ventricle is returned to its normal shape and is able to contract more efficiently.
9. *Cardiac transplantation* may be necessary if medical therapy does not relieve patient symptoms.

Hypertrophic Cardiomyopathy

The management of the patient with hypertrophic cardiomyopathy focuses on promoting myocardial relaxation and decreasing left ventricular obstruction.

1. *Decrease myocardial contractility:* Use beta-blockers to decrease heart rate, contractility, and myocardial oxygen consumption.
2. The following medications are usually *contraindicated* in patients with hypertrophic cardiomyopathy:
   - *Diuretics*, because a decrease in fluid volume decreases ventricle filling pressures and CO.
   - *Inotropes* (eg, dobutamine, milrinone), because an increase in contractility contributes to an increase in the left ventricular outflow obstruction.

- *Vasodilators* (eg, nitroglycerin, nitroprusside), because they decrease end-diastolic volume, leading to an increase in left ventricular outflow obstruction.

3. *Reduce physical and psychological stress:* Patients with hypertrophic cardiomyopathy are at an increased risk for sudden cardiac death, which may occur during stressful periods. Strenuous physical activity and psychological stress should be limited. In addition, sudden changes in position are avoided, because the heart cannot respond to fluid shifts created by sudden position changes. Valsalva maneuver should also be avoided. Teach patients strategies to enhance self-relaxation. Relaxation therapy may include rhythmic breathing, biofeedback, and imagery.

4. *Cardiac surgery:* Myectomy may be indicated for individuals who do not respond to medical management and have severe left ventricular outflow obstruction. Myectomy involves removal of a portion of the enlarged intraventricular septum in an attempt to decrease left ventricular outflow obstruction and improve myocardial functioning.

5. *Ethanol septal ablation:* Ethanol septal ablation involves instilling absolute alcohol (98% ethanol) into selected septal perforator branches of the left anterior descending coronary artery, resulting in a therapeutic MI. The result is reduced left ventricular outflow obstruction and improved CO. The procedure is performed in the cardiac catheterization laboratory by the interventional cardiologists. This procedure is less risky than myectomy because it is less invasive.

Restrictive Cardiomyopathy

Decrease preload: Diuretics, sodium and fluid restrictions, and vasodilators decrease ventricular end-diastolic volumes. The rigid ventricle is very sensitive to small fluid changes, significantly increasing ventricular end-diastolic pressure.

Facilitate Coping

For most patients, cardiomyopathy is a chronic, potentially life-threatening disease. Patients and their families often face an uncertain long-term prognosis. Emotions may vacillate as the family struggles to cope with the implications of the disease and its effect on lifestyle. Emphasis is placed on assisting the patient to remain active and to cope with a progressive disease. Involvement of the family unit in symptom management is also important. Relaxation therapy can benefit not only the patient but also the family. Goals of care discussions that include options for palliative and hospice care are essential components of patient management when the prognosis is poor or treatment options are limited.

Preventing and Managing Complications

1. *Dysrhythmias:* Continuous ECG monitoring; observe for potential side effects of cardiac medications and provide support for strict adherence. Encourage family to learn cardiopulmonary resuscitation (CPR).

2. *Hemodynamic instability:* Pulmonary artery pressure (PAP) monitoring; manage patient based on trends in hemodynamic parameters (ie, RA, PAS, PAD, and PAOP pressures; CO; CI; SVR; and PVR).

3. *Thromboembolic event:* Anticoagulation is necessary for patients with severely compromised left ventricular function and for patients with AF. In both circumstances, thrombi may develop due to increased fluid volume and stasis.

4. *Endocarditis:* Antibiotic prophylaxis is recommended for patients with valve involvement. Prophylaxis is provided prior to dental work, surgery, or other invasive procedures.

Valvular Heart Disease

Heart valve disorders result from both congenital and acquired causes. Valves on the left side of the heart are more commonly affected because they are constantly exposed to higher pressures. Normally, when a valve opens, there are no pressure gradients, or differences, between the chambers or vessel above and below the valve. As heart valve disease progresses, pressure gradients between the two structures develop.

Heart valve disorders are commonly classified as valve stenosis or valve insufficiency. A *stenotic valve* has a narrowed opening, that is, it does not open fully thereby reducing the amount of blood flowing forward through it. An *insufficient valve* does not close properly, thus permitting some blood to flow backward instead of forward. Heart valve insufficiency is also referred to as valve regurgitation. Heart valve disease may affect one or more valves.

The development of heart valve disease is usually a gradual process. As the case study below illustrates, the patient's valve problems began with a bacterial endocarditis 15 years prior to the onset of her symptoms of mitral valve insufficiency.

Etiology and Pathophysiology

Both congenital and acquired diseases can cause heart valve disorders (Table 19-2). Congenital valve disorders may affect any of the four valves and cause stenosis or insufficiency. An example of a congenital valve disorder is an aortic valve with only two, instead of three, cusps. The bicuspid valve is associated with an increase in turbulence as blood flows through the narrowed orifice. The individual may become symptomatic later in life when fibrotic tissue and calcium deposits form on the abnormal valve, leading to stenosis. This is often referred to as *senile aortic stenosis.*

There are three types of acquired valve disorders: degenerative disease, rheumatic disease, or infective endocarditis. Degenerative disease may occur as the valve is damaged over time due to constant mechanical stress. This may occur with aging, or may be aggravated by conditions such as hypertension. Hypertension places significant pressure on the aortic valve, often causing insufficiency.

TABLE 19-2. ETIOLOGY OF VALVULAR DISORDERS

Mitral Stenosis
- Rheumatic disease
- Endocarditis
- Degenerative process

Mitral Insufficiency
- Dilated cardiomyopathy
- Rheumatic disease
- Congenital
- Endocarditis
- Mitral valve prolapse
- Papillary muscle dysfunction
- Chordae tendineae dysfunction

Aortic Stenosis
- Rheumatic disease
- Congenital (bicuspid valve)
- Degenerative process

Aortic Insufficiency
- Rheumatic disease
- Congenital
- Hypertension
- Endocarditis
- Marfan syndrome

Tricuspid Stenosis
- Rheumatic disease
- Congenital
- Endocarditis

Tricuspid Insufficiency
- Rheumatic disease
- Dilated cardiomyopathy
- Marfan syndrome
- Endocarditis
- Ebstein anomaly
- Congenital
- Secondary to left-sided valve disease
- IV drug use

Pulmonic Stenosis
- Rheumatic disease
- Congenital
- Endocarditis

Pulmonic Insufficiency
- Primary pulmonary artery hypertension
- Secondary to left-sided valve disease
- Marfan syndrome
- Endocarditis

Individuals who develop rheumatic fever often experience valvular disease years later. Rheumatic disease contributes to gradual fibrotic changes of the valve, in addition to calcification of the valve cusps. Shortening of the chordae tendineae also may occur. Rheumatic fever commonly affects the mitral valve.

Infective endocarditis may occur as a primary or secondary infection. The infectious organism destroys the valve tissue. Table 19-2 lists other conditions that cause heart valve disease.

Pathophysiology of Mitral Stenosis

Several processes occur that together cause stenosis or narrowing of the mitral valve orifice. Gradual fusion of the commissures (the valve leaflet edges) and fibrosis of the valve leaflets are common. In addition, calcium deposits may invade the valve leaflets, further impeding their movement. As the mitral valve becomes increasingly stenotic, the left atrium has to generate significant amounts of pressure to propel blood forward through the mitral valve and into the left ventricle. Left atrial pressures are commonly increased, with left atrial dilation occurring as the stenosis worsens. Increased left atrial pressures may lead to increased pulmonary vascular pressures (pulmonary hypertension) contributing to the development of right ventricular failure (see Figure 19-2).

Pathophysiology of Mitral Insufficiency

Adequate closure of the mitral valve is important so that blood is ejected forward into the aorta, not backward into the left atrium, during ventricular systole. Damage to the mitral valve can affect the valve's ability to close properly (Figure 19-3). During ventricular systole, as blood is ejected forward into the aorta, blood is also ejected backward through the insufficient mitral valve. This abnormal blood flow contributes to an increase in left atrial volume, pressure, and eventually dilation. Increased left atrial pressures may cause increased pulmonary vascular pressures and right heart failure. The left ventricle usually dilates and hypertrophies over time as end-diastolic volumes increase and CO decreases.

ESSENTIAL CONTENT CASE

Heart Valve Disorder

A 48-year-old woman was admitted to the coronary care unit with increasing shortness of breath and fatigue. She had bacterial endocarditis 15 years ago, which resulted in mitral valve insufficiency. On admission, she was in normal sinus rhythm with frequent premature atrial contractions and a blood pressure (BP) of 150/94 mm Hg. Chest auscultation revealed crackles in the left lower lung field. Hemodynamic parameters included:

RAP	12 mm Hg
PAP	35/25 mm Hg
PAOP	24 mm Hg
CO	4.8 L/min
CI	1.9 L/min/m^2
SVR	2100 dynes/s/cm^5

Case Question. The initial priority for medical management of this patient will be to:
(A) Improve oxygen delivery to the tissues
(B) Consider initiation of an inotrope
(C) Initiate a sodium nitroprusside infusion to reduce the blood pressure
(D) Decrease preload

Answers
1. D is the correct answer. The crackles in the left lower lung field and associated increased RAP and PAOP indicated an increased preload. The initial goal will be to reduce the cardiac preload.

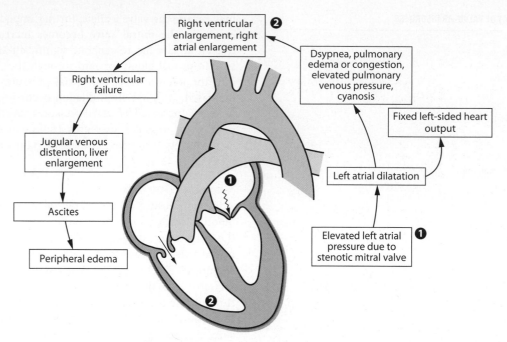

Figure 19-2. Cardiovascular effects of mitral stenosis.

Mitral insufficiency is often associated with dilated cardiomyopathy. As the left ventricle dilates, the papillary muscles are stretched and no longer able to maintain closure of the mitral valve during ventricular systole. Acute mitral insufficiency may occur due to dysfunction or rupture of the papillary muscles. Papillary muscle contraction contributes to preventing the valve leaflets from everting back into the left atrium during ventricular systole. Papillary muscles may rupture during an acute MI if blood supply to the tissue is diminished or absent during the infarct. Loss of a papillary muscle causes sudden, severe insufficiency of the mitral valve, resulting in rapid increase in both left ventricular and atrial volumes and pressures. The high left-sided pressures affect the pulmonary vascular system leading to acute pulmonary edema. Unlike chronic mitral insufficiency, in acute mitral insufficiency, there is no time

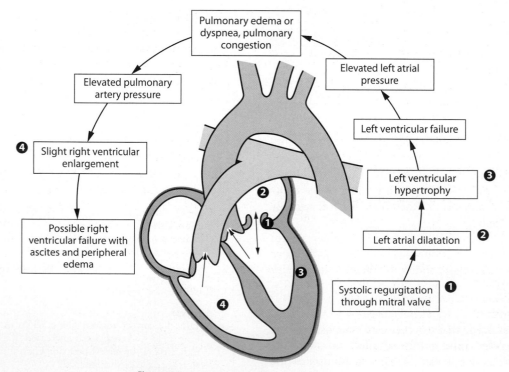

Figure 19-3. Cardiovascular effects of mitral insufficiency.

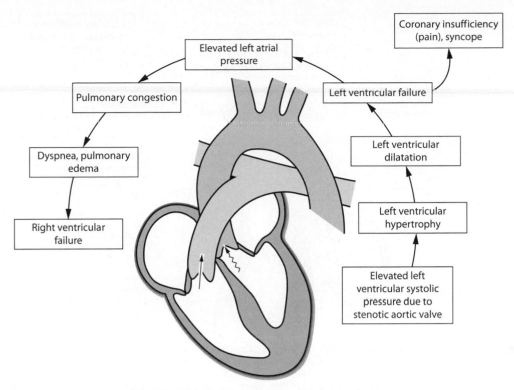

Figure 19-4. Cardiovascular effects of aortic stenosis.

for the heart to compensate for the sudden increases in volume and pressure.

Pathophysiology of Aortic Stenosis

A similar process occurs in aortic stenosis as occurs in mitral stenosis (Figure 19-4). Fusion of the commissures, fibrosis of the valve leaflets, and calcium deposits may occur on the aortic valve leaflets, impeding their movement. When aortic stenosis is present, the left ventricle has to generate a significant amount of pressure to propel blood forward through the aortic valve into the aorta. Increased left ventricular pressure contributes to left ventricular dilation and hypertrophy, as well as decreases in CO. Left atrial volume and pressure increase as the left atrium must generate more pressure to eject blood into the left ventricle. Left atrial dilation may eventually occur. The elevated left-sided pressures are reflected back into the pulmonary vascular system and to the right side of the heart, eventually causing right heart failure.

Pathophysiology of Aortic Insufficiency

A similar process occurs in aortic insufficiency as occurs with mitral insufficiency (Figure 19-5). Adequate closure of the aortic valve is even more important than adequate closure of the mitral valve. If the aortic valve does not close properly, blood flows backward from the aorta into the left ventricle during diastole. This can seriously affect forward blood flow into the aorta, and thus CO. This causes significant increases in the volumes and pressures of the left ventricle,

contributing to the gradual development of left ventricular dilation and hypertrophy. As with other left-sided valve disease, pulmonary vascular pressures increase contributing to the development of right heart failure.

Pathophysiology of Tricuspid Stenosis

Fused commissures or fibrosis of the valve leaflets may also narrow the tricuspid valve orifice. Right atrial pressures increase as the right atrium attempts to propel blood forward into the right ventricle. Eventually, RA dilation occurs and the increased RA pressure is reflected back into the venous system.

Pathophysiology of Tricuspid Insufficiency

Damage to the tricuspid valve that prevents complete closure during ventricular systole causes the abnormal ejection of blood through the tricuspid valve into the right atrium. Right atrial volumes and pressures increase, eventually leading to dilation and possible decreases in CO. Tricuspid insufficiency commonly occurs with dilated cardiomyopathy. As the right ventricle dilates, the papillary muscles are stretched and are unable to maintain closure of the valve during ventricular systole. This frequently accompanies mitral insufficiency.

Pathophysiology of Pulmonic Stenosis

Pulmonic stenosis develops as the pulmonic valve orifice becomes narrowed. Right ventricular pressures increase as the right ventricle attempts to eject blood forward into the pulmonary artery. Over time, right ventricular dilation may

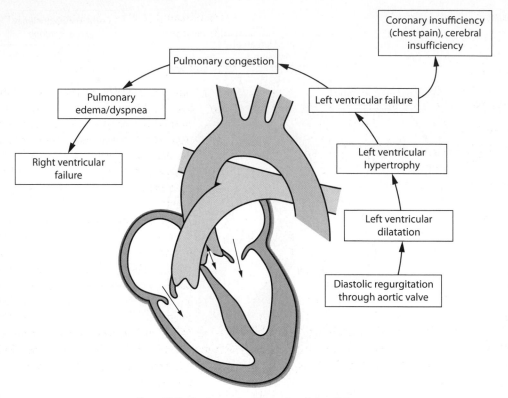

Figure 19-5. Cardiovascular effects of aortic insufficiency.

occur, with decreases in right-sided CO. The increased pressure may back up into the right atrium, causing an increase in volume and pressure, and eventually leading to dilation. This can lead to volume and pressure increases in the venous system.

Pathophysiology of Pulmonic Insufficiency

Closure of the pulmonic valve prevents blood from backing up from the pulmonary artery into the right ventricle during diastole. An insufficient pulmonic valve permits blood to flow backward into the right ventricle during diastole. Right-sided CO decreases as blood flows backward instead of forward into the pulmonary vascular bed. An increase in right ventricular volume and pressure occurs, which may eventually lead to dilation. The increased pressures may be reflected back into the right atrium and the venous system. Pulmonic stenosis and insufficiency are rarely seen in adults and are much more common in children, where they are usually the result of a congenital defect.

Clinical Presentation

Mitral and Aortic Disease

The following signs and symptoms are found in all of the valvular disorders of the left side of the heart:

- Dyspnea
- Fatigue
- Increased pulmonary artery pressures (PASs, PAD, PAOP)
- Decreased CO

Mitral Stenosis

- Palpitations
- Hemoptysis
- Hoarseness
- Dysphagia
- JVD
- Orthopnea
- Cough
- Diastolic murmur
- Atrial dysrhythmias (PACs, AF)
- Elevated A wave on PAOP pressure waveform

Mitral Insufficiency

- Paroxysmal nocturnal dyspnea
- Orthopnea
- Palpitations
- S_3 and/or S_4
- Crackles
- Systolic murmur
- Atrial dysrhythmias
- Elevated V wave on PAOP pressure waveform

Aortic Stenosis

- Angina
- Syncope
- Decreased SVR
- S_3 and/or S_4
- Systolic murmur
- Narrowed pulse pressure

Aortic Insufficiency

- Angina
- S_3
- Diastolic murmur
- Widened pulse pressure
- de Musset's sign (nodding of the head)

Tricuspid and Pulmonary Valve Disease

The following signs and symptoms are found in all of the valvular disorders of the right side of the heart:

- Dyspnea
- Fatigue
- Increased RA pressures
- Peripheral edema
- Hepatomegaly
- JVD

Tricuspid Stenosis

- Atrial dysrhythmias
- Diastolic murmur
- Decreased CO
- Elevated A wave on RA pressure waveform

Tricuspid Insufficiency

- Conduction delays
- Supraventricular tachycardia
- Systolic murmur
- Elevated V wave on RA pressure waveform

Pulmonic Stenosis

- Cyanosis
- Systolic murmur
- Elevated A wave on RA pressure waveform

Pulmonic Insufficiency

- Diastolic murmur
- Elevated A wave on RA pressure waveform

Diagnostic Tests

- *Chest x-ray:* Shows specific cardiac chamber enlargement, pulmonary congestion, presence of valve calcification
- *12-lead ECG:* Useful in the diagnosis of right ventricular, left ventricular, and left atrial hypertrophy
- *Echocardiogram:* Demonstrates the size of the four cardiac chambers, presence of hypertrophy, specific valve dysfunction, ejection fraction, and amount of regurgitant flow, if present
- *Radionuclide studies:* Identify abnormal ejection fraction during inactivity and activity
- *Cardiac catheterization:* Determines cardiac chamber pressures, ejection fraction, regurgitation, and pressure gradients, if present

Principles of Management for Valvular Disorders

The primary objectives in the management of valvular disorders are to maximize cardiac function, improve symptoms and prevent complications associated with valvular disease.

Maximize Cardiac Function: Medical Management

1. *Improve oxygen delivery:* As ventricular dilation occurs, there is an increase in ventricular wall tension, myocardial workload, and oxygen consumption. Oxygen therapy is initiated, as necessary, to increase oxygen saturation. Pulse oximetry, mixed venous oxygenation saturation (SVO_2), and arterial blood gases are helpful in guiding sufficient oxygen therapy.
2. *Decrease preload:* Diuretics decrease excess fluid and ventricular end-diastolic volumes. Fluid and sodium restrictions also may be necessary. (*Exception:* Preload reduction is not part of the management of patients with aortic insufficiency, because decreased left ventricular end-diastolic volumes may adversely affect CO by increasing backward flow.)
3. *Decrease afterload:* Afterload reduction may be indicated for patients with increased SVR and impaired left ventricular function (eg, aortic stenosis or mitral insufficiency).
4. *Improve contractility:* Inotropic agents (eg, milrinone, dobutamine) increase myocardial contractility and improve CO.
5. *Modify activity:* Activity limitation helps reduce myocardial oxygen consumption. Teach patients the importance of alternating periods of activity with periods of rest.
6. *Balloon valvuloplasty* may be an option for stenotic mitral or aortic valves. A percutaneous catheter is inserted via the femoral artery under fluoroscopy and the balloon is inflated at the stenotic lesion in an effort to force open the fused commissures and improve valve leaflet mobility.

Maximize Cardiac Function: Surgical Management

Cardiac surgery is indicated when medical management does not alleviate patient symptoms. Patients may have better surgical outcomes if surgery is done prior to left ventricular dysfunction.

1. *Valve repair:* An increasing trend is to have dysfunctional valves repaired instead of replaced. The hemodynamic function of the inherent valve is superior to any prosthetic valve. In addition, the risks associated with valve replacement are avoided. An open commissurotomy may be performed to relieve stenosis of any of the four heart valves. During open commissurotomy, the fused commissures are incised, thus mobilizing the valve leaflets. Valve leaflet reconstruction also may be done to patch tears in valve leaflets using pericardial patches for the repair. Chordae tendineae reconstruction may

be performed to elongate fibrotic tendineae or to shorten excessively stretched tendineae. An annuloplasty ring may also be inserted to correct dilation of the valve annulus.

2. *Prosthetic valve replacement:* Replacement of the native valve with a prosthetic, or artificial, valve is done for severely damaged valves or when repair is not possible. The entire native valve is removed and replaced with a mechanical or biological (porcine, bovine, or allograft [homograft or autograft]) prosthetic valve.

3. *Postoperative management* after cardiac surgery is similar to coronary artery bypass surgery management (see Chapter 9, Cardiovascular System). Special considerations for patients having valve repair or replacement include the following:

   - *Maintain adequate preload:* Patients with heart valve disease, particularly aortic insufficiency and mitral insufficiency, usually are accustomed to increased end-diastolic volumes. Although the valve is repaired, the heart needs time to adjust to the hemodynamic changes. Generally fluids are adjusted based on patient weight postoperatively as well as pulmonary symptoms, chest x-ray, and vital signs.

   - *Monitor for conduction disturbances:* The mitral, tricuspid, and aortic valves lie in close proximity to conduction pathways. Temporary or permanent cardiac pacing may be needed to manage postoperative conduction disorders.

   - *Initiate anticoagulation therapy:* Anticoagulation therapy is usually initiated for patients having valve replacement.

4. *If the patient had AF or flutter preoperatively*, the surgeon may perform a Maze procedure, ablating the area around the pulmonary veins in an effort to prevent return of the atrial dysrhythmia postoperatively.

5. *Transcatheter aortic valve replacement (TAVR).* Technological advances have allowed for the development of a minimally invasive approach to aortic valve replacement. In this approach, a prosthetic tissue valve is placed via a stent-like introducer catheter. The valve may be inserted through the femoral artery or axillary artery and placed across the native aortic valve. Preprocedure evaluation includes identifying the best insertion site. Another approach that is rarely used today is called transapical where a small incision is made in the anterior chest wall and the device is deployed through the left ventricular apex into the aortic valve position. All of these approaches avoid the use of cardiopulmonary bypass (CPB). Initially this procedure was limited to patients who were older (eighth or ninth decade) and were too frail to tolerate the traditional surgical approaches to aortic valve replacement. The patient often experiences near immediate relief of symptoms and is discharged home within a couple of days.

6. *Another method is the use of a transaortic approach.* In this approach, a mini-sternotomy is performed and the valve is accessed via the aorta. The benefit of this approach may include a decreased risk of postoperative bleeding compared to the transapical approach. A valve-in-valve procedure is another recently developed approach. This involves introducing a prosthetic tissue valve, using the transcatheter approach, into a previously implanted prosthetic tissue valve. The valve-in-valve TAVR approach was trialed in the PARTNER 2 study and found to have positive outcomes in those individuals who had a surgically implanted valve earlier that required replacement but the patient was no longer a surgical candidate. The PARTNER studies include randomized clinical trials over 10 to 12 years comparing outcomes in the surgical approach versus the transcatheter procedure. The PARTNER 3 Trial reported results favoring TAVR in patients with aortic stenosis who are considered to be low risk, so this procedure is now offered to a larger population.

Clinical trials are underway using the transcatheter approach for mitral valve and tricuspid valve replacement. Expect this to take a longer time to perfect due to the complexity of the mitral valve anatomy.

Improve Symptoms
Teach the patient relaxation techniques. Deep breathing or imagery may help alleviate anxiety especially when symptoms of valve dysfunction occur.

Discuss the impact of symptoms and strategies for managing them, such as alternating periods of activity and rest. Provide education to patients' identified support system so they can help the patient interpret and manage symptoms.

Preventing and Managing Complications
1. *Dysrhythmias:* Maintaining continuous ECG monitoring promotes early recognition of cardiac dysrhythmias. The onset of atrial fibrillation within 24 to 48 hours postoperatively is common, especially if the patient was in atrial fibrillation preoperatively. If an ablation procedure for atrial fibrillation was performed perioperatively, there is an increased risk for AV blocks to develop requiring pacemaker support.

2. *Hemodynamic instability:* Hemodynamic monitoring may be invasive using a pulmonary artery catheter, minimally invasive using a central venous catheter and/or arterial pressure monitoring, or completely noninvasive. Whichever method is employed, monitoring trends in hemodynamic measures is essential.

3. *Thromboembolic event:* Anticoagulation is necessary for patients with severely compromised left ventricular function or AF, and after valve surgery. Lifelong anticoagulation therapy is indicated for patients after mechanical valve replacement. Short-term anticoagulation therapy is usually initiated for patients having a biological valve replacement.

4. *Endocarditis:* Antibiotic prophylaxis is recommended for patients with valve disorders and for patients with prosthetic valves. Prophylaxis is provided prior to dental work, surgery, or other invasive procedures. Prior to discharge, teach the patient and family the importance of prophylaxis.

5. *Prosthetic valve dysfunction:* Biological valve dysfunction usually develops slowly with gradual signs and symptoms (eg, presence of a new murmur, dyspnea, syncope). Mechanical valve dysfunction may occur slowly or suddenly. Rapid valve dysfunction requires emergency intervention as the patient presents with signs and symptoms of acute cardiac failure (hypotension, tachycardia, low CO/CI, heart failure, cardiac arrest).

Pericarditis

Pericarditis is a chronic or acute inflammation of the pericardial lining of the heart. Acute pericarditis usually occurs secondary to another disease process and usually resolves within 6 weeks. Chronic pericarditis, however, may last for months.

Pericarditis may lead to pericardial effusion or cardiac tamponade. Pericardial effusion occurs as fluid builds up within the pericardial sac. Cardiac tamponade can occur as the pericardial fluid compresses the heart, restricts ventricular end-diastolic filling, and compromises cardiac function.

The case study on pericarditis is an example of the importance of accurate diagnosis of patients with chest pain. The pain of pericarditis may be similar to anginal pain, but the treatment is very different.

Etiology and Pathophysiology

A number of different conditions and situations can cause pericarditis (Table 19-3). Common causes include MI, infections, neoplasm, radiation therapy, collagen vascular disease, and uremia.

TABLE 19-3. ETIOLOGY OF PERICARDITIS

Idiopathic
Infections (viral/bacterial)
Myocardial infarction
Cardiac surgery
Neoplasm
Radiation therapy
Rheumatic disease
Lupus erythematosus
Scleroderma
Uremia
Medication induced

Normally, the pericardial sac contains a small amount of clear serous fluid, typically less than 50 mL. This fluid lies between the visceral and parietal pleura and lubricates the surface of the heart as it expands and contracts. An inflammation of the pericardium causes friction between the visceral and parietal pleura.

Inflammation of the pericardium causes an increase in pericardial fluid production, with increases of up to 1 L or more. A gradual buildup of fluid may have little compromising effect on the heart as the pericardium expands and normal hemodynamics are not altered. A sudden increase in pericardial fluid, however, dramatically impairs the hemodynamic status.

Chronic pericarditis causes fibrotic changes within the pericardial lining. The visceral and parietal pleura eventually adhere to each other, restricting the filling of the heart. This condition may be referred to as *constrictive pericarditis*. The pressure created by the constricted pericardium affects the heart's ability to distend properly, causing decreases in end-diastolic volume and CO. These changes may contribute to increases in ventricular end-diastolic pressures and atrial pressures, leading to increases in pulmonary vascular and venous system pressures.

ESSENTIAL CONTENT CASE

Pericarditis

A woman had an acute anterior MI 7 days ago. She was readmitted to the critical care unit (CCU) with sharp, substernal chest pain worsening with inspiration, shortness of breath, and ST-segment elevations in the precordial leads and in leads I, II, and III. The chest pain was unrelieved with nitroglycerin. Her pain was decreased after receiving 4 mg of morphine IV. The pain went away completely when she sat up and leaned forward so that her nurse could auscultate posterior breath sounds.

Case Question 1: A classic sign of pericarditis is:
(A) Sharp pain on inspiration relieved by leaning forward
(B) Distended neck veins
(C) Narrow pulse pressure
(D) Cough

Case Question 2: An important nursing action for this patient is to:
(A) Continue to administer morphine for pain
(B) Encourage patient to ambulate as much as possible
(C) Alleviate anxiety by informing patient this is not another heart attack
(D) Encourage deep breathing exercises to expand the lung

Answers
1. A is the correct answer. A sharp pain on inspiration relieved by leaning forward is a classic sign of pericarditis. Neck vein distention may accompany pericarditis but is not always present.
2. C is the correct answer. Many patients believe the onset of chest pain indicates they are having another MI. It is important to inform the patient that it is not.

Clinical Presentation
Acute Pericarditis

- Sharp, stabbing, burning, dull, or aching pain in the substernal or precordial area, which increases with movement, inspiration, or coughing, or when the patient is in a recumbent position
- Pericardial friction rub
- Fever
- Sinus tachycardia
- Dyspnea, orthopnea
- Cough
- Fatigue
- Narrowed pulse pressure
- Hypotension
- Dysrhythmias
- Elevated cardiac pressures (PA, PAOP, RA)
- Decreased CO
- Peripheral edema
- JVD

Chronic Pericarditis

- Dyspnea
- Anorexia
- Fatigue
- Abdominal discomfort
- Weight gain
- Activity intolerance
- JVD
- Peripheral edema
- Hepatomegaly
- Kussmaul sign (increase in RA pressure during inspiration)

Diagnostic Tests

- *Chest x-ray:* Normal or enlarged heart; chronic pericarditis may reveal a decrease in heart size.
- *ECG:* ST-segment elevation in precordial leads (V leads) and leads I, II, or III; T-wave inversion after ST-segment returns to isoelectric line; decrease in QRS voltage.
- *Echocardiogram:* Presence of increased fluid in pericardial sac; chronic, constrictive pericarditis may demonstrate a thickened pericardium and diminished ventricular contractility.
- *Laboratory:* Elevated sedimentation rate and elevated WBC; causative organisms may be identified from blood cultures.
- *CT/MRI scan:* Detects a thickened pericardium for patients with chronic pericarditis.

Principles of Management for Pericarditis
The primary principles of management of pericarditis are to correct the underlying cause, relieve pain and promote comfort, relieve pericardial effusion, and prevent and manage complications associated with pericarditis.

Promoting Comfort and Relieving Pain

1. *Decrease pain:* Teach the patient that chest pain may be decreased or relieved by sitting up and/or leaning forward. Analgesics, colchicine, and nonsteroidal anti-inflammatory agents administered around the clock assist in pain relief.
2. *Promote relaxation:* Teach the patient relaxation techniques such as progressive muscle relaxation and visualization. This may assist the patient to cope. Relaxation techniques that include deep breathing are avoided because pericardial pain usually increases with deep inspiration.
3. *Limit activity:* This is especially important during the acute period of inflammation. Activity can be gradually increased as fever and chest pain decrease. Assist patients to find a position of comfort. Patients often are more comfortable sitting up and leaning slightly forward.

Correcting the Underlying Cause

1. *Decrease pericardial inflammation:* Nonsteroidal anti-inflammatory agents (eg, indomethacin, ibuprofen) decrease inflammation of the pericardium and the associated pain and the first several doses are given as standing doses, not as needed. Chronic, recurrent pericarditis may require corticosteroid therapy.
2. *Eliminate infection:* If the cause of the pericarditis is an infectious process, appropriate medications, including antibiotic therapy, are necessary.

Relieving Pericardial Effusion

1. *Pericardiocentesis:* A needle or small catheter is introduced subxiphoid into the pericardial sac. Fluid is withdrawn via the needle or is attached to a catheter and drained into a vacuum bottle. This procedure is performed to remove fluid from the pericardium and improve myocardial function. Culture specimens of the drained fluid can be obtained and sent to the laboratory for analysis. The drain may be left in for several days until the volume of drainage is minimal.
2. *Pericardiotomy/pericardial window:* This is a surgical procedure in which a section of the pericardium is removed in an effort to decrease pericardial pressure on the heart and to allow pericardial fluid to drain more readily. A drain may be inserted into the pericardium and tunneled down across the diaphragm into the peritoneal cavity. This permits the excess fluid to drain continuously into the peritoneal space where it is eventually absorbed into the lymph system. It may be performed for recurrent pericardial effusions.
3. *Pericardiectomy:* This involves surgically removing the entire pericardium. This may be necessary for chronic pericarditis that is refractory to other interventions.

Preventing and Managing Complications

1. *Monitor for signs and symptoms of acute heart failure:* These include hypotension, tachycardia, increased respiratory rate (RR), dyspnea, decreased oxygen saturation, decreased peripheral pulses, and decreased urinary output. Oxygen therapy and inotropic agents assist in improvement of myocardial contractility. Assessment of the need for surgical intervention for pericarditis may be indicated.

2. *Cardiac tamponade:* Monitor for signs and symptoms of cardiac tamponade. These include hypotension, tachycardia, tachypnea, dyspnea, pulsus paradoxus, narrowed pulse pressure, muffled heart sounds, and distended neck veins. Another sign of tamponade is equalization of pressures, when hemodynamic assessment reveals PAS, PAD, PAOP, and CVP that fall within a close range. Emergency pericardiocentesis is necessary to prevent further hemodynamic compromise.

Aortic Aneurysm

An *aortic aneurysm* is an area of aortic wall dilation. Aneurysms are most prevalent in men, commonly occurring during their early 50s to late 60s. Without treatment, mortality associated with thoracic aortic aneurysms is high.

Aneurysms frequently are classified by types (Figure 19-6). A *fusiform aneurysm* is characterized by distention of the entire circumference of the affected portion of the aorta. A *saccular aneurysm* is characterized by distention of one side of the aorta. The distention of a saccular aneurysm resembles a bulging sac. Aneurysms may also be classified according to their location (Figure 19-7):

- *Ascending:* Between the aortic valve and the innominate artery
- *Transverse:* Between the innominate artery and the left subclavian artery
- *Descending:* From the left subclavian artery to the diaphragm
- *Thoracoabdominal:* From above the diaphragm to the aortic bifurcation

Aneurysms have the potential to dissect or rupture. *Dissection* occurs when the intimal aortic wall is disrupted or torn and blood extends into the aortic vessel layers (Figure 19-6C and 19-6D). *Rupture* occurs when all three layers of the aorta are torn and massive hemorrhage occurs. Both dissection and rupture are life-threatening events. The case study demonstrates the sudden onset of signs and symptoms associated with aortic rupture and the emergent need for life-saving interventions.

Etiology and Pathophysiology

Aortic aneurysms are caused by a variety of conditions, including atherosclerosis, genetic link, congenital abnormality, hypertension, Marfan syndrome, and trauma to the chest.

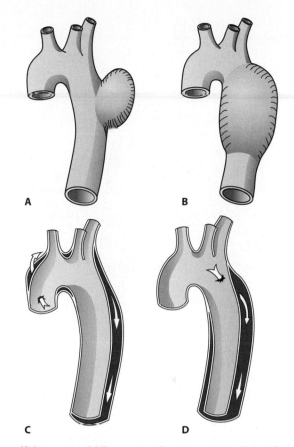

Figure 19-6. Diagram of different types of aortic aneurysms. **(A)** Saccular aneurysm. **(B)** Fusiform aneurysm. **(C, D)** Two aortic dissections. (*Reproduced with permission from Underhill SL, Woods SL, Sivarajan ES, et al. Cardiac Nursing. Philadelphia, PA. JB Lippincott; 1982.*)

The aorta is composed of three layers: the intima, media, and tunica adventitia. Aneurysm development is initiated by degeneration of smooth muscle cells and elastic tissue in the medial layer of the aorta. This weakens the vessel wall, potentially leading to dilation of all layers of the aorta. The aortic wall may be further weakened with age, as well as from hypertension.

As the aortic aneurysm gradually expands, there is an increase in the risk for aortic dissection. Dissection begins with a tear in the intima. Blood leaves the central aorta via the intimal tear and flows through the medial layer of the aorta (Figure 19-6C and 19-6D). This creates a false lumen. As the amount of blood increases in the medial layer, the pressure in the false lumen increases, compressing the central aorta (Figure 19-6D). This compression may decrease or totally obstruct blood flow through the aorta and/or its arterial branches. Dissections are classified as acute if they have occurred less than 2 weeks since the onset of symptoms. They are classified as chronic if they occurred more than 2 weeks since the onset of symptoms.

Two additional classifications exist for identifying the location of aortic dissections (Figure 19-8). The first (Stanford Classification) classifies the dissection as type A, involving the ascending aorta, or type B, involving the

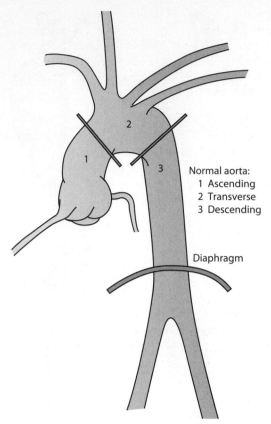

Figure 19-7. Classification of aortic aneurysms according to location. (*Reproduced with permission from Seifert PC. Cardiac Surgery. St Louis, MO: Mosby Yearbook; 1994.*)

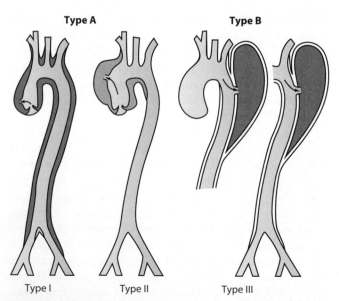

Figure 19-8. Classification for the location of aortic dissections. The Stanford system classifies aortic dissections based on involvement (type A) of the ascending aorta or noninvolvement (type B). The DeBakey system classifies dissections into types I, II, or III. (*Reproduced with permission from DeBakey ME. Surgical management of dissecting aneurysms of the aorta. J Thorac Cardiovasc Surg. 1965;49:131; adapted with permission from Seifert PC. Cardiac Surgery. St Louis, MO: Mosby Yearbook; 1994.*)

descending aorta (distal to the left subclavian artery). Type A requires immediate surgical intervention whereas type B is managed medically until surgery is deemed necessary. Another classification system for aortic dissection has three categories for the dissection: type I, the original intimal tear begins in the ascending aorta and the dissection extends to the descending aorta; type II, the original intimal tear begins and is contained in the ascending aorta; and type III, the original intimal tear begins and is contained in the descending aorta.

Clinical Presentation

Patients rarely demonstrate early signs of an aortic aneurysm. Diagnosis is commonly made during a routine physical examination or chest x-ray. Signs and symptoms of an aortic aneurysm occur as the aneurysm enlarges and compresses adjacent organs, structures, and/or nerve pathways.

Thoracic Aneurysm

- Symptoms of dissection include a ripping, tearing, or splitting pain, located at the anterior chest or posterior chest between the scapulas, of an intense or excruciating nature
- Oftentimes, thoracic aneurysm is asymptomatic until the growing aneurysm puts pressure on surrounding nerves and organs
- Chest pain
- Back pain
- Dysphagia
- Hoarseness, cough
- Dyspnea
- Different blood pressures when comparing right and left arms
- Different pulses when comparing right and left peripheral pulses

Abdominal Aneurysm

- Dull, constant abdominal or low back or lumbar pain
- Abdominal mass
- Pulsations in the abdomen
- Reduced lower extremity pulses
- Nausea and/or vomiting

Aortic Dissection

- Sudden intense pain in chest or back (or sudden increase in the intensity of pain)
- Dyspnea
- Syncope
- Abdominal discomfort or bloating
- Extremity weakness
- Oliguria or hematuria
- Hemiparesis, hemiplegia, or paraplegia
- Speech or visual disturbances
- Decreased hemoglobin and hematocrit
- Loss of consciousness

Aortic Rupture

- Sudden cessation of pain
- Reoccurrence of pain
- Signs and symptoms of shock, with the exception of blood pressure (high in rupture), including tachycardia, increased respiratory rate, pallor, moist skin, and restlessness

Diagnostic Tests

- *Chest x-ray:* Shows the dilated aorta, widening of the mediastinum, and mediastinal mass.
- *CT/MRI scan:* Determines the size of the aorta, size of the aneurysm, extent of a dissection, involvement of additional arterial branches, lumen diameter, and wall thickness.
- *Echocardiogram:* Can sometimes visualize the location and size of an aneurysm. Transesophageal echo (TEE) may be more helpful, particularly in visualizing thoracic aneurysms and when dissection is suspected.
- *Aortography:* Determines the origin, size, and location of the aneurysm and involvement of additional arterial branches.

Principles of Management for Aortic Aneurysm

The primary objectives in the management of aortic aneurysm are relieving pain and anxiety, lowering BP and thereby decreasing stress on the aneurysm, surgical repair if necessary, patient teaching, and prevention of complications.

Relieving Pain and Anxiety

Administer narcotics (eg, morphine) as necessary. Unrelieved pain is likely to increase anxiety, tachycardia, and hypertension, all of which may aggravate the condition. Relaxation therapy, with deep breathing exercises or imagery, may be extremely helpful.

Decreasing Stress on Aneurysm Wall

1. *Decrease afterload:* Vasodilators (eg, nitroprusside, nicardipine, esmolol) may be prescribed to lower blood pressure and thus pressure on the aneurysm. Blood pressures are maintained as low as possible (systolic blood pressure 90-120 mm Hg), without compromising perfusion to vital organs.
2. *Decrease preload:* Limit oral and IV fluids, decrease sodium intake, and administer diuretics as indicated. A decrease in preload decreases the circulating blood volume, thus decreasing pressure at the site of the aneurysm.
3. *Decrease myocardial contractility* with beta-blockers (eg, esmolol, labetalol). A decrease in the strength of each cardiac contraction decreases the pulsatile pressure on the aneurysm.

Patient and Family Teaching

1. *Follow-up:* If the patient is to be medically managed, follow-up chest x-rays, CT scans, MRI scans, and/or ultrasounds will be needed at 6-month intervals to

---

ESSENTIAL CONTENT CASE

Aortic Aneurysm

A 62-year-old man was admitted to the intensive care unit (ICU) with substernal chest pain. The chest pain was unrelieved by nitroglycerin. The pain decreased in intensity after 8 mg of morphine sulfate. His admitting ECG was normal. His chest x-ray revealed a widened mediastinum, and an aortogram demonstrated a thoracic aneurysm. He has nitroprusside infusing at 1.0 mcg/kg/min to maintain his systolic blood pressure below 100 mm Hg. Suddenly, the patient yells out, "The pain, the pain . . . it's back . . . it's even worse than before." A rapid assessment reveals the following:

BP	190/100 mm Hg
HR	110 beats/min
RR	30 breaths/min
Color	Gray
Skin	Moist and cool
Pain	Rated 10 on a 0 to 10 scale, described as tearing in the middle of his chest and between his shoulder blades

Case Question 1: Following relief of the patient's pain with morphine and notification of the physician, the nurse anticipates the patient will need:
(A) STAT chest x-ray
(B) STAT CT scan of the chest
(C) Cardiac catheterization
(D) STAT MRI

Case Question 2: Based on the description of the location of the pain, the nurse suspects the dissection is located in the:
(A) Ascending thoracic aorta
(B) Transverse thoracic aorta
(C) Descending thoracic aorta
(D) Abdominal aorta

Case Question 3: Medical management of a thoracic aortic aneurysm is focused on:
(A) Maintaining the systolic BP less than 120 mm Hg
(B) Maintaining the diastolic BP less than 40 mm Hg
(C) Maintaining the heart rate less than 100 beats/min
(D) Reducing the CO to less than 2.0 L/min

Answers
1. B is the correct answer. The CT will reveal the location and extent of the aneurysm.
2. C is the correct answer. Chest pain is a common symptom associated with a dissection of the descending thoracic aorta.
3. A is the correct answer. It is important to maintain the systolic pressure at 120 or below to prevent further dissection or rupture of the aneurysm.

assess the status of the aneurysm. The importance of these studies is stressed.

2. *Diet modification:* Teach the patient and family the importance of following a low-sodium diet. Consult a nutritionist for recipes and tips for food preparation.

3. *Smoking cessation:* Assist patient with programs available to help with smoking cessation.

4. *Physical/psychological stress modification:* Teach the patient and family the hazardous effects of stress and the importance for modification. Discuss activity limitations and relaxation therapy.

5. *Medications:* Teach the patient and family the importance of adherence to the medication regimen. Stress that the medications are essential even though the patient may be asymptomatic.

Surgical Management

Surgery is indicated for acute aneurysm rupture, aortic dissection in the ascending aorta, aortic dissection refractory to medical therapy, and asymptomatic patients with a fusiform aneurysm 6 cm or more in diameter (normal diameter is 2.5-3 cm). In some nonemergent situations, aortic aneurysms can be repaired nonsurgically with endovascular stent grafting or endovascular aneurysm repair (EVAR). During this procedure, a catheter is placed into the femoral artery. The catheter is advanced into the aorta to allow for a stent graft to be placed inside the dilated portion of the vessel. With the placement of the stent, a hemostatic seal occurs between the stent and the aortic wall. When compared to conventional surgical repair, this approach decreases procedure time, length of hospital stay, and the risk of complications including paraplegia and renal failure.

1. During surgical repair, the aortic aneurysm is resected and a prosthetic graft is sutured in place. The original aortic wall may be wrapped around the prosthetic graft for additional support.

2. If an acute dissection or rupture occurs and the patient is waiting for the operating room team to arrive:
   - Administer narcotics for pain.
   - Titrate vasodilators to maintain the patient's blood pressure as low as possible (90-120 mm Hg if tolerated). This decreases the pressure on the aneurysm.
   - Administer fluids to prevent hypovolemia.
   - Administer blood replacement products to maintain adequate hemoglobin and hematocrit levels.
   - If rupture occurs, the chest/abdomen will be opened emergently. The patient has a high risk of mortality or complications, including cerebral anoxia, severe hypovolemic shock, and multiple organ dysfunction syndrome (MODS).

3. Postoperative management:
   - Same interventions as described to relieve pain and anxiety and decrease stress on the aorta wall.

It is important to decrease pressure on the repaired aorta so that suture lines can heal and bleeding is kept to a minimum.
- Continuous ECG and hemodynamic monitoring.
- Continuous spinal pressure monitoring (for surgical repair of descending thoracic aortic dissection) draining spinal fluid as necessary to maintain pressure at 10 mm Hg or less.
- Complete assessment (including a focused neurologic assessment) every 1 to 2 hours.
- Gradual rewarming to prevent postoperative shivering, which increases blood pressure and places additional stress on suture lines.
- Maintain adequate oxygenation through ventilator management.
- Progressive mobility according to institution standards and surgeon preference.
- Monitor renal function [urine output, blood urea nitrogen (BUN)], and creatinine, especially if the aorta was cross-clamped above the renal arteries.
- *Initiate anticoagulation:* Anticoagulation therapy is initiated for patients receiving prosthetic valves.

Preventing and Managing Complications

1. *Hemorrhage:* Hourly assessment of vital signs and hemodynamic parameters and daily assessment of hemoglobin and hematocrit.

2. *Dysrhythmias:* Continuous ECG monitoring; monitoring electrolytes and replacing as indicated.

3. *Hemodynamic instability:* Arterial and PAP monitoring; manage hemodynamic parameters based on trends.

4. *Altered perfusion:* Arteries originating from the aorta may be compromised, leading to MI, cerebral insufficiency/cerebrovascular accident, bowel necrosis, renal failure, paraplegia, and limb ischemia. Assess and monitor the patient for these conditions.

5. *Aortic insufficiency:* Aortic insufficiency may develop if the aneurysm is located in the ascending aorta. Enlargement or dissection of the aneurysm may dilate or damage the aortic valve, causing signs of acute heart failure and pulmonary edema.

Cardiac Transplantation

Cardiac transplantation has evolved since 1967 to a standard modality for the treatment of end-stage cardiac disease. When medical, surgical, or pharmacologic interventions have failed to improve quality of life and functional capacity, cardiac transplantation offers patients improved survival. The survival rate in the United States is 93.6% at 6 months, 92.1% at 1 year, 85.6% at 3 years and 79.9% at 5 years. The primary indications for cardiac transplantation include cardiomyopathies or ischemic heart disease. Other indications include heart valve disease, congenital heart disease, and myocarditis.

Candidate Selection

Candidates for cardiac transplant usually have a poor prognosis without cardiac transplant and are in New York Heart Association (NYHA) functional class III or IV or American Heart Association (AHA) stage D. Some patients require a cardiac assist device such as the intra-aortic balloon pump (IABP), VAD, or ECMO to maintain adequate hemodynamic stability while awaiting transplantation. Because of the shortage of available organs and the complexity of post-transplant care, the patient must undergo an extensive screening process to ascertain that they are appropriate for the candidate list (Table 19-4). They must demonstrate a commitment to the rigors of being a candidate and eventual recipient through adherence to their medical regimens.

The period of waiting for an available donor can be extremely stressful for patients and their families. It is important to explore their perceptions of the transplant process, what outcomes they anticipate, and what methods they have utilized to cope in the past. Support group participation or meetings with a therapist or psychiatric provider may be beneficial. Fear of death and critical illness may heighten the patient's anxiety. Family members may need proximity to the patient, and this may assist in alleviating anxiety. Incorporating their involvement in direct patient care may enhance their coping abilities.

TABLE 19-4. GENERAL INDICATIONS FOR CARDIAC TRANSPLANTATION

Criteria for Consideration of Heart Transplantation in Advanced Heart Failure
General Indications:
• Dilated cardiomyopathy
• Ischemic cardiomyopathy
• Congenital heart disease for which no conventional therapy exists or for which conventional therapy has failed
• Ejection fraction less than 20%
• Pulmonary vascular resistance of less than 2 Wood units
• Age younger than 70 years
• Ability to comply with medical follow-up care
• Absence of tobacco use
Updated Criteria:[a]
• An estimated 1-year survival of less than 80%, as calculated by the Seattle Heart Failure Model or Heart Failure Survival Score in high/medium risk range
• Right heart catheterization should be performed on all adult candidates in preparation for listing and periodically until transplanted
• After LVAD, reevaluation of hemodynamics should be done after 3 to 6 months to ascertain reversibility of pulmonary hypertension
• Recommend weight loss to achieve body mass index less than or equal to 35 kg/m²
• Severe symptomatic cerebrovascular disease
• Assessment of frailty (three of five possible symptoms: unintentional weight loss more than or equal to 10 lb within the past year, muscle loss, fatigue, slow walking speed, and low levels of physical activity)
• Re-transplantation is indicated for those patients who develop significant cardiac allograft vasculopathy with refractory cardiac allograft dysfunction, without evidence of ongoing rejection

[a]Data from Mehra MR, Hannan MM, Semigran MJ, et al. The 2016 International Society for Heart Lung Transplantation listing criteria for heart transplant: a 10-year update. J Heart Lung Transplant. 2016 Jan;35(1):1-23.

Pretransplant Process

The greatest delay for cardiac transplantation occurs because of the shortage of donors. When a brain-dead donor is identified, they are carefully managed to maintain cardiovascular stability and avoid electrolyte and renal complications. The United Network for Organ Sharing (UNOS) coordinates the allocation of organs based on a nationwide waiting list. The donor must be of a compatible ABO blood type to the recipient and of similar body size and weight. The recipient is tested for relative immunologic compatibility with the donor to avoid hyperacute rejection. Panel-reactive antibody screening is performed using the recipient's serum with a random pool of lymphocytes. If no lymphocyte destruction occurs, the cross-match is negative and the transplant may proceed. The donor's cardiac function must be normal as assessed by an echocardiogram, nuclear studies, or cardiac catheterization. The donor should have stable hemodynamic profiles on minimal inotropic support.

This process may take several hours, and it is imperative that the patient and family be frequently updated and made aware of the clinical plan of care. Pretransplant teaching is reviewed to clarify misconceptions and correct knowledge deficits. If CO is compromised, decreased cerebral perfusion may compromise the attention span. During this time, the recipient needs close monitoring to maintain cardiovascular stability. The recipient may require antiarrhythmic therapy, inotropes, diuretics, or afterload reduction agents to achieve major organ perfusion adequate for cellular function. Anticoagulation therapy may be instituted to decrease risk of embolization secondary to AF, reduced left ventricular function, or peripheral venous stasis.

Transplant Surgical Techniques

In the past, there were two surgical options for cardiac transplantation. Today, almost all are orthotopic transplants in which the recipient's heart is removed and replaced by the donor's heart in the normal anatomic position (Figure 19-9). The surgical approach is a median sternotomy; the recipient's heart is incised at the superior and inferior vena cavae, pulmonary artery, and aorta. The donor's and recipient's vena cavae, aortas, and pulmonary arteries are aligned and anastomosed. This technique is called the bicaval technique. Another technique, which is less common, is the biatrial technique. This method involves removing the native heart but leaving the superior/posterior aspects of both atria. This will leave the native SA node intact and may result in double P waves on the ECG tracing (see Figure 19-9). In both techniques, the donor's heart is denervated and therefore receives no sympathetic or parasympathetic influence from the recipient's nervous system. Changes in CO after heart transplant depend on noncardiac mediators.

The other surgical option was a heterotopic approach, which is interesting from a historical perspective. It was used in about 5% of cardiac transplants at one point and was also

ESSENTIAL CONTENT CASE

Cardiac Transplant

A 54-year-old man is admitted to the surgical ICU for idiopathic cardiomyopathy after an orthotopic heart transplant (OHT). He is orally intubated with a mediastinal chest tube draining 60 mL of sanguineous fluid per hour. Atrial and ventricular epicardial wires, a left radial arterial line, and a right subclavian pulmonary artery catheter are in place.

Temperature	35.8°C
BP	140/82 mm Hg
HR	90 beats/min
NSR without ectopy; remnant P wave present	
RR	18 breaths/min
Ventilator settings:	
–Assist control mode, rate of 14/min	
–0.50 Fio$_2$	
–TV of 700 mL	
–PEEP 5 cm H$_2$O	
CO	3.80 L/min
Urine	60 mL/h
CI	2.0 L/min/m^2
Mediastinal tube	60 mL/h
SVR	1800 dyne/s/cm^5
SVO$_2$	58%
SpO$_2$	96%
Neurologically intact and moving all extremities on command	

Case Question 1: Which of the following hemodynamic measurements would contribute to the CI of 2.0 L/min/m^2?
(A) Heart rate 90 beats/min
(B) SVR 1800 dynes/s/cm^5
(C) Svo$_2$ 58%
(D) Respiratory rate 18 breaths/min

Case Question 2: Which of the following treatments would be appropriate to increase the CO/CI?
(A) Dobutamine to improve ventricular contractility
(B) Dopamine to improve renal perfusion
(C) Sodium nitroprusside to reduce afterload
(D) Esmolol to control the heart rate

Answers
1. B is the correct answer. The increased SVR reflects an increased afterload on the left ventricle causing an increased cardiac workload.
2. C is the correct answer. Sodium nitroprusside is an arterial vasodilator and will reduce the SVR thereby reducing myocardial work.

known as a "piggyback" approach. The donor heart was placed to the right side of the pleural cavity and performed as an auxiliary pump for the native heart. This was used as an option in a size mismatch between donor and recipient or for severe pulmonary hypertension. This approach is rarely performed anymore.

Principles of Management for Cardiac Transplantation
The postsurgical care is similar to care following conventional open heart surgery (see Chapter 9, Cardiovascular System). The primary objectives in the early postoperative period include stabilizing cardiovascular function, monitoring altered immune response and graft protection, and providing post-transplant psychological adjustment.

Stabilizing Cardiovascular Function
1. *Cardiac denervation:* Postoperatively, there is loss of vagal influence, and the patient usually has a higher resting heart rate than normal.
   - The post-transplant patient requires more stabilization prior to exercise or position changes to avoid orthostasis due to these effects from denervation. With loss of vagal tone, if the sinus rate decreases, there is a stronger potential for junctional rhythms to result.
   - *Surgical manipulation and postoperative edema* may decrease donor SA node automaticity, and therefore the patient may require temporary pacing or isoproterenol (Isuprel) to increase the heart rate.
   - If *dysrhythmias* such as SVT occur, beta-blockers or calcium channel blockers are used to decrease heart rate in these circumstances. It is important to assess the patient for response to isoproterenol, because this medication can increase myocardial oxygen consumption.
   - *Denervation* creates a more long-term concern in these patients because the patient no longer experiences angina if the myocardium becomes ischemic. Pain impulses are not transmitted to the brain, so patients must be taught to report other signs of declining cardiac function (ie, decreased exercise tolerance). This is seen in chronic rejection where even with diffuse coronary artery disease, the patient does not experience angina. The patient transplanted for ischemic cardiac disease may find this difficult to comprehend.
2. *Ventricular failure:* Any element of pulmonary hypertension can result in right ventricular dysfunction and eventually compromise left ventricular function also. Inotropic and vasodilating agents may be required to enhance cardiac function. It is essential to rule out any cardiac injury during harvesting and implantation that may have an impact on cardiac function. Review of the operative procedure can help rule out reperfusion injuries or post-bypass problems.
3. *Bleeding:* Risk factors include cardiopulmonary bypass (CPB), altered coagulation factors, impaired hepatic function due to right ventricular failure compromise, and preoperative anticoagulation therapy. The recipient's pericardium may be enlarged from pretransplant

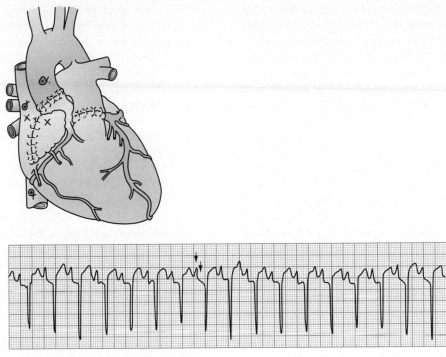

Figure 19-9. Orthotopic method of transplantation using biatrial approach. Both the donor and the recipient SA nodes are intact (x). This results in an ECG tracing as shown. Note the double P wave at independent rates (*arrows*). (*Reproduced with permission from Morton PG, Fontaine DK. Critical Care Nursing: A Holistic Approach. 9th ed. Philadelphia: Lippincott Williams & Wilkins; 2009.*)

cardiomegaly. With a smaller donor heart, there is more room for blood accumulation without early detection. If there is greater than 100 to 200 mL/h of bleeding for 2 hours, the patient may need to return to the operating room. All medications are reviewed for potential effect on platelet function and coagulation factors.

Monitoring Altered Immune Response and Graft Protection

After cardiac transplantation, the patient is pharmacologically managed with immunosuppressive treatment for graft protection, titrating for the best graft function with the least adverse effects. By virtue of these agents, patient survival has been tremendously enhanced, with a decrease in the need for retransplantation.

1. *Immunosuppression:* Most patients are maintained on triple-therapy immunosuppression: mycophenolate mofetil (Cellcept®), tacrolimus (Prograf®), and corticosteroids.
   - Tacrolimus (Prograf®), previously known as FK506, is indicated for both prevention of and management of organ rejection. It is classified as a calcineurin inhibitor, which inhibits the phosphate required for interleukin (IL)-2 production. The effect is limiting T-lymphocyte activation. Tacrolimus is used in combination with mycophenolate mofetil and is generally preferred over cyclosporine which has adverse effects including prolonging QTc intervals and producing and

producing hyperkalemia so that careful monitoring of potassium is required. Tacrolimus trough levels are measured to assess therapeutic dosages and avoid toxicity.
   - Cyclosporine creates a "selective immunosuppression" by selectively inhibiting T-cells. T-cells dependent on humoral immunity continue intact and no bone marrow suppression occurs. T-cell lymphocytes become unresponsive to IL-1, ultimately preventing maturation of helper and cytotoxic T-cells. Adverse effects include hypertension, nephrotoxicity, hepatotoxicity, hirsutism, tremors, and gum hyperplasia. When the first intravenous (IV) dose is administered, it is important to assess the patient closely for potential histamine-type reactions with cardiovascular collapse. This is related to the IV solution preparation and is not seen with the oral preparation. Cyclosporine trough levels are measured to assess therapeutic doses and avoid toxicity.
   - Basiliximab (Simulect) is an immunosuppressive agent that is an IL-2 antagonist. It is indicated for patients with renal insufficiency related to their chronic low CO because it is renal sparing. This medication is given preoperatively and then 2 to 4 days postoperatively.
   - Mycophenolate mofetil has potent cytotoxic effects on lymphocytes. It inhibits the proliferative responses of T and B lymphocytes to both myogenic and allospecific stimulation. It also

suppresses antibody formation against B lymphocytes. The adverse effects include gastrointestinal tract ulceration, nausea, vomiting, and diarrhea. It has severe neutropenic effects and can cause anemia, leukopenia, and thrombocytopenia.

- Corticosteroids are administered to both prevent and treat rejection. They are able to decrease antibody production and inhibit antigen-antibody production, as well as interfere with production of mediators IL-1 and IL-2. Both their anti-inflammatory and immunosuppressive properties offer the patient benefits. Immediately postoperatively, they are administered in high doses, and then tapered over the next 6 months. However, if the patient experiences two or more episodes of acute rejection, they remain on a maintenance dose. In situations of acute or chronic rejection, the patient may be "pulsed" with steroids. These doses are 500 to 1000 mg IV every day for 3 days, during which other steroids are discontinued. The patient then resumes the maintenance dose of steroids. Complications from steroid treatment are numerous and include infection, hyperlipidemia, diabetes, hypertension, osteoporosis, sodium and water retention, metabolic alkalosis, peptic ulceration, pancreatitis, increased appetite, adrenopituitary suppression, lymphocytopenia, opportunistic infections, and aseptic necrosis of femoral and humoral heads. The patient often receives ulcer prophylaxis with a histamine blocker or antacids. Strict fluid and electrolyte balance must be maintained, and close assessment must be maintained for glucose intolerance. The anti-inflammatory response may mask an infection; therefore, identification of malaise, anorexia, myalgias, and change in wound appearance, cough, or sore throat must be reported. With all these immunosuppressive agents, the patient has an intrinsic risk for malignancies and needs comprehensive teaching regarding this and all preventive therapies.
- Newer therapies offer further improvement in transplant outcomes. Muromonab-CD3 (Orthoclone OKT3), a monoclonal antibody, may be given to reverse acute rejection although it is rarely used. Antibodies that react with T_3 cells' surface antigens are produced, interfering with T-cell antigen recognition and making it more difficult for active T-cells to recognize the target organ. Muromonab-CD3 is administered for a 10- to 14-day course of therapy as a daily bolus dose of 5 to 10 mg IV. There is a danger of flash pulmonary edema, so patients receiving this medication are closely monitored, with emergency intubation equipment on hand, and often premedicated with steroids, acetaminophen, and diphenhydramine.

Cyclosporine is usually held during the period of Muronab-CD3 administration, and then titrated back up during the last 3 days of treatment. CD3 levels are monitored in the laboratory on the fourth and tenth days of therapy to assess effectiveness. Some centers utilize a monoclonal or polyclonal antibody for induction therapy in the immediate postoperative period. Others reserve medications such as Muromonab-CD3 for rescue therapy.

2. *Infection risk:* The immunosuppressive medications decrease the normal immune response, increasing the risk for nosocomial or suprainfections. Transplant patients are more susceptible to infection with common bacterial pathogens such as *Escherichia coli,* enterococci, staphylococcus, and streptococcus organisms. In addition, opportunistic infections such as cytomegalovirus (CMV) and pneumocystis pose a threat to patients who are immunocompromised. In the immediate post-transplant period, when steroid doses are highest, the patient is more vulnerable to these infections. Infections are a major cause of morbidity and mortality, and prevention and early detection are crucial.

The most challenging aspect of determining an infection is the clinical presentation, which is often masked by immunosuppressive therapy. The patient may not mount a fever or develop a high white blood cell (WBC) as rapidly because of this therapy. It is imperative to assess the individual trend in each patient and have a strong suspicion for infection if patients appear more fatigued, complain of sore throats, develop a new cough, or run low-grade temperatures. Bacterial, fungal, viral, and protozoal infections may compromise the post-transplant recipient.

Meticulous skin care to decrease dermal injuries, adequate nutrition and hydration, removing all invasive devices as soon as possible, and limiting unnecessary procedures may assist in reducing the risk for sepsis. Patients and families are provided thorough education regarding the risk of infection transmission. Antimicrobial therapy is instituted postoperatively while invasive devices are in place but their use is limited to avoid growth of antibiotic-resistant organisms. Thorough skin and oral assessments as part of the routine examination of the patient can help identify viral or fungal infections.

3. *Assessing for rejection:* Following transplant, patients undergo routine endomyocardial biopsy to rule out rejection (Figure 19-10). Under fluoroscopy, utilizing a cardiac bioptome via the right internal jugular vein into the right ventricle, multiple (three to five) samples are taken of the myocardium. If one or more of these samples demonstrates rejection, the patient is treated with the appropriate protocol

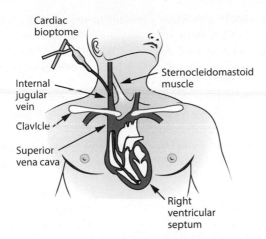

Figure 19-10. Endomyocardial biopsy technique. (*Reproduced with permission from Smith SL. Tissue and Organ Transplantation: Implications for Professional Nursing Practice. St Louis, MO: Mosby Yearbook, 1990.*)

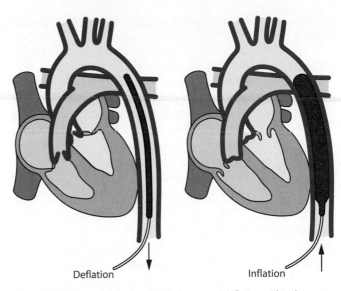

Figure 19-11. Counterpulsation. IABP inflation and deflation within the aorta.

(pulsed steroids or monoclonal antibodies). Other diagnostic procedures such as transesophageal echo-cardiogram and chest x-ray are often performed routinely as well. Cyclosporine levels or tacrolimus levels are routinely monitored. (See Chapter 7). These data provide further guidance for early detection of rejection.

Providing Post-transplant Psychological Adjustment

Many emotions impact the post-transplant patient. Often the patient and family have altered their roles and responsibilities during the illness. The post-transplant goal is to encourage role readjustment and resumption of pre-illness activities of daily living. The return to independence may frighten patients after the "security" of the hospital environment.

1. Involvement in a transplant support group may benefit the patient and family, reduce anxieties, and clarify misconceptions. Meeting other recipients may validate their feelings and enhance the patient's adjustments.
2. Some recipients experience body image concerns related to hirsutism and increased weight. Reviewing safe methods for dealing with these changes may decrease these concerns.
3. Weight loss may be enhanced through dietary counseling and participation in cardiac rehabilitation activities.
4. Discussions about quality-of-life with patients can heighten the positive side of transplantation.
5. Steroids may cause periods of mood swings from episodes of depression to euphoria. Counseling with the patient and family may reduce confusion over the cause of personality changes. During pulsed steroid therapy, it is very important to assess for cognitive

changes. Closer monitoring and reassurance during this therapy may assist in diminishing this side effect.

Intra-Aortic Balloon Pump Therapy

The IABP provides cardiac assistance by improving myocardial oxygen supply and reducing cardiac workload. The IABP catheter is inserted percutaneously or via a surgical incision into the femoral artery. It is advanced into the aorta and, when correctly positioned, lies below the subclavian artery and above the renal arteries.

The IABP works on the principle of counterpulsation. Gas (helium or CO_2) moves back and forth from the IABP console to the IABP catheter, causing the balloon to inflate and deflate (Figure 19-11). The balloon inflates during ventricular diastole, increasing intra-aortic pressure and blood flow to the coronary arteries. The balloon deflates just prior to ventricular systole, decreasing intra-aortic pressure. This pressure decrease reduces the resistance to left ventricular ejection or afterload.

Indications and Contraindications

IABP therapy may be used to treat angina refractory to medical therapy, left ventricular failure, cardiogenic shock, and failure to wean from CPB after cardiac surgery. Symptoms that indicate the need for IABP include signs of cardiogenic shock (tachycardia, systolic BP < 90 mm Hg, mean arterial pressure < 70 mm Hg, CI < 2.2-2.5 L/min/m^2, PAOP pressure < 18 mm Hg), decreased oxygenation, unstable angina, inadequate peripheral perfusion, and decreased urine output. The Thrombolysis and Counterpulsation to Improve Cardiogenic Shock Survival Trial demonstrated that augmentation of diastolic arterial pressure by IABP counterpulsation enhances thrombolysis and leads to faster reperfusion. Contraindications to IABP therapy include moderate to severe aortic insufficiency, aortic aneurysms, and severe peripheral vascular disease.

Intra-aortic Balloon Pump Timing

Balloon inflation and deflation are synchronized to left ventricular systole and diastole from the ECG signal and arterial pressure waveform. Accurate timing of the IABP is essential to avoid obstructing left ventricular ejection and severely compromising cardiac function. Proper timing of IABP requires extensive knowledge and skill development, which is beyond the scope of this book. Refer to specific IABP manufacturers' recommendations for timing guidelines.

Intra-aortic Balloon Pump Weaning

Weaning can be done by gradually, decreasing the frequency of the IABP ratio (1:1 to 1:3, depending on the balloon console) or by decreasing the IABP volume. Patients are ready to wean from the IABP when:

- Heart rate and rhythm are normal.
- Mean arterial pressure is greater than 70 mm Hg with minimal vasopressor support.
- CI is greater than 2.2 to 2.5 L/min/m^2.
- PAOP is less than 18 mm Hg.
- Oxygenation saturation is adequate.
- Urine output is adequate.

Principles of Management for Intra-aortic Balloon Pump Therapy

Intra-aortic Balloon Pump Maintenance

1. Monitor hemodynamic parameters to evaluate the effectiveness of IABP therapy and to identify the need to adjust prescribed vasoactive agents.
2. Frequently (every hour) monitor neurologic status and circulation to the extremity distal to the balloon catheter.
3. Limit activity to maintain proper catheter position.
   - Immobilize the affected leg so that the IABP catheter does not become dislodged or kinked.
   - Maintain head of bed according to insertion site manufacturer's recommendations.
   - Reposition patient l every 2 hours and perform range of motion for the affected extremity as appropriate.
4. Check the insertion site every hour, or per institution policy, for bleeding or hematoma formation.
5. Change the insertion site dressing daily using aseptic technique.

Intra-aortic Balloon Pump Removal

1. Discontinue anticoagulant therapy 4 to 6 hours prior to IABP removal.
2. Turn the IABP off just prior to removal.
3. Assist the provider with removal of the balloon.
4. Ensure that hemostasis is obtained after pressure is maintained on the insertion site for 30 to 45 minutes after balloon catheter removal.

5. Apply a pressure dressing to the insertion site for 2 to 4 hours.
6. Monitor vital signs and hemodynamic parameters every 15 minutes for 1 hour, every 30 minutes for 1 hour, and then every hour.
7. Assess peripheral perfusion to the affected extremity after catheter removal every hour for 2 hours, and then every 2 hours.
8. Restrict activity of the decannulated extremity and maintain bed rest with the patient's head of bed no greater than 45° for 24 hours.

Preventing and Managing Complications

1. *Intra-aortic balloon pump catheter misalignment:* If the IABP catheter is advanced too far, the brachial artery may become occluded; thus left arm (brachial, radial) pulses are diminished or absent and signs of limb ischemia are present. If the catheter is not in far enough, the mesenteric and/or renal arteries may be occluded. Signs of this include decreased or absent bowel sounds, increased abdominal girth, abdominal pain or firmness, and decreased urine output.
2. *Thromboemboli:* Anticoagulation is recommended to decrease the development of thromboemboli related to the indwelling IABP catheter. Fast flushing and withdrawing blood samples are avoided from the central aortic lumen of the IABP catheter. If this must be done, ensure that the IABP is on standby and that extreme care is taken to ensure that air bubbles are not introduced into the system. If the patient experiences asystole, turn the IABP console to the internal mode. In this mode, the catheter will flutter within the aorta so that thrombi formation is prevented. Refer to specific IABP manufacturer recommendations.
3. *Hemorrhage:* Monitor the central aortic pressure via the IABP catheter. This is connected to a transducer, a pressured flush system, and an alarm system. Accidental disconnection of the central aortic lumen could cause rapid exsanguination.
4. *Intra-aortic balloon rupture:* Signs of rupture include:
   - Loss of balloon augmentation.
   - Obvious blood or brown particles in the IABP catheter tubing.
   - Depending on the model of the IABP console, "a catheter problem" alarm may be activated.
   - Sudden hemodynamic instability.

If the intra-aortic balloon ruptures, turn the IABP console off, clamp the IABP catheter, notify the provider, and prepare for IABP removal or replacement. *Note:* the IABP should be removed within 30 minutes. Observe your patient's hemodynamic status and adjust vasoactive medications accordingly.

Ventricular Assist Devices

Ventricular assist devices provide greater support for a failing ventricle than the IABP, which only augments CO by 8% to 12%. When maximal medical therapy is inadequate, a VAD may be appropriate. The goals of utilizing a VAD are to reduce myocardial ischemia and workload, limit permanent cardiac damage, and restore adequate organ perfusion.

Indications

Patients with end-stage cardiac disease, patients who have recently come off CPB, and patients with cardiogenic shock following acute MI are candidates for VAD therapy. In some cases, insertion of a VAD is as a "bridge" until cardiac transplant takes place. The patient's status on the transplant list may or may not change once the VAD is in place. In other cases, such as post-MI, a patient may undergo VAD placement in the hope of myocardial recovery and eventual weaning from the device. This is often referred to as "bridge to recovery or decision." Once the VAD is inserted and the patient recovers, the patient is discharged home. Some patients experience myocardial recovery after VAD placement and can then undergo surgical removal. The VAD is removed when the myocardium has recovered to the point of consistently ejecting an adequate CO. After VAD removal, the patient is monitored closely for reoccurrence of heart failure symptoms. VAD is also used as "destination therapy" in which a nonsurgical/nontransplant candidate undergoes VAD placement with the expectation of ongoing dependence on the device. In those cases, the VAD remains in place until the patient dies or a decision is made to remove the device.

The appropriate selection of a candidate for these devices is based on hemodynamic criteria. If cardiovascular compromise persists despite increasing preload, reducing afterload, and instituting maximal medication doses, a VAD may be critical to achieve survival. Appropriate parameters to consider for VAD placement are:

- CI less than 2 L/min/m^2
- SVR more than 2100 dyne/s/cm^5
- Mean arterial pressure less than 60 mm Hg
- Left or right atrial pressure more than 20 mm Hg
- Urine output less than 30 mL/h
- PAOP more than 15 to 20 mm Hg

The exclusion criteria for use of a VAD include the following:

- Acute cerebral vascular damage
- Cancer with metastasis
- Renal failure (unrelated to cardiac failure)
- Severe hepatic disease
- Coagulopathy
- Sepsis, resistant to therapy
- Severe pulmonary disease
- Severe peripheral vascular disease
- Psychological instability

General Description of Ventricular Assist Device Principles

The VAD "unloads" the native ventricle or ventricles by way of artificial ventricles or a blood pump. CO is enhanced by blood circulating at a physiologic rate and by augmenting systemic and coronary circulation.

VAD support is predominately utilized for the left ventricle. However, if the right ventricle is compromised, support can be provided to both ventricles. This would necessitate separate VADs, yet the systems would function in tandem.

VADs can be used for postcardiotomy support as a bridge to recovery, a bridge to transplant, or as destination therapy. VADs can be nonpulsatile pumps (roller, centrifugal, or axial flow) or pulsatile pumps (pneumatically or electromagnetically driven). Previously, most VADs were inserted in the operating room but percutaneous placement is also an option, depending on the patient condition and the indication for VAD therapy. There are several approaches for cannula insertion depending on the type of device being used and whether support is needed for one or both ventricles.

There are smaller VADs that can be inserted in the cardiac catheterization laboratory using a percutaneous approach via the femoral vein and/or femoral artery. These include the Tandem Heart® and the Abiomed Impella® devices. The Tandem Heart® involves inserting a cannula into the right atrium via the femoral vein. The cannula is introduced across the fossa ovalis into the left atrium. Arterialized blood is removed from the left atrium, circulated through an axial flow device, and reintroduced into the arterial circulation via a cannula that has been inserted into the aorta via the femoral artery. The Abiomed Impella® is inserted percutaneously through the femoral artery and introduced across the aortic valve. The device is designed to augment the patient's CO. Blood is removed from the left ventricle and delivered into the ascending aorta. The Abiomed RP® supports the right ventricle. The device introduced via the femoral vein, introduced into the right ventricle, and advanced out into the pulmonary artery. Blood is removed from the right ventricle and ejected into the pulmonary artery.

VADs commonly used as a bridge to transplant are the HeartMate 3™ and HeartWare™ VAD. The older version HeartMate II™ is an axial flow device. The axial flow devices are usually not associated with a palpable pulse initially. Often, as the heart regains contractility over a period of several weeks, the pulse will return. The HeartWare™ and HeartMate 3™ are centrifugal continuous flow pumps. The HeartMate 3™ differs from the HeartWare™ in that the pump creates an intrinsic artificial pulse.

The HeartMate 3™ and the HeartWare™ VAD systems have both been Food and Drug Administration (FDA) approved for destination therapy. Destination therapy implies that the patient is not a candidate for transplant and will not be placed on the waiting list for a transplant.

The devices used as a bridge to transplant or for destination therapy are all left ventricular assist devices (LVADs). They all require an incision from the sternal notch to the umbilicus. A large cannula is inserted into the apex of the left ventricle and connected to the inflow port of LVAD with an outflow cannula inserted into the aorta. The LVAD is implanted outside the peritoneum just below the diaphragm. The drive line (power cord) is brought through the skin and connected to a power source. The drive line exit site requires meticulous care to prevent infection.

The LVAD has a monitor that provides the flow rate (similar to CO) and other information pertinent to the device. These devices can achieve flow rates that support adequate oxygen delivery to the tissues while reducing cardiac workload.

Weaning and Recovery

The plan for weaning depends on hemodynamic stability and the recovery of the patient's other organ systems following the period of poor perfusion. Assessment of CO, CI, SVR, PAOP pressure, mean arterial pressure, and SVO_2 guides decisions for initiating weaning. Pharmacologic support is maintained at a stable level with adequate major organ perfusion.

The arterial line waveform is assessed for the dicrotic notch appearance, evidence that there is adequate left ventricular pressure for aortic opening. The VAD is turned down at small increments to assess tolerance throughout the weaning process. Unfractionated heparin must be initiated before weaning and the device is never set at less than 2 L/min flow to avoid clot formation. At completion of weaning, the patient returns to the operating room for surgical removal.

Principles of Management for Ventricular Assist Device

The primary objectives in managing the patient with a VAD are to optimize CO, maximize coping, and prevent complications.

Optimizing CO

1. In the initial period after insertion, the risk of biventricular failure is still paramount and the patient must be closely evaluated. Cardiovascular profiles are measured every 2 to 4 hours and changes in the flow rate from the device reported to the physician. Pharmacologic support is titrated to achieve a stable mean arterial pressure and adequate SVO_2.
2. Assessing the VAD for proper function is essential to achieving an improved cardiovascular profile. As myocardial recovery occurs, more support occurs from the heart and less from the VAD. The patient can then support CO without as much mechanical support.

Maximizing Coping

The patient and family may be overwhelmed by the suddenness of the disease, the ICU environment, the equipment related to the VAD, and the threat of loss of life. Transplantation, if discussed, may significantly increase their stress. They may require intense information sharing and clarification of misconceptions.

1. Promote emotional and psychological adaptation, assess for nonverbal clues of fear or anxiety, and give frequent updates regarding goals for the day and the present plan of care. The advanced practice nurse and the patient's direct care nurse may coordinate this communication.
2. Provide realistic information related to prognosis. Twenty to forty percent of patients on VADs die awaiting a donor heart, and families need support to cope with this possibility. Early involvement with social work and chaplains also may assist patients and families. Closely assess for other situational stressors and review prior coping strategies the patient or family found helpful.

Preventing Complications

1. *Thromboembolism:* Anticoagulation therapy may include unfractionated heparin, dextran, or aspirin to reduce the risk for thromboembolism. Peripheral vascular impairment may occur secondary to vascular catheters. Frequent neurovascular checks are performed and any change reported immediately. Assess for the 5 Ps of vascular complications:
   - Pallor
   - Pain
   - Paresthesia
   - Paralysis
   - Pulselessness
2. *Bleeding:* Monitor hemoglobin, hematocrit, and coagulation factors frequently. Assess all catheter sites and wounds for oozing. For patients awaiting transplant, maintaining a narrow therapeutic range with anticoagulation is essential so that reversal of therapy can be achieved if a donor heart is available. Activated clotting levels should be appropriate for the device. The anticoagulation therapy may increase the propensity for cardiac tamponade to occur. This is a surgical emergency and may require reoperation for stabilization. Clues to this complication include the following:
   - Elevated atrial pressures/neck vein distention
   - Reduced CO as pump cannot fill properly
   - Elevated pulmonary pressures
   - Diastolic equalization
   - Reduced mean arterial pressure
   - Declining MvO_2
3. *Right ventricular failure:* Observe for development of elevated central venous pressure/neck vein distention combined with low to normal PAOP.
4. *Dysrhythmias:* Monitor ECG continuously. Patients may require antiarrhythmic medication or electrical cardioversion. Biventricular support may maintain nearly normal hemodynamics during dysrhythmias. Assess the effect of dysrhythmias on CO and augment the VAD accordingly. Treat all

electrolyte abnormalities aggressively to enhance contractility. Validate with physicians whether CPR may be performed for asystole, depending on the specific VAD.

5. *Decreased renal function:* Monitor renal function including BUN and creatinine daily, and urine output. Use nephrotoxic medications cautiously and ensure doses are based on creatinine clearance. Use vasopressor therapy to enhance renal perfusion, if appropriate. Maintain adequate fluid balance so preload is within normal limits. Monitor urinalysis for potential abnormalities, and avoid any period of hypotension as that will cause further injury to the kidneys.

6. *Infection:* Monitor closely for signs of infection as patients on VADs have large cannulas exiting the skin, which can be portals of entry for pathologic organisms. Patients on VAD support are also more prone to infections because of their underlying fragility. Patients awaiting transplant may become ineligible for the surgery, if they become septic. The best plan of action is prevention which includes:

   - Perform hand hygiene before and after all patient care activities
   - Use strict aseptic technique
   - Pan-culture for temperature more than 101°F (38.33°C)
   - Monitor wounds for erythema, exudate, or edema
   - Assess for leukocytosis or increase in bands on differential count

7. *Immobility:* Provide meticulous skin care and frequent position changes to reduce the risk of dermal injury during the patient's critical illness. Reduce the risk of catabolism by giving nutritional support. Collaborate with physical therapy to provide bedside exercise and ambulate as appropriate to prevent muscle loss. Apply foot splints to diminish the risk of foot drop.

8. *Poor device performance:* Evaluate the VAD performance routinely and with any change in the patient's clinical status. Dangers related to VAD mechanical problems include thrombus formation, in-flow obstructions, or device failures. Device failure may result in inadequate or no systemic perfusion, so emergency measures must be implemented rapidly (Table 19-5).

TABLE 19-5. EMERGENCY MEASURES FOR VAD FAILURE OR CARDIAC ARREST

- Backup VAD in place and ready for operation if mechanical failure occurs.
- CPR is usually not recommended. Should refer to manufacturer's guidelines.
- Assess availability of blood products should emergency transfusions be necessary.
- Have vascular clamps available for cannula disconnections.
- Educate all team members regarding emergency measures, if problem with VAD occurs.
- Patients can be safely cardioverted and defibrillated with VAD in place.
- Connect to emergency power outlets in case of an electrical outage.

ESSENTIAL CONTENT CASE

Thinking Critically

You are caring for a patient who just returned to the surgical intensive care unit (SICU) from cardiac surgery. He was admitted to the hospital with mitral insufficiency and today he had a mechanical valve inserted into the mitral position. Your assessment includes:

Temperature	36.28°C
HR	Temporarily atrial paced at 80 beats/min
BP	86/60 mm Hg
RR	Assist control of 12 on the ventilator
PAS	15 mm Hg
PAD	8 mm Hg
PAOP	4 mm Hg
RA	3 mm Hg
CO	4.9 L/min
CI	1.9 L/min/m^2
SVR	2200 dynes/s/cm^5

Case Question 1: What is the probable reason for his hypotension and low CO/CI?
(A) Hypervolemia
(B) Impaired myocardial contractility
(C) Hypovolemia
(D) Increased afterload

Case Question 2: What interventions should be immediately initiated to improve his cardiac status?
(A) Dobutamine to improve ventricular contractility
(B) Sodium nitroprusside to reduce afterload
(C) Increase heart rate to 90 beats/min
(D) Administer volume to increase preload

Answers
1. C is the correct answer. Hypovolemia is the most likely answer based on his low CVP and pulmonary artery pressures. The SVR is increased in response to the low CO/CI as a compensatory mechanism.
2. D is the correct answer. Administration of volume will normalize the pressures and improve the CO/CI.

SELECTED BIBLIOGRAPHY

General Cardiovascular

Fuster V, Harrington RA, Narula J, Eapan ZJ. *Hurst's The Heart.* 14th ed. New York, NY: McGraw Hill; 2017.

Good VS, Kirkwood PL. *Advanced Critical Care Nursing.* 2nd ed. St Louis, MO: Elsevier; 2018.

Hardin S, Kaplow R. *Cardiac Surgery Essentials for Critical Care Nursing.* 3rd ed. Sudbury, MA: Jones & Bartlett Publishing; 2020.

Morton PG, Fontaine DK. *Critical Care Nursing: A Holistic Approach.* 11th ed. Philadelphia, PA: Wolters Kluwer; 2017.

Zipes DP, Libby P, Bonow RO, Mann DL, eds. *Braunwald's Heart Disease: A Textbook of Cardiovascular Medicine.* 11th ed. Philadelphia, PA: Saunders Elsevier; 2018.

Cardiomyopathy

Bloom MW, Cole RT, Butler J. Evaluation and management of acute heart failure. In: Fuster V, Harrington RA, Narula J, Eapan ZJ, eds. *Hurst's The Heart*. 14th ed. New York, NY: McGraw Hill; 2017: chap 71. Accessed June 21, 2023. https://accessmedicine.mhmedical.com/content.aspx?bookid=2046&sectionid=176562062

Felker GM, Mann DL, eds. *Heart Failure: A Companion to Braunwald's Heart Disease*. 4th ed. St Louis: Elsevier; 2019.

Morton PG, Fontaine DK. *Critical Care Nursing: A Holistic Approach*. 11th ed. Philadelphia, PA: Wolters Kluwer; 2017, 378-381.

Siripanthong B, Nazarian S, Muser D, et al. Recognizing COVID-19-related myocarditis: the possible pathophysiology and proposed guideline for diagnosis and management. *Heart Rhythm*. 2020;17(9):1463-1471.

Heart Transplantation

Freeman R, Koerner E, Clark C, Halabicky K. Cardiac transplant: postoperative management. *Crit Care Nurs Q*. 2016;39(3):214-226.

Freeman R, Koerner E, Clark C, Halabicky K. The path from heart failure to cardiac transplant. *Crit Care Nurs Q*. 2016;39(3):207-215.

Jasiak NM, Park JM. Immunosuppression tips in solid organ transplantation: essentials and practical tips. *Crit Care Nurs Q*. 2016;39(3):227-240.

Kittleson MM, Patel JK, Kobashigawa JA. History and overview of cardiac transplantation. In: Fuster V, Harrington RA, Narula J, Eapan ZJ, eds. *Hurst's The Heart*. 14th ed. New York, NY: McGraw Hill Companies; 2017.

Mehra MR, Canter CE, Hannan MM, et al. The 2016 International Society for Heart Lung Transplantation listing criteria for heart transplantation: a 10-year update. *J Heart Lung Transplant*. 2016;35(1):1-23.

Valvular Disorders

Leeper B. Valvular disease and surgery. In: Good VS, Kirkwood PL, eds. *Advanced Critical Care Nursing*. 2nd ed. St Louis: Elsevier; 2018.

Leon MB, Mack MJ, Hahn RT, et al. Outcomes 2 years after transcatheter aortic valve replacement at low surgical risk. *J Am Coll Cardiol*. 2021;77:1149-1161.

Otto CM, Bonow RO, eds. *Valvular Heart Disease, A Companion to Braunwald's Heart Disease*. 5th ed. Philadelphia, PA: Saunders Elsevier; 2021.

Sorajja P, Moat N, Bradhwar B, et al. Initial feasibility study of a new transcatheter mitral prosthesis: the first 100 patients. *J Am Coll Cardiol*. 2019;73(11):1250-1260.

Pericarditis

Kloos JA. Characteristics, complications, and treatment of acute pericarditis. *Crit Care Nurs Clin North Am*, 2015;27(4):483-497.

Thoraco-Abdominal Aneurysms

Khan NR, Smalley Z, Nesvick CL, Lee SL, Michael LM. The use of lumbar drains in preventing spinal cord injury following thoracoabdominal aortic aneurysm repair: an updated systematic review and meta-analysis. *J Neurosurg Spine*. 2016;25(3):383-393.

Sidaway AN, Peria BA, eds. *Rutherford's Vascular Surgery and Endovascular Therapy*. 9th ed. Philadelphia, PA: Saunders Elsevier; 2018.

Intra-aortic Balloon Pump Therapy

Murks C, Juricek C. Balloon pumps inserted via the subclavian artery: bridging the way to heart transplant. *AACN Adv Crit Care*. 2016;27(3):301-315.

Quall SJ. *Comprehensive Intraaortic Balloon Pumping*. St Louis, MO: CV Mosby; 1984.

Ventricular Assist Devices

Doty D. Ventricular assist device and destination therapy candidates from preoperative selection through end of hospitalization. *Crit Care Nurs Clin North Am*. 2015;27(4):551-564.

Han JJ, Acker MA, Alturi P. Left ventricular assist devices: Synergistic model between technology and medicine. *Circulation*. 2018;138:2841-2851.

Puhlman M, Bingham A. Ventricular assist devices. In: Wiegand DL, ed. *AACN Procedure Manual for High Acuity, Progressive, and Critical Care*. 7th ed. St Louis, MO: Elsevier; 2017.

Rose EA, Moskowitz AJ, Packer M, et al. The REMATCH trial: rationale, design, and end points. *Ann Thorac Surg*. 1999;67:723-730.

Evidence-Based Practice/Guidelines

Baddour LM, Wilson WR, Bayer AS, et al. Infective endocarditis in adults: diagnosis, antimicrobial therapy, and management of complications: a scientific statement for healthcare professionals from the American Heart Association. *Circulation*. 2015. doi.org/10.1161/CIR.0000000000000296

Otto CM, Nishimura RA, Bonow RO, et al. 2020 Guideline for the management of patients with valvular heart disease. *Circulation*. 2021;143:e145-e171.

Cook JL, Colvin M, Francis G, et al. Recommendations for the use of mechanical circulatory support: ambulatory and community patient care. *Circulation*. 2017;135:e1145-1158.

Peura JL, Colvin-Adams M, Francis GS, et al. Recommendations for the use of mechanical circulatory support: device strategies and patient selection: a scientific statement from the American Heart Association. *Circulation*. 2012;126:2648-2667.

Yancy CW, Jessup M, Bozkurt B, et al. 2017 ACC/AHA/HFSA focused update on the 2013 ACCF/AHA/guideline for the management of heart failure: a report of the American College of Cardiology/American Heart Association Task Force on Clinical Practice Guidelines and the Heart Failure Society of America. *Circulation*. 2017. doi:10.1161/CIR.0000000000000509.

ADVANCED RESPIRATORY CONCEPTS: MODES OF VENTILATION

John J. Gallagher

20

KNOWLEDGE COMPETENCIES

1. Discuss the definition, patient selection process, application, assessment, and complications of pressure-targeted ventilation modes in critically ill patients.

2. Describe bilevel positive airway pressure, pressure-controlled/inverse ratio, volume-guaranteed pressure modes, airway pressure release ventilation (APRV), biphasic ventilation, adaptive support ventilation (ASV), proportional assist ventilation (PAV), and high-frequency ventilation used to support critically ill patients.

ADVANCED MODES OF MECHANICAL VENTILATION

New Concepts: Mechanical Ventilation

Mechanical ventilation is an essential support strategy for patients with respiratory failure. For years, volume ventilation was the dominant form of ventilation. With advancement in ventilator technology, numerous pressure modes emerged and are now commonly used in critical care units to ventilate patients from the acute phase of illness to weaning from the ventilator. Although selected characteristics of these pressure modes are attractive, some of the modes are not well understood and superior outcomes associated with their use have not been described. Results of studies of acute respiratory distress syndrome (ARDS) suggest that the long-held traditional approach to ventilation with larger tidal volumes was injurious to the lung. Thus, clinical applications aimed at lung protective ventilation have been undertaken to prevent ventilator-induced lung injury (VILI). These concepts are described here.

Mechanical Ventilation of Acute Respiratory Distress Syndrome

ARDS was previously described as the most severe presentation of acute lung injury (ALI), but the term ALI has been eliminated in favor of the labels "mild," "moderate," and "severe" ARDS. The Berlin Definition of ARDS consists of categories that identify the timing of the condition, chest imaging criteria, origin of lung edema, and oxygenation status. The severity stratification of mild, moderate, and severe are based on the Pao_2/Fio_2 score and positive end-expiratory pressure (PEEP) level. ARDS results from an acute insult to the body that may be direct (ie, specific lung condition such as pneumonia) or indirect (ie, condition outside the lung such as sepsis). The release of mediators and a host of other toxic substances affect the alveolar–capillary membrane adversely and result in a noncardiac pulmonary edema. Pathology includes decreased lung compliance, shunting, and refractory hypoxemia. Mortality rates once as high as 50% have been reduced over the years using lung protective and other organ support strategies. To date, there is no definitive treatment for ARDS. Therapy focuses on managing the underlying condition, optimizing mechanical ventilation, and providing supportive care until the lungs heal.

Studies of patients with ARDS show that large tidal volume delivery results in greater lung damage and higher mortality rates than low tidal volume ventilation, minimizing alveolar stretch due to excessive tidal volume (volutrauma), pressure (barotrauma), and the cyclic opening and collapse of diseased alveoli (atelectrauma). Although low tidal volume ventilation leads to hypoventilation and hypercapnia in the ARDS patient, mortality rates are lower with this approach.

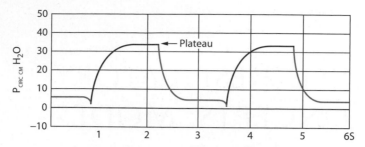

Figure 20-1. Square pressure waveform: pressure breath.

In addition, studies show that the use of PEEP decreases mortality in ARDS by opening collapsed lung units and preventing collapse during exhalation. This effect is called lung recruitment.

While results of recent studies have changed the management of patients with ARDS, during the acute phase, emerging information is further redefining the approach. In the last several years, additional components of "tidal energy" required for lung inflation have become the focus, with an increasing understanding of their contribution to VILI. These components collectively determine ventilation power and include the product of minute ventilation and the sum of the tidal pressure components: flow resistance, transpulmonary driving pressure, and PEEP. During delivery of the positive pressure breath, flow resistance is generated by the ventilator circuit, artificial and natural airways, and the alveoli. In the face of alveolar collapse, the flow rate (speed) at which the lung is inflated can contribute to shear injury, as aerated and collapsed alveoli will inflate at different rates, creating stress in the adjacent alveoli and interstitial lung tissue. Transpulmonary driving pressure is the difference between PEEP and the plateau pressure and may also contribute to lung injury.

Questions remain about whether pressure-targeted ventilation is the equivalent of low-volume ventilation, and how to best determine the optimal PEEP level. Additionally, data suggest that lower tidal volumes may be beneficial in patients who do not have ARDS but are at risk for lung injury. In these patients, larger tidal volumes may trigger inflammatory changes later resulting in lung injury.

Volume Control Versus Pressure Control Ventilation

Volume control ventilation (VCV) delivers a set tidal volume at a set flow rate with the peak inspiratory pressure (PIP) varying depending on the airway resistance and lung/chest wall compliance. As airway resistance increases and lung/chest wall compliance decreases, the PIP will increase. Conversely, a reduction in airway resistance or increase in lung/chest wall compliance will result in a decrease in PIP (see Chapter 5, Airway and Ventilatory Management). As a safety measure, a pressure limit may be set on the ventilator; if this limit is exceeded, the breath will be terminated before the full tidal volume is delivered to prevent lung injury from excessively high pressures.

In contrast, with pressure control ventilation (PCV), the inspiratory pressure level (IPL) is set, and the tidal volume varies with the selected IPL, airway resistance, and lung and chest wall compliance. As airway resistance increases or lung/chest wall compliance decreases, the set IPL will be achieved sooner, and the delivered tidal volume will decrease. Conversely, a reduction in airway resistance or increase in lung/ chest wall compliance will result in an increase in tidal volume for the set IPL. The square pressure waveform (Figure 20-1) and decelerating flow pattern (Figure 20-2) are characteristics of pressure control breath patterns and may improve gas distribution among collapsed alveoli. In contrast, VCV produces an ascending pressure waveform and square flow pattern providing a steady, yet fixed, gas flow throughout inspiration. (Figure 20-3). However, modern ventilators allow the VCV flow waveform pattern to be changed depending on the clinical need.

Flow patterns are important because they affect lung filling. Gas moving down the airways takes the path of least resistance and tends to preferentially fill alveoli that are open and compliant. Closed or partially open alveoli are less compliant and do not fill easily. With volume-targeted ventilation, gas flow can be quite turbulent (especially when short inspiratory times are used) and the distribution of gas is uneven; closed alveoli stay closed, while compliant alveoli receive the bulk of the fresh gases. With pressure-targeted ventilation, flow is high initially but slows toward the end of the breath; gas distributes more evenly. It is thought that this is because the slower end-inspiratory flow rate results in less turbulent gas flow (called laminar flow). A wide variety of pressure modes are available for application during the acute stage

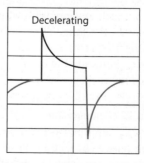

Figure 20-2. Decelerating flow waveform: pressure breath. (*©2023 Medtronic. All rights reserved. Used with the permission of Medtronic.*)

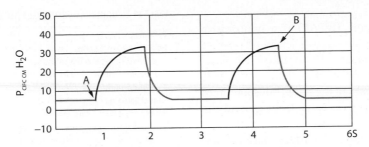

Figure 20-3. Ascending pressure waveform: volume breath.

of illness and for weaning. Descriptions are provided below. Specific information related to weaning with the modes is found in Chapter 5, Airway and Ventilatory Management.

Pressure Support Ventilation

PSV, first described in the early 1980s as a form of ventilation for the stable, spontaneously breathing patient during weaning, is now a popular mode of ventilation in most critical care units. The clinical success of pressure support resulted in the emergence of many other pressure modes.

PSV is designed for the spontaneously breathing patient but requires that the pressure support level be selected by the clinician. When the patient initiates a spontaneous breath, the ventilator senses the patient's breathing effort (sensitivity "trigger"). This trigger can be set to "pressure trigger," where the patient must generate negative pressure in the system to initiate the breath (usually set at −1 to 2 cm H_2O) or to "flow trigger" where the patient draws gas flow from the ventilator (usually 2-3 L) to initiate the breath. The ventilator then delivers a high flow of gas to the patient until the selected pressure level is reached early in inspiration. This pressure level is then maintained throughout the inspiratory phase. The ventilator cycles off and exhalation begins when flow decreases to approximately one-quarter of the original flow (the cycle-off mechanism varies with different ventilators). This occurs as the lungs fill toward the end of the inspiration. An important characteristic of PSV is that it enables the patient to determine inspiratory time, volume, and respiratory rate (RR). This characteristic is thought to explain why pressure support is a "comfortable" mode for spontaneously breathing patients. In addition, PSV decreases the work of breathing associated with circuits, high breathing rates, and small endotracheal tubes. Because the level of support can be gradually reduced, the mode is especially helpful for weaning. This method may be used in less stable patients as well, provided that the tidal volume is closely monitored. Patient selection, application, assessment, and potential complications are delineated in Table 20-1.

TABLE 20-1. PRESSURE SUPPORT VENTILATION

Definition
Pressure support ventilation (PSV) is a form of ventilation used to augment spontaneous respirations with a clinician-selected amount of positive airway pressure. There are two applications of PSV: (1) stand-alone mode and (2) mixed mode where a backup rate is set. Changes in compliance or resistance can result in changes in tidal volume and respiratory rate.

Patient Selection
1. Patients who are stable, ready to wean, and have a dependable ventilatory drive.
2. PSV helps overcome resistance associated with circuits and airways.
3. In less stable patients, close monitoring of tidal volume and respiratory rate is necessary.

Application
1. *Rest* (called PSV max): Adjust PSV level to obtain a respiratory rate of < 20 breaths/min, a tidal volume of 6-10 mL/kg, and an eupneic respiratory pattern.
2. *Work:* Decrease PSV level as tolerated. This varies between patients (from hours to days) and may be defined by a unit protocol. Respiratory rate may be higher and tidal volumes lower during work intervals. Monitor both parameters hourly and stop if the predetermined thresholds are exceeded.

Assessment
1. *Comfort:* The patient controls inspiratory and expiratory time, rate, and volume. The patient should be comfortable and without dyspnea.
2. *Secretions* can increase resistance and decrease tidal volume. Ensure airway patency with adequate humidification and suctioning as needed. If secretions are copious, pressure support may be contraindicated.
3. *Compliance changes:* Decreased lung compliance results in decreased tidal volume and often an increase in respiratory rate.
4. *Conditioning:* PSV is good for promoting endurance of the respiratory muscles by gradually increasing workload over time. For example, when the PSV level is set at a higher level, little effort (work) is required. The work is increased as the PSV level is gradually lowered. It is important to remember that when other activities are taking place (ie, sitting up in a chair, physical therapies) or when there are physical impediments to breathing (ie, ascites, obesity, distention), the PSV level may need to be increased. Use respiratory rate and tidal volume to determine optimal level of support.

Complications
1. Use caution when chest tube leaks and cuff leaks are present. Patients with large air leaks from chest tubes and/or endotracheal tube cuffs should not be placed on PSV. When a leak is present, the patient may not be able to control the parameters of inspiratory time, rate, or volume.
2. PSV should be used very cautiously in patients with asthma or in patients with rapidly changing physical status (ie, with acute bronchospasm there is an increase in airway resistance; a decrease in tidal volume; and increase in respiratory rate will result).

Bilevel Positive Airway Pressure

Bilevel positive airway pressure (BiPAP) is a noninvasive mode of ventilation that combines two levels of positive pressure (PSV and PEEP) by means of a full-face mask, nasal mask (most common), or nasal pillows. The ventilator is designed to compensate for leaks in the setup, but sometimes a chin strap is used to prevent excessive leaks around the mouth. Full-face mask ventilation is used cautiously because the potential for aspiration is high. If full-face mask ventilation is chosen, the patient should be able to remove the mask quickly if nausea occurs or vomiting is imminent. Obtunded patients and those with excessive secretions are not good choices for bilevel ventilation.

A number of options are available with BiPAP and include a spontaneous mode where the patient initiates all the pressure-supported breaths; a spontaneous-timed option, similar to PSV with a backup rate (some vendors call this A/C); and a control mode. The control mode requires the selection of a control rate and inspiratory time. High Fio_2 requirements are a relative contraindication for the use of BiPAP because generally, oxygen is bled into the system. Many ventilators have a noninvasive ventilation mode, allowing the machines to deliver BiPAP. This dual functionality provides flexibility when moving from invasive (intubated) to noninvasive (mask) ventilation.

BiPAP is used successfully in critical care patients to prevent intubation, and also to prevent reintubation following extubation. BiPAP may be especially helpful in patients with chronic obstructive pulmonary disease and with heart failure particularly, because these patients are often difficult to wean from conventional ventilation given their underlying disease processes. Study results suggest that noninvasive ventilation may improve outcomes in immunocompromised patients. Patient selection, application, assessment, and potential complications are delineated in Table 20-2.

Pressure Control and Pressure Controlled/Inverse Ratio Ventilation

Pressure controlled/inverse ratio ventilation (PC/IRV) is designed to ventilate patients with significant alveolar collapse such as occurs in ARDS. The pressure control option allows the clinician to control (or limit) the pressure during inspiration. Because the tendency of the stiff ARDS lung is to collapse, a prolonged inspiratory time may be used to recruit collapsed alveoli, while the shorter expiratory time may prevent alveolar closing (de-recruitment). In this mode of ventilation, inspiratory to expiratory ratios (I/E), which are normally 1:2 or 1:3, are increased to 1:1, 2:1, 3:1, or 4:1. The short expiratory time is generally sufficient for complete exhalation; however, in some cases, full exhalation may not occur before the next breath, generating auto-PEEP. In PC/IRV, auto-PEEP is desirable as it prevents end-expiratory collapse of alveoli between the ventilator breaths.

TABLE 20-2. NONINVASIVE BILEVEL POSITIVE AIRWAY PRESSURE (BiPAP)

Definition

BiPAP is pressure support with PEEP provided through a face mask, nasal pillows, or nasal mask (although it may also be provided through a tracheostomy tube, that application is rarely used in the critical care environment).

Patient Selection

Patients in whom invasive ventilation is not desired, for sleep apnea or hypoventilation syndrome, to prevent intubation or reintubation, and to treat heart failure. The mode should not be used in those who cannot protect their airway or in those with very high Fio_2 requirements.

Application

3. *Select mode* (names vary with the manufacturer): Spontaneous (PSV), spontaneous-timed (assist-control), or controlled.
4. *Spontaneous mode:* Select the level of pressure support (inspiratory pressure level) and the PEEP level (generally there must be at least 5 cm H_2O pressure difference between these).
5. *Spontaneous timed:* Pressure support level, PEEP, and backup rate are selected.
6. *Controlled:* Pressure support level, PEEP, rate, and inspiratory time are selected.
7. Fio_2 is adjusted by means of a flow meter and "bled" into the circuit to attain appropriate Sao_2 or Pao_2. The ventilator function is adversely affected if the flow rate is too high. Refer to manufacturers limits as this varies with the ventilator make and model. Some models are equipped with a dial to adjust Fio_2.

Assessment

1. *Rate and pattern of breathing:* The patient should look comfortable with no evidence of accessory muscle use and a reasonable respiratory rate.
2. Although ABGs are often obtained, Sao_2, in conjunction with assessment of rate and pattern of breathing, mental status, and vital signs, tells us much about how the patient is tolerating the mode.
3. This method of ventilation is labor intensive and requires that the nurse and respiratory therapist work together to determine the best settings for the patient.
4. A chin strap may be used if the patient cannot maintain a good seal by keeping his or her mouth closed.

Complications

1. Decreased mental status is a relative contraindication for BiPAP because the patient may not be able to protect the airway. Any acute change in mental status should be promptly reported and continued use of BiPAP carefully evaluated. Intubation may be necessary.
2. If the patient becomes nauseated, aspiration risk is increased. Make sure the patient can quickly remove the face or nasal mask if necessary.
3. Excessive secretions are a relative contraindication to the use of this mode unless the patient can adequately clear his/her airway.

The options of controlling pressure and prolonging inspiration, in conjunction with the decelerating flow pattern (see Figure 20-4), are beneficial aspects of this pressure mode. Use of PC/IRV frequently requires that the patient be heavily sedated and/or chemically paralyzed to ensure patient/ventilator synchrony. Generally, this mode option does not allow for spontaneous patient breathing through the inspiratory/expiratory cycles. Control is required to optimize the breath delivery. However, newer modes (see Airway Pressure Release Ventilation and Bilevel or Biphasic Ventilation described later in this chapter) are designed differently and allow for spontaneous breathing during the breath cycle. Guidelines for patient selection, application, assessment, and potential complications of PC/IRV are summarized in Table 20-3.

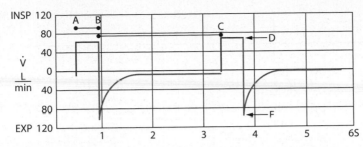

Figure 20-4. Square flow waveform: volume breath. (©2023 Medtronic. All rights reserved. Used with the permission of Medtronic.)

Volume-Guaranteed Pressure Modes of Ventilation

As noted earlier, a major drawback to the use of traditional pressure ventilation modes (ie, PSV, PC, and PC/IRV) is the inability to ensure consistent volume delivery. Delivered volume is dependent on compliance, resistance, and the selected pressure level. In severely ill patients, such as the patient with ARDS, changes in compliance can result in changes in volume delivery and ultimately acid-base disturbances. Ventilator manufacturers responded to this concern by designing mode options that guarantee a prescribed tidal volume while delivering the volume as a pressure breath (decelerating flow pattern, etc). These modes are often referred to as Volume-Guaranteed Pressure Modes or Dual Control Modes. The technology associated with these new mode options is sophisticated and characteristics vary between manufacturers. However, the inherent concepts are similar across manufacturers and can be applied in the clinical setting. Two different examples of volume-guaranteed pressure modes of ventilation are described as follows; however, others are available.

Pressure Augmentation

This mode option allows the clinician to select the desired tidal volume with a pressure option (called pressure augmentation). This option provides for all the delivered ventilator breaths to be pressure breaths unless it is determined (ie, by internal calculations of compliance, resistance, and flow during breath delivery) that the prescribed tidal volume goal will not be reached. If this occurs, the ventilator automatically delivers the rest of the inspiration as a volume breath (Dual Control "within" the breath) (Figure 20-5). The pressure waveforms vary and will change as the clinician adjusts the pressure level. This mode can be used as a control mode (rate selected) or a spontaneous mode (no rate).

Volume Support and Pressure-Regulated Volume Control

With these modes, the clinician selects the spontaneous option (VS) or the control option (PRVC) in addition to the desired tidal volume. Pressure limits are set in both. When VS is selected, the ventilator adjusts the pressure level on a breath-to-breath basis to maintain the desired volume (Dual Control "between" breaths). It is important to note that the minimum set volume is guaranteed, but the maximum is not. Increased patient effort may result in wide swings in tidal volume. The pressure waveforms (Figure 20-6) show step-wise changes in pressure levels as needed in the spontaneously breathing patient.

With PRVC, the same mechanism is in place to ensure that the desired tidal volume is delivered. A mandatory rate and inspiratory time are selected in the PRVC mode but the patient can also take spontaneous breaths. Thus, as noted above with VS, the maximum tidal volume may vary dependent on patient effort. There are generally two options for how the patient-initiated breaths are delivered. They can be set in the assist/control configuration (where spontaneous breaths are delivered at the PRVC-selected volume, or

TABLE 20-3.   PRESSURE CONTROLLED/INVERSE RATIO VENTILATION

Definition

PC/IRV combines PCV with an inverse breath ratio to lower peak airway pressure and improve gas distribution (and oxygenation).

Patient Selection

Patients with ARDS with $Pao_2 \leq 60$ mm Hg and increasing peak inspiratory and plateau pressures.

Application

1. *Select the inspiratory pressure level:* Generally this is around 30-35 cm H_2O initially. This can be lowered over time to ensure lower tidal volumes or plateau pressures.
2. Select inspiratory/expiratory ratio (1:1, 2:1, 3:1, and 4:1).
3. Select respiratory rate (this is usually high—in most cases > 20).
4. Set PEEP (the amount dialed in) may stay the same initially. However, with the prolonged inspiratory time secondary to inverse ratios, auto-PEEP may occur. Auto-PEEP may be a desirable outcome.
5. Fio_2 is initially high but can be decreased as oxygenation improves.
6. Patients placed on PC/IRV require sedation, and often, paralytic agents. This is because the inverse ratio is not physiologic and patient/ventilator asynchrony results in inadequate ventilation.

Assessment

1. Arterial blood gases, end-tidal CO_2, and pulse oximetry to monitor adequacy of oxygenation and ventilation.
2. With changing compliance or resistance (agitation, secretions, pneumothorax, bronchospasm, abdominal distention, fluid overload, etc), tidal volume is affected. Monitor tidal volume hourly and with any position change.
3. *Patient comfort/synchrony:* If paralytic agents are used, the appropriate use of sedatives and analgesics should be ensured.

Complications

1. A high index of suspicion for barotrauma: Acute changes in oxygenation, ventilation, tidal volume, and vital signs may herald a pneumothorax.
2. Acute changes in lung compliance and resistance affect tidal volume.
3. The use of paralytics and heavy sedation is commonly necessary to assure patient/ventilator synchrony with this mode.

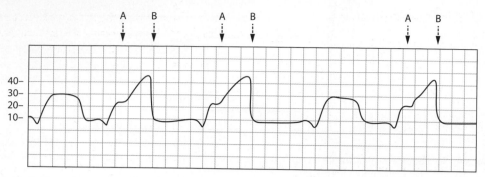

Figure 20-5. Pressure waveform of pressure augmentation: when desired tidal volume cannot be delivered, the ventilator supplies the remainder of the breath as a volume breath (A = beginning pressure breath [square pressure waveform], B = volume delivery [accelerating pressure waveform]).

they can be set in the SIMV mode configuration (where the spontaneous breaths are delivered at the patient-initiated volume). Table 20-4 summarizes the selection criteria, application, assessment, and potential complications associated with volume-guaranteed pressure modes (pressure augmentation, VS, PRVC, etc) of ventilation.

Airway Pressure Release Ventilation and Bilevel or Biphasic Ventilation

Airway pressure release ventilation (APRV) and bilevel positive airway pressure (bilevel or biphasic) ventilation are options available on some ventilators. Both options are commonly used for patients with ARDS. The APRV option employs a high level of continuous positive airway pressure (CPAP) to recruit the lung (ie, open alveoli and restore functional residual capacity [FRC]) and uses brief expiratory "releases" (no longer than 1.5 seconds and generally much shorter), provided at set intervals (similar to rate), to enhance CO_2 clearance.

In contrast, bilevel or biphasic modes use two different levels of CPAP called high-PEEP and low-PEEP. A rate and inspiratory time are set as in PC/IRV. A major difference between PC/IRV and both APRV and bilevel ventilation is that flow is available to the patient for spontaneous breathing at both pressure levels. Pressure support may also be added to decrease the work associated with spontaneous breathing. These features of unrestricted and parallel spontaneous breathing make the modes desirable in large part because the use of heavy sedation and paralytics may not be necessary. Table 20-5 summarizes the selection, application, assessment, and potential complications of these mode options.

TABLE 20-4. VOLUME-GUARANTEED PRESSURE MODES

Definition

Volume-guaranteed pressure modes (Dual Control Modes) provide spontaneous and controlled pressure ventilation mode options while ensuring that a predetermined tidal volume is delivered. The volume-guarantee characteristic is provided in one of two ways. Either the pressure level is automatically adjusted by the ventilator to attain the predetermined volume (ie, VS and PRVC), or the breath starts as a pressure breath but is completed as a volume breath (ie, pressure augmentation).

Patient Selection

1. *In weaning and/or stable patients*, spontaneous breathing options such as VS may be good options.
2. *In acutely ill and/or unstable patients*, selecting options that have a control rate (eg, "backup rate") such as PRVC may be used to assure adequate ventilation.

Application

Application varies with specific ventilators.

1. Volume desired is selected.
2. Pressure level automatically adjusts to attain desired volume in both VS and PRVC. A pressure limit may be set.
3. Respiratory rate is selected for controlled modes and as a backup if desired.
4. With PRVC, spontaneous breath options are also set.

Assessment

1. Clinical signs and symptoms, arterial blood gases, end-tidal CO_2, and pulse oximetry.
2. Monitor pressure waveforms to determine the need for pressure/volume adjustment (alarms also indicate when pressure limits are exceeded, indicating compliance and/or resistance changes).

Complications

1. Barotrauma is a potential complication of all mechanical ventilation.
2. These modes, if not understood, are difficult to assess. An understanding of the specific ventilator mode characteristics and the ability to interpret airway pressure waveforms are important to prevent errors in mode application.
3. Large variation in tidal volume is possible with these modes. The set tidal volume is the minimum volume that will be achieved, however, the patient may generate larger tidal volumes depending on inspiratory effort on a breath-to-breath basis.

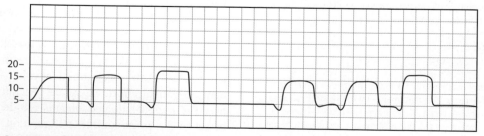

Figure 20-6. Pressure waveform of volume support: the pressure is increased in increments with each breath to attain the desired tidal volume.

TABLE 20-5. AIRWAY PRESSURE RELEASE VENTILATION AND BIPHASIC VENTILATION

Definitions
APRV: High level of CPAP provided with short releases at regular intervals.
Biphasic: Two levels of PEEP (high and low levels) with spontaneous
breathing allowed at both pressure levels.

Patient Selection
Patients with ARDS or with decreased lung compliance in whom lung
recruitment is desired.

Application
1. *APRV:* CPAP level, Fio_2 and pressure release interval (similar to frequency
   or rate), and duration (no more than 1.5 seconds; longer releases result in
   lung "de-recruitment" and are to be avoided). The frequency of pressure
   releases and their duration (time low) may be increased to lower CO_2.
2. *Bilevel or Biphasic:* This is similar to setting PC ventilation. Select a high
   PEEP level (this is like setting the inspiratory pressure level) and a low
   PEEP level (this is PEEP). Rate and inspiratory time are also selected.
3. Heavy sedation and paralysis should not be necessary because the
   patient can breathe at both levels of support. PSV may be set to assist
   with the patient's spontaneous breaths at the levels of support.

Assessment
Although comfort is a goal for the application of all mechanical ventilation,
patients on these modes may appear tachypneic yet be comfortable.

Complications
As per all modes of ventilation used in the acutely ill ventilated patient with
noncompliant lungs.

Adaptive Support Ventilation

Adaptive support ventilation (ASV) is also called as "intelligent ventilation." The mode assesses lung mechanics on a breath-to-breath basis (controlled loop ventilation) for both the spontaneous and the control settings. The clinician sets the desired minute ventilation based on the patient's predicted body weight (PBW) and the ventilator makes automatic adjustments in the inspiratory pressure (tidal volume), rate, and inspiratory/expiratory time ratios in order to minimize elastic and resistive workloads. Spontaneous breathing is promoted automatically. In this mode, the interactions required by the clinician are few (Table 20-6). The manufacturer suggests that this aspect of "intelligent ventilation" may decrease the potential for operator

TABLE 20-6. ADAPTIVE SUPPORT VENTILATION

Definition
ASV is designed to assess patient lung mechanics on a breath-to-breath basis
and adjust the tidal volume and respiratory rate to ensure that the work of
breathing is minimized. Spontaneous breathing is encouraged automatically.
The ventilator automatically minimizes auto-PEEP, prevents apnea and
tachypnea, and large breath size. Required ventilator parameters are few.

Patient Selection
Appropriate for all phases of ventilation from acute management to weaning.

Application
Set ideal body weight, %MinVol (minute volume) and high pressure limit.
Once these are set, ASV is started and %MinVol is adjusted if indicated.

Assessment
When the ventilator inspiratory pressure and frequency (fx) decrease, it is
evident that the patient requires minimal ventilatory support. Low to zero
levels may indicate the patient requires little to no inspiratory support and
is breathing entirely spontaneously.

Complications
As per all modes of ventilation used in the acutely ill ventilated patient.

error and save time, both desirable outcomes of any ventilator system. Built into the mode are algorithms that are "lung protective." These include strategies to minimize auto-PEEP and prevent apnea, tachypnea, excessive dead space, and excessively large breaths. Studies to date on ASV suggest the work of breathing may be decreased with the mode (see Table 20-6).

ESSENTIAL CONTENT CASE

Volume Support and Pressure-Regulated Volume Control

A 50-year-old man was admitted to the surgical intensive care unit (SICU) following repairs of multiple injuries resulting from a motor vehicle accident. His injuries included multiple leg fractures as well as blunt abdominal trauma. His legs were casted following repair and he was admitted for stabilization and to monitor his abdominal status. He was placed on PRVC (SIMV option) at a rate of 20 with a volume of 500 mL, PEEP of 5, and an Fio_2 of 60%. Within 3 hours of his admission to the SICU, his respiratory status deteriorated and his chest x-ray demonstrated pulmonary edema. His abdominal injuries were stable. ABGs were:

pH	7.25
$Paco_2$	67 mm Hg
Pao_2	55 mm Hg
RR (total)	35 breaths/min

The patient was given 20 mg of furosemide, his PEEP was increased to 10 cm H_2O and his control rate was increased to 25. His fentanyl infusion was maintained at 50 mcg/h and he was also given an additional bolus of 50 mcg.

The patient quickly recovered following the above interventions; oxygenation and ventilation improved and he slept well without further incidents. The next morning he was stable, alert, and anxious to get the "tube out." He was placed on VS with a selected tidal volume of 350 mL and an Fio_2 of 35%. Following this change, his Sao_2 was 98% and spontaneous RR was 20 and nonlabored. The team decided to extubate the patient. He did well and later that day was transferred to an acute care unit.

Case Question 1: In this example, the patient was set on PRVC (SIMV option). Instead of increasing the control rate to 25, what other option is available that may assure desired tidal volume in the PRVC mode?

Case Question 2: Why did the team select a tidal volume of 350 mL versus a higher tidal volume?

Answers
1. The PRVC mode may be adjusted to assure a stable volume delivery by using the assist/control option. With this option, the patient spontaneous effort to breathe results in a breath at the same guaranteed volume as the set or "control" breaths (ie, similar to how traditional A/C is designed).
2. Volume support is a spontaneous breathing mode that assures a selected tidal volume is delivered with each spontaneous breath. If the patient is weaning and stable, setting the selected tidal volume too high will deter weaning as the higher "selected volume" will be provided.

Proportional Assist Ventilation and Neurally Adjusted Ventilatory Assist

Proportional assist ventilation (PAV) is designed to prevent fatiguing workloads while still allowing the patient to spontaneously breathe. When activated, the mode automatically adjusts the pressure, flow, and volume proportionally to offset the resistance and elastance of the system with each inspiration (patient and circuit). Adjustments vary somewhat between the ventilators. This mode, like others discussed previously, may allow for more patient control, improved patient/ventilator synchrony, and ultimately better outcomes; however, studies to date are somewhat conflicting and it is clear that more research is needed to determine PAV's use in different populations.

Neurally adjusted ventilatory assist (NAVA) is a variation of PAV; however, a gastric tube with sensors is used to recognize the electrical activity of the diaphragm (EAdi) and generate a signal to the ventilator to initiate a breath. The concept is that the sensor activation system used with NAVA is more sensitive to patient effort because of the proximity of the gastric tube sensors to the diaphragm in comparison to traditional ventilator-triggering systems (ie, pressure and flow sensitivity at the patient/ventilator interface). The gastric tube is positioned just below the gastroesophageal junction and a waveform must be observed in order to ensure proper positioning (Table 20-7).

ESSENTIAL CONTENT CASE

Pressure Controlled/Inverse Ratio Ventilation and Airway Pressure Release Ventilation

A patient was admitted in respiratory distress. Her history included a flu-like illness that progressively got worse, necessitating a trip to the emergency room (ER). Her chest radiograph showed bilateral diffuse infiltrates in a honeycomb pattern consistent with ARDS. Once intubated, she was placed on assist control at a rate of 22/min and Vt of 500 mL. Her plateau pressure was very high (60 cm H_2O) and she required an Fio_2 of 1.0 and 10 cm H_2O of PEEP. ABGs on these settings were pH 7.23, $Paco_2$ 38 mm Hg, and Pao_2 52 mm Hg. She was agitated, thrashing, and asynchronous with the ventilator, despite a sensitivity setting of –1 cm H_2O, a short inspiratory time, and a high ventilator rate. The decision was made to sedate and paralyze the patient and place her on PC/IRV mode. Settings were:

PC level	30 cm H_2O (resulting in a Vt of 6 mL/kg)
RR	20 breaths/min
I:E ratio	2:1
Fio_2	0.6
PEEP	10 cm H_2O

ABGs after 30 minutes were:

pH	7.34
$Paco_2$	55 mm Hg
Pao_2	66 mm Hg

After 1 day of these ventilator settings, the team felt it would be best to stop the paralytic agents and decrease the sedation to allow for spontaneous breathing but still provide a high level of lung recruitment. Once the patient was awake and breathing spontaneously, the team switched the mode to APRV.

Settings were:

P_{hi} ($PEEP_{hi}$)	25 cm H_2O
P_{low} ($PEEP_{lo}$)	0 cm H_2O
T_{hi} ($Time_{hi}$)	5 seconds
T_{low} Release time	1.0 second
Fio_2	0.6
Spontaneous RR	28

ABGs after 30 minutes were:

pH	7. 35
$Paco_2$	56 mm Hg
Pao_2	70 mm Hg

Case Question 1: Are the pH of 7.34 and $PaCO_2$ of 55 obtained after changing the settings to PC/IVR appropriate for this patient?

Case Question 2: The team would like to decrease the patients CO_2 on APRV. What maneuver would be the next step?

Answers

1. The team felt that the laboratory results were positive and reflective of the improved gas distribution associated with the pressure ventilation and the use of sedation and paralytics. Further, decreasing or controlling the plateau pressure, which resulted in lower tidal volumes, lessened the risk of volutrauma. With lower volumes, the patient's CO_2 is expected to rise (and the pH will drop) and is called "permissive hypercarbia."

2. The team can increase the number of releases to help eliminate CO_2. The releases drop the system pressure to zero (or a low PEEP level) and do allow for more efficient CO_2 exchange. The time low can also be increased with each release to enhance CO_2 exchange.

Automatic Tube Compensation

Automatic tube compensation (ATC) is a ventilator option (not a mode) that is designed to overcome the work of breathing imposed by the artificial airway. ATC adjusts the pressure

(proportional to tube resistance) required to provide a variable fast inspiratory flow during spontaneous breathing. In this option, the size of the airway (endotracheal tube internal diameter (ETT ID) size) is entered along with the percentage

TABLE 20-7. PROPORTIONAL ASSIST VENTILATION AND NEURALLY ADJUSTED VENTILATORY ASSIST

Definition

These modes automatically adjust the pressure, flow, and volume proportionally to offset the resistance and elastance of the system with each inspiration. The concept is to prevent fatiguing workloads during spontaneous breathing. NAVA is an iteration of PAV in which it provides PAV but uses a gastric tube with sensors to recognize diaphragmatic activity and generate a signal to the ventilator to initiate a breath.

Patient Selection

Appropriate for all phases of ventilation from acute management to weaning.

Application (Differences in Names of Settings Are Manufacturer Dependent)

1. Set PEEP, Fio_2, and the proportion of assist (% assist) desired.
2. When NAVA is used, a special gastric tube with sensors must be placed to obtain an optimal signal from the diaphragm. Adjustments may be necessary over time.

Assessment

1. Comfortable breathing pattern should be noted.
2. With the use of NAVA, desired waveform must be observed.

Complications

As per all modes of ventilation used in the acutely ill patient population. If NAVA is used, complications related to gastric tube placement and manipulation must also be considered as potential complications.

of compensation desired (1%-100%). Some use the option during spontaneous breathing trials to offset the work related to tube resistance. While this is a useful ventilator adjunct, it is yet unclear how it works in combination with other modes of ventilation. Use of the option may increase auto-PEEP, if obstructive lung disease is present (Table 20-8).

High-Frequency Oscillation

High-frequency oscillation (HFO) has been suggested for use in ARDS patients. With HFO, a bias flow of gases is provided via an oscillator, which disperses the gases throughout the lung at very high frequencies. The bias flow, combined with oscillatory activity (extremely rapid pulses in a back-and-forth motion), results in the constant infusion of fresh gases and evacuation of old gases. The method provides

TABLE 20-8. AUTOMATIC TUBE COMPENSATION

Definition

ATC is a ventilatory option that is designed to overcome the work of breathing imposed by the artificial airway. Pressure is automatically adjusted to offset the resistance of the airway.

Patient Selection

Appropriate for all patients; however, it is unclear how effective the option is when used in combination with different modes.

Application

1. Enter endotracheal tube internal diameter.
2. Determine and enter percent of compensation desired.

Assessment

1. Some studies have suggested the mode may contribute to auto-PEEP if obstructive disease is present. Measure auto-PEEP to assess for auto-PEEP.
2. The addition of ATC to assist in decreasing resistive work during spontaneous breathing should result in a more comfortable rate and pattern of breathing.

Complications

Potential for increased auto-PEEP in patients with obstructive disease.

oscillation around a constant mean airway pressure, the lung is recruited, and a chest vibration ("wiggle") results. Some practitioners believe that this mode of ventilation may recruit alveoli and prevent tidal stress and lung injury.

The Multicenter Oscillatory Ventilation for Acute Respiratory Distress Syndrome Trial (MOAT) and the High Frequency Oscillation Ventilation in Early ARDS (Oscillate) Trial demonstrated that no substantial benefit in mortality rates was achieved with high-frequency oscillatory ventilation (HFOV) over conventional ventilation. Additional concern about HFOV rests with the fact that heavy sedation and often paralytics are necessary to assure compliance with the mode. These aspects, in addition to the fact that it is somewhat difficult to become proficient in the use of the mode, are limitations to its widespread applicability. Indications for, uses of, and associated complications are summarized in Table 20-9.

Multiple Patients on a Single Ventilator

During disaster conditions such as multi-casualty incidents and the recent COVID-19 pandemic, there is a potential for ventilator shortage. In addition to ongoing triage to guide ventilator allocation, the ventilation of multiple patients with a single ventilator has been proposed when no other option is available. While this approach has theoretical

TABLE 20-9. HIGH-FREQUENCY OSCILLATION

Definition

HFOs move in a back-and-forth motion (piston generated) and so have both active "inspiratory" and active "expiratory" phases. Fresh gas is supplied by a bias flow. Tidal volume is dependent on the oscillator displacement volume and the magnitude and location of the bias flow.

Patient Selection

1. Patients with large pulmonary air leaks (ie, bronchopleural fistulas) in whom a decreased pressure and improved gas distribution are desired (and in whom conventional modes have failed).
2. In lithotripsy, when a quiet thoracoabdominal wall is indicated.
3. Airway surgical procedures.
4. No benefit identified thus far over the use of more traditional ventilator modes. Some may use for severe cases of ARDS as a rescue therapy.

Application

1. *Bias flow:* In liters per minute (LPM); somewhere around 40-50 LPM).
2. *Oscillatory frequency (fx):* In hertz.
3. *Mean airway pressure:* Generally a bit above conventional ventilation to begin.
4. *ΔP:* The change in pressure or pressure amplitude (generally adjusted to achieve chest wall vibration).
5. *Fio_2 level:* As in conventional ventilation.
6. *% inspiratory time:* Controls the percentage of time the oscillator spends in the inspiratory phase.

Assessment

1. Arterial blood gases, pulse oximetry, and end-tidal CO_2 monitoring.
2. *Chest movement:* Generally the chest is seen to "wiggle." With adequate gas exchange, the patient may not initiate spontaneous breaths. Return of spontaneous effort may be indicative of increased $Paco_2$.

Complications

1. Adequate humidification is often difficult to attain, and airway obstruction is possible.
2. Barotrauma.

merit and has been evaluated in bench and animal models, mechanical and clinical limitations are significant. Mechanical ventilators are designed for the ventilation of a single patient, limiting the machines' ability to effectively deliver set parameters and monitor patient parameters/alarms without substantial modifications to the ventilator. Additionally, the pulmonary mechanics (lung compliance) of the patients connected to the single machine must be similar, or disparities in delivered ventilation will result. For this reason, the modified patient/ventilator system would require additional monitoring by experienced respiratory care providers. Equipment to perform these modifications should be prepared in advance as part of the facility disaster plan, along with education and simulation to ensure staff familiarity with the chosen operational protocol. Some examples of protocols are included in the *Additional Readings* for this chapter.

Conclusion

While the modes described in this chapter are sophisticated, none have demonstrated superiority over traditional volume control modes. (described in Chapter 5, Airway and Ventilatory Management). In addition to their complexity, the advanced modes of ventilation have names that vary by manufacturer and are not intuitive, which increases the risk for practice variation and miscommunication among team members. Understanding these modes of ventilation is not the role of a single person. If a healthcare team makes a commitment to implementing advanced modes of ventilation, education of the multi-professional team and resources to support consistent practice are essential.

The critical care nurse's role, to ensure the safe passage of the patient, requires interprofessional collaboration, recognition of the expertise that each member of the healthcare team brings, and an awareness of the resources available in their specific practice setting. In many cases, the best strategy for mechanical ventilation is the one that is most familiar to all members of the healthcare team and not the one that is most advanced. For further information, use the resources listed below.

SELECTED BIBLIOGRAPHY

Mechanical Ventilation: Modes

ARDS Definition Task Force, Ranieri VM, Rubenfeld GD, et al. Acute respiratory distress syndrome: the Berlin Definition. *JAMA.* 2012;307(23):2526-2533.

Ashworth L, Norisue Y, Koster M, et al. Clinical management of pressure control ventilation: an algorithmic method of patient ventilatory management to address "forgotten but important variables." *J Crit Care.* 2018;43:169-182.

Briel M, Meade M, Mercat A, et al. Higher vs lower positive end-expiratory pressure in patients with acute lung injury and acute respiratory distress syndrome: systematic review and meta-analysis. *JAMA.* 2010;303(9):865-873.

Brochard L, Harf A, Lorino H, et al. Inspiratory pressure support prevents diaphragmatic fatigue during weaning from mechanical ventilation. *Am Rev Respir Dis.* 1989;139:513-521.

Brochard L, Pluskwa F, Lemaire R. Improved efficacy of spontaneous breathing with inspiratory pressure support. *Am Rev Respir Dis.* 1987;136:411-415.

Brochard L, Slutsky A, Pesenti A. Mechanical ventilation to minimize progression of lung injury in acute respiratory failure. *Am J Respir Crit Care Med.* 2017;195(4):438-442.

Chatburn RL. Understanding mechanical ventilators. *Expert Rev Respir Med.* 2010;4(6):809-819.

Chatburn RL, El-Khatib M, Mireles-Cabodevila E. A taxonomy for mechanical ventilation: 10 fundamental maxims. *Respir Care.* 2014;59(11):1747-1763.

Conti G, Costa R. Technological development in mechanical ventilation. *Curr Opin Crit Care.* 2010;16(1):26-33.

Elsasser S, Guttmann J, Stocker R, Mols G, Prieve HJ, Haberthür C. Accuracy of automatic tube compensation in new-generation mechanical ventilators. *Crit Care Med.* 2003;31:2619-2626.

Fan E, Brodie D, Slutsky AS. Acute respiratory distress syndrome: advances in diagnosis and treatment. *JAMA.* 2018;319(7):698-710.

Fan E, Del Sorbo L, Goligher EC, et al. An official American Thoracic Society/European Society of Intensive Care Medicine/Society of Critical Care Medicine clinical practice guideline: mechanical ventilation in adult patients with acute respiratory distress syndrome. *Am J Respir Crit Care Med.* 2017;195:1253-1263.

Giannouli E, Webster K, Roberts D, Younes M. Response of ventilator-dependent patients to different levels of pressure support and proportional assist. *Am J Respir Crit Care Med.* 1999;159:1716-1725.

Grieco DL, Chen L, Dres M, Brochard L. Should we use driving pressure to set tidal volume? *Curr Opin Crit Care.* 2017;23(1):38-44.

Gurevitch MJ, Van Dyke J, Young ES, Jackson K. Improved oxygenation and lower peak airway pressure in serve adult respiratory distress syndrome. Treatment with inverse ratio ventilation. *Chest.* 1986;89:211-213.

Henderson WR, Chen L, Amato MBP, Brochard LJ. Fifty years of research in ARDS. Respiratory mechanics in acute respiratory distress syndrome. *Am J Respir Crit Care Med.* 2017;196(7):822-833.

Hickling KG, Walsh J, Henderson S, Jackson R. Low mortality rate in acute respiratory distress syndrome using low-volume, pressure-limited ventilation with permissive hypercapnia: a prospective study. *Crit Care Med.* 1994;22:1568-1578.

Kacmarek RM. Proportional assist ventilation and neurally-adjusted ventilatory assist. *Respir Care.* 2011;56(2):140-148.

Kallet RH. Patient-ventilator interaction during acute lung injury, and the role of spontaneous breathing: Part 2: airway pressure release ventilation. *Respir Care.* 2011;56(2):190-203.

Kang H, Yang H, Tong Z. Recruitment manoeuvres for adults with acute respiratory distress syndrome receiving mechanical ventilation: a systematic review and meta-analysis. *J Crit Care.* 2019;50:1-10.

Kirakli C, Ozdemir I, Ucar ZZ, Cimen P, Kepil S, Ozkan SA. Adaptive support ventilation for faster weaning in COPD: a randomised controlled trial. *Eur Respir J.* 2011;38(4):774-780.

Lellouche F, Brochard L. Advanced closed loops during mechanical ventilation (PAV, NAVA, ASV, SmartCare). *Best Pract Res Clin Anaesthesiol.* 2009;23(1):81-93.

Lim J, Litton E. Airway pressure release ventilation in adult patients with acute hypoxemic respiratory failure: a systematic review and meta-analysis. *Crit Care Med.* 2019;47:1794-1799.

Maitra S, Bhattacharjee S, Khanna P, Baidya DK. High-frequency ventilation does not provide mortality benefit in comparison with conventional lung-protective ventilation in acute respiratory distress syndrome: a meta-analysis of the randomized controlled trials. *Anesthesiology.* 2015;122(4):841-851.

Marini JJ. Evolving concepts for safer ventilation. *Crit Care.* 2019 Jun 14;23(Suppl 1):114.

Marini JJ, Rocco PRM, Gattinoni L. Static and dynamic contributors to ventilator-induced lung injury in clinical practice. Pressure, energy, and power. *Am J Respir Crit Care Med.* 2020;201(7):767-774.

Miller AG, Gentile MA, Davies JD, et al. Clinical management strategies for airway pressure release ventilation: a survey of clinical practice. *Respir Care.* 2017;62:1264-1268.

Mireles-Cabodevila E, Kacmarek RM. Should airway pressure release ventilation be the primary mode in ARDS? *Respir Care.* 2016;61:761-773.

Moerer O. Effort-adapted modes of assisted breathing. *Curr Opin Crit Care.* 2012;18(1):61-69.

Nichols D, Haranath S. Pressure control ventilation. *Crit Care Clin.* 2007;23(2):183-199.

Nieman GF, Gatto LA, Bates JHT, Habashi NM. Mechanical ventilation as a therapeutic tool to reduce ARDS incidence. *Chest.* 2015;148(6):1396-1404.

O'Croinin D, Ni Chonghaile M, Higgins B, Laffey JG. Bench-to-bedside review: permissive hypercapnia. *Crit Care.* 2005;9(1):51-59.

Pham T, Brochard LJ, Slutsky AS. Mechanical ventilation: State of the art. *Mayo Clin Proc.* 2017;92(9):1382-1400.

Rittayamai N, Katsios CM, Beloncle F, et al. Pressure-controlled vs volume-controlled ventilation in acute respiratory failure: a physiology-based narrative and systematic review. *Chest.* 2015;148:340-355.

Roberts KJ. 2018 year in review: adult invasive mechanical ventilation. *Respir Care.* 2019;64(5):604-609.

Santa CR, Rojas JI, Nervi R, Heredia R, Ciapponi A. High versus low positive end-expiratory pressure (PEEP) levels for mechanically ventilated adult patients with acute lung injury and acute respiratory distress syndrome. *Cochrane Database Syst Rev.* 2013;(6):CD009098.

Schmidt M, Kindler F, Cecchini J, et al. Neurally adjusted ventilatory assist and proportional assist ventilation both improve patient-ventilator interaction. *Crit Care.* 2015;19:56.

Slutsky AS. History of mechanical ventilation. From Vesalius to ventilator-induced lung injury. *Am J Respir Crit Care Med.* 2015;191(10):1106-1115.

Tharratt RS, Allen RP, Albertson TE. Pressure controlled inverse ratio ventilation in severe adult respiratory failure. *Chest.* 1998;94:755-762.

The Acute Respiratory Distress Syndrome Network. Ventilation with lower tidal volumes as compared with traditional tidal volumes for acute lung injury and the acute respiratory distress syndrome. *N Engl J Med.* 2000;342:1301-1307.

Turner DA, Rehder KJ, Cheifetz IM. Nontraditional modes of mechanical ventilation: progress or distraction? *Expert Rev Respir Med.* 2012;6(3):277-284.

Unoki T, Serita A, Grap MJ. Automatic tube compensation during weaning from mechanical ventilation: evidence and clinical implications. *Crit Care Nurse.* 2008;28(4):34-42.

Varelmann D, Wrigge H, Zinserling J, Muders T, Hering R, Putensen C. Proportional assist versus pressure support ventilation in patients with acute respiratory failure: cardiorespiratory responses to artificially increased ventilatory demand. *Crit Care Med.* 2005;33:1968-1975.

Vittacca M, Bianchi L, Zanotti E, et al. Assessment of physiologic variables and subjective comfort under different levels of pressure support ventilation. *Chest.* 2004;126:851-859.

Selected Vendor Web Pages

Drager. https://www.draeger.com/en-us_us/Hospital/Ventilators. Accessed August 25, 2021.

GE Healthcare. https://www.gehealthcare.com/products/ventilators/carescape-r860. Accessed August 25, 2021.

Getinge. https://www.getinge.com/us/products/hospital/mechanical-ventilation. Accessed August 25, 2021.

Hamilton Medical. https://www.hamilton-medical.com/en_US/. Accessed August 25, 2021.

Medtronic. https://www.medtronic.com/covidien/en-us/products/mechanical-ventilation.html. Accessed August 25, 2021.

Vyaire Medical. https://www.vyaire.com/products/vela-ventilator. Accessed August 25, 2021.

Evidence-Based Practice

Annane D, Orlikowski D, Chevret S, Chevrolet JC, Raphaël JC. Nocturnal mechanical ventilation for chronic hypoventilation in patients with neuromuscular and chest wall disorders. *Cochrane Database Syst Rev.* 2007;4:CD001941.

Antonelli M, Bonten M, Chastre J, et al. Year in review in intensive care medicine 2011: III. ARDS and ECMO, weaning, mechanical ventilation, noninvasive ventilation, pediatrics and miscellanea. *Intensive Care Med.* 2012;38(4):542-556.

Antonelli M, Conti G, Esquinas A, et al. A multiple-center survey on the use in clinical practice of noninvasive ventilation as a first-line intervention for acute respiratory distress syndrome. *Crit Care Med.* 2007;35:18-25.

Briel M, Meade M, Mercat A, et al. Higher vs lower positive end-expiratory pressure in patients with acute lung injury and acute respiratory distress syndrome: systematic review and meta-analysis. *JAMA.* 2010;303:865-873.

Burns KE, Adhikari NK, Keenan SP, Meade M. Use of non-invasive ventilation to wean critically ill adults off invasive ventilation: meta-analysis and systematic review. *BMJ.* 2009;338:b728.

Caples SM, Gay PC. Noninvasive positive pressure ventilation in the intensive care unit: a concise review. *Crit Care Med.* 2005;33:2651-2658.

Cortes I, Penuelas O, Esteban A. Acute respiratory distress syndrome: evaluation and management. *Minerva Anestesiol.* 2012;78:43-57.

Ip T, Mehta S. The role of high-frequency oscillatory ventilation in the treatment of acute respiratory failure in adults. *Curr Opin Crit Care.* 2012;18:70-79.

Nava S, Schreiber A, Domenighetti G. Noninvasive ventilation for patients with acute lung injury or acute respiratory distress syndrome. *Respir Care.* 2011;56:1583-1588.

Peter JV, Moran JL, Phillips-Hughes J, Graham P, Bersten AD. Effect of non-invasive positive pressure ventilation (NIPPV) on mortality in patients with acute cardiogenic pulmonary edema: a meta-analysis. *Lancet.* 2006;367:1155-1163.

Putensen C, Theuerkauf N, Zinserling J, Wrigge H, Pelosi P. Meta-analysis: ventilation strategies and outcomes of the acute respiratory distress syndrome and acute lung injury. *Ann Intern Med.* 2009;151(8):566-576.

The ARDS Definition Task Force, Ranieri VM, Rubenfeld GD, et al. Acute respiratory distress syndrome: the Berlin Definition. *JAMA.* 2012;307(23):2526-2533.

Unoki T, Serita A, Grap MJ. Automatic tube compensation during weaning from mechanical ventilation: evidence and clinical implications. *Crit Care Nurse.* 2008;28:34-42.

Additional Readings

Gallagher, JJ. Alternative modes of mechanical ventilation. *AACN Adv Crit Care.* 2018;29(4):396-404.

Multiple Patients/Ventilator Resources

Columbia University College of Physicians and Surgeons, New York Presbyterian Medical Center. Ventilator Sharing Protocol: Dual-Patient Ventilation with a Single Mechanical Ventilator for Use during Critical Ventilator Shortages. Ventilator-Sharing-Protocol-Dual-Patient-Ventilation-with-a-Single-Mechanical-Ventilator-for-Use-during-Critical-Ventilator-Shortages.pdf (gnyha.org). Accessed September 27, 2021.

U.S. Public Health Service Commissioned Corp. Optimizing-Ventilator Use During the COVID-19 Pandemic. optimizing-ventilator-use-during-covid19-pandemic.pdf (hhs.gov). Accessed September 27, 2021.

ADVANCED NEUROLOGIC CONCEPTS

John C. Bazil and DaiWai Olson

KNOWLEDGE COMPETENCIES

1. Compare and contrast the pathophysiology, clinical presentation, patient needs, and management approaches for the following conditions:
   • Subarachnoid hemorrhage
   • Traumatic brain injury
   • Acute spinal cord injury
   • Brain tumor
2. Describe the concept of cerebral oxygenation and brain tissue oxygen monitoring.

SUBARACHNOID HEMORRHAGE

Etiology, Risk Factors, and Pathophysiology

Subarachnoid hemorrhage (SAH) can result from trauma, aneurysm, or other vascular malformations. This discussion focuses on SAH due to the rupture of an intracranial aneurysm. Intracranial aneurysms usually occur near the circle of Willis at arterial bifurcations or trifurcations (Figure 21-1). Aneurysms vary in size and shape; saccular (also called berry) aneurysms are the most common and most amenable to treatment. When an intracranial aneurysm ruptures, blood is expelled. The blood takes the path of least resistance, which most often is into the subarachnoid space. Subsequently, a clot may form in the ventricular system or in the brain parenchyma. In some patients, blood in the subarachnoid space causes hydrocephalus by obstructing cerebrospinal fluid (CSF) flow through the ventricles or by clogging the arachnoid granulations (or arachnoid villi) that reabsorb CSF. Although the mechanism is not well understood, arterial narrowing, commonly referred to as "vasospasm" or "cerebral artery vasospasm," occurs in a significant number of patients in the days following aneurysm rupture and can cause delayed cerebral ischemia (DCI) or delayed ischemic neurological deficit (DIND). There are several scales used to grade the severity of aneurysmal SAH (aSAH). The Hunt and Hess scale and World Federation of Neurological Surgeons (WFNS) scale (Table 21-1) are most commonly used.

Risk factors for intracranial aneurysm formation include smoking, hypertension, bacteremia, family history of intracranial aneurysm, and certain genetic disorders (autosomal dominant polycystic kidney disease, Ehlers-Danlos syndrome). Roughly 10% to 15% of patients have multiple aneurysms. Risk factors associated with aneurysm rupture include size of the aneurysm, hypertension, smoking, age (risk increases with age, peaking at age 50-60), and the use of stimulants (cocaine, amphetamines). Aneurysmal SAH is more common in men until the age of 50; the incidence is higher in women after age 50 and in the overall population.

Mortality and morbidity associated with aSAH is substantial but improving. Approximately 40% of individuals with aSAH will die either at the time of rupture or during hospitalization. Two-thirds of aSAH survivors are left with some type of neurological deficit. Predictors of outcome after aSAH include neurologic condition on admission, age, comorbidities, and the amount of blood on the initial computerized axial tomography (CT) scan.

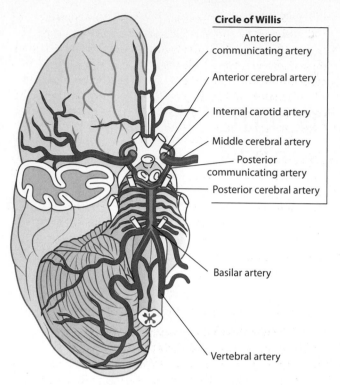

Figure 21-1. The circle of Willis as seen from below the brain. (*Reproduced with permission from Phipps WJ, Marek JF, Monahan FD, et al. Medical-Surgical Nursing: Health and Illness Perspectives. St Louis, MO: Mosby; 2003.*)

Clinical Presentation

Most patients are asymptomatic until the time of aneurysm rupture, but some have prodromal signs such as headache or visual changes. Upon aneurysm rupture, many patients experience a sudden, severe headache, sometimes described as "thunderclap," "explosive," or the "worst headache of my life." Transient or prolonged loss of consciousness may occur. Episodes of acute hypertension or intense physical activity may increase the pressure on an aneurysm and cause rupture. Bystanders may describe seizure-like activity; it is unclear whether this is an actual seizure or abnormal posturing related to a sudden increase in intracranial pressure (ICP).

Other common signs and symptoms include nausea and vomiting, stiff neck, vision changes, mental status changes, and photophobia. Focal deficits, such as hemiparesis, hemiplegia, or aphasia, may also occur.

Diagnostic Tests

Computerized Axial Tomography Scan

Patients with aSAH often present with signs and symptoms; therefore, a brain CT scan is first-line imaging used to rule-in aSAH and rule out thrombolytic therapy. The brain CT can also be useful to assess for hydrocephalus. CT scan will detect subarachnoid blood in almost all patients if performed within the first 3 days of symptom onset. As the blood in the subarachnoid space starts to break down, the sensitivity of CT scan decreases. CT angiography can be performed quickly at the time of the initial scan and may reveal aneurysm location. The amount of blood present on the initial CT scan as measured using the Fisher scale (see Table 21-1) is predictive of vasospasm risk.

Magnetic Resonance Imaging and Magnetic Resonance Angiogram

Magnetic resonance imaging (MRI) and magnetic resonance angiogram (MRA) are used to identify aneurysm location and look for other vascular abnormalities. These studies are especially useful in patients with a negative CT or negative CT angiogram and may also be considered in patients with renal impairment.

Lumbar Puncture

A lumbar puncture (LP) is performed when CT fails to demonstrate SAH in a patient with a history highly suspicious for SAH. LP is avoided in patients with signs or symptoms of elevated ICP due to the risk of cerebellar tonsillar herniation. LP is performed at least 6 to 12 hours after the onset of symptoms to allow red blood cells (RBCs) in the CSF to start to break down. This breakdown in RBCs gives a yellow tinge to the CSF after centrifugation. This pigmentation is called xanthochromia and will not be present if blood in the CSF is due to a traumatic LP.

TABLE 21-1. SEVERITY OF SUBARACHNOID HEMORRHAGE CLASSIFICATION SCALES

Grade	Hunt and Hess Based on Symptoms	World Federation of Neurological Surgeons Based on Assessment	Fisher Based on Diagnostic Imaging
0	Unruptured		
I	Asymptomatic or minimal headache, nuchal rigidity	Glasgow Coma Score = 15 Motor deficit = Absent	No blood detected on brain CT
II	Moderate to severe headache, nuchal rigidity, no neurological deficit other than cranial nerve palsy	Glasgow Coma Score = 13-14 Motor deficit = Absent	Diffuse thin layer of subarachnoid blood (vertical layers < 1 mm thick)
III	Drowsiness, confusion, mild focal deficit	Glasgow Coma Score = 13-14 Motor deficit = Present	Localized clot or thick layer of subarachnoid blood (vertical layers ≥ 1 mm thick)
IV	Stupor, moderate to severe hemiparesis, possible early decerebrate rigidity, and vegetative disturbances	Glasgow Coma Score = 7-12 Motor deficit = Present or absent	Intracerebral or intraventricular blood with diffuse or no subarachnoid blood
V	Deep coma, decerebrate rigidity, moribund appearance	Glasgow Coma Score = 3-6 Motor deficit = Present or absent	

ESSENTIAL CONTENT CASE

Subarachnoid Hemorrhage

A 54-year-old loan officer experienced the sudden onset of a severe headache while at work. She was taken to the emergency department of a local hospital where she described the pain as the "worst headache of my life." CT scan confirmed the diagnosis of SAH. Angiography revealed an aneurysm of the anterior communicating artery at the junction of the left anterior cerebral artery. The aneurysm was successfully coiled. Following the procedure, she was admitted to the intensive care unit (ICU).

Case Question 1: Describe nursing priorities of care for this patient.

On the fifth day post-bleed, the nurse noted that this previously neurologically intact patient was difficult to arouse and once awake had right upper extremity weakness and difficulty speaking.

Case Question 2: What actions should the nurse anticipate?

The patient was taken to radiology where a CT and computed tomography angiography (CTA) revealed normal postoperative changes and arterial narrowing, especially of the left middle cerebral artery. Her symptoms improved transiently with fluid resuscitation and induced hypertension but then recurred. Catheter angiography confirmed severe vasospasm of the left middle cerebral artery. Intra-arterial milrinone was infused with radiologic improvement in vasospasm.

Postprocedure, she was able to speak clearly (but unable to name objects accurately) and move her right arm, against resistance (4 out of 5 strength). Following several days in the ICU, she was transferred to the progressive care unit where she was monitored for new or worsening DIND. Her neurologic examination continued to improve, and she was discharged home on post-bleed day 14 with outpatient speech therapy to address occasional word-finding difficulty and subtle cognitive deficits.

Answers
1. In addition to routine post-angiogram care, nursing priorities include close monitoring of neurologic and volume status. Maintenance of euvolemia is important to decrease the risk of DCI due to vasospasm. Close monitoring of neurologic status allows prompt intervention if complications develop. Other priorities of care include pain management, encouraging mobility, and prevention of nosocomial complications.
2. The nurse prepares the patient for stat CT scan and potentially angiogram. Fluid balance is checked and fluid administration may be ordered. The cause of neurological decline is likely cerebral ischemia due to vasospasm. This will be treated initially by maintaining euvolemia and a normal to slightly elevated serum sodium level. It may be determined that permissive or induced hypertension is also appropriate. These interventions are important to prepare for potential endovascular interventions.

Cerebral Angiography

Although CTA done at the time of the initial CT scan detects many aneurysms, cerebral angiography remains the standard and may also be performed to identify the location, size, and shape of the aneurysm or other vascular anomalies. The initial angiogram may fail to reveal an aneurysm in approximately 10% to 20% of patients with SAH. Repeat angiogram approximately 1 week later will reveal an aneurysm in a small number of these patients. A negative angiogram with a distinct pattern of bleeding on CT scan may indicate a nonaneurysmal perimesencephalic SAH; patients with this diagnosis have an excellent prognosis.

For many patients in whom an aneurysm is detected, angiogram is used to guide endovascular treatment (described later). Angiogram is also used to detect arterial narrowing in patients with neurological decline in the days following aneurysm rupture. Angioplasty or directed medication injection may be used to treat the arterial narrowing. Nurses should know that vasospasm treatment is rapidly evolving and new treatments are likely to be identified and tested in the next few years.

Principles of Management of Aneurysmal Subarachnoid Hemorrhage

Patients who survive the initial rupture of a cerebral aneurysm are at risk for complications that increase their chances for morbidity and death. Primary central nervous system (CNS) complications include rebleeding, hydrocephalus, and DCI due to arterial narrowing. Arterial narrowing correlates temporally with the breakdown of subarachnoid blood and occurs because of a combination of arterial spasm and inflammatory changes that thicken the vessel wall. This phenomenon is commonly referred to as "vasospasm." Although "vasospasm" reflects an incomplete understanding of the pathophysiology leading to DCI, this terminology is commonly used in practice and will be used in this text to reflect arterial narrowing after aSAH.

Rebleeding

Prior to the aneurysm being secured with surgical clipping or intravascular coiling, the biggest risk to the patient is aneurysmal re-rupture (or "rebleed"). The probability of death is markedly increased by rebleed. This risk is highest within the first 24 hours. Signs and symptoms of rebleeding include a sudden reappearance or increase in headache, nausea, vomiting, decrease in the level of consciousness, and new focal neurologic deficits. Neurologic assessment is performed hourly (or more frequently if indicated) to promptly identify changes related to rebleeding or hydrocephalus. If an external ventricular drain is present, careful management is essential to prevent overdrainage of CSF, which can result in rebleeding due to a change in transmural pressure. The most definitive method to prevent rebleeding is to secure the aneurysm using surgical clipping or endovascular embolization.

In the interim between admission and definitive treatment, strategies such as blood pressure (BP) management and prevention of activities that increase blood pressure or ICP are used to decrease the risk of rebleeding. The goal of blood pressure management is to treat hypertension without dropping the blood pressure to a level that decreases cerebral perfusion. Systolic BP goals with an upper range of 150 to 160 mm Hg are common. The use of agents that can be titrated is recommended, particularly calcium channel blockers. Vasodilating agents are avoided. Bed rest is typically ordered prior to securing the aneurysm. Prophylaxis for venous thromboembolism (VTE), including sequential compression devices, is implemented. Stool softeners are used to prevent straining due to constipation. Pain is treated with analgesics, usually short-acting narcotics. Anxiety is decreased by providing explanations of care activities and psychological support.

Two management options exist to secure the aneurysm and prevent re-rupture: surgical clipping of the aneurysm via craniotomy and endovascular embolization of the aneurysm with catheter angiography. Management at a facility that offers both treatment modalities and frequently treats patients with aSAH is recommended to optimize outcomes. The decision to secure the aneurysm via open craniotomy versus an endovascular procedure is made on the basis of aneurysm location and morphology, comorbidities, and the severity of neurologic deficits on admission. When the aneurysm is amenable to treatment by either modality, endovascular management is generally performed.

The aneurysm is secured as soon as possible, prior to the period of time when patients are most at risk for vasospasm. With the aneurysm secured, standard management strategies for vasospasm can be implemented without the risk of causing additional hemorrhage. Aneurysm surgery is performed using a craniotomy incision. The surgeon carefully dissects tissue away from the aneurysm and places a titanium or titanium alloy clip across the base (Figure 21-2). Different sizes and shapes of clips are available. Following surgery, the patient returns to the ICU for continued management. Follow-up radiologic studies may be done, including CT scanning to look for bleeding at the operative site and angiography to evaluate clip position. Postoperative care includes frequent neurologic assessment (every 15 minutes initially), pain management, and prevention of postprocedure complications, that include monitoring of catheter insertion site for hematoma or bleeding, hemodynamic changes, and possible permissive hypertension. The postoperative neurologic assessment is compared to the preoperative assessment and any changes are reported to the neurosurgeon.

Endovascular embolization decreases rebleeding risk by preventing blood flow into the aneurysm. Using cerebral angiography, the interventional neuroradiologist threads the microcatheter into the aneurysm and then deploys one or more implantable devices (commonly called coils) to fill the space inside the aneurysm. Coils are typically made of a soft metal (platinum) and now come in a variety of shapes and sizes. The neck of the aneurysm must be narrow enough for the coils to be retained in the aneurysm instead of floating back out into the vessel lumen. Figure 21-3 depicts endovascular coil embolization of an aneurysm with a wide neck (berry or saccular aneurysm).

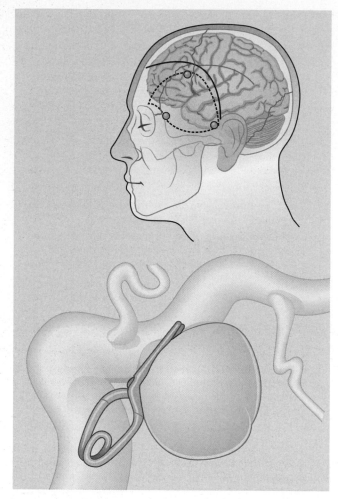

Figure 21-2. Clipping of a posterior communicating artery aneurysm. The clip is placed across the base of the aneurysm so that it can no longer fill with blood, but blood flow can continue through the parent artery.

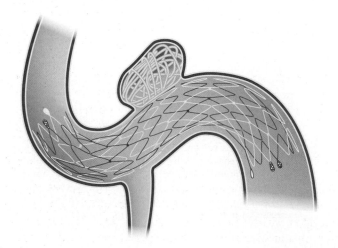

Figure 21-3. Stent-assisted coiling of a wide neck aneurysm. After the coils are placed and detached during an endovascular procedure, a stent is placed to keep the coils within the aneurysm sac.

If the neck is wide, special stents may be used to assist with coiling or to span the aneurysm. The coils fill the space inside the cavity of the aneurysm, preventing blood flow into the aneurysm and reducing the risk of rebleed. The primary risks associated with coil embolization are aneurysmal rupture during the procedure and ischemia related to clot formation in the vessel lumen. Postprocedure care for the patient who has received embolization is similar to that of a patient postsurgical clipping, with the addition of the postangiography care as described in Chapter 12, Neurologic System.

Hydrocephalus

SAH disrupts normal CSF flow through two mechanisms. Intraventricular blood may create a blockage in the ventricular drainage system and cause CSF to build up (obstructive or noncommunicating hydrocephalus). In addition, the arachnoid granulations that absorb CSF may become blocked with cellular debris. This results in decreased reabsorption of CSF and communicating (nonobstructive) hydrocephalus. Nurses may note signs and symptoms of acute hydrocephalus related to increased ICP. Acute obstructive hydrocephalus after SAH may be managed by external ventricular drainage or a ventriculoperitoneal (VP) shunt. Patients with continued hydrocephalus require placement of a ventricular shunt.

Late or chronic hydrocephalus can develop weeks after SAH. These patients present with headache, gait instability, incontinence, and cognitive decline. Treatment is placement of a ventricular shunt.

Delayed Cerebral Ischemia Due to Arterial Narrowing (Vasospasm)

Arterial narrowing occurs in many patients after aSAH and may cause decreased perfusion, potentially leading to DCI and infarction of cerebral tissue (ischemic stroke). As previously noted, several mechanisms contribute to arterial narrowing, commonly referred to as "vasospasm." Vasospasm typically develops 3 to 14 days after initial hemorrhage, with peak incidence around day 7, and is the biggest contributor to morbidity and mortality rates in patients with aSAH who survive to hospital admission. Approximately 30% of patients with aSAH will develop DINDs because of vasospasm, and another third will have angiographic evidence of arterial narrowing without neurologic decline. The amount of blood on initial CT scan is a good predictor of the risk of vasospasm and DCI. At many institutions, transcranial Doppler studies (TCDs) (see Chapter 12, Neurologic System) are used to monitor the development of vasospasm. TCDs assess blood flow velocity in selected arteries, which will become higher as vessels narrow. TCDs are noninvasive and can be done at the bedside, but accuracy varies based on patient and operator characteristics. CT angiography is also used to look for vasospasm, but catheter angiography remains a standard. Vasospasm is suspected in any patient who develops neurologic decline, especially a decrease in level of consciousness, agitation, or

paresis or paralysis of the face or limb on one side of the body, or aphasia. Early identification of neurologic deficits allows rapid intervention to improve cerebral perfusion and prevent infarction.

Maintenance of euvolemia is essential to decrease the risk of DCI. "Triple-H" therapy (hypervolemia, hypertension, and hemodilution) is no longer recommended. Careful attention to fluid balance is important and must include recognition of insensible fluid loss. Dehydration increases blood viscosity and decreases cerebral perfusion. SAH patients are at risk for dehydration because of cerebral salt wasting, in which excessive sodium is excreted, leading to increased water loss and hypovolemia. If serum sodium falls, volume restriction is contraindicated because of increased risk of DIND. Infusion of hypertonic saline (HTS) is commonly used to treat hyponatremia.

Blood pressure goals vary based on the patient response but are usually in the range of 160 to 200 mm Hg. Treatment goals are primarily based on improvement in neurologic examination instead of a strict range of hemodynamic values, but advanced monitoring is often utilized. Nimodipine, a calcium channel blocker, is prescribed for most patients with aSAH. Nimodipine does not decrease angiographic vasospasm but may improve 3-month outcomes after aSAH.

Vasospasm can also be treated using an endovascular approach with transluminal balloon angioplasty or with a direct infusion of a calcium channel antagonist or a phosphodiesterase 3 inhibitor into the artery in spasm.

Additional Management Strategies and Prevention of Complications

Prophylactic anticonvulsants may be given to patients for short periods (3-7 days) immediately following presentation. Patients who demonstrate clinical or electrographic seizures are treated according to standard seizure management (see Chapter 12, Neurologic System) and remain on anticonvulsants throughout hospitalization. Systemic complications of aSAH include myocardial dysfunction, cardiac arrhythmias, and neurogenic pulmonary edema. Cardiac complications are believed to be due to massive catecholamine release at the time of initial hemorrhage. Ventricular dysfunction occurs but typically returns to baseline over days to weeks. The most common electrocardiogram (ECG) changes associated with SAH are ST-segment abnormalities, T-wave inversion, and prolonged QTc interval but other dysrhythmias such as atrial fibrillation, ventricular tachycardia, and pauses can also occur. Neurogenic pulmonary edema is relatively rare and may result from a CNS-mediated increase in intravascular permeability, massive sympathetic discharge, or a combination of these factors. Neurogenic pulmonary edema occurs rapidly and presents with signs and symptoms similar to those of cardiogenic pulmonary edema. Treatment is supportive and often includes mechanical ventilation. Neurogenic pulmonary edema typically resolves within 72 hours. Patients are also at risk for complications of immobility such as infection and VTE.

TRAUMATIC BRAIN INJURY

Etiology, Risk Factors, and Pathophysiology

The major causes of traumatic brain injury (TBI) are falls, motor vehicle accidents (MVAs), and "struck by/against" events (eg, assault or falling debris). Together, these make up over 80% of all TBI-related admissions. While TBI from falls is more commonly the cause of TBI in the very young and elderly, MVA is more likely the cause for persons aged 15 to 44 years. The incidence of TBI is higher in males than females and higher in children aged 0 to 4 years compared to all other age groups. The rate of TBI admissions has steadily increased, but TBI-related deaths have been steadily declining. Rates of hospitalization and death are greatest in those 75 years and older. TBI ranges from mild (causing a brief change in consciousness) to very severe (causing prolonged unresponsiveness or even death).

Although a higher Glasgow Coma Scale (GCS) score is associated with better outcomes, a TBI does not have to be severe to cause long-term impact. TBI severity can be classified using the GCS (see Chapter 12, Neurologic System). Mild brain injury refers to patients with a GCS score of 13 to 15, moderate indicates a GCS score of 9 to 12, and patients with a score of 8 or less are categorized as having severe brain injury. Mild TBI can cause significant functional deficits that become apparent in the weeks and months following injury; however, these patients are not admitted to the ICU unless they have other injuries. Patients with moderate TBI are typically admitted for close monitoring and may require aggressive intervention. Patients with severe TBI are among the most challenging critical care patients and require frequent interventions to prevent secondary brain injury. The majority of this discussion is limited to moderate and severe TBI.

The damage that occurs following TBI is described as primary or secondary. Primary injury occurs due to the biomechanical effects of trauma on the brain and skull as a result of the initial insult. Prevention is the only way to avoid primary injury. Secondary brain injury (SBI) refers to the complications that result from pathophysiologic changes caused by the primary injury. There are many causes of SBI, including hypoxemia, hypotension, increased ICP, infection, and biochemical imbalances. These problems compromise the oxygen and nutrient supply necessary for adequate cerebral cell metabolism, result in the buildup of waste products, and contribute to cerebral ischemia and poor patient outcomes.

Mechanism of Injury

TBI occurs as the result of blunt trauma to the head, penetrating trauma (missile or impaled object), or blast injury.

Blunt trauma occurs as the result of:

- *Deceleration:* The head is moving and strikes a stationary object (eg, pavement).
- *Acceleration:* A moving object (eg, baseball bat) strikes the head.
- *Acceleration–deceleration:* The brain moves rapidly within the skull, resulting in a combination of injury-causing forces. This is common with MVA.

ESSENTIAL CONTENT CASE

Traumatic Brain Injury

A 30-year-old construction worker was involved in a single-vehicle, high-speed rollover accident. Upon the arrival of the emergency medical service (EMS), the patient displayed decorticate posturing and did not verbalize or open his eyes (GCS score of 5). He was intubated and transported by helicopter to the nearest Level 1 trauma center, where a CT scan revealed diffuse cerebral edema and some small (punctate) hemorrhages. The rest of his trauma evaluation was negative except for a broken right clavicle. An ICP monitor was placed to guide therapy and the patient was admitted to the ICU. Over the first 24 hours, his ICP ranges from 11 to 23 mm Hg on continuous infusions of fentanyl and midazolam. On postinjury day 3, the nurse notes that the patient's ICP is consistently ranging between 28 and 30 mm Hg.

Case Question 1: What independent nursing actions can be tried to decrease ICP?

With these interventions, the patient's ICP decreases to approximately 25. The patient is normothermic and his Paco$_2$ is in the desired range. The physician orders a dose of mannitol to be given.

Case Question 2: How does mannitol work to decrease ICP?

Following mannitol administration, the patient's ICP decreased to a range of 15 to 18 mmHg and remained well controlled for the next 2 days. The ICP monitor was discontinued and sedation was weaned. On the seventh day postinjury, he opened his eyes to painful stimulation and attempted to push the stimulus away with his right hand (localization). Tracheostomy and gastric tubes were placed the next day. About 3 weeks after his injury, the patient was opening his eyes spontaneously and following simple commands. He was transferred to a rehabilitation hospital. Two months after his accident, he was discharged to the care of his parents. He was able to perform activities of daily living (ADLs), but remained unable to work because of decreased judgment and cognitive skills.

Answers
1. The nurse optimizes jugular venous return by keeping the patient's head in the midline position, elevating the head of bed 30° to 45°, and ensuring that the cervical collar is applied correctly. Managing pain with fast-acting intravenous analgesics is also indicated.
2. Mannitol is an osmotic diuretic that is used to decrease cerebral edema. Because of its diuretic effect, it is important to maintain euvolemia to prevent hypotension. Hypertonic saline is fast becoming an accepted alternative to mannitol. The higher concentration of extracellular sodium in hypertonic saline creates an osmotic gradient that helps pull fluid from the interstitial tissues into the intravascular space (and thereby to the kidneys) thus decreasing cerebral edema.

- *Rotation:* Twisting motion of the brain occurs within the skull, usually due to side impact.
- *Deformation/compression:* Direct injury to the head changes the shape of the skull, resulting in compression of brain tissue.

In the United States, gunshot wound (GSW) is the most common type of penetrating brain trauma. The degree of injury caused by a GSW varies based on the type of firearm, bullet type, and trajectory of the bullet. Tissue is destroyed by the bullet, and shock waves and cavity formation occur along the bullet's path. Some bullets will ricochet once inside the skull, creating more tissue destruction. Other causes of penetrating brain injury include stab wounds and small bore flying debris (eg, nail gun). Surgical management of penetrating trauma to the brain differs from the management of closed injury, but many of the issues relevant to critical care nurses remain the same.

Awareness of TBI because of blast injury caused by an explosion has increased in recent years. The individual may be hit by flying debris or may be thrown by the force of the blast, causing blunt or penetrating trauma. The brain is also thought to be sensitive to the initial wave of pressurization, with damage occurring as the result of the diffuse impact of intense pressure on brain structures.

Skull Fractures

Skull fractures can result in injury to the underlying brain tissue, but can also occur in isolation. Skull fractures are classified as linear, depressed, or basilar.

- Linear skull fractures resemble a line or single crack in the skull. Generally, they are not displaced and require no treatment.
- Depressed skull fractures are characterized by an inward depression of bone fragments. Surgery to elevate the depressed bone may be required. In the case of an open fracture, the wound is also washed out in the operating room to decontaminate the area and decrease the risk of infection.
- Basilar skull fractures involve the base of the skull, including the anterior, middle, or posterior fossa. Clinical manifestations of a basilar skull fracture include periorbital ecchymosis (raccoon eyes), mastoid ecchymosis (Battle sign), rhinorrhea (CSF or blood leaking from the nose), otorrhea (CSF or blood leaking from the ears), hemotympanum (blood behind the tympanic membrane), conjunctival hemorrhage, and cranial nerve dysfunction. The presence of otorrhea or rhinorrhea indicates a dural tear which increases the risk of meningitis. Although most CSF leaks stop spontaneously, those that persist may require surgical repair. Management of CSF leak includes elevating the head of bed, antibiotics, and, occasionally, lumbar drainage of CSF to decrease pressure on the healing dura (Figure 21-4).

Primary Brain Injury

Primary injury occurs at the time of initial impact and causes focal or diffuse anatomic changes to the cerebral tissue or cerebral vasculature. Focal injury refers to one damage at the site of injury, while diffuse injury affects the whole brain. Focal injuries take up space, and can cause

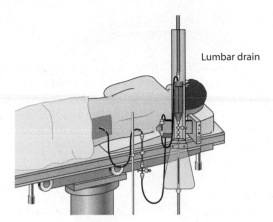

Figure 21-4. Lumbar drain.

tissue compression, increased ICP, brain shift, and herniation. Examples of focal injury include cerebral contusions and hematomas. Diffuse brain injuries involve microscopic damage to cells deep in the white matter. They occur as lateral head motion produces angular movement of the brain within the skull, causing shearing or stretching of axonal nerve fibers. Damage is variable and dependent on the amount of force transmitted to the brain. Focal and diffuse brain injuries do not typically occur in isolation; for example, a patient with a focal cerebral contusion is also likely to have some component of diffuse brain injury. Examples of primary injury follow.

- *Contusion:* Contusions are cortical bruises caused by the brain impacting the inside of the skull. They may be described as coup (occurring at the site of impact) or contrecoup (occurring opposite the site of impact). The frontal and temporal lobes are common sites of contusions. Clinical presentation depends on the site and extent of brain injury. Progressive focal edema and mass effect may result in neurologic deterioration. The severity of injury may not be apparent on the initial CT scan, because bleeding into the contused tissue often occurs later and results in intracerebral hematoma. Repeat CT scanning may be performed to evaluate for injury progression.
- *Epidural hematoma:* An epidural hematoma (EDH) (Figure 21-5) is bleeding located above the dura and below the skull. EDH is associated with skull fractures that lacerate an underlying artery, and is most common in the temporal region due to tearing of the middle meningeal artery. Patients may have a lucid interval, especially if the injury is very focal, and then deteriorate rapidly as the bleed expands, displacing brain structures and causing increased ICP. While a lucid interval suggests EDH, many patients do not follow this course. Symptoms of EDH include a decrease in consciousness, headache, seizures, vomiting, hemiparesis, and pupillary dilation. Management includes emergency surgery to evacuate the hematoma. Nursing care includes close monitoring of

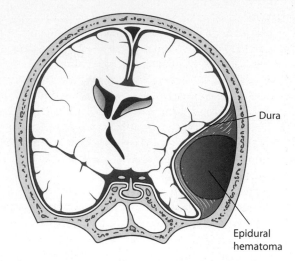

Figure 21-5. Schematic illustration of an epidural hemorrhage. (*Reproduced with permission from Waxman SG.* Clinical Neuroanatomy. *New York, NY: McGraw Hill; 2003.*)

neurological status, bed rest, and minimizing activities that increase BP to prevent re-bleed.

- *Subdural hematoma:* Subdural hematoma (SDH) is bleeding that occurs in the subdural space between the dura and arachnoid layer, creating direct pressure on the brain. SDH (Figure 21-6) results from rupture of the bridging veins between the brain and the dura, bleeding from contused or lacerated brain tissue, or extension from an intracerebral hematoma. SDH is described as acute if symptoms begin within the first 48 hours after injury. Many patients experience significant symptoms immediately following the injury or much sooner than 48 hours. Patients with acute SDH present with progressive decline in level of consciousness, headache, agitation, and confusion. Motor deficits, pupillary changes, and cranial nerve dysfunction may be seen, reflecting

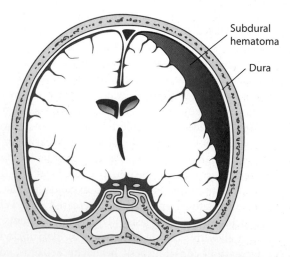

Figure 21-6. Schematic illustration of a subdural hemorrhage. (*Reproduced with permission from Waxman SG.* Clinical Neuroanatomy. *New York, NY: McGraw Hill; 2003.*)

the primary brain injury and compressive effects. Treatment of acute SDH consists of evacuation of the hematoma by craniotomy. Blood may also collect in the subdural space more slowly, over days to weeks (subacute SDH) or weeks to months (chronic SDH). Symptom onset is insidious because the brain can better compensate for this slow increase in mass. Symptoms include an increasingly severe headache, confusion, drowsiness, and possibly, seizures, pupillary abnormalities, or motor dysfunction. Predisposing conditions include advanced age, alcoholism, and disorders or treatments that result in prolonged coagulation times. Treatment of subacute or chronic SDH includes evacuation via burr holes or craniotomy or placement of a drain to allow egress of blood (eg, subdural evacuating port system or SEPS drain).

- *Traumatic subarachnoid hemorrhage:* Traumatic SAH can occur alone or in combination with other types of primary brain injury and may be present in up to one-third of severe TBI cases. The risk of vasospasm is less than that associated with aSAH, perhaps because the amount of blood seen in the subarachnoid space is typically less with traumatic SAH than when SAH is due to aneurysm rupture. In patients who present with traumatic SAH, the possibility that the patient experienced an aSAH (which then caused the traumatic event) should be investigated, especially if the events preceding the trauma are unclear.

- *Diffuse injury:* Diffuse TBI exists on a continuum from cerebral concussion to severe diffuse axonal injury (DAI). Cerebral concussion is a transient, temporary neurologic dysfunction caused by rapid acceleration-deceleration or by a sudden blow to the head. Symptoms include headache, confusion, disorientation, and amnesia. Most symptoms resolve without intervention. Patients with severe DAI typically experience an immediate and prolonged loss of consciousness and display abnormal posturing. The initial CT scan may appear normal, show signs of diffuse cerebral edema (decreased ventricle size, loss of differentiation between gray and white matter, and loss of sulci), or show very small areas of hemorrhage (punctate hemorrhage). The clinical course and outcome are dependent upon the severity of axonal injury.

Secondary Brain Injury

SBI is the ongoing neuronal damage that occurs following a TBI as the result of systemic and neurologic complications. The management of severe TBI focuses on minimizing SBI by improving the supply of oxygenated blood to the brain and decreasing cerebral metabolic demands. Major contributors to secondary injury include the following:

- *Hypoxemia:* The brain needs a constant supply of oxygen to function, and is very sensitive to systemic insults that create hypoxemia. Causes of hypoxemia in patients with TBI include pneumonia, atelectasis, chest trauma, neurogenic pulmonary edema, airway obstruction, and pulmonary embolus. Hypoxemia results in cerebral tissue hypoxia and anaerobic metabolism. Anaerobic metabolism produces less energy (ATP) than aerobic metabolism and results in a number of metabolic by-products. These metabolic by-products cause further cell damage.

- *Hypotension:* Hypotension resulting in decreased cerebral perfusion (MAP < 65-75 mm Hg) is associated with increased risk of mortality after TBI. Hypotension decreases cerebral blood flow (CBF), leading to tissue ischemia and buildup of waste products. Causes of hypotension following TBI include other injuries, the administration of sedating medications, and hypovolemia because of mannitol administration. Mortality risk increases with multiple episodes of hypotension.

- *Anemia:* Anemia may cause SBI by decreasing oxygen delivery to the brain. Controversy exists regarding the optimal hematocrit and use of transfusion in patients with cerebral insults, but minimizing avoidable blood loss such as with excessive drawing of labs is recommended.

- *Hypo- or hyperglycemia:* The brain cannot store glucose and is dependent on a constant supply to maintain metabolic function. Hypoglycemia must be avoided because it disrupts this supply and leads to cellular dysfunction. Significant hypoglycemia is uncommon following TBI but can occur in patients with diabetes who have taken antihyperglycemic medication prior to injury. Hyperglycemia is more common and significant hyperglycemia is associated with increased mortality; it is unclear whether elevated blood glucose is a marker of severity of injury or contributes to pathologic changes that increase mortality. Blood glucose monitoring and management is essential to the care of all ICU patients, but optimal glucose levels for patients in TBI are unknown.

- *Increased intracranial pressure:* Increased ICP (>22 mm Hg) may negatively affect cerebral perfusion and the viability of neurons. The major sources of increased ICP after brain injury are cerebral edema and expanding lesions, such as hematomas. Compression of blood vessels can result in ischemia and infarction of specific areas. Cerebral edema commonly contributes to elevations in ICP after severe TBI. Edema may be localized to the site of the injury or diffuse. The peak onset and the severity of edema vary but the range for maximum edema is 2 to 7 days after injury and it may last up to 2 weeks.

- *Loss of autoregulatory mechanisms:* As discussed in Chapter 12, Neurologic System, in the section on ICP, autoregulatory mechanisms in the uninjured brain maintain constant cerebral blood flow (CBF) over a wide range of mean arterial pressures (MAPs, between 60 and 160 mm Hg). When MAP decreases, cerebral vasodilation occurs to maintain CBF by increasing cerebral blood volume. When MAP increases, cerebral vasoconstriction occurs, maintaining CBF with a lower cerebral blood volume. The ability to autoregulate blood flow can be lost in the injured brain. CBF becomes dependent on changes in blood pressure. The extent of this autoregulatory loss varies in TBI patients. Because of the loss of cerebral autoregulation, the injured brain is more susceptible to ischemia caused by decreased blood flow.

- *Hypo- or hypercapnia:* Hypocapnia decreases CBF by increasing pH and causing cerebral vasoconstriction. CBF decreases, lowering ICP but creating a potentially ischemic state. Hypercapnia results in cerebral vasodilation and may increase CBF, but can also increase ICP.

- *Biochemical changes:* A number of biochemical changes occur following TBI, including the release of excitatory amino acids, free radical production, inflammation, and abnormal calcium shifts. A complete explanation of the processes underlying these changes is beyond the scope of this text. All factors contribute to changes in cellular function and can cause cell death.

- *Increased metabolic demands:* Fever, agitation, and seizures increase metabolic demand. Fever increases ICP and can be due to an infectious process or injury to the hypothalamus.

Clinical Presentation

Patients with TBI often present with external signs of trauma to the head such as ecchymosis, lacerations, and abrasions. Level of consciousness is the most important indicator of severity of injury and is assessed using the GCS. A decreasing GCS or changes in pupillary light reflex (PLR) indicate neurologic deterioration and warrant immediate provider notification. The type, location, and severity of TBI determine specific neurologic assessment findings. Patients may display hemiparesis, hemiplegia, language deficits, cognitive changes, or behavioral changes. If the injury is severe, the patient may display flexor or extensor posturing. Vital sign and PLR changes may reflect increased ICP or dysautonomia associated with severe DAI (eg, fever, tachycardia, or hypertension).

Patients with mild TBI, often referred to as post-concussive syndrome, may not display focal deficits such as hemiplegia or hemiparesis, but report a variety of physical, cognitive, and emotional symptoms. Signs and symptoms of mild TBI include headache, nausea/vomiting, dizziness, balance disturbance, visual problems, fatigue, and sensitivity to light or sound. Patients often report difficulty concentrating, decreased memory for recent events, slowed thought processes, irritability, anxiety, sadness, and increased emotion. Sleep disturbances are also common following mild TBI, and include both drowsiness/increased need for sleep and difficulty sleeping. Treatment and management for these patients may include speech therapy, occupational therapy, and physical therapy, under the supervision of physical medicine and rehabilitation services.

Diagnostic Tests

Brain CT is used to rapidly identify intracranial hematoma, traumatic SAH, contusions, skull fractures, and cerebral edema. MRI is useful in the detection of DAI, brainstem injury, and vascular injury and may aid prognostication. The diagnostic workup of the TBI patient includes a search for other injuries as appropriate to the mechanism of injury.

Principles of Management of Traumatic Brain Injury

Management priorities for patients with TBI vary based on the severity of injury but focus on SBI prevention. Patients with mild TBI do not usually require critical care unless required due to other injuries. TBI management in these patients focuses on assessment of neurologic status and education regarding post-concussive syndrome, including headaches, difficulty concentrating, dizziness, fatigue, irritability, decreased processing speed, and sleep disturbances. Resources for follow-up are provided to the patient and family. In most cases, the symptoms will resolve, but evaluation by a neuropsychologist or other rehabilitation professional is recommended if symptoms persist. Patients with moderate TBI pose a significant challenge to the healthcare team. While some patients will improve with minimal intervention, other patients with moderate TBI will decline and require aggressive management similar to those with severe TBI. The management of patients with severe TBI is focused on optimizing functional recovery by minimizing secondary brain injury. Supporting cerebral perfusion and preventing ischemia are the principal goals of treatment. General principles of management for the patient with severe TBI include:

Airway Management

Patients with a GCS <9 require intubation and mechanical ventilation. Patients with TBI are treated with spine precautions until injury to the spinal column can be ruled out, so manual in-line stabilization of the cervical spine is used during intubation. Endotracheal tubes are secured without causing pressure on the jugular veins to avoid increases in ICP due to decreased jugular venous return. In patients with severe TBI, a tracheostomy is often placed once the patient's condition has stabilized to allow faster ventilator weaning and facilitate rehabilitation.

Oxygenation

Hypoxemia worsens SBI. Patients with severe TBI may vomit and aspirate prior to airway placement, may have thoracic injuries, or may experience neurogenic pulmonary edema, complicating pulmonary management. The use of higher levels of positive end-expiratory pressure (PEEP) can increase ICP in some patients, but improves oxygenation; the improvement in oxygenation seen with PEEP typically outweighs the impact on ICP, provided elevations in ICP can be successfully managed. Suctioning and other airway clearance maneuvers may increase ICP, but are essential to maintaining adequate oxygenation. Premedication with a sedative agent may decrease the impact on ICP. Patients are suctioned when clinically indicated and preoxygenation is provided. If oxygenation is severely compromised, the use of sedation and paralytics may be considered. These options affect evaluation of neurological status but maintaining adequate oxygenation is the higher priority.

Ventilation

In general, the goal of management is to maintain a normal $PaCO_2$ and a normal $EtCO_2$. Hypoventilation causes cerebral vasodilation, which may increase ICP. Prolonged or prophylactic hyperventilation causes cerebral vasoconstriction and is not recommended.

Fluid and Volume Management

The goal of fluid management is euvolemia. Hypotonic solutions are avoided because they increase cerebral edema. Patients with injury to the hypothalamus or pituitary gland are at risk for diabetes insipidus (DI) or syndrome of inappropriate antidiuretic hormone (SIADH), further complicating fluid management. For more information on DI and SIADH, refer to Chapter 16, Endocrine System. In patients with agitation or autonomic instability due to DAI, high insensible losses because of diaphoresis and fever often occur in the post-acute management phase of care; these patients are at risk for significant dehydration.

Managing Increased Intracranial Pressure

Most patients with severe TBI undergo invasive ICP monitoring to guide treatment. Interventions to decrease ICP are typically initiated when ICP is sustained more than 22 mm Hg, although radiologic findings are also considered when determining the need for treatment. Nursing measures to prevent and manage elevations in ICP are discussed in Chapter 12, Neurologic System. In addition to surgical evacuation of hematomas, operative interventions to decrease ICP include resection of severely contused tissue and craniectomy (removal of a portion of the skull to decrease ICP and allow swelling external to the normal confines of the cranium). An external ventricular drain can be placed both for ICP monitoring and to permit drainage of CSF. Steroids are not used because they worsen outcomes after TBI. Osmotherapy is often used to decrease ICP after TBI. Mannitol is administered as a bolus dose of 0.25 to 1 g/kg in patients with signs of herniation even prior to ICP monitoring, and may also be used in patients with sustained ICP elevation. Mannitol is an osmotic diuretic, so careful attention to maintaining euvolemia and avoiding hypotension is required. hypertonic saline (HTS) is also used by many practitioners, either as a continuous infusion or bolus dose. The concentration for continuous infusion ranges from 1.8% NaCl to 5% NaCl and the bolus concentration is 23.4%. Higher concentrations should be administered via central line. HTS works by pulling fluid from the brain tissue into the intravascular space, thus decreasing cerebral edema. Sodium levels are closely monitored.

Supporting Cerebral Perfusion

Hypotension (SBP < 90 mm Hg) is associated with a poor outcome in TBI patients. Cerebral perfusion pressure (CPP) is calculated as MAP minus ICP. CPP is an indirect estimate of CBF. Goal CPP may vary based on clinical scenarios and other monitors of cerebral perfusion, but a CPP of less than 50 mm Hg is avoided because of cerebral ischemia. Once euvolemia is established, vasopressors (typically phenylephrine or norepinephrine) are used to raise MAP and thus CPP. Although requirements may vary by patient age, CPP augmentation to levels >70 mm Hg has been shown to increase the risk of acute respiratory distress syndrome (ARDS) without improving outcomes, probably due to the large amounts of fluids and vasopressors needed to achieve this goal. Measures of brain tissue oxygen, CBF, or brain metabolism may assist in determining the optimal CPP for individual patients; evidence is evolving.

Preventing Increased Cerebral Oxygen Demand

Seizures, fever, and agitation increase cerebral oxygen demand and are avoided. An anticonvulsant may be used to prevent posttraumatic seizures during the first 7 days after injury but is avoided after 7 days. Continued seizure prophylaxis does not impact the development of posttraumatic seizures and is not recommended. Patients with penetrating trauma are at higher risk for seizures than those with blunt injuries.

Fever is detrimental to the injured brain. Brain temperature is typically 0.5°C to 2.0°C higher than core temperature. For every 1°C increase in temperature, cerebral metabolism increases by approximately 6%. To prevent additional demands on the injured brain, fever is controlled using antipyretics, surface cooling, intravascular cooling, or a combination of methods. Because fever is eliminated, vigilance to other signs and symptoms of infectious complications is essential. It is important to manage shivering when treating fever because shivering markedly increases cerebral metabolic demand.

Agitation may increase cerebral oxygen demand. Strategies to reduce agitation include maintaining a calm, quiet environment (milieu therapy) and the use of anxiolytic and sedating medications. Both analgesics and sedatives are used in mechanically ventilated patients. In patients with moderate TBI who are not mechanically ventilated, care is taken to avoid respiratory depression, because $Paco_2$ may rise and

cause an increase in ICP. Propofol (a sedative-hypnotic) is commonly used in the care of neuroscience patients because of its short half-life. Care must be taken to avoid hypotension and decreased CPP, and the duration of use must be limited due to the risk of propofol infusion syndrome when used for more than 48 hours.

Additional Management Strategies

In patients with refractory intracranial hypertension, neuromuscular blocking agents may be used. The decrease in ICP with neuromuscular blockade may be related to the decreased intrathoracic pressure and improved ventilation. Induced hypothermia (goal temperature 32°C-34°C) has been studied in the management of severe TBI. Hypothermia decreases ICP but is associated with complications when maintained for greater than 48 hours. Current research supports maintenance of normothermia after acute TBI.

The use of high-dose barbiturates lowers ICP by decreasing cerebral metabolic demand and modulating neurochemical responses that cause edema, but has not been shown to improve outcomes. Complications of high-dose barbiturates include hypotension, myocardial suppression, and pupil dilation.

Preventing Secondary Complications

Common secondary complications include pneumonia and other infections, venous and pulmonary embolism, and pressure injury. Hypermetabolism and nitrogen wasting are common in patients with TBI. Nutritional support is initiated as soon as possible, with the goal of meeting full caloric needs by 7 days after injury. VTE prophylaxis is initiated on admission with pneumatic compression devices. Pharmacologic prophylaxis varies by practitioner and type of injury. If lower extremity deep venous thrombosis (DVT) develops and anticoagulation is contraindicated, an inferior vena cava (IVC) filter may be placed.

Coagulopathy is also a common problem following severe TBI. Coagulopathy occurs when injury to the brain tissue leads to release of tissue stores of thromboplastin, which creates a fibrinolytic state. Treatment is based on laboratory values and provider orders.

Complications of immobility are common in patients with TBI. Progression of activity is optimized with early spine clearance. Institutional protocols vary, but typically include a series of spine x-rays, CT scanning, and MRI to rule out injury to the bones and ligaments of the spine.

Promoting Recovery After Traumatic Brain Injury

Following acute stabilization, most patients with severe TBI progress through a series of recovery stages, during which they become more alert, then agitated, then purposeful, and more appropriate. Managing agitation is frequently challenging in patients with TBI. Environmental strategies are very important but should be individualized to the patient. Consistent staff members should be assigned to care for the patient.

All lines and tubes (indwelling bladder catheters, IVs) are removed as soon as possible. Medications are often prescribed as part of managing agitation in patients with TBI, but should be used in the smallest doses possible for the shortest time possible because they may slow recovery. No particular medication has demonstrated superiority in a large-scale trial. Restraints are avoided unless patient or staff safety is compromised.

The best care for patients with TBI includes multidisciplinary input. Physical therapy, occupational therapy, speech therapy, nutrition, and social work are consulted early in the patient's hospital course. Family members and other professionals may also be helpful, including the rehabilitation provider and neuropsychologist.

Family Education and Support

TBI alters the life of the injured individual and their family. The unpredictable nature of brain injury recovery is difficult to comprehend. Family members may feel that information provided by different staff is inconsistent, or that information is being withheld. Family members of patients with TBI often express the need to be involved in care—to be "*part of the team*." Critical care nurses can support family members by providing direct, honest communication (including acknowledging the difficulty of providing a definitive prognosis) and by recognizing their need for presence and involvement in care. The transition from the ICU to the progressive care unit or acute care floor can be a stressful time for family members. Critical care nurses can decrease family members' anxiety by collaborating with their colleagues in progressive and acute care to provide continuity of care and education about the stages of recovery.

TRAUMATIC SPINAL CORD INJURY

Etiology, Risk Factors, and Pathophysiology

Falls, MVAs, and acts of violence account for over 80% of all spinal cord injury (SCI) events. Sports-related injuries account for approximately 9% of SCI and medical or surgical procedures account for nearly 5% of SCI. Nearly 60% of SCIs involve the cervical cord and result in partial or complete tetraplegia (loss of function in all four limbs). The average age at time of injury is about 43 years and 78% are male. SCI results in varying degrees of paralysis and loss of sensation below the level of injury, and impacts physical, emotional, and social function. Similar to brain injury, deficits are due to both the initial impact (primary injury) and the ongoing physiologic changes (secondary injury).

The spinal column consists of stacked vertebrae joined by bony facet joints and intervertebral disks. Ligaments provide structure and support to prevent the vertebrae from moving. The ring-like structure of the stacked vertebrae creates a hollow canal through which the spinal cord runs. SCI occurs when something (eg, bone, disk material, or foreign object) enters the spinal canal and disrupts the spinal cord or

its blood supply. Mechanisms of injury include hyperflexion, hyperextension, axial loading/vertical compression, rotation, and penetrating trauma (Figure 21-7). Damage to the spinal cord can be characterized as concussion, contusion, laceration, transection, hemorrhage, or damage to the blood vessels that supply the spinal cord. Concussion causes temporary loss of function. Contusion is bruising of the spinal cord that includes bleeding into the spinal cord, subsequent edema, and possible neuronal death from compression by the edema or damage to the tissue; the extent of neurologic deficits depends on the severity of the contusion. Laceration is an actual tear in the spinal cord that results in permanent injury. Transection is a severing of the spinal cord resulting in complete loss of function below the level of the injury. The most obvious example of cord laceration or transection is a penetrating injury. Damage to the blood vessels that supply the spinal cord can result in ischemia and infarction, or hemorrhage due to vessel tearing.

Regardless of the type of primary injury, secondary insults occur from cellular damage to the spinal cord, vascular damage, structural changes in the gray and white matter, and subsequent biochemical responses. Blood flow to the spinal cord is decreased during the acute phase of injury, resulting in changes in metabolic function, destruction of cell membranes, and the release of free radicals. Patients may develop neurogenic shock following cervical or upper thoracic cord injury. Neurogenic shock occurs due to the loss of sympathetic nervous system influences from the T1 to L2 area of the spinal cord, which normally increases heart rate and constricts the blood vessel walls. Loss of sympathetic outflow results in bradycardia and decreased vascular resistance. Blood pools in the peripheral vasculature, resulting in hypotension and decreased cardiac output. Neurogenic shock contributes to hypoperfusion and secondary injury.

Clinical Presentation

Initial assessment of the patient with SCI begins with basic life support and immobilization of the spine to prevent further injury. The focus then shifts to obtaining a baseline assessment of motor and sensory function. Assessment of motor function and sensory level is performed at least every 4 hours during the acute postinjury period. Decreased motor function may be seen with swelling at the injury site, loss of vertebral alignment, or intrathecal hematoma formation. Changes in function warrant immediate provider notification.

The severity of deficits caused by SCI is determined by whether the injury is complete or incomplete and the level of the spinal cord affected. Acute SCI can result in the temporary suppression of reflexes controlled by segments below the level of injury, a phenomenon referred to as "spinal shock." Formal determination of complete versus incomplete SCI cannot be made until spinal shock is resolved. Complete SCI results in total loss of sensory and motor function below

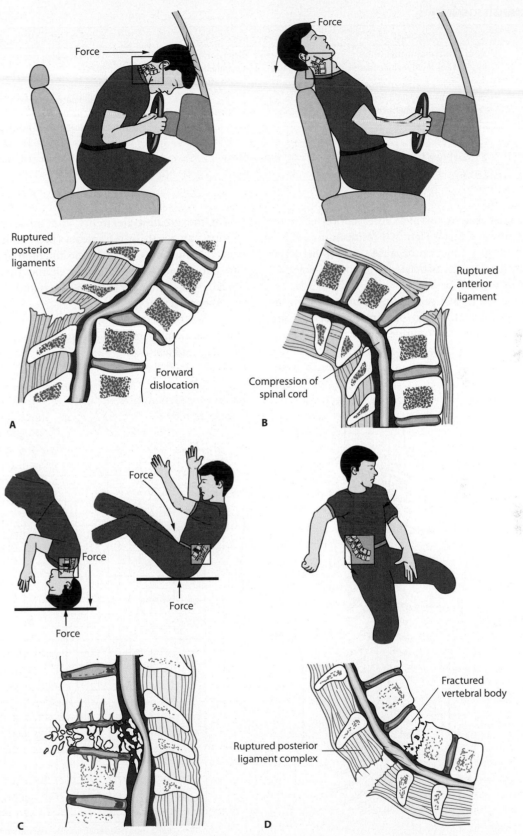

Figure 21-7. Mechanisms of spinal cord injury. **(A)** Hyperflexion. **(B)** Hyperextension. **(C)** Axial loading/vertical compression. **(D)** Rotation. (*Reproduced with permission from Phipps WJ, Marek JF, Monahan FD, et al. Medical-Surgical Nursing: Health and Illness Perspectives. St Louis, MO: Mosby; 2003.*)

TABLE 21-2. INCOMPLETE SCI SYNDROMES

Syndrome	Pathophysiology	Motor Function Below Level of Injury	Sensory Function Below Level of Injury
Central cord syndrome	Injury to central gray matter with preservation of outer white matter	Weakness/paralysis of upper extremities greater than lower extremities	Sensory loss greater in upper extremities than lower extremities
Anterior cord syndrome	Injury to anterior portion of spinal cord, disruption of blood flow through anterior spinal artery	Paralysis	Loss of pain and temperature with preservation of vibration and position sense
Posterior cord syndrome	Injury to posterior column	None	Loss of vibration and position sense with preservation of pain and temperature sensation
Brown-Séquard syndrome	Lateral injury to one side of the cord	Ipsilateral motor paralysis	Ipsilateral loss of vibration and position sense with contralateral loss of pain and temperature sensation

the level of injury due to complete interruption of motor and sensory pathways. Incomplete SCI results in mixed loss of motor and sensory function because some spinal tracts remain intact. Syndromes associated with incomplete SCI are described in Table 21-2.

Deficits caused by SCI relate to the level at which the injury occurs (cervical, thoracic, or lumbar). Cervical and lumbar injuries are more common because these areas

have the greatest flexibility and movement. A cervical injury can result in tetraplegia (previously called quadriplegia). Injuries to the thoracic and lumbar areas can result in paraplegia. The American Spinal Injury Association (ASIA) scale may be used to assess and document motor and sensory function.

Functional goals for patients with specific levels of injury are summarized in Figure 21-8.

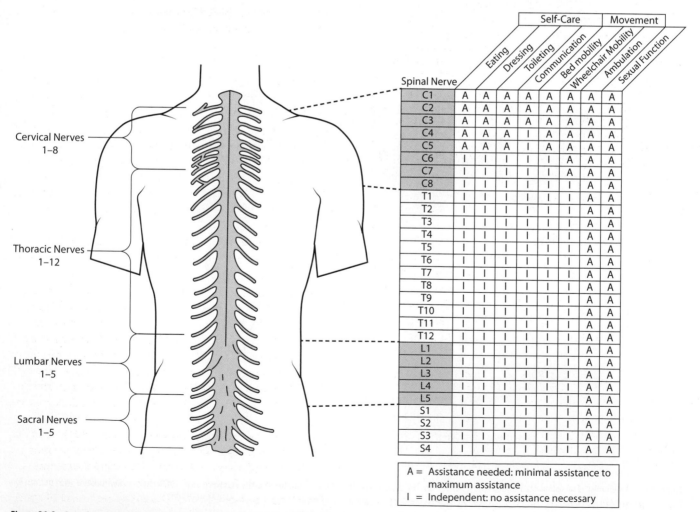

Figure 21-8. Spinal cord injury functional activity chart. (*Reproduced with permission from Monahan FD, Phipps WJ, Neighbors M, et al. Phipps' Medical-Surgical Nursing: Health and Illness Perspectives, 8th ed. Philadelphia, PA: Mosby Elsevier; 2006.*)

ESSENTIAL CONTENT CASE

Acute Spinal Cord Injury

A 39-year-old man was returning home from a party late one night when he struck another vehicle head on. He felt intense pain throughout his neck and body that was soon replaced with a burning sensation in his arms. When the paramedics arrived, he was unable to move his legs and had some gross motor movement of his arms. A CT scan and cervical spine x-rays revealed a C5-C6 subluxation with cord compression. His only other injury was a left wrist fracture. When the patient arrives in the ICU, his heart rate is 42, blood pressure 92/50 (MAP 64), and respirations 28 and shallow.

Case Question: In addition to maintaining spine immobilization, what are the initial priorities of care for this patient?

The patient was started on intravenous fluids and a norepinephrine infusion to keep his MAP greater than 85 mm Hg. He was placed in halo traction by the neurosurgeon with reduction of his subluxation, with plans for surgical fusion.

Answer

Because of the level of injury, the patient is at risk for respiratory failure and may require intubation. Close monitoring of the patient's airway and breathing is crucial so that intubation can take place in a controlled fashion. In addition, he is exhibiting signs of neurogenic shock. Fluid therapy and vasopressors should be anticipated.

Diagnostic Tests

Immobilization of the spinal column is maintained throughout the trauma evaluation to prevent additional injury. Cervical, thoracic, and lumbar spine x-rays identify the presence of injury to the vertebral column, although these tests are increasingly being replaced with specially constructed CT images. In addition to injury to the vertebral column, CT reveals any injury to the spinal cord itself, such as bleeding or significant compression. Most patients with suspected SCI require advanced imaging with MRI to reveal more subtle signs of injury to the cord and soft tissue, like injury to the supporting ligaments. Injury to the ligaments and spinal cord is possible even without bony abnormalities.

Principles of Management of Acute Spinal Cord Injury

As with brain injury, education is focused on primary injury prevention and critical care management is based on decreasing secondary injury and preventing complications. Priorities of management are covered below.

Immobilization and Prevention of Further Injury

Patients are immobilized with a rigid cervical collar and backboard in the prehospital environment and a rigid cervical collar and bed rest in the hospital until injury is ruled out or confirmed clinically and by radiograph. Rigid collars are temporary and should be replaced by soft collars if there is a delay in clearing the spine. If a rigid collar is not available, or adds to delay in treatment, a soft or temporary collar may be used. Some mattresses (such as air mattresses) do not provide adequate stability to the spinal column; follow manufacturer and institutional guidelines.

Airway Management

Loss of airway protection may be related to poor cough effort, concomitant brain injury, or facial trauma. Patients can develop neuromuscular respiratory failure and require an endotracheal tube and mechanical ventilation. Intubation is performed with careful attention to maintaining spine immobilization. Techniques include the use of manual in-line stabilization with direct laryngoscopy or fiber-optic awake intubation. The neuromuscular blocking agent succinylcholine is not used if more than 24 hours have elapsed since the time of injury. Succinylcholine administration in patients with denervated muscles can cause massive release of skeletal muscle potassium, resulting in serum hyperkalemia and potentially cardiac arrest. In patients with cervical or high thoracic SCI, tracheostomy is indicated to facilitate airway clearance and ventilator weaning.

Pulmonary Management

Altered respiratory function is a major concern for patients with high thoracic or cervical SCI. In the acute phase, impaired oxygenation contributes to secondary injury. The mnemonic "3, 4, 5, keep the lungs alive" helps to recall that the phrenic nerve, which supplies motor and sensory input to the diaphragm, arises from the C3 to C5. Patients with complete injuries at or above C2 require mechanical ventilation due to the loss of diaphragmatic innervation. The diaphragm is controlled by the phrenic nerve, which exits the spinal cord at the C3 to C5 level.

Patients with injuries below the level of diaphragmatic innervation will initiate breaths but still experience respiratory compromise owing to paralysis of the intercostal and abdominal muscles. Paralysis of the intercostal muscles causes the chest wall to be flaccid. Contraction of the diaphragm creates a negative pressure in the thoracic cavity and the intercostal muscles retract, decreasing lung capacity. Upright positioning creates further downward displacement of the diaphragm and increases intercostal retraction; flat positioning can improve respiratory function in patients with cervical or thoracic SCI. Abdominal binders can be useful, especially during physical activity (rehabilitation). With time, the intercostal muscles become spastic and the chest wall no longer collapses with inspiration, promoting improved ventilation and facilitating ventilator weaning.

Pulmonary function is closely monitored in patients with cervical and thoracic SCI. Ongoing assessment of maximal inspiratory pressure (MIP) and vital capacity allow early identification of impending respiratory failure. In general, a patient who is unable to generate an MIP of at least −20 cm H_2O or a vital capacity of greater than 10 to 15 mL/kg requires intubation and mechanical ventilation. No specific mode of mechanical ventilation is demonstrably superior in patients with SCI. Effective secretion clearance requires the ability to take a deep breath and then forcibly exhale against a closed glottis. Patients with cervical or thoracic SCI have decreased cough strength because of decreased intercostal and abdominal muscle strength. Pulmonary therapy is provided to both ventilated and nonventilated patients with cervical or thoracic injuries. After spine stabilization, manual cough assist ("quad-cough") is included unless contraindicated by other injuries. In addition, a mechanical cough assist device (in-exsufflator) can be used to clear secretions. This device imitates a physiologic cough by providing a deep breath via positive pressure followed by negative pressure. It is important to work closely with the respiratory therapist to optimize pulmonary care for SCI patients.

Hemodynamic Support

Neurogenic shock causes bradycardia and hypotension in many patients with injury above the midthoracic level. Because SCI can mask the signs and symptoms of other trauma, including abdominal or pelvic injury, hemorrhagic shock must be excluded in hypotensive patients with SCI. The normal tachycardic response to hemorrhagic shock may be blunted in the patient with SCI due to loss of sympathetic innervation. Bradycardia after SCI can be profound and may even progress to asystole in patients with high cervical injury. Bradycardia occurs more frequently during suctioning; the risk can be lessened but not eliminated by maintaining adequate oxygenation and ventilation. Symptomatic bradycardia is initially treated with atropine, although some patients may require temporary or permanent pacemaker placement.

Hypotension because of neurogenic shock reflects fluid displacement into the vasodilated periphery. As with all trauma patients, adequate volume resuscitation is indicated. Continued fluid administration will not correct hypotension and can lead to peripheral edema or pulmonary edema, especially in elderly patients or those with comorbidities. Norepinephrine is frequently used to counter the loss of sympathetic tone and provide inotropic and chronotropic support. Research suggests that blood pressure augmentation (MAP > 85 mm Hg) for up to 7 days after acute SCI may improve neurologic outcomes.

Neuroprotection

There are no approved neuroprotective agents that improve outcomes after SCI. Neuroprotection is an area of ongoing research, and includes both pharmacologic and nonpharmacologic strategies.

Decompression and Stabilization

Early management of SCI includes decompression of the spinal canal and stabilization of the spinal column. In patients with cervical injury, traction may be used to realign the spinal column and relieve pressure on the spinal cord. Traction devices include bed-based (ie, Gardner-Wells tongs) and personalized thoracolumbar sacral orthosis (TLSO) equipment. Nursing responsibilities during traction placement include patient monitoring, pain management, and administration of sedating agents. Decompression of the spinal cord can also be accomplished surgically. Rapid surgical intervention is indicated for patients with a worsening neurologic examination and ongoing spinal cord compression.

Stabilization of the spinal column does not improve neurologic function but enables the patient to be mobilized without causing additional damage to the spinal cord. In patients who require operative decompression of the spinal canal, the spinal column is stabilized at the time of surgery using rods, screws, or other hardware. For other patients, the timing of surgical stabilization varies. Surgery is commonly performed within 24 hours of injury if the patient's cardiorespiratory status is stable because early surgery decreases secondary complications and length of stay. Some fractures can be managed without surgery by immobilizing the spinal column and allowing the bones to heal. Immobilization is achieved using a cervical collar, halo vest, or other orthotic device. Skin care is a primary concern for these patients because pressure injury can occur at contact points with the brace, especially in patients with decreased sensation.

Bladder and Bowel Management

Areflexia caused by spinal shock leads to urinary retention. An indwelling catheter is placed on admission and maintained until the patient is hemodynamically stable and fluid intake is consistent. A program of scheduled intermittent catheterization is then initiated. A bowel program is started soon after admission and typically includes daily stool softeners and digital stimulation. For patients with injuries at or above T6, an anesthetic jelly is used to decrease the risk of autonomic dysreflexia (AD; also called autonomic hyperreflexia). The goal of the bowel program is for the patient to have a bowel movement at planned intervals, without incontinence between scheduled evacuations. An effective bowel program decreases constipation, limits incontinence, decreases pressure injury, and increases the patient's sense of control.

Pain Management

Pain following SCI impacts functional recovery and can be challenging to treat. During the immediate postinjury period, many patients experience musculoskeletal pain and neuropathic pain (described as a burning sensation, paresthesia, or hypersensitivity). Medications prescribed include opiates and muscle relaxants as well as neuropathic agents such as gabapentin and pregabalin. Antidepressants and anticonvulsants also are useful in the treatment of neuropathic pain. Some patients benefit from nonpharmacologic methods such as massage, music, visual imagery, and distraction.

Psychological Considerations

Fear, uncertainty, and anxiety are common following SCI. The psychological and emotional trauma of SCI can be overwhelming. Sudden paralysis does not allow patients or family to prepare for this major insult. Fear focuses on the injury and life-and-death issues. Anxiety results from the ICU environment, feelings of dependence, sensory deprivation, powerlessness, and uncertainty. A trusting relationship must be established between the patient and the healthcare team. For patients on mechanical ventilation, communication strategies are developed based on the individual patient's abilities and needs. Use of eye contact, patience, honesty, and consistency are reassuring to the patient. Encouraging self-care within the patient's abilities decreases feelings of complete dependence. Whenever possible, the patient is allowed choices within the daily care routine. The family and significant others are incorporated into the plan of care. The use of an ICU-diary may reduce post-intensive care syndrome.

Prevention and Management of Complications

The prevention and effective management of complications maximizes rehabilitation potential. Common complications include:

- *Respiratory complications:* Neuromuscular respiratory failure, atelectasis, and pneumonia occur frequently following SCI. In addition to the strategies previously described under respiratory management, standard measures to prevent nosocomial pneumonia are implemented.
- *Gastrointestinal problems:* Paralytic ileus is common immediately following injury. An orogastric or nasogastric tube is placed initially for decompression. The current recommendation is for early enteral nutrition. Patients with acute SCI may also have an increased risk for stress ulcers and require prophylactic medications.
- *Pressure injury:* The patient with SCI is at high risk for pressure injury due to decreased blood flow to the skin and decreased cutaneous response to focal pressure. Skin inspection is performed at least twice daily and pressure reduction strategies are implemented. Early in the hospitalization, the patient who requires assistance with repositioning is encouraged to request that assistance at scheduled intervals. This increases the patient's sense of control and self-care responsibility, which is associated with improved long-term outcomes.
- *Orthostatic hypotension:* Blood pools in the lower extremities owing to loss of sympathetic vascular tone. Nursing strategies to decrease orthostatic hypotension include application of gradient compression stockings and elastic wraps to the legs, hydration, and gradual progression to an upright position. If these measures are ineffective, medication to raise blood pressure may be ordered.
- *Altered thermoregulation:* Individuals with SCI at or above the T6 level are unable to conserve heat by vasoconstriction or shivering. Heat loss is compromised by the inability to sweat below the level of injury.
- *Venothromboembolism:* Recommended strategies for prevention during acute hospitalization include mechanical prophylaxis for all patients starting at the time of admission, followed by low-molecular-weight heparin or the combination of low-dose unfractionated heparin and intermittent pneumatic compression. To prevent pulmonary embolus, IVC filters can be placed in patients who cannot receive pharmacologic prophylaxis.
- *Spasticity:* During spinal shock, there is a total loss of motor function below the level of injury. Flaccid paralysis progresses to spastic paralysis as spinal shock resolves. Measures to decrease spasticity in the critical care phase include frequent range-of-motion exercises and medications. Occupational and physical therapy are consulted early in the course of hospitalization.
- *Autonomic dysreflexia:* AD is a life-threatening complication that occurs in individuals with SCI at or above T6 due to unopposed sympathetic response below the level of injury. It can occur any time after spinal shock has resolved. AD results from a variety of stimuli, including overdistended bladder (most common), full rectum, infection, skin stimulation, pressure injuries, and pain. The stimulus causes massive vasoconstriction that causes elevation of blood pressure (relative to the patient's baseline, which is often low after SCI). Other symptoms include severe headache, nasal congestion, shortness of breath, nausea, blurred vision, facial flushing, diaphoresis, piloerection, and anxiety, but for some patients, the only sign is elevated BP. Treatment of AD includes moving the patient into a sitting position immediately, then identifying and treating the underlying cause (eg, bladder distention, impaction). Blood pressure and pulse are monitored closely, and the provider is notified. A short-acting antihypertensive agent may be ordered, if symptoms continue. Long-acting antihypertensives are avoided because once the stimulus is identified and removed, the blood pressure will drop. Careful attention to bowel and bladder management aids in the prevention of AD.

Future Spinal Cord Injury Treatment

Research in SCI focuses on limiting the neuronal damage caused by secondary injury (neuroprotection), enhancing regrowth of neurons (nerve regeneration) and the benefits of increased activity on functioning neurons (synaptic plasticity).

The National Institutes of Health: http://www.clinicaltrials.gov is a vital resource for patients seeking to be involved in clinical trials.

BRAIN TUMORS

Etiology, Risk Factors, and Pathophysiology

The epidemiology of brain tumors varies widely based on tumor type. When all primary CNS tumors are grouped together, the incidence is higher in women than in men. This overall gender difference is attributed to the greater incidence of meningiomas in women. Prognosis varies based on age (younger patients have a better prognosis), tumor type and degree of differentiation, functional status at diagnosis, and tumor location. The most common brain tumors are meningiomas, gliomas, and metastatic lesions. Intracranial tumors are classified by distinguishing criteria.

Primary Versus Secondary

Primary intracranial tumors originate from the cells and structures in the brain. Secondary or metastatic intracranial tumors originate from structures outside the brain, such as primary tumors of the lung or breast.

Histologic Origins

During the early stage of embryonic development, two types of undifferentiated cells are found—neuroblasts and the glioblasts. The neuroblasts become neurons. The glioblasts form a variety of cells that support, insulate, and metabolically assist the neurons. The glioblasts are collectively referred to as glial cells and are subdivided into astrocytes, oligodendrocytes, and ependymal cells. This is the basis of a broad category of intracranial tumors called gliomas. Gliomas are subdivided into astrocytomas, oligodendrogliomas, oligoastrocytomas (also called mixed gliomas), and ependymomas. Gliomas are graded based on histologic criteria related to the degree of differentiation from the parent cell. Higher-grade tumors are more malignant. Glioblastoma multiforme (GBM) is a rapidly growing, poorly differentiated tumor. GBM is the most aggressive brain tumor and carries the worst prognosis.

A meningioma is a tumor that arises from the meninges. Meningiomas tend to grow slowly and compress rather than invade the brain. Prognosis is excellent if the tumor is in a surgically accessible location. Neuromas (also called Schwannomas) are noninvasive, slow-growing tumors that arise from the Schwann cells, which produce myelin. Pituitary adenomas, located in the pituitary gland, can be secretory or nonsecretory. Secretory tumors increase the production of hormones such as prolactin, growth hormone, adrenocorticotropic hormone, thyrotropin, or gonadotropin. Nonsecretory pituitary tumors cause symptoms through mass effect; patients commonly present with visual changes due to compression of the optic chiasm. Pituitary tumors are treated with pharmacologic agents, surgery, radiation

therapy, or a combination of these modalities. The tumors described here are the ones most likely to be encountered in practice; other less common types of brain tumors are beyond the scope of this text.

Anatomic Location

This refers to the actual site of the tumor, such as the frontal lobe, temporal lobe, pons, or cerebellum. Knowing the location of the tumor helps in predicting deficits based on the normal functions of that anatomic area. Anatomic location also can refer to the location of the tumor in reference to the tentorium. Supratentorial refers to tumors located above the tentorium (cerebral hemispheres), and infratentorial refers to tumors located below the tentorium (brainstem and cerebellum).

Benign Versus Malignant

The distinction between benign and malignant intracranial tumors is based on histologic examination. Tumors made up of well-differentiated cells are histologically "benign" and the prognosis is generally better than if cells are poorly differentiated. However, a histologically benign tumor can be surgically inaccessible. This "benign" tumor continues to grow and ultimately contributes to a decline in neurologic function and even death. Benign tumors may convert to more histologically malignant types as they develop.

Clinical Presentation

Brain tumors are space-occupy lesions that cause compression of brain structures, infiltration of tissue that controls functions, and displacement of normal tissue. Brain tumors may disrupt the blood-brain barrier and contribute to cerebral edema. CSF flow may be obstructed by the tumor or edema, leading to hydrocephalus. Tumors are often vascular and may bleed, causing additional neurologic deficits.

The most common presenting signs and symptoms of intracranial tumors are headache, seizures, papilledema, and vomiting. Headache is usually progressive in severity and worse after lying flat; for example, upon awakening from sleep. Clinical presentation may also include decreased level of consciousness, changes in the PLR, visual abnormalities, and personality changes. Additional signs and symptoms depend upon the area of the brain that is being compressed or infiltrated (Table 21-3).

Diagnostic Tests

Advanced imaging with CT and MRI are used to differentiate tumor from abscess and to identify tumor location and characteristics. Functional MRI (fMRI) detects physiologic changes using MRI scanning during physical and cognitive activity and is helpful in mapping language, sensory, and motor function. Magnetic resonance spectroscopy and positive emission tomography (PET) scans evaluate cerebral metabolism and are used to provide information about how aggressive a tumor is (a more aggressive tumor

TABLE 21-3. CLINICAL PRESENTATION OF BRAIN TUMORS RELATED TO LOCATION

Location	Clinical Presentation
Frontal lobe	Inappropriate behavior
	Inattentiveness
	Inability to concentrate
	Emotional lability
	Quiet but flat affect
	Expressive aphasia
	Seizures
	Headache
	Impaired memory
Parietal lobe	Hyperesthesia
	Paresthesia
	Astereognosis (inability to recognize an object by feeling it)
	Autotopagnosia (inability to locate or recognize parts of the body)
	Loss of left-right discrimination
	Agraphia (inability to write)
	Acalculia (difficulty in calculating numbers)
Temporal lobe	Psychomotor seizures
	Receptive aphasia
Occipital lobe	Visual loss in half of the visual field
	Seizures
Pituitary and hypothalamus region	Visual deficits
	Headache
	Hormonal dysfunction of the pituitary gland
	Water imbalance and sleep alterations in tumors of the hypothalamus
Ventricles	Symptoms of increased ICP associated with obstruction of CSF flow
Cerebellum	Ataxia
	Incoordination
	Symptoms of increased ICP associated with obstruction of CSF flow

will display higher metabolic activity) and to differentiate necrosis or scarring from tumor. Additional testing includes cerebral angiography, visual field and funduscopic examination, audiometric studies, and endocrine studies. If the lesion is suspected to be metastatic, further diagnostic tests are needed to locate the primary tumor site, if not already known. A biopsy of the lesion determines tumor type and degree of differentiation. Biopsy may be performed via a burr hole using stereotactic guidance or may be done as part of a craniotomy for tumor resection.

Principles of Management of Intracranial Tumors

Treatment modalities may be used alone or in any combination. When selecting the most appropriate treatment, the tumor team will consider the type of tumor, its location and size, related symptoms and the severity of those symptoms, and the general condition of the patient.

Corticosteroids

A corticosteroid, typically dexamethasone, is administered to decrease vasogenic cerebral edema. Steroids are started when the tumor is diagnosed and the presence of cerebral edema is noted. Significant improvements in neurologic status can be seen soon after initiation of therapy. Side effects of steroid therapy may include gastrointestinal irritation, mood swings, fluid retention, hyperglycemia, myopathy, insomnia, and increased risk of infection.

Surgery

The goal of surgery is to resect as much of the tumor as possible without harming normal tissue. In most cases, a craniotomy is done to provide access for the resection. Total resection can be curative for some tumor types. Some tumors cannot be completely removed because of their location or histologic type. A partial resection of the tumor mass is still considered helpful as this temporarily relieves the symptoms associated with mass effect. When present, obstruction of CSF flow is treated by placement of a shunt to reroute CSF from the ventricular system to another part of the body (usually the peritoneal space) where it can be reabsorbed. Transsphenoidal resection uses a special technique to reach pituitary tumors by going through the sphenoid sinus (Figure 21-9).

Several strategies are available to decrease the morbidity associated with surgery. Intraoperative MRI is available at an increasing number of centers and is most often used when the lesion is in or near eloquent cortical structures such as the motor strip, difficult to access, or small and potentially hard to locate. Intraoperative MRI can be used alone or in conjunction with cortical mapping techniques. With cortical mapping, the patient is anesthetized for the initial part of the surgery, then awakened, and asked to perform certain tasks, allowing the surgeon to avoid areas of the brain that control speech or motor function. Stereotactic techniques allow targeted biopsy or resection based on previously obtained images.

Most patients undergo elective operations for intracranial tumors and may be admitted to the critical care

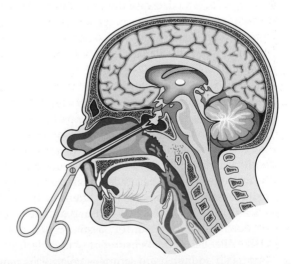

Figure 21-9. Transsphenoidal hypophysectomy. (*Reproduced with permission from Urden LD, Stacy KM, Lough ME. Thelan's Critical Care Nursing, 4th ed. St Louis, MO: Mosby; 2002.*)

unit postoperatively. Postoperative management includes monitoring with serial neurological exams, controlling pain, and preventing and managing complications. Potential complications in the immediate postoperative period include:

- *Hematoma formation:* Clinical signs include increasing headache, decreasing level of consciousness, and the development of new focal neurologic signs. If an intracranial bleed is suspected, a brain CT scan is obtained immediately. If significant bleeding is found, the patient is returned to the operating room for surgical removal of the hematoma and management of bleeding points.

- *Cerebral edema:* Postoperative cerebral edema may occur due to the long surgical procedure and/or the retraction of brain tissue to expose the operative area. Cerebral edema is suspected if the patient presents postoperatively with new deficit, or greater neurologic deficits than were present preoperatively. A CT scan is obtained and treatment initiated with mannitol or HTS to decrease edema. As noted previously, dexamethasone is useful in the management of tumor-related edema.

- *Infection:* Infection can occur following surgery because of contamination in the operating room or a defect in the dura, which allows communication of the CSF with the atmosphere. Patients who undergo trans-sphenoidal resection of pituitary tumors are at risk for CSF leak. Drainage from the nose can be collected and sent to the laboratory to be tested for tau transferrin, a protein present in CSF. The patient must not be suctioned nasally nor allowed to blow their nose. A nasogastric tube should never be inserted following trans-sphenoidal resection.

- *Venous thromboembolism:* Neurosurgical patients are at increased risk for deep vein thrombosis. Preventive measures to decrease this risk include the use of intermittent pneumatic compression devices, early progression of activity, and low doses of subcutaneous unfractionated heparin.

- *Diabetes insipidus:* DI is caused by a disturbance in the posterior lobe of the pituitary gland, which secretes antidiuretic hormone (ADH). If ADH is not secreted in sufficient amounts, the patient will produce large volumes of dilute urine with a low specific gravity. Significant fluid and electrolyte imbalances with dehydration can result. Management includes intravenous fluid resuscitation that correlates with urine output (or allowing the patient to drink fluids as needed to quench thirst) and administration of aqueous vasopressin or desmopressin acetate (DDAVP). The patient's hydration status, electrolytes (especially sodium), and serum osmolarity are monitored closely. DI is common following surgery for pituitary tumors.

Radiation Therapy

Radiation therapy preferentially destroys tumor cells because they are rapidly dividing, but affects normal cells also. The treatment dose depends on the histologic type, radio responsiveness, location of the tumor, and patient tolerance. Increased edema is a common complication of radiation therapy. Patients typically remain on dexamethasone throughout treatment. Special techniques, such as stereotactic radiosurgery or gamma knife radiation, focus concentrated radiation from many directions on the tumor site and reduce radiation to normal tissue.

Chemotherapy

Chemotherapy is used to slow or stop the proliferation of abnormal cells. One commonly used agent in the treatment of high-grade gliomas is temozolomide (Temodar). Temozolomide is administered orally and is generally well-tolerated by patients.

Prevention and Management of Seizures

The incidence of seizures in patients with brain tumors ranges from 20% to 50% in high-grade gliomas. Antiepileptic drugs are often given prophylactically to patients with supratentorial tumors. When seizures do occur, they are managed according to the guidelines described in Chapter 12, Neurologic System. Any seizure in the immediate postoperative period prompts an emergent CT scan to look for hematoma formation.

Transsphenoidal Resection of Pituitary Tumors

The surgical management of patients with pituitary tumors differs because a trans-sphenoidal approach may be used (see Figure 21-9). Transsphenoidal resection uses a special technique to reach pituitary tumors by going through the sphenoid sinus. An incision may be made under the patient's upper lip, or an endonasal approach may be used. Because the pituitary gland secretes a number of hormones, endocrine disturbances are common both before and after surgery. Care in the postoperative period is similar to that described for patients undergoing a craniotomy, but certain assessments are emphasized. Because the pituitary gland is located near the optic chiasm, visual acuity and visual field testing is essential. The patient is closely monitored for CSF leak, and is instructed not to blow his or her nose or lean over. Nasal packing, if present, is typically removed by the surgeon on the first or second postoperative day. Serum cortisol is monitored because the patient will no longer secrete adrenocorticotropic hormone if the anterior pituitary was resected.

Close monitoring of fluid balance and electrolytes is required because of the risk for DI caused by insufficient amounts of ADH. Significant fluid and electrolyte imbalances with dehydration can result. Intake and output are measured frequently (every hour initially). Electrolytes (especially sodium) and urine specific gravity are monitored frequently, typically every 4 hours. Serum and urine osmolality may also be monitored. Management of DI includes allowing the patient to drink fluids as needed to quench thirst. Management may also include IV therapy that correlates with urine output and administration of aqueous vasopressin or desmopressin acetate (DDAVP).

ADVANCED TECHNOLOGY

Invasive Monitoring of ICP

See Chapter 12.

Brain Tissue Oxygen Monitoring

As understanding of the pathophysiology of intracranial processes evolves, the search for improved monitoring techniques intensifies. A few of the modalities currently in use include CBF monitoring, continuous electroencephalography (cEEG), cerebral microdialysis catheters that sample the brain's extracellular fluid, and electrodes that measure the partial pressure of oxygen in the brain tissue. Of these strategies, brain tissue oxygen ($Pbto_2$) monitoring is the most widely used. The concept of brain tissue oxygenation is based on the understanding of cerebral metabolism and blood flow. As discussed throughout this chapter and Chapter 12, Neurologic System, the brain is dependent on a constant supply of oxygen and glucose. Anything that decreases cerebral perfusion or increases cerebral metabolic demand places brain cells at risk for hypoxia, ischemia, and eventual death. By measuring oxygen in the brain, therapies can be directed at avoiding or promptly treating tissue hypoxia. Tissue hypoxia and ischemia are due to intracranial or extracranial causes. Intracranial causes include elevated ICP, vasospasm, and seizures. Extracranial causes include anemia, hypotension, and hypoxemia. As discussed, $Paco_2$ also impacts the diameter of blood vessels and affects oxygen delivery to the tissues.

Brain tissue oxygen monitors are most commonly placed in patients with severe TBI or high-grade SAH. The probe is placed into the white matter of the brain via a burr hole. The probe measures regional oxygenation in the area into which it is inserted. In TBI patients, the probe can be placed near the area of injury or on the opposite side. In patients with SAH, the probe is most commonly placed in the vascular distribution believed to be at greatest risk for vasospasm. Low brain tissue oxygen partial pressure ($Pbto_2$) levels for extended periods are predictive of poor outcome and treatment is aimed at improving cerebral oxygenation. Examples of interventions to improve $Pbto_2$ include:

- Hemodynamic support (fluid volume resuscitation, MAP augmentation, correct anemia)
- Ventilation management: adjust Fio_2, PEEP to attain adequate oxygenation ($Pbto_2$, Pao_2, and Sao_2) and adjust tidal volume and rate to optimize $Pbto_2$, $Paco_2$, and $Etco_2$
- ICP management
- Decreasing metabolic demand (temperature management, sedation/analgesia, neuromuscular blockers)

The goal of therapy is early identification and treatment of conditions that increase the risk for secondary brain injury. While no randomized controlled trials have been published that link improved outcomes directly to $Pbto_2$ monitoring and treatment, several observational studies demonstrated improved outcomes in patients with TBI following implementation of treatment protocols that include management of cerebral oxygenation.

Cerebral Blood Flow Monitoring

Various elements of CBF monitoring can be accomplished using single photon emission CT (SPECT), positron emission tomography (PET), xenon-CT, TCD, and invasively with thermal dilution catheters. There are various advantages and disadvantages to each technology. While SPECT, PET, and xenon-CT provide global CBF, thermal dilution only provides regional CBF but has the advantage of being capable of continuous CBF monitoring. Similarly, TCD has the advantage of being portable and noninvasive, but is limited in the number of vessels that can be accurately insonated.

Cerebral Microdialysis

Cerebral microdialysis is performed using a tunneled fenestrated microcatheter with a solute infused slowly (0.3 µL/min) to allow for the diffusion of molecules into the catheter. The resulting perfusate is analyzed for select molecules. Typically, lactate, pyruvate, glucose, glutamate, and glycerol are the most frequently selected molecules. Changes in the absolute value and/or ratio of these molecules are indicative of changes in neuronal metabolism.

SUMMARY

Critical care nurses play a vital role in outcomes for patients with acute neurological illness or injury. Small changes in the neurological exam should not be overlooked. Serial assessments provide nurses with the ability to monitor small changes in status. While there are similarities across many different neurological diagnoses, there is a clear benefit to understanding the pathophysiology of illness.

SELECTED BIBLIOGRAPHY

Subarachnoid Hemorrhage

Boling B, Groves TR. Management of subarachnoid hemorrhage. *Critical Care Nurse.* 2019;39(5):58-67.

Delpirou Nouh C, Samkutty DG, Chandrashekhar S, et al. Management of aneurysmal subarachnoid hemorrhage: variation in clinical practice and unmet need for follow-up among survivors—a single-center perspective. *World Neurosurg.* 2020;139:e608-e617.

Liu X, Griffith M, Jang HJ, et al. Intracranial pressure monitoring via external ventricular drain: are we waiting long enough before recording the real value? *J Neurosci Nurs.* 2020;52(1):37-42.

Ortega-Perez S, Shoyombo I, Aiyagari V, et al. Pupillary Light reflex variability as a predictor of clinical outcomes in subarachnoid hemorrhage. *J Neurosci Nurs.* 2019;51(4):171-175.

Rao SS, Chung DY, Wolcott Z, et al. Intermittent CSF drainage and rapid EVD weaning approach after subarachnoid hemorrhage: association with fewer VP shunts and shorter length of stay. *J Neurosurg*. 2019:132(5):1583–1588.

Suarez JI, Sheikh MK, Macdonald RL, et al. Common data elements for unruptured intracranial aneurysms and subarachnoid hemorrhage clinical research: A National Institute for Neurological Disorders and Stroke and National Library of Medicine Project. *Neurocrit Care*. 2019;30(Suppl 1):4-19.

Traumatic Brain Injury

Carney N, Totten AM, O'Reilly C, et al. Guidelines for the Management of Severe Traumatic Brain Injury, Fourth Edition. *Neurosurgery*. 2017;80(1):6-15.

El Ahmadieh TY, Bedros N, Stutzman SE, et al. Automated pupillometry as a triage and assessment tool in patients with traumatic brain injury. *World Neurosurg*. 2021;145:e163-e169.

Olson DM, Parcon C, Santos A, Santos G, Delabar R, Stutzman SE. A novel approach to explore how nursing care affects intracranial pressure. *Am J Crit Care*. 2017;26(2):136-139.

Olson DM, Ortega-Perez S. The cue-response theory and nursing care of the patient with acquired brain injury. *J Neurosci Nurs*. 2018;51(1):43-47.

Ortega-Perez S, Amaya-Rey MC. Secondary brain injury: a concept analysis. *J Neurosci Nurs*. 2018;50(4):220-224.

Spinal Cord Injury

Hills TE. Caring for patients with a traumatic spinal cord injury. *Nursing*. 2020;50(12):30-40.

Hollenbach PM, Ruth-Sahd LA, Hole J. Management of the pregnant patient with a spinal cord injury. *J Neurosci Nurs*. 2020;52(2):53-57.

Ong B, Wilson JR, Henzel MK. Management of the patient with chronic spinal cord injury. *Med Clin North Am*. 2020; 104(2):263-278.

Rodger S, Bench S. Education provision for patients following a spinal cord injury. *Br J Nurs*. 2019;28(6):377-381.

Shank CD, Walters BC, Hadley MN. Management of acute traumatic spinal cord injuries. *Handbook of Clinical Neurology*. 2017; 140:275-298.

Brain Tumors

Cohen-Inbar O. Geriatric brain tumor management part II: Glioblastoma multiforme. *J Clin Neurosci*. 2019;67:1-4.

Hatiboglu MA, Akdur K, Sawaya R. Neurosurgical management of patients with brain metastasis. *Neurosurg Rev*. 2020;43(2):483-495.

Niranjan A, Monaco E, Flickinger J, Lunsford LD. Guidelines for multiple brain metastases radiosurgery. *Prog Neurol Surg*. 2019;34:100-109.

Reed ME, Anthony PP, Rosenfeld PB, Ligon BL, Doris EM, Fox SW. Reflections on 50 years of neuroscience nursing: neuro-oncology, moving forward by looking back. *J Neurosci Nurs*. 2018;50(3):124-128.

Saito J, Masters J, Hirota K, Ma D. Anesthesia and brain tumor surgery: technical considerations based on current research evidence. *Curr Opin Anaesthesiol*. 2019;32(5):553-562.

Schiff D, Alyahya M. Neurological and medical complications in brain tumor patients. *Curr Neurol Neurosci Rep*. 2020;20(8):33.

Suh JH, Kotecha R, Chao ST, Ahluwalia MS, Sahgal A, Chang EL. Current approaches to the management of brain metastases. *Nat Rev Clin Oncol*. 2020;17(5):279-299.

Advanced Technology: Multimodal Monitoring

Al-Mufti F, Lander M, Smith B, et al. Multimodality monitoring in neurocritical care: decision-making utilizing direct and indirect surrogate markers. *J Intensive Care Med*. 2019;34(6): 449-463.

Kebapçı A, Dikeç G, Topçu S. Interobserver reliability of Glasgow Coma Scale Scores for intensive care unit patients. *Crit Care Nurse*. 2020;40(4):e18-e26.

Khatibi K, Szeder V, Blanco MB, et al. Role of bedside multimodality monitoring in the detection of cerebral vasospasm following subarachnoid hemorrhage. *Acta Neurochir Suppl*. 2020; 127:141-144.

Musick S, Alberico A. Neurologic assessment of the neurocritical care patient. *Front Neurol*. 2021;12:588989.

Sacco TL, Davis JG. Management of intracranial pressure part II: nonpharmacologic interventions. *Dimens Crit Care Nurs*. 2019;38(2):61-69.

Zeiler FA, Ercole A, Czosnyka M, et al. Continuous cerebrovascular reactivity monitoring in moderate/severe traumatic brain injury: a narrative review of advances in neurocritical care *Br J Anaesth*. 2020;S0007-0912(19)30966-3.

Evidence-Based Guidelines

Lee JM, Moon JR, Kim HJ, Kwon DY, Shin JY. Evaluation of evidence-based guidelines for fever management in critically ill adult patients with brain injury. *J Neurosci Nurs*. 2020; 52(5):234-238.

Phillips SS, Mueller CM, Nogueira RG, Khalifa YM. A systematic review assessing the current state of automated pupillometry in the NeuroICU. *Neurocrit Care*. 2019;31(1):142-161.

Reuter-Rice K, Christoferson E. Critical update on the third edition of the guidelines for managing severe traumatic brain injury in children. *Am J Crit Care*. 2020;29(1):e13-e18.

Saherwala AA, Bader MK, Stutzman SE, et al. Increasing adherence to brain trauma foundation guidelines for hospital care of patients with traumatic brain injury. *Critic Care Nurse*. 2018; 38(1):e11-e20.

KEY REFERENCE
INFORMATION

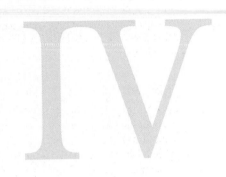

Normal Laboratory Reference Values

22

Sarah A. Delgado

Please note: The values listed below apply to the cases presented in this text. When evaluating patient data, please compare results to the laboratory's reference ranges to ensure appropriate interpretation.

Category	Abbreviation	Definition	Normal Value	Formula
Acid Base				
	pH		7.35-7.45	
	$Paco_2$	Partial pressure of arterial carbon dioxide	35-45 mm Hg	
	Pao_2	Partial pressure of arterial oxygen	75-100 mm Hg	
	Bicarbonate		18-22 mmol/L	
	Base deficit/ base excess		$(-3)-(+3)$	
	Lactate		0.5-1 mmol/L	
Cardiac and Hemodynamic				
	BSA	Body surface area	Meters squared (m^2)	Value obtained from a nomogram based on height and weight
	CI	Cardiac index	2.5-4.3 L/min/m^2	$CI\ (L/min/m^2) = \dfrac{cardiac\ output\ (L/min)}{body\ surface\ area\ (m^2)}$
	CK	Creatinine kinase	<120 mcg/L	
	CK-MB	Creatinine kinase MB band	<3 ng/mL	
	CO	Cardiac output	4-8 L/min	$CO = stroke\ volume \times heart\ rate$
	CVP	Central venous pressure	2-8 mm Hg	
	EF	Ejection fraction	Greater than 60%	$Ejection\ fraction = \dfrac{SV}{EDV}$
	HR	Heart rate	60-100 beats/min	
	LVSW	Left ventricular stroke work	8-10 g/m/m^2	$LVSW = SI \times MAP \times 0.0144$
	MAP	Mean arterial pressure	>70 mm Hg	$MAP\ estimate = \dfrac{(Systolic + 2\ Diastolic)}{3}$
	PAD	Pulmonary artery diastolic	8-15 mm Hg	
	PAS	Pulmonary artery systolic pressure	16-24 mm Hg	
	PAOP	Pulmonary artery occlusion pressure	8-12 mm Hg	PAOP obtained via Swan-Ganz catheter
	PVR	Pulmonary vascular resistance	100-250 dynes/s/cm^{-5}	$PVR = (dynes/s/cm^5) = \dfrac{PAM\ (mm\,Hg) - PAOP\ (mm\,Hg) \times 80}{cardiac\ output\ (L/min)}$

(continued)

Category	Abbreviation	Definition	Normal Value	Formula
	RVEDV	Right ventricular end-diastolic volume	100-160 mL	SV/EF
	RVSW	Right ventricular stroke work	51-61 g/m/m^2	$RVSW = SI \times MAP \times 0.0144$
	SV	Stroke volume	60-100 mL/beat	$CO/HR \times 1000$
	SVI	Stroke volume index	33-47 mL/m^2/beat	$SI\ (mL/min/m^2) = \dfrac{stroke\ volume}{body\ surface\ area}$
	SVR	Systemic vascular resistance	800-1200 dynes-s/cm^{-5}	$SVR = 80 \times (MAP-RAP)/CO$
	SVRI	Systemic vascular resistance index	1970-2390 dynes-sec/cm^{-5}/m^2	$80 \times (MAP - RAP)/CI$
	Myoglobin	Female	10-65 ng/mL	
	Myoglobin	Male	10-95 ng/mL	
	Troponin I	Troponin I	<0.4 ng/mL	
	Troponin T	Troponin T	<0.1 ng/mL	
Functional Hemodynamics	SPV	Systolic pressure variation SPV%	>10 mm Hg >10%	$SBP_{max} - SBP_{min}$ $[(SBP_{max} - SBP_{min})/(SBP_{max} + SBP_{min}/2)] \times 100$
	PPV	Pulse pressure variation	>12.5%	$[(PP_{max} - PP_{min})/PP_{max} + PP_{min}/2)] \times 100$
	SVV	Stroke volume variation	>12%	$[(SV_{max} - SV_{min})/SV_{max} + SV_{min}/2)] \times 100$
Endocrine	ACTH	Adrenocorticotropic hormone	10-50 pg/mL Levels are usually less than 20 pg/mL in afternoon Less than 5-10 pg/mL at midnight	
	ADH	Antidiuretic hormone	1-5 pg/mL	
	Cortisol	Cortisol	10-20 µg/dL in the early morning 3-10 µg/dL afternoon <5 µg/dL after usual bedtime Great deal of variation	
	T3	Serum triiodothyronine	80-180 ng/dL	
	T4	Serum thyroxine	4.6-12 µg/dL	
	TSH	Serum thyrotropin (thyroid-stimulating hormone)	0.5-6 mIU/L	
Hematology	RBC	Red blood count	Males: 4.2-5.4 million/µL Females: 3.6-5.0 million/µL	
	Retic count	Reticulocyte count	0.5%-1.5%	
	WBC	White blood cell count	4500-10,500/µL	
	WBC differential (% of total)	As below		
		Neutrophils *Segmented Bands*	50%-70% 56% 0%-3%	
		Eosinophils	0%-3%	
		Basophils	0.5%-1.0%	
		Monocytes	3%-7%	
		Lymphocytes	25%-40%	
		Platelet count	150,000-400,000/µL	
		Bleeding time	3-10 minutes	

(continued)

Category	Abbreviation	Definition	Normal Value	Formula
	INR	International normalized ratio *Therapeutic anticoagulation*	0.8-1.1 2.0-3.0	
	aPTT	Activated partial thromboplastin time *Therapeutic anticoagulation*	30-40 seconds 1.5-2.5 times the mean normal value	
	ACT	Activated clotting time Therapeutic anticoagulation	70-120 seconds 150-210 seconds	
	Fibrinogen	Fibrinogen	200-400 mg/dL	
	D-dimer	D-dimer	<1.37 nmol/L	
Immunology				
	IgA	Immunoglobulin A	60-400 mg/dL	
	IgG	Immunoglobulin G	700-1500 mg/dL	
	IgM	Immunoglobulin M	60-300 mg/dL	
	IgE	Immunoglobulin E	3-423 IU/mL	
Liver Function				
	Albumin		35-50 g/L	
	Total protein		6-8.3 g/dL	
	Bilirubin	Total Direct	2-20 µmol/L 0-6 µmol/L	
	ALP	Alkaline phosphatase	50-100 U/L	
	AST	Aspartate aminotransferase	5-30 U/L	
	ALT	Alanine aminotransferase	5-30 U/L	
Pulmonary				
	A-a gradient	Alveolar-arterial oxygen gradient	When on 100% Fio_2 A-a gradient ~75 mm Hg, on 21% Fio_2 A-a gradient ~10-15 mm Hg	A-a = gradient See formula for calculation of alveolar O_2. Arterial (Pao_2) obtained via arterial blood gas.
	$C(a-v)O_2$	Arteriovenous oxygen content difference	4-6 mL/100 mL	$C(a-v)O_2$ (mL/100 mL or vol%) $= Cao_2 - Cvo_2$ (calculation for Cao_2 and Cvo_2 are below)
	Cao_2	Arterial oxygen content	~20 vol%	Cao_2 (mL O_2/100 mL blood or vol%) $= (Hb \times 1.39) Sao_2 + (Pao_2 \times 0.0031)$
	Cvo_2	Mixed venous oxygen content	~15 vol%	Cvo_2 (ml O_2/100 mL blood or vol%) $= (Hb \times 1.39) Svo_2 + (Pvo_2 \times 0.0031)$
	Cdyn	Dynamic compliance	~30-40 mL/cm H_2O	$Cdyn = Vt/PIP - PEEP$
	Cstat	Static compliance	~50 mL/cm H_2O	$Cstat = VT/Plat - PEEP$
	FRC	Functional residual capacity	2400 mL (dependent on height)	Measured in a pulmonary function laboratory
	NIP	Negative inspiratory pressure (also called NIF or negative inspiratory force)	−75 to 100 cm H_2O (the more negative the number, the stronger the force of the inspiration)	Measured at bedside or in a pulmonary function laboratory
	O_2 extraction ratio	Oxygen extraction ratio	0.25	$O_2 \text{ extraction ratio} = \dfrac{C(a-v)O_2}{CaO_2}$
	Pao_2	Mean partial pressure of oxygen in alveolus	104 mm Hg	$Pao_2 = Fio_2 (Pbar - PH_2O) - Paco_2/RQ$
	$Paco_2$	Partial pressure of carbon dioxide in arterial blood	35-45 mm Hg	$Paco_2$ obtained via arterial blood gas
	Pao_2	Partial pressure of oxygen in arterial blood	Will vary with patient's age and the Fio_2. Pao_2 on room air: 80-100 mm Hg, on 100% Pao_2: ≥ 500 mm Hg	Pao_2 obtained via arterial blood gas
	$Pvco_2$	Partial pressure of carbon dioxide in mixed venous blood	38-55 mm Hg	$Pvco_2$ obtained from the distal port of the PA catheter

(continued)

Category	Abbreviation	Definition	Normal Value	Formula
	Pvo_2	Partial pressure of oxygen in mixed venous blood	35-45 mm Hg—will vary with the Fio_2, cardiac output, and oxygen consumption	Pvo_2 obtained from the distal port of the PA catheter
	Q_S/Q_T	Right-to-left shunt (percentage of cardiac output flowing past nonventilated alveoli or the equivalent)	5%-8%	$Q_s/Q_T(\%) = \dfrac{0.0031 \times P(A-a)O_2}{C(a-v)O_2 + (0.0031 \times P[A-a]O_2)} \times 100$
	RQ	Respiratory quotient	0.8	$RQ = \dfrac{Vco_2}{VO_2}$
	Sao_2	Percentage of oxyhemoglobin saturation of arterial blood	96%-100% (on room air)	
	VO_2	Oxygen consumption	~250 mL/min	
	Svo_2	Percentage of oxyhemoglobin saturation of mixed venous blood	60%-80% (on room air)	
	VO_2	Oxygen consumption	~250 mL/min	
	VC	Vital capacity	65-75 mL/kg	
	Vco_2	Carbon dioxide production	~200 mL/min	
	VC	Vital capacity	65-75 mL/kg	
	V_D/V_T	Dead space to tidal volume ratio	0.25-0.40	$VD/VT = \dfrac{Paco_2 - PEco_2}{Paco_2}$
	V_T	Tidal volume	6-8 mL/kg	
Renal	ACR	Albumin to creatinine ratio	More than 30 mg per gram	
	BUN	Blood urea nitrogen	7-20 mg/dL	
	Creatinine (serum)		Women: 0.6-1.1 mg/dL Men: 0.7-1.3 mg/dL	Note: Serum creatinine may vary with patient size
	CrCl	Creatinine clearance	88-128 mL/min for women and 97-137 mL/min for men	
	FENa	Fractional excretion of sodium	<1% in prerenal injury >1% in intrarenal injury	FENa = [Na (urine) × creatinine (serum)] / [(Na (serum) × creatinine (urine)] × 100
	FEUrea	Fractional excretion of urea	<35% indicates prerenal injury >35% indicates intrarenal injury	[Cr (serum) × Urea (urine)] / Urea (serum) × Cr (urine)] × 100
	GFR	Glomerular filtration rate	>90 mL/min/1.73 m^2	
	Microalbumin (urine)		>30 mg	Microalbumin (urine)
	Sosm	Osmolality (serum)	285-295 mOsm/kg	Sosm = (2 × serum Na, in mmol/L) + [glucose, in mg/dL]/18 + [blood urea nitrogen, in mg/dL]/2.8

23

IMPLEMENTING CRISIS STANDARDS OF CARE

Laura Webster

EXAMPLES OF CONVENTIONAL, CONTINGENCY AND CRISIS STANDARDS OF CARE

The table below lists examples of conventional, contingency and crisis strategies when implementing Crisis Standards of Care. Interventions are sequentially applied based on an accurate assessment of existing resources. Conventional measures (conserve or substitute) are applied first, and if resources do not meet demand, contingency measures (adapt or resuse) are applied. Crisis standards of care are applied only when all other efforts to manage resources are in place and demand for care can not be met. See Chapter 8 for further discussion of Crisis Standards of Care

		Conventional		Contingency		Crisis	
		Conserve	**Substitute**	**Adapt**	**Reuse/Expand Use**	**Allocate**	**Reallocate**
Space	Hospital beds	Decrease non-essential surgical admissions	Expand into overflow areas in the PACU, OR, etc.	Change postoperative/ admission management with in-home resources	Create additional temporary spaces	Crisis Standards of Care (CSC) determines which patients are admitted	CSC determines which patients can stay
				Rapid discharge protocols			
Stuff	PPE	Limit non-essential staff and visitors. Limit non-essential interventions that require the scarce PPE	Different brands ordered	Prolonged use of PPE	Don and doffing the same PPE	CSC determines which people get PPE	CSC determines which people keep PPE
	Dialysis	Shorten or reduce frequency of routine dialysis runs	Change mode of dialysis	Intensive medical management of sub-acute patients	Wash and reuse disposal equipment when not available	Apply CSC to all patients currently receiving dialysis. CSC determines which patients get dialysis	CSC determines which patients keep a circuit
		Maximize clearance with high-efficiency filters	Consider Peritoneal dialysis program				
		Diet and fluid restrictions					

(continued)

		Conventional		Contingency		Crisis	
		Conserve	Substitute	Adapt	Reuse/Expand Use	Allocate	Reallocate
	Mechanical ventilation	identify and honor patient wishes for mechanical ventilation	Use transport ventilators or operating room ventilators for ongoing mechanical ventilation of critically ill patients	Use non-invasive mechanical ventilation	Use of one ventilator for two patients—of note, not recommended by Critical Care Societies Collaborative	Apply standards established in CSC to all patients currently receiving mechanical ventilation to make determinations about allocation	CSC determines which patients receive mechanical ventilation
Staff	Hospital staff	Reduce meetings to increase staff availability, discharge stable patients to in-home care	Use similarly trained staff	Delegate ADLs to volunteers and family caregivers	Increase ratios	CSC determines which patients get staff's time	CSC determines which patients keep staff's time
		Focus on core clinical skills	Increase agency, per diem, float pool staff	Reduce charting	Incentives for additional or longer shifts		
Staff	Critical care	Redeploy OR staff to ICU settings	Provide just in-time training to staff not normally providing care in ICU	Transfer critically ill patients to a site with more resources	Employ a team model of care in which staff with critical care experience work with staff with other skills sets to meet patient needs	Apply CSC to all patients currently receiving care in a critical care unit to determine allocation	CSC determines who is admitted and cared for in ICU

EXAMPLES OF CONVENTIONAL AND CONTINGENCY MEASURES FOR EVERYDAY SURGE

		Conventional		Contingency		Crisis	
		Conserve	Substitute	Adapt	Reuse/Expand Use	Allocate	Reallocate
Space	Patient placement—ICU admissions	Delay admission as ED/floor boarder	Expand into boarders overflow areas	Send ICU/stat RN to provide care on floor	Double up patients in ICU rooms	N/A	N/A
Stuff	10 mL saline syringes	Limit to "essential" patients	Use smaller 3 mL	Draw saline from vial into syringes	N/A	N/A	N/A
Staff	Critical care RNs	Finishing charting at the end of shift	Float pool RNs come	Covering for another RNs break (increase in ratio)	Working a double shift	N/A	N/A

HEMODYNAMIC MONITORING TROUBLESHOOTING GUIDE

Elizabeth J. Bridges and Mary Jo Kelly

TABLE 24-1. PROBLEMS ENCOUNTERED WITH ARTERIAL CATHETERS

Problem	Cause	Prevention	Treatment
Hematoma after withdrawal of needle	Bleeding or oozing at puncture site	Maintain firm pressure on site during withdrawal of catheter and for 5-15 minutes (as necessary) after withdrawal.	Continue to hold pressure to puncture site until oozing stops.
		Apply elastic tape firmly over puncture site. Care should be taken not to encircle the extremity (avoid ischemia).	
		For femoral arterial puncture sites, leave a sandbag or other device approved by hospital on site for 1-2 hours to prevent oozing.	Apply sandbag or other device approved by hospital to femoral puncture site for 1-2 hours after removal of catheter.
		If patient is receiving unfractionated heparin, a longer duration of direct pressure may be required to achieve hemostasis, when the catheter is removed.	
Decreased or absent pulse distal to puncture site	Spasm of artery	Introduce arterial needle cleanly, non-traumatically.	Call provider to inject lidocaine locally and/or an approved lidocaine dose into arterial catheter.
	Thrombosis of artery	Use 1 U of unfractionated heparin/1 mL IV fluid.	Arteriotomy and Fogarty catheterization may be needed both distally and proximally from the puncture site—results in return of pulse in >90% of cases if brachial or femoral artery is used.
Bleedback into tubing or transducer	Insufficient pressure on IV bag	Maintain 300 mm Hg pressure on IV bag.	Replace transducer. "Fast flush" through system.
	Loose connections	Use Luer-Lock stopcocks; tighten periodically.	Tighten all connections.
Hemorrhage	Loose connections	Keep all connecting sites visible. Observe connecting sites frequently. Use built-in alarm system. Use Luer-Lock stopcocks.	Tighten all connections.
Emboli	Clot from catheter tip into bloodstream	Always aspirate and discard before flushing. Monitor waveform for distortion (overdamping).	Remove catheter.
		Use continuous flush device. Gently flush < 2-4 mL.	
Local infection	Forward movement of contaminated catheter	Carefully secure catheter at insertion site.	Remove catheter.
	Break in sterile technique	Always use aseptic technique.	Prescribe antibiotic if indicated.
	Prolonged catheter use	Leave dressing in place until catheter is removed, changed, or dressing becomes damp, loosened, or soiled.	
Sepsis	Break in sterile technique	Use percutaneous insertion. Always use aseptic technique.	Remove catheter.
	Prolonged catheter use		Prescribe antibiotic if indicated.

(continued)

TABLE 24-1. PROBLEMS ENCOUNTERED WITH ARTERIAL CATHETERS (CONTINUED)

Problem	Cause	Prevention	Treatment
	Bacterial growth in IV fluid	Change stopcocks, transducer, and tubing every 96 hours. The IV fluid bag is changed more frequently, follow institutional guidelines. Do not use IV fluid containing glucose. Use a closed-flush system rather than an open system. Carefully flush remaining blood from stopcocks after blood sampling.	

Data from Blackburn J, Walton B. Risks associated with arterial lines: time for a national safety standard? J Anesth Pract. 2016, Nov 10. Lough ME. Hemodynamic Monitoring: Evolving Technologies and Clinical Practice. St Louis, MO: Elsevier; 2016; Simon EM, Summers SM. Vascular access complications: an emergency medicine approach. Emerg Med Clin North Am. 2017;35(4):771-788. Wiegand DL. AACN Procedure Manual for High Acuity, Progressive, and Critical Care. 7th ed. St. Louis, MO: Elsevier.

TABLE 24-2. INACCURATE ARTERIAL PRESSURE MEASUREMENTS

Problem	Cause	Prevention	Treatment
Damped pressure tracing	Catheter tip against vessel wall	Usually cannot be avoided.	Call provider to pull back, rotate, or reposition catheter while observing pressure waveform.
	Partial occlusion of catheter tip by clot	Use continuous infusion under pressure. Briefly "fast flush" after blood withdrawal (2-4 mL).	Aspirate clot with syringe and flush with saline (<2-4 mL). Consider line removal.
	Clot in stopcock or transducer	Carefully flush catheter after blood withdrawal and reestablish IV infusion. Use continuous flush device.	Flush stopcock and transducer; if no improvement, change stopcock and transducer.
	Air bubbles in transducer or connector tubing	Carefully flush transducer and tubing when setting up system and attaching to catheter.	Check system; flush rapidly; disconnect transducer and flush out air bubbles.
	Compliant tubing	Use stiff, short tubing.	Shorten tubing or replace softer tubing with stiffer tubing.
Abnormally high or low readings	Change in transducer air-reference level	Maintain air-fluid reference port of transducer at phlebostatic axis for serial pressure measurements.	Recheck patient and transducer positions.
No pressure available	Transducer not open to catheter	Follow routine, systematic steps for setting up system and turning stopcocks.	Check system—stopcocks, monitor, and amplifier setup.
	Settings on monitor amplifiers incorrect—still on zero, cal, or off		
	Incorrect scale selection	Select scale appropriate to expected range of physiologic signal.	Select appropriate scale.

Data from Lough ME. Hemodynamic Monitoring: Evolving Technologies and Clinical Practice. St Louis, MO: Elsevier; 2016; Wiegand DL. AACN Procedure Manual for High Acuity, Progressive, and Critical Care. 7th ed. St. Louis, MO: Elsevier.

TABLE 24-3. PROBLEMS ENCOUNTERED WITH PULMONARY ARTERY CATHETERS

Problem	Cause	Prevention	Treatment
Phlebitis or local infection at insertion site	Mechanical irritation or contamination	Prepare skin properly before insertion. Use sterile technique during insertion and dressing change. Insert smoothly and rapidly. Use Teflon-coated introducer. Change IV fluid bag, transducer, stopcocks, and connecting tubing every 96 hours or according to hospital policy. Remove catheter or change insertion site.	Remove catheter. Apply warm compresses. Give pain medication as necessary.
Ventricular irritability	Looping of excess catheter in RA	Carefully secure catheter at insertion site; check chest film.	Call healthcare provider to reposition catheter and remove loop.
	Migration of catheter from PA to RV		Inflate balloon to encourage catheter floatation out to PA. Most hospitals do not allow nurses to advance catheters.
	Irritation of the endocardium during catheter passage	Position catheter tip in main right or left PA.	Pull catheter back until RA waveform on monitor.
		Keep balloon inflated during advancement; advance gently.	
Apparent wedging of catheter with balloon deflated	Forward migration of catheter tip caused by blood flow, excessive loop in RV, or inadequate suturing of catheter at insertion site	Check catheter tip by radiograph or fluoroscopy; position in main right or left PA. Carefully secure catheter at insertion site.	Aspirate blood from catheter; if catheter is wedged, sample will be arterialized and obtained with difficulty. If wedged, call healthcare provider to slowly pull back catheter until PA waveform appears. If not wedged, gently aspirate and flush catheter with saline; catheter tip can partially clot, causing damping that resembles damped PAOP waveform.

(continued)

TABLE 24-3.   PROBLEMS ENCOUNTERED WITH PULMONARY ARTERY CATHETERS (CONTINUED)

Problem	Cause	Prevention	Treatment
Pulmonary hemorrhage or infarction, or both	Distal migration of catheter tip	Check chest film immediately after insertion.	Deflate balloon (passively).
	Continuous or prolonged wedging of catheter	Leave balloon deflated.	Place patient on side (catheter tip down).
		Carefully secure catheter at insertion site.	Stop anticoagulation.
		Call healthcare provider to pull catheter back to PA, if it spontaneously wedges.	Consider "wedge" angiogram.
		Do not flush catheter when in wedge position.	
	Overinflation of balloon while catheter is wedged	Inflate balloon slowly with only enough air to obtain a PAOP waveform.	
	Failure of balloon to deflate	Do not inflate 7-Fr catheter with more than 1.25-1.5 mL air. Do not leave balloon inflated for longer than 10-15 seconds.	
		Monitor patients for signs and symptoms of pulmonary infarction/rupture.	
"Overwedging" or damped PAOP	Overinflation of balloon	Do not inflate if resistance is met. Watch waveform during inflation; inject only enough air to obtain PAOP pressure.	Deflate balloon; reinflate slowly with only enough air to obtain PAOP pressure.
		Do not inflate 7-Fr catheter with more than 1.25-1.5 mL air.	
	Eccentric inflation of balloon	Check inflated balloon shape before insertion.	
PA balloon rupture	Overinflation of balloon	Inflate slowly with only enough air to obtain a PAOP pressure.	Remove syringe to prevent further air injection.
		Monitor PAEDP pressure as reflection of PAOP and LVEDP.	Monitor PAED pressure.
		Allow passive deflation of balloon.	
	Frequent inflations of balloon		
	Syringe deflation damaging wall of balloon	Remove syringe after inflation.	

(waveform graph axis labels: 320-80, 240-60, 160-40, 80-20; "Overwedged catheter. STOP-DEFLATE IMMEDIATELY")

Complication	Cause	Interventions
Infection	Nonsterile insertion techniques Contamination via skin	Use sterile techniques. Use sterile catheter sleeve. Prepare skin with effective antiseptic (chlorhexidine). Replace gauze dressings every 2 days and transparent dressings every 7 days or when dressings become damp, loosened, or soiled. Reassess need for catheter after 3 days, and daily thereafter. Avoid internal jugular approach. Remove catheter. Use antibiotics if indicated.
	Contamination through stopcock ports or catheter hub	Use a closed-system flush system rather than an open system. Use sterile dead-end caps on all stopcock ports. Change tubing, continuous flush device, transducer, and flush solution every 96 hours, or in accordance with hospital policy. Do not use IV flush solution that contains glucose.
	Fluid contamination from transducer through cracked membrane	Check transducer for cracks. Change transducers every 96 hours. Do not use IV flush solution that contains glucose.
	Prolonged catheter placement	Change catheter and/or insertion site with any local signs of infection and for infections without an obvious source (should obtain cultures). Remove catheter as soon as clinically feasible.
Heart block during insertion of catheter	Mechanical irritation of bundle of His in patients with preexisting left bundle branch block	Catheter should be advanced expeditiously during insertion with balloon inflated. Insert transvenous pacing catheter before PA catheter insertion. Use temporary pacemaker or flotation catheter with pacing wire.
Pneumothorax	With insertion into internal jugular or subclavian vein	Check chest film immediately after insertion. Insert chest tube
Air embolism	Can occur with central line insertion	Head of bed tilted down with insertion/removal of central line. Have patient hold breath. Promptly place patient in Trendelenburg position and on left side to help trap air in apex of ventricle.

Abbreviations: LVEDP, left ventricular end-diastolic pressure; PA, pulmonary artery; PAEDP, pulmonary artery end diastolic pressure; PAOP, pulmonary artery occlusion pressure; RV, right ventricle.
Data from Lough ME. Hemodynamic Monitoring: Evolving Technologies and Clinical Practice. St Louis, MO: Elsevier; 2016; Wiegand DL. AACN Procedure Manual for High Acuity, Progressive, and Critical Care. 7th ed. St. Louis, MO: Elsevier.

TABLE 24-4. INACCURATE PULMONARY ARTERY PRESSURE MEASUREMENTS

Problem	Cause	Prevention	Treatment
Damped waveforms and inaccurate pressures	Partial clotting at catheter tip	Maintain adequate flush bag pressures. Flush with large volume after blood sampling.	Aspirate, then flush catheter with fast flush (not in PAOP position).
	Tip moving against wall	Obtain more stable catheter position.	Call provider to reposition catheter.
	Kinking of catheter	Restrict catheter movement at insertion site.	Reposition to straighten catheter if a kink is suspected. Replace catheter.
Abnormally low or negative pressures	Incorrect air-fluid reference level (above phlebostatic axis)	Remeasure level of transducer air-reference and reposition at phlebostatic axis; re-zero.	Remeasure level of transducer air-reference and reposition at phlebostatic axis; re-zero.
	Incorrect zeroing and calibration of monitor	Zero and calibrate monitor properly.	Recheck zero and calibration of monitor.
	Loose connection	Use Luer-Lock stopcocks.	Check all connections.
Abnormally high pressure reading	Pressure trapped by improper sequence of stopcock operation	Use Luer-Lock stopcocks. Turn stopcocks in proper sequence when two pressures are measured on one transducer.	Thoroughly flush transducers with IV solution (do not flush into patient); re-zero and turn stopcocks in proper sequence.
	Incorrect air-reference level (below plebostatic axis level)	Maintain transducer air-reference port at phlebostatic axis level; recheck and re-zero after patient position changes.	Check air-fluid reference level; reset at phlebostatic axis and re-zero.
Inappropriate pressure waveform	Migration of catheter tip (eg, in RV or PAOP instead of in PA)	Establish optimal position carefully when introducing catheter initially.	Review waveform; if RV, call provider to reposition catheter. Check position under x-ray and/or fluoroscopy after reposition.

Inappropriate pressure waveform

Port

PAP   Scale (0/20/40/60)

Right atrium (CVP) = 12 mm Hg
a c v

Right ventricle = 40/12 mm Hg

PAP   Scale (0/20/40/60)

Problem	Cause	Intervention
No pressure available	Transducer not open to catheter	Check system, stopcocks.
	Amplifiers still on cal, zero, or off	Follow routine, systematic steps for pressure measurement.
Noise or fling in pressure waveform	Excessive catheter movement, particularly in PA	Secure catheter at insertion site and tape catheter to patient's skin. Avoid excessive catheter length in ventricle. Reposition catheter
	Excessive tubing length	Use shortest tubing possible (<3-4 ft). Eliminate excess tubing.
	Excessive stopcocks	Minimize number of stopcocks. Remove air bubbles. Eliminate excess stopcocks.

Abbreviations: PA, pulmonary artery; PAOP, pulmonary artery occlusion pressure; RV, right ventricle.

Data from Lough ME. Hemodynamic Monitoring: Evolving Technologies and Clinical Practice. St Louis, MO: Elsevier; 2016; Wiegand DL. AACN Procedure Manual for High Acuity, Progressive, and Critical Care. 7th ed. St. Louis, MO: Elsevier.

CARDIAC RHYTHMS, ECG CHARACTERISTICS, AND TREATMENT GUIDE

Carol Jacobson

25

Rhythm	ECG Characteristics	ECG Sample	Treatment
Normal sinus rhythm (NSR)	• Rate: 60-100 beats/min. • Rhythm: Regular. • P waves: Precede every QRS; consistent shape. • PR interval: 0.12-0.20 seconds. • QRS complex: 0.04-0.10 seconds.	Lead V1 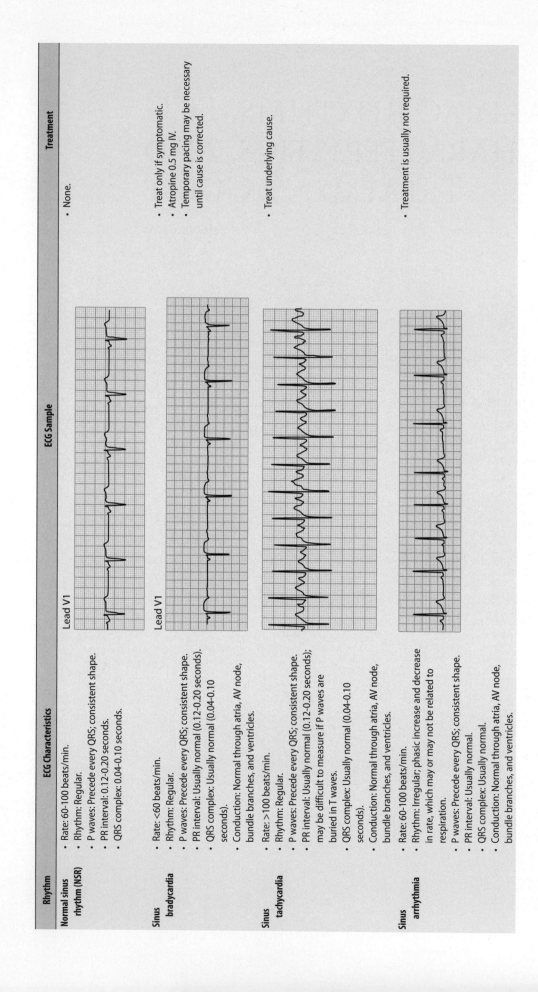	• None.
Sinus bradycardia	• Rate: <60 beats/min. • Rhythm: Regular. • P waves: Precede every QRS; consistent shape. • PR interval: Usually normal (0.12-0.20 seconds). • QRS complex: Usually normal (0.04-0.10 seconds). • Conduction: Normal through atria, AV node, bundle branches, and ventricles.	Lead V1	• Treat only if symptomatic. • Atropine 0.5 mg IV. • Temporary pacing may be necessary until cause is corrected.
Sinus tachycardia	• Rate: >100 beats/min. • Rhythm: Regular. • P waves: Precede every QRS; consistent shape. • PR interval: Usually normal (0.12-0.20 seconds); may be difficult to measure if P waves are buried in T waves. • QRS complex: Usually normal (0.04-0.10 seconds). • Conduction: Normal through atria, AV node, bundle branches, and ventricles.		• Treat underlying cause.
Sinus arrhythmia	• Rate: 60-100 beats/min. • Rhythm: Irregular; phasic increase and decrease in rate, which may or may not be related to respiration. • P waves: Precede every QRS; consistent shape. • PR interval: Usually normal. • QRS complex: Usually normal. • Conduction: Normal through atria, AV node, bundle branches, and ventricles.		• Treatment is usually not required.

Sinus pause/ arrest

- Rate: Usually within normal range, but may be in the bradycardia range.
- Rhythm: Irregular due to absence of sinus node discharge.
- P waves: Present when sinus node is firing and absent during periods of sinus arrest. When present, they precede every QRS complex and are consistent in shape. When only one sinus impulse is absent it is called a sinus pause. When more than one in a row is absent, it is called sinus arrest.
- PR interval: Usually normal when P waves are present.
- QRS complex: Usually normal when sinus node is functioning and absent during periods of sinus arrest, unless escape beats occur.
- Conduction: Normal through atria, AV node, bundle branches, and ventricles when sinus node is firing. When the sinus node fails to form impulses, there is no conduction through the atria.

- Treat underlying cause.
- Discontinue drugs that may be causative.
- Minimize vagal stimulation.
- For frequent sinus arrest causing hemodynamic compromise, atropine 0.5 mg IV may increase heart rate.
- Pacemaker may be necessary for refractory cases.

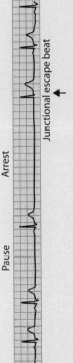

Pause Arrest

Junctional escape beat

III

Premature atrial contraction

- Rate: Usually within normal range.
- Rhythm: Usually regular except when PACs occur, resulting in early beats. PACs usually have a noncompensatory pause.
- P waves: Precede every QRS. The configuration of the premature P wave differs from that of the sinus P waves.
- PR interval: May be normal or long depending on the prematurity of the beat. Very early PACs may find the AV junction still partially refractory and unable to conduct at a normal rate, resulting in a prolonged PR interval.
- QRS complex: May be normal, aberrant (wide), or absent, depending on the prematurity of the beat.
- Conduction: PACs travel through the atria differently from sinus impulses because they originate from a different spot. Conduction through the AV node, bundle branches, and ventricles is usually normal unless the PAC is very early.

- Treatment is usually not necessary.
- Treat underlying cause.
- Drugs (eg, beta-blockers, disopyramide, flecainide, propafenone) can be used if necessary.

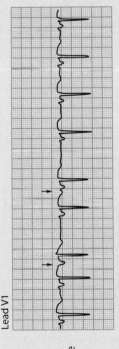

Lead V1

PACs conducted normally in the ventricle.

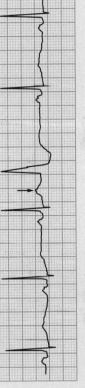

PAC with aberrant conduction

(continued)

Rhythm	ECG Characteristics	ECG Sample	Treatment
Wandering atrial pacemaker	• Rate: 60-100 beats/min. • Rhythm: May be slightly irregular. • P waves: Varying shapes (upright, flat, inverted, notched) as impulses originate in different parts of the atria or junction. At least three different P-wave shapes should be seen. • PR interval: May vary depending on proximity of the pacemaker to the AV node. • QRS complex: Usually normal. • Conduction: Conduction through the atria varies as they are depolarized from different spots. Conduction through the bundle branches and ventricles is usually normal.		• Treatment is usually not necessary. • Treat underlying cause. • For symptoms from slow rate, use atropine.
Multifocal atrial tachycardia	• Rate: Faster than 100. • Rhythm: Irregular. • P waves: Varying shapes (upright, flat, inverted, notched) as impulses originate in different parts of the atria or junction. At least three different P-wave shapes should be seen. Often misdiagnosed as atrial fibrillation. • PR interval: May vary depending on proximity of the pacemaker to the AV node. • QRS complex: Usually normal. • Conduction: Conduction through the atria varies as they are depolarized from different spots. Conduction through the bundle branches and ventricles is usually normal.		• Treat underlying cause, which is often COPD. Additional treatment may not be needed unless symptomatic or hemodynamic compromise. • Maintain normal Mg^{++} and K^+ levels. • Acute rate control: IV beta-blockers, IV verapamil. • Oral beta-blockers, verapamil, diltiazem. • AV node ablation with placement of a permanent pacemaker may be needed in select cases refractory to medication.
Atrial tachycardia	• Rate: Atrial rate is 120-250 beats/min. • Rhythm: Regular during tachycardia unless there is variable block at the AV node. • P waves: Differ in shape from sinus P waves because they are ectopic. Precede each QRS complex but may be hidden in preceding T wave. When block is present, more than one P wave appears before each QRS complex. • PR interval: May be shorter than normal but often difficult to measure because of hidden P waves. • QRS complex: Usually normal but may be wide if aberrant conduction is present. • Conduction: Usually normal through the AV node and into the ventricles. In atrial tachycardia with block, some atrial impulses do not conduct into the ventricles. Aberrant ventricular conduction may occur if atrial impulses are conducted into the ventricles while the ventricles are still partially refractory.		• Eliminate underlying cause and decrease ventricular rate. • Adenosine may be effective in some ATs. • IV beta-blockers, verapamil, or diltiazem can slow ventricular rate. • Flecainide, propafenone, amiodarone, sotalol, and dofetilide may be effective for ongoing management. • Cardioversion may be successful for reentry AT but not for automatic AT. • Radiofrequency ablation is often successful.

Atrial flutter	• Rate: Atrial rate varies between 250 and 350 beats/min, most commonly 300. Ventricular rate varies depending on the amount of block at the AV node. • Rhythm: Atrial rhythm is regular. Ventricular rhythm may be regular or irregular due to varying AV block. • P waves: Flutter waves (F waves) are seen, characterized by a very regular, "sawtooth" pattern. One F wave is usually hidden in the QRS complex, and when 2:1 conduction occurs, F waves may not be readily apparent. • FR interval (flutter wave to the beginning of the QRS complex): May be consistent or may vary. • QRS complex: Usually normal; aberration can occur. • Conduction: Usually normal through the AV node and ventricles.	• Cardioversion is preferred for markedly reduced cardiac output. • Beta-blockers, verapamil, or diltiazem for ventricular rate control if no pre-excitation. IV amiodarone can be used for rate control if systolic heart failure and no pre-excitation when beta-blockers ineffective or contraindicated. • Oral dofetilide or IV ibutilide for pharmacological conversion. • Amiodarone, dofetilide, or sotalol to maintain sinus rhythm; monitor QTc. • Radiofrequency ablation is usually successful.
Atrial fibrillation	• Rate: Atrial rate is 400–600 beats/min or faster. Ventricular rate varies depending on the amount of block at the AV node. In new atrial fibrillation, the ventricular response is usually quite rapid, 160–200 beats/min; in treated atrial fibrillation, the ventricular rate is controlled in the normal range of 60–100 beats/min. • Rhythm: Irregular. One of the distinguishing features of atrial fibrillation is the marked irregularity of the ventricular response. • P waves: Not present. Atrial activity is chaotic with no formed atrial impulses visible. Irregular f waves are often seen and vary in size from coarse to very fine. • PR interval: Not measurable; there are no P waves. • QRS complex: Usually normal; aberration is common. • Conduction: Conduction within the atria is disorganized and follows a very irregular pattern. Most of the atrial impulses are blocked within the AV junction. Those impulses that are conducted through the AV junction are usually conducted normally through the ventricles. If an atrial impulse reaches the bundle branch system during its refractory period, aberrant intraventricular conduction can occur.	• Eliminate underlying cause. • Cardiovert, if hemodynamically unstable. Anticoagulation is recommended prior to and after cardioversion if duration of afib is >48 our or is unknown. TEE can also be used to rule out left atrial and left atrial appendage thrombus prior to urgent cardioversion. • Calcium channel blockers and beta-blockers preferred for acute rate control if no pre-excitation. IV amiodarone in critically ill patients without pre-excitation. • Flecainide, cofetilide, propafenone, IV ibutilide, and amiodarone are used to convert to sinus. • Amiodarone, dofetilide, dronedarone, flecainide, propafenone, or sotalol are used for maintenance of sinus rhythm. • Radiofrequency ablation often successful.

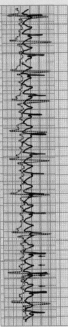
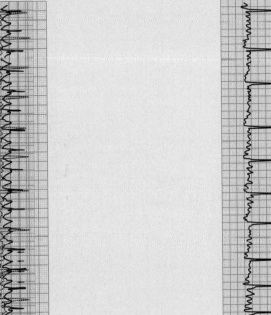
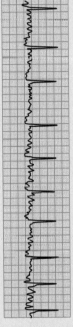
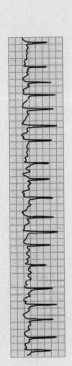

(continued)

Rhythm	ECG Characteristics	ECG Sample	Treatment
Premature junctional complexes	• Rate: 60-100 beats/min or whatever the rate of the basic rhythm. • Rhythm: Regular except for occurrence of premature beats. • P waves: May occur before, during, or after the QRS complex of the premature beat and are usually inverted in leads II, III, and AVF. • PR interval: Short, usually 0.10 seconds or less, when P waves precede the QRS. • QRS complex: Usually normal but may be aberrant if the PJC occurs very early and conducts into the ventricles during the refractory period of a bundle branch. • Conduction: Retrograde through the atria; usually normal through the ventricles.	 Lead II ↑ PJC	• Treatment is usually not necessary.
Junctional rhythm	• Rate: Junctional rhythm, 40-60 beats/min; accelerated junctional rhythm, 60-100 beats/min; junctional tachycardia, 100-250 beats/min. • Rhythm: Regular. • P waves: May occur before, during, or after QRS and are inverted in leads II, III, and AVF. • PR interval: Short, 0.10 seconds or less if P waves precede QRS. • QRS complex: Usually normal. • Conduction: Retrograde through the atria; normal through the ventricles.	 Junctional rhythm Accelerated junctional rhythm	• Treatment is rarely needed unless rate is too slow or too fast to maintain adequate CO. • Atropine is used to increase rate. • Verapamil, propranolol, or beta-blockers are used to decrease rate. • Withhold digitalis, if digitalis toxicity is suspected.
Premature ventricular complexes	• Rate: 60-100 beats/min or the rate of the basic rhythm. • Rhythm: Irregular because of the early beats. • P waves: Not related to the PVCs. Sinus rhythm is usually not interrupted by the premature beats, so sinus P waves can often be seen occurring regularly throughout the rhythm. • PR interval: Not present before most PVCs. If a P wave happens, by coincidence, to precede a PVC, the PR interval is short. • QRS complex: Wide and bizarre; >0.10 seconds in duration. May vary in morphology (size, shape) if they originate from more than one focus in the ventricles. • Conduction: Wide QRS complexes. Some PVCs may conduct retrograde into the atria, resulting in inverted P waves following the PVC.	 Unifocal PVCs Multifocal PVCs	• Eliminate underlying cause. • Drug therapy is not usually used, but, if desired, lidocaine, amiodarone, procainamide, beta-blockers may be effective.

Idioventricular rhythm	• Rate: <50 beats/min for idioventricular rhythm and 50–100 beats/min for accelerated idioventricular rhythm. • Rhythm: Usually regular. • P waves: May be seen but at a slower rate than the ventricular focus, with dissociation from the QRS. • PR interval: Not measured. • QRS complex: Wide and bizarre. • Conduction: If sinus rhythm is the basic rhythm, atrial conduction is normal. Impulses originating in the ventricles conduct via muscle cell-to-cell conduction, resulting in the wide QRS complex.	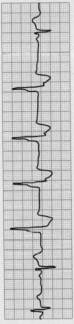 Idioventricular rhythm 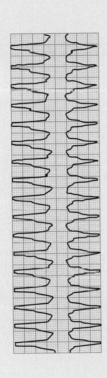 Accelerated idioventricular rhythm	• For ventricular escape rhythms, use atropine to increase sinus rate and overdrive ventricular rhythm. • Use ventricular pacing to increase ventricular rate if escape rhythm is too slow.
Monomorphic ventricular tachycardia	• Rate: Ventricular rate is faster than 100 beats/min. • Rhythm: Usually regular but may be slightly irregular. • P waves: P waves may be seen but will not be related to QRS complexes (dissociated from QRS complexes). If sinus rhythm is the underlying basic rhythm, regular P waves are often buried within QRS complexes. • PR interval: Not measurable because of dissociation of P waves from QRS complexes. • QRS complex: Wide and bizarre; >0.10 seconds in duration. • Conduction: Impulse originates in one ventricle and spreads via muscle cell-to-cell conduction through both ventricles. There may be retrograde conduction through the atria, but more often the sinus node continues to fire regularly and depolarize the atria normally.	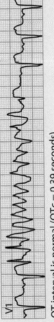	• Treatment depends on how rhythm is tolerated. • IV lidocaine, amiodarone, or procainamide should be given if patient is stable. • Cardioversion is preferred for hemodynamic instability. • Defibrillation should be performed if VT is pulseless. • Radiofrequency ablation is successful for some monomorphic VTs.
Ventricular tachycardia (polymorphic)	• Regularity: Irregular. • Rate: >100 beats/min, often very fast. • P waves: None associated with VT. • PR interval: None. • QRS width: >0.12 seconds, multiple shapes. • QT interval is normal (<0.47 seconds) for normal beats	V1 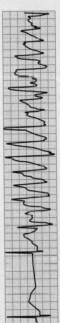 QT interval is normal (QTc = 0.39 seconds)	• Treat ischemia with beta-blockers, angioplasty/stent, or CABG. • IV amiodarone or lidocaine may be used. • Defibrillate if it becomes sustained with loss of consciousness.
Torsades de pointes (Polymorphic VT associated with prolonged QT interval)	• Regularity: Irregular. • Rate: >100 beats/min, often very fast. • P waves: None associated with VT. • PR interval: None. • QRS width: >0.12 seconds, multiple shapes, often appears to twist around the baseline. • QT interval for normal beats is prolonged; QTc > 0.50 seconds increases risk.	QT interval is very long (0.76 seconds)	• Discontinue causative drugs. • Correct electrolyte imbalances. • IV magnesium or overdrive pacing can be used until the cause is corrected. • Defibrillate if it becomes sustained with loss of consciousness.

(continued)

Rhythm	ECG Characteristics	ECG Sample	Treatment
Ventricular fibrillation	• Rate: Rapid, uncoordinated, ineffective. • Rhythm: Chaotic, irregular. • P waves: None seen. • PR interval: None. • QRS complex: No formed QRS complexes seen; rapid, irregular undulations without any specific pattern. • Conduction: Multiple ectopic foci firing simultaneously in ventricles and depolarizing them irregularly and without any organized pattern. Ventricles are not contracting.		• Immediate defibrillation. • CPR required until defibrillator is available. • Amiodarone, lidocaine, and magnesium are commonly used. • After conversion, use IV anti-arrhythmic that facilitates conversion to prevent recurrence.
Ventricular asystole	• Rate: None. • Rhythm: None. • P waves: May be present if the sinus node is functioning. • PR interval: None. • QRS complex: None. • Conduction: Atrial conduction may be normal if the sinus node is functioning. There is no conduction into the ventricles.		• Provide immediate CPR. • Give IV epinephrine. • Identify and treat cause.
First-degree AV block	• Rate: Can occur at any sinus rate, usually 60–100 beats/min. • Rhythm: Regular. • P waves: Normal; precede every QRS. • PR interval: Prolonged above 0.20 seconds. • QRS complex: Usually normal. • Conduction: Normal through the atria, delayed through the AV node. Ventricular conduction is normal.		• Treatment is usually not necessary.
Second-degree AV block type I (Wenckebach; Mobitz I)	• Rate: Can occur at any sinus or atrial rate. • Rhythm: Irregular. Overall appearance of the rhythm demonstrates "group beating." • P waves: Normal. Some P waves are not conducted to the ventricles, but only one at a time fails to conduct to the ventricle. • PR interval: Gradually lengthens in consecutive beats. The PR interval preceding the pause is longer than that following the pause. • QRS complex: Usually normal unless there is associated bundle branch block. • Conduction: Normal through the atria, progressively delayed through the AV node until an impulse fails to conduct. Conduction ratios can vary, with ratios as low as 2:1 (every other P wave is blocked), up to high ratios such as 15:14 (every 15th P wave blocked).		• Treatment depends on conduction ratio, ventricular rate, and symptoms. • Atropine is used for slow ventricular rate. • No treatment is given with normal ventricular rate. • Hold digitalis, beta-blockers, and calcium channel blockers. • Temporary pacemaker may be needed for slow ventricular rate.

Type	ECG	Characteristics	Treatment
Second-degree AV block type II (Mobitz II)		• Rate: Can occur at any basic rate. • Rhythm: Irregular because of blocked beats. • P waves: Usually regular and precede each QRS. Periodically a P wave is not followed by a QRS complex. • PR interval: Constant before conducted beats. The PR interval preceding the pause is the same as that following the pause. • QRS complex: Usually wide due to associated bundle branch block. • Conduction: Normal through the atria and through the AV node but intermittently blocked in the bundle branch system and fails to reach the ventricles. Conduction through the ventricles is abnormally slow owing to associated bundle branch block. Conduction ratios can vary from 2:1 to only occasional blocked beats.	• Pacemaker is often needed. • Atropine is not recommended.
High-grade (advanced) AV block		• Rate: Atrial rate < 135 beats/min. • Rhythm: Regular or irregular, depending on conduction pattern. • P waves: Normal; present before every conducted QRS, but two or more consecutive P waves are not followed by QRS complexes. • PR interval: Constant before conducted beats; may be normal or prolonged. • QRS complex: Usually normal in type I and wide in type II advanced blocks. • Conduction: Normal through the atria. Two or more consecutive atrial impulses fail to conduct to the ventricles. Ventricular conduction is normal in type I and abnormally slow in type II advanced blocks.	• Treatment is necessary if patient is symptomatic. • Atropine may increase ventricular rate. • Pacemaker is often required.
Third-degree AV block (complete)		• Rate: Atrial rate is usually normal; ventricular rate is <45 beats/min. • Rhythm: Regular. • P waves: Normal but dissociated from QRS complexes. • PR interval: No consistent PR intervals because there is no relationship between P waves and QRS complexes. • QRS complex: Normal if ventricles controlled by a junctional rhythm; wide if controlled by a ventricular rhythm. • Conduction: Normal through the atria. All impulses are blocked at the AV node or in the bundle branches, so there is no conduction to the ventricles. Conduction through the ventricles may be normal if a junctional escape rhythm occurs, and abnormally slow if a ventricular escape rhythm occurs.	• Pacemaker. • Atropine is usually not effective. • With severely decreased cardiac output, perform CPR until pacemaker available.

INDEX

Note: Page numbers by an "*f*" indicate figures; page numbers followed by a "*t*" indicate tables.

A

A-alpha (α) fibers, 167*f*, 176
A-beta (β) fibers, 176
A-delta (δ) fibers, 166, 167*f*, 176
AACN (American Association of
    Critical Care Nurses), 228
ABCDE acronym
  in admission assessment, 4*t*, 6
  in primary trauma survey, 456–457,
    456*t*
ABCDEF bundle
  for delirium prevention, 26, 26*t*
  in ICU Liberation Bundle, 179, 179*f*
  for weaning readiness, 150, 152*t*
Abciximab, 219, 260, 261*f*, 379*t*
Abdominal aneurysm, 538. *See also*
    Aortic aneurysm
Abdominal trauma, 464–466
Aberrancy, 505–506, 506*f*
ABG monitoring. *See* Arterial blood
    gas (ABG) monitoring
Abiomed Impella, 547
Absence seizure, 364. *See also* Seizures
Absorption atelectasis, 139
Accelerated idioventricular rhythm
    (AIVR), 59, 59*f*
Accelerated junctional rhythm, 57–58,
    58*f*
ACE (angiotensin-converting enzyme)
    inhibitors, 112*t*, 207, 272, 527
Acetaminophen
  antidote for, 331
  intravenous, 170
  overdose of, 330, 330*t*
  pharmacology of, 199
Acid-base analysis
  in arterial blood gas monitoring,
    125–127, 126*t*
  in diabetic ketoacidosis, 436, 436*t*
  normal values, 587*t*

Acidemia, 125, 126*t*
Acidosis, 422
Aciphex. *See* Rabeprazole
Acquired long-QT syndrome, 500
Activase. *See* Alteplase
Activated charcoal, 331
Activated coagulation time (ACT),
    370*t*, 372
Activated partial thromboplastin time
    (aPTT), 370*t*, 371–372
Acute colonic pseudo-obstruction, 404
Acute coronary syndromes. *See also*
    Myocardial infarction
  clinical presentation of, 257,
    258–259*t*
  definition of, 253, 484
  diagnostic tests for, 257, 259, 260*f*,
    260*t*, 269*t*
  ECG characteristics of, 485–487,
    485*f*, 486*f*
  etiology and pathophysiology of,
    253–255, 253*f*, 255*f*, 255*t*, 257*f*
  phases of, 484–485, 485*f*
  principles of management
    blood flow optimization, 260,
      260*t*
    complication prevention, 265
    medical, 260, 260*t*, 261*f*, 262*t*
    percutaneous coronary
      interventions, 262–263, 262*f*,
      263*f*
    surgical. *See* Coronary artery
      bypass grafting (CABG)
Acute hypoglycemia
  after traumatic brain injury, 571
  clinical presentation of, 445
  etiology, risk factors, and
    pathophysiology of, 443–444,
    443*t*
  principles of management, 446, 446*t*

Acute ischemic stroke
  clinical presentation of, 359–360,
    360*t*
  diagnostic tests for, 360
  etiology, risk factors, and
    pathophysiology of, 358–359
  principles of management, 360–362,
    361*t*, 362*t*
  recurrent, prevention of, 362–363
  secondary complications of, 362
Acute kidney injury (AKI)
  classification of, 417, 418*t*
  clinical phases of, 420
  clinical presentation of, 420
  diagnostic tests for, 420–421
  etiology, risk factors, and
    pathophysiology of, 417–419,
    418*f*
  overview of, 417, 418*f*
  physical assessment in, 420
  principles of management, 421–423,
    421*t*
Acute pancreatitis
  clinical presentation of, 400
  complications of, 400, 400*t*
  diagnostic tests for, 400–401
  etiology, risk factors, and
    pathophysiology of, 400
  overview of, 399–400
  principles of management, 401–402
Acute renal failure (ARF). *See* Acute
    kidney injury
Acute respiratory distress syndrome
    (ARDS)
  clinical presentation of, 297
  etiology, risk factors, and
    pathophysiology of, 296–297,
    296*t*
  mechanical ventilation for, 551–552
  overview of, 296